ELEVENTH EDITION

Handbook of Clinical Anesthesia Procedures of the Massachusetts General Hospital

ELEVENTH EDITION

Handbook of Clinical Anesthesia Procedures of the Massachusetts General Hospital

Senior Editor
Keith H. Baker, MD, PhD

Associate Editors
Edward A. Bittner, MD, PhD, MSEd
Hovig V. Chitilian, MD
Ryan J. Horvath, MD, PhD
Wilton C. Levine, MD
Jamie L. Sparling, MD

Department of Anesthesia, Critical Care, and Pain Medicine
Harvard Medical School
Massachusetts General Hospital
Boston, Massachusetts

Philadelphia • Baltimore • New York • London
Buenos Aires • Hong Kong • Sydney • Tokyo

Acquisitions Editor: Keith Donnellan
Senior Development Editor: Ashley Fischer
Editorial Coordinator: Ann Francis
Marketing Manager: Kirsten Watrud
Production Project Manager: Jennifer L. Harper
Manager, Graphic Arts & Design: Stephen Druding
Manufacturing Coordinator: Lisa Bowling
Prepress Vendor: Aptara, Inc.

11th edition

Copyright © 2026 Wolters Kluwer.

Copyright © 2022 Wolters Kluwer. Copyright © 2016 Wolters Kluwer. Copyright © 2010, 2007 Lippincott Williams & Wilkins, a Wolters Kluwer business. Copyright © 2002 Lippincott Williams & Wilkins. Copyright © 1998 Lippincott-Raven. Copyright © 1994 JB Lippincott. All rights reserved. This book is protected by copyright. No part of this book may be reproduced or transmitted in any form or by any means, including as photocopies or scanned-in or other electronic copies, or utilized by any information storage and retrieval system without written permission from the copyright owner, except for brief quotations embodied in critical articles and reviews. Materials appearing in this book prepared by individuals as part of their official duties as U.S. government employees are not covered by the above-mentioned copyright. To request permission, please contact Wolters Kluwer at Two Commerce Square, 2001 Market Street, Philadelphia, PA 19103, via email at permissions@lww.com, or via our website at shop.lww.com (products and services).

9 8 7 6 5 4 3 2 1

Printed in Mexico

Library of Congress Cataloging-in-Publication Data

ISBN-13: 978-1-9752-4298-5
Cataloging in Publication data available on request from publisher.

This work is provided "as is," and the publisher disclaims any and all warranties, express or implied, including any warranties as to accuracy, comprehensiveness, or currency of the content of this work.

This work is no substitute for individual patient assessment based upon healthcare professionals' examination of each patient and consideration of, among other things, age, weight, gender, current or prior medical conditions, medication history, laboratory data and other factors unique to the patient. The publisher does not provide medical advice or guidance and this work is merely a reference tool. Healthcare professionals, and not the publisher, are solely responsible for the use of this work including all medical judgments and for any resulting diagnosis and treatments.

Given continuous, rapid advances in medical science and health information, independent professional verification of medical diagnoses, indications, appropriate pharmaceutical selections and dosages, and treatment options should be made and healthcare professionals should consult a variety of sources. When prescribing medication, healthcare professionals are advised to consult the product information sheet (the manufacturer's package insert) accompanying each drug to verify, among other things, conditions of use, warnings and side effects and identify any changes in dosage schedule or contraindications, particularly if the medication to be administered is new, infrequently used or has a narrow therapeutic range. To the maximum extent permitted under applicable law, no responsibility is assumed by the publisher for any injury and/or damage to persons or property, as a matter of products liability, negligence law or otherwise, or from any reference to or use by any person of this work.

shop.lww.com

CONTRIBUTORS

Megan Abbott, MD
Resident
Department of Anesthesia, Critical Care and Pain Medicine
Massachusetts General Hospital
Boston, Massachusetts

Zachary Achen, MD, MPH
Resident
Department of Anesthesia, Critical Care and Pain Medicine
Massachusetts General Hospital
Boston, Massachusetts

Lauren Alderette, MD, MPH
Resident
Department of Anesthesia, Critical Care and Pain Medicine
Massachusetts General Hospital
Boston, Massachusetts

Lillye Anderson, MD
Resident
Department of Anesthesia, Critical Care and Pain Medicine
Massachusetts General Hospital
Boston, Massachusetts

Daniel Ankeny, MD, PhD
Anesthesiologist
Department of Anesthesia, Critical Care and Pain Management
Massachusetts General Hospital
Boston, Massachusetts

Susana Arango, MD
Resident
Department of Anesthesia, Critical Care and Pain Medicine
Massachusetts General Hospital
Boston, Massachusetts

Keith H. Baker, MD, PhD
Vice Chair for Education and Faculty Affairs
Department of Anesthesia, Critical Care and Pain Medicine
Massachusetts General Hospital
Boston, Massachusetts

Xiaodong Bao, MD, PhD
Anesthesiologist
Department of Anesthesia, Critical Care and Pain Medicine
Massachusetts General Hospital
Boston, Massachusetts

Victoria Bass, MD
Resident
Department of Anesthesia, Critical Care and Pain Medicine
Massachusetts General Hospital
Boston, Massachusetts

Christopher Bean, MD
Resident
Department of Anesthesia, Critical Care and Pain Medicine
Massachusetts General Hospital
Boston, Massachusetts

William Benedetto, MD
Anesthesiologist/Intensivist
Department of Anesthesia, Critical Care and Pain Medicine
Massachusetts General Hospital
Boston, Massachusetts

Edward A. Bittner, MD, PhD, MSEd
Anesthesiologist/Intensivist
Department of Anesthesia, Critical Care and Pain Medicine
Massachusetts General Hospital
Boston, Massachusetts

Scott Cao, MD
Resident
Department of Anesthesia, Critical Care and Pain Medicine
Massachusetts General Hospital
Boston, Massachusetts

Marvin G. Chang, MD, PhD
Anesthesiologist/Intensivist
Department of Anesthesia, Critical Care and Pain Medicine
Massachusetts General Hospital
Boston, Massachusetts

Hovig V. Chitilian, MD
Anesthesiologist
Department of Anesthesia, Critical Care and Pain Medicine
Massachusetts General Hospital
Boston, Massachusetts

James S. Cho, MD
Resident
Department of Anesthesia, Critical Care and Pain Medicine
Massachusetts General Hospital
Boston, Massachusetts

Parita A. Chowatia, PharmD
Pharmacist, Perioperative Services
Department of Pharmacy
Massachusetts General Hospital
Boston, Massachusetts

Jack Curtis, MD
Resident
Department of Anesthesia, Critical Care and Pain Management
Massachusetts General Hospital
Boston, Massachusetts

Julia M. Danford, MD
Resident
Department of Anesthesia, Critical Care and Pain Medicine
Massachusetts General Hospital
Boston, Massachusetts

Christopher Di Capua, MD, MBA
Resident
Department of Anesthesia, Critical Care and Pain Medicine
Massachusetts General Hospital
Boston, Massachusetts

Amy Du, MD, MS
Anesthesiologist
Department of Anesthesia, Critical Care and Pain Medicine
Massachusetts General Hospital
Boston, Massachusetts

Daniel Ellis, MD
Anesthesiologist
Department of Anesthesia, Critical Care and Pain Medicine
Massachusetts General Hospital
Boston, Massachusetts

J. Paul Fleming, MD
Anesthesiologist
Department of Anesthesia, Critical Care and Pain Medicine
Massachusetts General Hospital
Boston, Massachusetts

Timothy G. Gaulton, MD, MSc
Anesthesiologist/Intensivist
Department of Anesthesia, Critical Care and Pain Medicine
Massachusetts General Hospital
Boston, Massachusetts

Gregory E. Ginsburg, MD
Anesthesiologist
Department of Anesthesia, Critical Care and Pain Medicine
Massachusetts General Hospital
Boston, Massachusetts

Jeremy Goldfarb, MD
Associate Chief
Department of Anesthesia, Critical Care and Pain Medicine
Massachusetts Eye and Ear
Boston, Massachusetts

Christian Guay, MD
Clinical Fellow in Adult Cardiothoracic Anesthesia
Department of Anesthesia, Critical Care and Pain Medicine
Massachusetts General Hospital
Boston, Massachusetts

Ion A. Hobai, MD, PhD
Anesthesiologist
Department of Anesthesia, Critical Care and Pain Medicine
Massachusetts General Hospital
Boston, Massachusetts

Ryan J. Horvath, MD, PhD
Anesthesiologist/Intensivist
Post-Anesthesia Care Unit Director
Department of Anesthesia, Critical Care and Pain Medicine
Massachusetts General Hospital
Boston, Massachusetts

Zeyu Hu, MD
Resident
Department of Anesthesia, Critical Care and Pain Medicine
Massachusetts General Hospital
Boston, Massachusetts

Omar Hyder, MD
Anesthesiologist/Intensivist
Department of Anesthesia, Critical Care and Pain Medicine
Massachusetts General Hospital
Boston, Massachusetts

Ashwini Joshi, MD
Resident
Department of Anesthesia, Critical Care and Pain Medicine
Massachusetts General Hospital
Boston, Massachusetts

Rachel Padilla Judge, MD
Resident
Department of Anesthesia, Critical Care and Pain Medicine
Massachusetts General Hospital
Boston, Massachusetts

Adam W. Kaplon, MD
Resident
Department of Anesthesia, Critical Care and Pain Medicine
Massachusetts General Hospital
Boston, Massachusetts

Audrey Kennedy, PharmD
Pharmacist, Perioperative Services
Department of Pharmacy
Massachusetts General Hospital
Boston, Massachusetts

Brian J. Kinsman, MD, PhD
Resident
Department of Anesthesia, Critical Care and Pain Medicine
Massachusetts General Hospital
Boston, Massachusetts

Alexander S. Kuo, MD
Anesthesiologist/Intensivist
Department of Anesthesia, Critical Care and Pain Medicine
Massachusetts General Hospital
Boston, Massachusetts

Jean Kwo, MD
Anesthesiologist/Intensivist
Department of Anesthesia, Critical Care and Pain Medicine
Massachusetts General Hospital
Boston, Massachusetts

Johanna Lee, MD
Anesthesiologist
Department of Anesthesia, Critical Care and Pain Medicine
Massachusetts General Hospital
Boston, Massachusetts

Wilton C. Levine, MD
Executive Medical Director, Procedural Services
Department of Anesthesia, Critical Care and Pain Medicine
Massachusetts General Hospital
Boston, Massachusetts

Chang A. Liu, MD, PhD, FAAP
Anesthesiologist
Department of Anesthesia, Critical Care and Pain Medicine
Massachusetts General Hospital
Boston, Massachusetts

James Taylor Lloyd, MD
Anesthesiologist
Department of Anesthesia, Critical Care and Pain Medicine
Massachusetts General Hospital
Boston, Massachusetts

Ying Hui Low, MD
Anesthesiologist
Department of Anesthesiology
Dartmouth Hitchcock Medical Center
Lebanon, New Hampshire

Simona Iustina Lupu, MD
Anesthesiologist/Intensivist
Department of Anesthesia, Critical Care and Pain Medicine
Massachusetts General Hospital
Boston, Massachusetts

John J. A. Marota, MD, PhD
Anesthesiologist
Department Anesthesia, Critical Care and Pain Medicine
Massachusetts General Hospital
Boston, Massachusetts

Joseph L. McDowell, MD
Anesthesiologist
Department of Anesthesia, Critical Care and Pain Medicine
Massachusetts General Hospital
Boston, Massachusetts

Emily C. Mills, MD
Resident
Department of Anesthesia, Critical Care and Pain Medicine
Massachusetts General Hospital
Boston, Massachusetts

Rebecca D. Minehart, MD, MSHPEd
Division Chief, Obstetric Anesthesia
Department of Anesthesia, Critical Care and Pain Medicine
Massachusetts General Hospital
Boston, Massachusetts

Jeremi Mountjoy, MD, MSc, FRCPC
Anesthesiologist
Department of Anesthesia, Critical Care and Pain Medicine
Massachusetts General Hospital
Boston, Massachusetts

Alexander Nagrebetsky, MD, MSc
Anesthesiologist/Intensivist
Department of Anesthesia, Critical Care and Pain Medicine
Massachusetts General Hospital
Boston, Massachusetts

Emily Naoum, MD
Anesthesiologist/Intensivist
Department of Anesthesia, Critical Care and Pain Medicine
Massachusetts General Hospital
Boston, Massachusetts

John H. Nichols, MD
Division Chief of Pediatric Anesthesia
Director of Procedural Services, Massachusetts General for Children
Department of Anesthesia, Critical Care and Pain Medicine
Massachusetts General Hospital
Boston, Massachusetts

Ann Norris, MD
Resident
Department of Anesthesia, Critical Care and Pain Medicine
Massachusetts General Hospital
Boston, Massachusetts

Peter Ochieng, MD
Anesthesiologist
Department of Anesthesia, Critical Care and Pain Medicine
Massachusetts General Hospital
Boston, Massachusetts

Britlyn D. Orgill, MD
Anesthesiologist
Department of Anesthesia, Critical Care and Pain Medicine
Massachusetts General Hospital
Boston, Massachusetts

Lauren Peck, MD
Resident
Department of Anesthesia, Critical Care and Pain Medicine
Massachusetts General Hospital
Boston, Massachusetts

Carl Jn Pierre, MD
Resident
Department of Anesthesia, Critical Care and Pain Medicine
Massachusetts General Hospital
Boston, Massachusetts

Anastasia P. Piersa, MD, MDA
Resident
Department of Anesthesia, Critical Care and Pain Medicine
Massachusetts General Hospital
Boston, Massachusetts

Justin R. Porter, MD, PhD
Resident
Department of Anesthesia, Critical Care and Pain Medicine
Massachusetts General Hospital
Boston, Massachusetts

Jason Zhensheng Qu, MD
Anesthesiologist
Department of Anesthesia, Critical Care and Pain Medicine
Massachusetts General Hospital
Boston, Massachusetts

Neil Rens, MD, MBA, MSc
Resident
Department of Anesthesia, Critical Care and Pain Medicine
Massachusetts General Hospital
Boston, Massachusetts

David Rollins, MD
Resident
Department Anesthesia, Critical Care and Pain Medicine
Massachusetts General Hospital
Boston, Massachusetts

Katarina Ruscic, MD, PhD
Director of Anesthesia for Plastic, Reconstructive and Breast Oncology Surgery
Department of Anesthesia, Critical Care and Pain Medicine
Massachusetts General Hospital
Boston, Massachusetts

A. Sassan Sabouri, MD
Anesthesiologist
Department of Anesthesia, Critical Care and Pain Medicine
Massachusetts General Hospital
Boston, Massachusetts

Kendrick Shaw, MD, PhD
Anesthesiologist/Intensivist
Department of Anesthesia, Critical Care and Pain Medicine
Massachusetts General Hospital
Boston, Massachusetts

Andrew D. Siemens, MD
Resident
Department of Anesthesia, Critical Care and Pain Medicine
Massachusetts General Hospital
Boston, Massachusetts

Ken Solt, MD
Anesthesiologist
Department of Anesthesia, Critical Care and Pain Medicine
Massachusetts General Hospital
Boston, Massachusetts

Jamie L. Sparling, MD
Associate Director of Clinical Operations
Department of Anesthesia, Critical Care and Pain Medicine
Massachusetts General Hospital
Boston, Massachusetts

Peter Stefanovich, MD
Director, Regional Anesthesia and Perioperative Pain Medicine
Department of Anesthesia, Critical Care and Pain Medicine
Massachusetts General Hospital
Bostin, Massachusetts

Henry K. Su, MD
Anesthesiologist
Department of Anesthesia, Critical Care and Pain Medicine
Massachusetts General Hospital
Boston, Massachusetts

Matthew Thimm, MD
Resident
Department of Anesthesia, Critical Care and Pain Medicine
Massachusetts General Hospital
Boston, Massachusetts

A. Taylor Thomas, MD, MPH
Resident
Department of Anesthesia, Critical Care and Pain Medicine
Massachusetts General Hospital
Boston, Massachusetts

Alfredo Valdivia, MD, MPH
Resident
Department of Anesthesia, Critical Care and Pain Management
Massachusetts General Hospital
Boston, Massachusetts

Rafael Vazquez, MD
Director of Anesthesiology for Interventional Radiology
Department of Anesthesia, Critical Care and Pain Medicine
Massachusetts General Hospital
Boston, Massachusetts

Elisa C. Walsh, MD
Anesthesiologist/Intensivist
Department of Anesthesia, Critical Care and Pain Medicine
Massachusetts General Hospital
Boston, Massachusetts

Benjamin M. Weaver, MD
Resident
Department of Anesthesia, Critical Care and Pain Medicine
Massachusetts General Hospital
Boston, Massachusetts

Gabrielle White-Dzuro, MD
Anesthesiologist
Department of Anesthesia, Critical Care and Pain Medicine
Massachusetts General Hospital
Boston, Massachusetts

Hiu Ling (Karen) Wong, PharmD
Pharmacist, Perioperative Services
Department of Pharmacy
Massachusetts General Hospital
Boston, Massachusetts

Taylor A. Woo-Sekizaki, MD
Resident
Department of Anesthesia, Critical Care and Pain Medicine
Massachusetts General Hospital
Boston, Massachusetts

Fei Wu, MBBS
Resident
Department of Anesthesia, Critical Care and Pain Medicine
Massachusetts General Hospital
Boston, Massachusetts

Amanda Xi, MD, MSE
Director of Pre-Procedure Evaluation
Department of Anesthesia, Critical Care and Pain Medicine
Massachusetts General Hospital
Boston, Massachusetts

PREFACE

The publication of the 11th edition of *Clinical Anesthesia Procedures of the Massachusetts General Hospital* marks another milestone in our commitment to excellence in anesthesiology education. This handbook continues the legacy initiated by Dr. Richard Kitz who, in the 1970s, envisioned creating practical knowledge resources by those actively engaged in clinical practice. The collaborative model he established remains the cornerstone of our approach.

This edition features 40 comprehensive chapters and 3 valuable appendices that cover the full spectrum of anesthesia practice. Each chapter represents countless hours of dedication from resident physician authors who worked diligently to document current practices while faculty mentors provided guidance and expertise to ensure clinical accuracy and educational value. The pharmacists' contributions to the appendices have been invaluable, offering critical information on drug therapies that enhances patient safety and optimal care delivery.

I am extremely grateful to the other five associate editors (Drs. Ed Bittner, Hovig Chitilian, Ryan Horvath, Wilton Levine, and Jamie Sparling) who skillfully coordinated their sections, working tirelessly with authors to refine content and maintain cohesion throughout the handbook. Their commitment to excellence is evident in the quality of each chapter. The resident authors deserve special recognition for their exceptional contributions while balancing demanding clinical responsibilities. Similarly, the faculty mentors generously shared their expertise and time, embodying the educational mission that defines our institution.

The distinctive value of this handbook stems from its origins in daily clinical practice. Rather than presenting theoretical concepts alone, it offers practical approaches refined through decades of patient care at one of the world's leading medical institutions. This practical orientation makes it an essential resource for anesthesiologists, CRNAs, anesthesia assistants, medical students, anesthesia residents, and other health care professionals engaged in perioperative care. As with any book that summarizes and shortens more elaborate explanations, the information in this edition of the handbook should be augmented with consultation of other in-depth and peer-reviewed material which may include sophisticated online sources.

We stand proudly on the shoulders of those who contributed to the previous 10 editions, building upon their work while adapting to the evolving landscape of anesthesiology. My sincere appreciation goes to Dr. Seun Johnson-Akeju, our chairman, whose encouragement and support were instrumental in bringing this edition to fruition. Like most academic endeavors, this work was accomplished during evenings, weekends, holidays, and vacations—time otherwise spent with family and friends. Their understanding and support have been essential to completing this project. Of course, this entire endeavor hinged on the expertise that flowed from Wolters Kluwer and the superb team that was involved from the very start of this edition. I am especially grateful for the expert guidance and support from Keith Donnellan, Ashley Fischer, and Ann Francis.

As we present this 11th edition, we reaffirm our commitment to Dr. Kitz's original vision while embracing the innovations and advances that characterize modern anesthesiology practice. It is our hope that this handbook continues to serve as both a practical guide and an inspiration for excellence in patient care.

Keith H. Baker, MD, PhD
Boston, Massachusetts

CONTENTS

Contributors   v
Preface   xvi

PART I: EVALUATING THE PATIENT BEFORE ANESTHESIA   1

1 **Evaluating the Patient Before Anesthesia**   1
Jack Curtis and Amanda Xi

2 **Basics of Echocardiography and Lung Ultrasound**   21
Susana Arango and Alexander S. Kuo

3 **Specific Considerations for Cardiac Disease**   47
Peter Ochieng and Emily C. Mills

4 **Specific Considerations With Pulmonary Disease**   68
Benjamin M. Weaver and Timothy G. Gaulton

5 **Specific Considerations With Renal Disease**   78
Katarina Ruscic and Neil Rens

6 **Specific Considerations With Liver Disease**   98
Taylor A. Woo-Sekizaki and Ion A. Hobai

7 **Specific Considerations With Endocrine Disease**   113
Ion A. Hobai and Fei Wu

8 **Infectious Diseases and Infection Control in Anesthesia**   138
Ashwini Joshi and Jamie L. Sparling

PART II: ADMINISTRATION OF ANESTHESIA — 155

9 Safety in Anesthesia — 155
Britlyn D. Orgill and Rebecca D. Minehart

10 The Anesthesia Machine — 165
Zeyu Hu and Jeremi Mountjoy

11 Administration of General Anesthesia — 177
Matthew Thimm and Kendrick Shaw

12 Intravenous and Inhalation Anesthetics — 188
Justin R. Porter and Gregory E. Ginsburg

13 Airway Evaluation and Management — 205
Adam W. Kaplon and Jean Kwo

14 Neuromuscular Blockade — 227
Scott Cao and Simona Iustina Lupu

15 Monitoring — 243
Julia M. Danford and Elisa C. Walsh

16 Monitoring Anesthetic Brain States — 265
Christian Guay and Johanna Lee

17 Intra-anesthetic Problems — 280
Zeyu Hu, Ying Hui Low and Alexander Nagrebetsky

18 Perioperative Hemodynamic Control — 305
Victoria Bass and William Benedetto

19 Local Anesthetics — 323
Lillye Anderson and Ken Solt

20 Spinal, Epidural, and Caudal Anesthesia — 332
James S. Cho and Joseph L. McDowell

21	**Regional Anesthesia** David Rollins and A. Sassan Sabouri	357
22	**Anesthesia for Orthopedic Surgery** Megan Abbott and Amy Du	390
23	**Anesthesia for Neurosurgery** Daniel Ankeny and Gabrielle White-Dzuro	402
24	**Anesthesia for Spine Surgery** John J. A. Marota and Zachary Achen	423
25	**Anesthesia for Transplant Surgery** Lauren Alderette and James Taylor Lloyd	431
26	**Anesthesia for Abdominal Surgery** Scott Cao and J. Paul Fleming	446
27	**Anesthesia for Thoracic Surgery** Henry K. Su and Xiaodong Bao	465
28	**Anesthesia for Vascular Surgery** Ann Norris and James Taylor Lloyd	486
29	**Anesthesia for Cardiac Surgery** Brian J. Kinsman and Jason Zhensheng Qu	510
30	**Anesthesia for Head and Neck Surgery** Victoria Bass and Jeremy Goldfarb	544
31	**Anesthesia for Urologic Surgery** Lauren Peck and Daniel Ellis	557
32	**Anesthesia for Obstetrics and Gynecology** A. Taylor Thomas and Emily Naoum	566
33	**Anesthesia for Pediatric Surgery and Care of the Neonate** Christopher Bean and Chang A. Liu	589

34	**Non-Operating Room Anesthesia** Anastasia P. Piersa and Rafael Vazquez	632
35	**Anesthesia for Trauma and Burns** Carl Jn Pierre and Jamie L. Sparling	654
36	**Transfusion Therapy** Andrew D. Siemens and Marvin G. Chang	681

PART III: PERIOPERATIVE ISSUES — 705

37	**The Postanesthesia Care Unit** Alfredo Valdivia and Ryan J. Horvath	705
38	**Pain Management** Rachel Padilla Judge and Peter Stefanovich	725
39	**Adult, Pediatric, and Newborn Resuscitation** John H. Nichols and Christopher Di Capua	747
40	**Vascular Access** James S. Cho and Omar Hyder	772
	Appendix I: Drugs With Narrow Therapeutic Ranges and Potential for Harm Hiu Ling (Karen) Wong	777
	Appendix II: Commonly Used Drugs Audrey Kennedy	781
	Appendix III: Common Intravenous Antibiotics Parita A. Chowatia	800

Index — *805*

PART I: EVALUATING THE PATIENT BEFORE ANESTHESIA

Evaluating the Patient Before Anesthesia

Jack Curtis and Amanda Xi

I. INTRODUCTION

The clinic model for anesthesiologists' preoperative evaluation of patients is continuously evolving. Historically, prior to the day of surgery, a patient was evaluated in person at an office. The visit established rapport and allowed the anesthesiologist to become familiar with the patient's surgical illness, identify and medically optimize comorbidities, develop a perioperative management strategy, and obtain informed consent. Due to patient and hospital factors, this approach has been modified. Telemedicine consults arose as a cost- and time-saving method of accomplishing the same preoperative evaluation. Electronic consults, or eConsults, are also being used as a direct pathway of communication between the anesthesiologist and other patient providers. The anesthesiologist gathers clinical information through various health care systems and synthesizes an overall clinical picture to determine optimization and complete workup prior to surgery while actively communicating with the patient's surgical and medical providers. Physical examination and consent forms are completed on the day of surgery. Some centers with known low-risk patients and low-risk procedures defer the entire evaluation to the day of surgery. Regardless of the model of preoperative evaluation, the basic tenants remain the same.

II. HISTORY

Relevant information is obtained through chart review followed by corroboration with the patient interview. When the medical record is not available, a history is obtained from the patient and supplemented by the patient's other physicians.

- **A. History of presenting illness.** The anesthesiologist should review the symptoms of the present surgical illness, presumptive diagnosis, initial treatment, and diagnostic studies.
- **B. Medications.** The provider should establish the current dosing and schedules of all the patient's medications. Antihypertensive, antianginal, antiarrhythmic, anticoagulant, anticonvulsant, and specific endocrine (eg, insulin, hypoglycemics, SGLT2i, and GLP-1 receptor agonists [GLP-1RA]) medications are especially important. Deciding to continue medication during the preoperative period depends on the severity of the underlying illness, potential consequences of discontinuing treatment, half-life of the medication, and likelihood of deleterious interactions with anesthetic agents. Generally, most medications may be continued up through the time of surgery (see Section VI).

C. **Allergies and drug reactions.** True allergic reactions are relatively uncommon. Adverse reactions to perioperative medications are common, however, and may be reported by the patient. Therefore, it is important to obtain a careful description of the exact nature of the reaction.
   1. **True allergic reactions.** IgE-mediated reactions and anaphylaxis can be presumed based upon characteristic symptoms that occurred within a narrow timeframe after exposure to an allergen. Multiple organ systems can be affected, and common symptoms include pruritic rash, urticaria, angioedema, bronchospasm, shortness of breath, wheezing, hypotension, persistent vomiting, and intestinal cramping.
   2. **Antibiotic allergy.** Allergies to antibiotics, especially to sulfonamides, penicillins, and cephalosporin derivatives, are the most common drug allergies. While skin testing can help determine true penicillin allergy, 90% to 99% of patients with self-reported allergy have a negative skin test. Therefore, it should not be used as the sole predictor. In patients with a penicillin allergy, the major determinant of immunological reaction to a cephalosporin is the similarity between the side chain of first-generation drug rather than the β-lactam structure that they share. There is a 0.5% to 3% cross reactivity to first- and second-generation cephalosporins. Some institutions implement a test dose procedure prior to administering a therapeutic dose and monitor for adverse reactions. However, anaphylaxis is not dose dependent. For patients with a penicillin allergy, there is a threefold increased coincidental risk of reaction to even an unrelated drug. That is, they are more likely to react to any medication. A recent update to guidelines at MGH suggests that patients with known anaphylaxis to penicillin should not receive cefazolin unless an evaluation has been conducted by allergy/immunology.
   3. **Soybean oil and/or egg yolk allergy.** Propofol is commonly formulated as an emulsion containing soybean oil, egg lecithin, and glycerol which has created concerns regarding its use in patients with a history of associated food allergies. Egg allergies are predominantly to the ovalbumin protein found in the egg white, rather than the lecithin in the egg yolk. Similarly, soy allergy is typically to the soy protein rather than soy oil. Current data suggest low likelihood of adverse reaction to propofol in these patients.
   4. **Inhalational agent or succinylcholine "allergy."** A history of allergy to "anesthesia," inhalational agents, or succinylcholine, in the patient or any close relative, may represent a history of malignant hyperthermia (Chapter 17: Intra-anesthetic Problems) or atypical plasma cholinesterase.
   5. **Local anesthetic allergy.** Allergy to ester-type local anesthetics can be anaphylactic (see Chapter 19), while allergy to the amide-type local anesthetics is exceedingly rare. Tachycardia or palpitations associated with perivascular injection of local anesthetic mixed with epinephrine may be reported as an occurrence during regional anesthetics. A history of local anesthetic systemic toxicity (LAST) can uncover relevant neurological or cardiac sequelae and inform patient preferences but is unlikely to recur.
   6. **Shellfish or seafood allergy.** Patients with an allergy to shellfish, seafood, or topical antiseptic containing iodine are not at increased risk of adverse reaction to iodinated intravenous contrast. However, patients with a prior documented reaction to contrast are at risk if exposed to the same agent. It is important to note that there is no allergy cross reactivity between different classes of contrast, and alternate contrasts can typically be safely administered.

7. **Latex allergy or hypersensitivity reactions.** Latex allergy must be ascertained preoperatively to allow for preparation of a latex-free operating room. Additionally, banana, avocado, chestnut, kiwi, or papaya allergy should be elicited as 30% to 50% of individuals with these allergies have cross-reactive allergies to latex. Other risk factors for latex allergy include repeated exposure to latex (eg, health care workers or patients with multiple prior surgeries), atopy, and certain medical disorders, such as spina bifida. If these risk factors exist, and no prior skin or serologic tests have been conducted, it may be warranted to treat the patient as latex allergic.

D. **Anesthetic history.** It is crucial to question the patient about their prior experience with anesthesia. Common descriptions of anesthetic problems include postoperative nausea and vomiting (PONV), sore throat, neuropathy, difficult intubation, and prolonged emergence. Reviewing previous anesthetic records can shed light on other patient-specific considerations.
   1. **Response to medications.** Patient responses to sedative, analgesic, and anesthetic agents vary widely among individuals. Cognitive changes, such as memory loss, delirium, or dullness, are frequently described in elderly patients and can be minimized by avoiding burst suppression, anticholinergic drugs, and benzodiazepines. Intraoperative awareness may be reported. Describing to the patient the experience of procedural sedation versus general anesthesia may clarify a prior experience and provide reassurance. Those with true recall may require higher doses of hypnotic medication, modified electroencephalographic (EEG) assessment, and other mechanisms of confirming depth of anesthesia.
   2. **Vascular access and invasive monitoring.** Determining the need for ultrasound-guided IV placement or central access can help to avoid repeated attempts in a patient who is a "difficult stick." In morbidly obese patients, noninvasive blood pressure (BP) monitoring may be impossible due to the conical shape of the upper extremity and an arterial line may be required.
   3. **Airway management.** Determine past airway exams, ease of mask ventilation, view obtained on direct laryngoscopy, size and type of laryngoscope blade and endotracheal tube, and depth of endotracheal tube insertion. A prior history of a difficult intubation is the primary predictor of a difficult airway.
   4. **Perianesthetic complications.** Review prior records for complications such as adverse drug reactions, dental injury, protracted PONV, hemodynamic instability, respiratory compromise, postoperative myocardial infarction (MI), unanticipated admission to an intensive care unit (ICU), prolonged emergence, or need for reintubation.
   5. **Opioid requirements.** Opioid administration perioperatively can lend insight into future requirements and the need for alternative pain management strategies, such as neuraxial anesthetics, peripheral nerve blocks, multimodal pharmacology, and consideration of consultation with pain specialists.

E. **Family history.** A history of adverse anesthetic outcomes in family members should be assessed with open-ended questions, such as "Has anyone in your family experienced unusual or serious reactions to anesthesia?" Additionally, patients should be specifically asked about a family history of malignant hyperthermia.

F. **Social history and habits**
   1. **Smoking.** The perioperative period is a powerful time to provide counseling and support smoking cessation in patients and is associated

with a higher rate of success. Smoking cessation reduces postoperative complications, and evidence suggests that abstinence should be encouraged regardless of surgical interval timing. A history of exercise intolerance or the presence of a productive cough or hemoptysis may indicate the need for further evaluation.

2. **Drug and alcohol use.** Although self-reporting of drug and alcohol intake typically underestimates use, it is a helpful start to define the type of drugs used, routes of administration, frequency, and timing of most recent use. Stimulant abuse may lead to palpitations, angina, lowered thresholds for serious arrhythmias and seizures, and increased anesthetic requirements if used in the acute setting. Marijuana use can cause airway hyperreactivity and significantly increase the requirements of propofol and analgesics. Acute alcohol intoxication decreases anesthetic requirement and predisposes to hypothermia and hypoglycemia. Alcohol withdrawal may precipitate severe hypertension (HTN), tremors, delirium, and seizures and may markedly increase anesthetic and analgesic requirements. Risk of intraoperative awareness is also increased with chronic opioid or benzodiazepine use.

III. REVIEW OF SYSTEMS

The purpose of review of systems (ROS) is to elicit symptoms of occult disease and to determine the stability of current disease. Coexisting illnesses should be evaluated by an organ-systems approach with an emphasis on recent changes in symptoms, signs, and treatment (see Chapters 3–7). A minimum ROS should seek to elicit the following information:

A. Cardiovascular

1. **Coronary artery disease.** Preexisting coronary artery disease (CAD) may predispose the patient to spontaneous myocardial ischemia, demand ischemia, or ventricular dysfunction. Angina, dyspnea on exertion (DOE), paroxysmal nocturnal dyspnea, and reduced exercise capacity can help characterize the severity of disease.

2. **Pacemakers (permanent pacemaker, PPM) and implanted cardioverter-defibrillators (ICD).** ICDs should be interrogated within 6 months of surgery, PPMs within 12 months, and cardiac resynchronization therapy (CRT) devices within 3 to 6 months. The decision to deactivate functions of an ICD or change a PPM to asynchronous mode via transcutaneous magnet placement should be made based on the likelihood of electrocautery interference (ie, distance from the generator) causing unwanted shocks or failure to pace.

3. **HTN.** Baseline BP ranges should be established, and the perioperative goal should be to maintain pressures within 10% to 20% of the baseline. Poorly controlled HTN is frequently associated with marked preoperative HTN and labile intraoperative pressures. If the planned surgical position is prone or beach chair, the procedure may be delayed for BP optimization so the risk of blindness and stroke is minimized.

4. **DOE.** DOE is an important sign that can be caused by myriad underlying etiologies, including physical deconditioning, obesity, or cardiopulmonary pathology. If the DOE is acute or acute-on-chronic, the patient should be evaluated and referred for appropriate testing to determine etiology and treatment.

5. **Exercise capacity.** Assessment of functional capacity helps in risk stratification for predicting a perioperative cardiac event. Functional capacity is quantified in terms of metabolic equivalents of task (METs) rated on a scale of poor (<4 METs) to excellent (≥10). A METs of moderate

(≥4) or greater, such as the ability to climb two flights of stairs, is associated with reduced perioperative morbidity and mortality for those having noncardiac surgery. Metabolic equivalents are a central component of the ACC/AHA guidelines for perioperative cardiac assessment. Various assessment tools, such as the Duke Activity Status Index, can be utilized to estimate a patient's METs score.

B. Respiratory
1. **Upper respiratory infection (URI).** URI can predispose patients to bronchospasm and laryngospasm during induction and emergence from general anesthesia. In severe cases, this can lead to inability to oxygenate and ventilate. Therefore, the patient with active signs and symptoms of a URI (productive cough, rhinorrhea, sore throat, fever) should have elective procedures postponed for 4 to 6 weeks after recovery.
2. **Asthma.** Reactive airway disease may result in acute bronchospasm in the perioperative period. Specific questions about previous asthma-related hospitalizations, intubations, emergency room visits, and medication requirements (specifically, steroid use) can help delineate the severity of asthma.
3. **Obstructive sleep apnea (OSA).** Symptoms of OSA should be elicited as they may herald difficulty with bag-mask ventilation or episodes of perioperative hypoxia/hypercarbia. The STOP-BANG criteria helps rate the likelihood of having OSA. Long-standing and untreated OSA can lead to pulmonary HTN, and a transthoracic echocardiogram (TTE) can be used to confirm severity. (See Chapter 13 for additional details.)

C. Neurological.
Anesthetic agents may exacerbate underlying neurological disorders. It is important to evaluate the patient's current neurological state and for history of seizure disorder (presence of deep brain stimulator), stroke, amyotrophic lateral sclerosis (ALS), multiple sclerosis, myasthenia gravis, Lambert–Eaton syndrome, Parkinson disease (presence of deep brain stimulator), and cerebral palsy, among others. Baseline neurological deficits should be documented with precision to allow for accurate postoperative comparison and intervention. Neuromuscular blockade should be carefully considered prior to administration, as it may result in prolonged weakness or lethal hyperkalemia. Preexisting neurologic conditions should also be considered in the context of regional anesthetic techniques and must be evaluated on a case-by-case basis.

D. Renal.
Renal disease can be categorized according to severity, etiology, and acuity. All types affect perioperative management. Hemodialysis for end-stage renal disease (ESRD) should be performed 24 hours prior to surgical procedure to optimize electrolyte imbalances and volume status. Evaluation of creatinine, glomerular filtration rate (GFR), anemia, and electrolyte abnormalities are imperative. Nonsteroidal anti-inflammatory drug (NSAID) use should be avoided, and benzylisoquinolinium-type neuromuscular blocking agents such as cisatracurium are often a preferred neuromuscular blockade agent.

E. Endocrine
1. **Diabetes mellitus.** Diabetes is a risk factor for cardiovascular disease, nephropathy, neuropathy, and gastroparesis. The patient with autonomic nervous system dysfunction may have silent myocardial ischemia and endovascular disease. Endotracheal intubation may prove difficult secondary to arthritis of the temporomandibular joints and cervical spine as a result of glycosylation of synovium. Home blood glucose measurements, hemoglobin A1c level, and symptomatic swings in blood glucose may elucidate whether the diabetes is well controlled. It

is also important to distinguish between type 1 and type 2 diabetics due to the risk of diabetic ketoacidosis (DKA) and use of insulin pumps in the former group.
  2. **Thyroid disease.** Thyroid storm can lead to an intraoperative emergency and occurs in patients with thyrotoxicosis secondary to Graves disease and as well in those with untreated disease. Severe hypothyroidism can lead to slow metabolism of medication, hypothermia, and prolonged emergence from anesthesia.
- **F. Gastrointestinal**
  1. **Gastroesophageal reflux disease (GERD).** Symptoms of reflux with or without hiatal hernia increase the risk of pulmonary aspiration and may alter the anesthetic plan. An awake intubation or rapid sequence induction may be indicated. The patient should be asked specifically about chest pain/burning sensation, globus sensation, sour taste in the mouth after meals, frank regurgitation of food, or unexplained cough.
  2. **Dysphagia/odynophagia.** Those with subjective feelings of difficulty swallowing or pain with swallowing may have stricture, mass, or motility syndrome. They are poor candidates for transesophageal echocardiogram (TEE) and may require coordination of care to have an esophagogastroduodenoscopy (EGD) preoperatively in the presence of severe cardiac disease.
  3. **Motion sickness or PONV history.** A history of motion sickness and/or PONV increases the risk for PONV. Other factors associated with increased PONV risk include, but are not limited to, history of vertigo, female gender, nonsmoking status, gynecologic and laparoscopic procedures, strabismus surgery, and the need for large doses of perioperative or postoperative opioids. A different anesthetic technique, such as total intravenous anesthesia, may be warranted in the patient with multiple risk factors.
- **G. Musculoskeletal.** A history of radiation to the head or neck may increase the risk of distorted airway anatomy, reduce range of motion, and alter intubation technique. Rheumatoid arthritis and Down syndrome are associated with atlantoaxial instability, and ankylosing spondylitis may significantly reduce cervical spine range of motion. The patient should also be questioned about scoliosis when neuraxial anesthesia is being considered as well as joint pain for purposes of intraoperative positioning.
- **H. Obstetric/gynecologic.** Possibility of pregnancy and timing of last menses should be elicited in women of childbearing age as some medication may be teratogenic. Elective surgery should be postponed until the postpartum period. Maternal arterial pressures are directly proportional to uteroplacental perfusion, so sustained hypotension could result in fetal distress. For 2 weeks following nonobstetric surgery, the parturient is also at risk of preterm labor. Intraoperative fetal monitoring may be appropriate when the fetus is viable, monitoring is physically possible given the procedure, and emergent C-section would be considered if necessary. It can also provide useful information for maternal positioning during the case. The decision to utilize fetal monitoring should be coordinated among the anesthesia, surgical, and obstetric teams.
- **I. Hematologic.** A history of easy bruising, bleeding diathesis, heavy menses, or unprovoked blood clots warrants further questioning and workup. Idiopathic thrombocytopenia, von Willebrand disease, thalassemia, hemophilia, sickle cell disease, and inherited thrombophilias add a layer of complexity to peripheral nerve blocks, neuraxial anesthetics, planning for surgical blood loss, and need for anticoagulation postoperatively.

IV. THE PHYSICAL EXAMINATION

The physical examination should be thorough but focused. Special attention is directed toward evaluation of the airway, heart, lungs, and neurologic status. Assessment of the block site is warranted before a regional anesthetic. Patient devices, such as pacemakers, insulin pumps, and intrathecal pumps should also be evaluated and set to appropriate modes. This may require discussion with the patient and the devices' managing specialists.

A. Vital signs
1. **BP.** If the patient has aortic arch or significant vascular disease, BP measurement should be taken in both arms. Noninvasive BP measurements should be avoided on an extremity with an arteriovenous fistula. While there is controversial evidence for causing lymphedema with a BP cuff after axillary lymph node dissection or radiation, it is reasonable to avoid the limb for patient preference and assuaging anxiety. Arterial lines should, however, be avoided on the side of breast cancer surgery to reduce the risk of cellulitis causing lymphedema.
2. **Pulse.** Resting heart rate should be noted for regularity and rate.
3. **Respiratory rate.** Respirations should be observed for rate, depth, effort, and pattern.
4. **Oxygen saturation.** Etiology of a saturation less than 93% should be investigated.

B. Height and weight.
Height and weight measurements are necessary for determining drug dosages, fluid requirements, adequate urine output, and ventilator settings. Ideal body weight (IBW) should be calculated using the formula:
1. Males: IBW (kg) = 50 + 2.3 kg for each inch over 5 ft
2. Females: IBW (kg) = 45.5 + 2.3 kg for each inch over 5 ft

C. Head and neck.
During the basic preoperative examination, the anesthesiologist should evaluate the following:
1. **Maximal mouth opening**
2. **Ability to prognath.** Upper lip bite test.
3. **Mallampati classification** (see Chapter 13: Airway Evaluation and Management)
4. **Thyromental distance.** Thyromental distance is the distance between the tip of the chin and the thyroid notch. Approximately three fingerbreadths distance is considered normal.
5. **Dentition.** Evaluate teeth for those loose, chipped, or missing. Crowns, bridges, dentures, braces, retainers, and other dental appliances should be noted. Nonpermanent implants should be removed prior to entering the operating room.
6. **Facial hair.** A large beard or mustache may be taped with Tegaderm or shaved so as not to interfere with achieving a seal for bag-mask ventilation.
7. **Cervical spine.** Evaluate range of motion in flexion, extension, and rotation of the cervical spine.
8. **Superficial neck.** Check for tracheal deviation, cervical masses, and jugular venous distention. The presence of a carotid bruit is nonspecific but may suggest a need for evaluating carotid stenosis.
9. **Neck circumference.** A neck circumference measurement of 17 inches for men and 16 inches for women is associated with OSA and obstruction during bag-mask ventilation.

D. Precordium.
Auscultation of the heart may reveal murmurs, S3, S4, or a pericardial rub.

E. Lungs.
Auscultate for wheezing, rhonchi, or rales, which should be correlated with observations regarding the ease of breathing and the use of accessory muscles for respiration.

F. **Abdomen.** Any evidence of abdominal distention, masses, or ascites should be noted as these may predispose the patient to regurgitation or ventilatory compromise. Gastric ultrasound has shown to be highly sensitive and specific for evaluation of full stomach when presence of gastric content is in question.
G. **Extremities.** Evaluate for muscle wasting and weakness, distal perfusion, clubbing, cyanosis, edema, and the presence of any cutaneous infections (especially over sites of planned vascular cannulation or regional nerve block). Ecchymosis or unexplained injury, especially in children, women, and elderly patients, can be an indication of an abusive relationship.
H. **Back.** Note any deformity, scoliosis, bruising, rash, cellulitis, or skin condition that could lead to difficulty in patient positioning or performance of neuraxial analgesia.
I. **Neurologic examination.** Document mental status, cranial nerve function, cognition, and peripheral sensorimotor function.

V. LABORATORY STUDIES

Routine laboratory screening tests are generally not indicated. Tests should be selected based on the patient's medical condition and the proposed surgical procedure.

A. **Hematologic studies.** Hematologic studies are indicated if there are concerns regarding significant preexisting anemia, perioperative blood loss, or coagulopathy.
  1. **Recent hematocrit/hemoglobin level.** There is no universally accepted minimum hematocrit before anesthesia. The etiology and duration of anemia should be ascertained.
  2. **Platelet studies.** By history, platelet function can be assessed by easy bruising, petechiae, excessive bleeding from gums or minor cuts, and family history. Repeat complete blood count (CBC), smear, evaluation of liver function, autoimmune disease, and infectious etiology should be considered. A hematology consultation for etiology evaluation such as thrombotic thrombocytopenic purpura (TTP), immune thrombocytopenia (ITP), heparin-induced thrombocytopenia (HIT), von Willebrand disease (vWD), or malignancy may be pursued.
  3. **Coagulation studies.** Coagulation studies may be ordered to assess level of pharmacological anticoagulation, readiness for nerve block or neuraxial anesthesia after discontinuation of anticoagulant, synthetic liver function, and clinically relevant nutritional deficiency. Coagulation status of the patient on low–molecular-weight heparin may be monitored through measurement of anti–factor Xa levels.
  4. **Blood type/antibody screen.** Type and screen should be obtained if anticipating a significant intraoperative blood loss or if the patient has alloantibodies that are challenging to crossmatch.
B. **Serum chemistry.** A metabolic panel should be ordered in patients with risk factors for renal or hepatic disease that would affect their serum electrolytes, ability to metabolize drugs, and impact their response to fluid. It is also indicated for patients taking diuretics, digoxin, steroids, or aminoglycoside antibiotics.
  1. **Hypokalemia.** Low potassium levels are common in the patient receiving diuretics and are usually readily corrected by preoperative oral potassium supplementation. Mild hypokalemia (2.8 to 3.5 mEq/L) should not preclude elective surgery. Rapid correction with intravenous potassium may lead to dysrhythmias and cardiac arrest.

2. **Hyperkalemia.** Elevated potassium is often seen in the patient with ESRD. Mild elevations in serum potassium among those with already elevated baselines are well tolerated. Treatment of hyperkalemia is warranted if concentrations exceed 6 mEq/L or if electrocardiogram (ECG) changes occur, such as peaked T waves, prolonged PR interval, P-wave flattening, or widened QRS.
3. **Hyponatremia.** Serum sodium levels <135 mEq/L are an independent negative prognostic indicator for perioperative outcomes. Even mild hyponatremia in healthy patients undergoing nonemergent surgery is associated with an increased incidence of 30-day mortality, coronary events, pneumonia, wound infections, and hospital length of stay. The severity of hyponatremia corresponds to worse outcomes. Low serum sodium should be considered a surrogate marker for medical comorbidities, and perhaps not itself the cause of poor outcomes. The etiology should be determined, and if possible, severe abnormalities should be corrected preoperatively.

C. **ECG.** The most recent ACC/AHA guidelines for patients undergoing noncardiac surgery state that a preoperative ECG is not beneficial in asymptomatic patients undergoing low-risk procedures. Preoperative ECG is reasonable for patients with known severe arrhythmia, cerebrovascular disease, peripheral arterial disease, or structural or coronary heart disease undergoing greater than a low-risk surgical intervention. An ECG should not be done for the sole indication of advanced patient age; however, per the 2022 European Society of Cardiology Guidelines, in patients 65 years of age or older, ECG and biomarkers are recommended for intermediate and high-risk noncardiac surgery (Class 1). The Canadian Cardiovascular Guidelines recommend measuring BNP or NT-proBNP in this same age group in addition to patients aged 45 to 64 years with significant cardiovascular disease or with a Revised Cardiac Risk Index score ≥1. If elevated or unavailable, they recommend trending daily troponin for 48 to 72 hours postoperatively and obtaining an ECG in the PACU.

D. **Chest radiography.** A chest x-ray (CXR) should be obtained in the patient with signs or symptoms of acute or unstable chronic cardiopulmonary disease.

E. **Pulmonary function tests.** Pulmonary function tests (PFTs) are used to evaluate the severity of lung disease. They have a recognized role in the evaluation of patients undergoing lung resection surgery; however, they have not been shown to be predictive of postoperative pulmonary complications in surgeries other than lung resection (Chapter 4: Specific Considerations with Pulmonary Disease and Chapter 27: Anesthesia for Thoracic Surgery).

VI. PREOPERATIVE MEDICAL OPTIMIZATION

Preexisting medical conditions should be controlled or stabilized before surgery. Many of the complications associated with these conditions may be prevented by thoughtful administration of standard medications.

A. **HTN.** Untreated HTN can cause end-organ damage. Acute treatment of chronic HTN may be indicated in the patient with systolic BP greater than 20% of their baseline. If HTN persists despite treatment or if the BP is greater than 180/110 mm Hg, elective surgery should be postponed until the BP is better controlled. Angiotensin-converting enzyme inhibitors and angiotensin receptor–blocking agents may cause refractory vasoplegia and should be held the night before or on the day of surgery. β-Blockers, calcium channel blockers, and clonidine may be continued perioperatively.

B. CAD. In patients with a recent history of percutaneous coronary intervention or coronary artery bypass grafting on dual antiplatelet therapy (DAPT), careful consideration must be given to medication management and timing of surgical procedure. See the 2016 ACC/AHA Guideline focused update on duration of DAPT therapy in patients with CAD for comprehensive guidelines. Chapter 3: Specific Considerations for Cardiac Disease further outlines the stepwise approach to preoperative evaluation in patients with CAD.

Individuals on long-term β-blocker therapy should continue their medication in the perioperative period. Postoperative dose modification in the setting of bradycardia or hypotension is appropriate. Current literature does not support initiating prophylactic β-blockade immediately prior to or on the day of surgery, as this has been associated with increased all-cause mortality. Detailed recommendations for perioperative β-blocker administration are further outlined in the 2014 AHA/ACC Guideline on perioperative cardiovascular evaluation and management of patients undergoing noncardiac surgery.

With regard to aspirin, evidence reveals that the risks may outweigh the benefits for primary prevention, and some experts believe that particularly in the elderly, the bleeding risk outweighs the benefits. Guidelines at MGH state that aspirin (81 to 325 mg) be continued up to and including the day of surgery, except in the case of intracranial neurosurgical procedures, intramedullary spine surgery, surgery of the middle ear or posterior eye, and possibly prostate surgery. Complete reversal of aspirin effects requires 7 to 10 days for new platelet synthesis. Discontinuing aspirin in a patient receiving aspirin for secondary prophylaxis necessitates an explicit discussion with the patient's primary care physician, cardiologist, or vascular physician. The decision should weigh the cardiovascular risks of stopping aspirin versus the risk of bleeding from the surgery.

C. Anticoagulation therapy. Depending on the indication for anticoagulation, a patient on warfarin may need to be bridged with low–molecular-weight heparin or unfractionated heparin regimens prior to surgery. This decision should be made with the surgeon and physician prescribing the anticoagulation.

D. NSAIDs. The modest inhibition of platelet function caused by NSAIDs does not increase bleeding risk nor does it increase the risk of hematoma associated with spinal or epidural anesthesia. Celecoxib does not affect platelet function and therefore may be continued perioperatively in those who take it chronically. Some surgeons still hesitate to continue NSAIDs given data suggesting deleterious effects on bone healing; however, current data suggests that if used for less than 2 weeks, there is no significant risk of nonunion. Given the oppositional literature, a discussion with the surgeon regarding NSAID use is justified. As part of expedited recovery after surgery (ERAS) protocols, NSAIDs are often given as part of a preoperative cocktail. Caution should be taken with patients who have severe coronary disease, peptic ulcer disease, HTN, renal disease, and asthma.

E. Opioid tolerance. Usual doses of opioids should be continued in the perioperative period to avoid withdrawal. Multimodal analgesia and regional anesthetics should be pursued as determined by patients and surgical factors. A patient taking methadone should continue maintenance dosing through the day of surgery. A patient taking suboxone should have a plan formulated by their prescribing physician, surgeon, and anesthesiologist. Guidelines at MGH recommend patients on suboxone ≤8 mg/d (4 mg BID) continue their baseline regimen throughout the perioperative period. Higher daily dosage may require preoperative titration to optimize

surgical pain management. For inpatient procedures, the addiction services consult team should be consulted to assist in the postoperative titration of suboxone.
F. **Asthma.** A patient with moderate to severe asthma may require treatment with albuterol or ipratropium via metered dose inhaler immediately prior to airway instrumentation. A wheezing patient should be referred to a pulmonologist or internist for optimization and symptom control before surgery. All asthma medications—inhaled and oral—should be continued perioperatively.
G. **Diabetes mellitus.** A diabetic patient may present with hyperglycemia or hypoglycemia. A blood glucose level should be obtained by finger stick preoperatively and abnormal levels addressed (see Chapter 7: Specific Considerations with Endocrine Disease). Severe and acute hyperglycemia can lead to a hyperosmolar state that can result in impaired enzyme function, DKA, or a hyperosmolar hyperglycemic nonketotic state. Oral hypoglycemic agents and short-acting insulin should all be held on the day of surgery. Basal insulin should be continued, albeit many recommend a reduction of 20% to 50%, and blood glucose levels closely monitored. Two classes of diabetic medications that are of particular importance to anesthesiologists include sodium-glucose cotransporter-2 (SGLT2) inhibitors and (glucagon-like peptide-1) GLP-1RA.
  1. SGLT2 inhibitors work in the proximal convoluted tubule of the kidney, thereby reducing resorption of glucose and increasing its excretion. The primary concern with this class of medications in the perioperative period is the increased risk of euglycemic DKA when not appropriately held. The loss of glucose in conjunction with a state of fasting leads to an increase in the ratio of glucagon to insulin, resulting in ketogenesis. SGLT2 inhibitors should be held for 72 to 96 hours prior to surgery to minimize the risk of euglycemic DKA. If not held for the appropriate amount of time, MGH guidelines recommend preoperatively obtaining a BMP for evaluation of bicarbonate and anion gap and postoperatively repeating a BMP with the addition of checking β-hydroxybutyrate levels.
  2. GLP-1RA stimulate insulin and reduce glucagon secretion, slow gastric emptying, and promote satiety. The primary anesthetic consideration for patients taking this class of medication lies in the delayed gastric emptying, increasing the concern for full stomach and aspiration risk. Current ASA guidance recommends holding daily dosed GLP-1RA on the day of surgery and weekly dosed medications 1 week prior to surgery. However, recent data suggests that these hold parameters may not reverse the effects of delayed gastric emptying, and that longer cessation of the drug should be considered. The American Gastroenterological Association (AGA) issued a rapid clinical practice update in response to the ASA guidelines regarding patients taking GLP-1RA in the context of endoscopies. In this update, one strategy discussed was transitioning patients to a liquid diet the day prior to endoscopy instead of holding the medication, noting that gastric emptying of fluid is more rapid than emptying of solids and that endoscopists immediately suction liquid contents upon entering the stomach. Mass General Brigham (MGB) issued a guideline to hold long-acting GLP-1RA agents (eg, semaglutide, dulaglutide, tirzepatide) for at least one dose and adhere to a clear liquid diet. However, if not held appropriately, an individualized approach is required based on urgency of procedure, presence of gastrointestinal symptoms (nausea, vomiting, bloating), and findings on gastric ultrasound if available.

H. **High aspiration risk.** Guidelines to reduce the risk of pulmonary aspiration have been published by the ASA and include preoperative assessment risk factors, nil per os (NPO) status, and pharmacological agent recommendations. These precautions should be implemented for patients at high risk of aspiration, such as those with a hiatal hernia, difficult airway, ileus, obesity, poorly controlled diabetes, depressed sensorium, pregnancy, delayed gastric emptying, and acute trauma. The following medications can be administered to decrease gastric acid and/or decrease gastric volume: H_2 antagonists such as cimetidine, famotidine, and ranitidine reduce the volume and acidity of gastric secretions. Cimetidine inhibits the CYP P450 system and prolongs the elimination of many drugs, including theophylline, diazepam, propranolol, and lidocaine, potentially increasing the toxicity of these agents. Ranitidine has recently been withdrawn from the market due to FDA concerns over contamination. Proton-pump inhibitors are highly effective in reducing acid production but do not work quickly enough to be used in the immediate preoperative period; the greatest benefit is seen in patients on long-term therapy. Nonparticulate antacids, such as sodium citrate and citric acid (Bicitra), raise gastric pH. Metoclopramide enhances gastric emptying by increasing lower esophageal sphincter tone and simultaneously relaxing the pylorus. As with all dopamine antagonists, it may produce dystonia or other extrapyramidal effects. Metoclopramide is contraindicated in suspected bowel obstruction due to increased risk of perforation.
I. **Other medications.** In general, anticonvulsants, antiarrhythmics, steroids, and hormonal supplements may be continued through the perioperative period. Vitamins and herbal supplements should be discontinued a minimum of 7 days prior to surgery.

VII. ANESTHETIC ASSESSMENT AND PLAN
A. **ASA physical status class.** ASA class provides an overall impression of the severity of the patient's illness. The six physical classes are described in **Table 1.1**.
B. **Airway management.** Plan for a natural airway or placement of either a laryngeal mask airway (LMA) or endotracheal tube should take into consideration the patient's current airway examination, past airway management, aspiration risk, and the planned procedure, including positioning and estimated duration.
C. **Monitoring.** The healthy patient undergoing minimally invasive surgery needs only the standard ASA monitors. However, if the patient has significant cardiovascular disease, pulmonary disease, or is at risk for blood loss, invasive monitoring such as a central line and arterial line should be considered for the granularity of hemodynamic status and assessing blood gases and cell counts frequently.
D. **Anesthetic options.** Numerous methods are available for providing anesthesia, analgesia, and hemodynamic stability for any given type of surgery. General anesthesia, regional anesthesia, and combinations thereof should be reviewed and considered.

VIII. PATIENT DISCUSSION
The perioperative period is emotionally stressful for patients who frequently have fears about surgery, anesthesia, diagnoses, complications, and mortality. The anesthesiologist can alleviate much of this stress with a thoughtful discussion. Moreover, the anesthesiologist should explain the

TABLE 1.1 ASA Physical Status Classification System

ASA PS Classification	Definition	Adult Examples, Including, But Not Limited to
ASA I	A normal healthy patient	Healthy, nonsmoking, no or minimal alcohol use
ASA II	A patient with mild systemic disease	Mild diseases only without substantive functional limitations. Current smoker, social alcohol drinker, pregnancy, obesity (30 < BMI < 40), well-controlled DM/HTN, mild lung disease
ASA III	A patient with severe systemic disease	Substantive functional limitations; one or more moderate to severe diseases. Poorly controlled DM or HTN, COPD, morbid obesity (BMI ≥ 40), active hepatitis, alcohol dependence or abuse, implanted pacemaker, moderate reduction of ejection fraction, ESRD undergoing regularly scheduled dialysis, history (>3 mo) of MI, CVA, TIA, or CAD/stents
ASA IV	A patient with severe systemic disease that is a constant threat to life	Recent (<3 mo) MI, CVA, TIA, or CAD/stents, ongoing cardiac ischemia or severe valve dysfunction, severe reduction of ejection fraction, shock, sepsis, DIC, ARD, or ESRD not undergoing regularly scheduled dialysis
ASA V	A moribund patient who is not expected to survive without the operation	Ruptured abdominal/thoracic aneurysm, massive trauma, intracranial bleed with mass effect, ischemic bowel in the face of significant cardiac pathology or multiple organ/system dysfunction
ASA VI	A declared brain-dead patient whose organs are being removed for donor purposes	

ARD, acute respiratory distress; ASA, American Society of Anesthesiologists; BMI, body mass index; CAD, coronary artery disease; COPD, chronic obstructive pulmonary disease; CVA, cerebrovascular accident; DIC, disseminated intravascular coagulation; DM, diabetes mellitus; ESRD, end-stage renal disease; HTN, hypertension; MI, myocardial infarction; TIA, transient ischemic attack.

The addition of "E" denotes Emergency surgery: (An emergency is defined as existing when delay in treatment of the patient would lead to a significant increase in the threat to life or body part).

Excerpted from ASA Physical Status Classification System, 2020 of the American Society of Anesthesiologists. A copy of the full text can be obtained from ASA, 1061 American Lane Schaumburg, IL 60173–4973 or online at www.asahq.org

events of the perioperative period and give instruction and information on the following:

A. Perioperative procedures. Explanation of the procedures that will occur prior to induction—placement of intravenous, arterial, or epidural catheters, placement of routine monitors, preoxygenation—with reassurance that supplemental sedation and analgesia will be provided as necessary.

TABLE 1.2 ASA Practice Guidelines for Preoperative Fasting

Ingested Material	Minimum Fasting Period[a]
Chewing gum	No delay in surgery after confirming removal
Clear liquids	2 h
Breast milk	4 h
Infant formula, nonhuman milk, light meals	6 h
Full meal	8 h

[a]Healthy patients, elective cases.
ASA, American Society of Anesthesiologists.

- **B. Perioperative medication use.** If a necessary medication was forgotten on the morning of surgery, it should be given by the anesthesiologist. Preoperative oral medications, such as acetaminophen, gabapentin, and celecoxib, are commonly seen in patients getting multimodal pain control (see Section VI).
- **C. Preoperative fasting.** Specific instructions about fasting should be addressed. See **Table 1.2**. Several key updates were provided in the 2023 ASA Guidelines for Preoperative fasting: clear liquids containing carbohydrates decrease hunger compared to noncaloric liquids (with no benefit or harm observed with added protein); no procedural delay is recommended after removal of chewing gum; and particularly in pediatric patients, clear liquids should be allowed as close to 2 hours before procedures as feasible.
- **D. Postoperative recovery.** Explain the intended plan for postoperative recovery in the postanesthesia care unit or ICU.
- **E. Pain control.** Detail the plan for perioperative pain control.
- **F. Autologous blood donation.** Autologous donation may be considered in the stable patient scheduled for surgery in which blood transfusion is likely.

IX. INFORMED CONSENT

Informed consent involves discussing the anesthetic plan, alternatives, and potential complications. The patient must demonstrate decision-making capacity; that is, understanding, appreciation, reasoning, and choice. Consent must be voluntary, and free from coercion. Descriptions should be made in layman's terms and conducted in the patient's native language, using a trained medical interpreter when appropriate. Children should not be used as interpreters, although adult family members may serve as interpreters if the patient signs a waiver of disclosure stating they choose to waive access to a hospital-appointed translator.

- **A. Explanation of general anesthesia.** Many aspects of anesthetic management are outside the realm of common experience and must be explicitly defined. Examples of this include endotracheal intubation, mechanical ventilation, invasive hemodynamic monitoring, regional anesthesia techniques, blood product transfusion, and postoperative ICU care.
- **B. Alternatives.** Alternatives to the suggested, management plan should be presented as they may become necessary if the planned procedure fails or if there is a change in clinical circumstances.

C. **Risks.** Risks associated with anesthesia-related procedures should be disclosed in a manner that the average person would find helpful in decision making. The best-case/worst-case communication tool is useful to guide this discussion. Offering the most likely situation is clarifying for patients as well. The discussion should also include complications that occur with a relatively high frequency and those that are just remote risks.
   1. **Regional anesthesia.** The risks of regional and neuraxial anesthesia include infection, local bleeding, nerve injury, headache, drug reaction, and possible failure to provide adequate anesthesia. Certain regional anesthetic techniques may carry more specific risks, for example, pneumothorax after an infraclavicular nerve block, and should be weighed against the associated benefits specific to the patient. General anesthesia and its attendant risks should also be discussed as it could become necessary.
   2. **General anesthesia.** The risks of airway instrumentation include sore throat, hoarseness, and dental injury. The anesthetic agents may cause nausea and vomiting or produce an allergic reaction. The possibility of intraoperative awareness, pulmonary or cardiac injury, stroke, postoperative visual loss, postoperative cognitive dysfunction, postoperative intubation, ICU admission, or death should be discussed when appropriate.
   3. **Blood transfusion.** The risks associated with blood transfusion are fever, hemolytic reactions, and infection. Current data assessing blood donations demonstrates a prevalence of hepatitis B virus ~1:1 to 1.5 million donations, human immunodeficiency virus ~1:1.6 to 2.3 million donations, and hepatitis C viruses ~1:2 to 2.6 million donations.
   4. **Vascular cannulation.** The risks of intravenous catheters include injury of peripheral nerves, tendons, blood vessels, and site infection causing a phlebitis or cellulitis. Hemothorax, pneumothorax, and central line bloodstream infection are risks associated with central venous access.
D. **Extenuating circumstances.** Anesthetic procedures may proceed without informed consent in emergency situations as consent is assumed under dire circumstances.

X. DAY OF SURGERY PREMEDICATION
A. **Sedatives and analgesics.** The goal for administering sedatives and analgesics before surgery is to allay the patient's anxiety, decrease pain during administration of regional anesthesia or preoperative line placement, and facilitate smooth induction of anesthesia. The dose of sedatives and analgesics should be reduced or withheld for the elderly, debilitated, or acutely intoxicated patient. The dose should also be decreased in a patient with upper airway obstruction, central apnea, neurologic deterioration, or severe pulmonary disease.
   1. **Benzodiazepines**
      a. **Midazolam.** Midazolam, 1 to 3 mg intravenously or intramuscularly, is a short-acting benzodiazepine that provides excellent anterograde amnesia and anxiolysis. It plays a role in preventing PONV. It is known to cause delirium in the elderly and to be synergistic with opioids in causing respiratory depression. There is ongoing research assessing the risks and benefits of benzodiazepine use in the elderly. One recent study in patients aged 65 to 80 found no difference in patient satisfaction scores with preoperative oral midazolam; however, the data also showed no difference in incidence of postoperative delirium.

b. **Lorazepam.** Lorazepam, 1 to 2 mg orally or intravenously, may cause more prolonged amnesia and postoperative sedation than midazolam.
  2. **Opioids.** Opioids may be given preoperatively to a patient who has, or is anticipated to have, significant pain or to a patient who is opioid dependent. The opioid-dependent patient should receive sufficient premedication to overcome tolerance and prevent perioperative withdrawal. Intravenous fentanyl is ideally dosed at least 2 to 5 minutes prior to airway instrumentation so that its effect blunts the reaction from laryngoscopy.
 B. **Anticholinergics.** Anticholinergics are not frequently used for premedication. Glycopyrrolate, 0.2 to 0.4 mg intravenously for adults and 10 to 20 μg/kg for pediatric patients, may be given in conjunction with ketamine as an antisialagogue. Occasionally, this antisialagogue effect is desirable during oral surgery, bronchoscopy, fiberoptic intubation, or to treat secretions related to recent smoking cessation.
 C. **Antiemetics.** Antiemetics may be given prior to induction or intraoperatively to prevent PONV (see Chapter 37: The Post-Anesthesia Care Unit). Adequate prophylaxis includes the use of at least two antiemetics with differing mechanisms of action (see **Table 1.3**).
 D. **Aspiration risk-mitigating agents.** Aspiration risk-mitigating agents may be warranted on the day of surgery in the at-risk patient (see Section VI.H).

TABLE 1.3 Antiemetic Agents

Antiemetic Agent	Mechanism of Action	Side Effects	Dose
Ondansetron	Serotonin (5-HT$_3$) receptor antagonist	Dizziness, headache, and QTc prolongation	4 mg intravenously
Droperidol[a]	Dopamine (D$_2$) receptor antagonist	Dystonia, prolonged QTc, and decreased seizure threshold	0.5–1.25 mg intravenously
Haloperidol	D$_2$ receptor antagonist	Dystonia, prolonged QTc, and decreased seizure threshold	1 mg intravenously
Dexamethasone	Unknown	Anal/vulvar pruritus and hyperglycemia	4 mg intravenously
Metoclopramide	Dopamine receptor antagonist	GI upset with abdominal cramping and dystonia	10 mg intravenously
Promethazine	Antihistamine	Sedation and decreased seizure threshold	6.25 mg intravenously
Scopolamine	Anticholinergic	Dry mouth, blurred vision, confusion, and urinary retention	1.5 mg transdermally

[a]The Food and Drug Administration requires 2 to 3 h of electrocardiogram (ECG) monitoring following administration given the risk of QTc prolongation and torsades de pointes.

XI. DELAYING SURGICAL PROCEDURES

Occasionally, it is in the best interest of the patient to delay elective surgical procedures for further medical evaluation and optimization. Some conditions can significantly increase morbidity and mortality if not appropriately evaluated and treated.

  A. Recent MI. If the patient has had a recent MI that was managed medically, then elective noncardiac surgery should be delayed for 60 days. If the patient underwent percutaneous coronary intervention, surgery should be delayed in accordance with antiplatelet therapy recommendations. See Chapter 3: Specific Considerations for Cardiac Disease for further details.

  B. New dysrhythmia. New-onset atrial fibrillation, atrial flutter, supraventricular tachycardia, sustained ventricular tachycardia, and second-degree, type II, or third-degree heart block must be evaluated with an ECG, rhythm strip, electrolyte replenishment, and a cardiology consultation. Surgery should be postponed until workup and treatment are complete and stability is established.

  C. Coagulopathy. Coagulopathies can predispose the patient to massive intraoperative blood loss. As such, surgery should be postponed until all possible etiologies have been thoroughly investigated and treated.

  D. Hypoxia. If hypoxia is of unclear etiology, surgery should be postponed until the cause is investigated and the patient optimized. V/Q mismatch, dead space, shunt, decreased fraction of inspired oxygen (FiO_2), and inadequate respiratory rate/effort should be considered. Workup should begin with a physical examination and evaluation of vital signs. Diagnostic studies such as a CXR, computed tomography (CT) scan, or arterial blood gas may be ordered as needed.

  E. New cardiovascular symptoms. Unstable angina and new shortness of breath or DOE are concerning symptoms. Surgery should be postponed until they can be fully evaluated by an appropriate specialist. New ECG changes, especially those indicative of silent MI, such as bifascicular block or new Q waves, must be evaluated prior to elective procedures.

  F. New murmurs. New heart murmurs may be indicative of a change in valvular pathology and should be evaluated by echocardiography and/or a cardiologist before proceeding with elective surgery.

  G. Hypertension/hyperglycemia. Many patients present with hypertension due to medication holds or anxiety. Additionally, hyperglycemia is common due to underlying poor control or instruction for reduced doses of insulin while the patient is NPO. In these instances, a discussion with the surgical team is warranted prior to cancellation.

XII. ETHICAL CONSIDERATIONS IN PATIENT CARE

A highly valued ethical principle that guides patient care in the United States is the concept of **patient autonomy.** Adult patients with decision-making capacity can and may choose to accept or refuse life-sustaining medical therapies in accordance with their own morals and beliefs. Respect for patient autonomy is demonstrated in the physician's ethical responsibility of attaining informed consent and including the patient in the medical decision-making process whenever possible.

  A. Advance directive. Also referred to as a **living will**, is a legal document written by a patient that outlines instructions for medical care should the patient become unable to communicate their wishes in the future. It often designates a surrogate decision maker.

  B. A health care proxy or **durable power of attorney for health care** is a designated surrogate who has legal charge to execute the patient's wishes should they

become unable to do so. If a representative has not been designated by the patient, the next of kin may become the de facto surrogate.
- C. **Physician orders for life-sustaining treatment (POLST).** Patients who have been diagnosed with a serious, life-limiting medical condition can create an advanced set of **portable medical orders** that are signed by their health care provider and placed in their medical record.
- D. **The pediatric patient** deserves special consideration when ethical issues are confronted. Legally, such decisions are deferred to the parents. Ethically, the child may participate in these decisions depending on their developmental level and decision-making capacity.
- E. **Religious/personal beliefs.** Certain personal beliefs and desires may warrant special consideration prior to surgery. The Jehovah's Witness patient undergoing elective surgery should have a clear plan that is understood and agreed to by the patient and the entire surgical team; specifically, their consent or refusal to use blood subfractions or contiguous autotransfusion should be documented. The same considerations apply to the patient with a preexisting DNR/DNI order where further discussion should guide suspending those directives versus proceeding with goal-directed resuscitation.
- F. **Ethical issues for the anesthetist.** The ethical and moral beliefs of the anesthetist must be taken into consideration for elective procedures. It is within the right of the individual to refuse to participate in the care of, for example, a therapeutic abortion, or a patient who is DNR. Additionally, physicians are not bound to provide care that they deem futile. Involving palliative care physicians in patient and family meetings is often critical to determining a patient's thought process and highlighting their ultimate goals.

ACKNOWLEDGMENTS

We gratefully acknowledge the contributions of previous edition authors, Michelle Dyrholm and Kate Cohen, as portions of those chapters have been retained in this revision.

Suggested Readings

Al Farii H, Farahdel L, Frazer A, Salimi A, Bernstein M. The effect of NSAIDs on postfracture bone healing: a meta-analysis of randomized controlled trials. *OTA Int.* 2021;4(2):e092.

American Society of Anesthesiologists. Consensus-based guidance on preoperative management of patients (adults and children) on glucagon-like peptide-1 (GLP-1) receptor agonists. June 29, 2023.

American Society of Anesthesiologists. Ethical guidelines for the anesthesia care of patients with do-not-resuscitate orders or other directives that limit treatment. Approved October 17, 2001, reaffirmed October 17, 2018.

American Society of Anesthesiologists Task Force on Perioperative Management of patients with obstructive sleep apnea. Practice guidelines for the perioperative management of patients with obstructive sleep apnea: an updated report by the American Society of Anesthesiologists Task Force on perioperative management of patients with obstructive sleep apnea. *Anesthesiology.* 2014;120(2):268–286.

Apfelbaum JL, Hagberg CA, Caplan RA, et al; American Society of Anesthesiologists Task Force on Management of the Difficult Airway. Practice guidelines for management of the difficult airway: an updated report by the American Society of Anesthesiologists Task Force on Management of the Difficult Airway. *Anesthesiology.* 2013;118(2):251–270.

Baron TH, Kamath PS, McBane RD. Management of antithrombotic therapy in patients undergoing invasive procedures. *N Engl J Med.* 2013;368:2113–2124.

Bittl JA, Baber U, Bradley SM, Wijeysundera DN. Duration of dual antiplatelet therapy: a systematic review for the 2016 ACC/AHA guideline focused update on duration of dual antiplatelet therapy in patients with coronary artery disease: a report of the American

College of Cardiology/American Heart Association Task Force on clinical practice guidelines. *J Am Coll Cardiol.* 2016;68:1116–1139.

Blumenthal KG, Peter JG, Trubiano JA, Phillips EJ. Antibiotic allergy. *Lancet.* 2019; 393(10167):183–198.

Blumenthal KG, Shenoy ES, Varughese CA, Hurwitz S, Hooper DC, Banerji A. Impact of a clinical guideline for prescribing antibiotics to inpatients reporting penicillin or cephalosporin allergy. *Ann Allergy Asthma Immunol.* 2015;115(4):294–300.e2.

Committee on Standards and Practice Parameters; Apfelbaum JL, Connis RT, Nickinovich DG, et al. Practice advisory for preanesthesia evaluation: an updated report by the American Society of Anesthesiologists Task Force on preanesthesia evaluation. *Anesthesiology.* 2012;116(3):522–538.

Crossley GH, Poole JE, Rozner MA, et al. The Heart Rhythm Society (HRS)/American Society of Anesthesiologists (ASA) Expert Consensus Statement on the perioperative management of patients with implantable defibrillators, pacemakers and arrhythmia monitors: facilities and patient management. *Heart Rhythm.* 2011;8:1114–1154.

Dodd RY, Crowder LA, Haynes JM, Notari EP, Stramer SL, Steele WR. Screening blood donors for HIV, HCV, and HBV at the American Red Cross: 10-year trends in prevalence, incidence, and residual risk, 2007 to 2016. *Transfus Med Rev.* 2020;34(2):81–93.

Douketis JD, Spyropoulos AC, Spencer FA, et al. Perioperative management of antithrombotic therapy: antithrombotic therapy and prevention of thrombosis, 9th ed: American College of Chest Physicians evidence-based clinical practice guidelines. *Chest.* 2012; 141(2 suppl):e326S–e350S.

Duceppe E, Parlow J, MacDonald P, et al. Canadian Cardiovascular Society Guidelines on perioperative cardiac risk assessment and management for patients who undergo noncardiac surgery. *Can J Cardiol.* 2017;33(1):17–32.

Fihn SD, Gardin JM, Abrams J, et al; American College of Cardiology Foundation/American Heart Association Task Force. 2012 ACCF/AHA/AATS/PCNA/SCAI/STS guideline for the diagnosis and management of patients with stable ischemic heart disease: a report of the American College of Cardiology Foundation/American Heart Association Task Force on practice guidelines, and the American College of Physicians, American Association for Thoracic Surgery, Preventive Cardiovascular Nurses Association, Society for Cardiovascular Angiography and Interventions, and Society of Thoracic Surgeons. *Circulation.* 2012;126(25):e354–e471.

Fleisher LA, Fleischmann KE, Auerbach AD, et al. 2014 ACC/AHA guideline on perioperative cardiovascular evaluation and management of patients undergoing noncardiac surgery: executive summary: a report of the American College of Cardiology/American Heart Association Task Force on practice guidelines. *Circulation.* 2014;130: 2215–2245.

Halvorsen S, Mehilli J, Cassese S, et al; ESC Scientific Document Group. 2022 ESC Guidelines on cardiovascular assessment and management of patients undergoing non-cardiac surgery. *Eur Heart J.* 2022;43(39):3826–3924.

Hashash JG, Thompson CC, Wan AY. AGA rapid clinical practice update on the management of patients taking GLP-1 receptor agonists prior to endoscopy: communication. *Clin Gastroenterol Hepatol.* 2024;22(4):705–707.

Hlatky MA, Boineau RE, Higginbotham MB, et al. A brief self-administered questionnaire to determine functional capacity (the Duke Activity Status Index). *Am J Cardiol.* 1989;64(10):651–654.

Joshi GP, Abdelmalak BB, Weigel WA, et al. 2023 American Society of Anesthesiologists Practice Guidelines for Preoperative Fasting: carbohydrate-containing clear liquids with or without protein, chewing gum, and pediatric fasting duration—A modular update of the 2017 American Society of Anesthesiologists practice guidelines for preoperative fasting. *Anesthesiology.* 2023;138:132–151.

Kowark A, Keszei AP, Schneider G, et al; I-PROMOTE Study Group. Preoperative midazolam and patient-centered outcomes of older patients: the I-PROMOTE randomized clinical trial. *JAMA Surg.* 2024;159(2):129–138.

Kruisselbrink R, Gharapetian A, Chaparro LE, et al. Diagnostic accuracy of point-of-care gastric ultrasound. *Anesth Analg.* 2019;128(1):89–95.

MGH Guidelines for perioperative aspirin administration. Consensus Statement from the Departments of Anesthesia, Medicine, Cardiology, and Surgery. 12/2011.

Nonobstetric surgery during pregnancy. ACOG Committee Opinion No. 775. American College of Obstetricians and Gynecologists. *Obstet Gynecol.* 2019;133:e285–e286.

Piccolo R, Windecker S. Low-dose aspirin to reduce the risk for myocardial infarction among patients with coronary stents undergoing noncardiac surgery. *Ann Intern Med.* 2018;168(4):289–290.

Practice advisory for the perioperative management of patients with cardiac implantable electronic devices: pacemakers and implantable cardioverter–defibrillators 2020: an updated report by the American Society of Anesthesiologists Task Force on perioperative management of patients with cardiac implantable electronic devices: Erratum. *Anesthesiology.* 2020;132:225–252.

Practice guidelines for preoperative fasting and the use of pharmacologic agents to reduce the risk of pulmonary aspiration: application to healthy patients undergoing elective procedures: an updated report by the American Society of Anesthesiologists Task Force on preoperative fasting and the use of pharmacologic agents to reduce the risk of pulmonary aspiration. *Anesthesiology.* 2017;126(3):376–393.

Prins KW, Neill JM, Tyler JO, Eckman PM, Duval S. Effects of beta-blocker withdrawal in acute decompensated heart failure: a systematic review and meta-analysis. *JACC Heart Fail.* 2015;3:647–653.

Ridker PM. Should aspirin be used for primary prevention in the post-statin era? *N Engl J Med.* 2018;379(16):1572–1574.

Rosenstock J, Ferrannini E. Euglycemic diabetic ketoacidosis: a predictable, detectable, and preventable safety concern with SGLT2 inhibitors. *Diabetes Care.* 2015;38(9):1638–1642.

Steele WR, Dodd RY, Notari EP, et al; Transfusion-Transmissible Infections Monitoring System (TTIMS). HIV, HCV, and HBV incidence and residual risk in US blood donors before and after implementation of the 12-month deferral policy for men who have sex with men. *Transfusion.* 2021;61(3):839–850.

Stern T, Cifu AS. Perioperative beta-blocker therapy. *J Am Med Assoc.* 2015;313(24):2486–2487.

Wijeysundera DN, Duncan D, Nkonde-Price C, et al. Perioperative beta blockade in noncardiac surgery: a systematic review for the 2014 ACC/AHA guideline on perioperative cardiovascular evaluation and management of patients undergoing noncardiac surgery: a report of the American College of Cardiology/American Heart Association Task Force on practice guidelines. *J Am Coll Cardiol.* 2014;64(22):2406–2425.

Wu F, Smith MR, Mueller AL, et al. Association of glucagon-like peptide receptor 1 agonist therapy with the presence of gastric contents in fasting patients undergoing endoscopy under anesthesia care: a historical cohort study. *Can J Anesth.* 2024;71(7):958–966.

Basics of Echocardiography and Lung Ultrasound

Susana Arango and Alexander S. Kuo

INTRODUCTION
Echocardiography is the use of ultrasound (US) to image the heart and associated structures. It allows real-time assessment of the cardiac structure, cardiac function, and hemodynamic parameters. There are two primary modalities of echocardiography, transthoracic (TTE) and transesophageal (TEE). This chapter will focus on the basic principles of TTE and the use of cardiac point-of-care ultrasound (POCUS) for clinical monitoring.

I. CARDIAC POINT-OF-CARE ULTRASOUND (POCUS)
As smaller and more cost-effective US machines have become available, the use of echocardiography by noncardiologists has increased across all phases of patient care. Cardiac POCUS can be defined as the use of US by the treating clinician, who obtains and interprets the images at bedside to rapidly assist in clinical decision making and management. While POCUS can aid with initial patient management, patients found to have abnormal findings not previously recorded on echocardiography should be referred for a comprehensive echocardiographic examination.

II. CLINICAL USES OF POCUS
A. Purpose
The purpose of POCUS is to provide timely diagnostic information at the point of care when a clinical question arises. It is useful in the acute setting to narrow differential diagnosis, initiate or guide therapy, or trigger further diagnostic workup. In the following section we will review clinical applications of POCUS.

B. Technical aspects
The ideal probe for cardiac POCUS is a small, phased-array cardiac probe that allows optimal imaging between the ribs. Abdominal US transducers are not ideal but can be considered when no other probes are available. The most useful acoustic windows used in POCUS are the parasternal long axis (PLAX), parasternal short axis (PSAX) at the level of the midpapillary muscles, apical four-chamber (A4C), subcostal inferior vena cava (IVC), and subcostal four-chamber views. Other views that can be useful for hemodynamic measurements include apical five-chamber (A5C).

C. Obtaining the views
During cardiac POCUS, the US probe is applied to the chest or upper abdomen. It can be technically difficult to obtain images because of intervening structures such as the chest wall, ribs, or lung. Cardiac POCUS exam should be brief and focused to prevent delay in medical management. There are six different views that are used predominantly for cardiac POCUS interrogation.

1. **Parasternal long-axis (PLAX) view:** allows for evaluation of left ventricular (LV) size and systolic function, limited assessment of right ventricular (RV) size and function. Useful to evaluate presence of pericardial

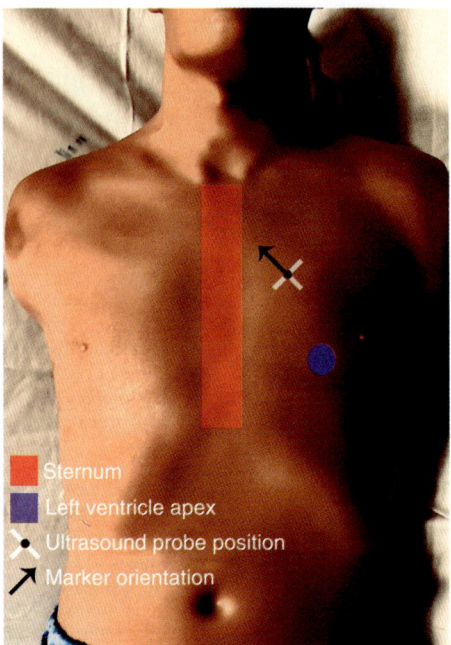

FIGURE 2.1 Parasternal long-axis transthoracic echocardiogram probe position.

effusion and differentiate pericardial versus pleural effusion. To obtain the view: position the transducer in the second, third, or fourth intercostal space at the left parasternal border with the marker oriented toward the right shoulder (**Figure 2.1**). Place the mitral valve and aortic valve in the center of the image (**Figure 2.2**).

2. **Parasternal short-axis (PSAX) view:** allows for evaluation of ventricular size, systolic function, and estimation of RV pressure/volume overload by assessing the interventricular septum. To obtain this view: position the transducer in the second, third, or fourth intercostal space at the left parasternal border with the marker oriented toward the left shoulder (**Figure 2.3**). If you are in the parasternal LAX view, the SAX can be obtained by rotating the probe 90 degrees counterclockwise. Tilt or slide the transducer slightly inferiorly and laterally toward the LV apex until both the papillary muscles can be visualized attaching to the LV wall (**Figure 2.4**).

3. **Apical four-chamber (A4C) view:** allows for assessment of LV and RV size and systolic function, atrial dilation, presence of pericardial effusion, presence of RV/right atrial collapse, and Doppler measurements through the mitral valve. To obtain this view: position the transducer in the fourth or fifth intercostal space between the anterior and midaxillary lines, along the point of maximal pulsation (apex) with the direction marker pointing toward the left axilla (**Figure 2.5**). Move the probe laterally so the interventricular septum is in the center of the image and vertical (**Figure 2.6**). If atria cannot be appreciated, tilt the probe face anteriorly. If ventricles appear too spherical, move the transducer inferiorly, or move down one rib interspace.

Chapter 2 Basics of Echocardiography and Lung Ultrasound

FIGURE 2.2 Parasternal long-axis transthoracic echocardiographic image.

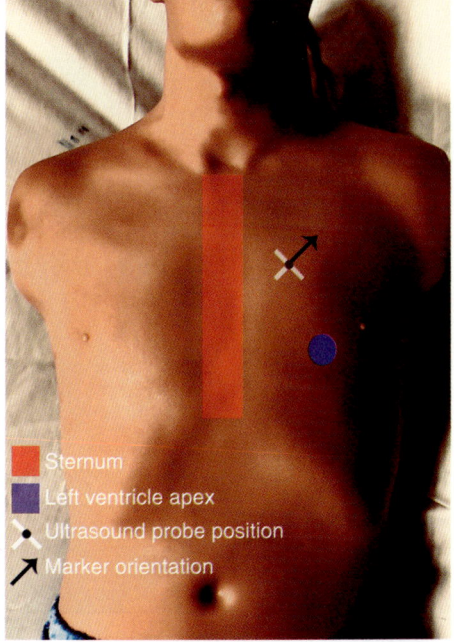

FIGURE 2.3 Parasternal short-axis probe position.

FIGURE 2.4 Parasternal short-axis midpapillary transthoracic echocardiographic image.

4. **Apical five-chamber (A5C) view:** important for estimation of cardiac output. To obtain this view: obtain the A4C view. Tilt the transducer face anteriorly along the chest wall to visualize the aortic valve and left ventricle outflow tract (LVOT) in the center of the image (**Figure 2.7**).

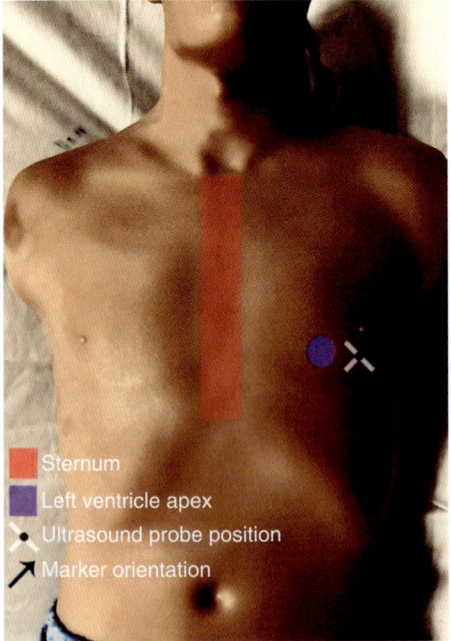

FIGURE 2.5 Apical four-chamber probe position.

Chapter 2 Basics of Echocardiography and Lung Ultrasound

FIGURE 2.6 Apical four-chamber transthoracic echocardiographic image.

Consider moving the transducer superiorly, up a rib interspace, or more laterally to align the LVOT.
5. **Subcostal four-chamber (S4C)** view: allows imaging of the atria, ventricles, and pericardial space. Useful for assessing pericardial effusion and overall assessment of biventricular systolic function. To obtain

FIGURE 2.7 Apical five-chamber transthoracic echocardiographic image.

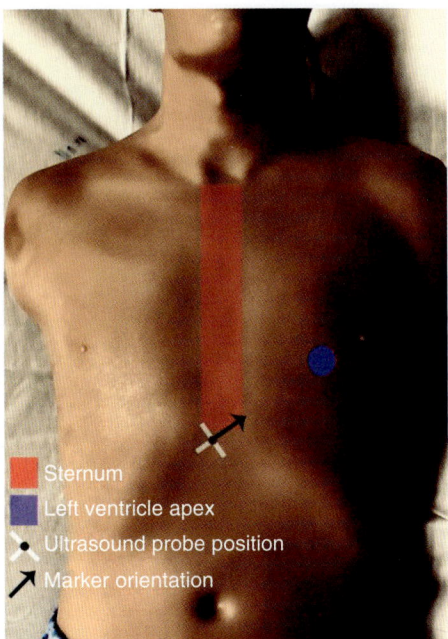

FIGURE 2.8 Subcostal four-chamber probe position.

this view: position the transducer in the subxiphoid region of the abdomen, at a flat angle parallel to the skin surface, with the index marker directed toward the left flank (**Figures 2.8** and **2.9**). Consider moving the probe slightly right of the patient's midline to utilize the liver as an echogenic window.

6. **Subcostal inferior vena cava (IVC) view:** allows for assessment of IVC size, estimation of central venous pressures (CVPs), and fluid responsiveness. To obtain this view: obtain the S4C view. Rotate the transducer 90 degrees counterclockwise so the index marker is oriented toward the patient's head, while keeping the right atrium (RA) in the center of the image (**Figure 2.10**). Visualize the junction of the IVC and RA by tilting the probe face inferiorly (**Figure 2.11**). Attempt to make the IVC appear more horizontal and appreciate hepatic veins draining into IVC. Ensure that the IVC is nonpulsatile (aorta is pulsatile).

III. TRANSESOPHAGEAL ECHOCARDIOGRAPHY (TEE)

TEE requires insertion of a US probe into the esophagus and stomach. It is a more invasive procedure that often requires sedation or intubation of the patient. With TEE there is risk of oral–dental injuries, bleeding, or even rarely perforation of the esophagus or stomach. Therefore, it is important to ensure that the patient does not have a history of abnormal anatomy, prior surgeries, or radiation to the esophagus or stomach that can increase the risk of these injuries. TEE offers superior imaging of the cardiac structures due to the proximity of the heart to the esophagus. The performance of a TEE exam is beyond

Chapter 2 Basics of Echocardiography and Lung Ultrasound 27

FIGURE 2.9 Subcostal four-chamber transthoracic echocardiographic image.

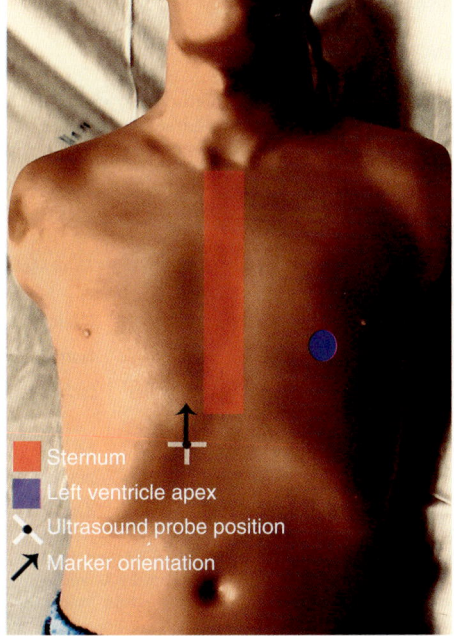

FIGURE 2.10 Subcostal inferior vena cava probe position.

FIGURE 2.11 Subcostal inferior vena cava transthoracic echocardiographic image.

the scope of this chapter, but the same views and measurements described here can also be obtained by TEE.

IV. CARDIAC FUNCTION ASSESSMENT
A. Left Ventricular (LV) Assessment
There are multiple quantitative methods to evaluate the LV, including Simpson biplane method, fractional area of change (FAC), strain, and 3D assessment, however, these methods can be time consuming (**Table 2.1**). Further qualitative evaluation of the LV is frequently sufficient for point-of-care clinical evaluation.

TABLE 2.1 Standard Grading System for Left Ventricle Wall Motion

Qualitative Descriptor	Systolic Thickening and Motion	Clinical Implication
1. Normal/Hyperkinetic	Thickens and shortens	Normal
2. Hypokinetic	Reduced thickening and shortening	Ischemia or dysfunction
3. Akinetic	Does not thicken or shorten	Myocardial scar, infarction, hibernating
4. Dyskinetic	Thins or elongates	Aneurysm

Derived from Lang RM, Badano LP, Mor-Avi V, et al. Recommendations for cardiac chamber quantification by echocardiography in adults: an update from the American Society of Echocardiography and the European Association of Cardiovascular Imaging. *J Am Soc Echocardiogr.* 2015;28(1):1–39.e14.

1. **LV size:** The assessment of the left ventricle should begin with an evaluation of the architecture of the chamber, noting whether it is dilated or hypertrophied. The most common echocardiographic views for the assessment of the left ventricle size are the A4C, the PLAX, and the PSAX.
2. **Global LV function:** Visual estimation of LVEF is a quick and simple method. By assessing myocardial thickening and endocardial motion in the PLAX, SAX, and A4C, one can classify LV function into four discrete categories: (1) normal, (2) hyperdynamic, (3) reduced, and (4) severely reduced. In patients with normal LV systolic function, the myocardium can be seen thickening in all segments and the endocardium moving toward the center of the LV chamber in systole. Hyperdynamic LV function is characterized by excessive inward motion and myocardial thickening, leading to complete or near-complete obliteration of the LV cavity at the end of systole. This is often a marker of decreased preload or severely decreased afterload. Conditions that can present with hyperdynamic LV function include hypovolemia, sepsis, massive pulmonary embolism (PE), severe mitral regurgitation, or cardiac tamponade.
3. The PLAX and A4C views allow visualization of only the LV anteroseptal and inferolateral, and anterolateral and inferoseptal walls, respectively. This can lead to overestimation of LV systolic function if regional wall motion abnormalities are present elsewhere, while the PSAX at the midpapillary level provides a circumferential view of all LV walls and is the best view for appreciating global LV function. Decreased excursion and myocardial thickening are seen in patients with decreased systolic LV function.
4. **E-point septal separation (EPSS):** Using the PLAX, EPSS is measured as the smallest distance between the anterior mitral valve leaflet and the interventricular septum early diastole. A distance greater than 7 mm is a marker for LV ejection fraction less than 30%. Mitral valve stenosis or aortic regurgitation can cause decreased excursion of the anterior mitral leaflet and when present can underestimate ejection fraction. Conversely, acute LV dysfunction may present with preserved mitral valve excursion.
5. **Regional LV function:** POCUS can also be used to assess regional wall motion. The American Society of Echocardiography (ASE) recommends a grading system that ranges from (1) normal, (2) hypokinetic, (3) akinetic, and (4) dyskinetic (**Table 2.1**).

    It is important to evaluate each wall segment for both myocardial thickening and endocardial motion. Wall segments with normal function may "pull on" adjacent nonfunctioning wall segments, creating an illusion of normal function. It may be helpful to visually isolate each segment to avoid this bias. The parasternal SAX is particularly useful for appreciating gross regional wall motion abnormalities corresponding to the coronary circulation. Typically, the left anterior descending artery perfuses the anterior portion of the left ventricle and provides perfusion to the anterolateral papillary muscle; the circumflex artery perfuses the lateral portion of the left ventricle and also provides perfusion to the anterolateral papillary muscle; and the right coronary artery perfuses the inferior portion of the ventricle (**Figures 2.12** and **2.13**) and the posteromedial papillary muscle.

B. Right Ventricular (RV) Assessment

The RV has a complex geometry, and thus no single POCUS view can offer a comprehensive assessment of function. When viewed in a PSAX, it has

FIGURE 2.12 Coronary artery distribution in relation to ventricle wall segments.

a crescent shape and when viewed from the A4C view it has a triangular shape. Assessing RV function is useful for diagnosing and treating shock and respiratory failure in critically ill patients.

1. **RV size:** The normal RV chamber is approximately two-thirds the size of the LV chamber. The most common method to assess RV enlargement is direct comparison of RV and LV size performed at end diastole from the A4C view. If the RV extends to the apex of the heart or its size is equal or larger than the LV, then the RV is likely significantly enlarged. RV enlargement can also be seen on the SAX view, when the normal RV crescent shape becomes more circular.
2. **RV wall thickness:** Increased wall thickness of the otherwise thin-walled RV suggests RV hypertrophy, which can result from chronic pulmonary

FIGURE 2.13 Standard left ventricular myocardial segmentation for tomography.

hypertension or chronic RV volume overload. RV lateral wall thickness is best measured using the S4C. The measurement is made at end diastole at the level of the tip of the anterior tricuspid valve (TV) leaflet. The RV wall is normally less than 5 mm thick. An RV wall thickness >10 mm is highly suggestive of a chronic disease. Of note, increases in RV wall thickness can occur within 48 hours of sudden increases in pulmonary artery pressure, as seen in patients with PE.

3. **Interventricular septal morphology:** It is important to evaluate the shape of the interventricular septum when evaluating the right ventricle since the geometry of this anatomic structure significantly contributes to RV pressure and function. During RV overload, the interventricular septum flattens causing the left ventricle to become "D" shaped. Ultimately, this change in shape will impair RV function and LV filling.

    a. **Volume overload:** The interventricular septum will flatten during diastole if the right ventricle is volume overloaded with restoration of normal shape during systole. Circumstances that would cause the right ventricle to experience volume overload include tricuspid regurgitation and left-to-right shunts such as atrial or ventricular septal defects.

    b. **Pressure overload:** The interventricular septum will flatten during systole and restore normal shape during diastole if the right ventricle is pressure overloaded. Pathologic conditions that would increase pressure include pulmonary hypertension and PE.

    c. **Volume and pressure overload:** If the right ventricle experiences both pressure and volume overload, the interventricular septum will be flattened throughout the entire duration of the cardiac cycle.

4. **RV systolic function:** In contrast to the LV that contracts concentrically, the RV contraction is complex and occurs in phases. It primarily contracts from base to apex (longitudinally). Therefore, the RV systolic function is best evaluated by assessing the TV annulus motion and the RV free wall in the A4C or S4C view.

    a. **FAC:** It is determined in the same manner as for the left ventricle. The A4C view is most useful for measuring right ventricle FAC by tracing the endocardium to the tricuspid annulus and comparing the area between end diastole and end systole before dividing by end-diastolic area. Normally, right ventricle FAC is >35%.

    b. **Tricuspid annular plane systolic excursion (TAPSE):** TAPSE is the distance the lateral annulus travels toward the apex during systole. In the A4C view, an M-mode beam is placed through the interventricular septum and lateral wall tricuspid annulus to measure the systolic excursion of the right ventricle in a longitudinal plane. Normal TAPSE is >16 mm; however, the major limitation of this measurement is that it only evaluates the free wall of the right ventricle in one plane of motion and does not evaluate the contributions of the interventricular septum and RV outflow tract. In addition, TAPSE may be limited in patients who have undergone TV replacement, repair, or those with restrictive or constrictive disease.

    c. **RV lateral annular systolic velocity** (S') can be obtained using tissue-Doppler and represents the highest systolic velocity of RV excursion. It should be measured on the basal segment of the free wall side of the RV on A4C view. A measurement of <10 cm/s is suggestive of abnormal RV systolic function. The limitations are similar to TAPSE.

C. Pulmonary Embolism (PE)

Computed tomography pulmonary angiography (CTPA) is the main modality for the diagnosis of PE. However, POCUS can be useful to identify hemodynamically significant PE in patients with persistent hypotension

or shock in which CTPA is not immediately available or is clinically contraindicated. No single echocardiographic sign is specific or sensitive for PE unless thrombus is directly visualized. However, the following echocardiographic findings can help support the diagnosis of PE and guide reperfusion therapy:
1. **RV dilatation, RV dysfunction, or septal flattening** (see previous section) can be appreciated and are due to increased afterload. These signs are nonspecific and can also be seen in patients with heart failure, right wall myocardial infarction, and chronic pulmonary hypertension.
2. **Distended IVC** with poor collapsibility (see section that follows)
3. **McConnell sign** is described as akinesia of the mid-RV free wall but normal motion at the apex. Although initially described in patients with PE, it is not specific and can also be found in acute chest syndrome, RV myocardial infarction, and acute respiratory distress syndrome.
4. **Normal or hyperdynamic LV** due to decreased preload from the RV.
5. **Visualization of thrombus in the RV or extending into the RV outflow tract into the pulmonary artery.** These findings are observed only in a minority of patients, however, when seen is confirmatory of an acute PE. A thrombus in transit has a high mortality without therapy, due to its propensity to cause immediate hemodynamic instability and therefore POCUS can have diagnostic and prognostic implications. A normal echocardiogram does not rule out a PE, however, in patients with hypotension or shock and absence of the above signs, hemodynamically significant PE is unlikely and other causes of shock should be investigated.

D. Pericardial Effusion and Cardiac Tamponade
1. **On US, pericardial fluid appears as an anechoic space between the two layers of the pericardium.** POCUS can be used to identify and estimate the size of a pericardial effusion and to evaluate the hemodynamic significance usually in the SC4C and the PLAX view. Effusions can be classified into trivial (seen only in systole), mild (<10 mm), moderate (10 to 20 mm), and severe (>20 mm). Notably, the volume of pericardial effusion does not necessarily correlate with clinical symptoms. Several conditions can mimic pericardial effusion.
   a. **Epicardial fat is located within the pericardial space and can be confused with a pericardial effusion.** Compared to fluid, fat appears more echogenic and more granular and is usually located along the front of the right ventricle. Hence, an isolated anterior pericardial separation is most likely to be epicardial fat.
   b. **A pericardial effusion can be mistaken with a pleural effusion.** In the PLAX, both pericardial and pleural effusions can be seen posterior to the left atrium and left ventricle. However, a pericardial effusion can also be seen anterior to the descending thoracic aorta, while a pleural effusion is more commonly seen posterior to the descending thoracic aorta.
   c. **In the SC4C, ascites can be mistaken with a pericardial effusion.** Corroborating an effusion in other echocardiographic views is always recommended.
2. **Tamponade is a clinical and physiologic diagnosis**; however, the following echocardiographic signs can be supportive of tamponade diagnosis.
   a. **RA systolic collapse:** The earliest finding of cardiac tamponade and one of the most sensitive signs is the inversion of the RA-free wall for more than one-third of the ventricular systole. Usually seen in the A4C or SC4C views.
   b. **RV diastolic collapse:** most specific findings. May not occur when the RV is hypertrophied or with elevated diastolic pressure. Best seen in

the PLAX view with dimpling of the RV outflow tract noted during mitral valve opening.
- **c. IVC dilation:** A plethoric IVC with minimal respiratory variation is very sensitive sign and has a high negative predictive value for cardiac tamponade in spontaneous breathing patients.

V. HEMODYNAMIC MEASUREMENTS

A. Doppler Ultrasound

US cannot directly measure pressures or blood flow, but using Doppler, blood flow velocity can be assessed, and pressure and flows inferred. Ideally, the Doppler is aligned along the direction of the US beam or as close to parallel as feasible. Velocity assessment is most accurate when the angle of the transducer beam is less than 20 degrees to the direction of blood flow. There are different modes of Doppler: continuous wave, pulse wave, color, and tissue.

1. **Continuous-wave (CW) Doppler** continuously transmits and receives Doppler signals. This allows measurement of the highest velocity of blood flow along the path of the beam and is useful for assessing high-velocity regurgitant jets or the flow through a stenotic aortic valve. However, unlike pulsed-wave (PW) Doppler, CW does not allow the position of the velocity measurement to be known.
2. **PW Doppler** allows velocity measurements at a specific location. However, due to the Nyquist limit, the maximum measurable velocity is limited by aliasing. Thus, only lower velocity flow can be measured, such as ventricular outflow ejection or mitral inflow.
3. **Color Doppler** allows visualization of flow overlaid on a 2D echo image. Like PW, it is also limited to measurements at lower velocities. It is a very useful tool to qualitatively evaluate flow patterns.
4. **Tissue-Doppler imaging (TDI)** measures the velocity of myocardial tissue motion. TDI can be performed in PW and color modes. TDI can be used to measure myocardial velocities to estimate longitudinal systolic function and myocardial relaxation.

B. Flow Measurements

Although US cannot measure blood flow directly, blood flow velocity can be measured and integrated over time, velocity–time integral (VTI), to determine distance traveled. Multiplying the VTI by the cross-sectional area of the structure through which the velocity is measured yields the rate of flow. A common application of this approach is the measurement of stroke volume (SV) and cardiac output.

1. **SV and cardiac output measurement:** This is performed by first measuring the LVOT diameter in the PLAX view. Assuming the LVOT is a circle, the area can be calculated, $LVOT_{area}$. Blood flow velocity in the LVOT is then measured from the A5C view PW Doppler. From the PW Doppler, the area under the curve of ejection is then measured to obtain the VTI. This VTI is then multiplied by $LVOT_{area}$ to give the SV. The SV can then be multiplied by the heart rate (HR) to give the cardiac output.

$$LVOT_{area} = (\pi/4) \times \left(LVOT_{diameter}\right)^2$$
$$\text{Stroke volume} = LVOT_{area} \times VTI_{LVOT}$$
$$\text{Cardiac output} = SV \times HR$$

C. Pressure Gradient Assessment

The difference in pressure between chambers can be assessed by measuring the velocity of blood flow between the two chambers. This relationship

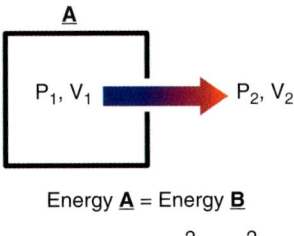

FIGURE 2.14 Bernoulli equation for calculating transvalvular gradients.

is given by simplified Bernoulli equation (**Figure 2.14**) where P2 to P1 is the difference in pressure between the two chambers in mm Hg and V is the velocity of the blood flow between the chambers in meters per second. A common usage of this equation is in the measurement of right ventricular systolic pressure (RVSP).

Simplified Bernoulli equation:

$$P_2 - P_1 (\text{mm Hg}) = 4V^2 (\text{m/s})$$

1. **RVSP measurement:** The tricuspid regurgitant jet is measured in the A4C or parasternal RV-inflow view using CW Doppler. The peak velocity is then inserted in the simplified Bernoulli equation. CVP is then added to the calculated pressure gradient since the calculated pressure difference is between the RV and the RA and not the absolute pressure.

$$RVSP = 4V^2_{\text{tricuspid regurg.}} + CVP$$

If the fluid is starting with a significant initial velocity, a slightly more accurate modified Bernoulli equation must be used to account for this. An example of this would be measurement of the aortic stenosis with high cardiac output since the LVOT would have significant velocity.

Modified Bernoulli equation:

$$P_2 - P_1 (\text{mm Hg}) = 4(V_2^2 - V_1^2)(\text{m/s})$$

VI. CARDIAC FILL STATUS ASSESSMENT
A. Inferior Vena Cava (IVC) Estimation of RA Pressure

The IVC can be readily assessed using POCUS. Imaging of the IVC is performed from the subcostal window to the right of midline in the sagittal plane to obtain LAX view of the IVC. The morphology of the IVC can provide insight into the filling pressures of the heart and provide supportive data for diagnoses of tamponade, hypovolemia, or heart failure.

1. **IVC diameter and CVP:** In spontaneously breathing patients, IVC diameter correlates to right atrial pressure (RAP) and can act as a surrogate for CVP. In euvolemic patients who are breathing spontaneously, inspiration leads to a reduction in intrathoracic pressure and a decrease in the size of the IVC. Hypovolemic patients can exhibit an exaggerated collapse of the IVC during inspiration. For accurate measurement, this assessment should be done with the patient supine and the diameter should be taken 1 to 2 cm away from the RA (see **Table 2.2**).

Inferior Vena Cava Diameter Correlation to Central Venous Pressure		
IVC Diameter	**Collapse With Sniff**	**Approximate CVP**
Less than 2.1 cm AND	Greater than 50%	Normal, 0–5 mm Hg
Greater than 2.1 cm AND	Less than 50%	Elevated, >15 mm Hg
Does not meet both conditions above		Indeterminate or intermediate

CVP, central venous pressure; IVC, inferior vena cava.

Derived from Lang RM, Badano LP, Mor-Avi V, et al. Recommendations for cardiac chamber quantification by echocardiography in adults: an update from the American Society of Echocardiography and the European Association of Cardiovascular Imaging. *J Am Soc Echocardiogr.* 2015;28(1):1–39.e14.

    a. If the IVC diameter is <2.1 cm AND collapses >50% with sniff, this indicates filling pressures are normal, CVP <5 mm Hg.
    b. If the IVC diameter is >2.1 cm AND collapses <50% with sniff, this indicates elevated filling pressures, CVP >10 to 20 mm Hg.
    c. If the IVC diameter is ≤2.1 cm AND collapses <50, or if >2.1 cm and >50%, this indicates a CVP of 5 to 10 mm Hg.
 2. **Limitations:** The IVC can be compressed during examination due to excessive pressure of the probe on the abdominal wall. Other factors that can affect the IVC diameter include significant tricuspid regurgitation, larger body surface area, masses, and elevated intrathoracic or intraabdominal pressures.
B. Left Atrial Pressure (LAP) Estimation
LAP can be estimated with echocardiography using the E/e' ratio. This ratio represents the relationship between early-diastolic mitral inflow velocity (E) and early-diastolic tissue-Doppler velocity of the mitral annulus (e'). In the A4C view, the PW-Doppler cursor is placed at the tip of the mitral valve leaflets and the peak velocity during early diastole (E) is measured. To calculate e', the TDI cursor is placed at level of the lateral mitral annulus and then the septal mitral annulus. The peak velocity during early diastole is calculated for both measurements and then averaged. The the E/e' is calculated by dividing the E velocity by the average e' velocity. A ratio >14 has been correlated with elevated left atrial filling pressures (pulmonary capillary wedge pressure >15 mm Hg) with modest accuracy. Limitations include heavy mitral annular calcification, mitral valve, pericardial disease, and patients with regional wall motion abnormalities.
C. Fluid Status and Fluid Responsiveness
 1. **Assessment of intravascular volume in the perioperative and critically ill patient is foundational for guiding volume resuscitation and diuresis.** Echocardiography can be used to estimate intravascular volume status by measuring fluid responsiveness and identifying signs of volume overload.
 2. **Fluid responsiveness is defined by a 10% to 15% increase in SV after receiving a 500 mL fluid bolus over 10 to 15 minutes.** Conceptually, administering additional fluid will only increase SV if it increases stressed blood volume and if both ventricles are volume-responsive and functioning on the ascending portion of the Frank–Starling curve. It is important to consider that a heart with impaired systolic function can respond to an increase in fluid; however, the overall response will be relatively reduced.

3. **Echocardiographic parameters** to assess volume status can be divided into static and dynamic indicators. Dynamic indicators are significantly more effective in predicting volume responsiveness.
4. **Static echocardiograph parameters:** measurements obtained at a specific point in time that are surrogates for right or LV preload. Fluctuations in these indices may only manifest in clear cases of hypervolemia and hypovolemia. Static parameters often require baseline measurements for comparison and may not be applicable to critically ill patients with multiple comorbidities or complex hemodynamic profiles.
5. **Left ventricular end-diastolic area (LVEDA)** is best measured in the PSAX view at the midpapillary level. Overall, LVEDA <10 cm^2 has been associated with severe hypovolemia, and conversely, >20 cm^2 has been associated with volume overload. However, LVEDA measure can be significantly confounded by other conditions including LV hypertrophy and constrictive pericarditis.
6. **Left ventricular end-systolic area (LVESA)** is best measured in the PSAX view at the midpapillary level. Particular attention should be paid to the positioning of the papillary muscles. The classical teaching is that contact between opposing papillary muscles at the end of systole ("kissing papillary muscles") is indicative of severe hypovolemia. There are various other factors that can also cause a small LVESA, including distributive shock, hyperdynamic left ventricle, RV failure, acute mitral regurgitation, or cardiac tamponade.
    a. **LAP:** See previous section on LAP assessment.
    b. **IVC diameter:** See previous section on IVC assessment.
7. **Dynamic echocardiographic parameters:** These parameters assess fluid responsiveness by assessing the hemodynamic effect (alterations in SV) of preload-altering maneuvers (such as a mechanical breath, leg raise, fluid administration). These hemodynamic effects are exaggerated in states of low circulating volume and attenuated in patients with volume overload or when the ventricle is failing. There is more evidence supporting dynamic indices for determining fluid responsiveness relative to static measurements.
8. **Stroke volume variation (SVV):** This assesses changes in the SV induced by changes in intrathoracic pressure throughout the respiratory cycle. To calculate SVV, an A5C view is obtained to determine the blood flow through the LVOT using PW Doppler. Placing the marker through the LVOT will produce a series of VTIs, and SVV is calculated by subtracting the maximum velocity by the minimum velocity divided by the average of the two velocities. Changes >12% correlate with a likelihood of fluid responsiveness; however, this technique has only been validated for patients in sinus rhythm who are mechanically ventilated without spontaneous respiratory effort and receiving a tidal volume of 8 mL/kg. A major limitation of this method is that patients with arrhythmias, valvular abnormalities, elevated abdominal pressures, abnormal lung and chest compliance, can have SVV can cause variations in SV of their volume status.

$$SVV = \frac{SV_{Max} - SV_{Min}}{SV_{average}}$$

9. **IVC diameter variation** is measured in a manner similar to the static assessment of IVC diameter (see above). In the subcostal IVC view, the M-mode beam is sited approximately 1 to 2 cm proximal to the

cavoatrial junction and used to measure the change in maximum diameter (at the end of positive pressure inspiration) and minimum diameter (at the end of positive pressure expiration). A value greater than 12% after calculating the difference between the maximum and minimum diameters divided by the mean of each has been shown to predict fluid responsiveness to an 8 mL/kg intravenous (IV) volume bolus (**Table 2.3**). Although this technique has only been validated in mechanically ventilated patients, with no respiratory effort, IVC diameter variation does

TABLE 2.3 Quantitative Methods for Echocardiographic Assessment of Left Ventricular Function

Parameter and Method	Technique	Advantages	Limitations
Fractional shortening (FS)	Based on 2D or M-mode derived measurements (during PSAX or PLAX) of the LVEDD and LVESD. FS = LVEDD − LVESD/LVEDD × 100%.	Uses routine echo views. Measurements are simple and easy to obtain.	The major limitation occurs in patients with regional wall motion abnormalities. Based on geometric assumptions to calculate an area from linear dimensions. Highly preload and afterload dependent.
Fractional area of change (FAC)	Similar to FS, however, instead of diameter is based on circumferential area by tracing the wall of the endocardium in the PSAX view. FAC = (LVEDA − LVESA)/LVEDA × 100%.		
Left ventricular ejection fraction (LVEF) using Simpson's biplane method	Based on calculation of LV volume by manually tracking the LV endocardial border in the A4C and the apical two-chamber views. LV ejection fraction (LVEF) = (EDV − ESV)/EDV.	Is the currently recommended 2D method to assess LVEF.	Requires training in obtaining comprehensive echocardiography views. Requires adequate endocardial definition.
LVEF using 3D echocardiography	Allows acquisition of the entire LV volume in a single volumetric data set and calculation of LVEF.	Strong correlation with cardiac MRI.	Requires special training and equipment. Requires adequate endocardial definition.
Global longitudinal strain	Measures the relative change in length of the LV myocardium between end diastole and end systole using speckle-tracking echocardiography.	Useful in the assessment of regional wall motion abnormalities and scar tissue.	Requires special equipment and training. Require adequate endocardial definition.

LV, left ventricle; LVEDA, left ventricular end-diastolic area; LVEF, left ventricle ejection fraction; LVESA, left ventricular end-systolic area; LVEDD, left ventricular end-diastolic diameter; LVESD, left ventricular end-systolic diameter; PLAX, parasternal long axis; PSAX, parasternal short axis.

not require sinus rhythm, unlike SVV. Conditions that affect intrathoracic pressure [positive end expiratory pressure (PEEP)], impede venous returns (tamponade, right heart failure, tricuspid regurgitation), and IVC compression (masses, thrombosis) decrease the accuracy of this test.

10. **PLR** test is a reversible preload challenge that translocates approximately 300 mL of blood from the lower extremities by changing a semirecumbent-positioned patient into a supine position with leg elevation. The maximal cardiac response to PLR occurs within 2 minutes of the change in positioning. Like conventional SVV, a sonographer will calculate the LVOT velocity in the A5C view, both before and after the maneuver. An increase in the velocity by 10% to 15% corresponds with likelihood of fluid responsiveness. A meta-analysis of studies of PLR found the diagnostic value of this technique to be excellent. A particular advantage of this approach is the lack of requirement for mechanical ventilation, sinus rhythm, or normal pulmonary compliance. It is not a reliable test in patients with increased abdominal pressures. One of the major limitations of this method is that positional changes are typically not feasible during surgery.

11. **Fluid challenge:** A final method is to measure CO before administration of an IV fluid bolus and then measure the CO after. If the cardiac output does not increase with the fluid challenge, the patient is presumed not to be fluid responsive and no further IV fluids are administered until there has been a change in physiologic state. Measurement of CO using echocardiography is described the above in the section on *"Flow measurement"*.

VII. LUNG ULTRASOUND (LUS)

LUS facilitates rapid diagnosis of pulmonary pathology at the bedside. Compared with chest radiography, lung US has higher sensitivity and specificity for the detection of pleural effusion, pneumonia, pneumothorax, and pulmonary edema. This chapter focuses on the basics of LUS technique and the interpretation of normal and pathologic findings.

LUS images reflect the relative amounts of air and fluid in the lung. In healthy lungs, the elevated air content prevents US wave propagation through the parenchyma. As a result, in an expanded lung, structures deep into the pleura cannot be directly visualized. Instead, image interpretation is based on the detection and evaluation of imaging artifacts. These artifacts will vary depending on the ratio of air and fluid in the lungs.

A. Lung Ultrasound Examination

1. **Any probe can be used for LUS, however the low-frequency curvilinear transducer (3 to 6 MHz) is the most widely used.** Microconvex transducers have a smaller footprint and fit better between ribs, especially in pediatric patients. High-frequency linear transducers (7 to 12 MHz) allow better visualization of superficial structures and therefore are better for visualizing lung sliding and A-lines.

2. **The exam can be performed with the patient in a seated, supine, or prone position.** The probe should be positioned on the patient's chest wall, vertically, perpendicular to the long axis of the ribs with the probe indicator pointing toward the patient's head (**Figure 2.15**).

   The probe should be scanned along the anterior lung fields in the midclavicular line, superior to inferior. Then along the posterior lung fields in the midaxillary line, again, superiorly to inferiorly. Multiple exam protocols have been proposed. A common approach is the Bedside Lung Ultrasound in Emergency (BLUE) protocol which is based on three-point examination of each lung. This has been widely studied in patients with

Chapter 2 Basics of Echocardiography and Lung Ultrasound

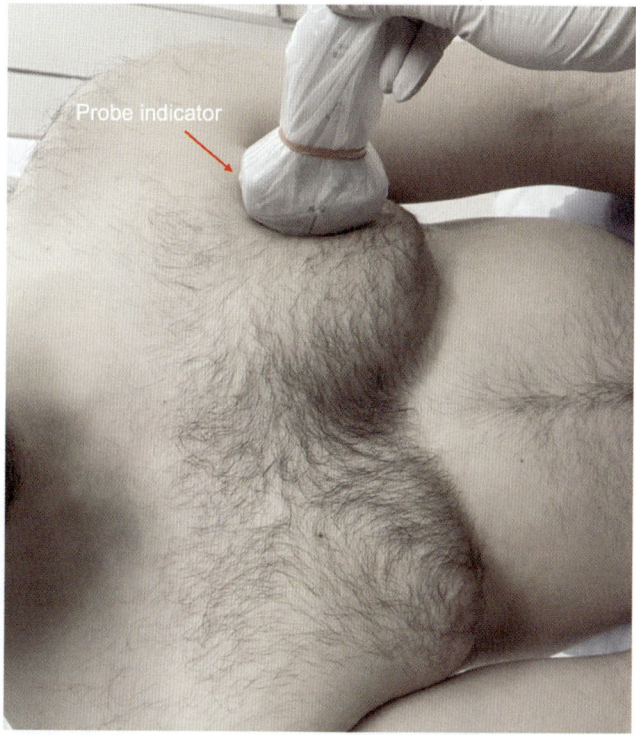

FIGURE 2.15 Curvilinear probe positioned vertically along the longitudinal axis of the chest wall during lung ultrasound with the probe indicator pointing toward the patient's head.

acute respiratory failure and has been proven to be easy to perform with high accuracy. Other common approaches include the division of each hemithorax into six segments (**Figure 2.16**). If available, the lung preset setting on the US device should be selected to optimize the images.

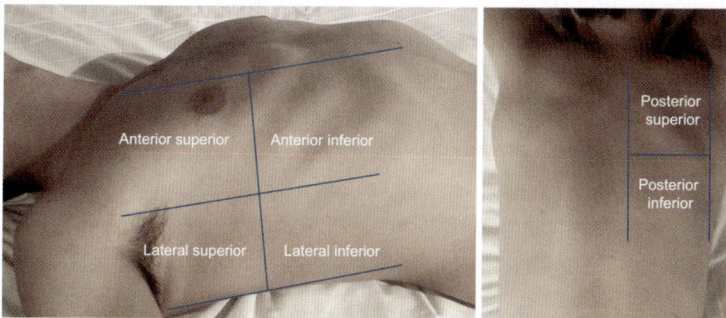

FIGURE 2.16 Anterior, lateral, and posterior segments for lung ultrasound.

FIGURE 2.17 Normal lung image demonstrating "bat sign" (*red line*), hyperechoic pleura (*arrow*), and ribs on either side.

B. Lung Ultrasound Findings
When placing the probe on the chest, the pleura appears as a hyperechoic horizontal line about 0.5 cm below two adjacent ribs. The acoustic shadowing caused by the two adjacent ribs is called the bat sign (**Figure 2.17**). Healthy lungs have the following characteristics on LUS: lung sliding, a visibly smooth and hyperechoic pleural line; and visible A-lines.

C. A-lines
Under normal conditions, the lungs are mostly filled with air that reflects the US waves back to the transducer at the air-tissue interface. This generates evenly-spaced repeating horizontal artifacts called A-lines. The distance between A-lines is equal to the distance between the skin surface

FIGURE 2.18 Lung ultrasound demonstrating the pleura and A-lines.

and the pleural line (**Figure 2.18**). A-lines can be seen both in the normal lung and in the presence of a pneumothorax.
- D. Lung Sliding
    1. **Under normal conditions, the visceral and parietal pleura are in direct contact and slide over each other.** This is seen on LUS as a shimmering or crawling artifact of the pleural line, referred to as "lung sliding." It also creates a grainy, constantly shifting artifact below the pleural line. In M-mode, this appears as the "seashore sign," where the area above the pleura shows stable horizontal lines (sky and ocean), and below it looks grainy (sand) due to lung sliding (**Figure 2.19**).
    2. **Lung sliding decreases with low tidal volumes or hyperinflated lungs** and is absent in conditions in which the pleura are not directly opposed (pneumothorax or effusion), are adherent (pneumonia complicated by adhesions or

FIGURE 2.19 M-mode of a normal lung pattern demonstrating the seashore sign with superficial layers representing the waves, and the deeper layers representing the sand.

pleurodesis) or in the absence of spontaneous or mechanical ventilation (pneumonectomy, one lung intubation). In these cases, M-mode shows only horizontal lines, called the "stratosphere" or "barcode sign."

E. B-lines

B-lines are reverberation artifacts that arise from the pleural line as a result of increased lung density due to fluid or fibrosis. They are long, vertical, and hyperechoic streaks that extend to the periphery of the image resembling "comet tails" or "lung rockets" (**Figure 2.20**). B-lines efface A-lines and move with lung sliding. Up to two B-lines between adjacent ribs can be seen in normal lungs (especially at the bases). Three or more are considered pathologic.

F. Consolidation

Lobar pneumonia, pulmonary contusion, and lobar atelectasis can lead to consolidation of lung tissue and near-complete loss of aeration allowing US waves to travel through the tissue. Consolidated lung can appear as dense liverlike tissue, a phenomenon known as hepatization of the lung. Air bronchograms can also be seen in consolidated lung as hyperechoic punctiform or tubular structures within lung tissue.

G. Pleural Effusion

1. **Effusions tend to accumulate in caudal posterior areas due to gravity and therefore are best seen in the basal posterior fields of the lung.** Three elements should be visualized to identify the location of the pleural fluid: the pleural cavity, the diaphragm, and an abdominal organ, either the liver or the spleen. Atelectatic lung can often also be seen floating in the pleural fluid (**Figure 2.21**).
2. **Spine sign:** In healthy lung, the spine is obscured by air in the lung and is not visible past the diaphragm. In patients with pleural effusions, US

FIGURE 2.20 B-lines radiating down between two ribs.

can travel through the pleural fluid allowing the spine to be seen above the diaphragm.
3. **Curtain sign:** Occurs when the lungs are full of air and expanded obstructing the view of the diaphragm underneath. This will move back and forth with respirations, obstructing the view like a curtain. A large enough pleural effusion will prevent this obstructing to US transmission.

H. **Alveolar–Interstitial Syndromes**

These are characterized by heterogeneous conditions that lead to decreased air in the lungs and increased lung density resulting in diffuse B-lines. In severe cases, multiple B-lines can fuse creating a pattern called "white lung." The differential diagnosis includes pulmonary edema, acute

FIGURE 2.21 Right lung ultrasound showing a hypoechoic area representing a pleural effusion bordered by atelectatic lung to the left and separated from the liver by the diaphragm.

respiratory distress syndrome (ARDS), interstitial pneumonia or pneumonitis, and diffuse parenchymal lung disease such as pulmonary fibrosis. The pattern and distribution of B-lines can help point toward a specific condition. Multiple B-lines of 7 mm correlate with thickened interlobular septa as seen in interstitial edema and B-lines of 3 mm or less apart correlate with ground-glass opacities seen in alveolar edema. There is a correlation between the number of B-lines and the degree of disease severity.

1. **Cardiogenic pulmonary edema**: Homogeneous B-lines distribution, no spared areas, normal-appearing pleura, normal lung sliding, and associated bilateral pleural effusions.
2. **ARDS**: Nonhomogeneous B-lines distribution, spared areas of normal lung, irregular thickened pleura, with reduced or absent lung sliding,

subpleural and posterior consolidations. More severe in dependent areas.
3. **Pulmonary fibrosis:** Diffuse distribution, irregular thickened pleura.
4. **B-lines can be seen in focal areas** not meeting criteria for alveolar–interstitial syndrome in conditions like pneumonia, atelectasis, pulmonary contusion, pulmonary infarction, and neoplasia.

I. Limitations of Lung Ultrasound

US is operator dependent and requires training. Morbid obesity, subcutaneous emphysema, medical devices, and the position of the patient can limit access to specific areas of the chest. Various medical conditions can produce similar or identical US findings. B-lines, for example, may appear in patients with diseases such as cardiac or noncardiogenic pulmonary edema, ARDS, or fibrosis. Although LUS can help detect a pneumothorax at the bedside, determining its size can be difficult and decisions to treat it should be based on clinical condition.

VIII. CONCLUSION

The use of point-of-care echocardiography with LUS by noncardiologists is an established and growing clinical tool. This allows the clinician at the bedside to rapidly and repeatedly evaluate a patient. It supplements physical examination and obviates the potential risk involved in waiting for or transporting an unstable patient for, additional forms of diagnostic testing. A POCUS examination does not replace the role of a comprehensive echocardiographic examination and care must be taken to practice within the limitations of one's own expertise. Consultation with an expert echocardiographer is recommended when there is any question or complex diagnosis. However, cardiac POCUS is a powerful diagnostic and monitoring tool for the bedside clinician, and the applications will continue to develop in the future.

Suggested Readings

Beigel R, Cercek B, Luo H, Siegal RJ. Noninvasive evaluation of right atrial pressure. *J Am Soc Echocardiogr.* 2013;26(9):1033–1042.

Bouhemad B, Zhang M, Lu Q, Rouby J-J. Clinical review: bedside lung ultrasound in critical care practice. *Crit Care.* 2007;11(1):205.

Boussier J, Lemasle A, Hantala N, et al. Lung ultrasound score on postoperative day 1 is predictive of the occurrence of pulmonary complications after major abdominal surgery: a multicenter prospective observational study. *Anesthesiology.* 2024;140(3):417–429.

Buda N, Mendrala K, Skoczyński S, et al. Basics of point-of-care lung ultrasonography. *N Engl J Med.* 2023;389(21):e44.

Cherpanath TGV, Hirsch A, Geerts BF, et al. Predicting fluid responsiveness by passive leg raising: a systematic review and meta-analysis of 23 clinical trials. *Crit Care Med.* 2016;44(5):981–991.

Feissel M, Michard F, Faller JP, Teboul JL. The respiratory variation in inferior vena cava diameter as a guide to fluid therapy. *Intensive Care Med.* 2004;30:1834–1837.

Feissel M, Michard F, Mangin I, Ruyer O, Faller JP, Teboul JL. Respiratory changes in aortic blood velocity as an indicator of fluid responsiveness in ventilated patients with septic shock. *Chest.* 2001;119(3):867–873.

Labovitz AJ, Noble VE, Bierig M, et al. Focused cardiac ultrasound in the emergent setting: a consensus statement of the American Society of Echocardiography and American College of Emergency Physicians. *J Am Soc Echocardiogr.* 2010;23:1225–1230.

Lang RM, Badano LP, Mor-Avi V, et al. Recommendations for cardiac chamber quantification by echocardiography in adults: an update from the American Society of Echocardiography and the European Association of Cardiovascular Imaging. *J Am Soc Echocardiogr.* 2015;28(1):1–39.e14.

Lichtenstein DA, Mezière GA. Relevance of lung ultrasound in the diagnosis of acute respiratory failure: the BLUE protocol. *Chest.* 2008;134(1):117–125.

Luis SA, Chan J, Pellikka PA. Echocardiographic assessment of left ventricular systolic function: an overview of contemporary techniques, including speckle-tracking echocardiography. *Mayo Clin Proc.* 2019;94(1):125–138.

Martelli G, Congedi S, Lorenzoni G, et al. Echocardiographic assessment of pulmonary capillary wedge pressure by E/e' ratio: a systematic review and meta-analysis. *J Crit Care.* 2023;76:154281.

McKaigney CJ, Krantz MJ, La Rocque CL, Hurst ND, Buchanan MS, Kendall JL. E-point septal separation: a bedside tool for emergency physician assessment of left ventricular ejection fraction. *Am J Emerg Med.* 2014;32(6):493–497.

Miller A. Practical approach to lung ultrasound. *BJA Educ.* 2016;16(2):39–45.

Monnet X, Marik PE, Teboul JL. Prediction of fluid responsiveness: an update. *Ann Intensive Care.* 2016;6(1):111.

Nasser MF, Jabri A, Limaye S, et al. Echocardiographic evaluation of pulmonary embolism: a review. *J Am Soc Echocardiogr.* 2023;36(9):906–912.

Panoulas VF, Daigeler A-L, Malaweera ASN, et al. Pocket-size hand-held cardiac ultrasound as an adjunct to clinical examination in the hands of medical students and junior doctors. *Eur Heart J Cardiovasc Imaging.* 2013;14(4):323–330.

Perel A. Using dynamic variables to guide perioperative fluid management. *Anesthesiology.* 2020;133(4):929–935.

Pérez-Casares A, Cesar S, Brunet-Garcia L, Sanchez-de-Toledo J. Echocardiographic evaluation of pericardial effusion and cardiac tamponade. *Front Pediatr.* 2017;5:79.

Spencer KT, Kimura BJ, Korcarz CE, Pellikka PA, Rahko PS, Siegel RJ. Focused cardiac ultrasound: recommendations from the American Society of Echocardiography. *J Am Soc Echocardiogr.* 2013;26:567–581.

Vetrugno L, Biasucci DG, Deana C, et al. Lung ultrasound and supine chest X-Ray use in modern adult intensive care: mapping 30 years of advancement (1993–2023). *Ultrasound J.* 2024;16(1):7.

Wetterslev M, Haase N, Johansen RR, Perner A. Predicting fluid responsiveness with transthoracic echocardiography is not yet evidence based. *Acta Anaesthegiol Scan.* 2013;57(6):692–697.

Mielnicki W, Dyla A, Zawada T. Utility of transthoracic echocardiography (TTE) in assessing fluid responsiveness in critically ill patients—a challenge for the bedside sonographer. *Med Ultrason.* 2016;18(4):508–514.

Zaidi A, Knight DS, Augustine DX, et al; Education Committee of the British Society of Echocardiography. Echocardiographic assessment of the right heart in adults: a practical guideline from the British Society of Echocardiography. *Echo Res Pract.* 2020;7(1):G19–G41.

3 Specific Considerations for Cardiac Disease

Peter Ochieng and Emily C. Mills

I. GENERAL CONSIDERATIONS

It is estimated that 48.6% of American adults have one or more types of cardiovascular disease (CVD). Heart disease remains the leading cause of death in the United States.

II. CORONARY ANATOMY

The coronary arteries perfuse the myocardium. The left and right coronary arteries originate from the ascending aorta, just distal to the aortic valve. The left main coronary artery (LMCA) branches into the left anterior descending artery (LAD) and the left circumflex artery (LCX) to supply most of the left ventricle (LV), interventricular septum (IVS), and the left atrium (LA). The right coronary artery (RCA) supplies the right atrium (RA) and right ventricle (RV), as well as the posterior one-third of the IVS, including the sinoatrial (SA) and atrioventricular (AV) nodes (**Figure 3.1**). In approximately 70% of the population, the posterior descending artery (PDA) is supplied by the RCA. This circulation is described as "right dominant." The remainder of the

FIGURE 3.1 Coronary anatomy.

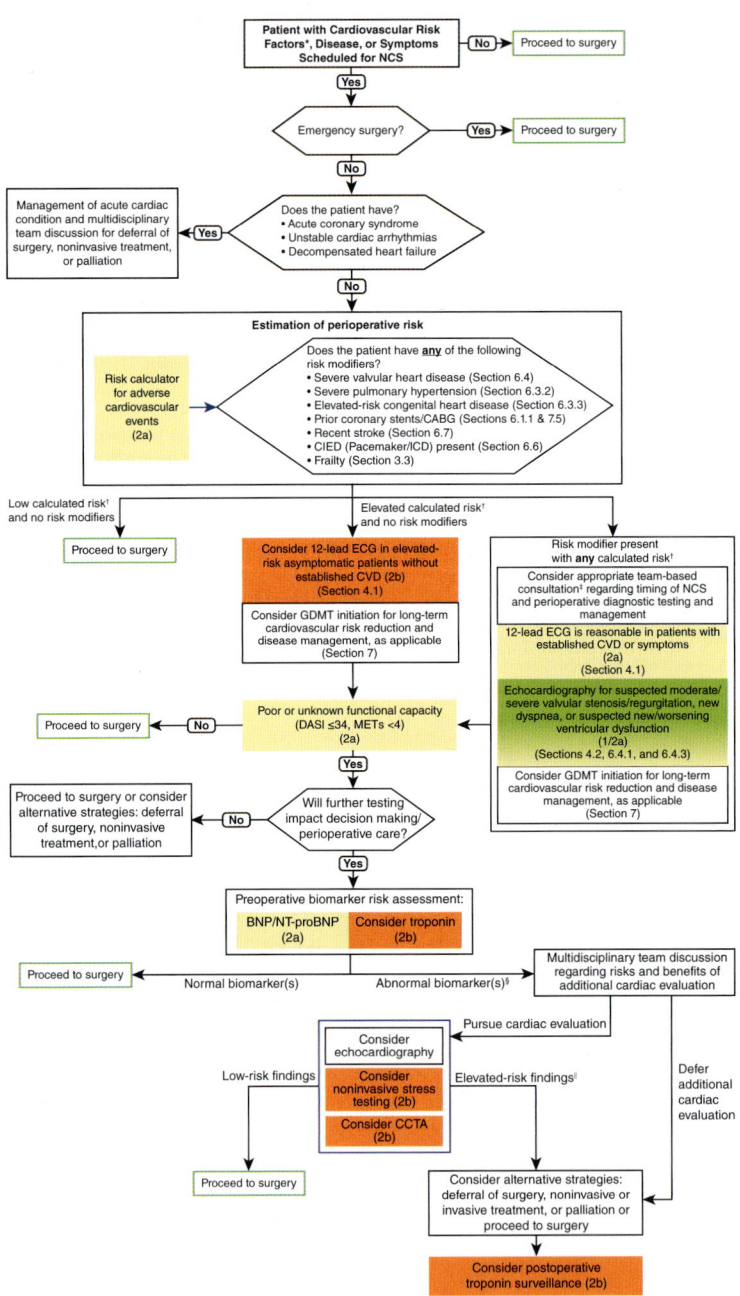

FIGURE 3.2 Stepwise approach to perioperative cardiac assessment. *Cardiovascular risk factors: hypertension, smoking, high cholesterol, diabetes, women age >65 years; men age >55 years; obesity; family history of premature CAD. †Determining elevated calculated risk depends on the calculator used. Traditionally, RCRI >1 or a calculated risk of MACE with any perioperative risk calculator >1% is used as a threshold to identify patients at elevated risk. §Abnormal biomarker thresholds: troponin >99th percentile URL for the assay; BNP >92 ng/L, NT-proBNP ≥300 ng/L. ‡Conditions that pose additional risk for MACE. ‖Noninvasive stress testing or CCTA suggestive of LM or multivessel CAD. Colors correspond to Class of Recommendation. BNP, B-type natriuretic peptide; CABG, coronary artery bypass grafting; CAD, coronary artery disease; CCTA, coronary computed tomography angiography; CIED, cardiovascular implantable electronic device; CVD, cardiovascular disease; DASI, Duke Activity Status Index; ECG, electrocardiogram; GDMT, guideline-directed management and therapy; ICD, implantable cardioverter-defibrillator; LM, left main; MACE, major adverse cardiovascular event; METs, metabolic equivalents; NCS, noncardiac surgery; NT-proBNP, N-terminal pro B-type natriuretic peptide; RCRI, Revised Cardiac Risk Index; URL, upper reference limit. Sections referenced in the figure can be found in the original paper. (From Thompson A, Fleischmann KE, Smilowitz NR, et al.; Peer Review Committee Members. 2024 AHA/ACC/ACS/ASNC/HRS/SCA/SCCT/SCMR/SVM guideline for perioperative cardiovascular management for noncardiac surgery: a report of the American College of Cardiology/American Heart Association Joint Committee on clinical practice guidelines. *Circulation.* 2024;150(19):e351–e442. Erratum in: *Circulation.* 2024;150(21):e466. Figure 1.)

population is either "left dominant," with the PDA emerging from the LCX (10% of the population), or "codominant," with the PDA receiving contributions from both the LCX and RCA (20% of population).

III. PREOPERATIVE CARDIOVASCULAR EVALUATION FOR NONCARDIAC SURGERY

In 2014, the American College of Cardiology and the American Heart Association (ACC/AHA) published updated guidelines for the preoperative cardiovascular evaluation and management of patients undergoing noncardiac surgery. The initial evaluation consists of the patient's history, a focused physical examination, and routine laboratory investigation. Based on the patient's history, cardiac risk factors, functional status, and the nature of the surgical procedure, the ACC/AHA guidelines provide a stepwise approach to identifying patients who may benefit from further cardiovascular testing (**Figure 3.2**).

A. Initial screening

1. The need for **emergency surgery** preempts further cardiac workup. The ACC/AHA guidelines define an emergency procedure as one in which life or limb is threatened, and thus started within 6 hours. As there is little to no time, the case must proceed with no or very limited clinical preoperative evaluation. Emergent surgery should proceed with appropriate patient monitoring and management strategies based on the patient's clinical risk factors for coronary artery disease (CAD). Bedside transthoracic echocardiography can be performed to rule out life-threatening cardiac conditions such as tamponade, aortic dissection, or myocardial infarction (MI) to help with perioperative management in the emergent setting.

2. If the **surgery is not emergent**, determine whether the patient has an acute coronary syndrome (ACS). An ACS is an unstable angina or an MI. The patient may present with chest pain, shortness of breath, diaphoresis, or nausea. The electrocardiogram (ECG) may show ST-segment depressions or elevations. If the patient has an ACS, the surgical procedure should be postponed, and the patient should immediately undergo further cardiac evaluation and guideline-directed medical

therapy (GDMT). If the patient does not have an ACS, then proceed with an assessment of the patient's perioperative risk for a major adverse cardiac event (MACE), defined as MI, cardiac arrest, or cardiac death.
- B. **Risk of MACE.** The patient's risk of MACE should be determined based on clinical characteristics and the surgical procedure. Clinical risk factors for MACE include a history of heart failure, CAD, cerebrovascular disease, diabetes, and chronic kidney disease. Validated risk prediction tools, such as the Revised Cardiac Risk Index (RCRI) and the American College of Surgeons National Surgical Quality Improvement Program (ACS NSQIP) Surgical Risk Calculator (riskcalculator.facs.org), can be used to help predict the risk of perioperative MACE.
  1. If the patient has a **low risk of MACE** (<1%), then **no further testing** is needed, and the patient may **proceed to surgery.**
  2. If the patient has an **elevated risk of MACE** (≥1%), then the **functional capacity** should be determined. **Functional capacity** can be expressed as metabolic equivalents (METs). A single MET represents oxygen consumption at rest. If the patient has moderate or excellent functional capacity without cardiac symptoms, then the patient may proceed to surgery without further evaluation. **Moderate or excellent functional capacity** is defined as an **exercise capacity greater than or equal to 4 METs.** Activities that correspond to moderate functional capacity include climbing two flights of stairs, walking on level ground at 4 mph, running a short distance, scrubbing floors, or playing golf without a cart. The ability to participate in strenuous sports such as swimming, singles tennis, or football generally corresponds to excellent functional capacity.
  3. If the patient has poor or unknown functional capacity, then further testing may be indicated if the results will change a patient's management. **Poor functional capacity** is defined as an **exercise capacity of less than 4 METs.** Examples include the inability to walk more than two blocks on level ground without stopping due to symptoms and activity limited to eating, dressing, and walking indoors. Further testing may include exercise or pharmacologic stress testing. If abnormal, coronary angiography and revascularization may be considered. The patient can then proceed to surgery with GDMT. Testing may not be necessary if the results will not alter patient management.
- C. **Supplemental cardiac evaluation.** Supplemental cardiac evaluation should be performed when indicated to measure functional capacity, identify the presence of cardiac dysfunction, and provide an estimate of the perioperative cardiac risk.
  1. **Preoperative resting 12-lead ECG** should be considered for patients with known coronary heart disease, significant arrhythmia, peripheral arterial disease, cerebrovascular disease, or other structural heart diseases, except for those undergoing low-risk surgery. Routine preoperative ECG is not indicated for asymptomatic patients undergoing low-risk surgery.
  2. **Rest echocardiography** may be used to evaluate ventricular function in patients with a history of heart failure or dyspnea of unknown origin. It is also useful to assess valvular pathology in patients with a history of valvular disease or a newly identified heart murmur.
  3. **Stress testing** is recommended for patients with elevated risk of MACE and poor or unknown functional capacity if the outcome will change management. This means the patient would be both amenable to revascularization and the intended noncardiac surgery would

be compatible with postcatheterization anticoagulation requirements. Routine screening with stress testing is not useful for patients undergoing low-risk noncardiac surgery.

   a. **Exercise stress testing** provides an objective measure of functional capacity. It is the preferred modality in patients who are capable of achieving adequate workloads. Sensitivity and specificity for multivessel CAD are 81% and 66%, respectively. Exercise stress tests are highly predictive when ST segment changes are characteristic of ischemia (>2 mm, sustained into recovery, and/or associated with hypotension). The risk of perioperative cardiac events is increased significantly in patients who have abnormal exercise ECGs at low workloads. Radionuclide imaging or echocardiography can be combined with exercise stress testing for patients whose baseline ECGs render interpretation invalid.

   b. **Pharmacologic stress testing** can be conducted with either an agent that increases myocardial oxygen demand (dobutamine) or dilates coronary arteries and causes coronary steal from diseased vessels (ie, dipyridamole or adenosine). Pharmacologic stress tests are suitable for patients who are unable to exercise due to physical limitations. Dobutamine stress testing is typically combined with echocardiography to detect wall motion abnormalities elicited by the increased myocardial workload. Dipyridamole or adenosine stress tests are typically combined with radionuclide imaging to detect areas of myocardium that are at risk. Pharmacologic vasodilation has the risk of a false-negative test in patients with multivessel CAD where all vessels are already maximally vasodilated. In both cases, perioperative cardiac risk is directly proportional to the extent of myocardium that is found to be at risk on imaging.

4. **Cardiac catheterization** is considered the "gold standard" for evaluating CAD. Information obtained includes coronary anatomy with visualization of direction and distribution of flow, hemodynamics, and overall function of the heart. Routine preoperative coronary angiography is not recommended. Revascularization before noncardiac surgery is recommended in circumstances in which revascularization is indicated according to existing clinical practice guidelines.

5. **Noninvasive imaging** including cardiac MRI (CMR) and coronary computed tomography angiogram (CCTA) have emerged as reasonable options for preoperative cardiac evaluation. CMR is usually reserved for patients after first-line imaging (echocardiography) is either inconclusive or indeterminant; it is generally reserved for patients with complex diseases. Contraindications to CMR include the presence of implants or cardiovascular implantable electronic devices (CIEDs) that are not MRI safe. CCTA can be utilized to rule out obstructive CAD in low- to medium-risk patients, but it is not advised for high-risk patients; coronary catheterization remains the gold standard for high-risk patients. Contraindications to cardiac CTA include renal failure or allergy to contrast.

6. **Cardiac consultation** may be helpful in determining which tests will be useful and in interpreting the results. The consultant can help optimize the patient's preoperative medical therapy and provide follow-up in the postoperative period. Such follow-up is crucial with the initiation of new drug therapies and often for patients with pacemakers and implantable cardioverter-defibrillator (ICD) devices (see Section XI).

D. Indications for preoperative coronary revascularization with either **percutaneous coronary intervention (PCI)** or **coronary artery bypass grafting (CABG)** are, in general, the same as in the nonoperative setting. Surgery, in and of itself, is not an indication of coronary revascularization, regardless of extent of vessel disease or left ventricular dysfunction.

IV. PREANESTHETIC CONSIDERATIONS

A. Patients are likely to be anxious. Reassurance during the preoperative consultation has been shown to be useful in decreasing anxiety. **Anxiolytics** may blunt rises in sympathetic tone and can be invaluable.

B. **Cardiac medications** are usually continued perioperatively. Possible exceptions include angiotensin-converting enzyme inhibitors (due to prolonged vasodilation), sustained-release or long-acting medications, and diuretics.

  1. **β-Blockers.** There is a consensus that patients already taking β-blockers should continue them in the perioperative period. For patients not already on β-blockers, multiple studies have shown an increased risk of perioperative stroke, hypotension, bradycardia, and mortality when started within 24 hours of surgery. For this reason, **they should not be started on the day of surgery in all patients.** However, in patients with moderate to high risk of perioperative myocardial ischemia or with three or more RCRI risk factors (eg, diabetes mellitus, HF, CAD, renal insufficiency, cerebrovascular accident), it may be reasonable to start β-blockers before surgery. When possible, β-blockers should be started days to weeks before elective surgery and titrated cautiously.

  2. **Statins.** Patients taking statins should continue to receive statins perioperatively. Preoperative initiation of statin therapy is reasonable in patients undergoing vascular surgery as well as in patients with standard clinical indications for statin therapy who are undergoing elevated-risk procedures.

  3. **Aspirin.** The efficacy of aspirin for the secondary prevention of MI in patients with ischemic heart disease has been well documented. Data on the risk of discontinuing antiplatelet therapy in patients with coronary stents have strongly suggested continuing aspirin in the perioperative period. The data on continuing aspirin in patients undergoing elective noncardiac, noncarotid surgery who have not had previous coronary stenting, however, is controversial. Some publications recommend that aspirin should routinely be continued in the perioperative period, while a recent systematic review and meta-analysis suggests that aspirin has no significant effect on overall survival, cardiovascular mortality, or arterial ischemic events, while reducing venous thromboembolic events at the expense of increased risk of major bleeding.

C. **Timing of elective surgery in the setting of previous PCI** presents a special challenge. Management decisions should be made in consultation with the patient's cardiologist and surgeon.

  1. **Balloon angioplasty without stent placement.** The ACC/AHA recommends that elective noncardiac surgery should be **delayed 14 days** after balloon angioplasty. Aspirin therapy should be continued in the perioperative period.

  2. **Bare-metal coronary stents (BMS).** Current recommendations are to **delay elective noncardiac surgery for 30 days** following PCI with BMS. This time period allows for the completion of thienopyridine therapy and the endothelialization of the stent. The risk of ischemic events is greatest within 30 days of PCI, significantly lower at 30 to 90 days, and lowest after 90 days. Aspirin therapy should be continued perioperatively.

3. **Drug-eluting stents (DES).** Thrombosis of DES can occur months after placement and is often related to the discontinuation of dual antiplatelet therapy (DAPT) perioperatively. The current consensus recommendation is to **defer elective surgery for at least 3 months, and optimally 6 months**, following placement. Aspirin therapy should be continued perioperatively. Elective noncardiac surgery after DES implantation **may be considered after 3 to 6 months** if the risk of further delay is greater than the expected risks of ischemia and stent thrombosis.
4. Should an urgent or emergent noncardiac surgical procedure be required while a patient is on DAPT following PCI, both aspirin and thienopyridine should be continued. If bleeding risk necessitates the discontinuation of thienopyridine therapy, aspirin therapy should be continued and thienopyridines restarted as soon as possible.

D. **Supplemental oxygen** should be provided to all patients who have a significant risk of ischemia.

E. **Monitoring** is discussed in Chapter 15: Monitoring.

F. **Anesthetic technique.** There is no data to support the superiority of one particular anesthetic technique over another in the management of patients at risk for perioperative cardiac events. The anesthetic technique should be selected based on patient and surgical factors. The use of MAC, local, or neuraxial anesthesia can sometimes be more hemodynamically stable compared to general anesthesia but can present challenges with regard to anticoagulation status, level of consciousness, and pain control (tachycardia and hypertension). For major open abdominal aortic surgery, it has been shown that epidural anesthesia with general anesthesia improved pain control while reducing postoperative respiratory failure and MI; however, there was no observed difference in mortality.

V. ISCHEMIC HEART DISEASE

An estimated 30% of patients undergoing surgery in the United States have CAD. Risk factors for CAD include increasing age, hypercholesterolemia, male gender, hypertension, cigarette smoking, diabetes mellitus, obesity, and family history of ischemic heart disease. CAD is a risk factor for perioperative cardiac complications, including MI, unstable angina, congestive heart failure (CHF), and serious dysrhythmias.

A. **Pathophysiology.** Myocardial ischemia occurs when oxygen demand exceeds oxygen delivery. The heart demonstrates the highest per-gram oxygen consumption of any organ, extracting about 70% to 80% of delivered oxygen, even at rest. Therefore, the myocardium is exquisitely sensitive to coronary blood flow.

B. **Supply.** The myocardium is supplied via the coronary arteries. Myocardial oxygen delivery depends on coronary artery diameter, LV diastolic pressure, aortic diastolic pressure, and arterial oxygen content.
   1. **Coronary blood flow** is dependent on the aortic root-to-downstream coronary pressure gradient. Most **coronary blood flow occurs during ventricular diastole**. Coronary artery blood flow is controlled primarily through local mediators. The coronary arteries of patients with significant CAD may be maximally dilated at rest.
   2. **Heart rate** is inversely proportional to the length of diastole. Faster heart rates decrease the duration of maximal coronary perfusion.
   3. **Blood oxygen** content is determined by hemoglobin concentration, oxygen saturation, and dissolved oxygen content. Increasing inspired oxygen fraction and/or hemoglobin concentration increases blood oxygen content.

C. **Demand.** Myocardial oxygen consumption (MVO_2) is a function of ventricular wall tension, heart rate, and, to a lesser degree, contractility.
   1. **Ventricular wall tension** is modeled by Laplace law: wall tension is directly proportional to the ventricular transmural pressure and the ventricular radius and inversely proportional to the ventricular wall thickness. Changes in these parameters affect oxygen demand.
   2. **Heart rate.** Tachycardia is well tolerated in normal hearts. Atherosclerotic coronary arteries may not adequately dilate to meet increased demands of faster heart rates.
   3. **Contractility** increases with the increased chronotropy, myocardial stretch, calcium, and catecholamines. Increasing contractility increases oxygen consumption.
D. **Supply and demand balance.** Atherosclerosis is the most common etiology for supply–demand imbalances. Conditions such as aortic stenosis, systemic hypertension, and hypertrophic cardiomyopathy, which are characterized by marked ventricular hypertrophy and high intraventricular pressures, may also increase MVO_2. These conditions may create imbalances, even in the setting of normal coronary arteries. The goal of treatment is to improve the myocardial oxygen supply–demand balance.
   1. **Management to increase supply**
      a. **Increase coronary perfusion pressure** with the administration of volume or α-adrenergic agonists to increase aortic root diastolic pressure.
      b. **Increase coronary blood flow** with nitrates to dilate coronary arteries.
      c. **Increase oxygen content** by raising hemoglobin concentration or oxygen partial pressure.
   2. **Management to decrease demand**
      a. **Decrease heart rate** either directly with β-adrenergic antagonists or indirectly by treating underlying causes of tachycardia (eg, pain, anxiety).
      b. **Decrease ventricular size** (decrease wall tension) by decreasing preload with nitrates, calcium channel blockers, or diuretics. Occasionally, increasing inotropy may decrease demand by decreasing ventricular size and wall tension.
      c. **Decreasing contractility** may decrease MVO_2 if ventricular size and wall tension do not increase excessively. Calcium channel blockers and volatile anesthetics decrease contractility.
      d. **Intra-aortic balloon counter pulsation** increases coronary perfusion pressure by augmenting diastolic pressure. It also reduces resistance to LV ejection, thereby reducing LV size and wall tension.

VI. VALVULAR HEART DISEASE
A. Aortic stenosis
1. **Etiologies include** progressive narrowing secondary to calcification (most common), congenital (bicuspid/unicuspid valves), or rheumatic heart disease. Echocardiography severity is defined by valve area and mean gradient (mild, greater than 1.5 cm^2 or less than 25 mm Hg; moderate, between 1.0 and 1.5 cm^2 or between 25 and 40 mm Hg; and severe, less than 1.0 cm^2 or greater than 40 mm Hg, respectively). Beyond this, patients are classified as either high gradient (>40 mm Hg) or low gradient (<40 mm Hg), normal flow (Stroke volume index [Svi] >35 mL/m^2) or low flow (Svi <35 mL/m^2), and normal (>50%) or reduced LVEF (<50%).
2. **Symptoms** include exertional dyspnea, angina, syncope, and heart failure late in the disease process.

3. **Pathophysiology.** The **LV** becomes **hypertrophied** and stiff in response to the increased afterload. Coordinated atrial contraction becomes critical to maintaining adequate ventricular filling and stroke volume. The ventricle is susceptible to ischemia due to increased muscle mass and decreased coronary perfusion in the setting of increased intraventricular pressure.
4. **Anesthetic considerations.** Aortic stenosis is the only valvular lesion associated with an increased risk of perioperative ischemia, MI, and death. In patients with severe AS undergoing elective noncardiac surgery, management of the lesion, with either surgical aortic valve replacement or transcatheter aortic valve replacement (TAVR), may be warranted prior to proceeding.
    a. **Normal sinus rhythm** and adequate **volume status** should be maintained.
    b. **Avoid systemic hypotension.** Hypotension should be treated immediately and aggressively with an α-agonist such as phenylephrine to maintain adequate coronary perfusion pressure.
    c. **Avoid tachycardia.** Tachycardia results in increased oxygen demand along with a shorter period of diastole leading to decreased coronary perfusion and reduced cardiac output. Severe bradycardia can lead to reduced cardiac output and should be avoided as well. **Cardiac pacing** capabilities should be considered to treat severe bradycardia. Supraventricular tachydysrhythmias should be treated aggressively with direct current cardioversion.
    d. **Nitrates** and **peripheral vasodilators** should be administered with extreme caution.
    e. The **treatment of ischemia** in these patients is directed at increasing oxygen delivery by raising coronary perfusion pressure and decreasing oxygen consumption (by increasing blood pressure and lowering heart rate).

B. Aortic regurgitation

1. **Etiologies** include calcification, rheumatic heart disease, endocarditis, trauma, collagen vascular diseases, and processes that dilate the aortic root (eg, aneurysm, Marfan syndrome, and syphilis).
2. **Pathophysiology**
    a. Acute aortic regurgitation may cause sudden LV volume overload with increased LV end-diastolic pressure and pulmonary capillary occlusion pressure. Manifestations include decreased cardiac output, CHF, tachycardia, and vasoconstriction.
    b. Chronic aortic regurgitation leads to LV dilation and eccentric hypertrophy. Symptoms may be minimal until late in the disease process when left-sided heart failure occurs.
3. **Anesthetic considerations**
    a. Maintain a normal to slightly increased heart rate to minimize regurgitation and maintain aortic diastolic and coronary artery perfusion pressure.
    b. Maintain adequate volume status.
    c. Improve forward flow and decrease LV end-diastolic pressure and ventricular wall tension with vasodilators.
    d. Avoid peripheral arterial vasoconstrictors, which may worsen regurgitation.
    e. Consider pacing. These patients have an increased incidence of conduction abnormalities.
    f. Intra-aortic balloon counter pulsation is generally **contraindicated** in the setting of aortic regurgitation.

C. Mitral stenosis
1. **The etiology** is almost always rheumatic. Severe MS is defined as a valve area of less than 1.5 cm^2.
2. **Pathophysiology**
   a. Increased left atrial pressure and volume overload increase left atrial size and may cause **atrial fibrillation** and **pulmonary edema.**
   b. **Elevated left atrial pressure** increases pulmonary venous pressure and pulmonary vascular resistance. In turn, right ventricular pressure is increased for a given cardiac output. Chronic pulmonary hypertension produces pulmonary vascular remodeling. **Pulmonary hypertension** may lead to tricuspid regurgitation, RV failure, and decreased cardiac output.
3. **Anesthetic considerations**
   a. **Avoid tachycardia.** Tachycardia is poorly tolerated because of decreased diastolic filling time leading to decreased cardiac output and increases in left atrial pressure. Control ventricular response pharmacologically or consider cardioversion for patients with atrial fibrillation. Continue digoxin, calcium channel blockers, and β-adrenergic blockers perioperatively.
   b. **Avoid pulmonary hypertension.** Hypoxia, hypercarbia, acidosis, atelectasis, and sympathomimetics increase pulmonary vascular resistance. Oxygen, hypocarbia, alkalosis, nitrates, prostaglandin E_1, and inhaled nitric oxide decrease pulmonary vascular resistance.
   c. **Hypotension** may indicate RV failure. Inotropes and agents that decrease pulmonary hypertension may be useful (eg, dobutamine, milrinone, nitrates, prostaglandin E_1, and inhaled nitric oxide). It is also important to avoid hypervolemia.
   d. **Pulmonary artery catheter** may assist in the perioperative evaluation of volume status, intracardiac pressures, and cardiac output.
   e. **Premedication** should be adequate to prevent anxiety and tachycardia. Exercise caution in patients with hypotension, pulmonary hypertension, or low cardiac output.

D. Mitral regurgitation
1. **Etiologies** include mitral valve prolapse, ischemic heart disease, endocarditis, and post-MI papillary muscle rupture.
2. **Pathophysiology.** Mitral regurgitation allows blood to be ejected into the LA during systole. The amount of regurgitant flow depends on the ventricular-atrial pressure gradient, size of the mitral orifice, and duration of systole.
   a. **Acute mitral regurgitation** usually occurs in the setting of MI. Acute volume overload of the left side of the heart leads to LV dysfunction, LA pressure/volume overload, and resultant pulmonary edema.
   b. **Chronic mitral regurgitation** causes gradual left atrial and LV overload and dilation with compensatory eccentric hypertrophy.
   c. **Measurement of ejection fraction** does not accurately reflect forward flow, because the incompetent valve permits immediate bidirectional ejection with systole.
3. **Anesthetic considerations**
   a. **Relative tachycardia** is desirable to decrease ventricular filling time and ventricular volume.
   b. **Afterload reduction** is beneficial. Increased systemic vascular resistance will increase regurgitation.
   c. **Maintain preload and contractility.**

VII. CONGESTIVE HEART FAILURE

Heart failure results from impairment of ventricular systolic or diastolic function. Heart failure manifests as dyspnea, fatigue, decreased exercise tolerance, and pulmonary or peripheral edema. Heart failure can be classified into two categories: (1) heart failure with reduced ejection fraction (HFrEF) that is associated with variable degrees of LV enlargement and depressed ventricular ejection and (2) heart failure with preserved ejection fraction (HFpEF) in which diastolic dysfunction predominates.

- **A. Etiologies** include ischemic cardiomyopathy; hypertension; valvular heart disease; endocrine and metabolic causes such as diabetes, thyroid disease, and acromegaly; toxic cardiomyopathies due to alcohol, cocaine, or chemotherapy; nutritional causes such as carnitine deficiency; infective causes such as viral myocarditis, human immunodeficiency virus (HIV) infection, and Chagas disease; iron overload states; amyloidosis; sarcoidosis; and catecholamine-induced takotsubo.
- **B. Pathophysiology** of heart failure is the culmination of progressive changes in myocyte architecture that result in changes in ventricular shape, chamber size, ventricular wall thickness, and stiffness that lead to reduced myocardial function and cardiac output.
- **C. Anesthetic considerations.** Hemodynamic goals aim to preserve cardiac output and minimize myocardial work. Medical management should be optimized preoperatively.
    1. **Maintain preload but with caution.** Patients with impaired LV function depend on preload to maintain cardiac output; however, they are at risk of pulmonary edema with fluid overload.
    2. **Avoid tachycardia** to minimize myocardial work and preserve ventricular filling during diastole.
    3. **Aggressively treat arrhythmias** as they may lead to reduction in cardiac output. The absence of coordinated atrial contractions (such as in atrial fibrillation) can lead to significant compromise of ventricular preload.
    4. **Preserve contractility.** Patients with heart failure may rely on increased sympathetic tone to maintain cardiac output. As a result, they can become profoundly hypotensive following induction or even after analgesic or anxiolytic therapy. Inotropic support may be required.
    5. **Afterload reduction** is favorable as it reduces myocardial work. If vasopressors are needed, they should be used with caution.
- **D. Anesthetic considerations for durable ventricular assist devices (VADs)**
Approximately 20% to 30% of patients with durable VADs will present for noncardiac surgery. The two most commonly implanted VADs are the HeartMate 3 (Abbott, Abbott Park, IL) and the HeartWare HVAD (Medtronic, Dublin, Ireland). These are both considered continuous centrifugal flow assist devices and are FDA approved for bridge-to-transplant or destination therapy that is a final intervention for patients who are poor heart transplant candidates. Hemodynamic goals should focus on maintaining adequate preload and preserved afterload. Patients with VADs may not be good candidates for regional techniques due to anticoagulation but should be considered for local or MAC techniques when indicated.
    1. **Preoperative considerations**
        a. Perform a **system controller history review** and contact the institutional or patient's **VAD care team**. Device settings (including device type, implantation date, pump speed, pump flow, pump power, and pulsatility index) should be documented. Adequacy of the VAD's current function as well as any previous device-related problems should be reviewed with the VAD care team.

b. Review pertinent laboratory studies and physical examination to assess for other sequelae of end-stage heart failure (progression of kidney or liver disease).
c. Discuss any current home **inotropic** medications, **anticoagulation**, and/or presence of **CIEDs**. Most VAD patients will have had a CIED placed prior to VAD implantation due to their reduced EF and risk for sudden cardiac death.

2. **Intraoperative considerations**
   a. **Ensure reliable AC power and/or backup battery power** for the VAD.
   b. VAD parameters should be monitored throughout by a provider with expertise in the device. Due to the continuous flow from the device, often noninvasive blood pressure monitors and pulse oximeters do not function. Consider the use of an invasive arterial line or cerebral oximetry as alternative monitors. A pulmonary artery catheter for monitoring pulmonary artery pressure and central venous pressure should be considered depending on procedure type and patient status. Transesophageal echocardiography is not mandatory but should be available to assist in troubleshooting hemodynamic events.
   c. Induction of anesthesia should be focused on adequate preoxygenation, **avoidance of significant reductions in afterload, maintenance of heart rate** and **rhythm**, and optimizing fluid balance.
   d. Patient can be positioned in the usual fashion including prone and lateral with caution to avoid compression of the VAD driveline.
   e. Administer surgical site infection prophylaxis with antibiotics in the usual fashion; however, close attention should be paid to proper sterile technique around the driveline site.
   f. Target a **mean arterial pressure of 65 to 80 mm Hg**, to be maintained with either **volume resuscitation or afterload support** (vasopressin preferred due to reduced effect on PVR). If continued hemodynamic instability is observed, consider increasing VAD pump speed.
   g. **Maintenance of right ventricular function** and **reduction of pulmonary artery pressure** is crucial. Care should be taken to prevent hypoxia, hypercarbia, acidosis, and arrhythmia. For additional reduction in pulmonary artery pressure, consider the use of pulmonary vasodilators such as inhaled epoprostenol, nitric oxide, or milrinone.
   h. If mechanically ventilating, strategy is aimed at mitigating hypoxia and hypercarbia with an **avoidance of excessive positive end-expiratory pressure (PEEP)** or high tidal volumes, which can result in a hemodynamically significant reduction in preload.
   i. Intraoperative challenges specific to VAD patients include:
      1. **Suction events**
         a. Occurs when the **IVS is shifted** toward the inflow cannula located in the LV leading to **obstruction of the inflow cannula** and resultant hypotension, arrhythmias, and pump flow reductions. This can stem from hypovolemia, increased PVR, and/or increased VAD pump speeds. Treatment depends on the etiology but can include fluid bolus or transfusion, vasopressor therapy (phenylephrine or vasopressin bolus), and lowering the VAD pump speed.
      2. **Power failure**
         a. This can occur when there is a disconnection of the driveline from the system controller or when the system is unplugged from AC power with inadequate backup battery. The best way

to avoid this is to secure alternative AC power sources and to ensure backup batteries are charged.
3. **VAD pump thrombosis**
    a. This critical event rarely occurs intraoperatively but can lead to **complete pump failure and hemodynamic collapse.** This occurs when thrombus forms inside the VAD pump due to inadequate anticoagulation, acute increases in afterload, or dramatic reductions in pump speeds. Signs of pump thrombosis include sudden increases in pump power without resultant increases in pump flow and speed. Treatment usually involves replacement of the VAD.
3. **Postoperative considerations**
    a. Recovery of VAD patients can be performed in the postanesthesia care unit (PACU) but may require intensive care unit (ICU)-level care depending on the intraoperative course.
    b. Attention should be paid to any preoperative programming changes of a patient's CIED; it is advised to reverse these changes in the postoperative period prior to discharge.
    c. Reinitiate anticoagulation therapy in coordination with the surgical team.

VIII. HYPERTROPHIC CARDIOMYOPATHY

Hypertrophic cardiomyopathy is a genetic disorder characterized by **asymmetric LV hypertrophy and impaired relaxation in diastole.** Although most patients with hypertrophic cardiomyopathy do not have an increased LV outflow tract gradient at rest, many of them develop **dynamic outflow tract obstruction** with decreased filling and increased contractility. Under these conditions, as flow accelerates through the narrowed LV outflow tract, it creates drag, which pulls the anterior leaflet of the mitral valve toward the septum. This systolic anterior motion (SAM) of the anterior mitral leaflet leads to further outflow obstruction and mitral regurgitation.

A. Anesthetic considerations. Factors that **worsen the outflow obstruction** include decreased arterial pressure, decreased intraventricular volume, increased contractility, and increased heart rate.
   1. **Maintain normal volume status.**
   2. **Avoid tachycardia.** Continue β-adrenergic and calcium channel blocker therapy for heart rate control.
   3. **Maintain normal sinus rhythm.** Consider cardioversion for supraventricular tachycardia.
   4. **Avoid hypotension.** Correct vasodilation with α-adrenergic agonists to avoid tachycardia and marked changes in contractility. Use nitrates and peripheral dilators with extreme caution.
   5. **Use inotropes with caution.** Increased inotropy may exacerbate the outflow obstruction.

IX. CONGENITAL HEART DISEASE

With improvement in the survival of congenital heart disease (CHD) patients, anesthesiologists are encountering them with greater frequency as adults in noncardiac surgical settings. Depending on the underlying lesion, an adult with a history of CHD (ACHD) may have an **uncorrected** lesion or may have undergone a **reparative** or **palliative** procedure in the past. As the medical and surgical management of these conditions continues to evolve, different patients with the same original congenital defect may present having undergone significantly different procedures and, as a result, may differ in their anatomy and physiology. Transferring patient care to institutions with extensive experience in managing these disorders should be considered.

A. General considerations

1. A thorough understanding of the patient's **cardiac anatomy, physiology,** and **functional status** along with the **physiologic stresses** associated with the surgical procedure is essential.
2. **Myocardial dysfunction** may be present as a long-term consequence of the physiology of the original lesion or from the subsequent reparative or palliative procedure. It may also be a consequence of chronic hypoxemia.
3. **Dysrhythmias** are common and may be due to the pathophysiology of the cardiovascular defect or scarring from prior surgery. Intra-atrial reentrant tachycardia and ventricular tachycardia are commonly encountered in this patient population.
4. **Cyanotic patients** are often polycythemic and at risk for stroke and thrombosis. Intravenous hydration is important. Hemodilution may be considered in the instance of a preoperative hematocrit greater than 60%. **Abnormal hemostasis**, usually mild in severity, has been noted in patients with cyanotic CHD.
5. **Systemic air emboli** are a constant danger in the presence of bidirectional or right-to-left shunts. Intravenous lines must be purged of air bubbles, and air filters should be used.
6. **Infective endocarditis prophylaxis.** Some CHD patients require antibiotic prophylaxis for infective endocarditis with certain procedures. See Chapter 8: Infectious Diseases and Infection Control in Anesthesia.
7. A complete discussion of the specific lesions common in ACHD patients is beyond the scope of this chapter. For a more thorough treatment of the subject, please refer to the Suggested Readings.

X. CARDIAC TRANSPLANT PATIENT

Globally, more than 5500 cardiac transplants are performed each year. The 1-year survival rate is approximately 90%, and the 5-year survival rate is approximately 70%. These patients are increasingly encountered in the noncardiac surgical setting.

A. Physiology of the transplanted heart

1. Sympathetic reinnervation may occur over time. Parasympathetic reinnervation is not thought to occur; however, bradycardia related to the administration of neostigmine has been reported.
2. Transplanted hearts exhibit accelerated graft atherosclerosis and are at increased risk for myocardial ischemia.
3. **Hemodynamics of the transplanted heart**
   a. Cardiac impulse formation and conduction are normal, although the resting heart rate is increased to the range of 90 to 130 BPM.
   b. The Frank–Starling mechanism remains intact. Transplanted hearts respond normally to circulating catecholamines.
   c. Autoregulation of coronary blood flow is intact.
   d. Due to autonomic denervation, the transplanted heart meets the demand for increased cardiac output initially by increasing stroke volume and subsequently by increasing heart rate in response to circulating catecholamines.
4. **Drug effects**
   a. Drugs that act via the autonomic system (eg, atropine, and ephedrine) are ineffective.

b. Direct-acting agents are effective. Isoproterenol, dopamine, or epinephrine may be used to increase heart rate. Norepinephrine or phenylephrine may be used to increase blood pressure.
c. β-Adrenergic receptors are intact and may be present in increased density.
d. Traditional teaching dictates that anticholinesterases have no effect on the rate of a denervated heart; however, over time, other receptor-related mechanisms may take over and allow anticholinesterases to exert bradycardic effect. A muscarinic antagonist should always be co-administered to block the cardiac and other muscarinic side effects.

B. Anesthetic considerations
1. The patient's activity level and **exercise capacity** should be determined. A cardiology consultant may provide data concerning cardiac function and anatomy as measured by echocardiography and catheterization.
2. Underlying **CAD may be asymptomatic.** Evidence of ischemia may include a history of dyspnea, signs of reduced cardiac function, and dysrhythmias.
3. A baseline 12-lead ECG should be obtained and may demonstrate multiple P waves and right bundle branch block.
4. To assess the effect of immunosuppression and concomitant drug therapy, baseline laboratory studies should include complete blood count, serum electrolytes, blood urea nitrogen, serum creatinine, glucose, and liver function tests.
5. Strict aseptic technique is required for all interventions (eg, intravenous access), because the patient may be receiving long-term immunosuppression.
6. **Monitoring.** Invasive monitoring is used when indicated by the patient's cardiopulmonary status and the surgical procedure. The right internal jugular vein is often the access site for repetitive endocardial biopsies and may need to be reserved for this purpose.
7. **Anesthesia**
   a. General, regional, and spinal anesthesia have been administered to cardiac transplant patients. Selection of a specific anesthetic technique should be guided by considerations other than the patient's history of cardiac transplantation.
   b. Hemodynamic goals
   1. Maintain preload.
   2. Avoid sudden vasodilation. Initial compensatory changes in cardiac output depend on the Frank–Starling mechanism to increase stroke volume because of the delayed heart rate response.
   3. If sudden hypotension occurs, administer volume and direct-acting vasopressors such as phenylephrine and norepinephrine.

XI. CARDIAC IMPLANTABLE ELECTRONIC DEVICES: PACEMAKERS AND IMPLANTABLE CARDIOVERTER-DEFIBRILLATORS
A. CIEDs
1. Easing numbers of patients with permanent pacemaker (PPM) and ICD devices are undergoing noncardiac surgery. Familiarity with the indications, functions, and perioperative management of these devices is essential.
2. PPMs are utilized in a variety of conditions where the patient's native conduction is compromised or inadequate, including structural or ischemic heart disease, infiltrative diseases, and postprocedural alterations in conduction pathways, among many others.

3. ICDs have significantly improved the mortality of patients at high risk for sudden cardiac death. The four key ICD functions are **antitachycardia pacing** (ATP), **cardioversion**, **defibrillation**, and **backup pacing**. The conventional ICD is implanted in the upper chest and is connected to one or two defibrillating transvenous leads that also have sensing and pacing capabilities.
4. Current PPM and ICD devices include traditional subcutaneous generators with transvenous leads that have single- or dual-chamber sensing and pacing and possibly antitachycardia therapies (ie, cardioversion–defibrillation, ATP), as well as newer technologies including leadless pacemakers and subcutaneous ICDs (see below).
5. **Indications for PPM**
    a. Symptomatic bradycardia.
    b. Third-degree (complete) AV block.
    c. Type II, second-degree AV block.
    d. Cardiac resynchronization therapy. Biventricular pacing to synchronize RV and LV depolarization in patients with symptomatic HFrEF (left ventricular ejection fraction [LVEF] ≤35%) with sinus rhythm and interventricular conduction abnormality (left bundle branch block [LBBB], QRS ≥150 ms).
6. **Indications for ICD**
    a. **Primary prevention** in patients at high risk for sudden cardiac death (LVEF ≤35%, at risk for ventricular tachyarrhythmias).
    b. **Secondary prevention** in patients with prior sudden cardiac death or unstable ventricular arrhythmias.

B. Pacemaker nomenclature
1. A standard five-letter code is used to describe pacemaker settings and function. The first letter designates the **chamber paced** (O, none; A, atrium; V, ventricle; D, dual [both atrium and ventricle]).
2. The second letter describes the **chamber sensed** (O, none; A, atrium; V, ventricle; D, dual).
3. The third letter describes the **pacemaker's response** to sensed events (O, none; I, inhibition of pacemaker output; T, triggering of pacemaker output; D, dual response: spontaneous atrial and ventricular activity inhibit atrial and ventricular pacing and atrial activity triggers a ventricular response).
4. The fourth letter indicates the presence or absence of **rate modulation** (O, no rate modulation; R, rate modulation present).
5. The fifth letter specifies the presence and type of multisite **pacing** (O, none; A, more than one stimulation site in either atrium, stimulation sites in each atrium, or a combination of the two; V, more than one stimulation site in either ventricle, stimulation sites in each ventricle, or a combination of the two; D, any combination of A and V).
6. For example, a **VVI** pacemaker will sense and pace the ventricle yet will be inhibited and will not fire if an R wave is detected. A **DDD** pacemaker senses and paces both the atrium and ventricle. A VVIRV pacemaker has ventricular inhibitory pacing with rate modulation and multisite ventricular pacing. This mode is often used in patients with heart failure, chronic atrial fibrillation, or intraventricular conduction delay. A **DDDRD** pacemaker has dual-chamber pacing with rate modulation and multisite pacing in both the atrium (or atria) and ventricle(s).

C. Considerations for magnet application to CIEDs
1. **Applying a magnet to most pacemakers** (excluding leadless pacemakers) will cause them to function in an **asynchronous mode** (eg, VOO),

which may be desirable in the pacing-dependent patient undergoing a procedure with possible electromagnetic interference (EMI). However, **the magnet response of a pacemaker is most reliably determined by device interrogation.** The clinician should be aware of the pacemaker's type, current device settings, the patient's pacemaker dependence, and the device's default mode and rate when the magnet is in place. If used, the magnet should be placed directly over the pacemaker. It is best to tape the magnet in place to avoid inadvertent dislodgment. Typically, normal pacemaker function is restored upon removal of the magnet. **Magnet application should be used with caution,** as asynchronous pacing has the potential to cause unstable arrhythmias through the R-on-T phenomenon if ventricular pacing output occurs during the relative refractory period of cardiomyocyte repolarization.
2. All ICDs are exquisitely sensitive to EMI associated with electrocautery above the level of the umbilicus. EMI can be interpreted by an ICD as ventricular fibrillation leading to **inappropriate shocks.** Inappropriate shocks can be difficult to detect in an anesthetized and paralyzed patient and can lead to battery depletion.
3. Most ICDs are designed to **suspend antitachycardia therapies in response to a magnet** application and resume function upon removal of the magnet. Some models of St. Jude and Boston Scientific ICDs can be programmed to ignore magnet application. It is **best to have ICD function interrogated preoperatively** to determine its settings and response to magnet application.
4. **Indiscriminate use of magnets for ICDs is best avoided.** It is preferable to reprogram and disable antitachycardia therapies while taking steps to prepare for prompt treatment of any unstable arrhythmia as described below. Also, magnet application to ICDs **does not change pacing to an asynchronous mode**, and pacing-dependent patients should have the device reprogrammed to an asynchronous mode if indicated.

D. Leadless pacemakers
1. Leadless pacemakers, including the AVEIR (Abbott Medical) and the Micra (Medtronic) are beginning to have more widespread use. They are comprised of a small generator with contained sensing and pacing electrodes, which are **implanted (and removed) directly into the RV** via a femoral transcatheter approach. The battery life is approximately 8 to 12 years.
2. This system **eliminates the need for transvenous leads** and subcutaneous pockets, reducing risks of infection and lead-related problems, which can lead to perforation, venous occlusion, tricuspid regurgitation, oversensing, and infection. Major risks of the device itself include perforation, dislodgement and embolization, and tamponade.
3. The leadless system is designed predominantly for bradyarrhythmias with different models allowing for either single- or dual-chamber pacing modes. These devices are considered "MRI-conditional."
4. There are currently no consensus societal guidelines on the perioperative management of such devices, but the same general principles for other CIEDs described below should apply, with the following unique considerations:
    a. The Medtronic Micra leadless system does not have a Hall sensor; thus, it **cannot detect the presence of a magnet** and will not switch to an asynchronous mode if a magnet is applied. It **requires the use of the leadless programmer to change the settings** of the device.

b. The Abbott AVEIR **does respond to the presence of a magnet.** The magnet should be placed above the center of the heart, and it defaults to VOO at a rate from 85 to 100 BPM depending on the remaining battery life of the device.
   c. Therefore, consultation with a specialist with the knowledge, equipment, and ability to interrogate the device and reprogram it to an appropriate setting for the given clinical circumstance is necessary.
  5. Wireless ultrasound endocardial pacing, a system that involves a subcutaneous generator and endocardial receiver used with a traditional CIED, is another system that may be seen more in noncardiac surgery patients.
E. **Subcutaneous ICDs (S-ICDs)**
  1. New devices that include a subcutaneous generator implanted in the left lateral chest with a tunneled subcutaneous parasternal lead are available for patients with indications for an ICD who have inadequate vascular access, very high risk of infection, or for very young people with a long life expectancy. These devices avoid the complications associated with transvenous leads. S-ICDs have a battery life of approximately 7 years, can withstand external cardiopulmonary resuscitation (CPR), and can be implanted under monitored anesthesia care.
  2. Limitations include the absence of bradycardia pacing, ATP, or cardiac resynchronization therapies. Unlike traditional ICDs, the S-ICD does not contain any PPM functions except a 30-second backup pacing function immediately following a shock (VVI at 50 BPM). The generator is larger than traditional ICDs and delivers a higher-energy shock of 80 J. It is susceptible to the same oversensing problems from EMI as traditional ICDs, which could lead to inappropriate shocks.
  3. Currently available S-ICDs respond to external magnet application by temporarily suspending shock therapy while the magnet is applied, with resumption of the permanent settings on removal of the magnet. However, the lateral location of the device (midaxillary) and off-centered placement of the magnet may make magnet application more challenging than traditional anteriorly located ICD generators.
F. **Preoperative evaluation and preparation**
  1. Determine if a CIED is present by conducting a focused history and physical examination and reviewing any available imaging or cardiology reports.
  2. Determine the **type, manufacturer, primary indication, and if the patient is pacing dependent** (eg, prior AV nodal ablation, no spontaneous ventricular activity noted on prior interrogation, or concerning history such as syncope related to symptomatic bradycardia).
  3. Determine the **current device settings** and **status** (ie, properly functioning generator, leads if present, and battery life) by patient history, electrophysiology records, and ECG. Device interrogation is the only reliable method for determining the settings and battery function of the device.
  4. If the information is not readily available, the manufacturer and model number may be obtained from a radiograph of the generator. The manufacturer of the device must be identified in order to be able to program the pacemaker, as each manufacturer has a unique programming device. Determine whether rate modulation is active. Also, determine the response of the device to a magnet.
  5. Determine if EMI is likely (sources include: monopolar electrosurgery or radiofrequency ablation superior to the umbilicus, transcutaneous

electrical nerve stimulation, lithotripsy, magnetic resonance, radiofrequency identification devices, and electroconvulsive therapy [ECT]).
  a. If EMI is likely, reprogram to asynchronous pacing in patients who are pacing dependent, and suspend any antitachycardia therapies if an ICD is present. Rate-responsive mode should also be disabled to prevent inappropriate tachycardia.
  b. Continuously monitor the patient and ensure that temporary backup pacing and/or defibrillating methods are immediately available.

G. Intraoperative management
  1. Modern pacemakers are extremely resistant to EMI. If interference does occur, the pacemaker output may be inappropriately inhibited or the pacemaker may be reset to a committed pacing mode (ie, DOO or VOO).
  2. **Resetting of pacemakers** by EMI will produce asynchronous pacing that can be noted on the ECG.
  3. Intraoperative exposure of the device to EMI can be reduced by placing the current return pad (**"grounding pad"**) in a location on the patient such that the **current path** from the electrocautery or radiofrequency ablation catheter **does not pass near the pulse generator or leads.** Other measures include the use of **short, intermittent, irregular bursts** at the lowest possible energy level and the use of a **bipolar electrocautery** system or an **ultrasonic (harmonic) scalpel.** During lithotripsy, the beam should not be focused near the generator.
  4. **Monitor heart rate** during EMI with a pulse oximeter, arterial line, precordial or esophageal stethoscope, or a finger on the pulse.
  5. For procedures or diagnostic **tests involving MRI**, it is essential to **follow institutional protocols**, and in the event that an external defibrillator, device programmer, or any other MRI unsafe equipment is necessary, the **patient should be removed from the MRI area prior to use of these devices.**
  6. Prior to any MRI scan in patients with MRI conditional devices, the device should be interrogated as described above, antitachycardia therapies should be suspended, and asynchronous pacing should be activated in pacing-dependent patients.
  7. **Avoid using radiofrequency identification devices** in close proximity to CIEDs and ensure continuous monitoring for signs of EMI to allow for prompt discontinuation if interference is noted.
  8. For **ECT**, take the same considerations as above including suspending antitachycardia therapies and switching to an asynchronous mode in pacing-dependent patients, while being prepared to promptly manage any sinus tachycardia or ventricular arrhythmias that can be associated with ECT.
  9. **Postoperative evaluation of pacemaker function** is recommended by most manufacturers if electrocautery is used or if settings are changed perioperatively.

H. Temporary perioperative pacing and cardioversion–defibrillation options
  1. **Transcutaneous.** External pacing and cardioversion–defibrillation can be performed via large pads placed on the anterior and posterior thorax. This is an easy and inexpensive method of ventricular pacing and antitachycardia therapy. Avoid placing pads directly over subcutaneous generators.
  2. **Transvenous**
     a. A temporary pacing electrode can be inserted via a central vein into the heart.

b. Various pulmonary artery catheters with pacing options exist (see Chapter 15: Monitoring).
   3. Transesophageal. The LA can be paced with a pacing probe placed in the esophagus. Transesophageal pacing requires intact AV nodal conduction.
I. Emergency external cardioversion or defibrillation
   1. If unstable arrhythmias occur and a magnet is being used to disable antitachycardia therapies of an ICD, immediate steps should be taken to terminate the source of EMI and remove the magnet from the ICD, which should resume antitachycardia therapies usually within 10 seconds.
   2. If after removal of the magnet, there is no prompt restoration of antitachycardia therapies with appropriate response to any arrhythmia, or if the antitachycardia therapies were suspended by device interrogation preoperatively, advanced cardiac life support (ACLS) guidelines including external defibrillation should be followed.
   a. If possible, avoid placing pads directly over the generator to minimize current flow through the generator and the leads.
   b. Use the clinically appropriate energy level regardless of the presence of a CIED.
   c. Any device should be immediately interrogated after external cardioversion/defibrillation, as device reset or malfunction is possible after external electrical therapy.
J. Postoperative management
   1. Ongoing monitoring of rate and rhythm with ECG and pulse oximetry should continue in the immediate postoperative period.
   2. If the device was reprogrammed periprocedurally, ensure that backup pacing and cardioversion–defibrillation methods are readily available if indicated until permanent settings are restored.
   3. Have the device interrogated immediately if there is any concern for inappropriate or unreliable device settings or function (eg, emergency surgery without thorough preoperative evaluation, concern for disabled rather than suspended antitachycardia therapy from magnet application in an older device, observed or suspected shocks from device intraoperatively, or any concern for malfunction from EMI, physical disruption, or large fluid shifts).

ACKNOWLEDGMENTS

We gratefully acknowledge the contributions of previous edition authors, Adam A. Dalia and Casey Hamilton, as portions of those chapters have been retained in this revision.

Suggested Readings

Al-Khatib SM, Stevenson WG, Ackerman MJ, et al. 2017 AHA/ACC/HRS guideline for management of patients with ventricular arrhythmias and the prevention of sudden cardiac death: a report of the American College of Cardiology/American Heart Association Task Force on clinical practice guidelines and the Heart Rhythm Society. *Circulation.* 2018;138:e272-e391.

American Society of Anesthesiologists. Practice advisory for the perioperative management of patients with cardiac implantable electronic devices: pacemakers and implantable cardioverter–defibrillators 2020: an updated report by the American Society of Anesthesiologists Task Force on perioperative management of patients with cardiac implantable electronic devices. *Anesthesiology.* 2020;132(2):225-252.

Blasco LM, Parameshwar J, Vuylsteke A. Anaesthesia for noncardiac surgery in the heart transplant recipient. *Curr Opin Anaesthesiol.* 2009;22:109-113.

Cardiac implantable electronic device management [corrected]. *Anesthesiology.* 2020;132(2): 225–252.

Dalia AA, Cronin B, Stone ME, et al. Anesthetic management of patients with continuous-flow left ventricular assist devices undergoing noncardiac surgery: an update for anesthesiologists. *J Cardiothorac Vasc Anesth.* 2018;32(2):1001–1012.

Devereaux PJ, Mrkobrada M, Sessler D, et al; POISE-2 Investigators. Aspirin in patients undergoing noncardiac surgery. *N Engl J Med.* 2014;370:1494–1503.

Epstein AE, DiMarco JP, Ellenbogen KA, et al; American College of Cardiology Foundation; American Heart Association Task Force on Practice Guidelines; Heart Rhythm Society. 2012 ACCF/AHA/HRS focused update incorporated into the ACCF/AHA/HRS 2008 guidelines for device-based therapy of cardiac rhythm abnormalities: a report of the American College of Cardiology Foundation/American Heart Association Task Force on Practice Guidelines and the Heart Rhythm Society. *J Am Coll Cardiol.* 2013;61:e6–e75.

Fleisher LA, Fleishmann KE, Auerbach AD, et al; American College of Cardiology; American Heart Association. 2014 ACC/AHA guideline on perioperative cardiovascular evaluation and management of patients undergoing noncardiac surgery: a report of the American College of Cardiology/American Heart Association Task Force on practice guidelines. *J Am Coll Cardiol.* 2014;64(22):e77–e137.

Hawn MT, Graham LA, Richman JR, et al. The incidence and timing of noncardiac surgery after cardiac stent implantation. *J Am Coll Surg.* 2012;214:658–666.

Hindler K, Shaw AD, Samuels J, Fulton S, Collard CD, Riedel B. Improved postoperative outcomes associated with preoperative statin therapy. *Anesthesiology.* 2006;105:1260–1272.

Kertai MD. Preoperative coronary revascularization in high-risk patients undergoing vascular surgery: a core review. *Anesth Analg.* 2008;106:751–758.

Lei Lei E, Heggie J. Adult congenital heart disease and anesthesia: an educational review. *Paediatr Anaesth.* 2021;31(2):123–131.

Levine GN, Bates ER, Bittl JA, et al. 2016 ACC/AHA guideline focused update on duration of dual antiplatelet therapy in patients with coronary artery disease: a report of the American College of Cardiology/American Heart Association Task Force on clinical practice guidelines. *J Am Coll Cardiol.* 2016;68:1082–1115.

Lloyd-Jones DM, Allen NB, Anderson CAM, et al; American Heart Association. Life's Essential 8: updating and enhancing the American Heart Association's construct of cardiovascular health: a presidential advisory from the American Heart Association. *Circulation.* 2022;146:e18–e43.

Mahmoud KD, Sanon S, Habermann EB, et al. Perioperative cardiovascular risk of prior coronary stent implantation among patients undergoing noncardiac surgery. *J Am Coll Cardiol.* 2016;67:1038–1049.

Otto CM, Nishimura RA, Bonow RO, et al. 2020 ACC/AHA guideline for the management of patients with valvular heart disease: a report of the American College of Cardiology/American Heart Association Joint Committee on clinical practice guidelines. *Circulation.* 2021;143(5):e72–e227.

POISE Study Group; Devereaux PJ, Yang H, Yusuf S, et al. Effects of extended-release metoprolol succinate in patients undergoing non-cardiac surgery (POISE trial): a randomised controlled trial. *Lancet.* 2008;371:1839–1847.

Stout KK, Daniels CJ, Aboulhosn JA, et al. 2018 AHA/ACC guideline for the management of adults with congenital heart disease: a report of the American College of Cardiology/American Heart Association Task Force on clinical practice guidelines. *J Am Coll Cardiol.* 2019;73:e81–e192.

Thomas H, Plummer C, Wright IJ, Foley P, Turley AJ. Guidelines for the peri-operative management of people with cardiac implantable electronic devices: guidelines from the British Heart Rhythm Society. *Anaesthesia.* 2022;77(7):808–817.

Vouliotis AI, Roberts PR, Dilaveris P, Gatzoulis K, Yue A, Tsioufis K. Leadless pacemakers: current achievements and future perspectives. *Eur Cardiol.* 2023;18:e49.

Wijeysundera DN, Duncan D, Nkonde-price C, et al; ACC/AHA Task Force Members. Perioperative beta blockade in noncardiac surgery. A systematic review for the 2014 ACC/AHA guideline on perioperative cardiovascular evaluation and management of patients undergoing noncardiac surgery: a report of the American College of Cardiology/American Heart Association Task Force on Practice Guidelines. *Circulation.* 2014;130(24):2246–2264.

Wolff G, Navarese EP, Brockmeyer M, et al. Perioperative aspirin therapy in non-cardiac surgery: a systematic review and meta-analysis of randomized controlled trials. *Int J Cardiol.* 2018;258:59–67.

Specific Considerations With Pulmonary Disease

Benjamin M. Weaver and Timothy G. Gaulton

I. OVERVIEW
The focus of this chapter is on lung physiology and its interaction with anesthesia. Important concepts related to the care of patients at high risk of postoperative pulmonary complications including obesity, asthma, chronic obstructive pulmonary disease (COPD), and acute respiratory distress syndrome (ARDS) are described.

II. PULMONARY FUNCTION
Anesthetics and associated surgical procedures impair pulmonary function through direct impact on the lungs and indirect action on associated systems.

A. Alveolar ventilation decreases with exposure to volatile inhaled anesthetics, opiates, and intravenous sedatives in a dose-dependent manner through the disruption of different aspects of ventilatory control and ventilation-perfusion (V/Q) mismatch. Volatile anesthetics reduce tidal volumes (Vt) at concentrations greater than 1 minimum alveolar concentration (MAC) yet can stimulate respiratory centers and preserve respiratory drive. Propofol and barbiturates decrease Vt and respiratory drive in a dose dependent manner. Ketamine, etomidate, and dexmedetomidine cause less pronounced effects on respiratory drive and muscle tone, however, concurrent use of other sedatives and anesthetic drugs can result in clinically significant respiratory depression. Opiates reduce respiratory rate and increase tidal volume variability.

B. Functional residual capacity (FRC) universally decreases with anesthetic administration. FRC is a critical determinant of oxygen reserves and the propensity for ventilator-induced lung injury. FRC decreases primarily due to an increase in external forces on the lung parenchyma and a decrease in respiratory muscle tone (eg, intercostal muscles). This results in lung collapse, or atelectasis. In the supine position, a greater amount of pressure is transmitted from the abdomen to the thorax and the diaphragm shifts cephalad. FRC can decrease by more than one-third in the supine position. The decrease in respiratory muscle tone from anesthetics and/or neuromuscular blocking agents decreases the overall cross-sectional area of the chest wall and further contributes to decreased FRC. Dependent parts of the lung are the most susceptible to collapse. As the lung is tethered together in a network of bronchioles and alveoli, lung collapse compresses adjacent small airways and further impairs gas-exchange. Conditions that decrease the airway tone (eg, COPD, older age) or increase external pressure (eg, obesity) increase the risk of airway collapse. Restoring FRC is feasible through application of positive end-expiratory pressure (PEEP) in spontaneous and controlled breathing, recruitment maneuvers, and upright positioning. In some cases, FRC can be increased through prone positioning.

C. Gas exchange

Anesthesia increases V/Q mismatch across the lung. Shunt, or the absence of ventilation, is the primary type of mismatch resulting from atelectasis and reduces arterial oxygenation. Dead-space, or the absence of perfusion, also occurs under anesthesia due to the addition of instrumental dead space (eg, tracheal tube, heat and moisture exchanger), disruption of global (eg, decreased cardiac output) or local (eg, pulmonary thrombus, venous air emboli) perfusion, or alveolar overdistention (eg, excessive PEEP). In response to decreases in alveolar oxygen content, the pulmonary vasculature vasoconstricts, termed hypoxic pulmonary vasoconstriction (HPV), and diverts blood flow away from alveoli with reduced or absent ventilation. Anesthetic gases inhibit HPV, while intravenous anesthetics have a less pronounced effect. Antihypertensive drugs (eg, sodium nitroprusside, nitroglycerin, nicardipine) cause nonselective pulmonary vasodilation and may worsen shunt in the presence of atelectasis.

D. Respiratory reflexes
1. Minute ventilation increases linearly with arterial carbon dioxide content (P_aCO_2). Inhaled and intravenous anesthetics diminish this ventilatory response to hypercapnia and hypoxemia in a dose-dependent manner by decreasing the sensitivity of chemoreceptors at the carotid and aortic bodies. Opiates result in a right-shift of the P_aCO_2–ventilation response curve and a higher resting P_aCO_2.
2. Volatile anesthetics reduce airway resistance through bronchodilation and are a treatment for refractory cases of reactive airway disease in the intensive care unit. Pungent volatile agents (eg, desflurane, isoflurane) can result in increased airway irritability, breath-holding, and coughing when administered during spontaneous breathing. They should be avoided for inhalational inductions due to the risk of laryngospasm and bronchospasm. At high doses, desflurane can increase airway tone.
3. Intravenous anesthetics, especially propofol and ketamine blunt airway reflex bronchoconstriction, although to a lesser degree than volatile anesthetics. Upper airway reflexes are also reduced, facilitating laryngoscopy when used for induction but increase the risk of upper airway obstruction and aspiration.

E. Ciliary function. Volatile anesthetics and nitrous oxide reduce ciliary beat frequency, slowing the rate of mucous clearance from the airways. Likewise, barbiturates, dexmedetomidine, and benzodiazepines reduce ciliary beat frequency. In contrast propofol and ketamine can stimulate this process. Data examining the effect of opioids on ciliary beat frequency is conflicted. During mechanical ventilation, nonhumidified gasses are often delivered at high flow rates that dry secretions and damage the respiratory epithelium. Artificial airways bypass the nasopharynx that plays a critical role in airway humidification. Passive humidification can occur with use of a heat and moisture exchanger.

F. Coughing. Effective coughing for airway clearance requires adequate inspiratory and forced expiratory effort and the engagement of accessory muscles. Certain procedures (abdominal, thoracic, and spine surgeries) restrict adequate coughing due to splinting from pain. In high-risk patients, ineffective coughing leads to further atelectasis and mucous plugging. Strategies to provide adequate analgesia and avoid oversedation, including regional and neuraxial techniques, should be used when possible. Respiratory devices such as incentive spirometry or positive expiratory pressure devices can augment effort in inspiration yet require patient compliance and coordination.

III. EFFECTS FROM SURGICAL PROCEDURE
A. Pneumoperitoneum during laparoscopy changes the conformation of the chest wall and decreases chest wall compliance. Lung compliance is

mostly unaltered apart from the separate effects of body position and body weight.
- **B. Trendelenburg position.** A head-down position at 15° or more is often required for laparoscopic surgery. Trendelenburg positioning augments the pressure transmitted from the abdomen on the thorax. End-expiratory lung volume is further decreased in this position.
- **C. Acute acidosis** can transiently and profoundly increase pulmonary artery pressures resulting in acute right heart strain. Special care should be taken to support patient hemodynamics in circumstances where acute acidemia is expected (eg, release of cross clamp or tourniquet).
- **D. Prone positioning** can increase ventilation to dorsal lung regions, especially in patients with obesity. Respiratory system compliance does not change due to a decrease in chest wall compliance. Application PEEP (>5 cmH_2O) can shift perfusion away from dorsal lung regions and increase V/Q mismatch.

IV. ASTHMA

- **A. Background.** Asthma is a chronic and heterogeneous inflammatory disease characterized by bronchial hyperresponsiveness. Asthma affects more than 300 million people worldwide. A common endotype of asthma involves eosinophilic inflammation associated with Th2 response that responds to inhaled steroids. Other endotypes, including late-onset asthma, are less responsive to immunomodulating therapies and are associated with obesity and female sex.
- **B. Perioperative considerations**
  1. Standard asthma treatment includes the use of inhaled long-acting muscarinic antagonists (LAMAs), and long-acting beta agonists (LABAs). Severe asthma can often be recognized by treatment regimens that include anti-IgE (omalizumab) utilized in patients with persistent asthma on high-dose inhaled corticosteroids (ICS), anti-IL-5 (mepolizumab and reslizumab) for persistent eosinophilic asthma, and treatment with ICS in combination with LABAs.
  2. Preoperative assessment should include a review of recent asthma exacerbations, ongoing viral illnesses, recent increases in rescue inhaler use, any oral steroid use, overall functional capacity, a review of cardiopulmonary symptoms, and lung auscultation. Delaying elective procedures should be considered if a patient has an ongoing exacerbation/infection given their high potential for postoperative complications. Perioperative management should be discussed with a pulmonologist for severe cases of asthma.
  3. Asthma medications should be continued through the perioperative period.
  4. Bronchospasm occurs in about 9% of asthmatics undergoing anesthesia and is often related to an inadequate depth of anesthesia during stimulation (eg, intubation, surgical incision). Management of bronchospasm involves pharmacologic augmentation of bronchodilation through inhaled or intravenous beta-agonists (albuterol, epinephrine), inhaled anti-cholinergics, anesthetics (inhaled agents, ketamine, propofol), and other bronchodilators (magnesium).

V. CHRONIC OBSTRUCTIVE PULMONARY DISEASE

- **A. Background.** COPD is a leading cause of death worldwide and is associated with exposure to tobacco, biomass, and pollution. Major symptoms of COPD include dyspnea, cough, and/or sputum production. COPD is associated with an increased risk of invasive mechanical ventilation in the postoperative setting. The severity of COPD can be categorized by the Global Initiative for Chronic Obstructive Lung Disease (GOLD) criteria, involving symptom burden, exacerbation history, and forced expiratory volume (FEV_1).

B. Perioperative Considerations
1. Patients should continue their inhalers on the day of surgery. As with asthmatic patients, pulmonary symptoms (eg, dyspnea), frequency of rescue inhaler use, and recent exacerbations and steroid use need to be assessed. In patients with severe COPD, right heart function via transthoracic echocardiography should be evaluated prior to surgery, as right heart dysfunction and pulmonary hypertension (PH) significantly increases postoperative risk and is more prevalent in this patient population.
2. Patients with COPD are at risk of developing intrinsic PEEP (iPEEP) due to prolonged respiratory time and airway collapse. iPEEP occurs when alveoli incompletely empty at the end of exhalation, resulting in alveolar overdistention and an increase in airway pressure. iPEEP is difficult to quantify on anesthesia ventilators but is likely present when the expiratory flow-time tracing does not return to zero prior to inspiration.
3. iPEEP can be minimized by prolonging expiration (eg, reducing respiratory rate or set expiratory time) and avoiding large Vt and PEEP that increase lung volume beyond FRC. During assisted ventilation, iPEEP increases work of breathing and ventilator asynchrony. Application of external PEEP can reduce the work required to initiate a breath yet should not exceed iPEEP, otherwise overdistention will occur.
4. In patients with evidence of chronic hypercarbia (severe COPD, elevated serum bicarbonate), minute ventilation should not be adjusted to maintain a normal end-tidal CO_2.
5. Patients with COPD may require supplemental oxygen after surgery. In high-risk patients or in the event of postoperative respiratory insufficiency, noninvasive ventilation should be applied as first line therapy provided patient effort and mental status allow. High-flow nasal cannula is as an alternative therapy to decrease the work of breathing and increase alveolar ventilation. Narcotics should be used with caution.

VI. OBESITY

A. Background. Obesity is chronic condition characterized by excess adipose tissue and is associated with several comorbid conditions including diabetes, obstructive sleep apnea, and hypertension. Obesity is commonly defined by a body mass index (BMI) ≥ 30 kg/m^2. Severe obesity is defined by a BMI ≥ 40 kg/m^2. Obesity impairs respiratory function and increases risk of postoperative complications.

B. Respiratory pathophysiology
1. Excess adipose tissue results in compression of the lung parenchyma and upper airway obstruction resulting in a restrictive pattern of pulmonary pathology
2. Respiratory pathology in a patient with obesity is further characterized by:
   a. elevated pleural/intrathoracic pressures
   b. reduced FRC
   c. atelectasis and shunting
   d. small airway closure, air trapping, and iPEEP
   e. increased work of breathing
   f. obstructive apnea

C. Preoperative evaluation

1. Complications are increased in patients with truncal (central) rather than peripheral adiposity. Truncal adiposity has a more direct effect on the lung parenchyma and is associated with metabolic dysfunction.
2. Patients should be screened for the presence of obstructive sleep apnea (OSA) as it is highly co-prevalent and often underdiagnosed in patients with obesity. Patients with OSA who use continuous positive airway pressure (CPAP) at home should continue this therapy during the perioperative period. Always consider that the obese patient may have sleep-disordered breathing (Chapter 1: Evaluating the Patient Before Anesthesia).
3. Airway examination and history of previous airway management are important to evaluate risk of difficult intubation and/or mask ventilation.
4. Thorough cardiopulmonary assessment is important to assess perioperative risk in patients with obesity. Signs that may indicate an increased risk include:
   a. Baseline SpO_2 with arterial blood gas analysis if SpO_2 <95% on room air.
   b. Evidence of daytime hypercarbia (eg, elevated serum bicarbonate on basic metabolic panel) suggesting obesity hypoventilation syndrome
   c. Decreased functional capacity

D. Intraoperative considerations

1. **Airway.** The risk of difficult mask ventilation is elevated in obese patients. Due to a decreased FRC, oxygen desaturation can be rapid with the induction of anesthesia. Considerations for prevention of hypoxemia include:
   a. Ensuring complete denitrogenation with 100% FIO_2 administration.
   b. Applying CPAP during preoxygenation to increase end-expiratory lung volume. For patients with known OSA, CPAP should be applied at their home pressures level if known. If the pressure level is not known or there is no diagnosis of OSA, at least 10 cmH_2O should be applied to prevent lung collapse. For patients undergoing intubation in the intensive care unit who are unable to tolerate CPAP, high flow nasal cannula (HFNC) is better tolerated and will provide low amounts of PEEP and extend the time until desaturation.
   c. Positioning the patient with their head elevated (>30°) and off their chest will optimize positioning for laryngoscopy while increasing FRC. Reverse Trendelenburg combined with a back-up position on the bed can be used to facilitate a ramping position where the auditory meatus is in line with the sternal notch.

E. Maintenance of anesthesia

1. **Pharmacology.** Obesity may alter the pharmacokinetics of anesthetic drugs. Optimal methods for weight-based dosing in obesity are unclear and vary by drug class. Patients with obesity should be monitored closely throughout the perioperative period and drugs that decrease respiratory drive (eg, opiates) should be titrated carefully. Administration of large doses based on total body weight in patients with obesity can be dangerous. To mitigate risk, the following can be considered:
   a. The use of intraoperative depth of anesthesia monitoring is recommended, particularly when total intravenous anesthesia is administered.
   b. Assessment of neuromuscular blockade by train-of-four monitoring, preferably acceleromyography, is essential for the maintenance of adequate depth of paralysis and its complete reversal prior to emergence.

c. The use of maintenance anesthetics that have low fat-blood solubility coefficients (sevoflurane, desflurane) and are less lipophilic will facilitate quicker emergence.
d. The administration of long-acting opioids should be limited, and ideally spared. If used, patients should be monitored postoperatively with pulse oximetry and capnography.

2. Mechanical ventilation
a. Patients with obesity are more susceptible to lung and small airway collapse during mechanical ventilation due to increased transpulmonary pressures.
b. The mass load on the lungs from truncal adipose tissue requires high levels of counteracting airway pressure throughout the respiratory cycle to prevent lung collapse. Patients with obesity are less prone to alveolar overdistention, even when high airway pressure and recruitment maneuvers are applied, due to elevations in pleural pressure.

c. Ventilator settings
1. Either pressure (PCV)- or volume (VCV)-controlled modes can be used during controlled ventilation. With PCV, the inspiratory pressure needs to be set sufficiently high to overcome airway collapse, otherwise, inadequate alveolar ventilation can occur and plateau/driving pressures will be overestimated.
2. Patients with obesity benefit from ventilatory approaches that maintain end-expiratory lung-volume and prevent lung collapse. For most patients with mild to moderate obesity, a PEEP of 6 to 8 cmH_2O is appropriate.
3. In patients with severe obesity, higher levels PEEP and recruitment maneuvers may be required. A recruitment maneuver, or transient increase in mean airway pressure, should be applied prior to PEEP titration, targeting a plateau pressure up to 50 cmH_2O. Recruitment maneuvers can help to restore FRC.
4. Patients with obesity may benefit from advanced respiratory monitoring. Pleural pressure can be estimated using an esophageal pressure catheter. PEEP can be titrated to maintain a transpulmonary pressure (PEEP – end-expiratory esophageal pressure) of 0 to +2 cmH_2O.
5. Electrical impedance tomography (EIT) is a noninvasive, radiation-free imaging technique that measures regional ventilation based on variation in the electrical conductivity of the thorax. EIT can measure regional lung collapse and overdistention and may be a useful tool for PEEP titration.

F. Emergence. Multiple factors can be manipulated to optimize emergence. Extubation should occur with the patient in upright position to maximize FRC. For patients with severe obesity, CPAP should be administered after extubation. CPAP can be applied via a portable ventilator or a Boussignac mask. CPAP should be continued in the postanesthesia care unit until the patient is fully awake. Patients should be closely monitored after extubation and narcotics should be administered sparingly given the increased risk for postoperative respiratory depression.

VII. ACUTE RESPIRATORY DISTRESS SYNDROME
A. Background. ARDS represents a sudden and diffuse injury to the lungs that results in profound hypoxemia. Several conditions predispose patients to ARDS (**Table 4.1**). ARDS is defined by pulmonary imaging, acuity, risk factors, and hypoxemia severity (**Table 4.2**). Hypoxemia can be defined by

TABLE 4.1 Direct and Indirect Conditions That Place Patients at Risk of Developing ARDS

Conditions Precipitating ARDS

Direct	Indirect
• Pneumonia (bacterial, viral, mycobacterial, fungal, parasitic) • Aspiration pneumonitis • Pulmonary contusion • Inhalational injury • Near drowning	• Nonthoracic trauma • Pancreatitis • Burns • Transfusion-associated lung injury • Hematopoietic stem cell transplant • Cardiopulmonary bypass • Reperfusion injury after lung transplant or embolectomy • Medications (chemotherapy, amiodarone, radiation) • Immunologic response to viruses (COVID-19)

ARDS, acute respiratory distress syndrome.

the partial pressure of oxygen (PaO_2) or oxygen saturation (SpO_2), which is valuable in resource-limited settings. The diagnosis of ARDS is often missed, however, and associated with high mortality.

B. Preoperative considerations

1. Patients with ARDS or who are at risk of ARDS (eg, trauma, pancreatitis, sepsis) may require surgery before pulmonary function can be optimized. Many patients with ARDS require high levels of PEEP to maintain FRC. Care should be taken when transferring between transport ventilators and ICU/operating room ventilators to avoid the loss of PEEP. A clamp can be placed on the tracheal tube to prevent loss of pressure during circuit disconnection.

TABLE 4.2 Clinical Diagnosis and Severity Grading Criteria for ARDS

Criteria for ARDS

Risk factors and origin of edema	Precipitated by an acute predisposing risk factor. Hypoxemia is not primarily attributable to cardiogenic pulmonary edema or atelectasis			
Timing	New/worsening respiratory symptoms within 1 week of a known clinical insult			
Chest imaging	Bilateral opacities on imaging (not fully explained by effusions, lobar/lung collapse, nodules)			
	Nonintubated ARDS	**Intubated ARDS (PEEP of 5 cmH$_2$O)**		
		Mild	Moderate	Severe
Oxygenation	P:F < 300 on HFNC or CPAP/NIV with 5 cmH$_2$O of PEEP	200 < P:F ≤ 300	100 < P:F ≤ 200	P:F ≤ 100

ARDS, acute respiratory distress syndrome; CPAP, continuous positive airway pressure; NIV, Noninvasive ventilation; PEEP, positive end-expiratory pressure.

2. Close communication with the ICU team and respiratory therapist should occur prior to the OR. Information on respiratory mechanics, current ventilator settings, use of adjunct therapies, and patient trajectory should be defined to allow for adequate preparation.
C. Intraoperative considerations
1. **Lung protective ventilation** is a priority in ARDS. Ventilation should be set to limit the stress and strain applied to the lung. As with patients with severe obesity, consideration should be given to advanced respiratory monitoring (eg, esophageal pressure, EIT) in the OR. Anesthesia ventilators often overestimate plateau pressures as the inspiratory pause is not long enough to allow for static conditions. The following are techniques to limit further lung injury:
   a. Vt of 6 to 8 mL/kg based on predicted body weight (PBW) rather than actual weight should be used to minimize ventilator-induced lung injury. Vt should be adjusted to achieve a plateau pressure of <30 cmH$_2$O and driving pressure (Pplat-PEEP) <15 cmH$_2$O.
   b. Respiratory rate with goal <35 breaths/min to maintain adequate minute ventilation. Attention should be paid to avoid excessive air trapping and high airway pressures at high respiratory rates.
   c. Elevated P$_a$CO$_2$ may be tolerated to limit ventilator induced lung injury
   d. FIO_2 should be minimized to keep SpO$_2$ 90% to 95%. Hyperoxia can cause increased oxidative stress with sequelae of endothelial inflammation, mitochondrial dysfunction, and direct lung injury.
   e. PEEP should be adjusted to minimize lung collapse. Patients with moderate to severe ARDS may require high PEEP (12 to 15 cmH$_2$O). Overdistention with increased PEEP even with lung-protective plateau pressures can increase intrathoracic pressure and reduce cardiac output.
   f. There is no benefit of PCV versus VCV in ARDS. Measures of lung protection (plateau pressure, driving pressure, respiratory system compliance) can be measured in VCV through the addition of a brief (0.2 to 1 s) end-inspiratory pause.
2. The treatment of severe hypoxemia includes recruitment maneuvers and inhaled pulmonary vasodilators (eg, nitric oxide). Prone positioning increases dorsal lung aeration yet may not be feasible depending on the type of surgery. In refractory cases of hypoxemia, extracorporeal membrane oxygenation (ECMO) is a potential bridge to recovery.
3. **Fluid management.** Fluid management strategies depend on the subphenotype of ARDS. ARDS characterized by high inflammatory levels, vasopressor use, and hypotension, such as in sepsis, may benefit from more liberal administration of fluid to maintain organ perfusion. Regardless, measures of perfusion must be followed closely as excessive fluid administration can worsen alveolar edema and oxygenation.
D. Postoperative considerations.
Transport of patients with severe hypoxemia from the OR to the ICU can be perilous. Use of a transport ventilator is preferred over ventilation via an Ambu Bag or Mapelson circuit. Communication of intraoperative events to the ICU team ensures adequate hand-off.

VIII. OTHER PULMONARY CONDITIONS
A. Pulmonary contusion is common in blunt thoracic trauma cases that present emergently to the OR. Imaging findings of pulmonary contusion may lag behind the clinical manifestations. Bedside lung ultrasound can be used to

evaluate evolving pulmonary injury more rapidly than imaging modalities such as CT or CXR with a high sensitivity and specificity. Disruption of the alveolar capillary endothelium leads to intraparenchymal and alveolar hemorrhage and/or edema, increasing the shunt fraction. The inflammatory response provoked can lead to ARDS.
- **B. Rib fractures** are a frequent complication of blunt force trauma. Splinting due to pain associated with rib fractures or pleuritic pain results in more atelectasis. Neuraxial techniques such as epidural, paravertebral, or erector spinae plane catheters improve pain control and respiratory effort while minimizing the sedating effects of opiates.
- **C. Pneumonia and pneumonitis** can result in inflammation and endothelial leak that result in impaired gas exchange. It can precipitate severe hypotension when combined with the decrease in systemic vascular resistance caused by IV and volatile anesthetic agents.
- **D. PH** is defined by elevated pulmonary arterial pressures (mean pulmonary artery pressure >20 mmHg). It is associated with right ventricular strain and failure and increases the risk of perioperative complications such as arrhythmias, hypotension, and hypoxemia. PH often coexists with other conditions (eg, COPD, left heart dysfunction). Careful preoperative assessment, anesthetic management including avoidance of hypotension and hypercarbia, maintenance of FRC, and use of inhaled pulmonary vasodilators, and postoperative monitoring are crucial to mitigate these risks.
- **E. Interstitial lung disease (ILD)** is a heterogeneous group of disorders characterized by reduced lung compliance and total lung capacity, predisposing patients to hypoxia and hypercarbia with anesthesia. Pulmonary function tests can clarify the type and severity of respiratory impairment.

ACKNOWLEDGMENTS

We gratefully acknowledge the contributions of previous edition authors, Riccardo Pinciroli, Jeanine P. Wiener-Kronish, and Rachel Steinhorn, as portions of those chapters have been retained in this revision.

Suggested Readings

Agustí A, Celli BR, Criner GJ, et al. Global initiative for chronic obstructive lung disease 2023 report: GOLD executive summary. *Am J Respir Crit Care Med.* 2023;207(7):819–837.

Amato MB, Meade MO, Slutsky AS, et al. Driving pressure and survival in the acute respiratory distress syndrome. *N Engl J Med.* 2015;372(8):747–755.

Barrot L, Asfar P, Mauny F, et al; LOCO2 Investigators and REVA Research Network. Liberal or conservative oxygen therapy for adult respiratory distress syndrome. *N Engl J Med.* 2020;382:999–1008.

Casthely PA, Lear S, Cottrell JE, Lear E. Intrapulmonary shunting during induced hypotension. *Anesth Analg.* 1982;61:231–235.

Castillo JR, Peters SP, Busse WW. Asthma exacerbations: pathogenesis, prevention and treatment. *J Allergy Clin Immunol Pract.* 2017;5:918–927.

De Santis Santiago R, Teggia Droghi M, Fumagalli J, et al; Lung Rescue Team Investigators. High pleural pressure prevents alveolar overdistension and hemodynamic collapse in acute respiratory distress syndrome with class III obesity. A clinical trial. *Am J Respir Crit Care Med.* 2021;203(5):575–584.

Del Sorbo L, Goligher EC, McAuley DF, et al. Mechanical ventilation in adults with acute respiratory distress syndrome. Summary of the experimental evidence for the clinical practice guideline. *Ann Am Thorac Soc.* 2017;14(suppl 4):S261–S270.

Evgenov OV, Liang Y, Jiange Y, Blair JL. Pulmonary pharmacology and inhaled anesthetics. In: Gropper M, Eriksson L, Fleisher L, Wiener-Kronish J, Cohen N, eds. *Millers Anesthesia.* 9th ed. Elsevier; 2020:541.

Famous KR, Delucchi K, Ware LB, et al. Acute respiratory distress syndrome subphenotypes respond differently to randomized fluid management strategy. *Am J Respir Crit Care Med.* 2017;195(3):331–338.

Futier E, Constantin JM, Pelosi P, et al. Noninvasive ventilation and alveolar recruitment maneuver improve respiratory function during and after intubation of morbidly obese patients: a randomized controlled study. *Anesthesiology.* 2011;114:1354–1363.

Gleason JM, Christian BR, Barton ED. Nasal cannula apneic oxygenation prevents desaturation during endotracheal intubation: an integrative literature review. *West J Emerg Med.* 2018;19(2):403–411.

Grieco DL, Anzellotti GM, Russo A, et al. Airway closure during surgical pneumoperitoneum in obese patients. *Anesthesiology.* 2019;131(1):58–73.

Hignett R, Fernando R, McGlennan A, et al. A randomized crossover study to determine the effect of a 30° head-up versus a supine position on the functional residual capacity of term parturients. *Anesth Analg.* 2011;113:1098–1102.

LaGrew JE, Olsen KR, Frantz A. Volatile anesthetic for treatment of respiratory failure from status asthmaticus requiring extracorporeal membrane oxygenation. *BMJ Case Rep.* 2020;13:e231507.

Lipson DA, Crim C, Criner GJ, et al. Reduction in all-cause mortality with fluticasone furoate/umeclidinium/vilanterol in COPD patients. *Am J Respir Crit Care Med.* 2020; 201:1508–1516.

Lumb AB. Pre-operative respiratory optimization: an expert review. *Anaesthesia.* 2019; 74(suppl 1):43–48.

Lumb AB, Slinger P. Hypoxic pulmonary vasoconstriction: physiology and anesthetic implications. *Anesthesiology.* 2015;122:932–946.

Lumb AB, White A. Breathing in the prone position in health and disease. *BJA Educ.* 2021;21(8):280–283.

Neligan PJ, Malhotra G, Fraser M, et al. Continuous positive airway pressure via the Boussignac system immediately after extubation improves lung function in morbidly obese patients with obstructive sleep apnea undergoing laparoscopic bariatric surgery. *Anesthesiology.* 2009;110(4):878–884.

Pandit JJ. Effect of low dose inhaled anaesthetic agents on the ventilatory response to carbon dioxide in humans: a quantitative review. *Anaesthesia.* 2005;60:461–469.

Robba C, Ball L, Pelosi P. Between hypoxia or hyperoxia: not perfect but more physiologic. *J Thorac Dis.* 2018;10(suppl 17):S2052–S2054.

Rothen HU, Sporre B, Engberg G, Wegenius G, Hedenstierna G. Airway closure, atelectasis and gas exchange during general anaesthesia. *Br J Anaesth.* 1998;81:681–686.

Saraswat V. Effects of anaesthesia techniques and drugs on pulmonary function. *Indian J Anaesth.* 2015;59(9):557–564.

Satoh D, Kurosawa S, Kirino W, et al. Impact of changes of positive end-expiratory pressure on functional residual capacity at low tidal volume ventilation during general anesthesia. *J Anesth.* 2012;26:664–669.

Soldati G, Testa A, Silva FR, Carbone L, Portale G, Silveri NG. Chest ultrasonography in lung contusion. *Chest.* 2006;130(2):533.

Specjalski K, Niedoszytko M. MicroRNAs: future biomarkers and targets of therapy in asthma? *Curr Opin Pulm Med.* 2020;26:285–292.

Vuyk J, Sitsen E, Reekers M. Intraveous anesthetics. In: Gropper M, Eriksson L, Fleisher L, Wiener-Kronish J, Cohen N, eds. *Millers Anesthesia.* 9th ed. Elsevier; 2020:664.

Writing Group for the Alveolar Recruitment for Acute Respiratory Distress Syndrome Trial (ART) Investigators; Cavalcanti AB, Suzumura ÉA, Laranjeira LN, et al. Effect of lung recruitment and titrated positive end-expiratory pressure (PEEP) vs low PEEP on mortality in patients with acute respiratory distress syndrome: a randomized clinical trial. *J Am Med Assoc.* 2017;318(14):1335–1345.

Zhan Q, Sun B, Liang L, et al. Early use of noninvasive positive pressure ventilation for acute lung injury: a multicenter randomized controlled trial. *Crit Care Med.* 2012;40:455–460.

Specific Considerations With Renal Disease

Katarina Ruscic and Neil Rens

I. GENERAL CONSIDERATIONS
Approximately 15% of the population has renal disease, with a trend toward increasing prevalence with age. Perioperative renal dysfunction complicates patient management and results in increased morbidity and mortality. Aside from optimizing intravascular volume status, there is no definite consensus on prophylaxis for the development of acute kidney injury (AKI).

II. PHYSIOLOGY
The kidneys regulate intravascular volume, osmolality, acid–base and electrolyte balance, produce hormones, and excrete the end products of metabolism and drugs.

A. Fluid regulation
1. The kidney plays an important role in fluid regulation via neurohumoral interactions as outlined below.
    a. **Renin–angiotensin–aldosterone system** (RAAS). The juxtaglomerular apparatus of the kidney secretes **renin** in response to renal hypoperfusion, decreased sodium chloride delivery to the distal nephron, and increased sympathetic activity. Renin cleaves angiotensinogen to form angiotensin I, which is then converted to angiotensin II by angiotensin-converting enzyme (ACE) in the lung and other tissues.
    b. **Angiotensin II** produces arteriolar vasoconstriction and stimulates aldosterone release.
    c. **Aldosterone** is a mineralocorticoid released by the adrenal cortex in response to angiotensin II, increased potassium levels, decreased sodium content, and adrenocorticotropic hormone. Aldosterone acts on the distal tubules to increase reabsorption of sodium in exchange for potassium and protons.
    d. **Antidiuretic hormone (ADH)**, also known as arginine vasopressin (AVP), is released by the posterior pituitary gland in response to increased osmolality, decreased extracellular volume, positive-pressure ventilation, and surgical stimuli, including pain. ADH increases the permeability of the collecting duct to water through insertion of aquaporin water channels. Thus, ADH conserves water and concentrates urine.
    e. **Atrial natriuretic peptide** is a hormone released from the atrial myocytes during atrial stretch and contributes to a natriuretic response largely by decreasing RAAS activity. The resultant increase in renal sodium and water excretion decreases blood volume.
    f. **Kinins** are converted from kininogens by kallikreins and are regulated by salt intake, renin release, and hormone levels. They cause vasodilatation and natriuresis.

B. Electrolyte balance
1. **Disorders of sodium homeostasis**
    a. **Hyponatremia.** Plasma sodium concentration less than 134 mEq/L.

1. **Clinical features** vary with the degree of hyponatremia and the rapidity of onset. Symptoms generally do not appear until the sodium concentration falls below 125 mEq/L.
   a. **Moderate hyponatremia or gradual onset.** Confusion, muscle cramps, lethargy, anorexia, and nausea.
   b. **Severe hyponatremia or rapid onset.** Seizures and coma.
2. **Treatment.** Generally, acute normalization of the serum [Na$^+$] is not necessary unless the patient has severe symptoms. **Correct no more than 8 mEq/L in the first 24 hours** until 120 mEq/L is reached to prevent complications from rapid correction (osmotic demyelination syndrome [formerly central pontine myelinolysis] and seizures). At this point, the patient should be out of danger, and the [Na$^+$] should be normalized slowly over a period of days. Treatment depends on the volume status of the patient. In some cases, desmopressin can be preemptively coadministered to slow the rate of [Na$^+$] rise, preventing unintended overcorrection.
   a. **Hypervolemic hyponatremia** due to renal failure, congestive heart failure, cirrhosis, pregnancy, transurethral resection of prostate/hysteroscopy syndrome, or nephrotic syndrome is treated by sodium and water restriction and possibly with diuresis.
   b. **Hypovolemic hyponatremia** from renal losses (diuretics, especially thiazides, renal tubular acidosis with bicarbonaturia, salt wasting nephropathy, mineralocorticoid deficiencies), gastrointestinal losses (vomiting, bowel obstruction, bowel preparations), or sweating is treated with normal saline. Renal versus nonrenal etiology can be determined by the urine sodium (>20 mmol/L if renal loss, or appropriately low if extrarenal). For severe hypovolemic hyponatremia, the [Na$^+$] may be partially corrected over 6 to 8 hours with 3.5% hypertonic saline. Hypertonic saline is dangerous in volume-expanded salt-retaining states such as congestive heart failure.
   c. **Normovolemic hyponatremia** from the syndrome of inappropriate ADH (most commonly from malignancy), hypothyroidism, drugs that impair renal water excretion, or water intoxication is treated by fluid restriction.
   d. **Pseudohyponatremia** from hyperglycemia, hyperlipidemia, or hyperproteinemia (multiple myeloma) should be ruled out to avoid mistreatment. Corrected [Na$^+$] = measured [Na$^+$] + (glucose − 100) × 0.024, where [Na$^+$] is in mEq/L and glucose is in mg/dL.
b. **Hypernatremia.** Plasma sodium concentration greater than 144 mEq/L. It is usually caused by impairment of thirst or the ability to obtain water. In inpatients, it can be seen after aggressive use of loop diuretics for several days.
   1. **Clinical features** vary with the degree of hypernatremia and rapidity of onset, ranging from tremulousness, weakness, irritability, and mental confusion to seizures and coma.
   2. **Treatment** depends on determining the volume status of the patient, treating the underlying cause, and correcting the potential water deficit. Rapid correction can induce cerebral edema (with the feared complication of uncal herniation), seizures, permanent neurologic damage, and death, though these are rare in the adult population. Plasma [Na$^+$] should be corrected at a

maximum rate of 0.5 mEq/L/h. The water deficit, if present, can be calculated as follows:

Volume to be replaced (L) = ($n \times$ body weight (kg))
$$\times [([Na^+] - 140)/140]$$

$n = 0.6$ for adult males
$n = 0.5$ for adult females, elderly females, and elderly males

- a. **Hypervolemic hypernatremia** occurs secondary to Na^+ overload from mineralocorticoid excess, dialysis with hypertonic solutions, or treatment with hypertonic saline or sodium bicarbonate ($NaHCO_3$). The excess total body Na^+ (ie, volume) may be removed by dialysis or with diuretic therapy, and the blood $[Na^+]$ is gently decreased with intravenous isotonic water such as 5% dextrose (D5W).
- b. **Hypovolemic hypernatremia** occurs secondary to water loss exceeding Na^+ loss (eg, diarrhea, vomiting, heat injury, and diuresis) or inadequate water intake (eg, impaired thirst mechanism and altered mental status). If **hemodynamic instability or evidence of hypoperfusion** is present, replenish volume with Lactated Ringer's solution (which has $[Na^+]$ 130 mEq/L). **After volume replenishment,** the remaining free water deficit can be replaced gently with D5W to decrease the $[Na^+]$.
- c. **Normovolemic hypernatremia** is typically the result of diabetes insipidus (central or nephrogenic). Other causes include increased mineralocorticoid (primary hyperaldosteronism), increased glucocorticoid, or ectopic ACTH. Therapy consists of treating the underlying etiology, correcting the free water deficit with D5W, and exogenous vasopressin in central diabetes insipidus.

2. **Disorders of potassium homeostasis**
  a. **Hypokalemia.** Plasma $[K^+]$ less than 3.5 mEq/L.
    1. Serum $[K^+]$ is a poor index of **total body potassium** stores as 98% of body potassium is located intracellularly. Thus, large total K^+ deficits may be present before causing a decrease in serum $[K^+]$.
    2. **Etiologies**
      a. **Total body K^+ deficit** due to $[K^+]$ losses
        i. **Gastrointestinal tract** (eg, vomiting, diarrhea, fistula, nasogastric suctioning, chronic malnutrition, or obstructed ileal loops).
        ii. **Kidney** (eg, diuretics, some antibiotics, mineralocorticoid and glucocorticoid excess, and some types of renal tubular acidosis). Magnesium depletion increases renal K^+ loss.
      b. **Shifts in distribution** of K^+ (extracellular to intracellular)
        i. Alkalosis (H^+ shifts to the extracellular fluid and K^+ moves intracellularly). Thus, rapid correction of acidosis, by hyperventilation or $NaHCO_3$ administration, may produce undesirable hypokalemia.
        ii. Insulin therapy.
        iii. Beta-2 agonists.
    3. **Clinical features** rarely appear unless $[K^+]$ is less than 3 mEq/L or the rate of decrease is rapid.
      a. **Signs** include weakness, augmentation of neuromuscular block, ileus, and disturbances of cardiac contractility.

b. Hypokalemia **increases excitability** and predisposes the patient to **arrhythmias**. Electrocardiographic (ECG) changes include flattened T waves, U waves, increased PR and QT intervals, ST segment depression, and atrial and ventricular dysrhythmias.

c. Serum [K$^+$] less than 2.0 mEq/L is associated with vasoconstriction and rhabdomyolysis.

4. **Treatment.** Rapid replacement of K$^+$ may cause more problems than hypokalemia. There is some evidence that there is no need to correct chronic hypokalemia ([K$^+$] ≥2.5 mEq/L) before induction of anesthesia.

b. **Hyperkalemia.** Plasma [K$^+$] >5.5 mEq/L.
  1. **Etiologies**
     a. **Decreased excretion** (eg, renal failure and hypoaldosteronism).
     b. **Increased production/extracellular shift** (eg, acidosis, catabolic stress, ischemia, rhabdomyolysis, tumor lysis syndrome, administration of blood, gastrointestinal [GI] bleeding). Acidosis increases the serum [K$^+$] by 0.6 mEq (with wide variability) for every 0.1 unit decrease in the pH.
     c. **Drugs.** Succinylcholine, nonsteroidal anti-inflammatory drugs (NSAIDs), ACE inhibitor (ACEI), angiotensin receptor blocker (ARB), potassium-sparing diuretics, heparin, and β-blockers.
     d. **Pseudohyperkalemia** from a hemolyzed specimen, erythrocytosis, or thrombocytosis.
  2. **Clinical features** are more likely with acute changes.
     a. **Signs and symptoms** include muscle weakness, paresthesias, and cardiac conduction abnormalities, which become dangerous with levels >6.5 mEq/L. Bradycardia, ventricular fibrillation, and cardiac arrest may result.
     b. Hyperkalemia suppresses electrical conduction. **ECG findings** include peaked T waves, ST segment depression, prolonged PR interval, loss of the P wave, diminished R-wave amplitude, QRS widening, prolongation of the QT interval, and appearance of a sine wave ("preterminal" rhythm).
  3. **Treatment** depends on the nature of ECG changes and serum levels.
     a. **Rapidly acting therapies in the setting of clinical symptoms**
        i. Slow IV administration of 0.5 to 1.0 g of **calcium chloride** stabilizes the membrane of cardiac myocytes. The dose may be repeated in 5 minutes if changes persist.
        ii. **Insulin** shifts K$^+$ intracellularly. Ten units of regular insulin are given IV simultaneously with 25 g of glucose IV (one 50-mL ampule of a 50% solution) over 5 minutes. Check the glucose level 30 minutes later to avoid hypoglycemia.
        iii. **Hyperventilation and NaHCO$_3$** administration shift K$^+$ intracellularly. Between 50 and 100 mEq of NaHCO$_3$ may be given IV over 5 minutes, with a repeated dose in 10 to 15 minutes.
        iv. **Beta-2 agonists** (eg, albuterol nebulizer treatment) can lower serum K$^+$ by 0.5 to 1.0 mEq/L.
     b. **Definitive treatment**
        i. Diagnose and treat the underlying etiology.
        ii. Potassium elimination (decrease total body potassium).
        iii. Diuretics (loop and thiazide) waste potassium in the urine. Depending on the volume status of the patient, concomitant fluid resuscitation may be required.

iv. Cation exchange resins (sodium polystyrene sulfonate [Kayexalate], 20–50 g with sorbitol) given orally or rectally will remove K^+ through the intestinal route.
v. Serum $[K^+]$ can also be lowered by dialysis (ideally intermittent hemodialysis with high blood and dialysis flow rates, low $[K^+]$ and [high HCO_3^-] dialysate).

C. Extrarenal regulatory and metabolic functions
1. **Erythropoietin** is produced by the kidney to stimulate red blood cell production. Treatment of patients with exogenous recombinant erythropoietin can combat the anemia due to chronic kidney disease (CKD).
2. **Vitamin D** is converted to its most active form, 1,25-dihydroxy-cholecalciferol, by the kidney.
3. **Parathyroid hormone** acts on the kidney to conserve calcium, waste phosphate, and increase formation of 1,25-dihydroxycholecalciferol.
4. **Metabolization of protein hormones**, for example, insulin, accounts for the generally decreased insulin requirements as renal failure progresses.

III. RENAL FAILURE
A. Acute kidney injury (AKI)
1. **Epidemiology.** Estimated to occur in 12% of hospital admissions, 18% of patients undergoing major surgery, and 50% or greater of intensive care unit (ICU) patients. Risk increases with age. Perioperative acute kidney injury is common, accounting for 30% to 40% of all in-hospital cases of AKI. Development of postoperative AKI is associated independently with increased morbidity and mortality.
2. **Etiology**
   a. **Traditional categorization** is by the anatomical groups of prerenal, intrarenal, and postrenal.
      1. **Prerenal.** Due to decreased circulating blood volume (hypovolemia) or a perceived decrease in circulating volume (decreased cardiac output or hypotension). Early correction of the underlying cause usually results in rapid reversal of renal dysfunction, but continued renal hypoperfusion may result in intrinsic renal damage.
      2. **Intrarenal.** The most common cause is ATN due to ischemia. Other causes include toxins, acute glomerulonephritis, and interstitial nephritis.
      3. **Postrenal.** Obstructive lesions result in disrupted emptying and can be caused by renal calculi, neurogenic bladder, prostatic disease, or an encroaching tumor. Unilateral obstruction rarely causes AKI.
   b. **Modern description** favors describing specific syndromes (eg, hepatorenal, cardiorenal, nephrotoxic, sepsis-associated AKI) that do not always fit the traditional classification scheme, since each has a unique treatment.
      1. **Cardiorenal syndrome.** Inflammation and neurohormonal activation affect blood flow autoregulation, impairing compensation for the abnormal kidney perfusion pressure caused by low cardiac output and/or renal vein congestion.
      2. **Hepatorenal syndrome.** Hepatic dysfunction causes systemic vasodilation, triggering a high level of activation of the RAAS and subsequent renal dysfunction. Portal hypertension-induced splanchnic vasodilation seems to play a central role. Profound oliguria and sodium retention result.

3. **Classification.** There are three widely used classification systems for AKI (**Table 5.1**):
    a. The **RIFLE** criteria classify three levels of kidney injury (*r*isk, *i*njury, or *f*ailure) and two outcomes (*l*oss and *e*nd-stage renal disease [ESRD]) based upon (1) the increase in serum creatinine over 7 days or (2) a decrease in urine output (UOP).
    b. The **AKIN** criteria modify the RIFLE criteria by including absolute increases in serum creatinine and limiting the period of injury to a 48-hour window.

TABLE 5.1 Criteria for Acute Kidney Injury

	RIFLE	**AKIN**	**KDIGO**
Diagnostic criteria	Increase in SCr of 50% or UOP <0.5 mL/kg/h for 6 h	Increase in SCr of ≥0.3 mg/dL or ≥50% within 48 h OR UOP <0.5 mL/kg/h for >6 h	Increase in SCr of ≥0.3 mg/dL within 48 h or ≥50% within 7 d OR UOP <0.5 mL/kg/h for >6 h
Staging Criteria			
Risk (RIFLE) AKIN/KDIGO **stage 1**	Increase in SCr to ×1.5 baseline OR UOP <0.5 mL/kg/h for 6–12 h	Increase in SCr of ≥0.3 mg/dL or to 150–200% baseline OR UOP <0.5 mL/kg/h for 6–12 h	Increase in SCr of ≥0.3 mg/dL or ×1.5–1.9 baseline OR UOP <0.5 mL/kg/h for 6–12 h
Injury (RIFLE) AKIN/KDIGO **stage 2**	Increase in SCr of ×2 baseline OR UOP <0.5 mL/kg/h for 12–24 h	Increase in SCr to 200–300% baseline OR UOP <0.5 mL/kg/h for 12–24 h	Increase in SCr to ×2.0–2.9 baseline OR UOP <0.5 mL/kg/h for 12–24 h
Failure (RIFLE) AKIN/KDIGO **stage 3**	Increase in SCr to ×3 baseline OR Increase in SCr by 0.5 mg/dL to >4.0 mg/dL OR UOP <0.3 mL/kg/h for <24 h or anuria for >12 h OR Initiation of RRT	Increase in SCr to >300% baseline OR SCr ≥4.0 mL/dL with an acute increase of >0.5 mg/dL OR UOP of <0.3 mL/kg/h for >24 h or anuria for >12 h OR Initiation of RRT	Increase in SCr to ≥3.0 times baseline OR Increase in SCr to ≥4.0 mg/dL OR Urine output of <0.3 mL/kg/h for ≥24 h or anuria for >12 h OR Initiation of RRT
Loss (RIFLE)	Need for RRT >4 wk		
End-stage (RIFLE)	Need for RRT >3 mo		

AKIN, Acute Kidney Injury Network; ESRD, end-stage renal disease; KDIGO, Kidney Disease: Improving Global Outcomes; RIFLE, risk, injury, failure, loss, ESRD; SCr, serum creatinine.

Derived from Palevsky PM. Definition of acute kidney injury. In: Curhan GC, ed. *UpToDate*. UpToDate. Accessed June 2024. https://www.uptodate.com/contents/definition-and-staging-criteria-of-acute-kidney-injury-in-adults

TABLE 5.2 Urine and Serum Diagnostic Indexes

	Prerenal	Renal	Postrenal
FE_{Na}	<1%	>2%	>2%
FE_{Urea}	<35%	>50%	>50%
Serum (BUN)/creatinine	>20	10	10

BUN, blood urea nitrogen; FE_{Na}, fractional excretion of sodium.

    c. The **Kidney Disease. Improving Global Outcomes (KDIGO)** criteria fuse the RIFLE and AKIN criteria.
4. **Diagnosis.** History and physical examination, in particular assessing the patient's volume status, help determine etiology. Pertinent laboratory tests should include urinalysis, serum creatinine level, and fractional excretion of sodium (FE_{Na}), or fractional excretion of urea (FE_{Urea}) if the patient has been exposed to diuretics. Imaging studies can help rule out obstruction (**Table 5.2**).
5. **Clinical features.** Depending on the severity, the condition may be silent. It can present with hypervolemia due to an impaired ability to excrete water and sodium with resultant hypertension, cardiac arrhythmia, pulmonary edema, and peripheral edema. In the setting of underlying heart failure, this volume overload can precipitate rapid decompensation. Uremia can affect cognitive function and platelet efficacy. Urinary tract obstruction might present with pain. Inability to concentrate the urine can present with hypovolemia. AKI also can cause electrolyte derangements, impaired excretion of drugs and toxins, and potential progression to CKD. Two-thirds of cases of AKI resolve within 7 days, cases that do not resolve are associated with 47% hospital mortality.
6. **Prevention.** Mainly based on tradition and extrapolation from animal models. A modest goal is to keep UOP greater than 0.5 mL/kg/h and to avoid hypotension, hypoxia, renovascular constriction, and maintenance of renal vasodilation and renal tubular blood flow along with attenuation of renal ischemic reperfusion injury. N-acetylcysteine (NAC) and bicarbonate do not provide benefit beyond fluid hydration.
7. **Management**
    a. **Medications.** Although medications such as diuretics, dopamine, and fenoldopam can increase UOP, treat hypertension, and manage electrolyte, fluid, and acid–base disturbances, they have not been proven to prevent or treat AKI.
    b. **Optimization.** Remove toxic drugs, renally dose medications, and favor medications that do not require renal clearance. Avoid hydroxyethyl starch, especially in septic shock. Normal saline has a higher risk for composite death, dialysis, and renal dysfunction compared with more physiologic solutions (eg, Lactated Ringer's). Recent evidence suggests iodinated contrast does not cause AKI, though it is still reasonable to minimize use in patients with preexisting kidney disease. Control inflammation, correct anemia (hemoglobin >7 g/dL), optimize cardiac output, and correct volume status. This may require invasive hemodynamic monitoring. If adequately intravascularly replete, vasopressors may be needed to maintain mean arterial pressure (MAP) >65 mmHg.

c. **Specific syndromes.** In addition to the above optimization, address the underlying condition.
d. **Renal replacement therapy (RRT).** Incidence of patients with postoperative AKI requiring RRT varies depending on the underlying surgical operation (eg, coronary artery bypass grafting 3.0% vs general surgery 0.6%). Indications for RRT in AKI and CKD include hyperkalemia, acidosis, volume overload, and uremic complications (pericarditis, tamponade, and encephalopathy). Best timing for RRT initiation remains controversial.
   1. **Hemodialysis** uses an artificial semipermeable membrane that separates the patient's blood from the dialysate and allows the exchange of solutes by **diffusion** along a gradient. Vascular access (via central venous catheters or a surgically created arteriovenous fistula) and systemic or regional anticoagulation are often required. Hemodialysis is typically performed three times a week, and serum electrolyte and volume abnormalities are corrected by adjusting the dialysis bath fluid. Blood samples taken immediately after dialysis will be inaccurate, because redistribution of fluid and electrolytes takes approximately **6 hours.** Complications include arteriovenous fistula infection or thrombosis, dialysis disequilibrium or dementia, hypotension, pericarditis, and hypoxemia.
   2. **Ultrafiltration** and **hemofiltration** allow for the removal of volume with minimal removal of waste products. These techniques are useful in volume-overloaded patients. As with standard hemodialysis, anticoagulation is usually required.
      a. **Ultrafiltration** uses hemodialysis equipment to create a hydrostatic driving force across the membrane without a dialysate on the opposing side. Thus, an ultrafiltrate of serum is removed, and this volume is not replaced. If large volumes of fluid are removed rapidly, hypotension may ensue.
      b. **Hemofiltration** uses the same principle as ultrafiltration; however, replacement fluid is given to the patient either before or after the membrane filter and solutes/electrolytes are removed by convection. Volume shifts are minimized so that patients can tolerate longer periods of continuous filtration.
   3. **Continuous renal replacement therapy (CRRT)** refers to any continuous mode of extracorporeal solute or fluid removal. Slower blood flow rates with CRRT have been theorized to reduce hemodynamic instability compared with regular hemodialysis, but a 2007 Cochrane review found no difference in hemodynamic instability, hypotension episodes, or mortality.
B. **CKD** is defined by kidney damage manifested as abnormalities in the composition of blood or urine, abnormalities in imaging tests, or a glomerular filtration rate (GFR) <60 mL/min/1.73 m^2 for ≥3 months.
   1. **Epidemiology.** CKD affects 14% of adults (**Table 5.3**).
   2. **Etiology.** Common causes include diabetes mellitus (single largest cause of ESRD in the United States), hypertension, glomerulonephropathies, tubulointerstitial disease, renovascular disease, polycystic kidney disease, and obesity.
   3. **Clinical features**
      a. **Hypervolemia and hypertension,** sometimes resulting in congestive heart failure and edema.
      b. **Accelerated atherosclerosis** and **hypertriglyceridemia,** which may increase the risk of coronary artery disease.

Table 5.3 National Kidney Foundation Classification of CKD

Stage	Description	GFR	US Prevalence (%)
I	Normal	≥90	3.3
II	Mild	60–89	3.0
III	Moderate	30–59	4.3
IV	Severe	15–29	0.2
V	Failure	<15	0.1

      c. **Uremic pericarditis and pericardial effusions**, which may cause cardiac tamponade.

      d. **Hyperkalemia, hypermagnesemia,** and **hyponatremia** may occur.

      e. **Hypocalcemia** and **hyperphosphatemia** due to elevated parathyroid hormone, resulting in renal osteodystrophy.

      f. **Metabolic acidosis** due to retained sulfates and phosphates and an inability to excrete products of metabolism.

      g. **Chronic anemia,** secondary to decreased erythropoietin production and decreased red blood cell survival.

      h. **Platelet dysfunction,** secondary to uremia, which can be temporarily treated with desmopressin acetate.

      i. **Gastrointestinal dysfunction** is common as a result of accumulated urea that may result in inflammation of the entire GI tract. Increased gastric volume, acid production, and delayed gastric emptying result in an increased risk of regurgitation and aspiration during anesthesia.

      j. Increased **susceptibility to infection** due to leukocyte and immune dysfunction from uremia, malnutrition, and inflammatory reaction to dialysis.

      k. **Central nervous system changes** range from mild changes in mentation to severe encephalopathy and coma. Peripheral and autonomic neuropathies are common.

      l. **Glucose intolerance.**

    4. **Management.** When needed, approximately 88% of patients receive hemodialysis and 12% receive peritoneal dialysis. Transplantation is the preferred method of treatment for most patients with ESRD.

      a. **Hemodialysis** (see Section III.A.7.d).

      b. **Peritoneal dialysis** uses the capillaries of the peritoneum as a semipermeable exchange membrane with the dialysate infused into the peritoneal cavity via an indwelling peritoneal catheter. Advantages over hemodialysis include less hypotension or disequilibrium and no need for heparin treatment. However, peritoneal dialysis is less efficient and limited in catabolic states compared with hemodialysis. Complications include infection, hyperglycemia from the dextran in the dialysate, and increased protein loss in the dialysate.

IV. ANESTHETIC MANAGEMENT

  A. Preoperative assessment. The etiology of renal disease should be elucidated (eg, diabetes mellitus, hypertension). Elective surgery should be postponed in the setting of an acute, unoptimized disease process (eg, new type 1 hepatorenal syndrome). The degree of residual renal function is

best estimated by creatinine clearance (see Section IV.A.3.b). A thorough, systems-based history and physical should be performed (see Chapter 1: Evaluating the Patient Before Anesthesia).
1. **History**
    a. **Signs and symptoms** can be varied depending on the cause of renal failure but may include polyuria, polydipsia, dysuria, edema, dyspnea, arrhythmia, and mental status changes.
    b. **Relevant medications** should be detailed: diuretics, antihypertensives, potassium supplements, digitalis, and nephrotoxic agents (NSAIDs, aminoglycosides, exposure to heavy metals, and recent radiographic dye).
    c. **Schedule of hemodialysis** should be noted for coordination with procedures. Dry weight should be confirmed.
2. **Physical examination**
    a. Patients should be thoroughly examined for the stigmata of renal failure as described in Section III.B.3.
    b. **Arteriovenous fistulas** should be evaluated for patency (by the presence of a thrill or bruit). Intravenous access and blood pressure determinations should be performed on the opposite limb to preserve the fistula.
    c. **Avoid peripherally inserted central venous catheters** in patients with CKD given the risk of upper-extremity venous thrombosis and central venous stenosis, which impairs future RRT vascular access.
    d. For **central lines** in CKD, if clinically appropriate, choose smaller-bore catheters to preserve the veins. Internal jugular vein sites rather than subclavian veins are also less prone to thrombose or permanently damage vessels.
3. **Laboratory studies**
    a. **Serum creatinine (SCr)** is normally 0.6 to 1.2 mg/dL but is affected by the patient's skeletal muscle mass and activity level. SCr concentration is inversely proportional to GFR; thus, a doubling of SCr generally corresponds to a 50% reduction in GFR. In pregnancy, a physiologic increase in GFR and expansion of extracellular fluid volume mean normal SCr is 0.4 to 0.8 mg/dL (thus SCr of 1.0 mg/dL in pregnancy may mean renal failure, the etiology of which must be investigated).
    b. **Creatinine clearance** is used to estimate GFR and provides the best estimate of renal reserve. It is normally 80 to 120 mL/min. A gross estimate of creatinine clearance can be calculated by: {[140-age (years)] × weight (kg)}/[72 × serum creatinine (mg/dL)]. Multiply by 0.85 for women. Ideal body weight should be used in obesity. This formula is invalid with gross renal insufficiency or changing renal function. Medications such as trimethoprim, H_2 receptor antagonists, and salicylates block the secretion of creatinine and may elevate serum creatinine and decrease creatinine clearance.
    c. **Cystatin C** is often a more accurate measure of kidney function than creatinine, especially in patients with low muscle mass, advanced age, female sex, higher reported $eGFR_{cr}$ and albuminuria, and more comorbid conditions. However, it can be falsely elevated in chronic inflammation, obesity, smoking, and hyperthyroidism.
    d. **Blood urea nitrogen** is an insensitive measure of GFR because it is influenced by volume status, cardiac output, diet, and body habitus. The ratio of blood urea nitrogen to creatinine is normally 10 to 20:1; disproportionate elevation of the blood urea nitrogen may reflect

hypovolemia, low cardiac output, gastrointestinal bleeding, or steroid use.
  e. **Electrolytes.** Serum Na^+, K^+, Cl^-, and HCO_3^- concentrations will usually be normal until renal failure is advanced. Careful consideration of the risk and benefit of proceeding with elective surgery should be made if $[Na^+]$ is less than 131 or greater than 150 mEq/L, or if $[K^+]$ is less than 2.5 or greater than 5.9 mEq/L, because these abnormalities may exacerbate arrhythmias and compromise cardiac function. Serum Ca^{2+}, PO_4^-, and Mg^{2+} concentrations are altered in renal failure.
  f. **Urinalysis** provides a qualitative assessment of general renal function.
     1. Findings suggestive of renal disease include abnormal pH, proteinuria, pyuria, hematuria, and casts.
     2. The kidney's ability to concentrate urine is often lost before other changes become apparent. A specific gravity of 1.018 or greater after an overnight fast suggests that concentrating ability is intact. However, radiographic dye and osmotic agents will elevate specific gravity and invalidate this test.
  g. **Urine electrolytes**, osmolality, urine creatinine, and urine urea can help determine volume status and concentrating ability and are used to help differentiate between prerenal and intrarenal diseases (see **Table 5.2**).
  h. **Hematologic studies** should assess anemia and coagulation abnormalities.
  i. **ECG** may reveal myocardial ischemia or infarction, pericarditis, and the effects of electrolyte abnormalities (see Section II.B).
  j. **Imaging** may show evidence of fluid overload, pericardial effusion, infection, uremic pneumonitis, or cardiomegaly.
4. **Risk assessment for postoperative renal dysfunction**
  a. **Patient factors**
     1. Preoperative. Preexisting kidney dysfunction, diabetes, cardiac dysfunction, age >50 years, sepsis, volume depletion, hepatic failure, crush injury, exposure to nephrotoxins.
     2. Intraoperative. Hypotension, hypovolemia, kidney ischemia, inflammation, increased intra-abdominal pressure, decreased cardiac output, vasodilation, exposure to nephrotoxins, embolism.
     3. Postoperative. Intraoperative factors plus urinary obstruction, acute lung injury, mechanical ventilation.
  b. **Potential nephrotoxins**
     1. NSAIDs. Associated with increased risk of perioperative AKI in patients with underlying risk factors (age, higher burden of comorbidity). Consider avoiding or dose reducing.
     2. ARB/ACEI. Angiotensin II increases efferent arteriolar vasoconstriction to maintain glomerular filtration pressure. However, in patients taking ACEI or ARB, this compensatory mechanism may be decreased, which could cause a decrease in renal perfusion pressure and urine production. RCTs have failed to replicate mortality or cerebrovascular benefits from holding ARB/ACEI. Consider stopping these on the day of surgery.
     3. Antibiotics. Aminoglycosides, multitherapy versus monotherapy.
     4. Contrast media. These may cause a decrease in O_2 supply by causing intrarenal vasoconstriction, decreased medullary blood supply, and an increase in O_2 demand. The osmotic load increases work to the medullary nephrons.

Chapter 5 Specific Considerations With Renal Disease   **89**

      c. High-risk surgery. Renal artery surgery, thoracic and abdominal aortic surgery, nonrenal organ transplantation, surgery with large blood loss, and prolonged (>3 hours) cardiopulmonary bypass.
  5. Preoperative optimization
      a. Patients on hemodialysis should be dialyzed before surgery, allowing time between dialysis and surgery to permit equilibration of fluids and electrolytes. Blood samples taken immediately after hemodialysis may be inaccurate owing to redistribution of fluid and electrolytes. Equilibration may take up to 6 hours.
      b. If the patient is on CRRT, the decision to continue intraoperatively must be based on the underlying reason for the CRRT, the duration of the procedure, and the type of procedure. Most patients will be able to tolerate discontinuation of CRRT before surgery and reinstitution afterward.
      c. It may be prudent to postpone major elective vascular surgery for a few days after contrast media exposure. Some evidence exists for pretreatment with isotonic crystalloid for volume expansion, but there is no consensus on rate or duration. There is poor evidence for pretreatment with N-acetylcysteine (1200 mg PO every 12 hours for 2 days) or sodium bicarbonate infusion (three ampules of 50 mEq in 1 L D5W or free water).
B. Intraoperative management. There are limited data comparing general and regional anesthesia in terms of renal protection; currently, there is no benefit of one over the other. When regional anesthesia is considered, coexisting neuropathies should be determined (and documented) and the coagulation profile checked for coagulopathies.
  1. Premedication should be administered carefully because patients with renal failure may have an increased sensitivity to central nervous system depressants, especially if significant uremia is present (see Section VI.A.1).
  2. The dose of **induction agents** may need to be reduced and their rate of administration slowed to avoid hypotension (see Section VI.A.1). Serum potassium should be checked before administering succinylcholine.
  3. Many anesthetics cause peripheral vasodilation and myocardial depression necessitating the use of **vasopressors.** Current clinical data are insufficient to recommend one vasoactive agent as superior to another in preventing AKI. Appropriate use of vasoactive agents can improve kidney perfusion and should not be withheld from the patient in distributive shock owing to concern over kidney perfusion.
  4. Adequate **hemodynamic management,** in particular maintenance of adequate MAP, is vital in ensuring adequate renal perfusion pressure. Data suggest intraoperative hypotension is associated with postoperative AKI. Maintain at least MAP >65 mmHg. There is evidence that targeting an individualized systolic blood pressure (SBP) within 10% of the patient's baseline SBP decreases postoperative organ dysfunction.
  5. Surgical stimulation results in an increase in circulating catecholamines, catabolic hormones, and cytokines that increase ADH, resulting in sodium/water retention, potassium loss, and decreased UOP. Narcotics also increase ADH release, which may further reduce UOP (see Section V.B.3).
  6. Positioning should be done carefully. Patients with CKD are prone to fractures secondary to renal osteodystrophy.
  7. Ventilation with excessive positive-pressure ventilation can impair venous return by reducing preload, causing a resultant reduction

in renal perfusion pressure. Avoidance of hypoxia, hypercarbia, and ventilator-induced lung injury through the use of lung protective ventilation may help reduce inflammatory AKI risk factors. Determine optimal PEEP by oxygenation and compliance.

8. **Fluid management** should consider maintenance fluid requirements, evaporative/insensible losses (eg, open abdominal procedures with losses up to 10 mL/kg/h), extravasation/third-space losses of fluids, and intravascular/blood loss.

   a. Fluid replacement should proceed cautiously with balanced crystalloids. Liberal versus restrictive perioperative fluid management is a much-debated topic, though some studies show increased renal injury with a more restrictive approach. A goal-directed, patient-specific approach is recommended.

   b. Crystalloids may only stay intravascular for 20 to 80 minutes whereas colloids may stay intravascular for 2 to 3 hours. Intravascular persistence is affected by a variety of factors including inflammation impacting the glycocalyx.

   c. Large volumes of 0.9% sodium chloride administration may result in a hyperchloremic metabolic acidosis. Data suggests that Lactated Ringer's solution is associated with less metabolic acidosis and hyperkalemia, especially in patients undergoing renal transplant surgery.

   d. For more extensive procedures, arterial line waveform analysis, bedside point-of-care ultrasound, central venous pressure, or pulmonary artery catheter may help guide fluid management (see Chapter 3: Specific Considerations for Cardiac Disease).

   e. **Urine output** in patients who are neither oliguric nor anuric can be a helpful marker of adequate resuscitation with goal of 0.5 mL/kg/h (although this should be adjusted for the individual case and patient).

9. **Rhabdomyolysis** is skeletal muscle breakdown with release of nephrotoxic breakdown products, such as myoglobin. It may result from suboptimal positioning, compartment syndrome, tourniquet use, prolonged procedures, hypotension, neuroleptic malignant syndrome, and malignant hyperthermia. High BMI is an additional risk factor. Diagnose with serum creatinine kinase >5000 U/L. Treat the underlying source and concomitant electrolyte abnormalities and give generous volumes of crystalloid fluids (classically NS, although recent data suggest LR is equivalent). Urine alkalinization through sodium bicarbonate administration showed some benefit in a case series, though the benefit may be purely from volume expansion.

10. **Hematologic disturbances** are common in CKD, including anemia, leukocyte dysfunction, and coagulopathy. Accordingly, these patients are at an increased risk for intraoperative bleeding. Interventions to reduce bleeding include:

    a. **Recombinant erythropoietin** corrects anemia, normalizes starting hemoglobin, and may restore platelet function.

    b. **DDAVP** improves platelet function by stimulating release of von Willebrand–Factor VIII complex from the endothelium into the plasma where it binds and activates platelets. Effects are seen 1 to 2 hours postinfusion and last approximately 6 to 12 hours.

    c. **Cryoprecipitate** contains von Willebrand–Factor VIII complex, which corrects prolonged bleeding in about 50% of cases. However, there is a risk of bloodborne infection.

d. **Conjugated estrogens** may reduce bleeding and have a longer duration of action than DDAVP.
   e. Heparin-free or low-dose heparin hemodialysis.
   f. Tranexamic acid reduces mortality from traumatic bleeding in places lacking advanced trauma systems (CRASH trials). However, effects in severe kidney disease (CrCl <30 mL/min) are unknown.
   11. **Specific considerations for renal transplantation.** Recipients have ESRD and generally have hypertension and/or diabetes mellitus, are at increased risk for cardiac disease, and may have disturbances in electrolytes, acid–base balance, platelet function, and volume status. Specific considerations:
      a. IV access may be limited, and placement in extremities with fistulas or shunts should be avoided. The benefits of additional invasive monitors (central venous or arterial lines) should be weighed against the risks of catheter-related infections in functionally immunosuppressed patients.
      b. Patients may have delayed gastric emptying from diabetes, uremic neuropathy, and preoperative opioids, so a rapid sequence induction may be indicated. Succinylcholine is safe to use in ESRD, provided serum potassium is normal as the increase in plasma potassium is no greater than in the general population. If a rapid sequence induction is not indicated, either a benzylisoquinoloid or aminosteroid may be used (see VI.A.7 and VI.A.8).
      c. Graft function depends on adequate intravascular volume before and after vascular anastomosis to maintain perfusion to the transplanted kidney. Crystalloid and albumin are useful volume expanders. If pharmacologic support is necessary, inotropes may be preferable to α-agonists, but data are limited.
      d. Most patients receive immunosuppressants to prevent graft rejection, including induction therapy with antithymocyte globulin that can induce an anaphylactic reaction.

C. Postoperative management
   1. **Postoperative fluid management**
      a. Repletion should take into account effusions, drainage tube losses, and mobilization of third-space fluid back into the vascular compartment.
      b. Replacement fluid should consist of balanced crystalloids and dextrose until the patient is able to take adequate fluid orally.
      c. Postoperative oliguria can be a normal physiologic response to pain and surgical stress. Remembering this can avoid overzealous fluid administration that may be harmful.
   2. **Hypertension** is a common postoperative problem and is aggravated by fluid overload. For those not on dialysis, diuretics and short-acting antihypertensives are effective. For those on dialysis, postoperative dialysis may be required.

V. PHARMACOLOGY AND THE KIDNEY
A. Pharmacologic interventions for renal protection in the perioperative period
At present, no convincing evidence indicates that any of these measures are of benefit.
   1. **Diuretics** are used to facilitate management of fluid balance and manage electrolyte and acid–base disturbances (**Table 5.4**). However, the KDIGO guidelines 2012 recommend against use of diuretics specifically to prevent or treat AKI, except in management of volume overload.

Table 5.4 Diuretics

	Primary Site of Action	Primary Effect	Side Effects	Comments
Nonosmotic				
Loop (furosemide, **ethacrynic** acid, and bumetanide)	Thick ascending loop of Henle and $Na^+/K^+/Cl^-$ symporter	Moderate to severe natriuresis and chloruresis	Hypokalemia, alkalosis, and volume contraction	Interferes with both urinary concentration and dilution
Thiazides (chlorothiazide, and metolazone)	Distal tubules and Na^+/Cl^- symporter	Mild to moderate natriuresis	Hyponatremia, hypokalemia, alkalosis, and volume contraction	Interferes with urinary dilution and tends to be ineffective in renal failure and CHF
Carbonic anhydrase inhibitors (acetazolamide)	Proximal tubule and carbonic anhydrase	Mild natriuresis	Hyperchloremia, hypokalemia, and metabolic acidosis	Used primarily for ophthalmology; self-limiting renal effect
Potassium sparing (spironolactone, triamterene, and amiloride)	Collecting duct and ENaC channel or aldosterone receptor	Mild to moderate natriuresis	Hyperkalemia	Used in conjunction with K^+ losing diuretics or in hyperaldosterone states
Osmotic				
Mannitol	Proximal tubule, descending loop of Henle, and collecting duct	Moderate to severe diuresis	Early: vasodilation and volume expansion; Late: hyperosmolality and volume contraction	Draws intracellular fluid into intravascular space

CHF, congestive heart failure.

There is no evidence that use of diuretic therapy reduces severity or mortality in AKI. In fact, it may precipitate AKI.

2. **Dopamine** dilates renal arterioles, increases renal blood flow, and augments natriuresis and the GFR. Low-dose dopamine (0.5 to 3 μg/kg/min) has been proposed to prevent and treat AKI, but efficacy has never been demonstrated.

3. **Fenoldopam** is a specific dopamine-1 receptor agonist. Emerging data suggest decreased length of stay and rates of AKI but no effect on all-cause mortality.

4. **Natriuretic peptides.** There are currently no definitive trials to support use of ANP, BNP, or nesiritide.

B. **Anesthetic effects on the kidney.** Patients with normal kidney function experience transient postanesthetic alterations in renal function. These alterations may occur despite insignificant changes in blood pressure and cardiac output, suggesting that changes in intrarenal distribution of blood flow are responsible. With brief exposures to anesthesia, the observed changes in renal function are reversible (renal blood flow and GFR return to baseline within a few hours). With extensive surgery and prolonged anesthesia, impaired ability to excrete a water load or concentrate urine may last for several days.

1. All inhalational agents and many induction agents cause myocardial depression, hypotension, and a mild to moderate increase in renal vascular resistance, leading to a decreased renal blood flow and GFR.
2. Compensatory catecholamine secretion causes redistribution of renal cortical blood flow.
3. ADH release increases with the onset of surgical stimulation. Hydration before the induction of anesthesia attenuates the rise in ADH produced by painful stimuli.
4. Spinal and epidural anesthesia produce decreases in renal blood flow, GFR, and UOP.
5. There are historical concerns regarding adverse renal effects of some fluorinated volatile agents, in particular sevoflurane. Strong bases in CO_2 absorbents can theoretically accumulate at low fresh gas flow (FGF), degrading sevoflurane to the nephrotoxic by-product, Compound A. However, current data show that renal effects of low-flow (≤1 L/min) sevoflurane are no different from low-flow isoflurane. Package inserts in the United States currently recommend sevoflurane exposure should not exceed 2 MAC hours at flow rates of 1 to 2 L/min and that FGF <1 L/min is not recommended.
6. The VAPOR-1 trial suggests possible longer-term benefits in recipients receiving sevoflurane (vs propofol) during renal transplantation, with lower acute rejection rate after 2 years.

VI. PHARMACOLOGY AND RENAL FAILURE
A. Common anesthetic drugs
1. Many common anesthetic drugs may be affected by renal dysfunction owing to the changes that follow.
   a. Volume of distribution and electrolytes.
   b. **pH** (resulting in a higher percentage of nonionized drug).
   c. **Decreased serum protein concentration** resulting in increased bioavailability of protein-bound drugs, impaired biotransformation, and decreased rates of excretion (**Table 5.5**).
   d. **Loading doses** do not need to be altered significantly in CKD as the duration of action of drugs administered by bolus is **determined by redistribution,** not elimination. With repeated dosing or long-term infusion, the duration of action is dependent on elimination, and maintenance doses of drugs with significant renal excretion should be reduced.
2. **Lipid-soluble drugs** are generally poorly ionized and must undergo metabolism by the liver to water-soluble forms before elimination by the kidney. With few exceptions, the metabolites have little biologic activity.
3. **Benzodiazepines** are metabolized in the liver to both active and inactive compounds, which are then eliminated by the kidney. Benzodiazepines are 90% to 95% protein bound. Great care must be taken in using diazepam because of its long half-life and its active metabolites. Accumulation of benzodiazepines and their metabolites may occur in

Table 5.5 Pharmacologic Considerations for Perioperative Drugs Used in Patients With Chronic Renal Insufficiency

Drug Class	Pharmacokinetics	Considerations
Volatile anesthetics	Pulmonary metabolism	Sevoflurane produces compound A, a potentially nephrotoxic metabolite.
Lipid Soluble		
Barbiturates	Free fraction of induction dose is almost doubled in patients with CKD.	May induce exaggerated hypotension and other clinical effects in CKD. Consider reducing induction dose
Benzodiazepines	Increased free fraction in CKD	Potentiates clinical effects in CKD. Active metabolites accumulate with repeated dosing.
Propofol	Rapid, extensive hepatic metabolism. Pharmacokinetics unchanged in CKD	Conflicting evidence on pharmacodynamics
Etomidate	Increased free fraction in CKD	CKD may increase risk of toxic reactions
Ketamine	Redistribution and hepatic metabolism largely responsible for termination of anesthetic effects. Minimal change in free fraction in CKD	CKD does not alter clinical effects.
Opioids	Metabolized in liver	May have increased and prolonged effect in CKD. Active metabolites may prolong action with chronic administration: Morphine-6-glucoronide (morphine) has potent analgesic and sedative effects. Normeperidine (meperidine) has neurotoxic effects. Hydromorphone-3-glucoronide (hydromorphone) can cause cognitive dysfunction and myoclonus. Fentanyl has no active metabolite.
Ionized Drugs		
Muscle relaxants	Standard dose of succinylcholine increases serum K^+ by 0.5–0.8 mEq/L in CKD. Many nonpolarizing NMBs result in prolonged effects due to reliance on renal excretion	Succinylcholine is not contraindicated in CKD if serum K^+ is not elevated. Cisatracurium, mivacurium, and rocuronium are preferable in CKD.

TABLE 5.5 Pharmacologic Considerations for Perioperative Drugs Used in Patients With Chronic Renal Insufficiency (*continued*)

Drug Class	Pharmacokinetics	Considerations
Cholinesterase inhibitors	Decreased elimination in CKD, and half-life is prolonged	Half-life prolongation is similar to or greater than the duration of blockade from long-acting NMB so recurarization is rarely seen.
Digoxin	Excreted in urine	Increased risk of toxicity in CKD.
Vasoactive Drugs		
Catecholamines		Catecholamines with α-adrenergic effects constrict renal vasculature and may reduce renal blood flow.
Sodium nitroprusside	Metabolized by the kidney and excreted as thiocyanate	Toxicity from thiocyanate accumulation is more likely in CKD.
Antibiotics		
Penicillin, cephalosporins, aminoglycosides, and vancomycin	Predominately dependent on renal elimination	Loading dose is unchanged, but maintenance doses need adjustment.

severe renal failure. Benzodiazepines are not appreciably removed by dialysis.

4. **Barbiturates, etomidate, and propofol** are highly protein bound, and in hypoalbuminemic patients, a much greater proportion will theoretically be available to reach the receptor sites. Acidosis and changes in the blood–brain barrier may further reduce induction requirements. However, there is no high quality pharmacodynamic evidence for barbiturates and etomidate, and the studies on propofol have yielded conflicting results. Use clinical judgment.

5. **Opioids** are metabolized in the liver but may have a more intense and prolonged effect in patients with renal failure, particularly in hypoalbuminemic patients in whom protein binding will be reduced. Active metabolites of morphine and meperidine may prolong their actions, and accumulation of normeperidine may cause seizures. The pharmacokinetics of fentanyl, sufentanil, alfentanil, and remifentanil are unchanged in renal failure.

6. **Ionized drugs.** Drugs that are highly ionized at physiologic pH tend to be eliminated unchanged by the kidney, and their duration of action may be prolonged by renal dysfunction.

7. **Depolarizing neuromuscular blockers (NMBs).** Succinylcholine can be used safely in ESRD provided the potassium concentration is <5.5 mmol/L and repeated doses are avoided. An increase of ~0.5 mmol/L in serum potassium is observed both in ESRD and in healthy subjects.

8. **Nondepolarizing NMBs.** Traditionally, benzylisoquinolinium muscle relaxants (such as cisatracurium) are preferable in ESRD given their organ-independent metabolism. However, their metabolism is pH dependent, and acidosis in ESRD may prolong their effects. Rocuronium (an

aminosteroid NMB) is excreted primarily in bile, and ~33% is excreted in urine resulting in prolonged action in renal failure. Sugammadex is a modified gamma-cyclodextrin that binds to and encapsulates aminosteroid neuromuscular blocking agents. Although it is excreted in urine, its efficacy as a reversal agent appears to be independent of excretion of the cyclodextrin-NMB complex. In ESRD, excretion of the cyclodextrin-NMB complex is prolonged but no evidence of recurarization has been reported in studies. No known adverse side effects of delayed excretion are known; however, more study in this area is warranted. Reassuringly, the cyclodextrin-NMB complex can be removed by dialysis.
   a. **Cholinesterase inhibitors.** With impaired renal function, elimination of the reversal drugs is decreased and their half-lives are prolonged.
   b. **Digoxin** is excreted in the urine, and patients with renal failure are at increased risk of digitalis toxicity.

VII. FUTURE CONSIDERATIONS FOR IDENTIFICATION OF PATIENTS AT RISK OF PERIOPERATIVE AKI

Neither SCr nor urine output are direct markers of kidney injury. In addition, both are delayed and insensitive biomarkers affected by many variables. Several novel potential biomarkers have been identified that show promise, including kidney injury molecule 1 (KIM-1), interleukin 18, liver-type fatty acid-binding protein (L-FABP), **tissue inhibitor of metalloproteinase-2 (TIMP-2), insulin-like growth factor binding protein 7 (IGRBP7), and neutrophil gelatinase-associated lipocalin (NGAL).** Only TIMP-2 and IGRBP7 have entered routine clinical practice. These show great potential in identifying AKI early, which may allow for timely intervention and change the course and progression of the disease. With regards to intraoperative diagnostic technologies, research is ongoing into development of real-time GFR monitoring using novel fluorescent GFR tracer agents.

ACKNOWLEDGMENT

We gratefully acknowledge the contributions of previous edition author, Cliodhna Ashe, as portions of those chapters have been retained in this revision.

Suggested Readings

Abuelo JG. Normotensive ischemic acute renal failure. *N Engl J Med.* 2007;357:797–805.

Bito H, Ikeuchi Y, Ikeda K. Effects of low-flow sevoflurane anesthesia on renal function: comparison with high-flow sevoflurane anesthesia and low-flow isoflurane anesthesia. *Anesthesiology.* 1997;86(6):1231–1237.

Bugaj JE, Dorshow RB. Pre-clinical toxicity evaluation of MB-102, a novel fluorescent tracer agent for real-time measurement of glomerular filtration rate. *Regul Toxicol Pharmacol.* 2015;72(1):26–38.

Cammu G, Van Vlem B, van den Heuvel M, et al. Dialysability of sugammadex and its complex with rocuronium in intensive care patients with severe renal impairment. *Br J Anaesth.* 2012;109(3):382–390.

Colson P, Ryckwaert F, Coriat P. Renin angiotensin system antagonists and anesthesia. *Anesth Analg.* 1999;89:1143–1155.

Craig RG, Hunter JM. Recent developments in the perioperative management of adult patients with chronic kidney disease. *Br J Anaesth.* 2008;101:296–310.

Futier E, Lefrant JY, Guinot PG, et al. Effect of individualized vs standard blood pressure management strategies on postoperative organ dysfunction among high-risk patients undergoing major surgery: a randomized clinical trial. *J Am Med Assoc.* 2017;318(14):1346–1357.

Gropper M, et al. Chapter 17: Renal anatomy, physiology, pharmacology, and evaluation of function. In: *Miller's Anesthesia.* 9th ed. Elsevier; 2019.

Hahn RG, Lyons G. The half-life of infusion fluids: an educational review. *Eur J Anaesthesiol.* 2016;33(7):475–482.

Khwaja A. KDIGO clinical practice guidelines for acute kidney injury. *Nephron Clin Pract.* 2012;120(4):c179–c184.

Marcucci M, Painter TW, Conen D, et al. Hypotension-avoidance versus hypertension-avoidance strategies in noncardiac surgery: an international randomized controlled trial. *Ann Intern Med.* 2023;176(5):605–614.

Massoth C, Zarbock A, Meersch M. Risk stratification for targeted AKI prevention after surgery: biomarkers and bundled interventions. *Semin Nephrol.* 2019;39(5):454–461.

Mazze RI, Jamison RL. Low-flow (1 l/min) sevoflurane: is it safe? *Anesthesiology.* 1997;86(6):1225–1227.

McKinlay J, Tyson E, Forni LG. Renal complications of anaesthesia. *Anaesthesia.* 2018;73(1):85–94.

Nieuwenhuijs-Moeke GJ, Nieuwenhuijs VB, Seelen MAJ, et al. Propofol-based anaesthesia versus sevoflurane anaesthesia for living donor kidney transplantation: results of the VAPOR-1 randomized controlled trial. *Br J Anaesth.* 2017;118(5):720–732.

Ong Sio LCL, Dela Cruz RGC, Bautista AF. Sevoflurane and renal function: a meta-analysis of randomized trials. *Med Gas Res.* 2017;7(3):186–193.

PATCH-Trauma Investigators and the ANZICS Clinical Trials Group; Gruen RL, Mitra B, Bernard SA, et al. Prehospital tranexamic acid for severe trauma. *N Engl J Med.* 2023;389(2):127–136.

Petroni KC, Cohen NH. Continuous renal replacement therapy: anesthetic implications. *Anesth Analg.* 2002;94:1288–1297.

Prowle JR, Forni LG, Bell M, et al. Postoperative acute kidney injury in adult non-cardiac surgery: joint consensus report of the Acute Disease Quality Initiative and PeriOperative Quality Initiative. *Nat Rev Nephrol.* 2021;17(9):605–618.

Rabindranath KS, Adams J, Macleod AM, Muirhead N. Intermittent versus continuous renal replacement therapy for acute renal failure in adults. *Cochrane Database Syst Rev.* 2007;(3):CD003773.

Ronco C, Bellomo R, Kellum JA. Acute kidney injury. *Lancet.* 2019;394(10212):1949–1964.

Schmid S, Jungwirth B. Anaesthesia for renal transplant surgery: an update. *Eur J Anaesthesiol.* 2013;29:552–558.

Shlipak MG, Matsushita K, Ärnlöv J, et al. Cystatin C versus creatinine in determining risk based on kidney function. *N Engl J Med.* 2013;369(10):932–943.

Staals LM, Snoeck MM, Driessen JJ, Flockton EA, Heeringa M, Hunter JM. Multicentre, parallel-group, comparative trial evaluating the efficacy and safety of sugammadex in patients with end-stage renal failure or normal renal function. *Br J Anaesth.* 2008;101(4):492–497.

Sterns RH. Disorders of plasma sodium – causes, consequences, and correction. *N Engl J Med.* 2015;372(1):55–65.

Suneja M, Kumar AB. Obesity and perioperative acute kidney injury: a focused review. *J Crit Care.* 2014;29:694.e1–694.e6.

Thapa S, Brull SJ. Succinylcholine-induced hyperkalemia in patients with renal failure: an old question revisited. *Anesth Analg.* 2000;91(1):237–241.

Wagener G, Brentjens TE. Anesthetic concerns in patients presenting with renal failure. *Anesthesiol Clin.* 2010;28:39–54.

Zarbock A, Koyner JL, Hoste EAJ, Kellum JA. Update on perioperative acute kidney injury. *Anesth Analg.* 2018;127(5):1236–1245.

6 Specific Considerations With Liver Disease

Taylor A. Woo-Sekizaki and Ion A. Hobai

Patients with liver disease, especially those with liver failure, pose some of the most complex challenges for anesthesiologists due to the multisystem comorbidities associated with the condition. The reported mortality rates for patients with cirrhosis undergoing various elective, noncardiac, and nontransplant surgical procedures range from 6% to 27%, compared to just 1.1% for noncirrhotic patients.

I. ANATOMY, PHYSIOLOGY AND PATHOLOGY OF THE LIVER
A. Liver anatomy

The adult liver weighs approximately 2 kg. It is anatomically divided into two main lobes (left and right) and two accessory (caudate and quadrants) lobes, which are in turn divided into a total of eight segments. Also known as Couinaud segments, (**Figure 6.1**), they each have their own dual vascular inflow, biliary drainage, and lymphatic drainage and are thus anatomically and functionally independent. Hepatocellular carcinoma and liver metastases do not show a true segmental preference in location; variations in occurrence are primarily related to the relative volume of each liver segment. The liver thus comprises only 2% to 3% of the total body mass, but it receives 20% to 25% of the cardiac output. The hepatic artery supplies 25% of the blood flow to the liver and 50% of the liver's oxygen requirement. The portal vein drains the stomach, spleen, pancreas, and intestine. It supplies 75% of the hepatic blood flow and 50% of hepatic oxygen. The right,

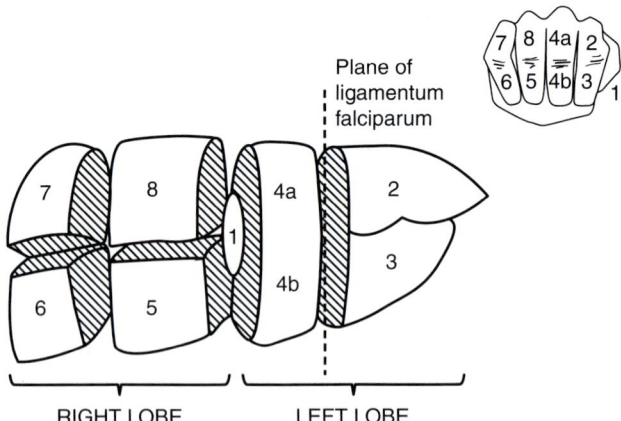

FIGURE 6.1 Liver lobes and segments, and a "handy" mnemonic (insert). Illustration by Spencer Hobai.

middle, and left hepatic veins drain independently of each other into the inferior vena cava.

B. Liver physiology

The liver plays crucial roles in the metabolism of proteins, carbohydrates, lipids, and hemoglobin, as well as the inactivation of many hormones and drugs.

1. **Proteins.** The normal adult liver produces 12 to 15 g of protein per day including albumin, coagulation factors, pseudocholinesterase, and α1-acid glycoprotein. Albumin and α1-acid glycoprotein are important drug-binding proteins, and their deficiency in liver disease may lead to an increase in the free, active fraction of drug. All proteinaceous clotting factors are produced in the liver except factor VIII, which is produced in the vascular endothelium. Synthesis of factors II (prothrombin), VII, IX, and X as well as proteins C, S, and Z, is vitamin K dependent; deficiency of vitamin K or disturbances of liver function may lead to deficiencies of clotting factors and excess bleeding. Pseudocholinesterase is responsible for the degradation of succinylcholine, and its deficiency in liver disease may increase the duration of action of succinylcholine and prolonged muscle relaxation. The liver is the major site of protein degradation where amino acids are broken down through a process that generates urea for the elimination of ammonia. Patients with liver disease may lack the ability to form urea, resulting in rapidly rising plasma ammonia levels and hepatic encephalopathy.

2. **Carbohydrates.** The liver is the principal site of carbohydrate storage (as glycogen) and production during periods of fasting (glycogenolysis and gluconeogenesis).

3. **Lipids.** Most of the body's lipoproteins, as well as cholesterol and phospholipids, are formed in the liver. Cholesterol is degraded principally by the liver, and its by-products serve as substrates for the production of bile salts, steroid hormones, and cell membranes. The liver also serves as the major site of steroid hormone degradation, and hepatic failure results in steroid excess. The resulting elevations of serum aldosterone and cortisol result in increased resorption of sodium and water, and loss of potassium in the urine, contributing to the edema, ascites, and electrolyte abnormalities frequently seen with liver disease. Decreased metabolism of estrogens and impaired conversion to androgens causes other clinical stigmata of liver disease including spider angiomata, gynecomastia, palmar erythema, and testicular atrophy.

4. **Hemoglobin catabolism and bile.** The liver is the primary erythropoietic organ of the fetus and continues to be a major site of hematopoiesis until approximately 2 months of age. In healthy adults, the liver is responsible for 20% of heme production. Abnormalities in heme synthesis can result in porphyria. In addition, the liver metabolizes hemoglobin degradation products, such as bilirubin, that undergo conjugation with glucuronic acid, forming water-soluble products that are excreted within the bile and are eliminated via the feces or urine.

5. **The bile.** The liver forms approximately 800 mL of bile per day. Bile salts are detergents that aid in absorbing, transporting, and excreting lipids. Bile also carries metabolic waste products and drug metabolites to the intestine from the liver. As an emulsifier, bile facilitates fat absorption by the small intestine. Failure to produce or release bile causes jaundice and an inability to absorb fat and fat-soluble vitamins (A, D, E, and K) and can result in steatorrhea, vitamin deficiencies, and coagulopathy.

6. **Drug metabolism.** The liver is the primary organ responsible for the degradation and detoxification of exogenous substances. **Phase I**

reactions change a compound's structure via oxidation, reduction, or hydrolysis, primarily via **cytochrome p450 enzymes**. In some cases, the resulting products may be still metabolically active and may further undergo **phase II reactions**, which consist of enzymatically enhanced conjugations with glucuronide, sulfate, taurine, or glycine. The resulting water-soluble metabolites are finally excreted via urine. Certain drugs such as barbiturates, ethanol, and phenytoin induce cytochrome p450 enzymes, resulting in apparent tolerance to drugs that are metabolized by the system. Drugs that have a high affinity for the p450 complex (eg, ciprofloxacin) may decrease the metabolism of concurrently administered drugs. Liver disease can be associated with decrease in drug–protein binding and an increase in the volume of distribution. In addition, portal–systemic shunting permits orally administered drugs to bypass the liver, reducing the first-pass liver metabolism of the drug.

C. Liver pathology

1. **Acute hepatocellular injury** has many etiologies, including viral infection (hepatitis A, B, C, D, and E; Epstein–Barr virus; cytomegalovirus; herpes simplex virus; ECHO virus; and coxsackievirus), shock, hepatic venous congestion from right heart failure, toxicity from drugs, chemicals and poisons (including alcohol, halothane, phenytoin, propylthiouracil, isoniazid, tetracycline, and acetaminophen), and inborn errors of metabolism (eg, Wilson disease and α1-antitrypsin deficiency).

2. **Chronic parenchymal insults** such as chronic active hepatitis, alcoholism, hemochromatosis, primary biliary cirrhosis (PBC), and congenital disorders may lead to hepatic dysfunction and **cirrhosis**. End-stage hepatic fibrosis causes significant resistance to portal blood flow, leading to portal hypertension and esophageal varices. Further complications from the combination of portal hypertension and decreased hepatic function include ascites, coagulopathy, gastrointestinal bleeding, and encephalopathy.

3. **Cholestasis** occurs most frequently in cholelithiasis and cholecystitis. PBC and primary sclerosing cholangitis also begin as cholestatic diseases, leading to parenchymal damage and liver failure. Hyperbilirubinemia is an important marker of hepatobiliary disease. The degree of conjugation of bilirubin can provide insight into the etiology of hepatic dysfunction such as in the case of impaired uptake of unconjugated bilirubin (Gilbert syndrome) versus elevated conjugated bilirubin in hepatobiliary disease (PBC, Dubin–Johnson syndrome) and obstructive processes.

II. ANESTHETIC CONSIDERATIONS IN PATIENTS WITH LIVER DISEASE

Liver disease, particularly end stage liver disease (ESLD) is associated with dysfunction of numerous other organ systems, which pose specific challenges during anesthesia.

A. Central nervous system

1. **Hepatic encephalopathy.** Although the exact pathogenesis is unclear, impaired neurotransmission, presence of intrinsic γ-aminobutyric acid-ergic substances, and altered cerebral metabolism may be involved in its pathogenesis. Ammonia levels are often elevated in encephalopathic patients but do not correlate with the severity or outcome of encephalopathy. The West Haven criteria (I to IV) is a grading system used to categorize severity of hepatic encephalopathy, ranging from mild covert nonreproducible symptoms like mood changes and changes in attention (I) to obvious clinical manifestations like asterixis,

stupor, and eventually coma (IV). Assessing the patient's capacity for informed consent in the setting of hepatic encephalopathy is a crucial step in preoperative evaluation.
2. **Patients with altered mental status due to hepatic encephalopathy** are at increased risk of oversedation when administered standard doses of benzodiazepines. This heightened risk is attributable to several factors. Benzodiazepines have low hepatic extraction ratios and are metabolized by hepatic enzymes which are compromised in patients with liver dysfunction. Hypoalbuminemia further leads to a greater potency of benzodiazepines due to an increased unbound free form of the drug. Consequently, oversedation can result in respiratory depression and an impaired ability to protect the airway. In severe liver failure, rapidly progressive encephalopathy may be associated with cerebral edema and increased intracranial pressure, which must be managed aggressively to prevent cerebral ischemia. Patients in this condition are typically intubated for airway protection.
3. **Interventions** to monitor and reduce intracranial pressure, such as ventricular drains, carry a bleeding risk due to the underlying coagulopathy. Repeated neuroimaging is essential to monitor cerebral edema progression and assess the need for interventions. Without timely liver transplantation, the prognosis is grave, and recovery is rare.

B. Cardiovascular system
1. **Hyperdynamic circulatory state.** Patients with advanced liver disease exhibit decreased systemic vascular resistance, increased venous return, and elevated cardiac output with increased myocardial contractility and resting tachycardia. Systemic vasodilation occurs with elevated levels of nitric oxide, glucagon, and prostaglandins. Due to arteriolar vasodilation, the effective intravascular volume in central compartments is reduced despite increases in total body plasma volume. In these low arteriolar pressure states, the renin–angiotensin–aldosterone system is activated resulting in augmented renal sodium and water retention manifesting as hyponatremia, ascites, and generalized edema/anasarca. Furthermore, patients with cirrhosis have reduced vascular arteriolar responsiveness to vasoconstrictors. The clinical effect of this cardiovascular state is the potential for profound hypotension with the induction of anesthesia and the need for invasive monitoring and adequate access.
2. **Cardiomyopathy.** Cirrhotic cardiomyopathy is characterized by an impaired systolic response to physical stressors, abnormal diastolic relaxation, and electrophysiologic changes such as prolonged QT interval. This condition occurs in advanced liver disease without the presence of other cardiac diseases. A history of alcohol-related cirrhosis necessitates evaluation for alcohol-induced cardiomyopathy which is a separate entity from cirrhotic cardiomyopathy. Several mechanisms have been proposed to explain the impaired systolic function observed in these patients. One key mechanism is the reduced response to β-adrenergic stimuli, which is a result of prolonged sympathetic overactivity in the high-output cardiac state associated with advanced liver disease. Additionally, endogenously secreted cannabinoids and nitric oxide (NO) are believed to act as myocardial depressants. Management of cirrhotic cardiomyopathy is like that of other etiologies of heart failure, though reduction in afterload is limited by frequently low arteriolar blood pressures.

C. Respiratory system
1. **Airway protection** is a major concern for patients with liver disease. The combination of encephalopathy, obtundation, respiratory failure, and

the risk of aspiration necessitates careful titration and monitoring of respiratory depressants, particularly preoperative anxiolytics.
2. **Risk of pulmonary aspiration.** Liver failure is a recognized cause of gastroparesis. This condition, coupled with increased abdominal pressure from ascites and the presence of encephalopathy, significantly heightens the risk of aspiration. This risk is present in the immediate preoperative period, during intubation, and following extubation. Consequently, full stomach precautions, including rapid sequence intubation and immediate access to oral suctioning are typically warranted.
3. **Respiratory failure and chronic hypoxemia** in patients with advanced liver disease are commonly mechanical in nature. The presence of ascites and pleural effusion lead to atelectasis and restrictive lung physiology. Preoperative respiratory optimization may necessitate draining ascitic fluid and pleural effusions through paracentesis and thoracentesis. Other contributing factors may include portopulmonary hypertension, impaired hypoxic pulmonary vasoconstriction (resulting in ventilation-perfusion mismatch), and hepatopulmonary syndrome. These conditions are more challenging to correct perioperatively and must be considered in postoperative planning. In symptomatic patients, arterial blood gas analysis may reveal a significant arterial–alveolar gradient.
4. **Hepatopulmonary syndrome** is manifested as platypnea-orthodeoxia: dyspnea and hypoxemia occur when upright, and improve upon lying down. Thought to be the result of significant intrapulmonary shunting, the syndrome can be debilitating in everyday life and constitutes a common reason for exception points for patients on liver transplantation waiting lists. However, apart from that, it has minimal implications in anesthetized patients, since they are generally supine.
5. **Portopulmonary hypertension** develops in patients with portal venous hypertension and is physiologically and histologically distinct from pulmonary arterial hypertension. Screening Doppler transthoracic echocardiography and right heart catheterization can provide quantitative data to make the diagnosis, which is particularly important for patients undergoing liver transplantation, as it confers significantly worse morbidity and mortality. Patients with severe portopulmonary hypertension who are nonresponsive to pulmonary vasodilator treatment are not candidates for liver transplantation. Portopulmonary hypertension is associated with right ventricular dysfunction and progression of the disease can lead to right heart failure and death.
6. **Impaired hypoxic pulmonary vasoconstriction.** Patients with advanced liver disease have impaired hypoxic pulmonary vasoconstriction response leading to ventilation–perfusion mismatch and intrapulmonary shunting. This can be particularly evident in anesthetics that require single-lung ventilation. Attention to proper positioning of the double lumen tube, PEEP titration, or advanced maneuvers, such as applying CPAP to the nonventilated lung may be necessary.

D. Gastrointestinal system
1. **Portal hypertension** is associated with splenomegaly, splanchnic venous congestion, and increased collateral circulation, which manifest as hemorrhoids, esophageal varices, and dilated abdominal wall veins (caput medusae). These conditions present an increased risk of hemorrhage, due to either spontaneous rupture or surgical interventions in the abdomen.
2. **Esophageal varices.** Screening for esophageal varices by means of esophagogastroduodenoscopy (EGD) is recommended for patients

with cirrhosis. According to the American Association for the Study of Liver Diseases, esophageal varices should follow a simple two-grade classification system; small or large (>5 mm) and should note the presence or absence of red signs (red wale marks or red spots). Older classification (Paquet) differentiates varices in grade I (only slightly elevated above the mucosal level), grade II (project one-third into the lumen and are noncompressible by air), and grade III varices (extend up to 50% into the luminal diameter and touch each other). Prophylactic management of varices includes beta-blockers, endoscopic ligation, and banding. Transesophageal echocardiography (TEE) may be safely performed in patients with small varices but should be evaluated on a case-by-case basis. Management of upper gastrointestinal bleeding due to esophageal variceal rupture represents a well-recognized anesthesia challenge, as detailed below.

3. **Ascites.** Ascites is due to splanchnic venous congestion coupled with hypoalbuminemia and decreased oncotic pressure. Ascites may increase the risk of abdominal wound dehiscence, abdominal wall herniation, and respiratory compromise. Ascites can be managed with diuretics, with careful attention to electrolytes and renal function. If a large volume of ascites is uncontrolled prior to surgery, paracentesis may be advisable. After large volumes paracentesis, resuscitation with albumin, colloids, or blood products is advisable to reduce the risk of hepatorenal syndrome (HRS).

4. **Nutritional deficiency,** as manifested as protein-energy malnutrition, such as marasmus and kwashiorkor, can be part of liver disease, especially in patients with heavy alcohol use. Nutritional deficiency is a risk factor for increased morbidity and mortality postoperatively and should be treated with supplementation high in carbohydrate/lipid content and low in amino acid content to prevent worsening of hepatic encephalopathy. Nutritional supplementation is especially important in alcoholics and should include vitamin B1 supplementation. If surgery is not urgent, nutritional status should be optimized preoperatively. Due to the low risk of intravenous thiamine, it should be administered before any dextrose in patients presented with any concern for nutritional deficiency.

E. **Renal system**
  1. **Hepatorenal syndrome (HRS).** In many liver failure patients, intravascular volume depletion may produce a degree of prerenal azotemia. The blood urea nitrogen level may be deceptively low because of the liver's inability to synthesize urea from ammonia. This condition is treated by correcting the patient's volume status, typically with a combination of albumin and crystalloid solutions. However, in severe and/or long-standing disease, renal failure can develop as a result of HRS. HRS is characterized by increased renal vascular resistance and oliguria, and can be precipitated by infection and nephrotoxic compounds, such as nonsteroidal anti-inflammatory medications, aminoglycosides, and radiologic contrast. Unrecognized development of HRS can lead to a decreased elimination and overdosing of medications such as opioids and beta blockers, which is frequently a presenting feature. Diagnosis is clinical and based on exclusion of alternative causes of kidney injury. Two subtypes of HRS are defined: Type 1 is characterized by a two-fold increase in serum creatinine (greater than 2.5 mg/dL) in a period of less than 2 weeks, accompanied by significant oliguria. Type 2 is less severe and usually presents as resistance to diuretics. Treatment of

HRS includes blood pressure augmentation to achieve higher mean arterial pressure, fluid resuscitation with albumin, and discontinuation of diuretics, antihypertensives, and beta blockers. Normal renal function may return after liver transplantation or if liver function improves.
 2. **Risk of hyperkalemia in patients with HRS requiring massive transfusion.** Patients with HRS, especially those on dialysis, are a particular challenge for the anesthesiologist during surgical operations complicated by massive bleeding and blood transfusions, because of the development of refractory hyperkalemia. It must be kept in mind that massive blood transfusions induce an increase in serum K, whose usual treatment with forced diuresis will not be possible in patients with renal failure. A careful surgical approach and avoidance of accidental overtransfusion are essential preventive measures. In the event of hyperkalemia, diuretic administration is usually the most effective immediate treatment, but in patients with HRS, this is not an option. Administration of insulin and glucose, along with epinephrine, are effective temporary measures. Prompt correction of metabolic acidosis using sodium bicarbonate, hyperventilation, and calcium administration are essential. Renal replacement therapy or continuous venovenous hemofiltration may be acutely indicated. Should these interventions fail to prevent hyperkalemia-induced cardiac arrest, typically manifested as atrioventricular block and asystole, rapid establishment of transcutaneous ventricular pacing is indicated. A pacer/defibrillator should be quickly available, and the external pads could be attached in advance.

F. Serum electrolytes and pH
 1. **Hyponatremia**, may occur despite total body sodium overload and may lead to seizures and worsening of hepatic encephalopathy. Hyponatremia is typically corrected with fluid restriction and discontinuation of diuretics. Caution should be used as rapid correction may lead to central pontine myelinolysis (Chapter 5: Specific Considerations With Renal Disease).
 2. **Hypo/hyperkalemia.** Since many patients with ascites and esophageal varices are managed with diuretics, they are prone to chronic hypokalemia. This poses the risk of exacerbating the QT-prolonging effect of many drugs, and thus of ventricular tachycardia. However, rapid preoperative correction must be avoided, because of the significant risk of hyperkalemia in ESLD patients undergoing massive transfusions, as explained above.
 3. **Alkalosis/acidosis.** Similarly, although ESLD is usually associated with respiratory, hypoalbuminemic, or metabolic alkalosis, development of metabolic acidosis is common during surgery, especially if complicated by massive bleeding and transfusion.

G. Blood and coagulation
 1. **Anemia and thrombocytopenia.** Patients with ESLD are frequently anemic as a result of decreased production and recognized or occult gastrointestinal bleeding. Similarly, thrombocytopenia may result from bone marrow failure, increased platelet consumption, and hypersplenism. Checking a complete blood count should be considered before most surgical operations, followed by correction by means of blood transfusions. Depending on the risk of bleeding during surgery and patient comorbidities, reasonable preoperative targets are a blood hemoglobin of 8 to 10 mg/dL and platelet count of 50,000 to 80,000/mm^3.
 2. **Coagulopathy.** Coagulopathy in liver failure has multiple etiologies, including impaired synthesis of clotting factors II, VII, IX, and X, as well as altered production of endogenous anticoagulants, such as proteins

C, S, and Z. Vitamin K deficiency may also be present, as a result of decreased intestinal production in the setting of frequent antibiotic use, decreased absorption due to cholestasis, or poor nutritional status. Checking a prothrombin time/international normalized ratio (PT/INR) is essential before surgical operations. Preoperative correction of clotting abnormalities can be achieved with vitamin K administration, keeping in mind that the effect may take several days until production of coagulation factors recovers and INR normalizes. For emergent surgeries, reversal of coagulation abnormalities is best achieved with administration of fresh frozen plasma (FFP) and/or prothrombin complex concentrates. Compared to FFP, administration of prothrombin complex concentrates offers several advantages, including less volume administration and no need for cross-matching, leading to a more rapid normalization of INR and reduced risk of transfusion-related lung injury (TRALI). Although not mechanistically justified, the use of cryoprecipitate, DDAVP (1-desamino-8-d-arginine vasopressin), and factor VIIa should be considered for refractory situations.
3. **Procoagulant states and risk of venous thrombosis.** In addition to elevated risk of bleeding, patients with ESLD are also at risk of thromboembolism due to impaired synthesis and abnormal function of endogenous vitamin K–dependent antithrombotic agents like protein C and S, endothelial dysfunction, and increased venous stasis. Increased awareness is thus necessary for early recognition of intraoperative acute pulmonary embolism, which is usually manifested as severe decreases in blood pressure and end-tidal CO_2, and may lead to a pulseless electrical activity (PEA) arrest. Postoperative mental status changes warrant investigation for cerebrovascular accident (CVA).
4. **Disseminated intravascular coagulation (DIC).** It is still unclear whether ESLD is associated with an increased incidence of DIC, compared to the risk inherently associated with major abdominal operations with high blood loss. Manifested as a combination of intravascular thrombosis (such as pulmonary embolism and right ventricular thrombus) and coagulopathic bleeding, it offers limited therapeutic options and an almost invariably lethal outcome.
5. **Bleeding risk.** Coagulopathy, thrombocytopenia, abdominal venous congestion, and the potential development of DIC can lead to the danger of massive blood loss during surgery, especially abdominal surgery. Apart from preoperative correction of coagulation factors and platelets, adequate venous access, invasive monitoring including arterial and possibly central lines, the availability of blood products for transfusion, and adequate postoperative disposition to an intensive care unit should be considered. Regional anesthesia including neuraxial anesthesia may not be appropriate in the setting of liver failure or anticipated liver failure, due to coagulopathy. The potential for postoperative coagulopathy should be considered before placing an epidural.

H. Endocrine system
1. **Hypoglycemia.** Glycemic control depends heavily on the liver. Severe hepatic insufficiency leads to diminished glycogen stores, requiring gluconeogenesis to maintain normoglycemia. Gluconeogenesis is also impaired in severe liver disease and heavy alcohol use. Hypoglycemia may occur in end-stage hepatic insufficiency, during the anhepatic phase of liver transplantation, or in liver failure that may accompany an episode of severe circulatory shock. Close monitoring of blood glucose levels should be performed, and glucose-containing solutions should be administered as necessary.

I. Skin
1. **Skin trauma.** Patients with ESLD have very fragile skin, that is prone to tears even after minor trauma and spontaneous formation of blisters. Increased attention is needed during the removal of the adhesive tape used to secure intravenous catheters and lines and protective eye covers.

III. PHARMACOLOGY IN SEVERE LIVER DISEASE
A. Altered metabolism of anesthetics
Although both propofol and etomidate are metabolized by the liver, their actions are terminated by redistribution, making them reasonable anesthetics to use in patients with liver disease. Benzodiazepines, barbiturates, and most opioids however may have prolonged effects, as a result of both decreased clearance and an increase in the free active fraction of these drugs, in patients with marked hypoalbuminemia. Remifentanil clearance is not affected by liver dysfunction.

B. Neuromuscular blocking agents
Patients with liver disease often need a higher initial dose of nondepolarizing neuromuscular blockers, probably because of increased volume of distribution or increased neuromuscular receptors. However, for some, a slower elimination time may decrease the requirement for maintenance dosing. Vecuronium and rocuronium are highly dependent on hepatobiliary excretion and metabolism and show a decreased clearance and a prolonged effect in patients with liver disease. Cisatracurium and atracurium are degraded via Hofmann elimination and are unaffected by liver disease. Succinylcholine and mivacurium (not available in the United States) are completely metabolized in the plasma by pseudocholinesterase, which may be depressed in severe liver disease, prolonging their duration of action.

C. Acetaminophen and Nonsteroidal Anti-inflammatory Drugs
Acetaminophen is deemed safe in total daily doses of less than 2000 mg. Nonsteroidal anti-inflammatory drugs (NSAIDs) may exacerbate risk of surgical bleeding, gastrointestinal bleeding, and renal injury but should be utilized on a case-by-case basis.

IV. POSTOPERATIVE HEPATIC DYSFUNCTION
Once being relatively common and associated with the use of halothane, postoperative aggravation of hepatic dysfunction is today rare, and attributed mostly to episodes of perioperative hepatic ischemia, due either to systemic hypotension or to surgical manipulation of the liver.

V. ANESTHETIC MANAGEMENT OF PATIENTS WITH LIVER DISEASE
In summary, the anesthetic management of patients with liver disease is a remarkably complex challenge. A careful preoperative assessment is essential and must include the evaluation of the severity of liver dysfunction and other associated organ dysfunctions, bearing in mind that a relatively well-compensated dysfunction at baseline can manifest when the patient is subjected to the stresses of surgery. Check laboratory data, in particular Na^+, K^+, BUN/creatinine, hematocrit, platelets, coagulation tests, and albumin levels. Regional and neuraxial anesthesia may be contraindicated due to coagulopathy and thrombocytopenia. The induction of general anesthesia may need to be performed with full stomach precautions. Prepare for marked hypotension on induction, as well as possible massive bleeding: two large bore IVs, and an arterial line should be carefully considered for most surgical operations apart from the most minor. A central line may be necessary for

TABLE 6.1 Modified Child–Pugh Score

Parameter	Points 1	Points 2	Points 3
Albumin (g/dL)	>3.5	2.8–3.5	<2.8
Bilirubin (mg/dL)[a]	<2.0	2.0–3.0	>3.0
Ascites	Absent	Slight	Moderate
Encephalopathy	Absent	Grades I and II	Grades III and IV
PT prolongation (s)	<4.0	4.0–6.0	>6.0

Class A, 5–6 points; class B, 7–9 points; class C, 10–15 points.

PT, prothrombin time.

[a]For primary biliary cirrhosis: 1 point for bilirubin <4.0 mg/dL, 2 points for bilirubin 4–10 mg/dL, and 3 points for bilirubin more than 10 mg/dL.

advanced hemodynamic monitoring and vasopressor administration. Expect an altered pharmacodynamics, an exaggerated effect of sedatives, a higher initial requirement for neuromuscular blockers, and a prolonged effect of these and opioids as well as the need for postoperative ICU admission.

VI. RISK ASSESSMENT AND CLASSIFICATION

Two preoperative risk assessment tools have been developed to predict perioperative and nonoperative survival in liver dysfunction patients.

- **A. The Child–Turcotte–Pugh (CTP) classification** was designed to evaluate the risk of surgical portosystemic shunt procedures and was subsequently found to predict long-term survival in patients with cirrhosis. This risk stratification system includes ascites, bilirubin level, albumin level, nutritional status, encephalopathy, and PT (**Table 6.1**). CTP is considered to be the best prognostic indicator for overall mortality.
- **B. The model for end-stage liver disease (MELD)** is a prognostic scoring system originally designed for predicting 3-month mortality following transjugular intrahepatic portosystemic shunt (TIPS) insertion. It was later found useful for predicting mortality of patients on the liver transplantation waiting list and is therefore used for their ranking. The score is calculated based on a patient's serum bilirubin, serum creatinine, and INR (**Table 6.2**). A newer refinement to the MELD scoring system, MELD-sodium (MELD-Na), has been shown to be better at predicting overall 1-year mortality compared to both CTP and MELD scores.
- **C. Other predictors of perioperative risk** include type of surgery, presence of sepsis, reoperation, and elective versus emergent surgery. Procedures involving a laparotomy (associated with a greater reduction in hepatic arterial blood flow) or other intra-abdominal procedures (open cholecystectomy, gastric surgery, and colectomies), cardiac surgery, or those associated with increased blood loss have particularly high mortality rates.

VII. COMMON PROCEDURES IN PATIENTS WITH LIVER DISEASE
A. Management of esophageal varices
Esophageal varices are a common complication of portal hypertension, splanchnic vasodilatation, and portosystemic collateral formation in

TABLE 6.2 MELD Score and MELD-Na

MELD = 3.78[Ln Serum Bilirubin (mg/dL)] + 11.2[Ln INR] + 9.57[Ln Serum Creatinine (mg/dL)] + 6.43

MELD-Na = MELD − Na − (0.025 × MELD × (140 − Na)) + 140

In interpreting the MELD score in hospitalized patients, the 3-month mortality is:
- 40 or more—100% mortality
- 30–39—83% mortality
- 20–29—76% mortality
- 10–19—27% mortality
- <10—4% mortality

In interpreting the MELD-Na score in hospitalized patients, the 3-month mortality is:
- 32 or more—65–66% mortality
- 27–31—27–32% mortality
- 23–26—14–15% mortality
- 21–22—7–10% mortality
- 17–20—3–4% mortality
- <17—less than 2% mortality

The maximum score given for MELD is 40. All values higher than 40 are given a score of 40. If the patient has been dialyzed twice within the last 7 d, then the value for serum creatinine used should be 4.0. Any value <1 is given a value of 1 (ie, if bilirubin is 0.8, a value of 1.0 is used).

INR, international normalized ratio; MELD, model for end-stage liver disease; MELD-Na, MELD-sodium.

---

severe liver disease. Approximately 50% of patients with cirrhosis develop esophageal varices. The yearly incidence of variceal bleeding in this population is 5% to 20%. All patients with severe liver disease should undergo screening EGD to assess the development and progression of esophageal varices. EGD can be performed under nurse-administered sedation (with midazolam and fentanyl), monitored anesthesia care (MAC, usually with a propofol infusion and natural airway), or general endotracheal anesthesia (GETA). Patients judged to be at risk for intraprocedural variceal bleeding or at risk for aspiration should receive general anesthesia with rapid sequence induction (RSI) to secure the airway.

B. Management of acute variceal bleeding

Rupture of esophageal varices can be rapidly lethal, necessitating emergent interventions under anesthesia. These procedures include balloon tamponade and EGD for esophageal sclerotherapy, banding, or stenting. For patients with active hemorrhage requiring airway protection or procedures:

1. RSI should be performed to secure the airway.
2. Multiple suction catheters should be readily available for laryngoscopy.
3. The patient should be positioned upright to minimize the risk of pulmonary aspiration.
4. Direct laryngoscopy may be preferred over video laryngoscopy, as bleeding may impair indirect visualization.
5. Ensure adequate venous access in the form of large-bore peripheral IVs. Prepare for possible massive transfusion.
6. Resuscitation should include transfusion threshold Hb >7.0 g/dL.
7. Rapid transfusion devices with warming capability should be available. If using a rapid transfusion device, dedicated venous access in

a large central venous catheter or in a visible part of the extremity is preferable to prevent inadvertent extravasation and compartment syndrome. Monitor for high pressure and impedance of flow.
8. Arterial line placement should be considered for patients at risk for hemodynamic instability, those requiring large-volume transfusion, and for frequent laboratory monitoring [arterial blood gas (ABG), complete blood count, and coagulation studies].
9. Consider intraoperative administration of somatostatin analogues.
10. Administer prophylactic antibiotics perioperatively.
11. Consider postprocedure ICU admission.

C. Management of portal hypertension—transjugular intrahepatic portosystemic shunt (TIPS) procedures

TIPS is a radiologic procedure in which a prosthetic stent is placed to create a direct connection between the hepatic vein and the portal vein. This shunt reduces the pressure in the portal venous system, thereby decreasing the risk of variceal bleeding and alleviating refractory ascites. The primary drawback of bypassing the liver is an additional reduction in blood detoxification and worsening encephalopathy. TIPS typically requires general anesthesia with endotracheal intubation to secure the airway and facilitate controlled ventilation for optimal surgical conditions as the procedure is complex, may be prolonged, and requires precise positioning of multiple intravascular and intrahepatic sheaths.

D. Anesthetic considerations for TIPS procedures
1. Preoperative baseline mental status should be evaluated so the development of post-TIPS hepatic encephalopathy can be assessed objectively. A severe baseline impairment may reduce capacity of informed consent.
2. RSI should be considered for patients with high risk of aspiration.
3. Ensure adequate venous access for possible transfusion.
4. Arterial line placement should be considered for patients at risk for hemodynamic instability, those requiring large-volume transfusion, and for frequent laboratory monitoring (complete blood count and coagulation studies).

E. Complications of TIPS procedures
1. **Hemorrhage.** Bleeding can occur during the procedure due to puncture of the liver or surrounding structures. Inadvertent arterial puncture is rare but can occur. The inadvertent puncture of the extrahepatic portal vein may result in intraperitoneal bleeding.
2. **Hepatic encephalopathy.** The direct communication of portal vein to systemic circulation can result in the accumulation of toxins in the bloodstream, causing hepatic encephalopathy. If severe hepatic encephalopathy occurs that does not improve with traditional medical management including lactulose therapy and dietary protein restriction, TIPS revision to reduce portal–systemic circulation may be necessary.
3. **Acute liver failure.** Though rare, patients with low liver function before the procedure are at risk for acute liver failure potentially due to hepatic ischemia related to reduced portal venous flow, compromised hepatic artery perfusion, and hepatic venous congestion if the stent occludes a shared hepatic vein origin.
4. **Biliary injury.** The procedure carries a risk of puncturing or compressing the bile ducts, leading to complications like biliary-venous fistulas, bilomas, and biliary obstruction, which can result in cholangitis, infection/sepsis, and liver dysfunction.

5. **Stent-related complications.** These include stent occlusion, thrombosis, malposition, or migration, which may require reintervention to maintain patency.
6. See additional reading list for American Association for Study of Liver Disease guidelines on TIPS.

VIII. LIVER RESECTION
A. Indications
Indications for liver resection include primary hepatobiliary carcinoma, metastatic disease, benign liver lesions, liver donation, and occasionally trauma. The liver receives a substantial proportion (25%) of the cardiac output at all times, making liver resections a procedure with potential for high blood loss.

B. Anesthetic considerations for hepatectomy
1. Ensure adequate venous access in the form of multiple large-bore peripheral IVs in anticipation of possible massive transfusion.
2. Rapid transfusion devices with warming capability should be available in case of hemorrhage.
3. Invasive arterial blood pressure monitoring is typically indicated for close hemodynamic observation, frequent lab tests, and glucose monitoring.
4. Central venous access may be necessary, especially if a low CVP strategy is employed. This access allows for CVP transduction and the administration of vasopressors. Inotropic medications may also be needed for patients with reduced cardiac function.
5. Monitor temperature; lower body temperature worsens coagulopathy and predisposes to bleeding.
6. Monitor for hypoglycemia.
7. Thoracic epidurals can be considered for postoperative analgesia if there is no underlying coagulopathy and no anticipated development of coagulopathy. Epidural analgesia provides excellent pain relief and may reduce postoperative complications.

IX. METHODS TO REDUCE BLOOD LOSS IN LIVER RESECTION
A. Excessive bleeding and transfusion requirements
Excessive bleeding and transfusion requirements have been correlated with increased postoperative morbidity. Management must focus on the balance between reducing blood loss and maintaining adequate liver perfusion. Surgical techniques for hepatic resection and other procedures on the liver have been developed to decrease blood loss. Total hepatic vascular exclusion, the Pringle maneuver, low central venous pressure anesthesia, and venovenous bypass are four such techniques.

B. Total hepatic vascular exclusion
Total hepatic vascular exclusion consists of clamping the hepatic inflow vessels (portal vein and hepatic artery) to the liver as well as the outflow vessels (inferior vena cava). The latter can have profound deleterious effects on venous return and the hemodynamics of the patient. This method also results in a significant amount of warm ischemic time to the liver, a hemodynamically complex reperfusion syndrome on unclamping, and may increase the incidence of postoperative hepatic dysfunction.

C. The Pringle maneuver
The Pringle maneuver consists of intermittent clamping of the hepatic inflow vessels (portal vein and hepatic artery) causing intermittent hepatic ischemia. There can be significant back bleeding through the hepatic veins and vena cava. A recent meta-analysis did not demonstrate a difference in

blood loss using the Pringle maneuver in patients undergoing liver resection; however, previous older studies have shown a reduction in blood loss. This difference is thought to be attributed to newer surgical techniques that limit blood loss without occluding the hepatic inflow vessels.

D. Low CVP

A low CVP (ie, <5–10 mmHg) facilitates control of bleeding from hepatic veins and the inferior vena cava during parenchymal dissection. Low CVP anesthesia has been demonstrated to reduce blood loss; however, it has not been demonstrated to reduce postoperative morbidity. Caveats for CVP monitoring with liver resection include increased risk of AKI and a shorter time available to react in case of accidental bleeding. After resection and hemostasis are achieved the patient should be resuscitated with crystalloid and colloid.

E. Venovenous bypass

Venovenous bypass consists of a circuit that diverts venous blood from large-bore cannulas placed in the common femoral vein and potentially the portal vein to a cannula in either the internal jugular or axillary vein. This allows for caval interruption of the liver during surgery for control of hemorrhage without a significant decrease in preload. The placement of the cannulas should only be performed by an experienced team since it is particularly hazardous. To date, no study has shown a benefit to this technique, so clinical judgment is essential on a case-by-case basis.

X. LIVER TRANSPLANTATION

Liver transplantation is the only potentially curative intervention for patients with end-stage liver disease. Anesthetic considerations for this complex surgery are covered in Chapter 25: Anesthesia for Transplant Surgery; additional sources include the American Association for Study of Liver Disease practice guidelines on pretransplant evaluation.

XI. ENHANCED RECOVERY AFTER SURGERY

Enhanced recovery after surgery (ERAS) protocols for liver resections were first released in 2016 and updated in 2022 and have been shown to decrease morbidity and duration of postoperative admissions after liver resections. Guidelines highlight ensuring adequate preoperative nutritional status and avoiding long-acting anxiolytics preoperatively, maintaining low-CVP anesthesia with balanced crystalloids, and the use of abdominal wound catheters and intrathecal opioids instead of epidural anesthesia. Minimally invasive surgery is recommended when appropriate. Postoperative considerations include early oral intake, mobilization, and a strong recommendation for multimodal analgesia. While there is strong evidence for many of the ERAS recommendations for perioperative nutrition and early mobilizations, the data for some of the other recommendations are equivocal particularly for low CVP anesthesia and epidural analgesia as discussed in the previous sections.

ACKNOWLEDGMENTS

We gratefully acknowledge the contributions of previous edition authors, Mark Abraham and Jerome Crowley, as portions of those chapters have been retained in this revision.

Suggested Readings

Diaz GC, O'Connor MF, Renz JF. Anesthesia for patients with concomitant hepatic and pulmonary dysfunction. *Anesthesiol Clin.* 2016;34(4):797–808.

Huntington JT, Royall NA, Schmidt CR. Minimizing blood loss during hepatectomy: a literature review. *J Surg Oncol.* 2014;109(2):81–88.

Joliat GR, Kobayashi K, Hasegawa K, et al. Guidelines for perioperative care for liver surgery: Enhanced Recovery After Surgery (ERAS) Society Recommendations 2022. *World J Surg.* 2023;47(1):11–34.

Krige A, Kelliher LJS. Anaesthesia for hepatic resection surgery. *Anesthesiol Clin.* 2022;40(1):91–105.

Lee EW, Eghtesad B, Garcia-Tsao G. AASLD Practice Guidance on the use of TIPS, variceal embolization, and retrograde transvenous obliteration in the management of variceal hemorrhage. *Hepatology.* 2024;79(1):224–250.

Martin P, DiMartini A, Feng S, Brown R Jr, Fallon M. Evaluation for liver transplantation in adults: 2013 practice guideline by the American Association for the Study of Liver Diseases and the American Society of Transplantation. *Hepatology.* 2014;59(3):1144–1165.

Mcclain RL, Ramakrishna H, Aniskevich S III, et al. Anesthetic pharmacology and perioperative considerations for the end stage liver disease patient. *Curr Clin Pharmacol.* 2015;10(1):35–46.

Moreau R, Gao B, Papp M, Bañares R, Kamath PS. Acute-on-chronic liver failure: a distinct clinical syndrome. *J Hepatol.* 2021;75(1):S27–S35.

Newman KL, Johnson KM, Cornia PB, Wu P, Itani K, Ioannou GN. Perioperative evaluation and management of patients with cirrhosis: risk assessment, surgical outcomes, and future directions. *Clin Gastroenterol Hepatol.* 2020;18(11):2398–2414.e3.

Ostojic A, Mahmud N, Reddy KR. Surgical risk stratification in patients with cirrhosis. *Hepatol Int.* 2024;18(3):876–891.

Spring A, Saran JS, McCarthy S, McCluskey SA. Anesthesia for the patient with severe liver failure. *Adv Anesth.* 2020;38:251–267.

Van Eldere A, Pirani T. Liver intensive care for the general intensivist. *Anaesthesia.* 2023;78(7):884–901.

Specific Considerations With Endocrine Disease

Ion A. Hobai and Fei Wu

In this chapter, we will summarize the primary anesthesia-related concerns for diseases of the endocrine system. In addition, for the endocrine diseases that have surgical treatment, we will present the main considerations regarding the respective operations or point to the chapters where these are covered in this manual.

I. DIABETES MELLITUS

A. Pathophysiology, diagnosis, and management

1. Insulin is synthesized in pancreatic β-cells and secreted in response to feeding and/or hyperglycemia. Among various endocrine functions, insulin is responsible for glucose transport into cells to serve as metabolic substrate. Diabetes mellitus (DM) is a chronic systemic disease characterized by an absolute or relative lack of insulin. As of 2021, 14.7% of US adults (>18 years old) had DM, out of which 3.4% were unaware of their diagnosis. DM is the most common endocrinopathy encountered in the perioperative period.

2. There are two main types of DM. Around 5% of DM cases are type 1 (DM1) is caused by autoimmune destruction of pancreatic β-cells resulting in an absolute insulin deficiency. Patients are usually diagnosed at a young age and are not obese. The great majority of DM (95%) is type 2 (DM2), characterized by peripheral insulin resistance with or without impaired insulin secretion. Patients are typically diagnosed in adulthood and are frequently obese. In addition to DM1 and DM2, gestational DM complicates approximately 7% of pregnancies. Secondary DM is due to other causes of absolute or relative insulin insufficiency. Insulin hyposecretion is seen with pancreatic destruction due to cystic fibrosis, pancreatitis, hemochromatosis, cancer, or pancreatic surgery. Glucose intolerance may result from a glucagonoma or pheochromocytoma, thyrotoxicosis, acromegaly, or glucocorticoid excess.

3. Usually asymptomatic and diagnosed incidentally, DM may present in severe cases with glycosuria, polyuria, and polydipsia. Management for DM1 is primarily insulin replacement. For DM2, diet and exercise, oral hypoglycemic agents, insulin sensitizers, and insulin formulations are all used on an individual basis.

4. Acute complications of DM, including diabetic ketoacidosis (DKA, mostly in DM1), and hyperglycemic hyperosmolar state (HHS, mostly in DM2) represent medical emergencies. Chronic sequelae include vasculopathy (cardio-, cerebro-, or peripheral), nephropathy, neuropathy, and retinopathy.

B. Anesthesia management of diabetic patients

Given the complex and multifaceted nature of DM, we will organize the main anesthesia–related concerns into: (1) concerns related to the basic mechanisms of disease (which would apply to all patients with the diagnosis, such as hyperglycemia and DKA, for example), (2) concerns related to the common sequelae of the disease (which are usually in the back of your mind, but not necessarily applying to all patients, such as silent ischemia, for example), and (3) concerns related to the medications used to treat the disease (which only apply to patients using the specific medications, such as hypoglycemia in patients using insulin).

C. **Considerations related to the primary pathophysiology**
   1. **Perioperative hyperglycemia and glycemic targets.** Even a previously well-controlled diabetic patient may develop severe perioperative hyperglycemia, or acute complications, such as HHS and DKA, due to surgical stress and/or emergencies such as trauma, bleeding, or infection. Although perioperative hyperglycemia has been almost invariably associated with increased morbidity and mortality, it is unclear how much of this is due to its direct effect, as opposed to it being a marker of increased severity of DM and associated comorbidities. In addition, aggressive glycemic control increases the incidence of accidental hypoglycemia, which is, arguably, even more dangerous. With no consensus between medical societies, a cautious approach is to accept a moderate degree of hyperglycemia perioperatively, targeting a glucose level between 140 and 180 mg/dL. Treatment of perioperative hyperglycemia is usually accomplished with intravenous insulin. A reasonable dose is given by the formula Insulin units = (blood glucose, mg/dL)/40. The onset of action is immediate, and the duration of action is ~1 hour. Therefore, treatment must be continued, with regular glucose checks. For longer cases, transition to an infusion equivalent may be worthwhile, with the rate adjusted based on at least hourly checks.
   2. **Acute complications of DM.** No elective surgery should be performed on a patient presenting in HHS or DKA. However, as mentioned above, these conditions could be triggered by the stress of surgery or the acute conditions that warrant emergency surgery. Because of that, your ability to recognize them early and familiarity with the principles of management are crucial, as well as the ability to work in collaboration with your local intensivist colleagues.
   3. **Diabetic ketoacidosis (DKA).** In DKA, an absolute insulin deficiency leads to hyperglycemia and decreased intracellular glucose, which shifts metabolism from glucose based to ketogenic. Uncontrolled production of ketone bodies causes high anion gap metabolic acidosis, osmotic diuresis, hypovolemia, and severe electrolyte abnormalities. Clinical manifestations of DKA include nausea, vomiting, abdominal pain, polyuria, polydipsia, weakness, deep rhythmic (Kussmaul) breathing with a fruity odor, and mental status changes. It is associated with depressed myocardial contractility and decreased vascular tone. Patients are often profoundly hypovolemic owing to hyperglycemia-related osmotic diuresis, emesis, and reduced oral intake. Total body potassium (K^+) is depressed, but serum levels are spuriously normal or elevated at presentation because acidemia shifts K^+ out of cells via transcellular hydrogen (H^+)–K^+ exchange. Serum sodium (Na^+) concentrations may be spuriously low because hyperglycemia causes osmotic shifts of water from the intracellular to the extracellular space, leading to a relative dilutional hyponatremia. Hypophosphatemia and hypomagnesemia from osmotic diuresis are common. Treatment of DKA is based on the principles of volume replacement (fluid deficit in adult DKA averages 6 to 9 L), insulin therapy, correction of electrolyte abnormalities (most importantly potassium replacement), identification and treatment of

underlying stressors or precipitants, and supportive care. DKA management protocols often vary by institution. Goal for initial stabilization is resolution of ketosis and normalization of anion gap.
4. **Hyperosmolar hyperglycemic state (HHS).** HHS is primarily a complication of DM2, the result of severe hyperglycemia. It is often associated with serum glucose levels exceeding 600 mg/dL, precipitating significant osmotic diuresis and profound hypovolemia. Patients present with CNS dysfunction (depressed sensorium, seizure, coma), blurred vision, neurologic deficits, weight loss, leg cramps, polydipsia, polyuria, and electrolyte abnormalities. Mortality in HHS may be as high as 20%. Treatment of HHS is similar to the treatment of DKA, with an emphasis on volume repletion, insulin therapy, correction of electrolyte abnormalities, and diagnosis and treatment of underlying precipitants. Intubation should be considered if there is a concern for lack of airway protection owing to altered mental status. Volume repletion is generally more aggressive in HHS owing to a higher fluid deficit (8 to 10 L in the average size adult), and initial target glucose level is higher than DKA (250 to 300 mg/dL in HHS, 200 mg/dL in DKA). This is to prevent rapid correction of serum osmolality and subsequent cerebral edema.

D. **Considerations related to sequelae of DM.** Macrovascular disease (coronary artery, cerebrovascular, and peripheral vascular) and microvascular disease (retinopathy, neuropathy, and nephropathy) occur in diabetic patients more frequently and at an earlier age than in the general population.
1. **Cardiovascular disease and silent coronary ischemia.** Diabetic patients with ischemic heart disease are more likely to be asymptomatic or have atypical anginal symptoms. Continuation of aspirin and β-blockade are essential, as is a high index of suspicion for perioperative cardiac ischemic events.
2. **Peripheral vascular disease.** Diabetic patients frequently have atherosclerosis in various peripheral arteries. Consider checking that blood pressure cuff measurements are similar in both arms, if not, assume a degree of arterial stenosis and rely on the higher measurement. Arterial access, especially distal small arteries (eg, radial, dorsalis pedis) can be more challenging and may warrant ultrasound guidance and the use of specialized (micropuncture) guiding wires.
3. **Nephropathy.** DM is the most common cause of chronic and end-stage renal disease. Maintaining adequate mean arterial pressure as well as avoiding intraoperative hypovolemia is key for keeping kidney perfusion, thus preventing further kidney injury. Nephrotoxins, such as aminoglycoside antibiotics, IV radiologic contrast medium, or NSAIDs should be avoided or used judiciously.
4. **Neuropathy. Peripheral neuropathy** may cause pain and/or numbness. Patients with peripheral neuropathy may be more vulnerable to positioning injuries and should be positioned and padded carefully. Document existing neuropathies in the anesthesia preoperative evaluation, especially before regional anesthesia. **Diabetic autonomic neuropathy** can be present even in patients with well-controlled DM. It has widespread effects, including decreased lower esophageal sphincter tone, gastroesophageal reflux disease, gastroparesis, bladder atony, sexual dysfunction, orthostatic hypotension, and labile blood pressure. It is associated with an increased risk for silent myocardial ischemia, renal failure, stroke, obstructive sleep apnea, and overall mortality among patients with DM. Patients may be at higher risk for

intraoperative hypothermia, more susceptible to aspiration owing to higher residual gastric volumes, and less able to compensate for the sympathectomy from neuraxial anesthesia. Signs of cardiac autonomic neuropathy include resting tachycardia, orthostatic hypotension, and decreased beat-to-beat variability with deep breathing.

5. **Gastroparesis** merits special consideration. Although diabetes has been shown to cause delayed gastric emptying reliably, there is conflicting evidence on whether diabetic patients have a higher incidence of a full stomach condition when presenting for surgical procedures after fasting. Some of the common medications used to treat DM, such as insulin and glucagon-like peptide 1 receptor agonists (GLP-1 RA) have also been shown to cause gastroparesis, independent of diabetes. Although there are no current recommendations to treat all fasting DM patients as full stomach, increased vigilance is warranted. The use of point-of-care ultrasound may help with risk stratification. More information on this can be found below, in the discussion of GLP-1 RA-related concerns.

6. **Airway management**

    Obesity, sleep apnea, and redundant pharyngeal tissue are common in patients with metabolic syndrome and DM2, which can lead to difficult mask ventilation. Diabetic "stiff joint syndrome" can lead to decreased mobility of temporomandibular and atlanto-occipital joint, which can lead to difficult laryngoscopy (reported to be 20% to 30% in DM). This may be predicted by signs of other joint stiffness, such as incomplete approximation of one or more digits when attempting to approximate palmar surfaces (prayer sign).

E. **Considerations related to diabetes medications**

   Many antidiabetic medications need careful perioperative dosing adjustment.

   1. **Insulin**
      a. **Insulin treatment of diabetes** usually includes a mixture of compounds with different duration of action. Regular insulin (Humulin R, Novolin R) is classified as short acting. After subcutaneous injection, it has an onset of action of 0.5 to 1 hour, peak effect in 2 to 4 hours, and duration of action of 6 to 10 hours. Rapid-acting insulins like Lispro (Humalog) and Aspart (NovoLog) exert their effect within 15 minutes, with a duration of 2 to 4 hours. Short-acting and rapid-acting insulins are either given just before meals to prevent postprandial hyperglycemia or administered continuously via a subcutaneous pump. Intermediate-acting (NPH, with a duration of action of 12 to 18 hours) and long-acting insulins (Glargine [Lantus], with a duration of action of 20 to 24 hours) are given one to two times a day to mimic basal insulin secretion. The liver and kidney metabolize insulin. As a result, renal insufficiency and hepatic impairment may produce clinically significant prolongation of insulin action and reduce insulin requirements.
      b. **Perioperative management of insulin therapy** depends on the type of diabetes. Patients with DM1 must always receive insulin to prevent ketoacidosis, even in the setting of low or normal glucose levels. Simultaneous infusion of a glucose-containing solution may be necessary to prevent hypoglycemia. Patients receiving intensive regimens of three or more daily insulin injections are best managed in collaboration with the patient's endocrinologist.
      c. **Patients with insulin-dependent DM2** should continue insulin therapy through the night before surgery. If the patient has a history of hypoglycemia, the dose should be reduced to half to two-thirds of the patient's routine evening dose. DM2 patients should receive

approximately half of their routine morning dose of intermediate- or long-acting insulin. Rapid- and short-acting insulins should not be given.
  d. **Fixed-ratio insulin combinations** are prescribed for the outpatient management of some diabetics. In consultation with the physician managing the diabetes, these patients should be switched to preparations of individual insulins in the immediate preoperative period. An appropriately reduced dose (approximately 50%) of only the long-acting insulin can then be taken on the morning of surgery as described above.
  e. **If glucose drops below 120 mg/dL, consider starting a glucose infusion.** If glucose rises above 180 mg/dL consider starting insulin. IV insulin should be used if the patient (1) is expected to be hemodynamically unstable, (2) expected to have fluid shifts or temperature changes, (3) has an operative duration >4 hours, (4) is critically ill, or (5) has poorly controlled DM at home. If insulin is started, check blood sugars and potassium levels at least every 1 to 2 hours.
  f. **Insulin pump**
      1. For the **patient with an insulin pump**, the following information should be obtained preoperatively: pump identification, settings, insertion site, blood sugar measurements, plans for correction dosing, pump failure plan, and diabetes provider contact. The anesthesia provider needs to know how to operate the pump in case settings need to be changed intraoperatively. The usual basal rates can be reduced by 10% to 20% while the patient is nil-per-os (NPO) to avoid hypoglycemia. Only use insulin pumps intraoperatively if (1) the site does not interfere with the surgery, (2) there is no plan for MRI or other radiation, (3) the pump is out of the path of the electrocautery return circuit, and (4) there is minimal risk of needing defibrillation. Blood glucose levels should be checked frequently with target glucose level of 120 to 180 mg/dL, which is typically more liberal than home management. This may require turning basal rate down to 80% of home regimen.
      2. **Protamine/insulin cross reactivity.** One additional aspect to be considered in patients using NPH or NPL (Humalog mix) insulin is that they are at increased risk for protamine reactions because they contain protamine.
2. **Other diabetes medication.** Chronic diabetes management may include a variety of oral agents, some of which pose distinct perioperative risks.
  a. **Metformin** and other biguanides decrease hepatic glucose production, inhibit intestinal glucose absorption, and increase peripheral glucose uptake and utilization. Metformin has a very low risk of associated hypoglycemia; however, a risk of lactic acidosis has been reported, especially in patients with perioperative exacerbation of renal dysfunction (reduced drug clearance), hepatic dysfunction (reduced lactate clearance), or heart failure. Some authors (but not all) recommend that the morning dose of metformin should be held. At MGH, we recommend that metformin should be held from the day of surgery until normal postoperative renal function has been confirmed.
  b. **Sulfonylureas**, such as glyburide and glimepiride increase pancreatic insulin release, and can therefore be associated with increased risk of perioperative hypoglycemia for more than 24 hours after administration. Sulfonylureas also increase the effectiveness of thiazide

diuretics, barbiturates, and anticoagulants by displacing these drugs from albumin.

c. **Thiazolidinediones**, including rosiglitazone and pioglitazone, increase insulin sensitivity and decrease hepatic glucose production. Risk of perioperative hypoglycemia is low when used as monotherapy. Thiazolidinediones, especially rosiglitazone, have been associated with edema and heart failure exacerbation.

d. **Glucagon-like peptide-1 receptor agonists (GLP-1RA)** enhance glucose-dependent insulin secretion, reduce inappropriate postprandial glucagon secretion, and reduce appetite partially by delaying gastric emptying. Initially developed for DM, GLP1-RA have proven to cause weight loss, by suppressing appetite, and to ameliorate many complications of DM and obesity, such as obstructive sleep apnea, heart failure, and kidney dysfunction. They have also been shown to increase the incidence of procedural patients presenting with residual food in their stomachs despite adequate perioperative fasting, but it is still controversial whether this is associated with increased risk of pulmonary aspiration during anesthesia. Which precautionary measures (if any) are indicated is also controversial (see text box). At the time of this writing, and consistent with the most recent multi-society consensus guideline, at MGH we recommend that patients using GLP-1RA observe a prolonged, 24 h clear fluid diet preoperatively. The older recommendation of holding the GLP-1RA preoperatively for one dose is not currently advised. Alternative solutions are evaluation of stomach contents by gastric ultrasound or performing the case with full stomach precautions.

e. **Dipeptidyl peptidase IV (DPP-4) inhibitors** prevent the breakdown of endogenous GLP-1, thereby enhancing insulin secretion and decreasing glucagon secretion in a glucose-dependent manner. They are not associated with significant gastrointestinal side effects or risk of hypoglycemia. There is a potential increased risk of heart failure with some DPP-4 agents in susceptible patients.

f. **Sodium–glucose cotransporter 2 (SGLT2) inhibitors**, such as empagliflozin, decrease renal glucose reabsorption by inhibiting renal SGLT2, which is responsible for more than 90% of renal glucose reabsorption. Use of SGLT2 inhibitors has rapidly expanded due to recent emerging evidence of its cardiovascular and renoprotective benefits. SGLT2 inhibitors do not usually cause hypoglycemia because they induce glucosuria in a plasma glucose–dependent manner. Adverse effects include an increased risk of genitourinary infection, osmotic diuresis leading to volume depletion, and orthostatic hypotension. A feared perioperative complication specifically from SGLT2 inhibitors is euglycemic (glucose <250 mg/dL) diabetic ketoacidosis (eDKA), partially due to prolonged fasting preoperatively. This happens when relative hypoglycemia (as a result of glucosuria and fasting) is coupled with relative hypoinsulinemia (worsened insulin resistance during surgical stress), which causes the body to shift to ketones for alternative energy source. eDKA shares similar pathophysiology, clinical signs, and symptoms with regular DKA, but the relatively low glucose level can delay diagnosis. Current society and FDA guidelines recommend holding SGLT2 inhibitors for 3 to 4 days before surgery. For patients who did not hold this medication properly or presented for emergent procedures, perioperative lab works including basic metabolic panel and blood gas can be sent for close monitoring.

> **BOX 7.1 Current Controversies in Anesthesia: GLP-1 Receptor Agonists and the Risk of Intraprocedural Pulmonary Aspiration**
>
> *Several case reports (including a pioneering one from our department), and retrospective and prospective studies have demonstrated that procedural patients using GLP-1RA have an increased risk of presenting with residual food in the stomach (ie, "full stomachs") despite adhering to the usual 8 hours of preoperative fasting. At least in endoscopy patients, the risk is around fivefold, compared to patients not on GLP1-RA, to an actual incidence of around 20%, even after accounting for other factors that could cause gastroparesis. Whether this is associated with an increase in the incidence of postoperative pulmonary aspiration is controversial, with some authors reporting an increase and others not. Whether the potentially increased risk can be mitigated by either a prolonged, 24 hours nil-per-os for solids period and/or holding the drug preoperatively is currently unclear, although both measures have been proposed. Also unclear is whether all GLP-1RA using patients have the same increased risk, or the risk is higher in patients taking higher doses or/and at the beginning of the therapy. Despite their different opinions, all authors agree that more data is needed to clarify this controversy, and more research will likely appear in the near future. Until then, at MGH, we recommend a modified version of the most recent multi-society guidance, as mentioned in the text.*

   g. **Other less commonly used drugs** include meglitinides and D-phenylalanine derivatives (which act via a nonsulfonylurea receptor pathway to rapidly increase insulin release), α-glucosidase inhibitors (which prevent intestinal absorption of glucose). These drugs can be safely continued in the perioperative period. Amylin analogues, which suppress inappropriate postprandial glucagon secretion and also delay gastric emptying, should be held on the day of surgery (**Box 7.1**).

II. HYPOGLYCEMIA

A. Unexpected delayed emergence or a pre- or postoperative seizure

Any patient who experiences an unexpected delayed emergence or a pre- or postoperative seizure should be investigated for hypoglycemia. A common cause is an inappropriate continuation of insulin and other antidiabetic medication in patients who are fasting preoperatively. Other causes include sepsis, liver failure, a spectrum of pancreatic diseases, including pancreatitis and rarely, an insulinoma, some malignancies, hypopituitarism, adrenal insufficiency, and renal failure in patients who receive insulin (reduced insulin clearance). Signs and symptoms include irritability, tremulousness, headache, confusion, stupor, and tachycardia, palpitations, and hypertension. General anesthesia masks the signs and symptoms of hypoglycemia. Patients with long-standing DM and previous episodes of hypoglycemia often lose sympathetic responses to hypoglycemia, a condition termed hypoglycemic unawareness. In a patient in whom hypoglycemia is suspected, it is imperative to regularly check blood glucose levels, by finger sticks, arterial or venous blood analysis. Glucose boluses will correct a temporary hypoglycemic episode, which, if repeated, can be followed with a continuous glucose infusion.

B. Insulinomas

Insulinomas are insulin-secreting intrapancreatic neuroendocrine tumors. Most insulinomas are benign and present as one solitary tumor in the fourth or fifth decade of life. Anesthetic management during surgical resection of insulinomas presents the challenge of sequentially managing hypoglycemia during the exposure and manipulation of the tumor and hyperglycemia after the resection is completed. Frequent monitoring of blood glucose levels is essential.

III. THYROID DISEASE
A. Overview
1. **Thyroid-stimulating hormone (TSH)** from the anterior pituitary stimulates the thyroid gland to produce triiodothyronine (T3) and L-thyroxine (T4); T3 is more potent than T4, and 80% of serum T3 is produced by peripheral conversion from T4. Both are extensively (>99%) bound to plasma proteins and only the free (unbound) thyroid hormone is biologically active. Thyroid hormones regulate overall body metabolism.
2. **Thyroid disease** is common in the US adult population, with a higher prevalence among women and with increasing age. Serum TSH is the best screening test for determining thyroid function in ambulatory population, with which it is inversely related: High TSH levels are indicative of hypothyroidism, whereas low levels indicate hyperthyroidism.
3. **Hyperthyroidism and hypothyroidism** are thyroid dysfunctions that can arise from a variety of etiologies and have distinct symptomatology and impact on anesthesia management. For both, common principles include:
   a. **Hypo- and hyperthyroid patients** should be adequately treated and made euthyroid before any elective operation.
   b. Only **emergent surgery** should be considered in patients with myxedematous coma or thyroid storm, which represent extreme cases of thyroid dysfunction, and medical emergencies with high mortality.

B. Anesthesia management of hypothyroid patients
1. Currently, **common causes of hypothyroidism** include history of radioiodine therapy and/or thyroidectomy, as well as Hashimoto disease, a chronic autoimmune thyroiditis; in the past, iodine deficiency was more prevalent. Hypothyroidism can also be induced by medications such as amiodarone or lithium, or found in patients with other autoimmune conditions like DM1 or celiac disease and in patients with Down or Turner syndrome. In acute or chronic systemic illness, there is frequently reversible abnormal thyroid function, known as nonthyroidal illness syndrome. Fewer than 1% of cases are due to central TSH deficiency.
2. **Hypothyroidism causes a hypometabolic state**, which could be manifested by depression, cold intolerance, extreme fatigue, muscle aches, irregular menses, constipation, and weight gain. Neck swelling (goiter) and nonpitting edema (myxedema) can be found on exam. Cardiovascular signs include reduced cardiac output due to decreased contractility and heart rate, pericardial effusion, reversible cardiomyopathy, conduction abnormalities, and diminished baroreceptor reflexes. Treatment is titrated thyroid hormone replacement. T4 (available both oral and intravenous) is administered once daily and requires 7 to 10 days to have initial effects; 3 to 4 weeks of therapy are needed to achieve a stable state. T3 is not routinely used as therapy because of its short half-life.
3. **Anesthesia considerations**
   a. Patients should continue their thyroid hormone replacement throughout the perioperative period.

b. Securing the airway may be difficult because of an enlarged tongue, tissue edema, relaxed oropharyngeal tissues, goiter, and delayed gastric emptying.

c. Patients may be prone to hypotension owing to hypovolemia, blunted baroreceptor reflexes, reduced myocardial contractility, and bradycardia.

d. Patients may be susceptible to hypoventilation owing to respiratory muscle weakness and impaired responsiveness to hypoxia and hypercarbia.

e. There may be an increased sensitivity to CNS depressant and paralytic medications.

f. Corticosteroid supplementation should be considered given increased incidence of adrenal insufficiency and reduced catecholamine response in this population.

g. There is an increased likelihood of heart failure, hypothermia, hypoglycemia, hyponatremia, and delayed emergence.

C. Myxedema coma

Myxedema coma is a rare complication in poorly controlled hypothyroidism. It can be triggered by infection, myocardial infarction, cold exposure, surgery, or the administration of sedative drugs, especially opioids. Patients show a global hypofunction, including altered mental status, hypothermia, hypoventilation, hypoglycemia, hyponatremia, decreased cardiac output, and hypotension.

1. Treatment of myxedema coma is with IV T3 and T4.
2. Patients are usually intubated for airway protection.
3. Stress-dose steroids are administered if concomitant primary or secondary adrenal insufficiency is suspected.
4. Electrolyte abnormalities are possible and should be corrected.
5. Management of hypotension and/or heart failure is usually instituted using vasopressors and positive inotropes. Advanced monitoring is therefore essential, should an emergent surgical operation be needed.
6. Pericardial and/or pleural effusions are not uncommon and may need to be drained if patients show persistent circulatory and/or respiratory dysfunction.
7. Passive rewarming is usually instituted and may cause hypotension in those patients who are hypovolemic with peripheral vasoconstriction.
8. Concomitant with patient stabilization, an active search for precipitating causes should be performed.

D. Anesthesia management of hyperthyroid patients

1. **Hyperthyroidism, also known as thyrotoxicosis,** can be caused by Graves disease, toxic multinodular goiter, and toxic adenoma. Excessive thyroid hormone production causes a hypermetabolic state, which leads to tremor, nervousness, insomnia, heat intolerance, hyperhidrosis, muscle weakness, irregular menses, diarrhea, and weight loss. Cardiovascular signs include an increase in cardiac output and pulse pressure, tachycardia, dysrhythmias, and high-output heart failure in predisposed patients.
2. **Diagnosis** is made by demonstration of increased T4 and low TSH levels. Euthyroid hyperthyroxinemia is a condition where total serum T4 concentrations are elevated but serum TSH levels are normal. This can be secondary to thyroid hormone–binding protein disorders or medications, such as propranolol, amiodarone, or amphetamine abuse.
3. **Treatment** consists of:
    a. Antithyroid medications, such as methimazole and propylthiouracil are used primarily. These drugs directly inhibit synthesis of

thyroid hormone but can take 6 to 8 weeks to achieve a euthyroid state. Common side effects of both medications include thrombocytopenia, aplastic anemia, and agranulocytosis; propylthiouracil can also cause fulminant liver failure and antibody-positive vasculitis.
- **b.** Pharmacologic iodine preparations (such as iopanoic acid and saturated solution of potassium iodide, SSKI) should be administered after the initial administration of antithyroid medication.
- **c.** A β-adrenergic blocker should be started in the elderly, patients with a resting heart rate over 90 bpm, or patients with coexisting cardiovascular disease. Calcium channel blockers like verapamil or diltiazem can also be used in patients who do not tolerate β-blockade.
- **d.** Glucocorticoids (hydrocortisone, dexamethasone) can further block thyroid hormone release and T3 to T4 conversion.
- **e.** In appropriate candidates, radioactive ablation or surgical resection is curative.

4. **Anesthesia considerations**
   - **a.** Patients should be euthyroid prior to elective surgery, this can take weeks if they are recently started on antithyroid drugs.
   - **b.** Antithyroid drugs, pharmacologic iodine, and β-blockers should be continued through surgery.
   - **c.** Avoid sympathetic stimulation (pain, anxiety, ketamine, and local anesthetics with epinephrine). Consider generous sedative premedication unless there is concern for airway compromise.
   - **d.** Regional anesthesia may be beneficial in thyrotoxic patients because it blocks sympathetic responses. The addition of epinephrine to the local anesthetic should be avoided owing to the risk of systemic uptake and worsening tachycardia and hypertension.
   - **e.** Thrombocytopenia sometimes occurs in thyrotoxicosis, or as a side effect of antithyroid medication. Consider checking the platelet count before initiating regional anesthesia.
   - **f.** Patients may be hypovolemic owing to hypertension, diarrhea, and perspiration. Postinduction hypotension should be anticipated and treated with vasoconstrictor agents and fluids.
   - **g.** Patients may present with symptoms of heart failure due to tachycardia-induced cardiomyopathy, exacerbation of subclinical ischemic cardiomyopathy, and, in Graves disease, pulmonary hypertension and right heart failure. For these reasons, invasive monitoring can be essential.
   - **h.** Drug metabolism and anesthetic requirements may be increased owing to thyrotoxicosis-related hypermetabolism.
   - **i.** Anesthesia for thyroid surgery is presented in Chapter 30: Anesthesia for Head and Neck Surgery.

E. **Thyroid storm**
   1. A feared **complication of poorly managed thyrotoxicosis is thyroid storm**, an endocrine emergency with around 20% mortality. Even in previously well-compensated patients, a thyroid storm can be triggered by infection, surgery, trauma, cessation of antithyroid medications, excess iodine, iodinated IV contrast agents, and amiodarone and may occur 6 to 18 hours postoperatively. Common signs include hyperpyrexia, altered mental status, tachycardia, hypotension, heart failure, or even circulatory collapse. Thyroid storm may mimic malignant hyperthermia, neuroleptic malignant syndrome, sepsis, hemorrhage, pheochromocytoma crisis, or transfusion/drug reaction.

2. Management principles
  a. Continuation of antithyroid medication and β-blockers is essential.
  b. Glucocorticoids may also be considered because they inhibit the peripheral conversion of T4 to T3 and treat a potentially reduced adrenocortical reserve.
  c. Active cooling, volume resuscitation, and electrolyte replacement should be instituted as needed. Meperidine can attenuate heat production from shivering.
  d. Invasive hemodynamic monitoring is essential.
  e. Postoperative admission to an ICU for ongoing care is usually necessary.

F. Anesthesia management of patients with euthyroid Graves disease
Graves disease is an autoimmune condition caused by the presence of thyroid-stimulating thyrotropin receptor antibodies. Patients usually present with exophthalmos, goiter, and hyper- or euthyroidism.
  1. Prior to a thyroidectomy for Graves disease, preoperative oral iodine solutions may decrease intraoperative blood loss by decreasing thyroid vascularity.
  2. Large goiters may displace and compress the trachea, compromising the airway. Emergency tracheostomy may be difficult in patients with goiter.
  3. Assure full eye protection, as proptotic eyes may not have complete lid closure.
  4. Approximately 65% of patients with Graves disease have pulmonary hypertension. Hypotension in a hypoxemic patient should be treated by rapidly improving oxygenation, and only secondarily with vasopressors.

IV. PARATHYROID DISEASE AND CALCIUM METABOLISM
A. Physiology
Almost every regulated cell process is at some point mediated by temporary spikes in intracellular calcium levels. Membrane excitation, manifested either as an action potential or as the activation of a membrane receptor, leads to a brief calcium entry into the cell, sometimes amplified by intracellular calcium release, which controls muscle contraction, synaptic neurotransmission, hormone secretion, and the activity of several enzyme. Because of that, extracellular calcium level is maintained within a very narrow range. Calcium homeostasis is achieved through the actions of the parathyroid hormone (PTH), vitamin D, and calcitonin. PTH is released when serum ionized calcium and magnesium are low and corrects it by increasing osteoclastic release of calcium and phosphorus from bone and decreasing renal clearance of calcium. PTH also activates vitamin D in the kidneys, which increases calcium absorption from the GI tract. In contrast, calcitonin lowers serum calcium by inhibiting osteoclast activity and renal reabsorption of calcium and phosphorus.

B. Calcium measurement
Serum calcium is found in both bound (primarily to albumin) and unbound forms, and only ionized calcium is physiologically relevant. Hypoalbuminemia produces a decrease in total calcium, and serum calcium levels should be corrected accordingly (0.8 mg/dL calcium per 1 g/dL albumin below normal). Acidemia increases and alkalemia decreases ionized calcium levels owing to hydrogen competing for albumin binding sites.

C. Hypercalcemia
  1. **Etiologies** of hypercalcemia include hyperparathyroidism, malignancy, immobilization, granulomatous diseases, vitamin D intoxication,

familial hypocalciuric hypercalcemia, thyrotoxicosis, drugs (lithium, thiazides, calcium, vitamin A, theophylline), Paget disease, renal disease, and adrenal insufficiency. Primary hyperparathyroidism is usually due to a parathyroid adenoma and is characterized by hypercalcemia and hypophosphatemia with an elevated PTH. Hypercalcemia of malignancy can be due to tumor release of PTH-related protein (a protein that binds the same receptor as PTH) or osteolytic metastases resulting in direct bony destruction and calcium release.

2. **Manifestation.** Mild hypercalcemia is usually asymptomatic. When total serum calcium (corrected for albumin level) is >13 mg/dL, there is an increased risk of end-organ calcification, renal calculi, and nephrocalcinosis. A total serum calcium level of >14 mg/dL is considered an endocrine emergency, as patients may experience uremia, coma, cardiac arrest, or death.

3. **Treatment** of hypercalcemia includes:
    a. Initial treatment for hypercalcemia is hydration with IV normal saline to maintain a urine output of 100 to 150 mL/h. The patient must be monitored for hypokalemia, hypomagnesemia, and fluid overload. Short of overt volume overload, routine administration of diuretics is not recommended.
    b. Calcitonin will lower serum calcium concentrations by 1 to 2 mg/dL in 4 to 6 hours, but its effect is transient (~48 hours) due to tachyphylaxis.
    c. Bisphosphonates decrease bone resorption and are the treatment of choice in severe or life-threatening hypercalcemia and in hypercalcemia of malignancy. The maximum effect occurs in 2 to 4 days. Side effects include renal insufficiency, fever, myalgias, uveitis, and osteonecrosis of the jaw. Lower bisphosphonate doses are used in patients with renal insufficiency.
    d. Denosumab and cinacalcet are alternative therapies for severe hypercalcemia with bisphosphonate intolerance, or resistance to other therapies.
    e. Glucocorticoid therapy is effective in some cases of multiple myeloma, vitamin D toxicity, and granulomatous diseases.
    f. In patients with renal or cardiac failure, dialysis should be considered.
    g. Efforts to find cause of hypercalcemia should be made after initial stabilization.

4. **Anesthetic considerations**
    a. Hypercalcemia >12 mg/dL warrants preoperative correction.
    b. Intravascular volume and other electrolyte abnormalities should be normalized and monitored.
    c. Hypercalcemia has an unpredictable effect on neuromuscular blockade, so muscle relaxants should be carefully titrated. Muscular weakness due to hypercalcemia may worsen respiratory function. Avoid hypoventilation because acidosis increases ionized calcium levels.
    d. Careful positioning is required because patients can be osteoporotic.
    e. Patients with hypercalcemia are predisposed to digitalis toxicity and may have conduction abnormalities. Shortened QTc and high-grade AV block have been described.
    f. Anesthesia for parathyroid surgery is presented in Chapter 30: Anesthesia for Head and Neck Surgery.

D. Hypocalcemia
1. Hypocalcemia is serum calcium <8.5 mg/dL in the absence of hypoalbuminemia or acid/base abnormalities.
2. **Etiologies** include hypoparathyroidism, vitamin D deficiency, chronic kidney disease, hyperphosphatemia, drug effects (furosemide, antiepileptics), and pancreatitis. Hypoparathyroidism is commonly due to destruction of parathyroid glands (surgery, autoimmune diseases, irradiation, infiltrative diseases) and less commonly due to PTH underproduction (sepsis, severe burns). Severe hypomagnesemia (<1 mg/dL) can also lead to PTH underproduction and may cause PTH resistance. In the operating room, hypocalcemia can be seen in hyperventilation leading to a respiratory alkalosis, as well as massive transfusion when citrate (an anticoagulant used in blood products) binds ionized calcium. Because the liver metabolizes citrate, hypocalcemia is often seen during the anhepatic phase of liver transplantation.
3. **Clinical features.** Patients are usually asymptomatic until total calcium is less than 7.0 mg/dL or ionized calcium is less than 2.8 mg/dL (0.7 mmol/L) especially if the onset is gradual.
4. **Chronic hypocalcemia** causes lethargy, muscle cramps, a prolonged QT interval, renal failure, cataracts, dementia, and personality changes.
5. **Acute hypocalcemia** produces neuromuscular irritability with muscle cramps and hand, foot, and circumoral paresthesia. Patients may demonstrate facial nerve irritability to percussion (Chvostek sign) or carpal spasm with tourniquet ischemia for 3 minutes (Trousseau sign).
6. **Severe acute hypocalcemia** results in stridor, laryngospasm, tetany, apnea, coagulopathy, hypotension with catecholamine resistance, psychosis/confusion, and seizures unresponsive to conventional therapy.
7. **Treatment.** Severe or symptomatic hypocalcemia should be treated with IV calcium. Calcium formulations cause chemical phlebitis; hence calcium should be administered centrally whenever possible. One gram of calcium gluconate contains 93 mg of elemental calcium; 1 g of calcium chloride contains 273 mg of elemental calcium. For urgent therapy, 1 to 2 g of calcium gluconate or 1 g of calcium chloride may be given IV over 10 to 20 minutes. Dilution may be needed depending on the available preparation of calcium gluconate or chloride. During parenteral therapy, calcium levels, creatinine, electrocardiogram (ECG), and hemodynamic status must be monitored. Therapeutic goals are a total serum calcium level near 8 mg/dL or an ionized calcium near 1.1 mmol/L in the setting of normal acid/base status. Evaluate and correct abnormalities in serum phosphorus, potassium, and magnesium levels. Treat elevated phosphorus levels with oral phosphate binders; treat low magnesium levels (<1 mg/dL) with parenteral magnesium sulfate.
8. **Management.** Mild to moderate hypocalcemia may be managed with oral calcium and activated vitamin D analogue. Patients require elemental calcium at 1.5 to 3 g/d (3750 to 7500 mg of calcium carbonate) and 1, 25-dihydroxyvitamin D (calcitriol, 0.25 to 3.0 μg/d) in four to six divided doses. For chronic replacement, patients receive calcitriol or vitamin D (ergocalciferol 50,000 IU, once/wk) in addition to calcium.
9. **Anesthetic considerations**
    a. Severe hypocalcemia should be corrected preoperatively. Central access or a large-bore IV is preferred for intravenous calcium administration. When sodium bicarbonate or other compounds are administered simultaneously, they should be given in different lines, because of the theoretical risk of precipitation.

b. Check for and correct hypomagnesemia to sustainably address hypocalcemia.
   c. Frequently check ionized calcium levels during massive transfusion, as the citrate in blood products will chelate calcium.
   d. Cardiovascular effects of hypocalcemia include hypotension with insensitivity to β-adrenergic agonists, a prolonged QT interval, atrioventricular block, and digitalis insensitivity.
   e. Respiratory alkalosis may cause a decrease in ionized calcium with no change in total calcium; consider the underlying cause of a low ionized calcium before treating.

V. ADRENAL CORTICAL DISEASE
A. Physiology
The adrenal glands consist of two functionally distinct areas: the adrenal cortex and the adrenal medulla. The adrenal cortex has three zones, each secreting a different hormone: mineralocorticoids, glucocorticoids, and androgens. The adrenal medulla secretes catecholamines which will be discussed next.

1. Mineralocorticoids

Aldosterone is the principal hormone of this class and a major regulator of extracellular fluid volume and potassium homeostasis. Its production is regulated by the renin–angiotensin–aldosterone system, blood K^+ concentration, and, to a lesser extent, pituitary adrenocorticotropic hormone (ACTH). Increased renin, as a result of decreased renal blood flow, decreased sodium level, or sympathetic activation, promotes the conversion of angiotensinogen to angiotensin I. Angiotensin-converting enzyme (ACE) cleaves angiotensin I to generate angiotensin II. Angiotensin II then stimulates aldosterone secretion. Aldosterone causes reabsorption of Na^+ and subsequently water, as well as excretion of K^+ and H^+ in the distal tubule of the nephron.

2. Glucocorticoids

Cortisol is the principal hormone of this class. It is produced daily in a diurnal manner in response to ACTH from the anterior pituitary, which can be augmented during stress. Cortisol has anti-inflammatory and immunosuppressive properties. It raises blood glucose levels by stimulating gluconeogenesis and promoting insulin resistance. It also has multiple effects on carbohydrate, protein, and fatty acid metabolism. Cortisol is required for converting norepinephrine to epinephrine in the adrenal medulla. Cortisol raises blood pressure by various mechanisms.

3. Androgens

Abnormalities in androgen secretion are rarely pertinent to anesthetic management.

B. Synthetic steroids are used mainly for their immunosuppressive effect in inflammatory diseases and exhibit different potencies, duration of action, and ratios of glucocorticoid to mineralocorticoid effect.

   1. Hydrocortisone (100 to 200 mg IV) is the name of the hormone cortisol as a medication and has the most balanced glucocorticoid to mineralocorticoid effect ratio.
   2. Fludrocortisone has 10 times more mineralo- than glucocorticoid effect and is used to reverse the electrolyte dysfunctions in patients with primary hypoaldosteronism.
   3. Other drugs, such as prednisone, prednisolone, methylprednisolone, and dexamethasone have a marked glucocorticoid anti-inflammatory effect. In the operating room, **methylprednisolone** (125 to 250 mg IV) and

dexamethasone (4 to 8 mg) are the most commonly used, to treat allergic reactions, bronchoconstriction, for immunosuppression during organ transplantation and (controversially) for stress-dose steroid supplementation. Dexamethasone, especially, is also routinely used to prevent postoperative nausea and vomiting (PONV), among other beneficial effects.

C. Primary hyperaldosteronism: Conn syndrome
1. Conn syndrome is **caused by either aldosterone-producing adrenal adenomas or from bilateral adrenal hyperplasia.** Clinical features include hypertension, mild hypernatremia, hypokalemic metabolic alkalosis, hypokalemia-related muscle weakness, and increased incidence of metabolic syndrome. The **recommended treatment** for unilateral aldosterone-producing adrenal adenoma or hyperplasia is adrenalectomy. The treatment for bilateral disease is with a mineralocorticoid receptor antagonist, such as spironolactone or eplerenone.
2. **Anesthesia considerations**
    a. Mineralocorticoid receptor antagonist therapy should be continued perioperatively.
    b. Consider checking serum sodium, potassium, and pH perioperatively. However, due to chronic nature, aggressive correction is rarely necessary.
    c. Avoid hyperventilation as this can worsen alkalosis.
    d. Ensure adequate reversal of neuromuscular blockade as hypokalemia increases effects of nondepolarizing neuromuscular blockers.

D. Glucocorticoid excess and Cushing syndrome
1. **Cushing syndrome is usually caused by excess exogenous steroid administration, excess pituitary ACTH secretion, ectopic ACTH secretion, and excess cortisol secretion.** Clinical features include truncal obesity, moon face, gastroesophageal reflux disease, peptic ulcers, hypertension, hypernatremia, hypervolemia, hyperglycemia, hypokalemia, red or purple cutaneous striae, poor wound healing, muscle wasting and weakness, osteopenia/porosis, hypercoagulability, mental status changes, emotional lability, aseptic osteonecrosis, pancreatitis, benign intracranial hypertension, cataracts, and glaucoma. Treatment includes surgical resection, in the case of ACTH-secreting tumor (pituitary or ectopic) or cortisol-secreting adrenal adenoma. Medical therapy with adrenal enzyme inhibitors (eg, ketoconazole, etomidate) and glucocorticoid receptor antagonists (eg, mifepristone) can be considered in nonresectable disease. In refractory cases, bilateral adrenalectomy is the definitive therapy.
2. **Anesthesia considerations**
    a. **Beware of difficult mask ventilation and intubation,** given central obesity and increased incidence of OSA.
    b. Patients often **exhibit hypertension refractory** to treatment.
    c. Unrecognized coronary artery disease is also **possible.** Consider preoperative cardiac evaluations.
    d. Patients may have **unrecognized insulin resistance.** Monitor serum glucose levels and treat as needed.
    e. Osteoporosis and skin fragility make **careful positioning necessary.**
    f. **Consider venous thrombosis prophylaxis** given hypercoagulability.
    g. **Glucocorticoid replacement should begin postoperatively** for both unilateral and bilateral adrenalectomies. Mineralocorticoid replacement is necessary only after bilateral adrenalectomy.
    h. **Excess ACTH secretion is treated by excision of the secreting tumor,** usually via transsphenoidal pituitary surgery (Chapter 30: Anesthesia for Head and Neck Surgery).

E. Adrenal cortical hypofunction and Addison disease
1. Adrenal cortical hypofunction may be due to dysfunction of the adrenal gland (primary, aka Addison disease), pituitary gland (secondary), or hypothalamus (tertiary), which have different pathologies, manifestations, and anesthesia concerns.
2. **Anesthetic considerations in patients with Addison disease**
   a. **Primary** adrenal insufficiency (Addison disease) is associated with low cortisol and aldosterone levels. In the United States, 80% of primary adrenocortical insufficiency results from autoimmune adrenalitis; other causes include tuberculosis (the most common cause worldwide), various viral conditions [HIV, cytomegalic virus (CMV)], hemorrhage (often from anticoagulants), tumor metastasis, and sepsis.
   b. The **main manifestations are hyponatremia and hyperkalemia**, which lead to psychiatric changes, weakness, fatigue, weight loss, nausea/vomiting, abdominal pain, myalgias, arthralgias, postural hypotension, salt craving, hyperpigmentation, and, frequently, anemia.
   c. **Acute adrenal insufficiency (adrenal crisis) primarily presents as shock and is a life-threatening emergency**. The precipitant is usually a physiologic stressor (eg, surgery, trauma, infection), but can also be inadequate daily doses of mineralocorticoid and/or glucocorticoid, a missed dose, or reduced drug absorption from vomiting or diarrhea.
   d. **Treatment of adrenal crisis** includes:
      1. Elective surgery should be delayed if there is concern for uncorrected adrenal insufficiency.
      2. Identification and correction of hyperkalemia, hyponatremia, and hypoglycemia
      3. Patients with adrenal hypofunction may exhibit marked sensitivity to sedative, anesthetic, or vasodilator drugs. Titrate drug doses carefully to avoid cardiovascular depression.
      4. Avoid etomidate given the potential for further adrenal suppression.
      5. Steroid replacement. Hydrocortisone 100 mg IV followed by 50 mg IV every 6 hours, usually no more than 200 mg daily are necessary; other parental glucocorticoids may be used in equivalent dosages. In primary adrenal insufficiency, daily fludrocortisone is required once the daily hydrocortisone dose is <50 mg.
      6. Stress-dose steroids. Surgery is a known activator of hypothalamic–pituitary–adrenal axis (HPAA) and physiologic cortisol production increases by 5- to 20-fold during surgery. An additional steroid dose (100 to 200 mg hydrocortisone) is probably indicated in patients with known primary adrenal insufficiency. It is controversial whether this is also necessary in patients with chronic high-dose steroid use, which, in principle may suppress HPAA, as discussed below.
      7. Unexplained or exaggerated episodes of intra- or postoperative hypotension should prompt further administration of hydrocortisone (keeping in mind, however, that the effect is nonspecific).
      8. It is important to aggressively identify and treat precipitating events (infection, organ ischemia, internal bleeding) that could be life threatening in themselves.
3. **Anesthetic considerations in patients with secondary and tertiary adrenal insufficiency**
   a. **Secondary and tertiary adrenal insufficiency are caused by pituitary or hypothalamic dysfunction, damage, or tumors and are rare.** Secondary

> **BOX 7.2   Current Controversies in Anesthesia: Stress-Dose Steroids**
>
> *It is controversial whether patients with chronic steroid use need a supplemental dose during surgery. The concept originated with several case reports in the 1950s, describing patients on chronic steroid therapy who developed severe hypotension and died postoperatively, with autopsy showing adrenal gland atrophy. A small number of small retrospective studies followed, as well as two prospective randomized trials totaling 37 relevant patients with and without steroid supplementation, a number too small to draw any conclusions. Despite that, doses of 100 to 200 mg hydrocortisone are well tolerated and commonly used in these patients. Theoretically, the 4 to 8 mg of dexamethasone that is commonly used for PONV prevention in most patients may cover this need as well, but there are currently no studies demonstrating this. Probably none will be performed either, given the lack of demonstrable adverse reactions to the additional doses of steroids. Investigation of the HPAA using ACTH suppression test was also proposed, but rarely used today, because of its poor predicting power. Other authors developed a differentiated strategy that considers steroid exposure and the severity of surgical trauma.*

adrenal insufficiency results in low cortisol levels and normal serum aldosterone because aldosterone production is relatively independent of ACTH. Patients may have panhypopituitarism with symptoms of low TSH, growth hormone (GH), and/or gonadotropin levels. Tertiary adrenal insufficiency is typically due to iatrogenic administration of glucocorticoids. In these patients, the basal steroid treatment should be continued perioperatively. It is controversial whether an additional "stress dose" is indicated in patients on chronic steroid therapy as discussed in the text box (**Box 7.2**).

VI. ADRENAL MEDULLARY DISEASE, PHEOCHROMOCYTOMA, AND PARAGANGLIOMAS

A. Physiology. Pheochromocytomas and paragangliomas are rare catecholamine-secreting neuroendocrine tumors derived from chromaffin cells located in the adrenal medulla and adjacent to sympathetic ganglia. Most tumors secrete epinephrine, norepinephrine, and dopamine, independent of neurogenic control. Pheochromocytomas arise from within the adrenal medulla and are more common (80% to 85% of cases), whereas extra-adrenal catecholamine-secreting tumors (15% to 20%) are referred to as paragangliomas. Pheochromocytomas are typically unilateral but can be bilateral, metastatic, or extra-adrenal. They are associated with an array of familial syndromic disorders, such as multiple endocrine neoplasia type 2, von Hippel–Lindau syndrome, and neurofibromatosis type 1. Many paragangliomas are found in the head and neck and are nonfunctioning. Most functional paragangliomas are found in the abdomen.

B. Manifestations. Clinical features are generally due to excess catecholamine release. The classic presentation includes palpitations, headache, and diaphoresis in an episodically hypertensive patient. Other symptoms include anxiety, flushing, tremor, orthostatic hypotension, hypovolemia, and weight loss. Plasma fractionated metanephrines or a 24-hour urine collection for catecholamines and their metabolites are the routine screening tests and usually show an increase of more than fourfolds from reference values. Borderline results can be confirmed with a clonidine suppression test prior to serum measurement of catecholamines and metanephrines.

Computed tomography (CT) or magnetic resonance imaging (MRI) are used for tumor localization. If metastatic disease is suspected, then functional imaging with 123I-metaiodobenzylguanidine, a radiolabeled norepinephrine analogue, can localize other tumor sites. **Surgery remains the definitive treatment of pheochromocytomas and paragangliomas**, and carries significant risk, especially in patients that cannot be medically optimized preoperatively.

C. Preoperative optimization. The goals of preoperative management are:
1. Adequate blood pressure control. α-receptor blockade is often started as an outpatient, using oral phenoxybenzamine, a long-acting, noncompetitive, nonspecific α-adrenergic blocker, or a shorter-acting, competitive α1-blocker (prazosin, doxazosin). A calcium channel blocker can be used as supplemental or alternative therapy, especially if the patient cannot tolerate α-blockers. Achieving adequate α-receptor blockade may require 7 to 14 days. Clinical endpoints suggesting adequate α-receptor blockade are known as the Roizen criteria and include no blood pressure readings >160/90 mmHg within 24 hours before surgery, postural hypotension (with standing blood pressure >80/45 mmHg), no more than one premature ventricular contraction every 5 minutes, and an ECG that is free of ST–T changes for >1 week. It is important to note that many centers consider preoperative alpha blockade not universally necessary (see **Box 7.3**).
2. Treating or preventing catecholamine-induced dysrhythmias, selective or nonselective β-blockers can be used, with dosing titrated to a heart rate of 60 to 80 bpm. β-Blockade should be instituted only after adequate α-blockade to prevent unopposed vascular α-receptor stimulation and catastrophic hypertensive crisis.
3. Assessing for catecholamine-induced cardiomyopathy. β-Blockade should be used with extreme caution in patients with catecholamine-induced cardiomyopathy.
4. Correcting other preoperative conditions, such as hypovolemia, hyperglycemia, and nausea/vomiting.
5. Comorbid endocrinopathies should be sought and treated.
6. The possibility of an intracranial hemorrhage should also be kept in mind.
7. Metyrosine can also be used for preoperative blood pressure management. It competitively inhibits tyrosine hydroxylase, the rate-limiting enzyme in the synthesis of catecholamines. It is less tolerated because of its side-effect profile.
8. After adequate α-receptor blockade, patients without heart failure or renal dysfunction are encouraged to start a high-sodium diet and increase fluid intake for volume expansion. This is done to attenuate catecholamine-induced volume contraction and prevent significant intraoperative hypotension.

D. Intraoperative management. The primary goal is to prevent and manage dramatic hemodynamic changes. Divided by the time of effluent vein clamping, there is an initial risk of hypertension and arrhythmias during induction and tumor manipulation, followed by hypotension due to the sudden drop of circulating catecholamines.
1. Arterial catheterization for continuous blood pressure monitoring is needed.
2. Central venous access is recommended for fast and definitive administration of vasoactive medications and preload monitoring. Preinduction placement should be considered.

> BOX 7.3 Current Controversies: Is Preoperative α-Blockade Universally Necessary in Pheochromocytoma?
>
> *In an 8-year retrospective study from a German center of excellence (Groeben et al., 2017), more than half of pheochromocytoma patients (n = 177) did not receive preoperative α-blockade, with no increased adverse events. The usual impression that these patients present hypovolemic was also challenged.*

3. A transesophageal echocardiogram and/or pulmonary artery catheterization may be necessary in patients with existing cardiac dysfunction.
4. Thoracic epidural can be considered; however, may lead to worse postoperative hypotension.
5. Avoid preoperative anxiety with generous sedation.
6. Ensure an adequate anesthesia level during induction and maintenance. Propofol and sevoflurane are the best choices, in case hypotension develops after tumor resection. Remifentanil, dexmedetomidine, and magnesium sulfate infusions can be useful additives. Adequately blunt sympathetic responses to induction, intubation, insufflation, incision, and surgical manipulation of the tumor.
7. Avoid sympathomimetic, vagolytic, dopamine-blocking drugs, or histamine-releasing drugs such as desflurane, ketamine, morphine, atracurium, pancuronium, ephedrine, glucagon, and metoclo-pramide.
8. Treat severe hypertension with labetalol, sodium nitroprusside, nitroglycerin, clevidipine, and nicardipine. Hydralazine has a long duration of action and could aggravate postresection hypotension.
9. Arrhythmias can be addressed with β-blockers, calcium channel blockers, and magnesium. Esmolol is preferred because of its rapid onset and short duration of action.
10. Volume loading prior to tumor resection may attenuate hypotension after effluent vein clamping, and treatment with a direct-acting vasopressor is usually necessary. Vasopressin may be particularly helpful as it does not act on adrenergic receptors.
11. Glucose should be monitored frequently. Hyperglycemia is common preoperatively owing to suppression of insulin release, and increased glucose mobilization. Hypoglycemia can be seen after tumor resection.
12. ICU care may be required in the postoperative period.
13. Endogenous catecholamine levels should return to normal shortly after tumor removal, but blood pressure may take much longer to normalize.
14. Patients undergoing bilateral adrenalectomy will require glucocorticoid and mineralocorticoid replacement therapy.
15. Magnesium has many intraoperative uses during pheochromocytoma resection. It has both antiarrhythmic and vasodilating properties owing to its ability to antagonize catecholamine receptors and function as a calcium channel blocker. It can be a useful adjunct but may potentiate the effects of nondepolarizing neuromuscular blocking agents (**Box 7.3**).

VII. ANTERIOR PITUITARY DISEASES
A. Physiology
1. The anterior pituitary regulates the thyroids, adrenals, ovaries, and testes, as well as growth and lactation through the production of TSH, ACTH, follicle-stimulating hormone (FSH), luteinizing hormone (LH), growth hormone (GH), and prolactin.

2. A negative feedback system mediated by peripheral hormones tightly controls anterior pituitary secretion.
3. Anterior pituitary adenomas may lead to hormone excess or hypopituitarism.
4. Macroadenomas (>1 cm in diameter) can compress adjacent structures producing visual disturbances, seizures, or increased intracranial pressure.

B. Anterior pituitary hyperfunction
1. **Pituitary adenoma is the most common cause of anterior pituitary hyperfunction.** Prolactinomas generally do not affect anesthetic management. The hyperthyroidism of a TSH-secreting adenoma and the hyperadrenalism of an ACTH-secreting adenoma are treated as described in the previous sections. The anatomic and physiologic changes seen with GH-secreting tumors are discussed in the sections that follow.

C. Acromegaly and gigantism
1. **Clinical features**
   a. GH stimulates bone, cartilage, and soft tissue growth leading to macrognathia, subglottic narrowing of the trachea, and soft tissue overgrowth of the lips, tongue, epiglottis, and vocal cords. Connective tissue overgrowth can cause recurrent laryngeal nerve paralysis, carpal tunnel syndrome, and other peripheral neuropathies.
   b. These patients often develop glucose intolerance, arthritis, osteoporosis, obstructive sleep apnea, hypertension, cardiomyopathy manifesting as diastolic dysfunction, and arrhythmias. They also have an increased incidence of valvular heart disease, coronary artery disease, and colon cancer.
   c. The primary treatment is surgical removal of the tumor. Medical management for persistent disease after surgery includes dopamine agonists (bromocriptine and cabergoline), somatostatin analogues (octreotide and lanreotide), GH receptor antagonists (pegvisomant), and radiation therapy. Excision of GH-secreting pituitary adenomas is often performed via the transsphenoidal approach.

2. **Anesthetic considerations**
   a. Patients should be evaluated for other endocrinopathies and cardiac disease preoperatively.
   b. Direct blood pressure measurement with an arterial line should be considered, given the risk of compensated cardiomyopathy. The need for additional invasive hemodynamic monitoring depends on the patient's medical status.
   c. Airway management may be challenging. Masking is often difficult, and endotracheal intubation can be challenging. Advanced airway and tracheostomy equipment should be available, and awake fiberoptic intubation should be considered. Small-diameter endotracheal tubes may be required for tight glottic opening.
   d. Serum glucose levels should be carefully monitored.
   e. Patients may be osteoporotic and have an increased susceptibility to peripheral neuropathies. Careful positioning is necessary.

D. Anterior pituitary hypofunction
1. **Etiologies.** Pituitary adenoma is also the most common cause of anterior pituitary hypofunction, if nonfunctional and compressing the rest of the gland. Other causes of pituitary failure include trauma, radiation, pituitary apoplexy, tumors, infiltrative disease, and surgical hypophysectomy. Sheehan syndrome is a condition of pituitary failure in which hemorrhagic shock causes vasospasm and subsequent pituitary necrosis in postpartum women.

2. Anesthetic considerations. Adrenal insufficiency develops over 4 to 14 days after destruction of the pituitary gland. Perioperative glucocorticoid supplementation may be necessary. Because the half-life of thyroid hormone is 7 to 10 days, symptomatic hypothyroidism does not occur until 3 to 4 weeks after pituitary surgery or apoplexy.

VIII. POSTERIOR PITUITARY DISEASES
A. Physiology
1. The posterior pituitary is composed of the nerve terminals of neurons originating in the hypothalamus.
2. Antidiuretic hormone (ADH, also known as vasopressin) and oxytocin are stored in the posterior pituitary.
3. ADH regulates plasma osmolarity and extracellular fluid volume by facilitating renal tubular resorption of free water. Intravascular hypovolemia, pain from trauma or surgery, nausea, and positive airway pressure stimulate ADH secretion. Oxytocin stimulates uterine contraction in labor and milk ejection during lactation.

B. Diabetes insipidus (DI)
1. **Etiologies.** DI results from insufficient ADH secretion by the posterior pituitary (central DI) or failure of the renal tubules to respond to ADH (nephrogenic DI). Causes of central DI include intracranial trauma, hypophysectomy, metastatic disease to the pituitary or hypothalamus, and infiltrative diseases. Causes of nephrogenic DI include hypokalemia, hypercalcemia, sickle cell anemia, obstructive uropathy, chronic renal insufficiency, and lithium therapy. Nephrogenic DI may be seen in the third trimester of pregnancy due to placental vasopressinase and may also be congenital.
2. **Clinical features** include polydipsia and polyuria. Urine output is greater than 2 L/d. The urine is inappropriately dilute, and serum osmolarity is high.
3. **Treatment.** Central DI may be treated with the synthetic vasopressin analogue desmopressin (DDAVP) at 1 to 2 μg subcutaneously or IV every 12 hours as needed (or with an infusion intraoperatively). Side effects of DDAVP include hyponatremia, hypertension, and coronary artery vasospasm. Nephrogenic DI is usually not responsive to DDAVP. Adequate oral or parenteral hydration must be assured. Inhibition of prostaglandin synthesis (by ibuprofen, indomethacin, or aspirin) or mild salt depletion with a thiazide diuretic may help reduce urine volume.
4. **In patients who cannot drink or do not have an intact thirst mechanism, hypernatremia can ensue.** Initial therapy should be with isotonic fluids (normal saline) to reverse shock. Then hypotonic fluids (half normal saline or dextrose) can be used if necessary to gradually correct hypernatremia. Careful monitoring and titration of urine output and plasma volume, sodium, and osmolarity are needed.

C. Syndrome of inappropriate antidiuretic hormone secretion (SIADH)
SIADH is represented by the persistent secretion of ADH in the absence of an osmotic stimulus. SIADH can be caused by malignancy, CNS disorders (stroke, trauma, infection, and tumor), pulmonary disorders (tuberculosis, pneumonia, positive-pressure ventilation, and chronic obstructive pulmonary disease), and many drugs (nicotine, amitriptyline, chlorpropamide, clofibrate, serotonin reuptake inhibitors, nonsteroidal anti-inflammatory drugs, haloperidol, amiodarone, ciprofloxacin, valproate, methotrexate, and some chemotherapies). Other etiologies include lupus, HIV, Guillain–Barré syndrome, hypothyroidism, Addison disease, heart failure, and cirrhosis. SIADH is associated with urine osmolality greater than serum

osmolality (with a low serum osmolality), urine sodium greater than 20 mEq/L, and serum sodium less than 130 mEq/L. If serum sodium falls below 110 mEq/L, cerebral edema and seizures may result.

Treatment includes addressing the underlying cause and fluid restriction (800 to 1000 mL daily) for the mild and/or asymptomatic hyponatremia of SIADH. Chronic hyponatremia is generally not treated unless it is associated with symptoms, or the serum sodium is <120 mEq/L. Treatments include oral salt tablets or hypertonic saline for severe cases. Classically, the teaching was that hyponatremia should be corrected no faster than 0.5 mEq/L/h because overly aggressive correction may produce central pontine myelinolysis, an irreversible neurologic disorder, however, this recommendation has been recently challenged. Demeclocycline antagonizes the effects of ADH on renal tubules and may be helpful. Vasopressin receptor antagonists (eg, tolvaptan), may also be helpful but are associated with a concerning safety profile.

IX. CARCINOID
A. Physiolopgy, pathology and management
1. **Carcinoid tumors are part of the group of neuroendocrine tumors**, together with pheochromocytomas, paragangliomas, and insulinomas, discussed in the previous section. Carcinoid tumors are derived from enterochromaffin or Kulchitsky cells and arise from different embryonic divisions of the gut: Foregut tumors occur in the lungs and bronchi (~25%) or stomach (10%), midgut carcinoid tumors are found in the small intestine (30%), appendix, and proximal large bowel; hindgut carcinoid tumors arise in the distal colon or rectum (20%).
2. The term "carcinoid" is misleading, because these tumors are veritable cancers that frequently metastasize, mostly to the liver. **The defining characteristic is their ability to secrete hormones, most commonly serotonin (which is synthetized from 5-hydroxytryptophan), but also histamine, dopamine, substance P, neurotensin, prostaglandins, kallikrein, and corticotrophin.** Most tumors are typically indolent, because hormones released from gastrointestinal tumors are metabolized in the liver, and lung tumors are less secretory than others; however in approximately 10% of patients (commonly with liver metastases), the unregulated release of hormones induces carcinoid syndrome. Characterized classically by the triad of flushing, diarrhea, and wheezing, the syndrome can also include tachy- or bradycardia, hypo- or hypertension, and hypo- or hyperglycemia.
3. **Carcinoid syndrome can be triggered by** tryptophan and tyramine-rich foods (such as cheeses, chocolate, and pickled vegetables), supplements, alcoholic beverages, catecholamines (released during exercise, pain, or anxiety), and histamine.
4. In the **perioperative period**, a severe life-threatening carcinoid crisis could be induced by endotracheal intubation or surgical stimulation of an inadequately anesthetized patient, episodes of hypotension, or direct surgical manipulation of the tumor. Diagnosis is made clinically and confirmed by increased levels of urinary 5-hydroxyindoleacetic acid (5-HIAA, a serotonin metabolite) and serum chromagraffin A (a glycoprotein secreted with other hormones).
5. **Treatment** is by removal of the tumor, either by surgery, embolization, or radiofrequency ablation. Patients with metastatic disease benefit from various chemotherapy agents. Symptomatic patients are treated with octreotide or lanreotide, somatostatin analogues that are administered

daily monthly subcutaneous injections. They can also be given as an IV bolus in carcinoid crisis. The drugs act by inhibiting the secretion of hormones, so they may prevent or minimize future symptoms, but have limited value in the emergent treatment of an established crisis.

6. **In addition to carcinoid syndrome, the tumors may exert obstructive effects, either pulmonary (as postobstructive pneumonias, usually) or gastrointestinal (as a partial small bowel obstruction).** In chronic disease, plaque-like deposits of fibrous tissue can form in the right heart, resulting in tricuspid regurgitation, pulmonic valve stenosis, and right ventricular failure. Left-sided valvular disease is unusual owing to inactivation of humoral substances by the lung. Rarely, high serotonin synthesis rates may lead to tryptophan depletion and niacin deficiency, which is associated with dermatitis, diarrhea, and dementia.

B. **Preoperative anesthetic considerations.** Patients with carcinoid tumors may present in three distinct situations:

1. **Patients with known, symptomatic carcinoid disease**, on chronic somatostatin analogue treatment. In these patients, somatostatin analogue therapy should be continued perioperatively. In conjunction with the surgeon and endocrinologist, high-risk patients may require preoperative admission for therapy augmentation with intravenous infusions. Despite these efforts, even in the absence of preoperative symptoms and increased serology markers, a carcinoid crisis may still be triggered by the stress of surgery, and a high index of suspicion must be kept pre-, intra-, and postoperatively. Right heart investigation with echocardiography is essential. In patients with severe diarrhea, hypovolemia, hypoproteinemia, and vitamin deficiencies should be corrected before surgery, most efficiently parenterally. Triggers of mediator release should be avoided, such as anxiety, pain, hypotension, hypoxia, hypercarbia, tumor compression, drugs that cause histamine or catecholamine release, or sympathetic stimulation. Advanced monitoring with arterial and potentially central venous lines may be necessary, as well as a postoperative admission to an ICU for close monitoring, at least for 48 to 72 hours. A large blood loss could be expected, since these tumors are vascular.

2. **Asymptomatic patients.** Most patients with one primary carcinoid tumor, most commonly in the small intestine, stomach, or lungs, are asymptomatic when they present for tumor resection. It is yet unclear whether all these patients should receive somatostatin analogues preoperatively. While some centers apply this preventive measure uniformly, it is rarely done at MGH, in asymptomatic patients. However, increased vigilance must be exercised for the development of carcinoid crisis perioperatively and some or all of the precautionary measures detailed above may be used.

3. **Accidental discovery of a carcinoid tumor.** It must be kept in mind that any solid tumors that do not have a histopathologic characterization may represent carcinoid. In these cases, patients are usually undergoing surgical resection or biopsy because of obstructive symptoms or after incidental findings of a solid tumor or enlarged lymph nodes. Any episodes of cardiovascular instability (hypo- or hypertension, brady- or tachycardia), wheezing, or skin flushing temporarily associated with surgical manipulation of the tumor, or with intubation may, in fact, represent a carcinoid crisis and should be differentiated from other etiologies and treated as described below.

BOX 7.4 Current Controversies in Anesthesia: Octreotide: First- or Second-Line Treatment in Carcinoid Crisis

It is still controversial whether carcinoid crisis should be treated first with octreotide or with direct agents targeted at the primary symptoms. Retrospective reviews have been published showing either strategy can effectively end crisis.

C. Carcinoid crisis

1. A carcinoid crisis may occur immediately preoperatively, intraoperatively, or in the immediate postoperative period. A high degree of vigilance is necessary, because many of the symptoms are nonspecific, at least initially. Differential diagnosis include anaphylaxis, malignant hyperthermia, serotonin release syndrome, myocardial infarction, asthmatic attack, or, intraoperatively, a reflex response to acute blood loss. In some patients, increased serotonin release can lead to a delayed emergence.
2. Flushing is usually a warning sign and should lead to administration of octreotide, in an attempt to prevent the development of a full crisis. Bronchoconstriction, bradycardia, tachycardia, hypotension, or hypertension are treated as usual (as detailed in Chapter 17: Intra-anesthetic Problems). The old recommendation to avoid β-agonists, out of concern that they can stimulate mediator release, has largely been refuted, and they are commonly used to treat bradycardia, hypotension or bronchoconstriction. In principle, vasopressin may be more desirable for treatment of hypotension. Octreotide boluses (20 to 50 μg, titrated to effect) or infusion (starting at 50 μg/h) should be administered for prevention of further hormone release, keeping in mind that this has little effect on already established symptoms. Postoperative disposition to an intensive care unit is usually necessary, especially if an octreotide taper is required (**Box 7.4**).

Suggested Readings

Fang F, Ding L, He Q, Liu M. Preoperative management of pheochromocytoma and paraganglioma. *Front Endocrinol (Lausanne).* 2020;11:586795.

Fernandez-Robles C, Carr ZJ, Oprea AD. Endocrine emergencies in anesthesia. *Curr Opin Anaesthesiol.* 2021;34(3):326–334.

Fraser CG, Preuss FS, Bigford WD. Adrenal atrophy and irreversible shock associated with cortisone therapy. *J Am Med Assoc.* 1952;149(17):1542–1543.

Groeben H, Walz MK, Nottebaum BJ, et al. International multicentre review of perioperative management and outcome for catecholamine-producing tumours. *Br J Surg.* 2020;107(2):e170–e178.

Himes CP, Ganesh R, Wight EC, Simha V, Liebow M. Perioperative evaluation and management of endocrine disorders. *Mayo Clin Proc.* 2020;95(12):2760–2774.

Kindel TL, Wang AY, Wadhwa A, et al. Representing the American Gastroenterological Association, American Society for Metabolic and Bariatric Surgery, American Society of Anesthesiologists, International Society of Perioperative Care of Patients with Obesity, and the Society of American Gastrointestinal and Endoscopic Surgeons. Multi-society clinical practice guidance for the safe use of glucagon-like peptide-1 receptor agonists in the perioperative period. *Surg Endosc.* 2025;39(1):180–183.

Kelly KN, Domajnko B. Perioperative stress-dose steroids. *Clin Colon Rectal Surg.* 2013;26(3):163–167.

Klein SR, Hobai IA. Semaglutide, delayed gastric emptying, and intraoperative pulmonary aspiration: a case report. *Can J Anaesth.* 2023;70(8):1394–1396.

Lewis L, Robinson RF, Yee J, Hacker LA, Eisen G. Fatal adrenal cortical insufficiency precipitated by surgery during prolonged continuous cortisone treatment. *Ann Intern Med.* 1953;39(1):116–126.

Liu MM, Reidy AB, Saatee S, Collard CD. Perioperative steroid management: approaches based on current evidence. *Anesthesiology.* 2017;127(1):166–172.

MacKenzie CR, Goodman SM. Stress dose steroids: myths and perioperative medicine. *Curr Rheumatol Rep.* 2016;18(7):47.

Maxwell JE, Naraev B, Halperin DM, Choti MA, Halfdanarson TR. Shifting paradigms in the pathophysiology and treatment of carcinoid crisis. *Ann Surg Oncol.* 2022;29(5):3072–3084.

McCully BH, Kozuma K, Pommier S, Pommier RF. Comparison of octreotide and vasopressors as first-line treatment for intraoperative carcinoid crisis. *Ann Surg Oncol.* 2024;31(5):2996–3002.

Naranjo J, Dodd S, Martin YN. Perioperative management of pheochromocytoma. *J Cardiothorac Vasc Anesth.* 2017;31(4):1427–1439.

Oleinikov K, Avniel-Polak S, Gross DJ, Grozinsky-Glasberg S. Carcinoid syndrome: updates and review of current therapy. *Curr Treat Options Oncol.* 2019;20(9):70.

Peramunage D, Nikravan S. Anesthesia for endocrine emergencies. *Anesthesiol Clin.* 2020;38(1):149–163.

Preiser JC, Provenzano B, Mongkolpun W, Halenarova K, Cnop M. Perioperative management of oral glucose-lowering drugs in the patient with type 2 diabetes. *Anesthesiology.* 2020;133(2):430–438.

Thiruvenkatarajan V, Meyer EJ, Nanjappa N, Van Wijk RM, Jesudason D. Perioperative diabetic ketoacidosis associated with sodium-glucose co-transporter-2 inhibitors: a systematic review. *Br J Anaesth.* 2019;123(1):27–36.

Urmson K. Stress dose steroids: the dogma persists. *Can J Anaesth.* 2020;67(2):276–277.

Wu F, Smith MR, Mueller AL, et al. Association of glucagon-like peptide receptor 1 agonist therapy with the presence of gastric contents in fasting patients undergoing endoscopy under anesthesia care: a historical cohort study. *Can J Anaesth.* 2024;71(7):958–966.

Yong SL, Marik P, Esposito M, Coulthard P. Supplemental perioperative steroids for surgical patients with adrenal insufficiency. *Cochrane Database Syst Rev.* 2009;(4):CD005367.

Infectious Diseases and Infection Control in Anesthesia

Ashwini Joshi and Jamie L. Sparling

I. INTRODUCTION

A. The Centers for Disease Control and Prevention (CDC) estimated that in the United States, there were approximately 687,000 nosocomial infections in 2015 which contributed to 72,000 deaths. In 2022, acute care hospitals reported over 23,000 central line–associated bloodstream infections, 32,000 ventilator-associated events, and over 22,000 surgical site infections. In addition to the morbidity and mortality, these complications cost billions of dollars annually.

B. **Infection control responsibilities of anesthesia providers**
  1. **Carefully adhere to infection control measures** to prevent transmission of infectious agents between patients and between patients and operating room (OR) personnel.
  2. **Avoid infectious complications associated with anesthetic procedures** such as central venous catheter (CVC) insertion and epidural placement.
  3. **Prevent surgical wound infections and antibiotic resistance** with timely and appropriate perioperative antibiotic administration and thoughtful antibiotic stewardship.

II. INFECTION CONTROL IN THE OR

A. **Methods of infection spread**
  1. **Contact** with a colonized person, an actively infected person, a host, or a fomite is the most frequent route of transmission in the OR.
  2. **Body fluids** (blood, urine, cerebrospinal fluid) are a method of transmission that depends on access to a mucosal surface or a break in the integrity of the skin barrier.
  3. **Droplet transmission** is the transfer of infectious particles via suspension in large fluid droplets such as those released during coughing or sneezing which travel short distances (ie, 3 to 6 feet).
  4. **Airborne transmission** is similar to droplet transmission with the exception that aerosolized particles are small enough to remain suspended in air and travel in air currents.

B. **Standard or universal precautions** constitute a minimum of acceptable guidelines that should be used for all patient populations regardless of infectious status.
  1. **Hand hygiene** has consistently been shown to be the single most important method for preventing nosocomial infections. An alcohol-based hand rub or hand washing with soap and water should be used for at least 15 seconds before and after any patient contact including any contact with equipment in the immediate vicinity of the patient. Observational studies of hand hygiene reveal that anesthetists have variable adherence to basic hand hygiene requirements including missed opportunities for hand hygiene, short duration of handwashing, and incomplete cleaning of all surfaces of the hands and fingers. Some providers advocate for performing hand hygiene approximately eight

times/h during anesthetic care in the OR, placing alcohol-based hand rub in strategic locations, and double gloving during laryngoscopy, with removal of the top gloves after intubation, to reduce the likelihood of patient and workspace contamination.
2. **Personal protective equipment (PPE)** including gloves, gowns, masks, eye protection, and face shields should be readily available. Gloves should be used any time there is potential for contact with body fluids, and additional protective gear should be used when indicated based on precaution requirements.
3. **Safe injection practices, respiratory hygiene/cough etiquette, and use of masks for neuraxial procedures** have recently been added to the CDC's definition of Standard Precautions. Of note, respiratory hygiene includes use of surgical masks when appropriate, covering the mouth and nose with a tissue while coughing or sneezing and timely disposal of the contaminated tissue, hand hygiene after contact with respiratory secretions, and spatial separation of >3 feet between individuals when possible.
4. **Appropriate OR attire** to prevent infectious spread includes clean scrubs that have not been worn outside of the OR, a cap or bouffant that covers all hair including beards, a mask, and either OR dedicated closed-toed shoes or shoe covers over general use closed-toed shoes. The use of cloth hats, compared with disposable bouffants, does not significantly impact SSI rates.

C. **Transmission-based precautions** are necessary in addition to standard precautions and are based on specific pathogens and their mode of transmission. Transmission-based precautions include contact precautions, droplet precautions, and airborne precautions. Steps for each type of precaution are listed in **Table 8.1**. Organisms with multiple routes of transmission may require multiple simultaneous transmission-based precautions. For example, at our institution, "enhanced respiratory isolation" for SARS-CoV-2 includes elements from both contact precautions and airborne precautions.
1. **Contact precautions** are applied to patients with pathogens that can be transmitted by direct or indirect contact. The most frequently encountered organisms are methicillin-resistant *Staphylococcus aureus* (MRSA), vancomycin-resistant Enterococcus (VRE), extended-spectrum beta-lactamase (ESBL) Enterobacteriaceae, multidrug-resistant organisms (MDRO), and vancomycin intermediate sensitivity (VISA) or vancomycin-resistant *Staphylococcus aureus* (VRSA). In recent years, many hospitals have discontinued contact precautions for MRSA due to its high penetration in the community; nevertheless, the CDC continues to recommend contact precautions for patients colonized or infected with MRSA. Routine screening via rectal (VRE) and nasal (MRSA) swabs has increased the identification of colonized patients, thus increasing the number of patients on contact precautions. Removal of contact precautions is hospital specific and organism specific. Typical standards include cessation of antibiotics for at least 48 hours, negative cultures from the infected site if applicable, and three negative cultures on different dates from the common site of colonization (MRSA—nasal, VRE—rectal).
2. **Contact precautions plus** is for patients with known or suspected infection with spore-forming or alcohol-resistant organisms that can be transmitted by direct or indirect contact. The most frequently encountered is *Clostridium difficile*. In addition to contact precautions, hands

TABLE 8.1 Transmission-Based Precautions

Transmission Type	Example Pathogens	Precautions	Transportation
Contact precautions	Methicillin-resistant *S. aureus* (MRSA), vancomycin intermediate sensitivity (VISA) or vancomycin-resistant *S. aureus*, vancomycin-resistant Enterococcus (VRE), extended-spectrum beta-lactamase (ESBL) Enterobacteriaceae, multidrug-resistant organisms (MDRO)	**Gloves and gowns** should be donned prior to entering and removed upon exiting the patient room. **Alcohol-based hand cleanser or hand washing** should occur prior to gowning and gloving and immediately following gowning and glove removal. Hands must be washed with water and soap after glove and gown removal if *Contact Plus*.	**Cover or contain** the infected or colonized areas of the patient's body. Policies regarding wearing PPE during transport vary according to institution. **Medical records** should be kept outside of the patient room and transported in a plastic bag.
Droplet precautions	Influenza, rhinovirus, adenovirus, *N. meningitidis*, *M. pneumoniae*, *B. pertussis*, Group A Streptococcus (if <24 h of antibiotic therapy)	**Disposable surgical masks** should be worn by providers when within 3 feet of the patient and should be disposed of immediately after exiting the room. **Hand hygiene** should be completed after disposing of the mask.	**Transportation** of the patient requires the patient to wear a surgical mask and to follow respiratory hygiene/cough etiquette.
Airborne precautions	*M. tuberculosis*, Varicella (chickenpox), Rubeola (measles)	**N95 respirators or powered air-purifying respirators (PAPRs)** should be worn whenever in the patient's room. These are specialized masks that require fit testing and training prior to use. **Negative pressure** isolation rooms are required, and doors should remain closed. If a negative-pressure room is unavailable, the patient is required to wear a mask.	**Transportation** of the patient requires the patient to wear a surgical mask and those providing direct care to wear an N95 respirator.

must be washed with water and soap after glove and gown removal. These precautions may be discontinued after completion of an appropriate antibiotic course and resolution of symptoms.
3. **Droplet precautions** are for patients with known or suspected infection with organisms that are transmissible via large respiratory droplets. The most frequently encountered organisms/diseases include meningococcal meningitis, Mycoplasma pneumonia, and influenza.
4. **Airborne precautions** are for patients with known or suspected infection with organisms that may remain suspended in the air and be dispersed by air currents. The most frequently encountered organisms include pulmonary tuberculosis and Varicella.

D. **OR hygiene standards**
1. **Bactericidal cleaning agents** should be used between all cases on the anesthesia machine, monitors, and workstation.
2. **Clean workstation standards** at MGH mandate that any item that has touched the anesthesia machine tray will be discarded between cases to prevent cross-contamination. Designated clean areas, such as the medication cart and the top of the anesthesia machine at MGH, are used for clean, readily available equipment and should not be contaminated with dirty items that have come into contact with a patient. Hand hygiene should be performed between touching items that are considered "dirty" and touching the clean areas of the workstation.
3. **Sterilization of reusable equipment** between uses is necessary (ie, laryngoscopes, reusable laryngeal mask airways [LMAs], bronchoscopes, reusable stylets). Alternatively, single-use, disposable laryngoscope blades and handles are available.
4. **Bacterial and viral contamination of the anesthesia machine** and the possibility of cross-contamination between patients is a controversial topic. Available data have shown no significant difference in postoperative pulmonary infection rate between reusable circuits that are appropriately cleaned and disposable circuits. The high oxygen content, metallic ions, and the shifts in temperature and humidity present within the machine are bactericidal. The COVID-19 pandemic resulted in universal application of viral filters between the airway and sampled gas, and between the expiratory limb of the breathing circuit and the anesthesia machine.
5. **Air exchanges** in the OR should occur at a minimum of 15 times per hour, and the OR should be maintained at a positive pressure relative to surrounding areas with few exceptions (ie, airborne precaution patient).

E. **Avoid anesthesia-associated infectious complications**
1. **Access-related complications**
   a. **Peripheral intravenous lines** should be placed after cleaning the insertion site with an approved cleaning solution (at MGH, these include 70% isopropyl alcohol, povidone-iodine, or 2% chlorhexidine/70% isopropyl alcohol) and covered with a transparent occlusive dressing. Care should be taken to ensure that the needle and catheter are not touched or contaminated during line placement.
   b. **Central venous catheters (CVC)** are a major source of potentially avoidable nosocomial infections. The most common sites of venous cannulation are the femoral, internal jugular, and subclavian veins. It was traditionally taught that femoral lines were the "dirtiest," and subclavian lines the "cleanest," but recent studies indicate that sterile technique in placement and daily assessment is more important

than site choice. Central line–associated blood stream infection (CLABSI) is a source of major morbidity and health care expenditure, but the adoption of prevention bundles has decreased the rate of CLABSI by 46% from 2008 to 2013. While rates of CLABSI rose by up to 325% at a single center during the height of the COVID-19 pandemic, rates have again declined between 2021 and 2022.

c. **Causes** include infection from skin flora at the site, contamination of infusions or catheter hubs, and seeding from distant sites. Emergency insertion, incomplete adherence to aseptic technique, long duration in situ, an increased number of lumens, multiple catheter manipulations, use for total parenteral nutrition, malnutrition, immunocompromise, obesity (BMI >40), long hospital stay prior to CVC insertion, prematurity, and challenging venous access heighten the risk of CLABSI. The most common pathogens are bacteria including Staphylococcus and Streptococcus spp. as well as Candida spp.

d. **Protocols** for placement and daily care have been shown in multiple studies to decrease CLABSI. Use of a checklist, all-inclusive catheter insertion kit, and dedicated monitoring personnel during placement ensures strict sterile technique including maximal barrier precautions, full draping of the patient, aseptic technique (hand prep, site prep, sterile gown and gloves, mask), appropriate dressing, and decontamination of hubs and caps. Use of a daily care checklist ensures site skin integrity, maintenance of a transparent occlusive dressing, and ongoing evaluation for necessity of central access as well as appropriateness of removal. Routine replacement of CVC has not shown any clinical benefit.

e. **Diagnosis** of CLABSI is based on clinical manifestations, ranging from localized signs of infection to septic shock, combined with laboratory culture data. Blood, sputum, and urine cultures as well as wound cultures if applicable should be obtained prior to antibiotic initiation. If further clarity is required, simultaneous quantitative blood cultures, one from a peripheral site and one from the CVC, should be obtained. A threefold higher colony count on the culture from the CVC or >2 hours earlier positive culture in a central line sample compared with a peripheral sample supports the diagnosis of CLABSI. Of note, the National Healthcare Safety Network (NHSN) defines CLABSI as any bloodstream infection in a patient who has had an indwelling CVC for >48 hours at the time of blood culture collection, if no other source is identified.

f. **Treatment** of CLABSI includes removal of the CVC and replacement at a new site. Changing the catheter over a guide wire should be avoided. Empiric antibiotic coverage is appropriate with narrowing of coverage as soon as Gram stain and culture data allow. Typical antibiotic courses for uncomplicated CLABSI are 7 to 14 days, but longer courses may be indicated for fungal infections and immunocompromised hosts.

g. **Aseptic technique for medication administration** via established vascular access reduces iatrogenic bacteremia and pathogen transmission. Best practices include cleaning medication vials with an alcohol wipe after removal of the dust cover, disinfecting injection ports with alcohol prior to access, use of disinfectant caps for ports not in use, and avoiding open lumens (uncovered stopcocks). Proper disinfection technique with alcohol involves scrubbing the

vial or port with 70% to 90% isopropyl alcohol with friction for 5 to 30 seconds and then allowing the port to air dry. All injection ports, IV tubing, and syringe tips should be kept off the floor. Each medication vial, fluid bag, tubing, connector, and syringe may be used for a single patient only. Syringe tips should be covered with a sterile cap or blunt-tip needle to avoid contamination by fingers or other surfaces.
- h. **Strict sterile techniques for other invasive procedures** including site cleaning, drapes, mask, and sterile gloves should be used for these procedures including epidural placement, spinals, arterial lines, and peripheral nerve blocks.
- i. **Reusable ultrasound equipment** has recently been recognized as a potential vector for nosocomial infections and has a wide range of clinical applications in anesthetic practice, including vascular access, guidance for neuraxial procedures, point-of-care transthoracic echocardiography or gastric ultrasound, and transesophageal echocardiography (TEE). Surface ultrasound near nonintact skin, ultrasound for vascular access, and TEE are considered "semicritical" infection risks by the Spaulding system. Use of a sterile probe cover and high-level disinfection are recommended.

2. **Airway-related complications**
   - a. **Postoperative pulmonary complications (PPCs)** include respiratory infection, respiratory failure, pleural effusion, atelectasis, pneumothorax, bronchospasm, and aspiration pneumonitis. The ARISCAT group found that acute respiratory infection, with fever and antibiotic treatment, in the month prior to surgery was an independent predictor for developing a PPC. While the postoperative pulmonary complication risk of active viral perioperative upper respiratory infections is not well quantified in the adult population, this may be a reasonable concern necessitating delaying elective surgery depending on other patient risk factors and the risk of delaying surgery. Specific pathogens, such as SARS-CoV-2 and influenza virus have been shown to increase perioperative mortality (see below). Pediatric patients, who have frequent upper respiratory infections, merit special consideration given their increased risk of perioperative respiratory events.
   - b. **Ventilator-associated events (VAEs)** include both infectious and noninfectious complications associated with mechanical ventilation and are broadly defined as worsening oxygenation (ie, increased PEEP or FiO_2 requirements) after 2 calendar days of respiratory stability or improvement while mechanically ventilated for at least 4 days. According to the CDC, most VAEs are due to potentially preventable etiologies of respiratory infection, acute respiratory distress syndrome, pulmonary edema, and atelectasis. Interventions to reduce the likelihood of developing a ventilator-associated event are most relevant to an intensive care unit setting and include avoiding intubation, minimizing duration of intubation and mechanical ventilation, lung-protective ventilation, daily spontaneous breathing trial, minimizing sedation, daily toothbrushing, judicious fluid administration, consideration of recruitment maneuvers, and prevention of aspiration.
   - c. **Aspiration pneumonitis and aspiration pneumonia** are potentially lethal anesthetic complications as a result of aspiration of oropharyngeal or gastric contents that can occur at any point when the airway is not secured. Microaspiration can also occur around the

endotracheal tube cuff and is shown to correlate with ventilator-associated pneumonia (VAP) in the ICU.
   1. **Aspiration pneumonia** indicates an actual infection resulting from aspiration of gastric contents while **aspiration pneumonitis** reflects a noninfectious chemical pneumonitis. Differentiation between the two can be challenging, and as such, antibiotic therapy should not be reflexively initiated for all aspiration events.
   2. **Risk factors for aspiration** include emergency surgery, insufficient fasting time prior to induction, pregnancy, gastroparesis or other functional obstruction, bowel obstruction, and severe gastroesophageal reflux.
   3. **Risk factors for aspiration pneumonia** include large volume of aspiration, aspiration of low pH content matter, aspiration of particulate matter, immunocompromised status, known colonization of secretions, and recent administration of GLP-1 receptor agonists.
   4. **Treatment** of aspiration pneumonia should target the most frequent bacteria encountered: *S. aureus*, *Escherichia coli*, *Pseudomonas aeruginosa*, *Klebsiella pneumoniae*, and anaerobes. Broad-spectrum antibiotics may be indicated if pneumonitis has not improved in the first 48 hours. Narrowing of antibiotics should be accomplished as soon as possible based on respiratory Gram stain and culture. Steroids are no longer routinely administered for aspiration pneumonia, and therapeutic bronchoalveolar lavage (BAL) should be avoided.
3. **Transfusion-transmitted infections** have been minimized by careful donor screening and by using stringent testing protocols for all donated blood products. Use of appropriate transfusion thresholds can decrease the frequency and quantity of transfusion to additionally decrease related infection rates. The most common transfusion-related infection is bacterial contamination (1 in 2000 to 2500 platelet transfusions, according to the CDC), most commonly with Gram-positive bacteria that is typically part of skin flora. Transmission of viruses such as Hepatitis B, Hepatitis C, and human immunodeficiency virus (HIV); tick-borne illness; and parasites is rare.

III. PERIOPERATIVE ANTIBIOTICS
A. Indications for administration of antibiotics in the OR
   1. **Continuation of ongoing treatment** for active infection
   2. **Prophylaxis against surgical site infection**
   3. **Prophylaxis against endocarditis**
B. Principles of prophylaxis
   1. Surgical site infections are the costliest hospital-acquired infection and increase hospital length of stay, morbidity, and mortality. In 2015, the CDC estimated that 110,800 surgical site infections occurred in the United States with an average prolongation of hospital stay by 9.7 days and up to 11-fold increased risk of mortality.
   2. **Surgical Care Improvement Project (SCIP)** is a national initiative to improve surgical outcomes. Antibiotic prophylaxis and stewardship are a major part of the measures.
      a. **SCIP-1.** Preoperative antibiotic dosed within 1 hour before incision time. Exceptions include vancomycin and fluoroquinolones, which require administration within 120 minutes of incision due to longer administration times. Of note, not all procedures warrant routine antibiotic prophylaxis.

TABLE 8.2 SCIP-Recommended Perioperative Prophylactic Antibiotics

Surgical Procedure/Site	SCIP-Approved Antibiotics
Coronary artery bypass grafting (CABG), other cardiac, or vascular	Cefazolin, cefuroxime, OR vancomycin[a] If β-lactam allergy: vancomycin[b] OR clindamycin
Hip/knee arthroplasty	Cefazolin, cefuroxime, OR vancomycin[a] If β-lactam allergy: vancomycin[b] OR clindamycin[b]
Colon	Cefotetan, cefoxitin, ampicillin/sulbactam, OR ertapenem[c] OR cefazolin OR cefuroxime *and* metronidazole If β-lactam allergy: clindamycin *and* aminoglycoside OR clindamycin *and* quinolone OR clindamycin *and* aztreonam OR metronidazole *and* aminoglycoside OR metronidazole *and* quinolone
Hysterectomy	Cefotetan, cefazolin, cefoxitin, cefuroxime, OR ampicillin/sulbactam If β-lactam allergy: clindamycin OR metronidazole

[a]Justification for vancomycin is acceptable with provider documentation.
[b]Cardiac, orthopedic, and vascular surgery, if patient is allergic to β-lactam antibiotics, vancomycin, or clindamycin are acceptable substitutes.
[c]Single dose only.

    b. SCIP-2. Prophylactic antibiotic must be SCIP recommended. See **Table 8.2** for SCIP-recommended regimens. For surgeries not included in SCIP, institutional guidelines and/or the joint guidelines from the American Society of Health-System Pharmacists (ASHP), the Infectious Diseases Society of America (IDSA), Surgical Infection Society (SIS), and Society for Healthcare Epidemiology of American (SHEA) should be followed. An update to these guidelines is currently in process.

    c. SCIP-3. Prophylactic antibiotics must be discontinued within 24 hours of the anesthetic end time (exception is 48 hours for cardiac surgery).

3. Timing and administration

    a. As noted in the previous section, **antibiotic administration must occur within 60 to 120 minutes of incision** to allow appropriate blood and tissue levels. Care must be taken to ensure this, as administration may occur in an inpatient unit, in the preoperative area, in the emergency department, or in the OR. The institutional guidelines for the correct dose of antibiotics should be followed.

    b. Repeated dosing is indicated for surgeries of long duration, surgeries with large blood loss (>1500 mL), or large fluid replacement. Redosing is antibiotic specific. Cefazolin is the most frequently used perioperative antibiotic with a typical redosing schedule of 4 hours intraoperatively.

    c. Parenteral administration is standard. Slow intravenous push is appropriate for some antibiotics (ie, cefazolin), and prolonged infusions are required for others (ie, vancomycin, fluoroquinolones). Clinicians should follow institutional guidelines regarding administration time.

d. Observation for **adverse reactions**
      1. Antibiotics are the second leading cause of anaphylaxis in the OR.
      2. Agent-specific hypersensitivity reactions may be encountered (ie, red man syndrome with vancomycin).
   e. As noted above, prophylactic antibiotics should be discontinued within 24 hours to prevent development of drug-resistant organisms.
4. Additional measures for prevention of surgical site infections that are primarily the anesthetist's responsibility include glycemic control (goal glucose <150 to 200; <200 on POD1 and POD2 in cardiac surgery patients per **SCIP-Inf-4**) and maintenance of normothermia via active warming and used of warmed forced air (goal temperature >36 °C; colorectal surgery patients with temperature >96.8 °F per **SCIP-Inf-7**). A single temperature measurement <35 °C may be an independent risk factor for development of SSI in some populations. Anesthetists can also play a role in encouraging smoking cessation.
5. At this time, there is no evidence to support inhalational anesthesia versus total intravenous anesthesia (TIVA) as factors that affect surgical site infection. Some studies have shown a decrease in SSI rates with hyperoxia without an increase in pulmonary complications; as such, the use of supplemental oxygen to prevent hypoxia is recommended, however, a specific FiO_2 is not supported by the current evidence.

C. Endocarditis prophylaxis. Patients with certain congenital and acquired cardiac conditions are at increased risk for infective endocarditis following specific surgical and dental procedures. In 2007, the American Heart Association significantly narrowed the list of both cardiac abnormalities and procedures for which endocarditis prophylaxis is indicated. The latest guidelines are reflected in the 2020 ACC/AHA Guideline for Management of Patients with Valvular Heart Disease and summarized below.
   1. **Prophylaxis for high-risk patients only.** High-risk patients include (i) prosthetic cardiac valves including transcatheter-implanted prostheses and homografts, (ii) prosthetic material used in cardiac valve repair, (iii) history of infectious endocarditis, (iv) specific congenital heart diseases (CHD): unrepaired cyanotic CHD including palliative shunts and conduits, or repaired CHD with residual shunts or valvular regurgitation at the site of or adjacent to the site of a prosthetic patch or prosthetic device, and (v) cardiac transplant recipients who develop valvulopathies. All other cardiac abnormalities do not need endocarditis prophylaxis.
   2. **Prophylaxis for high-risk procedures only.** High-risk procedures include dental procedures that involve manipulation of gingival tissue, periapical region of the teeth, or perforation of the oral mucosa. Even in high-risk patients, antibiotic prophylaxis is not recommended for nondental procedures. Specifically, gastrointestinal and genitourinary procedures including transesophageal echocardiogram (TEE), esophagogastroduodenoscopy (EGD), colonoscopy, cystoscopies, and ureteral stent placements, in the absence of active infection, are no longer considered high risk.

D. Surgical wound classification. Surgical wounds are classified based on risk of infection and help to guide antibiotic therapy.
   1. **Clean** wounds are uninfected, show no signs of inflammation, do not enter the respiratory, gastrointestinal, or genitourinary tracts, and are closed primarily. The biggest risk for postoperative infections is from skin-colonizing bacteria such as Staphylococcus and Streptococcus spp.
   2. **Clean-contaminated** wounds enter the respiratory, gastrointestinal, or genitourinary tracts without spillage of contents. Common

pathogens are site dependent. Common respiratory pathogens include *Streptococcus pneumoniae*, *K. pneumoniae*, *S. aureus*, and *P. aeruginosa*. Common gastrointestinal pathogens include *E. coli*, Proteus spp., Bacteroides spp., and Enterococcus spp. Common genitourinary pathogens include *E. coli*, Proteus spp., Klebsiella spp., and *Staphylococcus saprophyticus*.
3. **Contaminated** wounds include gross spillage of nonpurulent contents and those with breaks in sterile technique. Common pathogens are site dependent.
4. **Dirty** wounds include gross spillage of purulent contents, existing infection or perforation, and organisms known to be present prior to the procedure. Again, common pathogens are site dependent.

E. **Commonly encountered perioperative antibiotics**
1. **β-lactams** include penicillins, carbapenems, monobactams, and cephalosporins. The common mechanism of action is inhibition of cell wall synthesis. **Cefazolin**, a first-generation cephalosporin, is the most commonly administered perioperative antibiotic as it provides coverage of most of the gram-positive and many of the gram-negative bacteria that are seen with clean wounds. **Cefoxitin** and **cefotetan**, second-generation cephalosporins, extended coverage of gram-negative bacteria and anaerobic bacteria making them appropriate selections for clean-contaminated and contaminated wounds. **Ceftriaxone** and **ceftazidime**, third-generation cephalosporins, and **cefepime**, a fourth-generation cephalosporin, extend coverage further over gram-negative bacteria making them appropriate selections for dirty wounds in particular. **Adverse reactions** include (i) hypersensitivity reactions from rash to anaphylaxis, (ii) central nervous system toxicity (especially high-dose penicillin), (iii) hematologic (platelet dysfunction with piperacillin or ticarcillin and impairment of clotting factor production with cefotetan), and (iv) interstitial nephritis (especially with methicillin or nafcillin).
   a. **Penicillin and cephalosporin cross-reactivity.** Among patients who report penicillin allergy, between 1% and 4% will react if given a cephalosporin. Older retrospective studies likely overestimated cross-reactivity due to contamination of cephalosporins with trace amounts of benzylpenicillin.
2. **Clindamycin** inhibits protein synthesis at ribosomal subunits and is an appropriate alternative for β-lactam allergic patients. Coverage includes most gram-positive bacteria (including MRSA) as well as many anaerobes. **Adverse reactions** include (i) rash (anaphylaxis is rare), (ii) hypotension with rapid administration, (iii) gastrointestinal distress, (iv) *C. difficile* colitis, and (v) potentiation of neuromuscular blockade.
3. **Vancomycin** inhibits cell wall synthesis at a different site than the β-lactams. It covers most gram-positive bacteria including MRSA but provides no coverage of gram-negative bacteria, making it an appropriate selection for β-lactam allergic patients and patients colonized or infected with MRSA. In a recent RCT of arthroplasty patients, the addition of vancomycin to cefazolin was not superior to cefazolin + placebo in patients without MRSA. **Adverse reactions** include (i) red man syndrome and hypotension from histamine release with rapid administration, (ii) hypersensitivity reactions, and (iii) increased nephrotoxicity and ototoxicity when administered with other agents at risk for causing nephrotoxicity and ototoxicity.

4. **Aminoglycosides** include gentamicin, tobramycin, streptomycin, and amikacin. The mechanism of action is inhibition of protein synthesis at a ribosomal subunit different from clindamycin. Coverage includes gram-positive and gram-negative aerobes and Mycobacteria spp. making them appropriate choices for combination therapy in wounds other than clean. **Adverse reactions** include (i) nephrotoxicity especially in patients with baseline renal impairment or other risk factors for renal impairment, (ii) ototoxicity, and (iii) potentiation of neuromuscular blockade.
5. **Fluoroquinolones** include ciprofloxacin, levofloxacin, and moxifloxacin. Mechanism of action is inhibition of bacterial DNA replication. Coverage includes extensive gram-negative bacteria, many gram-positive bacteria, and atypical bacteria making them appropriate choices for combination therapy in wounds other than clean. **Adverse reactions** include (i) gastrointestinal distress, (ii) hepatotoxicity, (iii) central nervous system effects especially in the elderly, (iv) connective tissue effects, and (v) variable QT prolongation.
6. **Metronidazole** inhibits nucleic acid synthesis. Coverage includes most anaerobic organisms making it appropriate for combination therapy in wounds other than clean. Adverse reactions include (i) gastrointestinal distress, (ii) thrombophlebitis, (iii) hypersensitivity reactions, (iv) neurologic effects including peripheral neuropathy, and (v) disulfiram-like reaction when combined with alcohol.

IV. PATHOGENIC ORGANISMS OF ANESTHETIC CONCERN

The CDC (www.cdc.org) has current reviews of common pathogens, including all reviewed here.

A. Viruses

1. **Novel coronaviruses (MERS, SARS, SARS-CoV-2).** Novel coronaviruses have been responsible for worldwide outbreaks of the Middle Eastern respiratory syndrome (MERS, 2012), severe acute respiratory syndrome (SARS, 2003), and COVID-19 (caused by SARS-CoV-2, 2019). These viruses spread from an infected person's respiratory secretions via droplets and aerosols but may also spread via fomites contaminated with infectious droplets. The occupational risk for health care workers is believed to be high, for which the use of proper protective equipment is mandatory when treating these patients. In patients with active SARS-CoV-2 infection requiring surgery, the increased risk of PPCs and mortality is weighed against the risk of delaying surgery. A multicenter prospective cohort study found that mortality in patients undergoing elective and emergency surgery reverted to baseline risk after a delay of at least 7 weeks from SARS-CoV-2 diagnosis without ongoing symptoms.
2. **Influenza virus**
   a. **Transmission.** Influenza is transmitted via respiratory secretions in the droplet route. Anesthesia providers can acquire and spread influenza via their close involvement with respiratory secretions. Influenza is generally not life threatening in healthy individuals but may be life threatening in the immunocompromised, the chronically ill, and elderly patients. Active or recent (<14 days) influenza infection in patients undergoing surgery may increase the risk of postoperative complications including pneumonia.
   b. **Influenza vaccination.** Most health care facilities now require annual vaccinations for health care workers.

Chapter 8 Infectious Diseases and Infection Control in Anesthesia

3. **Human immunodeficiency virus (HIV)**
   a. **Transmission.** HIV is transmitted through percutaneous or mucosal exposure to infected blood or body fluids via needlestick or other sharps injury, blood transfusion, sexual contact, and perinatally from infected mother to neonate.
   b. **Occupationally acquired HIV.** Risk is low for occupationally acquired HIV in health care workers. Risk of seroconversion after percutaneous exposure to blood from an HIV-positive patient is 0.3%. Risk is increased with deep injury, visible patient blood on the injurious device, a needle that was within a vein or artery in the HIV-positive patient, patients with higher viral loads, and larger bore hollow needles.
   c. **Postexposure prophylaxis (PEP).** In case of exposure, the Occupational Health Service of the institution should be contacted. Frequently updated guidelines are available for management of exposed health care workers on the CDC Web site (www.cdc.gov) and from the National Clinicians' PEP Hotline (888-448-4911). PEP must be initiated within 3 days of exposure making immediate reporting of exposure to occupational health of paramount importance. The decision to initiate PEP and the choice and duration of the PEP regimen are based on numerous factors including type of exposure, volume of exposure, and sensitivity of the virus to antiretroviral agents. PEP is not 100% effective, and follow-up testing is necessary.
4. **Hepatitis B virus (HBV)**
   a. **Transmission.** HBV is transmitted through percutaneous or mucosal exposure to infected blood or body fluids via needlestick or other sharps injury, blood transfusion, sexual contact, and perinatally from infected mother to neonate.
   b. **Occupationally acquired HBV.** Risk depends on immunization status of the health care provider, hepatitis Be antigen (HBeAg) status of the HBV-positive patient, and quantity of inoculate. Risk is increased in unimmunized health care workers (currently most hospitals and health care facilities require HBV vaccination and antibody titers prior to employment), source patients who are HBeAg positive, and when percutaneous exposure is via a hollow large bore needle. Risk of clinical hepatitis from HBeAg-negative percutaneous exposure via needlestick is 1% to 6%, but is 22% to 31% with HBeAg-positive percutaneous exposure via needlestick. Ninety percent of acute HBV hepatitis resolves without sequelae; however, 10% become chronically infected and are at risk for chronic hepatitis, cirrhosis, and hepatocellular carcinoma.
   c. **HBV vaccination.** Recombinant vaccination consisting of three vaccinations over 3 months is effective at least 90% of the time. As the nonresponder rate is 10%, verification of antibody titers should be completed for those who will be in contact with blood or bloody body fluids. Per the Occupational Safety and Health Administration (OSHA), employers must provide Hepatitis B vaccination to employees free of charge.
   d. **PEP.** Exposure to blood or body fluids from patients who are known to be hepatitis B surface antigen (HBsAg) positive or patients with unknown status who are high risk for HBV may require PEP. Immediate reporting of the event is of utmost importance. Vaccinated health care workers who have appropriate levels of

hepatitis B surface antigen antibodies (HBsAb) (≥10 mIU/mL) require no treatment. Vaccinated health care workers who have low levels of HBsAb (<10 mIU/mL) and previously unvaccinated health care workers are treated with hepatitis B immunoglobulin (HBIg) and vaccination/revaccination.

5. Hepatitis C virus (HCV)
  a. Transmission. HCV is typically transmitted through large volume or repeated percutaneous exposure to blood, blood transfusion, perinatally from infected mother to neonate, and less commonly from sexual contact.
  b. Occupationally acquired HCV. HCV seroconversion from percutaneous exposure via needlestick or other sharps injury is approximately 1.8%. Of those infected with HCV, 80% become chronically infected and are at risk for chronic hepatitis, cirrhosis, and hepatocellular carcinoma.
  c. PEP. No PEP is currently recommended for HCV exposure. Close clinical and laboratory follow-up should continue to evaluate for necessity of treatment for chronic infection.

6. Herpes simplex virus (HSV) I and II
  a. Transmission. HSV is transmitted by direct contact between infected individuals, whether symptomatic or not, or infected secretions, mucosa, or damaged skin.
  b. Occupationally acquired HSV. Herpetic whitlow is HSV infection of the finger that can occur in the health care setting from contact with oral secretions of an infected individual. Symptoms include fever, painful and inflamed lesions, and localized lymphadenopathy. Persons with active herpetic whitlow can transmit HSV, so patient contact should be avoided.

7. Cytomegalovirus (CMV). CMV is a herpesvirus that in healthy patients is usually asymptomatic; however, it can be life threatening in immunocompromised patients and in utero. Transmission of CMV occurs via direct contact between a susceptible host (severely ill or immunocompromised) and infected source in the form of blood transfusion or organ transplantation. Infection can be acute or reactivation of a latent infection. To reduce this risk, CMV-negative immunosuppressed patients and CMV-negative pregnant patients should receive blood transfusions from CMV-negative donors if transfusion is required.

8. Varicella-zoster virus (VZV)
  a. Transmission. VZV (chicken pox and shingles) is transmitted via direct contact or airborne routes. Anesthesia providers can be exposed or expose others to VZV. Like CMV, VZV can be life threatening to immunocompromised patients and in utero.
  b. VZV vaccination. VZV vaccination is indicated for all nonimmune health care workers who may come into contact with high-risk patient populations. A history of chicken pox as a child and/or antibody titers may be required by health care facilities as pre-employment screening.

9. Ebola. Ebola virus is a genus of five species from the filoviridae family. Several outbreaks have been reported since 1976, most recently the Zaire virus in 2014–2016. All species in the genus are highly virulent and transmissible by direct contact with infected blood, secretions, tissues, organs, and other bodily fluids from dead or living infected persons. Transmission via fomites contaminated with infected bodily fluids is also possible.

Chapter 8 Infectious Diseases and Infection Control in Anesthesia **151**

10. **Mpox (also known as Monkeypox)** is a zoonotic orthopox virus endemic to Central and West Africa involved in its first global outbreak with human-to-human transmission in 2022 and 2023. This outbreak occurred primarily, but not only, in men who have sex with men with transmission thought to occur via close physical contact (direct contact with skin lesions), fomites, and respiratory droplets. Transplacental transmission is also possible. Patients are thought to be contagious between the onset of prodromal symptoms and until all lesions are scabbed over. Due to occupational risk and risk of disease progression, postponement of nonurgent surgeries in patients with mpox is recommended. Recommended PPE for healthcare providers includes gloves, isolation gown, surgical mask, and N95 during aerosol-generating procedures such as intubation. PEP, typically via vaccine administration, is offered based on exposure risk and PPE worn during the patient interaction.

B. Bacteria
1. **Mycobacterium tuberculosis.**
    a. **Transmission of tuberculosis (TB).** TB is transmitted via respiratory secretions via an airborne route. TB is often a latent or inactive disease that may be asymptomatic. Active TB most often occurs in immunocompromised and chronically ill patients.
    b. **Occupational TB.** Most health care facilities require annual testing of health care workers for TB via purified protein derivative (PPD) skin testing. Recent seroconversion warrants treatment with a course of isoniazid. Additionally, health care workers need to be fitted and trained for N95 respirators; health care workers who cannot tolerate an N95 respirator should use a powered air-purifying respirators (PAPR).
2. **Antibiotic-resistant bacteria** are a growing problem in medicine. The rate of growth in antibiotic-resistant bacteria is currently outpacing the development of new antimicrobial drugs. Poor antibiotic stewardship, prolonged hospitalizations, presence of indwelling catheters, and prolonged mechanical ventilation have contributed to the increase in antibiotic-resistant bacteria. Anesthesia providers can help prevent the transmission of and slow the rate of growth of antibiotic-resistant bacteria with strict infection control policies and antibiotic stewardship.

C. Prion Diseases
1. **Protein-containing infectious particles (prions)** cause diseases such as **Creutzfeldt–Jakob** and **kuru.** Transmission is from direct inoculation of infected material into a host, with most commonly reported transmission being from dura transplantation. Epidemiologic studies are limited due to the long incubation time and rarity of the disease. Although the occupational risk for health care workers is believed to be very low, following a surgical procedure of confirmed or suspected disease decontamination of equipment is per specific protocols.

V. OCCUPATIONAL EXPOSURE TO INFECTIOUS DISEASE
A. Prevention of exposure
1. Use **standard or universal precautions** as noted in the previous section.
2. **Observe needle safety.** The CDC estimate that 385,000 needlestick and other sharps-related injuries occur in health care workers each year. Many safety needle and needleless systems have been designed and should be used preferentially over standard needles. Needles should

never be recapped, and needles should be discarded in a labeled sharps container immediately after use.
B. Management of exposure
  1. **Wash exposed area.** Soap and water or sterile saline should be used to wash skin, and water or sterile saline should be used to flush mucous membranes. Specialized eye washing stations should be available.
  2. **Immediate reporting of exposure** to occupational health or the emergency room (if after normal work hours) to ensure initiation of protocols for testing, PEP, and counseling.

VI. SPECIAL PATIENT POPULATIONS
A. Immunocompromised patients are at increased risk for community-acquired, nosocomial, and opportunistic infections. Immunocompromise can be due to malignancy, chemotherapy, burns, HIV infection, corticosteroids, severe malnutrition, extremes of age, and immunosuppressive therapy for solid organ and bone marrow transplant recipients, or severe autoimmune disease.
  1. **Elective surgery** should be delayed if possible in the severely immunocompromised (ie, total neutrophil count <500 cells/mm^3).
  2. Strict adherence to **sterile technique** is essential.
  3. **Providers with respiratory infections** should not be involved in the care of severely immunocompromised patients. If unavoidable, the provider should wear a surgical mask during any contact with the patient.
  4. Patients may be on **neutropenic precautions** that include specific dietary and environmental restrictions as well as the wearing of masks during transport.
  5. **Antibiotic prophylaxis** is used in various immunocompromised patients for prophylaxis against postoperative wound infection and for long-term prophylaxis against opportunistic infections. It is important to verify which immunosuppressant drugs a patient is taking as many may interact with common perioperative medications. Cyclosporine, in particular, is associated with metabolism alteration and toxicity when combined with various antibiotics. Additionally, it is important to verify that patients presenting for organ transplantation have received the appropriate antibiotic prophylaxis against both surgical site infection and opportunistic infection. Appropriate regimens are determined by recipient factors, donor factors, organ-specific concerns, and planned immunosuppression.
B. Patients with sepsis may require urgent or emergent surgery for source control. Guidelines from the Surviving Sepsis Campaign were updated in 2021 and should be followed, including the recommendations below. While treatment may begin in the Emergency Department or ICU, continuity and ongoing management in the OR are essential.
  1. 30 mL/kg of IV crystalloid should be given within the first 3 hours of resuscitation.
  2. Empiric antimicrobials should be given without 1 hour of recognition of sepsis or septic shock. Empiric MRSA, multidrug-resistant gram negative, and fungal coverage depend on risk of these infections.
  3. Serum lactate and other dynamic markers of perfusion should be followed.
  4. Norepinephrine is recommended as the first-line vasopressor. If mean arterial pressure remains inadequate (MAP <65 mmHg), the addition of vasopressin is recommended.
  5. In patients with evidence of ARDS, lung-protective ventilation strategies are recommended.

6. Adequate access and postop disposition, likely to an ICU, must be considered.

ACKNOWLEDGMENT

We gratefully acknowledge the contributions of previous edition author, Diana Barragan-Bradford, as portions of those chapters have been retained in this revision.

Suggested Readings

American Society of Anesthesiologists. New guidance outlines recommendations for infection control in anesthesiology. Published December 11, 2018. Accessed March 10, 2024. https://www.asahq.org/about-asa/newsroom/news-releases/2018/12/shea-guidance

ASA Committee on Occupational Health and Wellness. Recommendations for Infection Control for the Practice of Anesthesiology: Preventing Infectious Transmission During Anesthesia Care. Revised February 2024. Last accessed 27 March 2025. https://www.asahq.org/standards-and-practice-parameters/resources-from-asa-committees#OH

Bratzler DW, Dellinger EP, Olsen KM, et al. Clinical practice guidelines for antimicrobial prophylaxis in surgery. *Am J Health Syst Pharm*. 2013;70(3):195–283.

Canet J, Gallart L, Gomar C, et al. Prediction of postoperative pulmonary complications in a population-based surgical cohort. *Anesthesiology*. 2010;113(6):1338–1350.

Centers for Disease Control and Prevention (CDC). III. Precautions to prevent transmission of infectious agents. Published online 2019. https://www.cdc.gov/infectioncontrol/guidelines/isolation/precautions.html#:~:text=B.-,Transmission%2DBased%20Precautions,interrupted%20using%20Standard%20Precautions%20alone

Centers for Disease Control and Prevention (CDC). Diseases and organisms. Published online 2022.

Centers for Disease Control and Prevention (CDC). Guideline for hand hygiene in healthcare settings: recommendations of the healthcare infection control practices Advisory Committee and the HICPAC/SHEA/APIC/IDSA Hand Hygiene Task Force. Published online 2022. https://www.cdc.gov/mmwr/PDF/rr/rr5116.pdf

Centers for Disease Control and Prevention. 2023 National and State Healthcare-Associated Infections Progress Report. Updated November 2024. Last accessed 27 March 2025. https://www.cdc.gov/healthcare-associated-infections/php/data/progress-report.html.

Centers for Disease Control and Prevention (CDC). Updated U.S. Public health service guidelines for the management of occupational exposures to HBV, HCV, and HIV and recommendations for postexposure prophylaxis. Last accessed 27 March 2025. https://www.cdc.gov/mmwr/PDF/rr/rr5011.pdf

Charnin JE, Hollidge M, Bartz R, et al. A best practice for anesthesia work area infection control measures: what are you waiting for? *APSF Newsletter*. 2022;37(3). Accessed March 10, 2024. https://www.apsf.org/article/a-best-practice-for-anesthesia-work-area-infection-control-measures-what-are-you-waiting-for/

Chaudhry SB, Veve MP, Wagner JL. Cephalosporins: a focus on side chains and β-lactam cross-reactivity. *Pharmacy*. 2019;7(3):103.

COVIDSurg Collaborative, GlobalSurg Collaborative. Timing of surgery following SARS-CoV-2 infection: an international prospective cohort study. *Anaesthesia*. 2021;76(6):748–758.

Desai SR, Tang L, Hwang NC. Infection control for perioperative ultrasonography and echocardiography. *J Cardiothorac Vasc Anesth*. 2022;36(12):4440–4448.

Fuglestad MA, Tracey EL, Leinicke JA. Evidence-based prevention of surgical site infection. *Surg Clin North Am*. 2021;101(6):951–966.

Harbath S, Frankhauser C, Schrenzel J, et al. Universal screening for methicillin-resistant Staphylococcus aureus at hospital admission and nosocomial infection in surgical patients. *JAMA*. 2008;299:1149–1157.

Klompas M, Branson R, Cawcutt K, et al. Strategies to prevent ventilator-associated pneumonia, ventilator-associated events, and nonventilator hospital-acquired pneumonia in acute-care hospitals: 2022 Update. *Infect Control Hosp Epidemiol*. 2022;43(6):687–713.

Kothari SN, Anderson MJ, Borgert AJ, et al. Bouffant vs skull cap and impact on surgical site infection: does operating room headwear really matter? *J Am Coll Surg*. 2018;227(2):198–202.

Kwanten LE. Anaesthetists and syringe hygiene: getting to the pointy end – a summary of recommendations. *Br J Anaesth.* 2019;123(4):e475–e479.

Lam F, Liao CC, Chen TL, Huang YM, Lee YJ, Chiou HY. Outcomes after surgery in patients with and without recent influenza: a nationwide population-based study. *Front Med.* 2023;10:1117885.

Loftus R, Brown J, Koff M, et al. Multiple reservoirs contribute to intraoperative bacterial transmission. *Anesth Analg.* 2012;114:1236–1245.

Loftus R, Koff M, Burchman C, et al. Transmission of pathogenic bacterial organisms in the anesthesia work area. *Anesthesiology.* 2008;109:399–407.

Long DR, Alverdy JC, Vavilala MS. Emerging paradigms in the prevention of surgical site infection: the patient microbiome and antimicrobial resistance. *Anesthesiology.* 2022;137(2):252–262.

Mandell L, Niederman M. Aspiration pneumonia. *N Engl J Med.* 2019;380:651–663.

Mundangepfupfu T, Nadler JW. Updates in prevention of surgical site infection: comment. *Anesthesiology.* 2023;138(4):446–447.

Munoz-Price LS, Bowdle A, Johnston BL, et al. Infection prevention in the operating room anesthesia work area. *Infect Control Hosp Epidemiol.* 2019;40(1):1–17.

O'Grady NP. Prevention of central line–associated bloodstream infections. *N Engl J Med.* 2023;389(12):1121–1131.

Parienti JJ, Mongardon N, Megarbane B. Intravascular complications of central venous catheterization by insertion site. *N Engl J Med.* 2015;373:1220–1229.

Peel TN, Astbury S, Cheng AC, et al. Trial of vancomycin and cefazolin as surgical prophylaxis in arthroplasty. *N Engl J Med.* 2023;389(16):1488–1498.

Seidelman JL, Mantyh CR, Anderson DJ. Surgical site infection prevention: a review. *JAMA.* 2023;329(3):244–252.

Tait AR, Malviya S, Voepel-Lewis T, Munro HM, Siewert M, Pandit UA. Risk factors for perioperative adverse respiratory events in children with upper respiratory tract infections. *Anesthesiology.* 2001;95(2):299–306.

Teo CT, Wu JS, Chan K, Ng SWB, Somani J, Loh W. What does the anesthesiologist need to know about monkeypox? *Can J Anaesth.* 2023;70(5):893–900.

The Joint Commission. Specifications manual for national hospital inpatient quality measures. https://www.jointcommission.org/-/media/tjc/documents/measurement/specification-manuals/hiqr_specsman_july2019_v5_6.pdf

Wilson RB, Farooque Y. Risks and prevention of surgical site infection after hernia mesh repair and the predictive utility of ACS-NSQIP. *J Gastrointest Surg.* 2022;26(4):950–964.

PART II: ADMINISTRATION OF ANESTHESIA

Safety in Anesthesia
Britlyn D. Orgill and Rebecca D. Minehart

I. OVERVIEW OF SAFETY IN ANESTHESIA

A. Anesthesiology has led the patient safety movement, and anesthesia-related adverse outcomes have drastically declined since the 1960s. Despite this decline, the risks of both general and regional anesthesia remain. Recent data suggest that anesthetic-related mortality is 0.5 to 1/100,000 in the developed world.

B. The World Health Organization (WHO) and the World Federation of Societies of Anesthesiologists (WFSA) developed International Standards for a Safe Practice of Anesthesia. These standards are intended to guide individuals and organizations in maintaining and improving safety and quality in anesthesia care.

C. Adverse events are injuries resulting from medical care. Many systems and human factors errors can contribute to adverse events. Reason's "Swiss cheese model" of adverse event causation describes that many layers of defense lie between hazards and adverse events, and there are gaps in each layer which if aligned, can allow an event to occur.

D. Errors can occur despite a practitioner's expertise, experience, and good intention. In the perioperative arena, errors can result from the following:
  1. **Organizational influences** including production pressure or improperly maintained equipment
  2. **Inadequate supervision**, which includes the unavailability of attending anesthesiologists to immediately assist trainees
  3. **Preconditions** for unsafe acts include fatigued clinicians or improper communication practices
  4. **Specific individual acts**

E. Prevention of adverse events relies on optimizing practitioners' understanding of the system and resources of their workplace, in addition to individual practice improvement. Strategies to create safer systems include the following:
  1. **Simplification**
  2. **Standardization**
  3. **Improving teamwork and communication**
  4. Developing an organizational culture that promotes **learning from past mistakes**
  5. Building **resilient recovery systems**

F. Resilience is the adaptability or capacity to recover quickly from difficulties or unforeseen complications and is critical for maintaining safety. Resilient systems do not wait for errors to occur so they can be analyzed, but rather focus on prevention, ensuring best performances, and quick recovery.

II. STANDARDS FOR SAFE ANESTHESIA CARE

The International Standards for a Safe Practice can be grouped in different categories:

- **A. Professional aspects**, such as anesthetists having high levels of knowledge and skills, professional training through formally accredited training institutions, ensuring adequate numbers of anesthetists to meet the needs of the surgical workforce, appropriate clinical supervision, and quality assurance mechanisms to implement improvements in care
- **B. Facilities and equipment**, which must allow for safe care, according to the environment (preoperative area, operating room [OR], and postanesthesia recovery area)
- **C. Available medications and intravenous fluids**, such as basic hypnotics, anxiolytics, opioids and other nonopioid analgesics, local anesthetics, dextrose solutions, normal saline, Ringer lactate, resuscitative medications and concentrated oxygen, and magnesium
- **D. Monitoring capabilities**, including visualizing respiration rate and quality (including breathing system bag movement) and assessing tissue oxygen and perfusion, auscultating breath and heart sounds, palpating pulse rate and quality, enabling audible signals and alarms at all times, and using continuous pulse oximetry, intermittent noninvasive blood pressure monitoring, a carbon dioxide detector for patients undergoing intubation, and temperature monitoring
- **E. Conduct of anesthesia**, such as a single anesthetist per patient who is responsible for preanesthetic evaluation, present throughout the anesthetic, and responsible for safe transport to the recovery area with adequate handoff. Preanesthetic checks and the WHO Safe Surgery Checklist procedures are highly recommended as well as appropriate record keeping.

III. TYPES OF ERRORS

Errors are acts of commission (doing something wrong) or omission (failing to do the right thing) that lead to an undesirable outcome. Anesthetists should be aware of and actively work to mitigate common types of errors.

- **A. Medication errors.** It is estimated that at least 5% of hospitalized patients experience an adverse drug event. The cost of preventable medication errors in US hospitals has been estimated at $16.4 billion annually.
    1. **Examples of medication errors** include administration of an inappropriate dose, administration through an inappropriate route, administration at an inappropriate rate, and administration to the incorrect patient. Some specific examples are as follows:
        - **a.** The rapid intravenous (IV) administration of undiluted phenytoin or undiluted potassium can cause cardiovascular collapse or death.
        - **b.** Neostigmine administered without a corresponding antimuscarinic drug can lead to severe bradycardia, asystole, and death.
        - **c.** Inadvertent administration of a medication to which a patient has a known allergy.
    2. **Strategies to decrease medication errors**
        - **a.** Have a thorough understanding of the pharmacokinetics, pharmacodynamics, and effects of each medication administered.

b. Exercise vigilance in drug administration. Double-check medications prior to administration and consider implementing the "Five Rights" checklist: right patient, right route, right dose, right time, and right drug prior to drug administration.

c. Have only **unit dosing** available in the patient care area. Unit dosing refers to packaging medications in quantities and concentrations that are safe and appropriate for administration without dilution.

d. Involve clinical pharmacists in perioperative care. Pharmacists can assist with drug dosing and help identify medication errors.

e. Perform careful medication reconciliation when transitioning care between the floor, ICU, and perioperative and procedural areas. Medical reconciliation is the process of reviewing a patient's complete medication regimen on both ends of care to avoid unintended inconsistencies.

f. Avoid confusing and potentially hazardous abbreviations. The Joint Commission has issued a list of high-risk "do not use" abbreviations. For example, write out "unit" instead of using "u" as an abbreviation which can be mistaken for the number zero, four, or cc. https://www.jointcommission.org/resources/patient-safety-topics/patient-safety/

g. Consider bar-coding technology to decrease medication identification errors by allowing medications to be "scanned" directly into the medical record.

B. Procedure errors

1. **Examples of procedure errors** include wrong-site surgery, retained instruments, and OR fires. Better outcomes are associated with higher volumes of specific surgeries or procedures being performed by a single physician or institution.

2. **Strategies to reduce procedure errors**

    a. "Universal Protocols" should be implemented including marking the site of surgery, using preprocedural time-outs, and using checklists.

    b. Intraoperative surgical instrument and sponge counts are used to prevent retained surgical instruments in the patient. If the instrument counts at the end of the procedure indicate that an instrument is missing, radiography of the operative field should be conducted in the OR to determine whether the instrument is in the patient. A wand with radiofrequency (RFI) detection can help aid in sponge counts.

    c. Recognize and avoid the fire triangle: ignition source (electrocautery, lasers) plus fuel source (gauze, drapes, endotracheal tube) plus oxidizers (oxygen, nitrous oxide) equals fire.

    d. The positive volume–outcome relationship for procedures argues for simulation training and specialization. Robust competency training should take place for procedures such as vascular catheterization, advanced intubation techniques, and bedside ultrasound use.

    e. Where possible, consider a model where stable teams work together frequently to achieve familiarity, as they have been shown to patient care outcomes, likely due to improved communication, anticipation, and planning.

C. Cognitive errors result from faulty thought processes and subconscious biases, which can lead to missed diagnoses and patient injury.

1. **Table 9.1** lists 14 common cognitive errors.

2. **Strategies to decrease cognitive errors**

    a. Use **Bayesian reasoning** and **iterative hypothesis testing.** In Bayesian reasoning, the probability estimate for a hypothesis is updated as

Table 9.1 Cognitive Error Catalog

Cognitive Error	Definition	Illustration
Anchoring	Focusing on one issue at the expense of understanding the whole situation	While troubleshooting an alarm on an infusion pump, you are unaware of sudden surgical bleeding and hypotension
Availability bias	Choosing a diagnosis because it is in the forefront of your mind due to an emotionally charged memory of a bad experience	Diagnosing simple bronchospasm as anaphylaxis because you once had a case of anaphylaxis that had a very poor outcome
Premature closure	Accepting a diagnosis prematurely, failure to consider reasonable differential of possibilities	Assuming that hypotension in a trauma patient is due to bleeding, and missing the pneumothorax
Feedback bias	Misinterpretation of no feedback as "positive" feedback	Belief that you have never had a case of unintentional awareness, because you have never received a complaint about it
Confirmation bias	Seeking or acknowledging only information that confirms the desired or suspected diagnosis	Repeatedly cycling an arterial pressure cuff, changing cuff sizes, and locations, because you "do not believe" the low reading
Framing effect	Subsequent thinking is swayed by leading aspects of initial presentation	After being told by a colleague, "this patient was extremely anxious preoperatively," you attribute postoperative agitation to her personality rather than low blood glucose
Commission bias	Tendency toward action rather than inaction. Performing unindicated maneuvers, deviating from protocol. May be due to overconfidence, desperation, or pressure from others.	"Better safe than sorry" insertion of additional unnecessary invasive monitors or access; potentially resulting in a complication
Overconfidence bias	Inappropriate boldness, not recognizing the need for help, tendency to believe we are infallible	Delay in calling for help when you have trouble intubating, because you are sure you will eventually succeed
Omission bias	Hesitation to start emergency maneuvers for fear of being wrong or causing harm, tendency toward inaction	Delay in calling for chest tube placements when you suspect a pneumothorax, because you may be wrong and you will be responsible for that procedure
Sunk costs	Unwillingness to let go of a failing diagnosis or decision, especially if much time/resources have already been allocated. Ego may play a role.	Having decided that a patient needs an awake fiberoptic intubation, refusing to consider alternative plans despite multiple unsuccessful attempts

Cognitive Error Catalog (*continued*)

Cognitive Error	Definition	Illustration
Visceral bias	Countertransference; our negative or positive feelings about a patient influencing our decisions	Not troubleshooting on epidural for a laboring patient, because she is "high maintenance" or a "complainer"
Zebra retreat	Rare diagnosis figures prominently among possibilities, but physician is hesitant to pursue it	Try to "explain away" hypercarbia when malignant hyperthermia should be considered
Unpacking principle	Failure to elicit all relevant information, especially during transfer of care	Omission of key test results, medical history, or surgical event
Psych-out error	Medical causes for behavioral problems are missed in favor of psychological diagnosis	Elderly patient in postanesthesia recovery area is combative—prescribing restraints instead of considering hypoxia

Reprinted from Stiegler MP, Neelankavil JP, Canales C, et al. Cognitive errors detected in anaesthesiology: a literature review and pilot study. *Br J Anaesth*. 2012;108(2):229–235. Copyright © 2012 Elsevier. With permission.

additional evidence is acquired. With iterative hypothesis testing, a list of differential diagnoses is modified and reranked as more information becomes available.

   b. Be aware of performance-shaping factors that may adversely affect diagnostic abilities: noise, distractions (including from inappropriate alarms or use of mobile devices), illness, aging, sleep deprivation and fatigue.
   c. Continually learn from experience: self-reflect, discuss with senior and peer clinicians, and participate in morbidity and mortality conferences.
D. **Human factors errors.** Human factors engineering is the applied science of systems design which focuses on the interplay between people and their work environments. Pioneering studies of human factors were integral to the redesign of anesthesia equipment which significantly reduced the risk of injury or death in the OR. Experts in this field perform usability tests and heuristic analyses to identify error-prone devices or systems before they lead to harm.
E. **Care transition and handoff errors**
   1. **Examples of handoff errors.** The most common errors which occur at the time of care transitions (handoffs) are medication errors and failure to follow up diagnostic results.
   2. **Strategies to decrease handoff errors:**
      a. Handoffs should occur at designated times and without distractions. The anesthetic record should indicate the time of the change in staff.
      b. If possible, care transitions should be avoided during short procedures. They should be used carefully in complex cases.
      c. During a handoff, the following information should be clearly and accurately presented:

1. **Prior clinical details.** The patient's diagnosis, surgical procedure, allergies, past medical and surgical history, relevant medications, and any pertinent laboratory values or studies.
2. **Intraoperative management.** Status of the surgical procedure, airway assessment and management techniques, anesthetic plan, current vital signs with an explanation for any apparent abnormalities or trends, details of IV access and monitoring, blood loss and volume status assessment, status of the patient's blood bank sample plus blood product availability, anticipated need for additional intraoperative, and plan for postoperative recovery of the patient.
3. Handoffs should also address likely clinical scenarios and contingency plans.
  d. A handoff checklist may be used to ensure that complete information is communicated to the next responsible clinician. For example, "I-PASS" (Illness severity, Patient summary, Action list, Situation awareness and contingency planning, and Synthesis by the receiver) is a common strategy for handoffs.
F. **Teamwork and communication errors.** The perioperative, procedural, and intensive care units are team environments. Teamwork enhances safety and can be essential for preventing or recovering from a critical situation.
  1. **Strategies to enhance teamwork and decrease communication errors:**
      a. Start each day with effective **introductions**, consider **briefings and check-ins** with team members, and end with **debriefings**.
      b. Well-functioning teams are characterized by appropriate authority gradients and hierarchies that allow for "**speaking up**." "Authority gradients" refer to the established or perceived power hierarchy within a team, and how power distribution is balanced. Concentration of power in one person or in overbearing team leaders leads to a steep authority gradient, which can discourage input from other team members. In contrast, **inclusive leadership**, where input from team members is invited and appreciated, allows for improved collaboration.
      c. Develop an **understanding of the responsibilities and functions** of the other team members. During a crisis, maintain awareness of the other team members' actions.
      d. Make requests and **delegate tasks** clearly and specifically by name. Delegate tasks and encourage confirmation that team members can perform tasks designated.
      e. Utilize **closed-loop communication** to avoid misunderstandings. When one individual gives a message, the receiver should repeat the message back to ensure it was heard correctly. Always **confirm** that critical interventions have been made as planned.
      f. **Communicate concerns** early and clearly.

IV. GENERAL SAFETY STRATEGIES
A. **Crisis resource management**
  1. In the early 1990s, the concept of Anesthesia Crisis Resource Management was introduced by Dr. David Gaba. It was adapted from the aviation industry and their Crew (originally "cockpit") Resource Management principles and has extended to other specialties and fields under the name of Crisis Resource Management (CRM). CRM is a strategy to optimally identify, organize, and apply resources to preserve safety and acceptable outcomes for patients. CRM key principles were

Crisis Resource Management (CRM) Principles

CRM Principle	Elaboration on Principle
Call early for help	Know your limitations and call for help when a difference can be made. Anticipate and call people with special skills if they may be needed.
Anticipate and plan	Plan for possible difficulties ahead and the unexpected. Use wisely the time during low workload periods to prepare.
Know your environment	Know where things are and how they work. Know the vulnerabilities and strengths of your environment
Use all available information	Use different sources to gather data and integrate them to have better understanding of patients and situations. Cross check your information.
Allocate attention wisely	Minimize distractions. Do not fixate on a single variable. Alternate focusing on details and the big picture.
Mobilize resources	Think of resources (people or equipment) and activate them to help with the crisis. Do not struggle alone.
Use cognitive aids	Flexibility can be helpful, but also a source of errors. Cognitive aids can help minimize such errors. Know their formats, location, and content.
Communicate effectively	All team members must understand the situation (ie, have "shared situational awareness"). All requests must be clear and confirmed (directed, "closed loop").
Distribute the workload	Team leaders must distribute tasks according to team members' abilities. Reassess distribution and identify overload or failure in tasks.
Establish role clarity	Responsibilities must be clear to each member. Roles must be concordant to skill and training.
Designate leadership	Clear leadership must be established. The leader plans and communicates effectively.

Reprinted from Gaba DM, Fish KJ, Howard SK, et al. *Crisis Management in Anesthesiology*. 2nd ed. Saunders; 2015. Copyright © 2015 Elsevier. With permission.

designed for team members to focus their attention on elements that can improve patient safety. See **Table 9.2** for more details.

2. A simple mnemonic "Name/Claim/Aim" integrates key CRM principles (see **Figure 9.1**):
   a. Name. The clinical problem/crisis must be identified and called out loud, including when the diagnosis is unknown. This requires effective communication as the entire team is made aware of the problem at hand.
   b. Claim. A leader (the "event manager") must be established, and other roles must be assigned (either by the event manager or self-designated; roles may change). The term "event manager" is encouraged instead of "team leader" since it attempts to flatten hierarchy, better facilitating "speaking up" by team members.

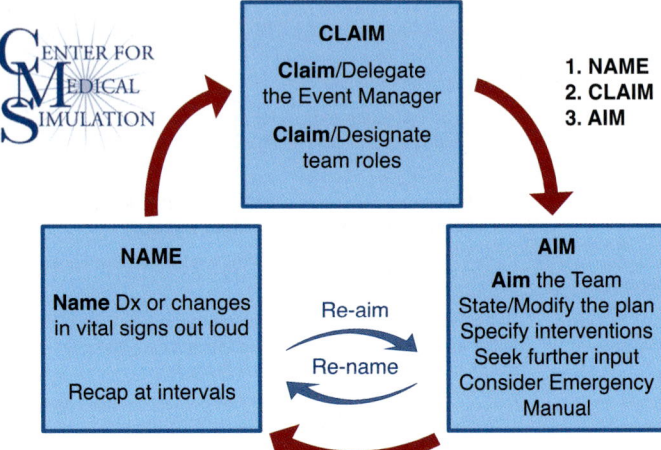

FIGURE 9.1 Name/Claim/Aim. This is an example of a tool to guide effective leadership, teamwork, and application of crisis resource management principles. (© Center for Medical Simulation, 2018.)

c. Aim. The team is aimed with a brief list of interventions, including diagnostic questions to resolve. This phase encompasses effective communication, mobilizing resources, using all available information, and using cognitive aids.

V. QUALITY ASSURANCE AND SAFETY IMPROVEMENT PROGRAMS

Institutional quality assurance programs should include a spectrum of activities aimed at maintaining and improving the quality of care and minimizing the risk of injury from anesthesia.

- **A. Just culture.** Health care organizations should strive to create a **just culture**. A just culture is one that recognizes that even competent professionals make mistakes and that individual practitioners should not be held accountable for system failings over which they have no control. A just culture does not tolerate the conscious disregard of clear risks to patients: reckless behavior or gross misconduct. Personnel should always feel comfortable disclosing their own errors while maintaining professional accountability.
- **B. Standards and guidelines.** Anesthetists should be aware of national and local safety policies and procedures. This includes policies for monitoring, response to adverse events, resuscitation protocols, perioperative testing protocols, and any special procedures or practices for the use of drugs, equipment, and supplies. The American Society of Anesthesiologists' standards and practice guidelines can be found at https://www.asahq.org/standards-and-practice-parameters.
- **C. Safety training.** Anesthetists should obtain training in fire safety, electrical safety, OR evacuation, infection control procedures, and crisis management. They should also be certified in advanced cardiac life support and, under certain circumstances, pediatric advanced life support and advanced trauma life support. Simulation techniques should be used wherever practical to allow practice under controlled conditions.

D. **Documentation.** Many systems depend on voluntary error reporting by anesthetists. A safety report or quality assurance incident report should be completed for any unusual occurrence, unforeseen outcome, patient injury, or near miss, especially if follow-up action may be required to prevent recurrence. Incidents are reviewed by the departmental quality assurance committee, which receives additional information from those involved in the event and may suggest compensatory mechanisms as systematic factors are identified. Cases with special educational value should be presented at departmental case conferences. There should be ongoing analysis of all adverse events to identify and assess system problems and developing patterns.
E. **Guidelines for action following an adverse anesthesia event.** Despite best efforts, errors may still occur. The objective of these guidelines is to limit patient harm from errors when they do occur, to ensure the causes of the event are identified, and to help prevent recurrence.
   1. **The anesthetist** involved in an adverse event should do the following:
      a. Continue to provide care for the patient.
      b. Notify the anesthesia OR administrator as soon as possible. If a resident or certified registered nurse anesthetist was involved in the event, they should notify the attending staff.
      c. Document events in the patient record. If appropriate, serial numbers or lot numbers of equipment or medication that was involved should be obtained.
      d. Do not alter the record.
      e. Stay involved with the follow-up care.
      f. Contact consultants as needed.
      g. Submit a follow-up report to the department quality assurance committee.
      h. Participate in apology and disclosure with the patient or patient's family.
      i. Obtain support as needed.

ACKNOWLEDGMENTS

We gratefully acknowledge the contributions of previous edition author, Miguel A. Patino Montoya, as portions of those chapters have been retained in this revision.

Suggested Readings

Agarwala AV, McCarty LK, Pian-Smith MC. Anesthesia quality and safety: advancing on a legacy of leadership. *Anesthesiology*. 2014;120(2):253–256.

American Society of Anesthesiologists. Accessed May 21, 2020. https://www.asahq.org/standards-and-practice-parameters

Anesthesia Patient Safety Foundation. Accessed May 21, 2020. www.asahq.org

Arriaga AF, Bader AM, Wong JM, et al. Simulation-based trial of surgical-crisis checklists. *N Engl J Med*. 2013;368:246–253.

Braz LG, Braz DG, da Cruz DS, Fernandes LA, Módolo NSP, Braz JRC. Mortality in anesthesia: a systematic review. *Clinics (Sao Paulo)*. 2009;64(10):999–1006.

Cooper JB, Gaba DM. A strategy for preventing anesthesia accidents. *Int Anesthesiol Clin*. 1989;27:148–152.

Cooper JB, Newbower RS, Kitz RJ. An analysis of major errors and equipment failures in anesthesia management: considerations for prevention and detection. *Anesthesiology*. 1984;60:34–42.

Gaba DM, Fish K, Howard S, Burden A. *Crisis Management in Anesthesiology*. 2nd ed. Saunders; 2015.

Gelb AW, Morris WW, Johnson W, et al; International Standards for a Safe Practice of Anesthesia Workgroup. World Health Organization-World Federation of Societies of Anaesthesiologists (WHO-WFSA) International Standards for a Safe Practice of Anesthesia. *Anesth Analg*. 2018;126(6):2047–2055.

Guohua L, Warner M, Lang BH, Huang L, Sun LS. Epidemiology of anesthesia-related mortality in the United States, 1999–2005. *Anesthesiology*. 2009;110:759–765.

Hallet J, Sutradhar R, Jerath A, et al. Association between familiarity of the surgeon-anesthesiologist dyad and postoperative patient outcomes for complex gastrointestinal cancer surgery. *JAMA Surg*. 2023;158(5):465–473.

Institute for Safe Medication Practice. Accessed May 21, 2020. www.ISMP.org

Kohn LT, Corrigan JM, Donaldson MS, eds. *To Err Is Human: Building a Safer Healthcare System*. National Academy Press; 1999.

Leape L, Berwick D, Clancy C, et al; Lucian Leape Institute at the National Patient Safety Foundation. Transforming healthcare: a safety imperative. *Qual Saf Health Care*. 2009;18:424–428.

Minehart RD, Foldy EG, Long JA, Weller JM. Challenging gender stereotypes and advancing inclusive leadership in the operating theatre. *Br J Anaesth*. 2020;124(3):e148–e154.

Oberfrank SM, Rall M, Dieckmann P, Kolbe M, Gaba DM. Chapter 6. Avoiding patient harm in anesthesia: human performance and patient safety. In: Gropper MA, Eriksson LI, Fleisher LA, Wiener-Kronish JP, Cohen NH, Leslie K, eds. *Miller's Anesthesia*. 9th ed. Elsevier Churchill Livingstone; 2020:105–178e.

Ostergaard D, Dieckmann P, Lippert A. Simulation and CRM. *Best Pract Res Clin Anaesthesiol*. 2011;25(2):239–249.

Pollard RJ, Hopkins T, Smith CT, et al. Perianesthetic and anesthesia-related mortality in a southeastern United States population: a longitudinal review of a prospectively collected quality assurance data base. *Anesth Analg*. 2018;127(3):730–735.

Reason J. Human error: models and management. *BMJ*. 2000;320(7237):768–770.

Shahian DM, McEachern K, Rossi L, Gino Chisari R, Mort E. Large-scale implementation of the I-PASS handover system at an academic medical centre. *BMJ Qual Saf*. 2017;26(9):760–770.

Smith AF, Plunkett E. People, systems and safety: resilience and excellence in healthcare practice. *Anaesthesia*. 2019;74(4):508–517.

Stiegler MP, Neelankavil JP, Canales C, Dhillon A. Cognitive errors detected in anaesthesiology: a literature review and pilot study. *Br J Anaesth*. 2012;108(2):229–235.

Watcher RM. *Understanding Patient Safety*. 2nd ed. McGraw Hill Medical Publishing; 2012.

The Anesthesia Machine

Zeyu Hu and Jeremi Mountjoy

I. OVERVIEW

The basic function of the anesthesia machine is to prepare a gas mixture of known and variable composition, and then deliver that gas to the patient. The machine regulates a controlled flow of oxygen, nitrous oxide, and air, to which anesthetic vapors are added. The gas mixture flows into a breathing system, from which the patient can breathe spontaneously. Alternatively, these gasses can be delivered via positive pressure ventilation using a mechanical ventilator or manual bag. The breathing system incorporates means for warming and humidification of gases, and for removal of carbon dioxide from the exhaled gasses. Anesthesia machines also provide a scavenger system to allow removal of waste gases from the immediate environment.

The anesthesia breathing system is unique among mechanical ventilators in that it is explicitly designed to allow patients to rebreath exhaled gases, so that the anesthetic agents can be conserved. To make rebreathing safe, several features are incorporated to ensure that the gas mixture delivered to the patient is safe. At minimum, anesthesia machines incorporate an oxygen sensor, to measure the oxygen concentration in the exhaled gas mixture. Many anesthesia machines now incorporate a sophisticated gas analysis system, capable of measuring oxygen, nitrous oxide, carbon dioxide, and anesthetic agents. Anesthesia machines also comply with a complex set of standards, with built-in monitors and sensors used to survey the functioning of the ventilation system, and detect equipment malfunctions.

II. THE GAS DELIVERY SYSTEM (FIGURE 10.1)

A. Medical gas supply

1. **Pipeline gas system.** Wall outlets deliver oxygen, nitrous oxide, and air, from a central supply source, at a pressure of 50 to 55 pounds/in^2 (psi). These outlets and the supply hoses to the machine are diameter-indexed and color-coded by gas type to safeguard against the administration of an incorrect or hypoxic gas mixture. This schema is referred to as the Diameter Index Safety System (DISS).

2. **Gas cylinders.** Gas cylinders are used as backup sources when wall delivery fails or as a primary gas source in locations where piped anesthesia gases are not available. Anesthesia machines use the size E cylinder. In a similar fashion to the gas supply hoses, cylinder colors are specific for each gas and pin indexed to prevent connection to the wrong regulator. This schema is referred to as the Pin Index Safety System (PISS). It is important to make sure that each anesthesia machine has a cylinder wrench to enable the flow of gas when piped gases are not available.

   a. **A full cylinder of oxygen,** color coded green (USA) or white (international), has a pressure of 2000 to 2200 psi and contains the equivalent of 660 L of gas at atmospheric pressure and room temperature. The oxygen cylinder pressure decreases in direct proportion to the amount of oxygen remaining in the cylinder.

FIGURE 10.1 Schematic of an anesthesia machine. There are many variations in the design depending on vintage and manufacturer.

- **b. A full cylinder of nitrous oxide,** color coded blue, has a pressure of 745 psi and contains the equivalent of 1500 L of gas at atmospheric pressure and room temperature. The nitrous oxide in the full cylinder is mainly in the liquid phase; the cylinder pressure does not decrease until the liquid content is exhausted, when about one-fourth of the total volume of gas remains.
- **c. A full cylinder of air** color coded yellow (USA) or black/white (international) has a pressure of 1800 psi and contains the equivalent of 630 L at atmospheric pressure and room temperature.
3. **Pressure regulators** in the anesthesia machine reduce the high pressures from each gas cylinder to 45 psi. This allows the flow valves to deliver a reliable flow from a cylinder, without constant adjustment as the internal pressure within the gas cylinder decreases as it empties. If an anesthesia machine is connected to a cylinder and pipeline of the same gas, gas is preferentially drawn from the pipeline because the pipeline has slightly higher pressure than the regulator. This pressure differential prevents flow from the cylinder unless pipeline pressures drop below that of the regulator. Without pipeline gas supply or if the pipeline gas supply fails, then the machine will draw from the gas cylinder until it is empty. It is important to note that despite this, when both a pipeline supply and cylinder of the same gas are connected to the anesthesia machine, fluctuations in the pipeline pressure can lead to gradual emptying of the cylinder. Therefore cylinders should be opened briefly to check pressure during the daily machine check, then kept closed, to preserve their contents in case of pipeline failure. If a pipeline supply failure occurs, the cylinder (tank) should then be opened and the corresponding hose disconnected from the anesthesia machine.
4. **Flow control valves and flowmeters** control and measure gas flows.
    - **a. A needle valve** controls the flow of each gas. Traditionally, anesthesia machines had manual knob for each gas. As a safety feature, the oxygen knob has a different texture and, occasionally, protrudes more than the nitrous oxide and air knobs. Many anesthesia machines now have electronically controlled valves, and the flow can be set by choosing a total flow and FiO_2. Flows can also be controlled electronically by algorithms within the anesthesia machine, in some machines.
    - **b. Flowmeters.** The traditional flowmeter is a calibrated tapered glass tube in which a bobbin or a ball float is used to indicate the flow of gas. Flowmeters with a ball float should be read in the middle of the ball. Meters with a bobbin should be read at the top of the bobbin. Newer anesthesia machines have electronic flowmeters and displays that often provide a digital readout, or a simulated bobbin. The oxygen flowmeter is always placed downstream in the series of flowmeters so that a leak will be less likely to result in delivery of a hypoxic gas mixture.

B. Vaporizers. Anesthesia machines are outfitted with one or more vaporizers, which are designed to add a precise concentration of anesthetic agent to the fresh gas flow. Anesthesia machines that allow mounting of two or more vaporizers have a mechanism that prevents more than one from being used at any one time. There are three main types of vaporizers:
1. Variable bypass. These vaporizers operate on the principle that a small proportion of the total gas mixture delivered to them is diverted into a vaporizing chamber, where it becomes fully saturated with anesthetic before it is added back to the main flow. The concentration of

anesthetic delivered by the vaporizer is therefore proportional to the amount of gas passing through the vaporizing chamber. Variable bypass vaporizers are available for sevoflurane and isoflurane. The setting on the vaporizer is controlled by a manual dial, typically labelled in units of %. However, in most vaporizers it is a partial pressure of gas that is being delivered. Variable bypass vaporizer set to 1% will deliver the same partial pressure of gas regardless of altitude. Because saturated vapor pressure additionally varies with temperature, a secondary mechanism alters the amount of gas diverted through the chamber to compensate for temperature changes. The vaporizers are calibrated for a specific anesthetic and have various indexed filling adapters to prevent inadvertent addition of an incorrect anesthetic to a vaporizer. The temperature of the vaporizing chamber is stabilized by a metal heatsink which mitigates the evaporative cooling of the anesthetic as it is vaporized.

2. Electronically controlled vapor cassettes have a physical and electronic interface with the anesthesia machine. These are currently marketed by GE Healthcare, for desflurane, isoflurane, and sevoflurane. The concentration of vapor is set by the user on the anesthesia machine interface. The valves at both the inlet and the outlet of the vaporizer are then electronically controlled to achieve the desired vapor concentration in the fresh gas mixture.

3. Heated Electronic Blenders are currently only used for desflurane which has a boiling point of 23 °C. If desflurane were used in a nonelectronic variable bypass vaporizer, and the temperature were to rise above 23 °C, the agent would boil and enter the fresh gas flow in uncontrolled quantities, an extremely dangerous situation. Desflurane is warmed and pressurized to create a predictable and controllable vapor pressure which can then be accurately and safely metered into the fresh gas flow. This also compensates for the extreme cooling that occurs when high concentrations are vaporized. A vapor pressure of approximately 2 atmospheres is created within the vaporizer regardless of ambient pressure. Subsequently, when desflurane is utilized at high altitude the partial pressure of gas ultimately delivered to the patient is less than at sea level. This means that to achieve a similar minimum alveolar concentration (MAC) at altitude, % set on the dial must be increased.

4. Some anesthesia machines are capable of automated control of gas flow and composition, including anesthetic agent. Some examples of this are the Draeger Zeus and the GE Aisys. These machines allow the user to set targets for FiO_2 and end-tidal anesthetic agent concentration; gas flow and anesthetic agent are then adjusted autonomously to achieve the prescribed levels quickly and efficiently.

C. **Oxygen flush valve.** One hundred percent oxygen at 45 to 55 psi comes directly from the high-pressure system to the common gas outlet. Oxygen flow can be as high as 40 to 60 L/min. Caution should be taken when using this valve in mechanically ventilated patients to prevent excessive volume delivery. Notable exceptions to this warning are Draeger anesthesia machines such as the Apollo, Primus, and Atlan, which use fresh gas flow isolation valves in their breathing systems to prevent excessive flow to the patient.

III. BREATHING SYSTEMS

The circle system is the most commonly used breathing system. The T-piece systems, often referred to as Mapleson circuits, are occasionally used in

infants because of low resistance and small dead space, but are extremely uncommon and are outside the scope of this chapter.
A. The **Circle System** incorporates a carbon dioxide absorber and prevents rebreathing of exhaled carbon dioxide. The system allows low fresh gas flows that conserve inhalation anesthetics and maintain humidity and temperature within the breathing circuit. The circle consists of an absorber, at least two one-way valves, a Y-piece adapter, a reservoir bag, and an adjustable pressure limiting (APL) valve (**Figure 10.2**).
  1. The **carbon dioxide absorber.** Soda lime ($CaOH_2$ + NaOH + KOH + silica) or Baralyme ($Ba[OH]_2$ + $Ca[OH]_2$) contained in the absorber combines with carbon dioxide, forming $CaCO_2$ and liberating heat and moisture (H_2O). A pH-sensitive dye changes to blue-violet, indicating exhaustion of the absorbing capacity. In older machines with a two-tiered canister system, the top canister should be changed when 25% to 50% of the pellets have changed color, although a second canister provides an additional margin of safety. The size of the container used should accommodate a patient's tidal volume for maximum efficiency.
  2. Two **one-way valves** (inspiratory and expiratory) ensure one way flow down the inspiratory limb to the Y-piece, and back through the expiratory limb. This both limits deadspace in the circuit and ensures that exhaled gas is not rebreathed without passing through the carbon dioxide absorber.
  3. The **Y-piece adapter** is used to connect the inspiratory and expiratory sides of the system to the patient.
  4. The **reservoir bag and APL valve** are located on the expiratory limb. The reservoir bag accumulates gas between inspirations. It is used to visualize spontaneous ventilation and to assist ventilation manually. Typically, a 3-L reservoir bag is used for adult patients; smaller bags may be appropriate for pediatric patients. The APL valve is used to control the pressure in the breathing system and allows excess gas to escape. The valve can be adjusted from fully open (for spontaneous ventilation, minimal peak pressure 1 to 3 cmH$_2$O) to fully closed (maximum pressure 70 cmH$_2$O). Dangerously high pressures that may produce barotrauma and hemodynamic compromise can occur if the valve is left unattended in the fully or partially closed position. Many anesthesia machines exclude both the reservoir bag and the APL valve from the circuit during mechanical ventilation. Draeger machines include the reservoir bag during mechanical ventilation, using it to accumulate fresh gas diverted by the fresh gas flow isolation valve, and as a visual confirmation of circuit integrity, since these machines lack a rising bellows.

IV. ANESTHESIA VENTILATORS

Modern anesthesia machines feature versatile **microprocessor-controlled ventilators**, which allow for sophisticated manipulation and monitoring of airway pressures (eg, variable positive end-expiratory pressure [PEEP]) and flow rates. Newer anesthesia machines are capable of multiple modes (such as pressure-regulated volume control, volume control, pressure control, pressure support, synchronized mandatory, and inverse ratio ventilation), thereby enabling the anesthetist to optimize ventilation, oxygenation, hemodynamics, and weaning.
  A. Many anesthesia machines are fitted with a mechanical ventilator that uses a **collapsible bellows** within a closed chamber. The bellows contains the anesthetic gas mixture intended to be delivered to the patient. It is

FIGURE 10.2 Representative circle breathing system with ventilator. The airway pressure gauge may sense on the patient side of the inspiratory valve. The PEEP valve may be integral to the ventilator. Other variations are possible depending on the manufacturer.

compressed pneumatically by a second gas, known as the driving gas, which is typically oxygen, which is directed into the chamber surrounding the bellows. This is known as a double-circuit design. These ventilators can be further subclassified into ascending bellows or descending bellows depending on whether the bellows ascend or descend with expiration. Most modern machines use ascending bellows, which are inherently safer, because failure of the bellows to reach the top of the chamber at the end of expiration allows for immediate recognition of a circuit leak. Gravity pulls on a descending bellows system which can entrain gas into the breathing system through a leak, preventing recognition of the leak. It is commonly thought that if there is a leak or tear of the bellow itself, the anesthetic gas mixture within the bellows could mix with the driving gas, however, literature has refuted this oft cited concern.

B. An alternative to the bellows ventilator is the **piston** ventilator, which uses an electronic motor instead of driving gas to deliver tidal volumes. In a piston ventilator design, the anesthetic gas mixture is propelled from a noncompressible cylinder by a piston which travels a prescribed distance within the cylinder to create a pressure gradient that will deliver a set volume to the patient. Compared to the bellows ventilator, the piston ventilator eliminates the need for a second driving gas, and potentially delivers more precise tidal volumes.

C. Servo-based anesthesia machines are now marketed by Getinge and MindRay. A servo is a small electronic device that is capable of metering out gas flow with great precision. Servo devices have been used in ventilators since the 1970s, but only recently have been incorporated into anesthesia machines. Unlike nonanesthesia ventilators, which use the servo to meter out the gas mixture the patient will breathe, servo-based anesthesia machines introduce a driving gas, oxygen, at the end of a long deadspace, which has a volume larger than the tidal volume. Gases leave the circuit during exhalation at the end of this deadspace. These gases do not mix with the gases in the circle system because of the long shape of this deadspace. This allows the patient to rebreathe from the circle, while receiving positive pressure ventilation from the servo (**Figure 10.3**).

V. SAFETY FEATURES

A. An **audible oxygen alarm** is fitted in the oxygen supply line of the high-pressure system. It consists of a pressure regulator and a reed or whistle that will sound when the pressure in the supply line is greater than 0 and less than about 25 psi.

B. A pressure-operated **"fail-safe" valve** in the high-pressure system of the nitrous oxide supply line opens only when oxygen pressure in the high-pressure system is above 25 psi. If the oxygen pressure falls below that, nitrous oxide will cease to flow. Because both the audible oxygen alarm and the fail-safe valve respond specifically to low pressure in the oxygen supply line of the high-pressure system, neither protects against the delivery of a hypoxic mixture downstream in the low-pressure system (eg, if the oxygen flow control valve is accidentally shut off).

C. **Oxygen ratio control**. Anesthesia machines are typically fitted with a device to control the proportion of oxygen delivered. This may take the form of a mechanical link between the oxygen and nitrous oxide flow control knobs that will not allow an FiO_2 of less than 25%. Alternatively, some machines incorporate a sensitive oxygen ratio controller which cuts off the flow of nitrous oxide if oxygen flows fall below a certain level.

Automatic ventilation insp./exp.

FIGURE 10.3 Getinge servo anesthesia–based schematic. (Courtesy of Getinge.) APL, adjustable pressure limiting; PEEP, positive end expiratory pressure.

D. **Pressure alarms** are incorporated into all anesthesia machines.
   1. A **low-pressure alarm** is triggered by a period of by a sustained pressure drop below atmospheric pressure. Low pressure may be caused by a disconnection or a large leak in the system. Negative pressure usually indicates a scavenging system malfunction or that the patient is inhaling against an obstruction.
   2. A **high-pressure alarm** may have a variable or a preset (eg, 65 cmH$_2$O) limit. A high-pressure alarm may indicate obstruction in the tubing or endotracheal tube or a change in the pulmonary compliance (eg, bronchospasm, pneumothorax, laparoscopic insufflation, or "light anesthesia").
   3. A **continuous pressure alarm** alerts the user in the event of high pressure being sustained for more than a few seconds. A blocked or kinked endotracheal tube, a closed pop-off valve, a malfunctioning ventilator pressure relief valve, or an obstruction in the scavenging system could create this condition.

VI. SCAVENGING

A scavenging system channels waste gases away from the operating room to a location outside the hospital building or a location where the gases can be discharged safely. The ambient concentration of anesthetic gases in the operating room should not exceed 25 parts per million (ppm) for nitrous oxide and 2 ppm for halogenated agents. Specific anesthetic gas-scavenging systems should be used routinely. These systems consist of a collecting system, a transfer system, a receiving system, and a disposal system.

A. The **collecting system** delivers waste gases to the transfer system. It collects gasses from the APL valve and the expiratory valve of the ventilator. In addition, waste gases may be collected from the gas analyzers.

B. The **transfer system** consists of tubing that connects the collecting and receiving systems.

C. The **receiving system** ensures that neither positive nor negative pressure builds at the patient end of the system. The system may be open or closed. An open system consists of a reservoir canister opened to atmosphere at one end. Suction usually is applied to the canister, exhausting the waste gas. A closed system consists of a reservoir bag with positive and negative pressure relief valves to maintain the pressure in the bag within an acceptable range.

D. The **disposal system** may be passive or active, although passive systems are inadequate for modern hospitals. A passive system consists of widebore tubing that carries gases directly to the exterior or into the exhaust ventilation ducts. Active systems can be powered by vacuum systems, fans, pumps, or Venturi systems.

VII. GAS ANALYSIS

Several methods are used to monitor concentrations of O_2, CO_2, and anesthetic gases in the breathing system. The oxygen analyzer is the most important monitor for detecting a hypoxic gas mixture. Capnography, the measurement of CO_2, has many uses, including monitoring the adequacy of ventilation, detecting breathing system faults, and it also provides conclusive evidence of cardiac output in a ventilated patient. Breath-to-breath monitoring of anesthetic concentrations provides information about anesthetic uptake and distribution. Most gas analyzers incorporate alarms. Among the techniques for measurement are the following:

A. **Mass spectrometry** was first used to provide rapid response measurement of the concentration of any gas. The major limitation was the large size of the device that required housing in a central location to serve multiple operating rooms. A sample of gas withdrawn through a side port in the breathing system near the Y-piece was carried through a nylon catheter to the mass spectrometer. After ionization in an electron beam, the resulting fragments are accelerated through a high-voltage field and then subjected to a deflecting magnetic field. The specific fragments are detected on collectors, and the relative concentration of each agent is determined. Calibration is performed automatically at the central system. By a switching system, the mass spectrometer can sample from numerous locations. The time between measurements in each room may be one or several minutes depending on the number of rooms "on line."

B. Infrared analysis uses spectrophotometry and Beer's law (the concentration of a solution is proportional to its light absorption) to provide continuous measurement of the concentration of gas or anesthetic in a gas mixture. Gases that have two or more different atoms in the molecule absorb infrared radiation; thus, infrared analysis can be used to measure concentrations of CO_2, N_2O, and halogenated anesthetics but not O_2. Typically, some gas is withdrawn from the breathing system at a steady rate (50 to 300 mL/min) and passed into a small measurement chamber in the instrument. Pulses of infrared energy at a wavelength that is absorbed only by the gas of interest are beamed through the gas, and the difference in energy absorbed is used to determine the gas concentration. In some capnographs, a miniaturized measurement chamber and sensor are placed in the breathing system. In most infrared instruments, only one preselected volatile anesthetic can be measured at a time.

C. Oxygen analyzers. Continuous measurements of oxygen concentrations in a mixture of gases can be provided by mass spectrometry; polarographic, galvanic, fuel cell analysis; or paramagnetic analysis.
  1. **Polarographic oxygen analyzers** are placed in the inspiratory limb of the circuit. The sensor consists of an anode and a cathode in an electrolyte solution with a polarizing voltage. Oxygen diffuses through a semipermeable membrane into the electrolyte solution. Subsequent cathode oxygen uptake creates a current that is measured and the partial pressure of oxygen is calculated. Sensors have a limited life span and should be placed in the upright position to avoid accumulation of moisture.
  2. **Galvanic or fuel cell analyzers** use a similar method to polarographic cell analyzers to ascertain oxygen content. However, different anode, cathode, and electrolyte materials are used, and no polarizing voltage is applied. This cell is similar to a battery that consumes oxygen.
  3. **Paramagnetic analyzers.** These analyzers are based on the principle that oxygen is paramagnetic and therefore attracted to a magnetic field, whereas most other gases are weakly diamagnetic and therefore repelled from a magnetic field. Modern miniaturized paramagnetic analyzers incorporate a rapidly oscillating magnetic chamber and are capable **of breath-to-breath analysis.** They are often combined with another gas analysis technique in an anesthetic agent monitor.

VIII. ANESTHESIA MACHINE CHECKOUT RECOMMENDATIONS

Advances in technology have dramatically changed the anesthesia machine checkout procedure. Integration and computerization have made troubleshooting difficult without advanced training in biomedical engineering. Manual calibration of oxygen sensors is often unnecessary and common gas outlets are often inaccessible to the user. It is no longer possible to describe a comprehensive machine checkout procedure that is adequate for all anesthesia machines. It is of primary importance to know and follow the manufacturer's recommended machine checkout and self-test procedure for the specific anesthesia machine being used. These procedures can be found in the anesthesia machine's instructions for use. Fortunately, many anesthesia machines now have on-screen instructions and checklists for checkout and self-test procedures. The following is a guideline that contains broad principles for an anesthesia machine checkout procedure. Users should refer to the operator's manual for the manufacturer's specific procedures for a machine check. (**Note:** If an anesthesia provider uses the same machine in successive cases, the steps denoted by an asterisk [*] in the section that follows may not need to be repeated and may be abbreviated after the initial checkout.)

A. **Emergency manual ventilator.** Verify that backup ventilation equipment is available and functioning.*
B. **Suction device.** Verify that a suction device is available and of adequate pressure to remove airway fluids.
C. **Gas supply**
   1. **Check oxygen cylinder supply.*** Verify oxygen cylinder pressure; a full tank has about 2000 psi
   2. **Check air and nitrous oxide cylinder supply.*** If applicable.
   3. **Check central pipeline supplies.*** Check if hoses are connected properly, and pipeline pressure gauges read approximately 50 psi.
D. **Scavenging system.** Check and adjust the scavenging system.*
E. **Low-pressure system**
   1. **Check initial status of low-pressure system.***
      a. Close flow control valves and turn vaporizers off.
      b. Check fill level and tighten vaporizers' filler caps, ensure vaporizers are securely attached to anesthesia machine.
   2. **Test flowmeters.*** Adjust flow of all gases through their full range, checking for smooth operation of floats and undamaged flow tubes, if present.
F. **Breathing system**
   1. **Calibrate O_2 monitor.** Verify that low O_2 alarm is enabled and functioning, if applicable.
   2. **Check initial status of the breathing system.**
      a. Check that breathing circuit is complete, undamaged, and unobstructed.
      b. Verify that CO_2 absorbent is adequate.
G. **Perform the manufacturer-prescribed self-test(s)** of the anesthesia machine. These will often encompass many elements of the systems listed in the previous section.
H. **Monitors.** Check function and alarm limits of all monitors.
I. **Preparation for use.** Check final status of the machine self-test to ensure proper operation.
   1. Vaporizers turned off
   2. APL valve open
   3. Breathing system set to manual ventilation
   4. All fresh gas flow turned off
   5. Other airway equipment prepared and ready

ACKNOWLEDGMENT

We gratefully acknowledge the contributions of previous edition author, Samuel Wood, as portions of those chapters have been retained in this revision.

Suggested Readings

Dorsch JA, Dorsch SE, eds. *A Practical Approach to Anesthesia Equipment.* Lippincott Williams & Wilkins; 2011.

Ehrenwerth J, Eisencraft J, Berry J, eds. *Anesthesia Equipment: Principles and Applications.* 2nd ed. Elsevier Saunders; 2013.

Lampotang S, Sanchez JC, Chen B, Gravenstein N. The effect of a bellows leak in an Ohmeda 7810 ventilator on room contamination, inspired oxygen, airway pressure, and tidal volume. *Anesth Analg.* 2005;101:151–154.

Olympio MA. Modern anesthesia machines offer new safety features. *Anesth Patient Saf Found Newsl.* 2003;18:17–32.

Sandberg WS, Urman RD, Ehrenfeld JM. *The MGH Textbook of Anesthesia Equipment.* Elsevier Saunders; 2011.

Administration of General Anesthesia

Matthew Thimm and Kendrick Shaw

The American Society of Anesthesiologists' (ASA) statement on the continuum of depth of sedation defines general anesthesia as "a drug-induced loss of consciousness during which patients are not arousable, even by painful stimulation." The goal of general anesthesia is to produce unconsciousness, amnesia, immobility, and analgesia while a surgical procedure is performed. To achieve this goal, patients under general anesthesia often require intervention to maintain a patent airway, ventilate adequately, and maintain appropriate cardiovascular function. In this chapter, we will summarize the indications for general anesthesia, preoperative evaluation, intraoperative management, and relevant side effects of general anesthesia in the intraoperative and postoperative periods.

I. INDICATIONS FOR GENERAL ANESTHESIA
A. Surgical Factors
Indications for general anesthesia generally fall into surgical or patient factors. Many surgical procedures require general anesthesia because they require complete patient immobilization for optimal surgical visualization and to prevent inadvertent injury due to patient movement. Examples include many open abdominal or pelvic procedures, laparoscopic procedures which require insufflation, and intrathoracic surgery. Some procedures require the patient to be in positions that a patient would find intolerable—for example, gynecologic surgery in steep Trendelenburg or prone positioning with the skull immobilized using pins for cervical spine surgery. Another factor is the duration of the procedure. While it may be possible to perform a procedure without general anesthesia, a patient may find it difficult to lay still for hours and thus prefer general anesthesia for a longer procedure. In addition, the urgency of a case may dictate the need for general anesthesia. In an urgent case, if a patient has not fasted long enough to reduce the risk of aspiration during sedation, it may be safer to perform general anesthesia and intubate the patient to protect their airway. In addition, in an emergency, inducing general anesthesia may be faster than neuraxial or regional techniques, for example, an emergent cesarean delivery in a patient with poorly functioning epidural. In other cases, conversion to general anesthesia may be required, for example, aspiration while under sedation. Other requirements for general anesthesia include specific monitoring such as sensory or motor evoked potentials during spine surgery.

B. Patient Factors
Relevant patient factors for general anesthesia include comorbidities and patient preference. Patients with significant comorbidities, especially significant cardiovascular or pulmonary comorbidities, may benefit from neuraxial or regional anesthesia compared to general anesthesia. However, even for procedures that could be performed under neuraxial or regional techniques, some patients have contraindications including

anticoagulation use and bleeding disorders, active infection, or abnormal anatomy that preclude safe administration of these techniques. Finally, patient preference is important, as some patients may refuse sedation or regional techniques and prefer general anesthesia (or vice versa).

II. PREOPERATIVE EVALUATION

A preoperative evaluation should be performed on every patient undergoing general anesthesia. A preoperative evaluation should include review of relevant medical history, patient interview, and physical examination. Even in emergent settings, it is usually possible to perform an abbreviated preoperative evaluation. (See Chapter 1: Evaluating the Patient Before Anesthesia.)

A. History and Interview

Review of the patient's medical history should include pertinent cardiovascular and pulmonary history, allergies, relevant medications, and any laboratory results. The patient interview should ascertain the last time the patient consumed anything orally. Inquiry about gastroesophageal reflux disease, gastroparesis, nausea/vomiting, or other factors that may impact airway management should also be made. Increasingly relevant is the use of glucagon-like peptide-1 agonists, which delay gastric emptying and may increase the risk of aspiration. In some circumstances, gastric ultrasound can be used to assess the contents of the stomach preoperatively to assess the risk of aspiration and guide the airway management plan. Prior anesthetics should be reviewed, including prior airway management, as well as any personal or family problems with anesthesia, for example a family history of malignant hyperthermia.

B. Physical Examination

The physical examination should at a minimum include assessment of the airway in an effort to predict difficulty with mask ventilation and/or intubation. Specific attention should be paid to the patient's Mallampati score, thyromental distance, mouth opening, cervical spine range of motion, dentition, presence of facial hair, prior surgery or radiation to the head or neck, and neck size. Assessment of the patient's cardiovascular and pulmonary system should also occur, typically through auscultation of the heart and lungs.

C. Airway Management

For a patient undergoing general anesthesia, typically an endotracheal tube or supraglottic airway (laryngeal mask airway [LAM]) is placed. When the airway exam is not reassuring, additional equipment including video laryngoscopy and/or fiberoptic bronchoscopy should be available. If there is concern for a difficult airway, additional preparation may be needed (eg, preparations for a potential emergent surgical airway) and consideration should be given for approaches that reduce the risk of hypoxia such as awake fiberoptic intubation.

D. Pain Management and Anxiolytics

Pain management is typically multimodal. Medications from different classes can be given preoperatively including acetaminophen, nonsteroidal anti-inflammatory drugs (typically selective COX-2 inhibitors), gabapentinoids, and opioids. For some procedures, neuraxial or regional anesthesia can be performed preoperatively or intraoperatively for postoperative pain control. An anxiolytic may be required preoperatively, especially for potentially painful procedures such as nerve blocks and epidural catheters. Typically, a short-acting benzodiazepine with or without an opioid can be used. Once given sedation, these patients should be monitored for potential respiratory depression. Children and those with cognitive disabilities may require oral or intramuscular anxiolytic or hypnotic agents preoperatively to allow for safe cooperation during induction of anesthesia.

E. Intravenous Access and Additional Monitors
Gaining adequate intravenous access is also necessary. The size and number of IVs depends on multiple factors including the surgical procedure, anticipated blood loss, and patient comorbidities. Additional monitors including an arterial line may be necessary in some cases—for example, patients with significant cardiovascular disease or surgeries that have the potential to cause significant hemodynamic changes. An arterial line can be placed before or after induction of anesthesia depending on the indication. A patient may require central venous access if they are expected to require significant vasopressor or inotrope support or if invasive monitoring such as a pulmonary artery catheter is planned.

F. Preoperative Huddle
A preoperative meeting should occur between anesthesia and surgical teams including the operating room staff to discuss the surgical and anesthetic plan, anticipated blood loss, and any specific concerns regarding airway management and the surgical procedure. Other concerns such as the need for additional equipment, medications, and blood products should also be discussed. A planned postoperative destination should also be determined preoperatively. For most patients, this is the postanesthesia recovery unit, however, some patients may require a higher level of care (such as an intensive care unit [ICU]) depending on specific patient or surgical factors.

III. INDUCTION OF GENERAL ANESTHESIA
The induction of general anesthesia involves administering anesthetic agents to induce unconsciousness, managing the airway, and patient positioning prior to the start of an operation.

A. Positioning and Preoxygenation
Following the preoperative evaluation, a patient is brought to the operating room and positioned on the operating room table. Typically, the patient is placed supine so that the anesthesiologist has adequate access to the airway. ASA standard monitoring is initiated including continuous oxygen saturation, electrocardiography, and serial blood pressure measurements. Preoxygenation is performed, where 100% oxygen is delivered to the patient, typically via a face mask that forms a good seal with the patient's face. Preoxygenation aims to increase the safe apnea time by replacing the nitrogen in the alveoli with oxygen. The functional residual capacity (FRC) of the lungs then provides a reservoir of oxygen to prevent desaturation during periods of apnea. For patients with reduced FRC, for example, obese or pregnant patients, a ramp or reverse Trendelenburg positioning may be used to elevate the thorax above the abdomen, therefore increasing the FRC and thus increasing safe apnea time. The goal of preoxygenation is to achieve an end tidal oxygen concentration of at least 80%, although 90% is achievable in most patients with tidal volume breathing over 3 minutes or eight vital capacity breaths in 1 minute. High-flow nasal oxygen can also be used for preoxygenation and to allow for apneic oxygenation in select patients who may desaturate quickly or are predicted to potentially have difficult airways.

B. Intravenous Induction
Once a patient is adequately preoxygenated, anesthesia can be induced. This typically involves intravenous administration of a hypnotic agent to

induce unconsciousness. Typical hypnotic agents include propofol, etomidate, and ketamine, although other agents may be chosen to facilitate the specific procedure being performed, such as methohexital for induction of anesthesia for electroconvulsive therapy. Often lidocaine is administered intravenously prior to reduce pain related to propofol or etomidate injection. Laryngoscopy and intubation are associated with tachycardia and hypertension so opioids like fentanyl and remifentanil or beta blockers can be administered to attenuate these sympathetic responses.

C. Inhalational Induction
In some circumstances, most commonly pediatric patients without intravenous access, anesthesia can be induced through inhalation. This involves administration of volatile anesthetic agents via mask. The concentration of these agents is increased until an adequate depth of anesthesia is reached to facilitate IV placement and/or airway manipulation. Inhalational inductions can also be used to maintain spontaneous ventilation in select patients.

D. Patient Positioning
Once the airway is secured, the patient can be positioned for the operation. Care should be made to pad pressure points to minimize the risk of peripheral nerve and pressure injuries. Special attention should be paid to covering the patient's eyes to prevent corneal abrasions (typically done before airway manipulation), keeping the patient's neck in a neutral position, and adequate padding of the upper extremities to avoid ulnar nerve compression or stretch injuries of the brachial plexus. Some positions pose unique challenges and risks to the patient, for example prone positioning requires careful positioning of the head and face to avoid pressure on the eyes. In addition, lithotomy can lead to lower extremity nerve injuries including femoral and common peroneal neuropathies. Safe positioning of the patient is a responsibility shared by the surgeons, anesthesiologists, and operating room staff.

IV. AIRWAY MANAGEMENT
Due to depressed airway reflexes and respiratory drive, the airway should be secured and mechanical ventilation initiated following induction of anesthesia. In most cases this is facilitated by an endotracheal tube or supraglottic airway (LMA). In some circumstances, spontaneous ventilation can be maintained during general anesthesia or, often only for short procedures, manual bag mask ventilation can be used to maintain ventilation.

A. Endotracheal intubation
Patients are typically positioned supine in "sniffing" position—where the neck is flexed and head extended—to facilitate endotracheal intubation. Visualization of the glottis and placement of the endotracheal tube can be achieved in many ways. Most commonly direct laryngoscopy is performed. However, video laryngoscopy or fiberoptic intubation can be performed if direct laryngoscopy is difficult or anticipated to be difficult. In situations where both mask ventilation and intubation are predicted to be difficult, an awake intubation can be performed using airway topicalization and minimal sedation.

For laryngoscopy, neuromuscular blockers are typically administered to facilitate optimal intubating conditions, by preventing movement or coughing in response to airway instrumentation. Neuromuscular blockers include depolarizing agents such as succinylcholine and non-depolarizing agents such as the aminosteroids (eg, rocuronium and vecuronium) and benzylisoquinoliniums (eg, cisatracurium and mivacurium).

Remifentanil can also be used to achieve adequate intubation conditions. High dose remifentanil is associated with hypotension and bradycardia and often ephedrine will be given with the remifentanil to reduce these effects. It is important to allow adequate time (typically 2 to 3 minutes) for a neuromuscular blocking agent to take effect before attempting intubation, and often a patient will be mask-ventilated during this time. When a patient is at high risk for aspiration, rapid sequence induction can be used to minimize the amount of time the airway is unprotected by proceeding with intubation as soon as possible following hypnotic administration. This typically involves administration of succinylcholine or higher doses of nondepolarizing neuromuscular blockers to allow for more rapid onset of muscle relaxation, avoiding positive pressure ventilation before the first attempt at laryngoscopy, and maintaining cricoid pressure from the onset of unconsciousness to the confirmation of endotracheal tube placement.

Following intubation, correct placement of an endotracheal tube should be confirmed by assessment of end-tidal CO_2 and auscultation of the lungs to assess for inadvertent placement in the right mainstem bronchus. A quantitative measurement of end-tidal CO_2 should be used while the patient is intubated.

B. Supraglottic Airway

Supraglottic airways, also known as LMAs, can also be used to maintain airway patency and facilitate mechanical ventilation. There are a variety of designs and sizes, including LMAs designed to facilitate intubation. Placement of an LMA typically does not require neuromuscular blockade and thus spontaneous ventilation can be maintained. LMAs are usually used for relatively short cases (<4 hours), as longer use can be associated with upper airway edema and injury. Other complications from LMAs include malposition and gastric insufflation. They should not be used in patients at high risk for aspiration. In addition, endotracheal intubation is often preferred in patients who will require higher airway pressures to facilitate ventilation, for example, morbidly obese patients or laparoscopic cases in Trendelenburg position. LMAs play an invaluable role in the difficult airway algorithm and can serve as a rescue device when a patient is difficult to mask ventilate.

V. MAINTENANCE OF ANESTHESIA

General anesthesia is typically maintained using volatile or intravenous anesthetics or both in combination. An anesthetic agent is usually continuously administered and the dose can be titrated based on surgical and patient factors. Depth of anesthesia can be assessed in many ways including patient responses to surgical stimulation like movement, respiratory changes, hypertension, tachycardia, sweating, or tearing. Awareness under anesthesia, defined as varying degrees of patient consciousness due to inadequate anesthesia, occurs infrequently, in approximately 0.1% to 0.2% of general anesthetics. In some surgical populations (cardiac surgery, trauma, and obstetrics), the risk of awareness under general anesthesia is higher. The use of neuromuscular blockers, total intravenous anesthesia (TIVA), and nitrous oxide use without other hypnotic agents increase the risk of awareness. Processed electroencephalography (EEG) technology (BIS or SedLine) can be used to assess depth of anesthesia, particularly when performing TIVA. However, processed EEG monitoring has not been shown to prevent awareness under anesthesia and its use for titration of volatile anesthetics remains controversial.

A. Inhaled Anesthetics

In the United States, the most commonly used volatile anesthetics include sevoflurane, isoflurane, and desflurane. These halogenated, potent inhaled anesthetics are delivered through the airway by the anesthesia machine and are typically titrated by targeting an end-tidal anesthetic concentration that is a chosen fraction of the minimal alveolar concentration (MAC). One MAC is defined as the alveolar concentration that prevents movement to surgical stimulation in 50% of patients. Many factors increase MAC including younger age, chronic alcohol or benzodiazepine use, and hyperthermia. Factors that decrease MAC include older age, acute alcohol or sedative intoxication, pregnancy, and hypothermia. When not using muscle relaxant, inhaled anesthetic concentration can be titrated to patient movement. With the use of neuromuscular blockers for immobility, delivering a concentration that is $0.7 \times MAC$ leads to a low risk of intraoperative awareness. Nitrous oxide can be used in combination with these potent inhaled anesthetics or with opioids to maintain general anesthesia. Using nitrous oxide allows for lower concentrations of volatile agents to be used while still maintaining an adequate depth of anesthesia. Nitrous oxide can cause rapid expansion of air-filled spaces, so its use is relatively contraindicated when this would create risk, such as in patients with pneumothorax or closed loop bowel obstruction. In addition, nitrous oxide inhibits methionine synthase, so its use should be avoided in patients with folate or vitamin B12 deficiencies. Notably, these inhaled anesthetics are also all greenhouse gases, with desflurane and nitrous oxide having the greatest global warming potential. Generally, using fresh gas flows of less than 1 to 2 L/min has been shown to be safe and to reduce anesthesia related greenhouse gas emissions.

B. Intravenous Anesthetics

TIVA is the use of intravenous agents alone to maintain general anesthesia. This typically involves an infusion of a hypnotic agent (eg, propofol) with or without opioids (eg, remifenantil infusion). TIVA is preferred in situations where it is difficult or impossible to deliver inhaled agents, for example, rigid bronchoscopy and airway surgery. TIVA is also associated with a reduced risk of postoperative nausea and vomiting (PONV) compared to inhaled agents. In situations where sensory and motor evoked potentials are being monitored, TIVA is often the preferred anesthetic, as propofol is associated with less reduction in amplitude and less latency prolongation of evoked potentials when compared to volatile agents.

C. Balanced Anesthesia

"Balanced" anesthesia is the use of a mixture of medications (which may include both volatile and intravenous components) to maintain general anesthesia. The premise is that when used in combination, lower doses of each can be used to maintain an adequate depth of anesthesia, thus reducing the risk of side effects or toxicities related to larger doses of a single agent. Additional adjuncts can be used including lidocaine, ketamine, dexmedetomidine, magnesium, opioids, and neuromuscular blockers. The use of regional techniques can reduce nociception and thus reduce anesthetic requirements.

VI. EMERGENCE, EXTUBATION, AND TRANSPORT

A. Emergence

At the end of most surgical procedures the goal is to awaken the patient from anesthesia and extubate. To achieve this, anesthetic agents should be discontinued at the appropriate time based on the pharmacokinetics of each agent. This strategy often involves reducing the volatile concentration and starting nitrous oxide. Some prefer to use propofol or other intravenous agents to allow for a reduction in inhaled anesthetic concentration toward the conclusion of the case. Recovery from neuromuscular blockade should be assessed using a quantitative measure like an accelerometer, to ensure a train-of-four ratio of at least 90%. Reversal of neuromuscular blocker should be administered if indicated. Adequate pain control should be ensured based on patient and surgical factors.

B. Extubation
Prior to extubation, the patient should be spontaneously breathing, with adequate ventilation to maintain normal gas exchange. Patients should also be normothermic with a normal acid base status. In some situations, a deep extubation may be preferred. This is removing the endotracheal tube while the patient remains deeply anesthetized. Deep extubation may be preferred following some surgical procedures where coughing or bucking could disrupt sutures or cause bleeding, for example, hernia or airway surgery, or for patients at high risk of bronchospasm or laryngospasm, for example, asthmatic patients or children. These risks must be carefully balanced against the risk of an unsecured airway during emergence. Following extubation, the ability to maintain a patent airway and ventilate adequately should be ensured. Some patients, especially those with reactive airways or children, are at higher risk of laryngospasm, which can lead to morbidity if not addressed promptly.

C. Transport and Disposition
The patient is then prepared for transport to the postanesthesia care unit (PACU) or ICU. Patients going to the PACU should have stable vital signs. Extubated patients should be ventilating spontaneously and be able to maintain a normal oxygen saturation. Patients requiring vasopressors or vasodilators should have hemodynamic monitoring during transport. Generally, all patients requiring an ICU level of care should be placed on basic monitors including pulse oximetry, blood pressure, and ECG during transport. Patients who are intubated should be connected to a transport ventilator and adequate ventilation should be ensured. When transporting patients who are unstable or remain intubated and sedated, emergency airway equipment and drugs should be available. Upon arrival in the PACU or ICU, report is given to the postoperative care team and bedside nurse which includes relevant history about the patient, details of the anesthetic including airway management and medications given, and pertinent intraoperative events. The patient should be monitored in the PACU or ICU with frequent assessment of their vital signs, ventilation, and level of consciousness until they are appropriate for discharge to a less closely monitored area.

VII. ADVERSE EFFECTS RELATED TO ANESTHESIA
Anesthetic agents can cause many adverse effects both intraoperatively and postoperatively. Intraoperatively respiratory, cardiovascular, and thermoregulatory effects are especially pertinent. Postoperatively adverse effects related to anesthesia include postoperative nausea/vomiting, cognitive dysfunction, hypotension, and upper airway obstruction.

A. Respiratory
Following administration of anesthetic agents, the patient's protective airway reflexes and their respiratory drive are both typically depressed. Furthermore, positioning, location of surgery (eg, intrathoracic surgery), and peritoneal insufflation can also impact respiratory function.

In most cases, management of this requires securing the airway with an endotracheal tube or LMA. Ventilation is initiated to maintain normal gas exchange, monitored through end-tidal CO_2 or $PaCO_2$. For cases where neuromuscular blockers are used, a controlled ventilation mode is necessary. When assisted ventilation is used, depth of anesthesia can be assessed based on respiratory pattern and respiratory rate. In addition, using assisted ventilation, the positive pressure can be minimized, which helps reduce gastric insufflation when an LMA is used. For laparoscopic procedures utilizing CO_2 insufflation, minute ventilation should be increased to counteract the increase in $PaCO_2$ related to CO_2 absorption. In some special circumstances (eg, craniotomies) the surgeon may request an increase in minute ventilation to decrease $PaCO_2$, reduce cerebral blow flow, and improve surgical exposure.

Once the airway is secured and ventilation is initiated, monitoring of airway pressures and inspiratory and expiratory flows in the ventilator can help detect and address potential problems. Low airway pressures may indicate a circuit disconnect or leak. High airway pressures may be related to obstruction at some point between the ventilator and alveoli or ventilator dyssynchrony. Kinking or obstruction of the endotracheal tube, related to positioning or biting, surgical compression, movement of the tube into the mainstem bronchus, change in level of sedation or muscle relaxant, bronchospasm, mucous plugging, and pneumothorax can all elevate airway pressures. Prompt evaluation of the patient, endotracheal tube, circuit, and ventilator is required to determine and address any potential problem.

B. Cardiovascular

The administration of most anesthetic agents is associated with hypotension. This is related to several factors including reduction in systemic vascular resistance and blunting of cardiovascular reflexes by anesthetic agents. Many anesthetics, including propofol and volatile agents, reduce myocardial contractility. In combination with this, many patients are relatively hypovolemic related to fasting or laxatives for bowel preparation. These factors lead to hypotension, which is may be more marked in older adults and those with poor cardiovascular reserve. Hypotension should be anticipated and treated promptly. Patients should be fluid resuscitated and vasopressors like phenylephrine may be needed to maintain normotension. For those with baseline cardiovascular dysfunction, ionotropes like norepinephrine or epinephrine may be needed.

C. Thermoregulation

Hypothermia is not uncommon during general anesthesia. Anesthetic agents cause an increased distribution of blood flow to the periphery, leading to immediate core temperature reduction. This heat loss can be mitigated by using forced air warmers preoperatively. Vasodilation by anesthetic agents promotes heat loss to the environment, the majority of which occurs through radiation. Other factors that contribute to heat loss include cooler room temperature, use of cold intravenous or irrigating fluids, larger surgical exposure, duration and type of surgery, BMI, and age. When significant temperature changes are anticipated, core temperature should be monitored. Common sites for temperature measurement include the nasopharynx, esophagus, bladder, axilla, and mixed venous blood. Strategies to mitigate temperature loss include using forced air warmers, reducing exposed areas, increasing the room temperature, and using warm intravenous and irrigating fluids. Hyperthermia is uncommon and usually only occurs in the context of a febrile illness, overwarming, or is related to the surgery, for example heated intraperitoneal chemotherapy following cytoreductive surgery.

D. Postoperative Nausea and Vomiting

PONV is the most frequent adverse side effect related to general anesthesia. While generally self-limited, there is the potential for significant impact on patient satisfaction and the duration of anesthesia recovery. The major risk factors for PONV include being female, being a nonsmoker, having a history of PONV or motion sickness, and the use of opioids postoperatively. A longer duration of surgery is associated with an increased risk and some surgeries themselves are independent risk factors (eg, strabismus surgery). Anesthetic factors that increase the risk of PONV include the use of nitrous oxide, volatile anesthetics, neostigmine, and opioids. TIVA is associated with a reduced risk compared to inhaled anesthetics. There are many agents that can be given to treat and/or prevent PONV including dexamethasone, ondansetron, scopolamine (typically transdermally), haloperidol, metoclopramide, promethazine, diphenhydramine, droperidol, and others. Propofol is also an antiemetic and can be used postoperatively in refractory cases. Most patients receive prophylaxis for PONV with at least one or two agents, and those at high risk should receive more.

E. Hypotension

Postoperative hypotension after anesthesia is not uncommon, especially among the elderly, those with poor cardiovascular reserve, and after surgeries of longer duration. These patients may require vasopressors in the postoperative period and should be adequately volume resuscitated. Care should be made to not miss other causes of hypotension when attributing hypotension to anesthesia.

F. Upper Airway Obstruction and Complications

Patients with obstructive sleep apnea or risk factors for it (high BMI, large neck, history of snoring) are at increased risk of upper airway obstruction postoperatively. For these patients, their level of consciousness and respiratory status should be monitored closely, and they may require positive pressure ventilation postoperatively. This is especially true of those with amyotrophic lateral sclerosis (ALS), even if they received minimal sedation.

Some patients may have airway complications related to laryngoscopy, intubation, LMA placement, or the surgery itself. The most common problems include sore throat, hoarseness, and minor injury to soft tissues of the oropharynx (eg, lips). More serious issues include dental injury, mucosal laceration, arytenoid dislocation, or vocal cord injury. Surgeries in the head and neck can cause injury to the recurrent laryngeal nerve (eg, thyroidectomy) or airway compression from bleeding or edema.

G. Neuromuscular Blockade Complications

Residual neuromuscular blockade has been documented in up to 50% of patients postoperatively. However, with the use of Suggamadex, this is less frequent than with neostigmine. Residual paralysis is associated with an increased risk of pulmonary complications including upper airway obstruction, atelectasis, and pneumonia. Patients who receive neuromuscular blockade should have quantitative monitoring before extubation. Reversal should be given if indicated (ie, if the train-of-four ratio is less than 0.9) and the train-of-four should be reassessed to ensure adequate reversal.

Succinylcholine can be associated with myalgias that are bothersome to patients. These myalgias typically resolve with time and respond well to nonsteroid anti-inflammatory drugs. The risk of myalgia can be decreased by giving a smaller dose of nondepolarizing neuromuscular blocker prior to succinylcholine administration.

H. Cognitive Side Effects

Emergence delirium is defined as hyperactivity with sensitivity to stimulation that occurs following a general anesthetic, usually within 30 minutes of emergence, and is typically self-limited. Emergence delirium can be upsetting to patients and their caregivers as well as significantly delay discharge from the recovery room. Emergence delirium occurs more commonly in children than adults, with reports ranging from 20% to 80% of pediatric general anesthetics. Risk factors include use of volatile agents (sevoflurane and desflurane), male gender, preschool age, and preoperative anxiety. Propofol is associated with reduced emergence delirium compared to sevoflurane. Other agents like alpha-2 agonists, potent opioids, benzodiazepines, and ketamine can be used as prevention and/or treatment.

Postoperative cognitive dysfunction (POCD) is a reduction in cognitive function including learning or memory following surgery. POCD and delirium are not uncommon following surgery with general anesthesia, especially among the elderly. The incidence of POCD may be as high as 30% in the week following surgery and declines to 1% by 1 year. Risk factors include older age, pre-existing dementia or cognitive deficits, lower educational level, alcohol abuse, longer duration of surgery, and cardiac surgery. POCD has the potential for significant morbidity, those with POCD are less likely to be able to function independently postoperatively and have reduced survival. No one anesthetic strategy has been shown to prevent POCD, but maintaining normotension, normothermia, normoglycemia, reducing sedating agents, and titrating the anesthetic based on EEG monitoring may help reduce the risk.

ACKNOWLEDGMENT

We gratefully acknowledge the contributions of previous edition author, Luca Zazzeron, as portions of those chapters have been retained in this revision.

Suggested Readings

American Society of Anesthesiologists Committee on Quality Management and Departmental Administration. Statement on continuum of depth of sedation: definition of general anesthesia and levels of sedation/analgesia. 2019. Accessed April 5, 2025. https://www.asahq.org/standards-and-practice-parameters/statement-on-continuum-of-depth-of-sedation-definition-of-general-anesthesia-and-levels-of-sedation-analgesia

Apfel CC, Korttila K, Abdalla M, et al; IMPACT Investigators. A factorial trial of six interventions for the prevention of postoperative nausea and vomiting. *N Engl J Med.* 2004;350(24):2441–2451.

Avidan MS, Jacobsohn E, Glick D, et al; BAG-RECALL Research Group. Prevention of intraoperative awareness in a high-risk surgical population. *N Engl J Med.* 2011;365:591–600.

Avidan MS, Zhang L, Burnside BA, et al. Anesthesia awareness and the bispectral index. *N Engl J Med.* 2008;358:1097–1108.

Brown EN, Pavone KJ, Naranjo M. Multimodal general anesthesia: theory and practice. *Anesth Analg.* 2018;127(5):1246–1258.

Cavallone LF, Vannucci A. Review article: extubation of the difficult airway and extubation failure. *Anesth Analg.* 2013;116(2):368–383.

Fleisher LA, Fleischmann KE, Auerbach AD, et al; American College of Cardiology; American Heart Association. 2014 ACC/AHA guideline on perioperative cardiovascular evaluation and management of patients undergoing noncardiac surgery: a report of the ACC/AHA Task Force on practice guidelines. *J Am Coll Cardiol.* 2014;64:e77–e137.

Joshi GP. Anesthetic considerations in adult patients on glucagon-like peptide-1 receptor agonists: gastrointestinal focus. *Anesth Analg.* 2024;138(1):216–220.

Kheterpal S, Vaughn MT, Dubovoy TZ, et al. Sugammadex versus neostigmine for reversal of neuromuscular blockade and postoperative pulmonary complications (STRONGER): a multicenter matched cohort analysis. *Anesthesiology.* 2020;132(6):1371–1381.

Kotekar N, Shenkar A, Nagaraj R. Postoperative cognitive dysfunction—current preventive strategies. *Clin Interv Aging.* 2018;13:2267–2273.

Lewis SR, Pritchard MW, Fawcett LJ, Punjasawadwong Y. Bispectral index for improving intraoperative awareness and early postoperative recovery in adults. *Cochrane Database Syst Rev.* 2019;9:CD003843.

Myles PS, Leslie K, McNeil J, Forbes A, Chan MTV. Bispectral index monitoring to prevent awareness during anaesthesia: the B-Aware randomised controlled trial. *Lancet.* 2004;363:1757–1763.

Plaud B, Debaene B, Donati F, Marty J. Residual paralysis after emergence from anesthesia. *Anesthesiology.* 2010;112(4):1013–1022.

Stanski DR, Shafer SL. Monitoring depth of anesthesia. In: Miller RD, ed. *Anesthesia.* 6th ed. Churchill Livingstone; 2005:1227–1264.

Willenkin RL, Polk SL. Management of general anesthesia. In: Miller RD, ed. *Anesthesia.* 4th ed. Churchill Livingstone; 1994:1045–1056.

World Alliance for Patient Safety. *WHO Surgical Safety Checklist and Implementation Manual.* 2009. https://www.who.int/teams/integrated-health-services/patient-safety/research/safe-surgery/tool-and-resources

Intravenous and Inhalation Anesthetics

Justin R. Porter and Gregory E. Ginsburg

I. PHARMACOLOGY OF INTRAVENOUS ANESTHETICS

Intravenous (IV) anesthetics are commonly used for the induction and maintenance of general anesthesia and for sedation. Propofol, thiopental (not available in the United States), and etomidate rapidly distribute into the **vessel-rich group** of highly perfused tissues (eg, brain, heart, liver, and kidneys), causing an extremely rapid onset of effect. Plasma concentrations decrease as the drug is taken up by the less well-perfused tissues (eg, muscle and fat), and the drug rapidly leaves the brain. This **redistribution** from the brain is responsible for the termination of effects; the **clearance** of the active drug occurs mainly by hepatic **metabolism** and renal **elimination. Elimination half-life** is defined as the time required for the plasma concentration of a drug to decrease by 50% during the elimination phase of clearance. **Context-sensitive half-time (CSHT)** is defined as the time required for a 50% decrease in the central compartment drug concentration after a steady-state infusion of specified duration (duration is the "context").

A. Propofol (2,6-diisopropylphenol) is used for the induction or maintenance of general anesthesia and for procedural sedation. In the United States, it is marketed as a 1% isotonic oil-in-water emulsion, which contains 10% soybean oil, 2.25% glycerol, and 1.2% purified egg phosphatide. Bacterial growth is inhibited by ethylenediaminetetraacetic acid, diethylenetri-amine pentaacetic acid, sulfite, or benzyl alcohol depending on the manufacturer. **Fospropofol**, a prodrug of propofol, is available as an aqueous formulation in some countries outside the United States.

1. **Mode of action.** Although complex and incompletely understood, propofol's primary mechanism is likely direct activation of inhibitory γ-aminobutyric acid type A ($GABA_A$) receptors in the central nervous system (CNS). Glycine, alpha-adrenergic, N-methyl-D-aspartate (NMDA), and cannabinoid receptors, as well as voltage-gated ion channels may contribute.

2. **Pharmacokinetics**
   a. After IV administration, these agents rapidly diffuse into the brain. They subsequently redistribute into fatty tissues.
   b. Hepatic as well as substantial (~30%) extrahepatic metabolism to inactive metabolites that are renally excreted.
   c. Although CSHT remains below 15 minutes following 2-hour infusion, CSHT can rise above 30 minutes for infusions lasting over 8 hours.

3. **Pharmacodynamics**
   a. **CNS**
      1. Induction doses rapidly produce unconsciousness (30 to 45 seconds). Emergence is also rapid and often accompanied by mood elevation. Low doses produce sedation and amnesia.
      2. Weak analgesia at hypnotic concentrations
      3. Weak akinesis at hypnotic concentrations

4. Decreases intracranial pressure (ICP) and also cerebral perfusion pressure (CPP) due to markedly decreased mean arterial pressure (MAP). Cerebral autoregulation and the vasoconstrictive response to hyperventilation are unaffected.
5. Anticonvulsant properties raise the seizure threshold.
6. Propofol-induced anesthesia is associated with frontal alpha oscillations (8 to 12 Hz), delta oscillations (1 to 4 Hz), and slow oscillations (0.1 to 1 Hz) electroencephalogram (EEG). Higher doses cause burst suppression and isoelectric EEG.
7. Depresses somatosensory-evoked potentials (SSEPs) and motor-evoked potentials (MEPs), but little effect on brainstem auditory–evoked potentials (BAEPs).
8. Has antiemetic effects, even at subhypnotic doses. Postoperative nausea and vomiting (PONV) is less frequent after propofol anesthetics compared with other techniques.

b. Cardiovascular system
1. Dose-dependent decreases in preload, afterload, and contractility lead to decreases in blood pressure (BP) and cardiac output. Hypotension may be marked in hypovolemic, elderly, or hemodynamically compromised patients.
2. Heart rate (HR) is minimally affected, and baroreceptor reflex is blunted.

c. Respiratory system
1. Dose-dependent decreases in respiratory rate (RR) and tidal volume (TV).
2. Ventilatory responses to hypoxia and hypercarbia are diminished.

4. Dosage and administration (Table 12.1)
  a. Titrate with reduced and incremental doses in hypovolemic, elderly, or hemodynamically compromised patients or if administered with other anesthetics.
  b. Relatively larger induction and maintenance doses are required in infants and small children.
  c. Propofol emulsion supports bacterial growth despite the addition of antimicrobials; prepare drug under sterile conditions, label with date and time, and discard unused propofol per your institutional protocol but not longer than **6 to 12 hours** to prevent inadvertent bacterial contamination.
  d. Target-controlled infusion pumps have been developed which, based on the patient's age and body weight, can titrate an initial bolus and variable infusion rate to achieve a desired plasma concentration (not available in the United States).
  e. Systems have also been developed to measure propofol concentration by mass spectrophotometry in exhaled gas or by IV electrodes, but these modalities are not used in common practice.

5. Adverse effects
  a. Venous irritation. May cause pain during IV administration, which is reduced by administration in larger veins. An alternative is to place a tourniquet proximal to the IV site and, with the tourniquet up, administer lidocaine (0.5 mg/kg, IV) 1 to 2 minutes before propofol injection. The tourniquet is released immediately before propofol injection.
  b. Lipid disorders. Propofol is a lipid emulsion and should be used cautiously in patients with disorders of lipid metabolism (eg, hyperlipidemia and pancreatitis).

TABLE 12.1 Dosages of Commonly Used IV Anesthetics and Induction Dose Onset and Duration

Drug	Induction (mg/kg)	Dose Maintenance (μg/kg/min)	Sedation (Titrate to Effect)	Onset (s)	Induction Dose Duration (min)
Propofol IV	1–3	100–150	25–75 μg/kg/min	<30	3–8
Midazolam IV	0.2–0.4	0.5–1.5	0.5–1.0 mg	30–60	15–30
Midazolam IM	—	—	0.07–0.1 mg/kg	—	—
Ketamine IV	1–2	15–90	0.1–0.8 mg/kg	45–60	10–20
Ketamine IM	5–10	—	2–4 mg/kg	—	—
Etomidate IV	0.2–0.4	10[a]	5–8 μg/kg/min[a]	<30	4–8
Dexmedetomidine IV	—	—	0.2–0.7 μg/kg/h[b]	—	—
Methohexital IV	1–1.5	—	0.5 mg/kg[c]	<30	4–7

IM, intramuscular; IV, intravenous.
[a]Off-label use, avoided due to risk of adrenal suppression.
[b]After loading dose of 0.5 to 1.0 μg/kg over 10 minutes.
[c]Off-label use, following initial loading dose of 0.75 to 1 mg/kg, redose every 2 to 5 minutes as needed.

    c. Myoclonus and **hiccups** can occur after induction doses, although less frequently than with methohexital or etomidate.

    d. Propofol infusion syndrome is a rare and potentially fatal disorder that occurs in critically ill patients (usually children) subjected to prolonged, high-dose propofol infusions. Typical features include rhabdomyolysis, metabolic acidosis, cardiac failure, and renal failure.

B. Barbiturates such as thiopental (unavailable in the United States since 2011) and methohexital rapidly produce unconsciousness (30 to 45 seconds) after IV administration, followed by rapid termination of effects due to redistribution. Barbiturate preparations for IV administration are highly alkaline (pH >10) and are usually prepared as dilute solutions (1.0% to 2.5%).

  1. Mode of action. Barbiturates facilitate inhibitory neurotransmission by enhancing $GABA_A$ receptor function, binding it at an allosteric site and increasing the duration of opening, prolonging Cl^- ion influx, leading to membrane hyperpolarization. At higher concentrations, they directly stimulate $GABA_A$ receptors. They also inhibit excitatory neurotransmission via glutamate and nicotinic acetylcholine receptors.

  2. Pharmacokinetics

    a. Hepatic metabolism. Methohexital has a much higher clearance than thiopental. Thiopental is metabolized to pentobarbital, an active metabolite with a longer half-life.

    b. Multiple doses or prolonged infusions may produce prolonged sedation or unconsciousness due to the reduced rate of redistribution, the return of the drug to the central compartment, and slow hepatic metabolism. The CSHT of thiopental is long, even after short infusions.

3. **Pharmacodynamics**
   a. **CNS**
      1. Dose-dependent CNS depression ranging from sedation to unconsciousness. Akinesis requires much higher doses.
      2. ICP and cerebral blood flow are reduced in a dose-dependent fashion due to cerebral vasoconstriction and decrease in cerebral metabolic rate ($CMRO_2$). Cerebral autoregulation is unaffected.
      3. At high doses, barbiturates all produce an isoelectric EEG. Methohexital, uniquely among barbiturates, reduces the seizure threshold at lower doses. Combined with its favorable pharmacokinetic profile, methohexital is often used during electroconvulsive therapy.
      4. Minimal effects on SSEPs or MEPs, but dose-dependent depression of BAEPs.
   b. **Cardiovascular system**
      1. Cause venodilation and depress myocardial contractility, leading to a dose-dependent decrease in BP and cardiac output, especially in patients who are preload dependent. Decrease in BP is less pronounced than with propofol.
      2. Baroreceptor reflexes remain largely intact; therefore, HR may increase in response to hypotension.
   c. **Respiratory system**
      1. Dose-dependent decreases in RR and TV. Ventilatory responses to hypoxia and hypercarbia are markedly depressed. Apnea may result 30 to 90 seconds after an induction dose.
      2. Laryngeal reflexes remain more intact relative to propofol; therefore, the incidence of cough and laryngospasm is higher.
4. **Dosage and administration (Table 12.1)**
   a. Doses should be reduced in hypovolemic, elderly, or hemodynamically compromised patients.
   b. May precipitate when mixed with drugs in lower pH solution (eg, succinylcholine) and cause the precipitation of other drugs (eg, vecuronium). Therefore, it is prudent to use a free-running IV and avoid simultaneous injection with other drugs.
5. **Adverse effects**
   a. **Allergy.** True allergies are unusual. Thiopental occasionally causes anaphylactoid reactions (ie, hives, flushing, and hypotension) due to histamine release.
   b. **Porphyria**
      1. **Absolutely contraindicated** in patients with acute intermittent porphyria, variegate porphyria, and hereditary coproporphyria.
      2. Barbiturates induce porphyrin synthetic enzymes such as δ-aminolevulinic acid synthetase; patients with porphyria may accumulate toxic heme precursors and suffer an acute attack.
   c. **Venous irritation and tissue damage**
      1. May cause pain at the site of administration due to venous irritation.
      2. Thiopental can cause severe pain and tissue necrosis if injected extravascularly or intra-arterially. If intra-arterial administration occurs, phentolamine (α-blocker), heparin, vasodilators, and regional sympathetic blockade may be helpful in treatment.
   d. **Myoclonus** and **hiccups** are often seen during induction with methohexital.

C. Benzodiazepines include midazolam, lorazepam, diazepam, and remimazolam (approved for use in the US in 2020). They are often used for sedation, amnesia, anxiolysis, or as adjuncts to general anesthesia. Midazolam is prepared in a water-soluble form at pH 3.5, while diazepam and lorazepam are dissolved in propylene glycol and polyethylene glycol, respectively. Remimazolam is distributed as a lyophilized powder which is reconstituted in normal saline before use.

1. **Mode of action.** Enhance inhibitory neurotransmission by increasing the affinity of $GABA_A$ receptors for GABA. In contrast to other agents (eg, barbiturates), benzodiazepines are unable to activate the $GABA_A$ receptor in the absence of GABA. Different clinical effects (eg, amnesia, sedation, and anxiolysis) appear to be mediated by different $GABA_A$ receptor subtypes, among which the benzodiazepines generally do not show selectivity.
2. **Pharmacokinetics**
   a. After IV administration, the onset of CNS effects occurs in 2 to 3 minutes for midazolam and diazepam (slightly longer for lorazepam). Effects are terminated by redistribution; therefore, durations of a single dose of diazepam and midazolam are similar. The effects of lorazepam are somewhat more prolonged.
   b. Midazolam, lorazepam, and diazepam are metabolized in the liver. Elimination half-lives for midazolam, lorazepam, and diazepam are approximately 2, 11, and 20 hours, respectively. The active metabolites of diazepam last longer than the parent drug and accumulate with repeated dosing. Hydroxymidazolam can accumulate and cause sedation in patients with renal failure.
   c. Remimazolam is hydrolyzed by plasma esterases to a carboxylic acid derivative with a 300-fold reduced affinity for the $GABA_A$. Compared to midazolam, it has a smaller Vd and faster, bodyweight-independent clearance. Its clearance is nonetheless reduced in liver failure, however.
   d. Diazepam, but not midazolam and lorazepam, show reduced clearance in the elderly. Obese patients may require higher initial doses of benzodiazepines, but clearance is similar.
3. **Pharmacodynamics**
   a. **CNS**
      1. Dose-dependent amnestic, anticonvulsant, anxiolytic, muscle relaxant, and sedative-hypnotic effects. Amnesia may last for up to 1 hour following a single premedication dose of midazolam. Sedation may be prolonged.
      2. Benzodiazepines alone do not inhibit the response to noxious stimulus sufficiently for surgical anesthesia.
      3. Do not produce significant analgesia.
      4. Dose-dependent reduction of cerebral blood flow (CBF) and $CMRO_2$.
      5. Do not produce burst suppression or isoelectric EEG pattern, even at very high doses.
   b. **Cardiovascular system**
      1. Mild systemic vasodilation and decrease in cardiac output. HR is usually unchanged, except with remimazolam, which modestly increases HR.
      2. Hemodynamic changes may be pronounced in hypovolemic or critically ill patients if rapidly administered in a large dose or with an opioid.

c. Respiratory system
1. Mild dose-dependent decreases in RR and TV. Some decrease in hypoxic ventilatory drive.
2. Respiratory depression may be pronounced if administered with an opioid, in patients with pulmonary disease or in debilitated patients.

4. Dosage and administration (see **Table 12.1** for midazolam)
   a. Incremental IV doses of diazepam (2.5 mg) or lorazepam (0.25 mg) may be used for sedation.
   b. Appropriate oral doses are 5 to 10 mg of diazepam or 2 to 4 mg of lorazepam.
   c. Remimazolam package insert suggests initial 5 mg bolus followed by 2.5 mg top-up doses.

5. Adverse effects
   a. Drug interactions. Administration of a benzodiazepine to a patient receiving the anticonvulsant **valproate** may precipitate a psychotic episode.
   b. Pregnancy and labor
   1. Experts generally do not recommend withholding routine anxiolysis in pregnant or laboring patients when otherwise indicated.
   2. There was historical concern for an association with cleft lip and palate in the first trimester. However, better-powered modern investigations have failed to reproduce this association.
   3. Although benzodiazepines cross the placenta, the risks of CNS depression in the neonate from routine anxiolytic doses appear to be limited even when given immediately prior to delivery.
   c. Superficial thrombophlebitis and injection pain may be produced by the vehicles in diazepam and lorazepam.

6. Flumazenil (imidazobenzodiazepine) is a competitive antagonist at the benzodiazepine binding site of $GABA_A$ receptors in the CNS.
   a. Reversal of benzodiazepine-induced sedative effects occurs within 2 minutes; peak effect at ~10 minutes. It does not completely antagonize the respiratory depressant effects of benzodiazepines.
   b. Half-life is shorter than the benzodiazepine agonists, thus repeated administration may be necessary.
   c. Metabolized to inactive metabolites in the liver.
   d. Dose of 0.3 mg IV every 30 to 60 seconds (to a maximum dose of 5 mg).
   e. Contraindicated in patients with tricyclic antidepressant (TCA) overdose (thought to be due to unmasking TCA-induced seizure activity) and in those receiving benzodiazepines for the control of seizures or elevated ICP. Use cautiously in patients who have had long-term treatment with benzodiazepines because acute withdrawal may be precipitated.

D. Etomidate is a benzylimidazole sedative-hypnotic agent most commonly used for IV induction of general anesthesia. It is supplied in a solution containing 35% of propylene glycol.
1. Mode of action. Facilitates inhibitory neurotransmission by enhancing $GABA_A$ receptor function.
2. Pharmacokinetics
   a. After an induction dose, times to loss of consciousness and return of consciousness are similar to that for propofol. Effects of a single bolus dose are terminated by redistribution.
   b. Very high clearance in the liver and by circulating esterases to inactive metabolites.

3. **Pharmacodynamics**
   a. **CNS**
      1. No analgesic properties.
      2. CBF, $CMRO_2$, and ICP decrease, while CPP is usually maintained. Cerebral vasoconstriction in response to hyperventilation is preserved.
      3. Induces burst suppression at high doses.
      4. Less depression of evoked potentials compared to that with propofol or thiopental. BAEPs are unaffected, while SSEPs are enhanced.
         a. Increases EEG activity in epileptogenic foci potentially precipitating with seizures.
   b. **Cardiovascular system**
      1. Minimal changes in HR, BP, and cardiac output. Often chosen to induce general anesthesia in hemodynamically compromised patients.
      2. Does not affect the sympathetic tone or the baroreceptor function. Will not effectively suppress hemodynamic responses to pain.
      3. Decreases myocardial oxygen consumption.
   c. **Respiratory system**
      1. Dose-dependent decreases in RR and TV; transient apnea may occur.
      2. The respiratory depressant effects of etomidate are less pronounced than those of propofol or barbiturates.
4. **Dosage and administration (Table 12.1)**
5. **Adverse effects**
   a. **Myoclonus** may occur after administration, particularly in response to stimulation. Can be avoided by premedication with benzodiazepines or opiates.
   b. **Nausea and vomiting** occur more frequently in the postoperative period than with other anesthetic agents.
   c. **Venous irritation and superficial thrombophlebitis** may be caused by the propylene glycol vehicle. Minimized by administration into a free-flowing IV carrier infusion. Pain at injection site has been described in 30% to 80% of patients.
   d. **Adrenal suppression.** Potent inhibitor of 11β-hydroxylase; a single induction dose suppresses adrenal steroid synthesis for up to 24 hours in elderly or debilitated patients. Clinical significance of this after a single dose is controversial, but prolonged ICU use has been associated with increased mortality.
   e. **Hiccups** and **nystagmus** are also relatively common side effects following induction with etomidate.
E. **Ketamine** is an arylcyclohexylamine (related to phencyclidine) sedative-hypnotic agent with potent analgesic properties. It is used for the induction of general anesthesia and for sedation and analgesia in the perioperative setting. It is a mixture of R+ and S– isomers. The S– isomer has higher potency and produces fewer side effects.
   1. **Mode of action.** Anesthetic effects are mainly attributed to noncompetitive antagonism of NMDA receptors in the CNS, while effects on opioid receptors, acetylcholine receptors, and voltage-gated sodium and calcium channels also have been reported.
   2. **Pharmacokinetics**
      a. Produces unconsciousness in 30 to 60 seconds after an IV induction dose. Effects are terminated by redistribution in 15 to 20 minutes.

After intramuscular (IM) administration, the onset of CNS effects is delayed for approximately 5 minutes, with peak effect at approximately 15 minutes.
- **b.** Metabolized rapidly in the liver to multiple metabolites, some of which have modest activity (eg, norketamine). Elimination half-life is 2 to 3 hours.
- **c.** Repeated bolus doses or prolonged infusions result in accumulation.

3. Pharmacodynamics
a. CNS
1. Produces a "dissociative" state accompanied by amnesia and profound analgesia. Analgesia occurs at much lower concentrations than hypnosis, so analgesic effects persist after the return of consciousness.
2. Increases CBF, ICP, and $CMRO_2$; cerebral vasoconstriction in response to hyperventilation is preserved.
3. Enhancement of SSEPs; depression of BAEPs and visual-evoked potentials.
4. Dose-dependent EEG changes that differ from other anesthetics; high doses do not produce an isoelectric EEG. Gamma oscillations (25 to 40 Hz) are often observed.

b. Cardiovascular system
1. Increases HR, cardiac output, and BP of systemic and pulmonary arteries by triggering the release of endogenous catecholamines.
2. Often used for inducing general anesthesia in hemodynamically compromised patients, particularly those for whom HR, preload, and afterload should remain high. Use with caution in CAD or pulmonary hypertension.
3. Direct negative inotrope and vasodilator, usually outweighed by a potent sympathomimetic effect. Sometimes acts as a cardiovascular depressant in cases of maximal sympathetic activity, autonomic blockade, and possibly catecholamine depletion.

c. Respiratory system
1. Usually depresses RR and TV only mildly and has minimal effect on CO_2 response.
2. Potent bronchodilator due to sympathomimetic effects.
3. Laryngeal protective reflexes are relatively well maintained, although aspiration can still occur. This also contributes to an increased risk of laryngospasm relative to other agents.

4. Dosage and administration (Table 12.1)
- **a.** Useful for IM induction in patients with no IV access (eg, children).
- **b.** A concentrated 10% solution is available for IM use only.

5. Adverse effects
- **a. Oral secretions** are markedly stimulated. The coadministration of an antisialagogue (eg, glycopyrrolate) may be helpful.
- **b. Emotional disturbance.** May cause agitation and unpleasant hallucinations during the early postoperative period. Incidence is higher with increased age, female gender, and dosages greater than 2 mg/kg but may be greatly reduced with the coadministration of a benzodiazepine or propofol. Children seem to be less troubled than adults by the hallucinations. Alternatives should be considered in patients with psychiatric disorders.
- **c. Muscle tone.** May lead to coordinated but apparently purposeless movements, especially in response to stimulation. Muscle tone is often increased.

d. **Increases ICP** and is relatively contraindicated in patients with head trauma or intracranial hypertension.
e. **Ocular effects.** May lead to mydriasis, vertical nystagmus, diplopia, blepharospasm, and increased intraocular pressure.
f. **Anesthetic depth may be difficult to assess.** Common clinical signs of anesthetic depth (eg, HR, BP, and RR) as well as EEG-based monitors of anesthetic depth are less reliable when ketamine is used.
g. **PONV**

F. **Dexmedetomidine.** Dexmedetomidine is a sedative agent with analgesic properties. It is used as an adjunct to general anesthesia and for sedation in the ICU and the OR. It is also used in regional anesthesia, in combination with local anesthetics to prolong the duration of the regional block, and for premedication of pediatric patients (nasal or oral). In some centers, it is used routinely for awake craniotomies, and also to treat shivering during c-sections performed under neuraxial anesthesia.

1. **Mode of action.** Highly selective α_2-adrenergic receptor agonist (α_2/α_1 1600:1). **Clonidine** is a less-selective and longer-acting α_2 agonist (α_2/α_1 200:1) with similar sedating and analgesic properties. Among anesthetic agents, its sedative effect is most similar to natural sleep: It decreases the inhibitory outflow from the locus coeruleus, causing an increase in the GABAergic outflow from the ventrolateral preoptic nucleus in the hypothalamus.

2. **Pharmacokinetics**
   a. Undergoes rapid redistribution after IV administration. Elimination half-life is approximately 2 hours.
   b. Metabolized extensively in the liver.

3. **Pharmacodynamics**
   a. **CNS**
      1. Elicits a sedated but arousable state similar to natural sleep.
      2. Potentiates CNS effects of propofol, volatile anesthetics, benzodiazepines, and opioids.
      3. Opioid sparing effect intraoperatively.
      4. Weak amnestic, lacking anticonvulsant properties.
         a. Low doses produce spindles on the EEG that are similar to those observed during non–rapid eye movement (REM) stage 2 sleep. Higher doses produce delta and slow oscillations similar to non-REM stage 3 sleep.
         b. Decreases the likelihood of emergence delirium in pediatric population.
   b. **Cardiovascular system**
      1. Decreases HR and BP, α_{2A} receptor–mediated decrease in catecholamine release.
      2. Transient hypertension may occur after an IV bolus, thought to be secondary to peripheral α_{2B} receptor activation.
      3. Baroreflex is well preserved.
   c. **Respiratory system**
      1. Minimal respiratory depression, although it may contribute to respiratory depressant effects of other anesthetics.
      2. Airway reflexes remain intact, making it useful for awake fiberoptic intubation.
      3. Associated with clinically significant reductions in coughing during and after extubation.
   d. **Endocrine system.** May decrease adrenal response to adrenocorticotropic hormone after prolonged infusions, although clinical significance is unclear.

4. **Dosage and administration** (Table 12.1)
   a. Decreased dosage should be considered in patients with significant hepatic dysfunction. Because the activity of dexmedetomidine metabolites has not been studied, decreased dosage may be prudent for patients with severe renal dysfunction.
   b. Indicated only for infusions of less than 24 hours.
5. **Adverse effects.** Antimuscarinic effects (eg, dry mouth and blurred vision) may occur due to α_2 adrenal receptor–mediated inhibition of acetylcholine release.

G. **Opioids.** Morphine, meperidine, methadone, hydromorphone, fentanyl, sufentanil, alfentanil, and remifentanil are opioids commonly used in general anesthesia. Their primary effect is analgesia; they are used to supplement other agents during the induction or maintenance of general anesthesia. In high doses, opioids are occasionally used as the primary anesthetic (eg, cardiac surgery). Opioids differ in their potencies, pharmacokinetics, and side effects.
   1. **Mode of action.** Bind to specific receptors in the brain, spinal cord, and on peripheral neurons. The opioids listed above are all relatively selective for μ-opioid receptors, and most of the analgesic and side effects of opioid medications are mediated by μ-opioid receptors. Additional mechanism of action for specific opioids includes NMDA antagonism, in the case of methadone, and inhibition of serotonin reuptake and α2b agonism, in the case of meperidine.
   2. **Pharmacokinetics**
      a. Pharmacokinetic data are presented in **Table 12.2**.
      b. After IV administration, the onset of action is within minutes for the fentanyl derivatives; hydromorphone and morphine may take

TABLE 12.2 Dose, Time to Peak Effect, and the Duration of Analgesia for Intravenous Opioid Agonists and Agonist–Antagonists[a]

Opioid	Dose (mg)[b]	Peak (minute)	Duration (h)[c]
Morphine	10	30–60	3–4
Meperidine	80	5–7	2–3
Hydromorphone	1.5	15–30	2–3
Oxymorphone	1.0	15–30	3–4
Methadone	10	5–10	—
Fentanyl	0.1	3–5	0.5–1
Sufentanil	0.01	3–5	0.5–1
Alfentanil	0.75	1.5–2	0.2–0.3
Remifentanil	0.1	1.5–2	0.1–0.2
Pentazocine	60	15–20	2–3
Butorphanol	2	15–20	2–3
Nalbuphine	10	15–20	3–4
Buprenorphine	0.3	<30	5–6

[a]Data for fentanyl derivatives are derived from intraoperative studies, the remainder from postoperative pain studies.
[b]Approximately equianalgesic doses (see text).
[c]Average duration of first single dose.

20 to 30 minutes for peak effect due to their lower lipid solubilities. The termination of effects for all opioids except remifentanil is by redistribution.
  c. Elimination is primarily by the liver and depends on hepatic blood flow. Remifentanil is metabolized by nonspecific esterases in tissues (primarily skeletal muscle). Morphine and meperidine have active metabolites, whereas hydromorphone and the fentanyl derivatives do not.
  d. Metabolites are primarily excreted in the urine. In patients with renal failure, the accumulation of morphine-6-glucuronide may cause prolonged narcosis and respiratory depression. Renal failure may also cause the accumulation of normeperidine, an active meperidine metabolite associated with seizure activity.
  e. CSHT of fentanyl derivatives: fentanyl > alfentanil > sufentanil > remifentanil

3. **Pharmacodynamics**
   a. **CNS**
      1. Produce sedation and analgesia in a dose-dependent manner; euphoria is common. Very large doses may produce amnesia and loss of consciousness, but opioids are not reliable hypnotics.
      2. Reduce the minimum alveolar concentration (MAC) of inhalational anesthetics and the requirements for IV sedative-hypnotic drugs.
      3. Decrease CBF and $CMRO_2$.
      4. Produce miosis by the stimulation of the Edinger–Westphal nucleus of the oculomotor nerve.
   b. **Cardiovascular system**
      1. All opioids except meperidine produce minimal changes in cardiac contractility. Baroreceptor reflexes are preserved.
      2. Systemic vascular resistance (SVR) usually is moderately reduced because of reduced medullary sympathetic outflow. Bolus doses of meperidine or morphine may reduce SVR secondary to histamine release.
      3. Produce bradycardia in a dose-dependent manner by the stimulation of the central vagal nuclei. Meperidine has a weak atropine-like effect and does not cause bradycardia.
      4. The relative hemodynamic stability offered by opioids often leads to their use in sedation or anesthesia for hemodynamically compromised or critically ill patients.
   c. **Respiratory system**
      1. Produce dose-dependent respiratory depression. RR decreases initially; TV decreases with larger doses. The effect is accentuated in the presence of sedatives, other respiratory depressants, or preexisting pulmonary disease.
      2. Decrease ventilatory response to hypercapnia and hypoxia. Effects are markedly increased if the patient falls asleep.
      3. Opioids dose-dependently decrease the cough reflex. Higher doses suppress tracheal and bronchial foreign body reflexes, so endotracheal intubation and mechanical ventilation are better tolerated.
   d. **Gastrointestinal system**
      1. Decrease gastric emptying and intestinal secretions. Colonic tone and sphincter tone increase and propulsive contractions decrease, resulting in constipation.

2. Increase biliary pressure and may produce biliary colic; the spasm of the sphincter of Oddi may prevent cannulation of the common bile duct. The incidence is lower with agonist-antagonist opioids.
4. **Dosage and administration.** Opioids are usually administered IV, either by bolus or by infusion. Appropriate dosages are presented in **Table 12.2**. Clinical dosing must be individualized and based on the patient's underlying condition and clinical response. Larger doses may be required in patients chronically receiving opioids. Opioids are also routinely utilized in neuraxial anesthesia techniques to optimize pain control.
5. **Adverse effects**
    a. **Allergic reactions** are rare, although anaphylactoid reactions may occur with morphine and meperidine secondary to histamine release.
    b. **Drug interactions.** The administration of meperidine or tramadol is contraindicated in patients taking monoamine oxidase inhibitor, as it may precipitate serotonin syndrome.
    c. **Nausea and vomiting** can occur because of the direct stimulation of the chemoreceptor trigger zone. Nausea is more likely if the patient is moving.
    d. **Muscle rigidity** may occur, especially in the chest, abdomen, and upper airway, resulting in the inability to ventilate the patient. The incidence increases with drug potency, dose, rate of administration, and presence of nitrous oxide. Rigidity may be reversed by administering neuromuscular relaxants but opioid antagonists may not be effective. Rigidity is less likely after pretreatment with a benzodiazepine or propofol.
    e. **Urinary retention** may occur because of increased tone in the vesical sphincter and inhibition of the detrusor (voiding) reflex. May also decrease awareness of the need to urinate.
6. **Naloxone** is a pure opioid antagonist that **reverses** opioid-induced effects such as respiratory or CNS depression.
    a. **Mode of action.** Competitive antagonist at opioid receptors in the brain and spinal cord.
    b. **Pharmacokinetics**
        1. Peak effects are seen within 1 to 2 minutes; a significant decrease in its clinical effects occurs after 30 minutes because of redistribution.
        2. Metabolized in the liver.
    c. **Pharmacodynamics**
        1. Reverses the pharmacologic effects of opioids such as CNS and respiratory depression.
        2. Crosses the placenta; administration to the parturient before delivery will decrease opioid-induced respiratory depression in the neonate.
    d. **Dosage and administration.** Perioperative respiratory depression in an adult can be treated with 0.04 mg IV every 2 to 3 minutes as needed. Therefore, **repeated administration may be necessary**.
    e. **Adverse effects**
        1. May lead to the abrupt onset of **pain** as opioid analgesia is reversed. This may be accompanied by sudden hemodynamic changes (eg, hypertension and tachycardia).
        2. May precipitate **pulmonary edema** and **cardiac arrest** in rare cases.

Table 12.3 Properties of Inhalation Anesthetics

Anesthetic	Vapor Pressure (mmHg, 20 °C)	Partition Coefficients Blood–Gas[a] (37 °C)	Brain–Blood (37 °C)	MAC (% With O_2 Only)
Isoflurane	238	1.4	1.6	1.28
Desflurane	664	0.45	1.3	6.0
Sevoflurane	157	0.65	1.7	2.05
Nitrous oxide	43,879	0.47	1.1	105

MAC, minimum alveolar concentration.

[a]The blood–gas partition coefficient is inversely related to the rate of induction.

II. PHARMACOLOGY OF INHALATION ANESTHETICS

Inhalation anesthetics are usually administered for the maintenance of general anesthesia, and also for "breathe-down" inhalation inductions. General properties of commonly used inhalation anesthetics are summarized in **Table 12.3**. Dosages of inhalation anesthetics are expressed as **MAC**. MAC is the concentration of agent as a sole agent at which, at 1 atm, 50% of patients do not move in response to a surgical stimulus. MAC is additive (eg, 0.5 MAC nitrous oxide + 0.5 MAC isoflurane = 1 MAC total).

A. Mode of Action

1. **Nitrous oxide.** Although exact mechanisms are unknown, anesthetic effects are mainly attributed to the antagonism of NMDA receptors in the CNS. It is the only inhaled anesthetic that directly produces analgesia.
2. **Volatile anesthetics.** Exact mechanisms are unknown. Various ion channels in the CNS involved in synaptic transmission (including $GABA_A$, glycine, and glutamate receptors) have been shown to be sensitive to inhalation anesthetics and may play a role.

B. Pharmacokinetics

1. **Determinants of the speed of onset and offset.** The alveolar anesthetic concentration (F_A) may differ significantly from the inspired anesthetic concentration (F_I). The rate of rise of the ratio of these two concentrations (F_A/F_I) determines the speed of induction of general anesthesia (**Figure 12.1**). Two opposing processes, anesthetic delivery to and uptake from alveoli, determine the F_A/F_I at a given time. Determinants of uptake include the following:
    a. **Blood–gas partition coefficient.** A lower solubility in blood will lead to lower uptake of anesthetic into the bloodstream, thereby increasing the rate of rise of F_A/F_I. The solubility of halogenated volatile anesthetics in blood is increased somewhat with hypothermia and hyperlipidemia.
    b. **Inspired anesthetic concentration.** This is influenced by the volume of the breathing circuit, fresh gas inflow rate, and the absorption of the volatile anesthetic by circuit components.
    c. **Alveolar ventilation.** Increased minute ventilation, without the alteration of other processes that affect anesthetic delivery or uptake, increases F_A/F_I. This effect is more pronounced with the more blood-soluble agents.

FIGURE 12.1 Ratio of alveolar to inspired gas concentration (F_A/F_I) as a function of time at constant cardiac output and minute ventilation.

- d. **Concentration effect.** As F_I increases, the rate of rise of F_A/F_I also increases. For a gas with a high F_I like nitrous oxide, a large amount is taken up into blood, causing noticeable reductions in total gas volume. The remaining nitrous oxide is thus "concentrated," and the addition of more anesthetic with the next breath will increase the concentration further. The uptake of a large gas volume also creates a void that draws more fresh gas into the alveoli, thereby increasing F_A and augmenting the inspired TV. The concentration effect explains why the rate of rise of F_A/F_I is faster for nitrous oxide than for desflurane (**Figure 12.1**), even though the blood–gas partition coefficient for desflurane is smaller.
- e. **The second gas effect.** This is a direct outcome of the concentration effect. When nitrous oxide and a potent inhalation anesthetic are administered together, the uptake of nitrous oxide concentrates the "second" gas (eg, isoflurane) and increases the input of additional second gas into the alveoli via the augmentation of inspired volume.
- f. **Cardiac output.** An increase in the cardiac output (and therefore pulmonary blood flow) will increase anesthetic uptake and thus decrease the rate of rise in F_A/F_I. A decrease in the cardiac output will have the opposite effect. This effect of cardiac output is more pronounced with nonrebreathing circuits or highly soluble anesthetics and is most prominent early in the course of anesthetic administration.
- g. **Gradient between alveolar and venous blood.** The uptake of anesthetic into the bloodstream will decrease as the anesthetic partial pressure gradient between the alveolar gas and the venous blood decreases. This gradient is particularly large early in the course of anesthetic administration.
2. **Distribution in tissues.** The rate of equilibration of anesthetic partial pressure between blood and a particular organ system depends on the following factors:
    a. **Tissue blood flow.** Equilibration occurs more rapidly in tissues receiving increased perfusion. The **vessel-rich group** of highly perfused organ systems receives approximately 75% of the cardiac output.

The remainder of the cardiac output perfuses predominantly into muscle and fat.
   b. **Tissue solubility.** For a given arterial anesthetic partial pressure, anesthetic agents with high-tissue solubility are slower to equilibrate. Solubilities of anesthetic agents differ among tissues. Brain–blood partition coefficients of inhalation agents are shown in **Table 12.3**.
   c. **Gradient between arterial blood and tissue.** Until equilibration is reached between the anesthetic partial pressure in the blood and a particular tissue, a gradient that leads to the uptake of anesthetic by the tissue exists. The rate of uptake will decrease as the gradient decreases.
3. **Elimination**
   a. **Exhalation.** This is the predominant route of elimination. After discontinuation, an anesthetic's tissue and alveolar partial pressures decrease by reversing the processes that occurred when the anesthetic was introduced.
   b. **Metabolism.** Significant biotransformation of nitrous oxide has not been demonstrated. Volatile anesthetics may undergo different degrees of hepatic metabolism.
   c. **Anesthetic loss.** Inhalation anesthetics may be lost both percutaneously and through visceral membranes, although such losses are probably negligible.

C. Pharmacodynamics
1. **Nitrous oxide**
   a. **CNS**
      1. Thought to act primarily by inhibiting NMDA receptors.
      2. Concentrations greater than 60% may produce amnesia, although not reliably.
      3. Because of its high MAC (105%), it is usually combined with other anesthetics to attain surgical anesthesia.
   b. **Cardiovascular system**
      1. Mild myocardial depressant and a mild sympathetic nervous system stimulant.
      2. HR and BP are usually unchanged.
      3. May increase pulmonary vascular resistance in adults.
   c. **Respiratory system.** Mild respiratory depressant, although less so than the volatile anesthetics.
2. **Volatile anesthetics**
   a. **CNS**
      1. Produce unconsciousness and amnesia at relatively low inspired concentrations (25% to 35% of MAC).
      2. At lower doses of halogenated ether anesthetics (isoflurane, sevoflurane, desflurane), alpha, delta, and slow oscillations are present. At higher doses, theta oscillations (4 to 8 Hz) appear, followed by burst suppression.
      3. Decreased amplitude and increased latency of SSEPs.
      4. Increase CBF and decrease $CMRO_2$; uncouple autoregulation of CBF.
   b. **Cardiovascular system**
      1. Produce dose-dependent myocardial depression and systemic vasodilation.
      2. HR tends to be unchanged, although desflurane can cause sympathetic stimulation, tachycardia, and hypertension at induction or when the inspired concentration is abruptly increased.

3. Sensitize the myocardium to the arrhythmogenic effects of catecholamines, which is of particular concern during the infiltration of epinephrine-containing solutions or the administration of sympathomimetic agents.
  c. **Respiratory system**
    1. Produce dose-dependent respiratory depression with decrease in TV, increase in RR, and increase in arterial CO_2 pressure.
    2. Produce airway irritation and, during light levels of anesthesia, may precipitate coughing, laryngospasm, or bronchospasm, particularly in patients who smoke or have asthma. The lower pungency of sevoflurane makes it more suitable for use as an inhalation induction agent.
    3. Equipotent doses of volatile agents possess similar bronchodilator effects, except for desflurane, which has mild bronchoconstricting activity.
    4. Inhibit hypoxic pulmonary vasoconstriction, which may contribute to pulmonary shunting.
  d. **Neuromuscular system**
    1. Dose-dependent decrease in skeletal muscle tone, often enhancing surgical conditions.
    2. May precipitate **malignant hyperthermia** in a susceptible patient.
  e. **Hepatic system.** May cause a decrease in hepatic perfusion. Rarely, a patient may develop hepatitis secondary to exposure to a volatile agent, most notably with halothane ("halothane hepatitis").
  f. **Renal system.** Decrease renal blood flow through either a decrease in MAP or an increase in renal vascular resistance.
D. **Adverse effects related to specific agents**
  1. **Nitrous oxide**
    a. **Expansion of closed gas spaces.** The predominant constituent in closed gas–containing spaces in the body is nitrogen. Because nitrous oxide is 35 times more soluble in blood than nitrogen, closed air spaces will expand as the amount of nitrous oxide diffusing into these spaces is greater than the amount of nitrogen diffusing out. Spaces containing air such as a pneumothorax, occluded middle ear, bowel lumen, or pneumocephalus will markedly enlarge if nitrous oxide is administered. Nitrous oxide will diffuse into the cuff of an endotracheal tube and may increase pressure within the cuff; this pressure should be assessed intermittently and, if necessary, reduced.
    b. **Diffusion hypoxia.** After discontinuation of nitrous oxide, its rapid elimination from the blood into the lung may lead to a low partial pressure of oxygen in the alveoli, resulting in hypoxia and hypoxemia if supplemental oxygen is not administered.
    c. **Inhibition of tetrahydrofolate synthesis.** N_2O inhibits methionine synthase, a vitamin B_{12}–dependent enzyme necessary for the synthesis of DNA. It should be used with caution in pregnant patients and those deficient in vitamin B_{12}.
  2. **Desflurane** can be degraded to carbon monoxide in carbon dioxide absorbents (especially Baralyme, now voluntarily withdrawn from the market). This is most likely to occur when the absorbent is new or dry.
  3. **Sevoflurane** can be degraded in CO_2 absorbents (especially Baralyme, now withdrawn) to fluoromethyl-2,2-difluoro-1-vinyl ether (**compound A**), produces renal toxicity in animals, and the package insert recommends >2 L/min fresh gas flows. However, there is no evidence of consistent

renal toxicity with sevoflurane usage in humans, and LiOH and Ca(OH)$_2$ absorbents without KOH or NaOH generate no or negligible compound A. Therefore, compound A most likely poses minimal risk to patients in routine clinical practice.

ACKNOWLEDGMENT

We gratefully acknowledge the contributions of previous edition author, Juan M. Cotte Cabarcas, as portions of those chapters have been retained in this revision.

Suggested Readings

Brown EN, Purdon PL, Van Dort CJ. General anesthesia and altered states of arousal: a systems neuroscience analysis. *Annu Rev Neurosci.* 2011;34:601–628.

Dershwitz M, Rosow CE. Intravenous anesthetics. In: Longnecker DE, Mackey SC, Newman MF, eds. *Anesthesiology.* 3rd ed. McGraw-Hill; 2017:636–649.

Eger EI. Uptake and distribution. In: Miller RD, ed. *Anesthesia.* 6th ed. Churchill Livingstone; 2005:131–153.

Forman SA, Benkwitz C. Inhalational anesthetics. In: Longnecker DE, Mackey SC, Newman MF, eds. *Anesthesiology.* 3rd ed. McGraw-Hill; 2017:551–570.

McPhee LC, Badawi O, Fraser GL, et al. Single-dose etomidate is not associated with increased mortality in ICU patients with sepsis: analysis of a large electronic ICU database. *Crit Care Med.* 2013;41(3):774–783.

Patel HH, Pearn ML, Patel PM, Roth DM. General anesthetics and therapeutic gases. In: Brunton LL, Hilal-Dandan R, Knollmann BC, eds. *Goodman & Gilman's: The Pharmacological Basis of Therapeutics.* 13th ed. McGraw-Hill; 2018:387–404.

Rosow C, Dershwitz M. Opioid analgesics. In: Longnecker DE, Mackey SC, Newman MF, eds. *Anesthesiology.* 3rd ed. McGraw-Hill; 2017:650–670.

Airway Evaluation and Management

Adam W. Kaplon and Jean Kwo

I. APPLIED ANATOMY

A. The pharynx is divided into the nasopharynx, the oropharynx, and the laryngopharynx.
1. The **nasopharynx** consists of nasal passages, including the septum, turbinates, and adenoids.
2. The **oropharynx** consists of the oral cavity, including the dentition and tongue.
3. The epiglottis separates the **laryngopharynx** into the larynx (leading to the trachea) and the **hypopharynx** (leading to the esophagus).

B. The larynx (see **Figure 13.1**)
1. The **larynx**, located at the level of the fourth to the sixth cervical vertebrae, originates at the laryngeal inlet and ends at the inferior border of the cricoid cartilage. It consists of nine cartilages: three unpaired (thyroid, cricoid, and epiglottis) and three paired (corniculates, cuneiforms, and arytenoids); ligaments; and muscles.
2. The **cricoid cartilage**, located just inferior to the **thyroid cartilage at the C5–6 vertebral level**, is the only complete cartilaginous ring in the respiratory tree. The **cricothyroid membrane** connects the thyroid and cricoid cartilages and measures 0.9×3.0 cm in adults. The membrane is superficial, thin, and devoid of major vessels in the midline, making it an important site for emergent surgical airway access (see Section VI.B.3).
3. **The laryngeal muscles** can be divided into two groups: muscles that open and close the glottis (lateral cricoarytenoid [adduction], posterior cricoarytenoid [abduction], and transverse arytenoid) and muscles that control the tension of the vocal ligaments (cricothyroid, vocalis, and thyroarytenoid).
4. **Innervation**
    a. **Sensory.** The **glossopharyngeal nerve** (cranial nerve IX) provides sensory innervation to the posterior one-third of the tongue, the oropharynx from its junction with the nasopharynx, including the pharyngeal surfaces of the soft palate, epiglottis, and the fauces, to the junction of the pharynx and esophagus. The **internal branch of the superior laryngeal nerve**, a branch of the vagus nerve (cranial nerve X), provides sensory innervation to the mucosa from the epiglottis to and including the vocal cords. The sensory fibers of the **inferior laryngeal nerve**, a branch of the recurrent laryngeal nerve (also a branch of the vagus nerve), provide sensory innervation to the mucosa of the subglottic larynx and trachea.
    b. **Motor.** The external branch of the **superior laryngeal nerve** provides motor innervation to the cricothyroid muscle. Activation of this muscle results in tensing of the vocal cords. The motor fibers of the **inferior laryngeal nerve** provide motor innervation to all other intrinsic muscles of the larynx. **Bilateral injury to the inferior laryngeal nerves** (eg, via injury to the recurrent laryngeal nerves) can produce

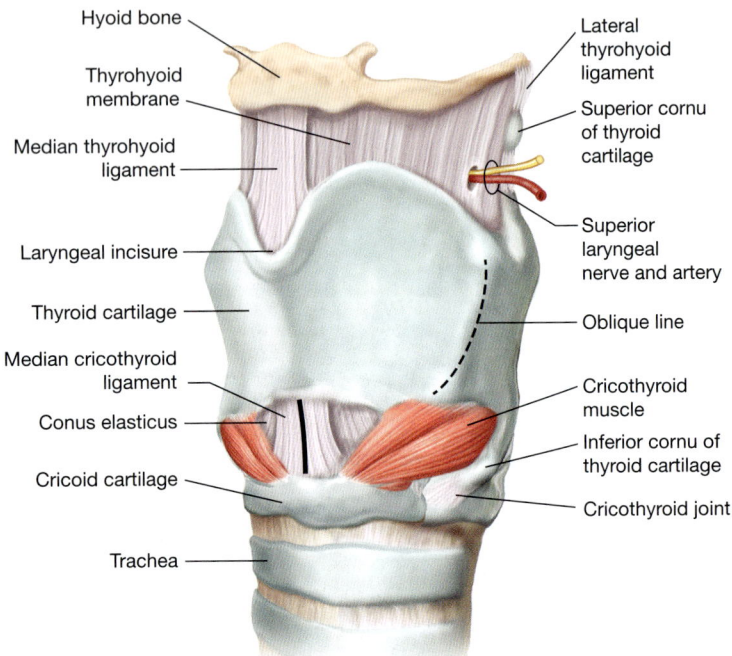

FIGURE 13.1 Laryngeal anatomy. (From Berning BJ, de Moya MA. Cricothyroidotomy. In: Hawn MT, ed. *Operative Techniques in Surgery*. 2nd ed. Wolters Kluwer; 2023:2502–2505. Fig. 7.40.1.)

unopposed activation of the cricothyroideus, leading to tensing of the vocal cords and airway closure.

C. The **glottis** is composed of the vocal folds (true and false cords) and the rima glottidis.
   1. The **rima glottidis** describes the aperture between the true vocal cords.
   2. The **glottis** is the narrowest point in the adult airway (more than 8 years of age), whereas the cricoid cartilage is the narrowest point in the infant airway (birth to 1 year of age). Of note, an MRI study showed the glottis is the narrowest portion of the airway in sedated, unparalyzed pediatric patients (2 months to 13 years).

D. **The lower airway** extends from the subglottic larynx to the bronchi.
   1. The subglottic larynx extends from the vocal folds to the inferior border of the cricoid cartilage (C6).
   2. The **trachea** is a fibromuscular tube that is 10 to 12 cm long with a diameter of approximately 20 mm in adults. It extends from the cricoid cartilage to the carina. The trachea is supported by 16 to 20 U-shaped cartilages, with the open end facing posteriorly. Noting the posterior absence of cartilaginous rings provides anterior–posterior orientation during fiberoptic exam of the tracheobronchial tree.
   3. The trachea bifurcates into the right and left main stem bronchi at the carina. The right main stem bronchus is approximately 2.5 cm long with a takeoff angle of approximately 25 degrees. The left main stem

bronchus is approximately 5 cm long with a takeoff angle of approximately 45 degrees. Because the right main stem bronchus branches at a less acute angle, aspiration and accidental bronchial intubation are more likely to occur on the right side.

II. EVALUATION

A. History. A history of difficult airway management in the past may be the best predictor of a challenging airway. Prior anesthetic records should be reviewed for the ease of intubation and ventilation (the ability to mask ventilate and whether adjuncts to mask ventilation were required, the number of intubation attempts, the type of laryngoscope blade used, the size of the endotracheal tube [ETT], or if any specialty airway equipment, ie, video laryngoscope or a bronchoscope were required). Importance should also be placed on diseases that may affect the airway. Specific symptoms related to airway compromise should be sought, including hoarseness, stridor, wheezing, dysphagia, dyspnea, and positional airway obstruction.

1. **Arthritis or cervical disk disease** may decrease neck mobility. Cervical spine instability and limitation of mandibular motion are common in rheumatoid arthritis. The temporomandibular and cricoarytenoid joints may also be involved. Aggressive neck manipulation in these patients may lead to atlantoaxial subluxation and spinal cord injury. The risk of atlantoaxial subluxation is highest in patients with severe hand deformities and skin nodules.

2. **Infections** of the floor of the mouth, salivary glands, tonsils, or pharynx may cause pain, edema, and trismus with limited mouth opening. **Epiglottitis** is a bacterial infection that causes an acute inflammation of the epiglottis and adjacent structures and can result in airway compromise. Because of routine vaccination against *Haemophilus*, epiglottitis has become more common in adults than children. In patients with airway compromise, intubation should be performed in the operating room with a specialist capable of performing rigid bronchoscopy or surgical airway on standby.

3. **Tumors** may obstruct the airway or cause extrinsic compression and tracheal deviation.

4. **Increased body mass index** (BMI >35) coupled with other anatomical findings (high Mallampati score, increased neck circumference, short thyromental distance) can be predictive for difficult mask ventilation and difficult tracheal intubation. The decreased functional residual capacity associated with an increased BMI can result in a precipitous oxygen desaturation with the apnea of induction.

5. A history of **snoring** or **obstructive sleep apnea** may be associated with difficult intubation.

6. **Trauma** may be associated with airway injuries, cervical spine injury, basilar skull fracture, or intracranial injury.

7. **Previous surgery, radiation, or burns** may produce scarring, contracture resulting in limited tissue mobility, and/or narrowed oral aperture.

8. The physiologic changes associated with **pregnancy** result in edema of the laryngeal and oral mucosa that can make obtaining a view of the glottis challenging, particularly at the end of the third trimester.

9. **Acromegaly** may cause mandibular hypertrophy and overgrowth and enlargement of the tongue and epiglottis. The glottic opening may be narrowed because of enlargement of the vocal cords.

10. **Scleroderma** may produce skin tightness and decrease mandibular motion and narrow the oral aperture.

11. **Patients with trisomy 21** may have atlantoaxial instability and macroglossia.
12. **Osteogenesis imperfecta and achondroplasia** may be associated with atlantoaxial instability and potentially difficult airway management because of mandibular hypoplasia (micrognathia).
13. **Other congenital anomalies** may complicate airway management, particularly in patients with craniofacial abnormalities such as Pierre Robin, Treacher Collins, Klippel–Feil, and Goldenhar syndromes. In contrast, children with isolated cleft palates are not specifically difficult to intubate if the condition is not associated with other airway or craniofacial abnormalities, but nasotracheal intubation should be avoided.

B. **Physical examination.** A normal airway exam does not completely exclude the likelihood of a difficult intubation.
  1. **Specific findings** that may indicate a difficult airway include the following:
     a. Inability to open the mouth or small mouth opening: distance between upper and lower incisors <5 cm
     b. Poor cervical spine mobility
     c. Receding chin (retrognathia): length between angle of jaw to tip of chin <9 cm
     d. Large tongue (macroglossia)
     e. Prominent incisors
     f. Short thick neck
     g. Short thyromental distance
     h. High Wilson score (**Table 13.1**)
  2. **Injuries** to the face, neck, or chest must be evaluated to assess their contribution to airway compromise.
  3. **Inhalational injury** to the airway due to direct thermal injury or chemical injury due to toxic gas inhalation can occur in patients with acute burns. The risk of inhalation injury increases with increased total body surface area burned. Upper airway swelling may not peak until 24 hours

TABLE 13.1 Wilson Score

	0	1	2
Weight	<90 kg	90–110 kg	>110 kg
Neck movement	>90 degrees	90 degrees	<90 degrees
Jaw mobility	Interincisor gap ≥5 cm or able to protrude lower incisors beyond upper incisors	Interincisor gap <5 cm or able to protrude lower incisors to meet upper incisors	Interincisor gap <5 cm or unable to protrude lower incisors to meet upper incisors
Receding mandible	Normal	Moderate	Severe
Prominent incisors	Normal	Moderate	Severe

An example of a composite score to predict difficult intubation. Score is calculated by totaling numbers of parameters (total possible score 10). A score of ≥2–3 is strongly predictive of a difficult intubation. However, a low score rate does not reliably rule out a difficult intubation.

Reprinted from Wilson ME, Spiegelhalter D, Robertson JA, et al. Predicting difficult intubation. *Br J Anaesth.* 1988;61(2):211–216. Copyright © 1988 Elsevier. With permission.

after the burn injury. Risk factors for impending airway obstruction include history of exposure to fire/smoke in an enclosed space, moderate to severe facial/oropharyngeal burns, circumferential neck burns, and evidence of airway injury on flexible nasoendoscopy.
4. **Head and neck examination**
   a. **Nose.** The patency of the nares or the presence of a deviated septum should be determined by occluding one nostril at a time and assessing ease of ventilation through the other nostril. This is especially important should nasotracheal intubation be required.
   b. **Mouth.** Identify macroglossia and conditions that reduce mouth opening (eg, facial scars or contractures, scleroderma, and temporomandibular joint disease). **Poor dentition** may increase the risk of tooth injury or avulsion during airway manipulation. Loose teeth should be identified preoperatively and protected or removed before initiation of airway management.
      1. The **upper lip bite test** (see **Figure 13.2**) assesses the range of motion of the mandible. Inability to bite upper lip with lower lip is associated with a 60% probability of difficult intubation.
   c. **Neck**
      1. A **thyromental distance** (the distance from the lower border of the mandible to the thyroid notch with the neck fully extended) of <6 cm (three to four finger breadths) is associated with difficulty visualizing the glottis. The mobility of laryngeal structures should be assessed. The trachea should be palpable in the midline above the sternal notch. Look for scars from previous neck surgery, an enlarged thyroid, other paratracheal masses, and indurated tissues suggestive of radiation therapy.
      2. **Cervical spine mobility.** Patients should be able to touch their chin to their chest and extend their neck posteriorly. Lateral rotation should not produce pain or paresthesia. Sternomental distance (measured from sternal notch to mandible) should be >12 cm at full neck extension.
      3. The presence of a healed or patent **tracheostomy** stoma may be a clue to subglottic stenosis or prior complications with airway management. Smaller diameter ETTs should be available for these patients.
      4. **Neck circumference** of >42 cm has been associated with difficult intubation.
      5. The **Mallampati classification** to predict difficult intubation is based on the finding that visualization of the glottis is impaired when the base of the tongue is disproportionately large. Assessment is made with the patient sitting upright, with the head in the neutral position, the mouth open as wide as possible, and the tongue protruded maximally without phonation. The modified classification includes the following four categories (**Figure 13.3**):
         a. **Class I.** Faucial pillars, soft palate, and uvula are visible.
         b. **Class II.** Faucial pillars and soft palate may be seen, but the uvula is masked by the base of the tongue.
         c. **Class III.** Only soft palate is visible. Intubation is predicted to be difficult.
         d. **Class IV.** Soft palate is not visible. Intubation is predicted to be difficult.
      6. There is no single best predictor of difficult airway management on the physical exam. **Multiple predictors** of difficult airway

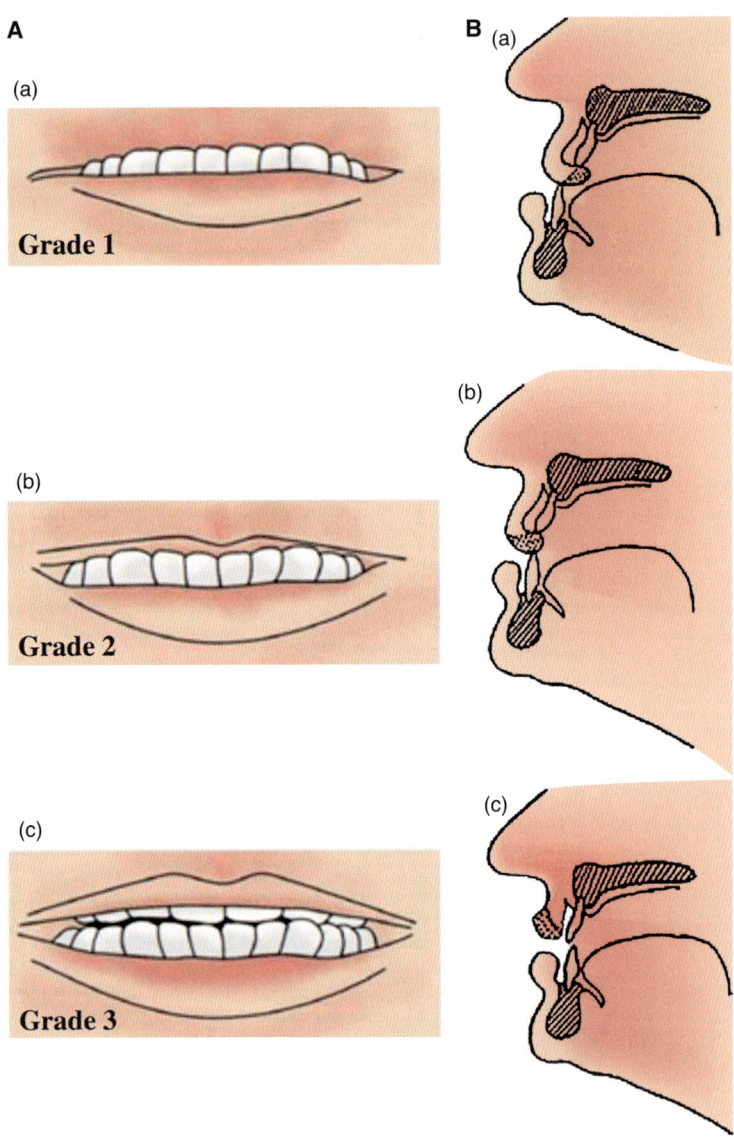

FIGURE 13.2 Frontal (**A**) and lateral (**B**) view of the upper lip bite test. Ask the patient to bite their upper lip with their lower incisors. (a) Class 1—lower incisors able to bite entire upper lip, lip mucosa barely visible. (b) Class 2—lower incisors bite upper lip partially, lip mucosa partially visible. (c) Class 3—lower incisors cannot bite upper lip at all. (A from Ma Y, Ibrahim Z, Davidson H. Advanced airway management: intubation. In: Rosen CA, ed. *Bailey's Head and Neck Surgery*. 6th ed. Wolters Kluwer; 2023:888–918. Figure 61.3. B from Khan ZH, Kashfi A, Ebrahimkhani E. A comparison of the upper lip bite test (a simple new technique) with modified Mallampati classification in predicting difficulty in endotracheal intubation: a prospective blinded study. *Anesth Analg*. 2003;96(2):595–599. Copyright © 2003 International Anesthesia Research Society.)

Class 1   Class 2   Class 3   Class 4

FIGURE 13.3 Mallampati classification of the oropharyngeal structures as modified by Samsoon and Young, as defined in a patient sitting upright with mouth maximally opened and tongue protruded without phonation. (From LaPree K. Preoperative cardiopulmonary risk stratification and prophylaxis. In: Brown DL, Adidharma W, Hespe GE, eds. *Michigan Manual of Plastic Surgery*. 3rd ed. Wolters Kluwer; 2024:128–134. Figure 12.1.)

will increase the specificity of the exam. A combination of high Mallampati class, short thyromental or sternomental distance, and impaired mandibular protrusion increases the likelihood of difficult intubation. Composite scores (eg, Wilson score—see **Table 13.1**) are of limited utility because while a higher score is predictive of difficult intubation, lower scores did not exclude difficult intubation.

C. Special studies. In most patients, a careful history and physical examination will be all that are needed to evaluate an airway. Useful adjuncts may include the following:
   1. **Laryngoscopy** (direct, indirect, video, or flexible fiberoptic bronchoscope) will provide information about the hypopharynx, laryngeal inlet, and vocal cord function. It can be performed in a conscious patient with topical anesthesia or nerve blocks.
   2. **Chest or cervical imaging** may reveal tracheal deviation or narrowing and bony deformities in the neck. Cervical spine films are important in trauma cases and should be performed in case of an injury above the clavicle or serious multiple traumatic injuries. In patients with altered mental status or distracting injuries, a normal cervical radiograph cannot rule out a significant ligamentous injury. Cervical spine precautions should be applied during intubation. Computed tomography (CT) or MRI scans may provide additional information. Lateral cervical spine films may be useful in symptomatic patients with rheumatoid arthritis or Down syndrome to assess for atlantoaxial subluxation.
   3. **Tracheal tomograms or CT** scan can delineate masses obstructing the airway.
   4. **Pulmonary function tests** and flow volume loops can help determine the degree and site of airway obstruction (see Chapter 1: Evaluating the Patient Before Anesthesia and Chapter 4: Specific Considerations With Pulmonary Disease).
   5. **Baseline arterial blood gas tensions** can indicate the functional consequences of airway abnormalities and alert the clinician to patients with chronic hypoxemia or hypercarbia.

6. **Airway ultrasound** is an emerging method for evaluation for preoperative difficult airway prediction; however, standardized practices are lacking.

III. MASK AIRWAY
A. Indications
1. To preoxygenate (denitrogenate) a patient before endotracheal intubation.
2. To assist or control ventilation as part of initial resuscitation before an ETT is placed.
3. To provide inhalation anesthesia in patients not at risk for regurgitation of gastric contents.

B. **Technique** involves placing a face mask and maintaining a patent airway.
1. **The mask** should fit snugly around the bridge of the nose, cheeks, and mouth. Clear plastic masks allow for observation of the lips (for color) and mouth (for secretions or vomitus).
2. **Mask placement.** The mask is held in the left hand so that the little finger is at the angle of the mandible, the third and fourth fingers are along the mandible, and the index finger and thumb are placed on the mask in the shape of the letter "C." The right hand is available to control the reservoir bag. Two hands may be required to maintain a good mask fit, necessitating an assistant to control the bag. Alternatively, two hands may be applied with the ventilator functioning in pressure mode if an assistant is not available. Head straps may be used to assist mask fit. Peak inspiratory pressures should be kept below 20 cm H_2O to minimize gastric insufflation. Some face masks have a Luer lock, which allows air to be injected or removed to aid in fit.
3. **Edentulous patients** may present a problem when attempting to achieve an adequate seal with the face mask because of decreased distance between the mandible and the maxilla. An oral airway will often correct this problem and the cheeks may be compressed against the mask to decrease leaks. Two hands may be required to do this. Alternatively, dentures may be left in place during mask ventilation and removed prior to intubation.
4. **Airway obstruction** during spontaneous ventilation may be recognized by a paradoxical "rocking" motion of the chest and abdomen. During spontaneous ventilation, if the upper airway is obstructed as the diaphragm contracts, the abdomen distends as it normally does for each breath, but the thorax collapses instead of being insufflated. Stridor is a high-pitched noise associated with extreme narrowing of the upper airway. It occurs with diseases like croup and can also be observed with **laryngospasm** after extubation. With airway obstruction, respiratory excursions in the reservoir bag will be decreased or absent, and peak airway pressures will be increased when positive-pressure ventilation is attempted.
5. **Airway patency** may be restored by the following:
   a. Neck extension
   b. Jaw thrust, by placing the fingers under the angles of the mandible and lifting forward
   c. Turning the head to one side or the other
   d. Insertion of an oral airway. An airway may not be tolerated if the gag reflex is intact. Complications from oral airways include vomiting, laryngospasm, and dental trauma. A misfitting oral airway may worsen obstruction. If the oral airway is too short, it may compress

the tongue and worsen obstruction; if it is too long, it may lie against the epiglottis. A proper fitting oral airway should extend from the midpoint of the incisors to the angle of the mandible when measured externally.
- **e.** A nasal airway helps maintain upper airway patency in a patient with minimal-to-moderate obstruction and is tolerated by awake or sedated patients. Nasal airways can cause epistaxis. Care should be taken when used with patients who are anticoagulated.
- **C. Difficult mask ventilation.** Obesity (BMI >30), edentulism, beards, higher Mallampati classification (III or IV), limited jaw protrusion, cervical arthritis, larger neck circumference (>42 cm), or snoring/obstructive sleep apnea is associated with difficult mask ventilation. Appropriate oral and nasal airways and laryngeal mask airways (LMAs) should be immediately available when difficult mask ventilation is anticipated.
- **D. Complications.** The mask can cause pressure injuries to soft tissues around the mouth, mandible, eyes, or nose. Mask ventilation does not protect the airway from aspiration of gastric contents. Loss of the airway may result from laryngospasm or vomiting. **Laryngospasm** is a tonic contraction of the laryngeal and pharyngeal muscles causing closure of the vocal cords and airway obstruction. It is relieved by jaw thrust and the application of constant positive airway pressure. If this fails, a small dose of succinylcholine (20 mg intravenously or intramuscularly in the adult) will relax the vocal cords and relieve the obstruction.

IV. LARYNGEAL MASK AIRWAY

- **A.** LMAs are supraglottic airway management devices that can be used as an alternative to both mask ventilation and endotracheal intubation in appropriate patients. The LMA plays a key role in the management of the difficult airway. When inserted appropriately, the LMA lies with its tip resting over the upper esophageal sphincter and the opening is directed toward the glottis (see **Figure 13.4**). Such positioning allows for effective ventilation with minimal inflation of the stomach. Some supraglottic airways have additional channels for suctioning the larynx or GI tract.
    1. **Indications**
        - **a.** As an alternative to mask ventilation or endotracheal intubation for airway management. The LMA is not a replacement for endotracheal intubation when endotracheal intubation is indicated.
        - **b.** In the management of a known or unexpected difficult airway.
        - **c.** In airway management during the resuscitation of an unconscious patient.
    2. **Contraindications**
        - **a.** Patients at risk of aspiration of gastric contents, such as patients with a full stomach.
        - **b.** Patients with decreased respiratory system compliance. The LMA cuff will leak at high inspiratory pressures resulting in gas entering the esophagus and gastric insufflation. Peak inspiratory pressures should be maintained at less than 20 cm H_2O.
        - **c.** Patients in whom long-term mechanical ventilatory support is anticipated or required.
    3. **Use**
        - **a.** LMAs are available in a variety of pediatric and adult sizes. Using the proper size maximizes the probability of appropriate cuff fit. There are many techniques for inserting the LMA. A common maneuver for insertion of the LMA is shown in **Figure 13.5**.

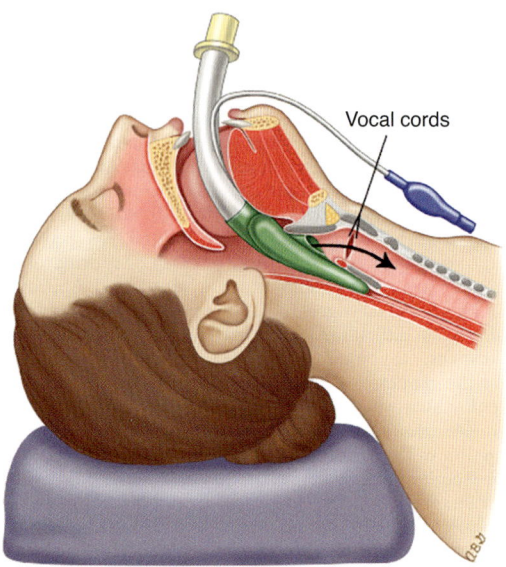

FIGURE 13.4 Position of properly inserted laryngeal mask airway. (Reproduced with permission from Doyle DJ. Supraglottic airways (SGAs) for airway management for anesthesia in adults. In: Connor RF, ed. *UpToDate*. Wolters Kluwer. Accessed March 13, 2025. Copyright © 2025 UpToDate, Inc. and/or its affiliates. All rights reserved.)

    b. The outer surface of the cuff may be lubricated to aid insertion. Lubrication of the LMA inner surface should be avoided.
    c. Follow usual preoxygenation and monitoring requirements.
    d. Ensure an adequate level of anesthesia and suppression of upper airway reflexes.
    e. Position the patient's head appropriately. The "sniffing" position used to optimize endotracheal intubation (see Section V.A.2.c) also typically provides the best positioning for LMA insertion.
    f. Insert the LMA (see **Figure 13.5**) and inflate cuff if necessary to obtain a seal (maintain cuff pressure less than 60 cm H_2O). Connect to anesthetic circuit and ensure adequate ventilation with chest rise, end-tidal CO_2. The LMA can be secured with tape if necessary.
    g. LMA removal. The LMA is generally tolerated by a patient emerging from general anesthesia if the cuff is not overinflated (cuff pressure less than 60 cm H_2O). The LMA can be removed by deflating the cuff once the patient has emerged from general anesthesia and has return of upper airway reflexes.
4. **Second-generation LMAs.** Classic LMAs consist of a cuff, valve, airway tube, and circuit connection. "Second-generation" LMAs have additional functionality for unique situations.
    a. Intubating LMAs are designed to facilitate intubation of the patient by passing an ETT through them, either blindly or with flexible bronchoscopic guidance.
    b. Flexible-reinforced LMAs have small, wire-reinforced airway tubes, which allow significant manipulation of the airway tube without interference with mask seal. These are particularly useful in

FIGURE 13.5 Technique for Insertion of laryngeal mask airway (LMA). **Top left:** Grasp the airway tube in the dominant hand and place the index finger between the tube and the deflated cuff of the mask. **Top right:** With the nondominant hand adjusting the head into the "sniffing" position, place the tip of the mask firmly against the palate and advance the LMA along the palate and into the posterior pharynx with the initial direction of force directed toward the operator's umbilicus. **Lower left:** The nondominant hand is then used to push the LMA further into the hypopharynx until resistance is encountered at the upper esophageal sphincter (UES). **Lower right:** Once inserted, the cuff of the LMA is insufflated with just enough air to create a seal. (From Egan B. Supraglottic airway devices. In: Chu LF, Traynor AJ, Kurup V, eds. *Manual of Clinical Anesthesiology*. 2nd ed. Wolters Kluwer; 2021:190–199 and adapted from Laurin E, Simon LV, Braude DA. Extraglottic devices. In: Brown CA III, ed. *The Walls Manual of Emergency Airway Management*. 6th ed. Wolters Kluwer; 2023:124–140. Figures 13.9, 13.10, 13.12, 13.13. From Brown CA III, Sakles JC, Mick NW, Mosier JM, Braude DA. *The Walls Manual of Emergency Airway Management*. 6th ed. Wolters Kluwer; 2023 and The Difficult Airway Course (www.theairwaysite.com). Used with permission.)

      procedures involving the head and neck where a classic LMA could obstruct the surgical field.
- c. Some LMAs have gastric access to allow passage of an orogastric tube or endoscope. These have been employed successfully in laparoscopic surgery and for upper endoscopy.
5. **Adverse effects.** The most common adverse effect of using an LMA is a sore throat with an estimated incidence of 10%. The primary major adverse event is aspiration, which occurs at an incidence comparable to mask or endotracheal anesthesia. LMAs have been associated with lingual, recurrent laryngeal, and hypoglossal nerve injuries. LMA use for a duration greater than 3 hours should be avoided.

V. ENDOTRACHEAL INTUBATION
A. Orotracheal intubation
1. **Indications.** Endotracheal intubation is required to provide a patent airway when patients are at risk for aspiration, when airway maintenance

by mask is difficult, and for prolonged controlled ventilation. Intubation also may be required for specific surgical procedures (eg, head/neck, intrathoracic, or intra-abdominal procedures).
2. **Technique.** Intubation is usually performed with a laryngoscope. The Macintosh and Miller blades are most commonly used.
   a. The **Macintosh blade** is curved and the tip is inserted into the vallecula (the space between the base of the tongue and the pharyngeal surface of the epiglottis) (**Figure 13.6A**). It provides a good view of the oropharynx and hypopharynx, thus allowing more room for passage of the ETT with decreased trauma to the epiglottis. Blade sizes are designated as No. 1 through 4, with most adults requiring a Macintosh No. 3 or 4 blade.
   b. The **Miller blade** is straight and it is passed so that the tip lies beneath the laryngeal surface of the epiglottis (**Figure 13.6B**). The epiglottis is then lifted to expose the vocal cords. The Miller blade provides excellent exposure of the glottic opening but provides a smaller passageway through the oropharynx and hypopharynx. Sizes are designated as No. 0 through 4, with most adults requiring a Miller no. 2 or 3 blade.
   c. The **sniffing position** is the classic intubation position with the occiput elevated by pads or folded blankets and the neck extended to achieve slight flexion of the lower cervical spine with extension of C1-C2. This improves the laryngoscopic view, although simple neck extension may be all that is needed in some patients. Neck flexion may make it more difficult to open the mouth.
   d. The laryngoscope is held in the left hand near the junction between the handle and blade. After propping the mouth open with a scissoring motion of the right thumb and index finger, the laryngoscope is inserted into the right side of the patient's mouth while sweeping the tongue to the left. The lips should not be pinched by the blade and the teeth should be avoided. The blade is then advanced toward the midline until the epiglottis comes into view. The tongue and pharyngeal soft tissues are then lifted to expose the glottic opening. The laryngoscope should be used to lift (see **Figure 13.6B**) rather than act as a lever (see **Figure 13.6A**) to prevent damage to the maxillary incisors or gingiva.
   e. An alternative to the classic sniffing position, the so-called **flexion–flexion** position, may be trialed if an appropriate glottic view cannot be obtained using conventional positioning. This technique involves first inserting the laryngoscope blade into the mouth as describe above. The head is then lifted, either using the anesthetist's right hand or the help of an assistant, and supported by the anesthetist's abdomen such that there is flexion both at the lower cervical level and at the atlantoaxial joint. The laryngoscope blade is then lifted such that the vector of force applied runs parallel to the body of the patient.
   f. An appropriate ETT size depends on the patient's age, body habitus, and type of surgery. A 7.0-mm ETT is used for most women, and a 7.5-mm ETT is used for most men. Larger tubes may be chosen to facilitate future bronchoscopy. The ETT is held in the right hand as one would hold a pencil and advanced through the oral cavity from the right corner of the mouth and then through the vocal cords. The anatomic view for visualization with a Macintosh laryngoscope is shown in **Figure 13.6C**. If visualization of the glottic opening

FIGURE 13.6 Anatomic relations for laryngoscopy and endotracheal intubation. **A,** Curved blade placement. **B,** Straight blade placement. **C,** Glottic exposure with curved blade placement.

is incomplete, it may be necessary to use the epiglottis as a landmark, passing the ETT immediately beneath it and into the trachea. External downward pressure on the cricoid and/or thyroid cartilage may aid in visualization. The proximal end of the ETT cuff is placed just below the vocal cords, and the markings on the tube are noted in relation to the patient's incisors or lips. The cuff is inflated just to the point of obtaining a seal in the presence of 20 to 30 cm H_2O positive airway pressure. Description of the visualization of the glottic opening should be recorded using the Cormack–Lehane scoring system (**Figure 13.7**).

   g. **Proper placement of the ETT** must be verified by the detection of carbon dioxide in end-tidal or mixed expiratory gas as well as inspection and auscultation of the stomach and both lung fields during positive-pressure ventilation. If an ETT is inserted too deeply, it usually passes into the right mainstem bronchus. When breath sounds are heard on only one side of the thorax, an endobronchial intubation should be suspected, and the ETT should be withdrawn until breath sounds are heard bilaterally. (In trauma patients, unilateral breath sounds may be indicative of a pneumothorax.) Listening for breath sounds high in each axilla may decrease the chances of being misled by transmitted breath sounds from the opposite lung. A high index of suspicion of an esophageal intubation should be maintained until adequate oxygenation and ventilation are ensured.
   h. The ETT should be fastened securely with tape, preferably to the skin overlying bony structures.
3. **Complications of orotracheal intubation** include injury of the lips or tongue, teeth, pharynx, or tracheal mucosa. Though rare, avulsion of arytenoid cartilage or damage to vocal cords or trachea can occur. High pressures in the cuff of the ETT can lead to ischemia of the tracheal

FIGURE 13.7 Cormack–Lehane grade for view on direct laryngoscopy. **Grade 1:** Full view of glottis. **Grade 2:** Partial view of glottis. **Grade 3:** Only epiglottis seen. **Grade 4:** Unable to visualize the glottis and epiglottis. (From Brown CA III, Sakles JC, Mick NW, Mosier JM, Braude DA. *The Walls Manual of Emergency Airway Management*. 6th ed. Wolters Kluwer; 2023 and The Difficult Airway Course (www.theairwaysite.com). Used with permission.)

mucosa. Ideally, the cuff pressure, measured with a manometer at the cuff inflation valve, should be between 20 and 30 cm H_2O.
B. Nasotracheal intubation
1. **Indications.** Nasotracheal intubations are uncommon but may be required in patients undergoing an intraoral or oral maxillofacial facial procedure. Compared with oral ETTs, the maximal diameter that can be accommodated nasally is usually smaller and therefore, the resistance to breathing may be higher. The nasotracheal route is rarely used for long-term intubation because of increased airway resistance and the increased risk of sinusitis.
2. **Contraindications.** Basilar skull fractures, especially of the ethmoid bone, nasal fractures, epistaxis, nasal polyps, coagulopathy, and planned systemic anticoagulation and/or thrombolysis (eg, patient with acute myocardial infarction) are relative contraindications to nasal intubation.
3. **Technique.** Topical anesthesia and vasoconstriction of the nasal mucosa may be achieved by applying a mixture of 2% lidocaine and 0.25% phenylephrine using cotton-tipped pledgets. If both nares are patent, the right side is preferred because this will direct the bevel of most ETTs toward the flat nasal septum reducing risk of damage to the turbinates. The inferior turbinates can interfere with passage and limit the size of the ETT. Usually, a 6.0- to 6.5-mm ETT is used for women and a 7.0- to 7.5-mm ETT is used for men. After it passes through the nares into the pharynx, the tube is advanced through the glottic opening. Intubation may be performed blindly on spontaneously breathing patients. In anesthetized and apneic patients, the tube can be passed using direct laryngoscopy assisted by Magill forceps or with bronchoscopic assistance.
4. **Complications** are similar to those described for orotracheal intubation (see Section V.A.3). In addition, epistaxis, submucosal dissection, and dislodgement of enlarged tonsils and adenoids may occur. Compared with orotracheal intubation, the nasotracheal route has been associated with an increased incidence of sinusitis and bacteremia.

C. Bronchoscopic intubation.
The flexible bronchoscope consists of either a camera or glass fibers that are bound together for the transmission of light and images. Bronchoscopes have working channels that can be used to administer topical anesthetics and provide suction or oxygen. The visual field can become limited as the bronchoscope nears the glottic opening due to secretions, blood, or fogging of the lens. Immersing the tip of the bronchoscope in warm water helps to prevent fogging.
1. **Standard equipment** for oral or nasal flexible bronchoscopic intubation includes an oral bite block or Ovassapian airway, topical anesthetics and vasoconstrictors, suction, and a sterile bronchoscope with a light source.
2. **Indications**
   a. The flexible bronchoscope can be used in both awake and anesthetized patients to evaluate and intubate their airways. It can be used for both nasal and oral endotracheal intubations and should considered as a first option in an anticipated difficult airway rather than as a "last resort."
   b. Initial flexible bronchoscopic intubation should be considered in patients with known or suspected cervical spine pathology, head and neck tumors, or a history of difficult mask ventilation or intubation.
3. **Technique.** An ETT is placed over a lubricated bronchoscope, suction or oxygen tubing is attached to the working port, and the control lever

is grasped with one hand while the scope is advanced or maneuvered with the other hand. The Ovassapian airway may be helpful for oral bronchoscopic intubation. It is well tolerated in awake patients, has a channel to guide the ETT midline, and can be removed after the ETT is placed. It is important to keep the bronchoscope in the midline to avoid entering the piriform fossa. The tip of the scope is positioned anteriorly when in the hypopharynx and advanced toward the epiglottis. If mucous or secretions impair the view, the scope should be retracted or removed to clean the tip and then reinserted in the midline. Oxygen attached to the suction port can be used to blow away secretions that may obstruct the view. As the scope slides beneath the epiglottis, the vocal cords are seen. The scope is advanced with the tip in a neutral position until the tracheal rings are noted. The scope is then stabilized within the trachea, and the ETT is advanced over it and into the trachea. If there is resistance to passage, turning the ETT 90 degrees counterclockwise to avoid the anterior commissure will often allow the ETT to pass through the vocal cords. "Flex-tip" ETTs have a tip that curves inward toward the lumen on the distal end that facilitates smoother passage through the vocal cords. The tracheal carina should be visualized prior to withdrawing the bronchoscope to ensure proper positioning of the tube.

D. Alternative intubation equipment and techniques

1. **Video laryngoscopy.** There are many specially designed laryngoscopes that incorporate a small video camera to further refine the concept of indirect visualization of the vocal cords on a video screen. These laryngoscopes include reusable systems that must be sterilized between each use and single-use systems, which involve a plastic sleeve that slips over a video wand that is discarded after use. Some systems consist of a laryngoscope and separate screen for viewing, while others consist of a blade with a small screen mounted at the base of the handle. These smaller portable systems may be more appropriate for use in remote locations outside of the operating room. When employed properly, all of these systems result in vocal cord visualization in nearly 100% of patients. Despite optimal visualization of the vocal cords, ETT advancement can still occasionally be difficult. Recent randomized controlled trials suggest greater first attempt success when using a hyperangulated video laryngoscope compared to direct laryngoscopy in adult patients.

    a. **Difficulty with ETT advancement** can occur because the laryngoscope occupies more space in the oropharynx than a conventional blade. One technique is to first advance the laryngoscope to obtain a glottic view and then partially withdraw the laryngoscope to allow the ETT to pass into the oropharynx. Then advance both the laryngoscope and ETT in parallel to visualize the ETT passing through the vocal cords.

    b. In cases where glottic visualization is achieved but there is significant difficulty in maneuvering the ETT through the cords, a **gum elastic bougie** (see Section V.D.2) may be easier to pass through the vocal cords. The ETT is then passed over the bougie and through the cords under direct visualization with the video laryngoscope.

    c. The different models of video laryngoscopes are all slightly different from each other. Proficiency with one model does not ensure proficiency with them all. Familiarization with the video laryngoscope by using it electively for intubations is recommended.

2. **The gum elastic bougie**, a 60-cm long, 15-French semirigid device with a slight J angle at its distal tip, exemplifies one of the various types of hollow and solid introducers that may facilitate passage of the ETT into the trachea when a partial view of the glottis is achieved with direct laryngoscopy. The bougie is advanced under the epiglottis under laryngoscopy and its angled end is directed anteriorly toward the glottic opening. If the bougie is inserted into the trachea, the tracheal rings can often be felt as a characteristic "clicking" sensation. The ETT is then advanced over the bougie and proper placement is confirmed as described above (see Section V.A.2.g). The bougie may also be used as an ETT exchanger.
3. **The light wand** consists of a malleable lighted stylet over which an oral ETT can be passed blindly into the trachea. To insert, the operating room lights are dimmed and the light wand and ETT are advanced following the curve of the tongue. A glow noted in the lateral neck indicates that the tip of the ETT lies in the piriform fossa. If the tip enters the esophagus, there is a marked diminution in the light's brightness. When the tip is correctly positioned in the trachea, a glow is noted in the anterior neck. At this point, the ETT is slid off the stylet and into the trachea.
4. **Retrograde tracheal intubation** can be performed when previously described techniques have been unsuccessful. It is performed in an awake or mildly sedated spontaneously breathing patient. For this technique, the cricothyroid membrane is identified, anesthetized with local anesthetic, and punctured in the midline with an 18-gauge intravenous (IV) catheter. An 80-cm, 0.025-inch guidewire is introduced and directed cephalad. A laryngoscope is used to visualize and retrieve the wire retrograde through the vocal cords. An ETT is then passed over the wire.

VI. THE DIFFICULT AIRWAY AND EMERGENCY AIRWAY TECHNIQUES

A. **Difficult airway.** The 2022 revision of the American Society of Anesthesiologists (ASA) algorithm for managing difficult airways is shown in **Figure 13.8**. Familiarity with this algorithm is crucial for anesthesiologists. Since its adoption in 1993, the number of death and brain death claims associated with airway-related events during induction of anesthesia has decreased significantly.
1. The difficult airway algorithm separates patients first into the awake intubation or postinduction intubation pathways.
2. **Awake intubation** should be considered if difficulty with tracheal intubation is known or suspected, if difficulty with ventilation with face mask or supraglottic airway is suspected, if the patient is at high risk for aspiration, or if the patient is at increased risk of rapid oxygen desaturation.
3. There is increased emphasis on limiting intubation attempts and early use of a supraglottic airway in situations where ventilation by face mask is adequate.
4. If intubation fails after the induction of general anesthesia, the pathway divides into emergency or nonemergency pathways depending on whether the patient can be ventilator either with a mask or supraglottic device.
5. **Nonemergency pathway**
    a. Patient can be ventilated either with mask or supraglottic device after general anesthesia is induced but cannot be intubated.
    b. Consider alternative intubation options (eg, video laryngoscopy, intubating LMA) or awakening patient for awake techniques or postponing surgery.

ASA DIFFICULT AIRWAY ALGORITHM: ADULT PATIENTS

FIGURE 13.8 American Society of Anesthesiologists (ASA) difficult airway algorithm. (Reprinted with permission from American Society of Anesthesiologists Task Force on Management of the Difficult Airway. Practice guidelines for management of the difficult airway: an updated report by the American Society of Anesthesiologists Task Force on Management of the Difficult Airway. *Anesthesiology.* 2022;136:31–81. Copyright © 2022 American Society of Anesthesiologists, Inc.)

6. **Emergency pathway**
   a. An airway in patients who cannot be intubated and cannot be ventilated.
   b. Call for help. Limit attempts at intubation and be aware of the passage of time.
   c. Attempt alternative intubation options while preparing for emergency invasive airway (eg, tracheostomy, cricothyrotomy).
7. The use of **regional anesthesia** to avoid the known or anticipated difficult airway deserves special mention. It must be kept in mind that the

regional block can fail, or the patient may require rapid conversion to a general anesthetic for other reasons. Regional anesthesia generally should not be selected for a patient with a known difficult airway if the surgery cannot be terminated rapidly (in case of failed or inadequate block) or access to the patient's airway is compromised.

B. Emergency airway techniques

1. **Percutaneous needle cricothyroidotomy** involves placing a 14-gauge IV catheter or 7.5-French introducer through the cricothyroid membrane into the trachea. Oxygen can be administered by connecting the breathing circuit to a 3-mm ID ETT adapter inserted directly into the IV catheter or to a 7.0-mm ID ETT adapter inserted into a 3-mL syringe barrel and connected to the IV catheter. Dedicated cricothyroidotomy catheters are preferred as the IV catheters have a very high rate of kinking and obstruction. Percutaneous needle cricothyroidotomy is a temporary maneuver until more stable airway access is achieved (tracheostomy or intubation). It is contraindicated in cases of complete upper-airway obstruction because severe barotrauma may result.

    a. **Oxygenation**, but not ventilation, can be achieved by administering oxygen through the catheter at flow rates of 10 to 12 L/min.

    b. **Some ventilation** may be achieved by pressing the oxygen flush valve for 1 second and allowing for passive exhalation over 2 to 3 seconds.

    c. Once in place, the catheter must be carefully and firmly held in position to **avoid dislodgment**, which can be life threatening.

    d. **Complications** include barotrauma, pneumothorax, subcutaneous emphysema of the neck and anterior chest, loss of the airway, aspiration, and death.

2. **Rigid bronchoscopy** by a surgeon or interventional pulmonologist may be necessary to support an airway partially obstructed by a foreign body, traumatic disruption, stenosis, or mediastinal mass. General anesthesia is usually required. A range of bronchoscope sizes (including pediatric sizes) should be available (see Chapter 27: Anesthesia for Thoracic Surgery).

3. **Cricothyroidotomy** is a rapid effective method for relieving severe upper airway obstruction. The cricothyroid membrane is an elastic tissue located between the inferior border of the thyroid cartilage and the superior border of the cricoid cartilage. With the neck extended, a small incision is made in this membrane in the midline. The handle of a scalpel or a Kelley forceps is used to separate the tissues, and a tube (eg, tracheostomy tube or ETT) is inserted. Alternatively, commercial kits are available, which allow cricothyroidotomy to be performed using Seldinger technique. An introducer needle is used to perforate the cricothyroid membrane and a guidewire is advanced through the needle. Next, a combined tissue dilator–airway catheter is advanced over the wire, the dilator is removed, and the airway catheter is left in the trachea.

4. **Tracheostomy** may be performed under local anesthesia before the induction of general anesthesia for a patient with a particularly difficult airway.

    a. **Technique.** After careful dissection of vessels, nerves, and the thyroid isthmus, a tracheal incision is made, usually between the third and fourth cartilaginous rings. Percutaneous dilational tracheostomy, using commercially available techniques and a modified Seldinger technique, may also be performed.

    b. **Complications** include hemorrhage, false passage, and pneumothorax.

VII. SPECIAL CONSIDERATIONS
A. Rapid sequence induction (RSI)
1. **Indications.** Patients at risk for aspiration include those who have recently eaten (full stomach), pregnant patients, and those with bowel obstruction, acute abdomen, recent use of GLP-1 agonists, or symptomatic gastroesophageal reflux.
2. **Technique.** RSI decreases the time between induction and placement of a cuffed ETT, decreasing the risk of aspiration.
   a. **Equipment** necessary for an RSI should include the following:
      1. Functioning suction with tonsil-tip (Yankauer) suction catheter
      2. Several different laryngoscope blades (Macintosh, Miller, or video laryngoscope)
      3. Several ETTs with stylets, including one that is of size smaller than normal
      4. An assistant who can apply cricoid pressure effectively
   b. The patient is **preoxygenated** using high flow rates of 100% oxygen for 3 to 5 minutes (denitrogenation). Four to five vital capacity breaths of 100% oxygen achieve nearly similar results when time is of the essence. The patient can also be placed in a head up, reverse Trendelenburg position during preoxygenation, which may delay the onset of desaturation upon apnea.
   c. The neck is extended so the trachea is directly anterior to the esophagus. The administration of an induction agent (eg, propofol or ketamine) is immediately followed by succinylcholine (1 to 1.5 mg/kg IV). High-dose nondepolarizing neuromuscular blockers or remifentanil (3 to 5 µg/kg) can be used as an alternative for muscle relaxation when succinylcholine is contraindicated. An assistant places firm downward digital pressure on the cricoid cartilage, effectively compressing and occluding the esophagus **(Sellick maneuver).** This maneuver theoretically reduces the risk of passive regurgitation of gastric contents into the pharynx and may bring the vocal cords into better view by displacing them posteriorly. It should not be used if the patient is actively vomiting, because high pressures could injure the esophagus. Of note, significant controversy exists regarding the use of cricoid pressure due to evidence showing that it may decrease lower esophageal sphincter tone and impair glottic view with unclear benefit in reducing aspiration. Regardless, cricoid pressure during RSI is commonly performed in anesthetic practice in the United States.
   d. There should be no attempt to ventilate the patient by mask. Cricoid pressure is maintained until successful endotracheal intubation is verified.
   e. Intubation should be performed within 30 seconds. If intubation attempts are unsuccessful, cricoid pressure should be maintained continuously during subsequent intubation maneuvers and while gentle mask ventilation is in progress.

B. Awake intubation
1. **Indications.** Awake oral or nasal intubation should be considered when there is:
   a. A difficult intubation anticipated in a patient at risk for aspiration
   b. Uncertainty about the ability to ventilate or intubate after induction of general anesthesia
   c. A need to assess neurologic function after intubation or positioning for surgery

2. **Technique**
   a. To perform an awake intubation, a 4% lidocaine gargle, followed by a lidocaine spray or nebulizer, is used to decrease upper airway sensation.
      1. **Superior laryngeal nerve block** may be used to anesthetize supraglottic structures. A 25-gauge needle is directed anterior to the greater cornu of the hyoid bone and inserted in the thyrohyoid membrane. After negative aspiration, 2 mL of 2% lidocaine is injected on each side.
      2. **Translaryngeal injection of local anesthetic** can anesthetize the glottis and upper trachea. A 25-gauge needle is inserted through the cricothyroid membrane in the midline. After aspiration of air to confirm placement within the tracheal lumen, 2 mL of 2% lidocaine is injected, and the needle is withdrawn. The patient will cough when local anesthetic is injected aiding in anesthetic spread. This block may increase the risk for aspiration in a patient with a full stomach or may be difficult in a patient with a large neck where precise palpation of the cricothyroid membrane is difficult.
      3. **Glossopharyngeal nerve block** may be useful in reducing the gag reflex during awake intubation. The tongue is swept to the opposite side, and a long 25-gauge needle is used to inject 2 mL of 2% lidocaine 0.5 cm deep just lateral to the base of the anterior tonsillar pillar.
   b. **Awake oral laryngoscopy** often allows one to assess the airway. Sedatives such as midazolam, propofol, dexmedetomidine, and fentanyl may be used in addition to the nerve blocks described above.
   c. **Awake (blind) nasal intubation** may be performed after adequate topical anesthesia and regional airway blocks.
      1. Incremental doses of sedatives are useful adjuncts.
      2. A well-lubricated ETT is passed into the nasopharynx with gentle pressure.
      3. Deep resonant breath sounds may be noted as the tube is advanced toward the glottis. An exaggerated sniffing position may be useful. The ETT is usually passed into the trachea during inspiration.
      4. Successful intubation is noted when the patient is unable to phonate, breath sounds and humidification within the ETT are noted with ventilation, and carbon dioxide is noted on the capnograph.
3. **Complications** are as described in Section V.A.3.
C. **ETT changes.** Occasionally, ETT cuff leaks or partial obstruction of the ETT necessitates changing an ETT in a patient with a difficult airway.
   1. The oropharynx is suctioned, and the patient is ventilated with 100% oxygen.
   2. A **tracheal tube exchanger** is a specialized stylet placed through the ETT and into the trachea. The depth of insertion is carefully measured. While one person holds the tube changer and assures that it does not pass too distally, the second anesthetist slides the original ETT off the changer and passes a new one over the stylet into the trachea. The risks of using this technique are pneumothorax if the tube changer enters a distal airway and failure to pass the ETT through the cords.
   3. A **flexible bronchoscope** can also be used for reintubation. An ETT is placed over the bronchoscope, the tip of which is passed into the trachea alongside the existing tube. The cuff of the existing ETT is deflated,

the bronchoscope is advanced, and tracheal rings are noted to confirm position. The existing ETT is removed (a tracheal tube changer may be left in its place), and the new one is advanced as described in Section V.C. The advantages of this technique are direct visualization of the trachea and oxygenation of the patient through the working port of the bronchoscope if there is difficulty passing the ETT through the vocal cords.
4. An **Aintree intubation catheter** is similar to a tracheal tube exchanger, but it has a large channel that allows it to slide over a flexible bronchoscope. It has a second, smaller channel that allows the anesthetist to deliver oxygen to the patient during the tube change.

ACKNOWLEDGMENT

We gratefully acknowledge the contributions of previous edition author, Gregory H. Foos, as portions of those chapters have been retained in this revision.

Suggested Readings

Adnet F, Baillard C, Borron SW, et al. Randomized study comparing the "sniffing position" with simple head extension for laryngoscopic view in elective surgery patients. *Anesthesiology.* 2001;95:836–841.

Apfelbaum JL, Hagberg CA, Connis RT, et al. 2022 American Society of Anesthesiologists practice guidelines for management of the difficult airway. *Anesthesiology.* 2022;136:31–81.

Biro P. Difficult intubation in pregnancy. *Curr Opin Anaesthesiol.* 2011;24:249–254.

Carsetti A, Sorbello M, Adrario E, Donati A, Falcetta S. Airway ultrasound as predictor of difficult direct laryngoscopy: a systematic review and meta-analysis. *Anesth Analg.* 2022;134(4):740–750.

Detsky ME, Jivraj N, Adhikari NK, et al. Will this patient be difficult to intubate?: The rational clinical examination systematic review. *J Am Med Assoc.* 2019;321:493–503.

Hansel J, Rogers AM, Lewis SR, Cook TM, Smith AF. Videolaryngoscopy versus direct laryngoscopy for adults undergoing tracheal intubation. *Cochrane Database Syst Rev.* 2022;4(4):CD011136.

Joffe AM, Aziz MF, Posner KL, Duggan LV, Mincer SL, Domino KB. Management of difficult tracheal intubation: a closed claims analysis. *Anesthesiology.* 2019;131(4):818–829.

Kheterpal S, Han R, Tremper KK, et al. Incidence and predictors of difficult and impossible mask ventilation. *Anesthesiology.* 2006;105:885–891.

Kheterpal S, Healy D, Aziz MF, et al; Multicenter Perioperative Outcomes Group (MPOG) Perioperative Clinical Research Committee. Incidence, predictors, and outcome of difficult mask ventilation combined with difficult laryngoscopy. *Anesthesiology.* 2013;119:1360–1369.

Lewis SR, Butler AR, Parker J, Cook TM, Schofield-Robinson OJ, Smith AF. Videolaryngoscopy versus direct laryngoscopy for adult patients requiring tracheal intubation: a Cochrane Systematic Review. *Br J Anaesth.* 2017;119:369–383.

Lin J, Bellinger R, Shedd A, et al. Point-of-care ultrasound in airway evaluation and management: a comprehensive review. *Diagnostics (Basel).* 2023;13(9):1541.

Riad W, Vaez MN, Raveendran R, et al. Neck circumference as a predictor of difficult intubation and difficult mask ventilation in morbidly obese patients: a prospective observational study. *Eur J Anaesthesiol.* 2016;33:244–249.

Samsoon GL, Young JR. Difficult tracheal intubation: a retrospective study. *Anaesthesia.* 1987;42:490–497.

Sellick BA. Cricoid pressure to control regurgitation of stomach contents during induction of anesthesia. *Lancet.* 1961;2:404–406.

Ushakumari DS, Sladen RN. ASA consensus-based guidance on preoperative management of patients on glucagon-like peptide-1 receptor agonists. *Anesthesiology.* 2024;140:346–348.

Neuromuscular Blockade

Scott Cao and Simona Iustina Lupu

The principal pharmacologic effect of **neuromuscular-blocking drugs (NMBDs)** is to interrupt transmission of synaptic signaling at **the neuromuscular junction (NMJ)** by interacting with **the nicotinic acetylcholine receptor (AChR).**

I. NEUROMUSCULAR JUNCTION

A. The NMJ (**Figure 14.1**) is a chemical synapse located in the peripheral nervous system. The NMJ is composed of **the neuronal presynaptic terminal,** where **acetylcholine (ACh)** is stored in specialized organelles known as **synaptic vesicles,** and the postsynaptic muscle cell **(motor endplate).**

B. In response to an action potential in the nerve, **voltage-dependent calcium channels** open and cause a rapid influx of calcium into the nerve terminal, increasing its intracellular concentrations. This influx of calcium induces fusion of synaptic vesicles with the plasma membrane to release stored ACh. ACh then diffuses across the synaptic cleft where two molecules of ACh bind to a single nicotinic AChR.

C. Postjunctional nicotinic AChRs are glycoproteins composed of five subunits (two α and one each of β, δ, and ϵ) with the two α-subunits constituting the binding sites for ACh and NMBDs. When two molecules of ACh are bound, the AChR undergoes a conformational change (activation) that allows influx of sodium and calcium into the muscle cell to depolarize the membrane and initiate contraction. Once depolarization occurs, repolarization begins with the efflux of potassium and the cessation of sodium and calcium entry. At this point, the AChR becomes inactivated. The amount of ACh released and the number of postsynaptic AChRs is much greater than that actually needed to induce contraction. This is termed the "safety factor" for neuromuscular transmission and plays a crucial role in certain pathologic conditions. After triggering depolarization, ACh diffuses into the synaptic cleft where it is rapidly hydrolyzed (within 15 ms) by **acetylcholinesterase (AChE)** into choline and acetate. Choline is subsequently recycled to synthesize new ACh in the motor nerve terminal.

D. Prejunctional nicotinic AChRs are located on the presynaptic nerve terminal and are responsible for augmenting depolarization of the nerve terminal during high-frequency stimulation, thereby enhancing ACh release. Antagonism of these receptors by nondepolarizing NMBDs is thought to be the mechanism by which these agents produce fade on the train of four (TOF).

II. GENERAL PHARMACOLOGY

A. Cholinergic receptors are categorized as **nicotinic** and **muscarinic** by their responses to the alkaloids nicotine and muscarine, respectively. There are two main classes of nicotinic cholinergic receptors: muscular (found at the NMJ) and neuronal (found in autonomic ganglia, at end-organ sites of parasympathetic nerves, and in the central nervous system). Since the cholinergic receptors have different subunit composition, most drugs

FIGURE 14.1 The neuromuscular junction. ACh, acetylcholine; AChE, acetylcholinesterase.

bind to them with different affinity and have different effects. Only ACh and drugs working by producing ACh (AChE inhibitors) are agonists at all of them.

B. There are well-described signaling systems that regulate the **distribution and density of AChRs** at the NMJ. Pathologic conditions that affect AChR distribution are quite common. For example, denervation, prolonged inactivity, or prolonged mechanical ventilation decreases the density of AChRs at the NMJ, whereas extrajunctional AChRs (often referred to as immature or fetal postjunctional nicotinic AChRs) proliferate over the surface of the muscle membrane. This **"upregulation" of AChRs** increases sensitivity to agonists such as ACh and succinylcholine (SCh), but it decreases the sensitivity to competitive antagonists such as nondepolarizing NMBDs. In contrast, increased sensitivity to antagonists and decreased sensitivity to agonists develop under conditions associated with **downregulation of AChRs**. This can occur when the NMJ is exposed to excess ACh (eg, following chronic use of AChE inhibitors).

C. NMBDs can be classified by the duration of effect: **ultrashort-acting** (<10 minutes; SCh), **short-acting** (<20 minutes; mivacurium [not available in the United States]), **intermediate-acting** (45 to 60 minutes; atracurium, cisatracurium, rocuronium [0.6 mg/kg dose], and vecuronium), and **long-acting** (>1 hour; pancuronium, rocuronium >0.9 mg/kg dose). Nondepolarizing NMBDs can be further classified by chemical class: **aminosteroid derivatives** (eg, pancuronium, rocuronium, and vecuronium)

TABLE 14.1 Comparative Clinical Pharmacology of Neuromuscular-Blocking Drugs[a]

	ED_{95} (mg/kg)[b]	Intubating Dose (mg/kg)[c]	Time to Intubation (minutes)[d]	Time to 25% Recovery (minutes)[e]	Infusion Rate (μg/kg/min)[f]	Elimination
Depolarizing drug						
Succinylcholine	0.25	1–1.5	1	4–6	60–100	Plasma cholinesterase
Nondepolarizing drugs						
Atracurium	0.25	0.4–0.6	2–3	20–35	4–12	Ester hydrolysis, Hofmann elimination
Cisatracurium	0.05	0.15–0.25	2–3	40–60	1–3	Hofmann elimination
Mivacurium	0.08	0.15–0.25	2–3	15–25	3–15	Plasma cholinesterase
Pancuronium	0.06	0.06–0.1	3–4	60–100	—	Kidneys (70–80%), biliary and hepatic (20–30%)
Rocuronium	0.3	0.6–1.2	1.5–3	30–150	4–12	Primarily by liver
Vecuronium	0.05	0.08–0.12	2–3	25–40	0.8–2	Biliary and hepatic (70–90%), kidneys (10–30%)

[a]There is a large variability in the response to all relaxants, especially at the extremes of age and with profound illness. Therefore, all patients should be carefully monitored as described in the text. Doses shown here are intended for intravenous administration in adult patients.

[b]An ED_{95} dose of a relaxant provides adequate surgical relaxation with nitrous oxide–opioid anesthesia.

[c]These are customary intubating doses and are not all equipotent. Neuromuscular blockade is potentiated by volatile anesthetics. For nondepolarizing agents, the intubating dose can be approximately double the ED_{95}.

[d]These times reflect the use of customary intubating doses and may be substantially altered by the depth of anesthesia. For a rapid sequence induction with nondepolarizing agents, onset time can be shortened by administering a priming dose 3 to 5 minutes before the full dose, although this causes its own side effects. Alternatively, a dose of a nondepolarizing agent four times higher than the ED_{95} dose can be used.

[e]Maintenance bolus doses to be given when the train-of-four count reaches 2 to 3 are generally 20% to 25% of the initial bolus dose.

[f]Continuous infusion should be initiated only after early evidence of spontaneous recovery from the initial bolus dose.

and **benzylisoquinolines** (eg, atracurium, cisatracurium, and mivacurium). NMBDs differ substantially in their onset, duration of blockade, metabolism, side effects, and interactions with other drugs (**Tables 14.1** and **14.2**).

TABLE 14.2 Cardiovascular Side Effects of Neuromuscular-Blocking Drugs

Drugs	Histamine Release[a]	Ganglionic Effects	Vagolytic Activity	Sympathetic Stimulation
Atracurium	+	0	0	0
Cisatracurium	0	0	0	0
Mivacurium	+	0	0	0
Pancuronium	0	0	++	++
Rocuronium	0	0	+	0
Succinylcholine	±	+	0	0
Vecuronium	0	0	0	0

[a]Histamine release is dose and rate dependent and, therefore, less pronounced if drugs are injected slowly.

III. NEUROMUSCULAR BLOCKADE
A. Depolarizing blockade

SCh, the only depolarizing NMBD in clinical use, is composed of two ACh molecules linked together via an acetyl moiety. SCh binds to the α-subunits of the nicotinic AChR leading to depolarization of the postjunctional membrane. Because SCh is not degraded by AChE as rapidly as ACh, it persistently depolarizes the motor endplate, leading to inactivation of the voltage-gated sodium channels in the perijunctional zone that are necessary for propagation of the depolarization. Intubating doses of SCh produce a rapid onset (about 1 minute) of a transient agonist effect (eg, muscle twitch) followed by skeletal muscle paralysis lasting 8 ± 2 minutes. These characteristics make SCh a common choice for facilitating rapid tracheal intubation.

1. SCh's neuromuscular-blocking effect terminates when the drug diffuses away from the AChRs and is rapidly hydrolyzed by **plasma cholinesterase** (produced in the liver and also referred to as pseudocholinesterase) to succinylmonocholine and then, more slowly, to succinic acid and choline. This enzyme is not the same as AChE and is not found in the synaptic cleft, therefore the action of SCh is terminated when it diffuses from the endplate to the extracellular fluid. Notably, inhibitors of AChE affect both enzymes to different degrees.
2. **Side effects of SCh** are related to its agonist effects at both the nicotinic and muscarinic AChRs. These include the following:
   a. **Myalgias**, especially in the muscles of the abdomen, back, and neck. It is attributed to muscle fasciculations and observed more frequently in females and younger patients after minor surgical procedures. Myalgias occur in about a third of patients.
   b. **Cardiac dysrhythmias.** SCh has no direct effect on the myocardium. However, ganglionic stimulation may increase heart rate and blood pressure in adults. Alternatively, SCh may stimulate muscarinic receptors at the sinus node, producing sinus bradycardia, a junctional rhythm, or even asystole, particularly in children, and following repeated exposure within a short time interval (within 5 minutes) or with the use of continuous infusions in adults. Pretreatment of

children with intravenous (IV) atropine immediately before SCh reduces the occurrence of bradyarrhythmias.
  c. **Elevated serum potassium.** SCh-mediated depolarization may raise serum potassium by 0.5 to 1.0 mEq/L by exaggerating the usual transmembrane ionic flux. However, life-threatening **hyperkalemia and cardiovascular collapse may occur** in patients with major burns, massive tissue injuries, extensive denervation of skeletal muscle, or upper motor neuron diseases. This effect is attributed to a proliferation of extrajunctional AChRs or damaged muscle membranes and a massive release of potassium upon stimulation. In patients with burns, the period of greatest risk is from 2 weeks to 6 months after the burn has been sustained. However, it is recommended to avoid SCh after the first 24 hours and for 2 years from the time of the injury. Patients with mild elevations of potassium related to renal failure are safe to receive SCh, especially if serum potassium is below 5 mEq/L.
  d. **Increased intraocular pressure,** by 5 to 10 mm Hg, which transiently occurs 2 to 4 minutes following SCh administration. The mechanism of this rise is not clear. The use of SCh in open eye injuries is still acceptable for rapid sequence inductions (Chapter 30: Anesthesia for Head and Neck Surgery).
  e. **Increased intragastric pressure (IGP)** results from fasciculations of abdominal muscles. The risk for aspiration is related to the balance between this pressure and the lower esophageal sphincter (LES) pressure. There have been limited human studies that demonstrate an increase in LES tone that is greater than the increase in IGP. There has not been clinical evidence of an increased aspiration risk with use of SCh for rapid sequence induction (RSI).
  f. **Increase in intracranial pressure,** but the magnitude and clinical importance of this are unclear (Chapter 23: Anesthesia for Neurosurgery). There have not been reports of cerebral herniation with use of SCh.
  g. **A history of malignant hyperthermia (MH) is an absolute contraindication to the use of SCh.** Some degree of masseter muscle spasm may be a normal response to SCh, but severe jaw rigidity increases the risk that a fulminant MH episode may follow. Generalized muscle rigidity, tachycardia, tachypnea, and profound hyperpyrexia after SCh should alert the clinician to MH (Chapter 17: Intra-anesthetic Problems).
  h. **Pretreatment with a subparalyzing dose of a nondepolarizing NMBD** (eg, cisatracurium 1 mg IV or rocuronium 3 mg IV) 2 to 4 minutes before SCh may blunt visible fasciculations but is not uniformly effective in attenuating the above mentioned side effects. Moreover, awake patients pretreated with a nondepolarizing NMBD may experience diplopia, weakness, or dyspnea. When pretreating for a rapid sequence induction, the subsequent IV dose of SCh should be increased to 1.5 mg/kg.
3. **Phase I blockade.** Neuromuscular blockade (NMB) produced by SCh can be separated into two phases. Phase I blockade (**Figure 14.2**) is the usual response to SCh as previously described and is characterized by the following:
  a. Transient muscle fasciculations followed by relaxation
  b. Absence of fade to tetanic or TOF stimulation (Section IV.C)
  c. Absence of posttetanic potentiation (PTP; Section IV.C)
  d. AChE inhibitors potentiate rather than reverse the block

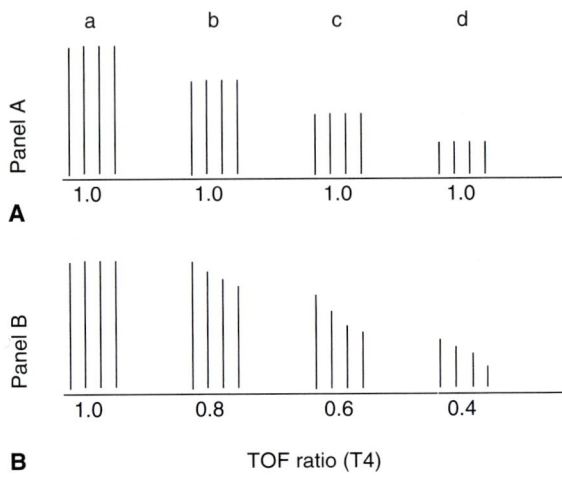

FIGURE 14.2 Schematic representation of train-of-four (TOF) responses to a depolarizing (**A**) and a nondepolarizing (**B**) muscle relaxant, showing the control response before the relaxant (a) and afterward (b, c, d). Note no fade with the depolarizing relaxant and progressive fade with the nondepolarizing relaxant.

4. **Phase II blockade** is most likely to occur after repeated or continuous administration of SCh when the total dose exceeds 3 to 5 mg/kg. Phase II blockade is thought to be secondary to repeated channel opening, causing distortion of the normal electrolyte balance and desensitizing the junctional membrane to further depolarization. It has some of the characteristics of a nondepolarizing blockade:
   a. Fade after tetanic or TOF stimulation (Section IV.C)
   b. Presence of PTP (Section IV.C)
   c. Tachyphylaxis (increasing dose requirement to achieve same depth of NMB)
   d. Prolonged recovery
   e. Partial or complete reversal by AChE inhibitors
5. **Prolonged blockade** following SCh may be caused by low levels of plasma cholinesterase, a drug-induced inhibition of plasma cholinesterase activity, or a genetically atypical enzyme.
   a. **Decreased plasma cholinesterase levels** are found in severe liver or kidney disease, starvation, carcinomas, hypothyroidism, burn patients, decompensated cardiac failure, the last trimester of pregnancy and several days postpartum, and after therapeutic radiation.
   b. **Inhibition of plasma cholinesterase** occurs with the use of organophosphorus compounds (eg, echothiophate eye drops and insecticides), AChE inhibitors (eg, neostigmine, pyridostigmine, and donepezil), chemotherapeutic agents (eg, cyclophosphamide and nitrogen mustard), oral contraceptives, glucocorticoids, esmolol, and monoamine oxidase inhibitors. Plasma cholinesterase levels are not usually altered by hemodialysis.
   c. **Several genetic variants of plasma cholinesterase** exist: normal (N), atypical (A), fluoride resistant (F), and silent (S). **Homozygous atypical cholinesterase** (A–A, prevalence 0.04%) results in prolonged (2 to

3 hours) skeletal muscle paralysis and respiratory insufficiency following a conventional dose of SCh. Heterozygous atypical cholinesterase (N–A, prevalence 4%) results in only modest prolongation of effect (20 to 30 minutes).

d. The **dibucaine number** is a laboratory assay used to characterize plasma cholinesterase abnormality. Normally, the local anesthetic dibucaine inhibits plasma cholinesterase activity by about 80% (dibucaine number of 80), whereas A–A plasma cholinesterase is inhibited by about 20% (dibucaine number of 20). In N–A, dibucaine numbers range from 30 to 65. The comparable **fluoride number** ranges from 0 to 60. N–F individuals (prevalence 0.005%) have slight prolongation of SCh effect, a normal dibucaine number, and a reduced fluoride number. A heterozygous silent N–S individual (prevalence 0.005%) has slightly prolonged effect, but dibucaine and fluoride numbers are normal. Homozygotes F–F and S–S are extremely rare.

e. Patients exhibiting prolonged blocks after a single administration of SCh require sedation and continued intubation until there is a return of twitches. The NMB at this point is similar to that seen with nondepolarizing NMBDs. Once fade with TOF is observed, reversal with neostigmine/glycopyrrolate is possible. Blood assays should be performed to determine total cholinesterase, dibucaine number, and fluoride numbers.

B. Nondepolarizing blockade is produced by reversible competitive antagonism of ACh at the α-subunits of the AChRs.
1. Nondepolarizing blockade is **characterized** by the following (**Figures 14.2** and **14.3**):
   a. Absence of fasciculations
   b. Fade during tetanic and TOF stimulation (Section IV.C)
   c. Presence of PTP (Section IV.C)
   d. Antagonism of depolarizing blockade
   e. Potentiation by other nondepolarizing NMBDs and volatile anesthetic agents
   f. Reversal by AChE inhibitors
2. **The clinical pharmacology** of the commonly used nondepolarizing NMBDs is outlined in **Table 14.1**. Synergistic blockade usually occurs when aminosteroid NMBDs are administered together with

FIGURE 14.3 A, Electromyographic response to repeated train-of-four (TOF) stimulation after injection of a nondepolarizing agent. Each vertical bar is composed of four individual twitch responses. Fade of TOF response eventually leaves only one twitch (approximately 90% blockade). **B,** Reversal of the blockade by neostigmine and atropine given 45 minutes later shows a progressive recovery of the TOF response and reduction in fade with a TOF ratio of 0.9.

benzylisoquinolines. When NMBDs with similar chemical class are combined, the effect is additive.

3. **Cisatracurium** is a benzylisoquinoline (see short description of fellow benzylisoquinolines atracurium and mivacurium in **Table 14.1**) of intermediate duration. High molar potency results in a relatively slow onset time (Section III.B.5). The drug is cleared primarily by Hofmann elimination, and its duration of action is largely independent of renal or hepatic function; it is, however, influenced by body temperature and pH given reliance on plasma enzymatic activity. Specifically, hypothermia may prolong duration of action, and hyperthermia may shorten duration of action.

4. **Vecuronium** is a lipophilic, aminosteroid NMBD that is readily taken up by the liver and excreted into the bile. One of the metabolites, 3-desacetylvecuronium, has neuromuscular-blocking properties (about 50% to 70% of the potency of vecuronium) and is eliminated by the kidneys. Vecuronium has a prolonged clinical effect in elderly patients and those with liver disease and renal failure, as a result of reduced clearance and extended elimination half-life. Vecuronium has no significant effects on heart rate and blood pressure, but it inhibits histamine N-methyltransferase and might potentiate effects such as flushing and hypotension when histamine is released by drugs such as morphine and vancomycin.

5. **Rocuronium** is an analogue of vecuronium that has lower potency. The large intubating dose results in a fast onset time because a larger number of molecules reach the NMJ per circulation time. At a dose of 0.6 mg/kg, maximal blockade can be achieved between 1.8 and 2.7 minutes in adults, per product packaging. Increasing the dose to 1.2 mg/kg (four times the ED_{95}) shortens the time even more but significantly prolongs the duration of action, which can be highly variable among patients. This drug is often chosen when a rapid sequence induction is required but SCh is contraindicated. Clearance of rocuronium occurs as unchanged drug in bile and through renal excretion. Administration of the drug to patients with renal failure may result in a longer duration of action, especially after repeated doses or continuous infusion, though this effect is unpredictable and varied.

6. The **cardiovascular side effects** of nondepolarizing NMBDs are summarized in **Table 14.2**.

IV. MONITORING OF NEUROMUSCULAR FUNCTION

A. There are several reasons to monitor neuromuscular function under anesthesia:
1. To facilitate timing of intubation
2. To provide an objective measurement of relaxation during surgery and degree of recovery before extubation
3. To titrate NMBD dosage according to patient response
4. To monitor for the development of phase II block when using SCh
5. To permit early recognition of patients with abnormal plasma cholinesterase activity
6. To prevent sequelae of residual postoperative NMB

B. **Peripheral nerve stimulators** use various patterns of stimulation: single twitch, tetanus, TOF, and double-burst stimulation as well as the "posttetanic count." The **adductor pollicis response to ulnar nerve stimulation** at the wrist is most often used because it is easily accessible, and the results are not confused with direct muscle activation. Cutaneous electrodes are placed at the wrist over the ulnar nerve and attached to a battery-driven pulse generator, which delivers a graded impulse of electric current at a specified frequency. For maximal twitch response, the negative pole (active) should be placed distally over the ulnar nerve at the wrist. Evoked muscle tension can be estimated by feeling for thumb adduction or measured by using a force transducer or accelerometer attached to the thumb. After administration of an NMBD, the developed tension and twitch height decrease with the onset of blockade. If the ulnar nerve is unavailable, other sites may be used (eg, facial, posterior tibial, peroneal, or lateral popliteal nerves). It is difficult to estimate twitch strength accurately by palpation, so significant residual muscular blockade may be missed by all these techniques. Qualitative TOF monitoring using stimulation of the facial nerve with monitoring of eye muscle response should be avoided, since it has been shown to result in a fivefold greater risk of residual NMB compared with similar monitoring at the adductor pollicis. Eye muscles are more resistant to NMBD effect. Currently, it is strongly recommended that quantitative monitoring should be used over qualitative monitoring or clinical assessment alone in the evaluation of reversal from NMB. When using quantitative monitoring, a TOF ratio of >0.9 at the adductor pollicis muscle needs to be confirmed prior to extubating.

C. The twitch response to various patterns of stimulation has been correlated with clinical end points, and these data are summarized in **Table 14.3**.

1. **Single twitch** is a supramaximal stimulus, typically lasting 0.2 ms at a frequency of 0.1 Hz (one impulse every 10 seconds). The height of the muscle twitch (its amplitude for a given load and peak tension) is determined as a percent of control. A supramaximal stimulus ensures recruitment of all muscle fibers, while a short duration prevents repetitive nerve firing. The stimulus frequency is important because it affects twitch height and degree of fade. Single twitch is not a sensitive measure of onset or recovery from blockade because 75% of AChRs must be

Clinical Assessment of Neuromuscular Blockade

Twitch Response	Clinical Correlate
95% suppression of single twitch at 0.15–0.1 Hz	Adequate intubating conditions
90% suppression of single twitch; TOF count of one twitch	Surgical relaxation with nitrous oxide–opioid anesthesia
75% suppression of single twitch; TOF count of three twitches	Adequate relaxation with volatile agents
25% suppression of single twitch	Decreased vital capacity
TOF ratio >0.75; sustained tetanus at 50 Hz for 5 s	Head lift for 5 s; vital capacity of 15–20 mL/kg; inspiratory force of −25 cm H_2O; effective cough
TOF ratio >0.9; sustained tetanus at 100 Hz for 5 s	Sit up unassisted; normal pharyngeal function
TOF ratio of 1.0	Normal expiratory flow rate, vital capacity, and inspiratory force; diplopia resolves

TOF, train-of-four.

blocked before twitch height begins to decrease, and 75% of the receptors may still be blocked when it returns to control height.
2. **Tetanic stimulus** frequencies vary from 50 to 200 Hz. All NMBDs reduce twitch height, but with nondepolarizing and phase II blockades, a tetanic fade is also demonstrated. This occurs when NMBDs bind to presynaptic receptors and decrease mobilization of ACh during high-frequency stimulation. A tetanic stimulus at 50 Hz for 5 seconds is clinically useful because a sustained tension at this frequency corresponds to that achieved with maximum voluntary effort. However, tetanic stimuli are painful and can speed up recovery in the stimulated muscle, thus misleading the clinician with respect to the degree of recovery in respiratory and upper airway muscles.
3. **Posttetanic single twitch** is measured by single-twitch stimulation 6 to 10 seconds after a tetanic stimulus. An increase in this twitch is called **PTP**, and it is due to increased mobilization and synthesis of ACh during and after tetanic stimulation. Both nondepolarizing and phase II blockade cause PTP, but depolarizing blockade does not.
4. **The TOF** is four supramaximal stimuli given at a frequency of 2 Hz (**Figure 14.2**). They could be repeated at intervals of at least 10 seconds. Responses at this frequency show fade during the onset and recovery of NMB. During nondepolarizing NMB, elimination of the fourth response corresponds to 75% depression of a single twitch. Disappearance of the third, second, and first responses correspond to 80%, 90%, and 100% depression of a single twitch, respectively. The ratio of the height of the fourth to the first twitch (**TOF ratio**) correlates with several clinical parameters (**Table 14.3**). However, clinicians often overestimate TOF ratios and are unable to detect fade when the TOF ratio is >0.4. Several commercially available TOF monitors quantify the TOF ratio using quantitative accelerometry, which measures the acceleration of muscle contraction in reaction to stimulus. These devices have been found to be much more reliable than clinical judgment alone. However, limitations do exist, such as hindered function when hands and arms are tucked in a fashion that prohibits motion. Functional impairment of the muscles of the upper airway may exist even with TOF ratios as high as 0.9, with a significant risk of regurgitation and aspiration. NMBDs may also impair the carotid body hypoxic response, even at a TOF ratio of 0.7. Nevertheless, TOF is a very useful method for clinical monitoring because it does not require a control measurement, it is less painful than tetanic stimulation, and it does not affect subsequent recovery. It provides a good measure of blockade required for surgical relaxation and is also very useful in assessing recovery from blockade. It is not helpful in quantifying the degree of depolarizing blockade because no fade will be evident. However, TOF monitoring may be used to detect fade, indicating the onset of phase II blockade during continuous or repeated administration of SCh.
5. **Posttetanic count** is used to quantify *deep* levels of nondepolarizing block. A 50-Hz tetanic stimulus is given for 5 seconds, followed 3 seconds later by repeated single stimuli at 1 Hz. The number of detectable responses predicts the time for spontaneous recovery. A response to posttetanic twitch stimulation precedes the return of TOF responses.
6. **Double-burst stimulation** uses a burst of two or three tetanic stimuli at 50 Hz followed 750 ms later by a second burst. A decrease in the second response indicates residual curarization. When using tactile

evaluation, fade in response to double-burst stimulation is more easily detected than fade in response to TOF stimulation. When quantitative measurements are used, there is no advantage to using double-burst over TOF stimulation.

V. REVERSAL OF NMB

A. Recovery from SCh-induced depolarizing blockade usually occurs within 5 to 10 minutes following a 1 mg/kg IV dose. Patients with atypical or inhibited plasma cholinesterase can have a greatly prolonged duration of blockade. Reversal of phase II blockade occurs spontaneously within 10 to 15 minutes in approximately 50% of patients. It is advisable to allow patients with prolonged blockade to recover spontaneously for 20 to 25 minutes and then reversal with an anticholinesterase agent may be attempted if there is no further improvement in twitch strength. Earlier reversal could potentiate the block.

B. Nondepolarizing blockade spontaneously recovers when the drug is no longer present at the NMJ. Reversal can be accelerated by administering agents that inhibit AChE, thereby increasing the ACh available to compete for binding sites, or by using encapsulating agents.

C. Historically, the most commonly used anticholinesterase drug has been **neostigmine** (0.03 to 0.07 mg/kg; maximum dose up to a total of 5 mg), which reaches its maximal antagonist effect in about 15 minutes after administration. This drug acts by increasing ACh levels, which competes with NMBDs at the NMJ level. Increased ACh produces both nicotinic and muscarinic effects. Bradycardia, bronchoconstriction, salivation, tearing, and miosis can be minimized by administering an antimuscarinic drug; glycopyrrolate (0.012 to 0.15 mg/kg) is used with neostigmine to mitigate muscarinic effects. A meta-analysis of 15 studies suggests there is no evidence of increased postoperative nausea and vomiting (PONV) with use of neostigmine compared with no use of neostigmine. However, a subsequent small randomized controlled trial (RCT) demonstrated a higher risk of PONV with use of neostigmine compared with sugammadex, suggesting a possible effect. However, the potential harm associated with lack of reversal far outweighs the risk of side effects.

D. Encapsulating reversal agents are muscle relaxant binding drugs that form tight water-soluble complexes with NMBDs, thereby reducing the amount of neuromuscular-blocking agent available to bind AChRs at the NMJ. **Sugammadex**, a modified γ-cyclodextrin, is the only such agent approved in the United States. Following IV administration, it binds aminosteroidal NMBDs in a 1:1 molar ratio (rocuronium > vecuronium >> pancuronium). Sugammadex should not be used to reverse benzylisoquinolinium NMBDs such as cisatracurium or atracurium. In clinical trials, sugammadex has demonstrated the ability to rapidly reverse rocuronium- or vecuronium-induced NMB. For reversal of moderate NMB (1 to 2 twitches by TOF), 2 mg/kg is recommended; for reversal of deep blockade (1 to 2 posttetanic counts), 4 mg/kg is recommended. If immediate reversal of rocuronium-induced RSI is required, a dose of 16 mg/kg is recommended. Sugammadex may not be ubiquitously available as cost may prohibit adoption depending on practice settings.

E. In patients with severe renal failure (creatinine clearance <30 mL/min), the excretion of sugammadex or the sugammadex–rocuronium complexes is delayed, but no signs of recurrent NMB are observed. If re-administration of rocuronium or vecuronium is required, a waiting time of 24 hours is recommended or significantly higher doses are required to paralyze the patient. Compared with neostigmine, sugammadex reverses blockade more quickly; it also was shown in a Cochrane review to be associated with 40% fewer adverse events than neostigmine, including decreased risks of bradycardia (relative risk [RR] 0.16), residual paralysis (RR 0.40), and PONV (RR 0.52). In addition, a blinded RCT of adults older than 70 years demonstrated a 40% reduction in residual neuromuscular block and a 10% reduction in 30-day hospital readmission rate when reversed with sugammadex versus neostigmine. Side effects of sugammadex include bradycardia, hypotension, bronchospasm, anaphylaxis (0.3% incidence rate), and alterations in partial thromboplastin time (PTT) and international normalized ratio (INR) (increases noted with doses of 16 mg/kg) which were found to be lab artifacts. The drug may also interfere with hormonal contraceptive medications; therefore, women of childbearing age should be advised to use alternative contraception for 7 days after use. Sugammadex can also encapsulate progesterone, therefore, its use in early pregnancy is not recommended, as progesterone is critical in the maintenance of pregnancy. In the pediatric population, there are no FDA dosing indications for children <2 years of age, and the 16 mg/kg dose is not indicated for any pediatric age group.

F. **Time to adequate reversal** is related to the degree of preexisting spontaneous recovery. Reversal may be more difficult with the use of long-acting NMBDs, large total doses, and high concentrations of inhalation anesthetics. Other factors that may prolong the blockade include hypothermia, antibiotics (particularly aminoglycosides, clindamycin, and tetracyclines), electrolyte disturbances (hypokalemia, hypocalcemia, and hypermagnesemia), and acid–base disturbances (alkalemia prolongs blockade, and acidemia impairs reversal with anticholinesterase drugs). Reversal with an anticholinesterase agent should not be attempted unless at least one response to TOF stimulation is present. Attempts to reverse a deep or resistant block with excessive doses of neostigmine may increase the degree of residual weakness due to excess ACh at NMJ terminals. If residual weakness is present after attempted reversal, the patient should remain sedated and the endotracheal tube should be left in place to provide adequate ventilation and airway protection. Currently, sugammadex is recommended over neostigmine for the reversal of deep, moderate, and shallow depths of NMB caused by aminosteroidal NMBDs to avoid residual weakness. Neostigmine continues to be a reasonable alternative when sugammadex is contraindicated or unavailable, for shallow depths of NMB, and for reversal of minimal blockade following administration of benzylisoquinolinium NMBDs.

G. **Evidence of neuromuscular recovery**
  1. The **TOF ratio corresponding to adequate neuromuscular recovery** is an objective standard for recovery, though the gold standard ratio has been a matter of debate. Historically, TOF ratios between 0.7 and 0.8 were deemed adequate; however, recent studies have demonstrated significant pharyngeal dysfunction associated with postoperative pulmonary complications at these TOF ratios. The current criterion, particularly for at-risk patients, is a TOF ratio of >0.9. A previously described multicenter, prospective observational study did not demonstrate decreased postoperative pulmonary complications (PPCs) when a TOF >0.9 cutoff was used. However, a post hoc analysis of the study suggested a significant risk reduction when using a cutoff of 0.95 compared to 0.9.
  2. **Clinical signs of adequate neuromuscular recovery** include maintenance of a patient airway without assistance, adequate ventilation and oxygenation, sustained grip strength, the ability to sustain head lift or

movement of an extremity without fade, the ability to clench down on an oral airway and prevent its withdrawal, and the absence of discoordinated muscle activity. While these signs have previously been cited as means of assessing recovery, they poorly correlate with objective degrees of reversal as defined by TOF ratio, thus conferring significant risk of residual blockade if used alone.

VI. EFFECTS OF NMB
   A. **Surgical conditions** have been rated as superior by surgeons in blinded studies for laparoscopic and open surgery when deep NMB (posttetanic count ≤1) was used compared with moderate block (1 to 2 twitches). Deep neuromuscular block has also been associated with more successful use of low-pressure pneumoperitoneum as well as reduced postoperative pain scores.
   B. **EEG monitoring** has been cited as a means of reducing the probability of intraoperative awareness by assessing the depth of anesthesia. However, the commercially available EEG monitors can be influenced by use of NMBs. Facial muscle activity may be necessary for the devices' proprietary algorithms to produce reliable assessments of EEG activity, such that **readings may provide false security** by suggesting an inaccurately deeper level of anesthesia when paralytics are administered.

VII. DISORDERS THAT INFLUENCE THE RESPONSE TO NMBDs
Certain illnesses, both those confined to the NMJ and those affecting more general systems, dramatically affect the response to and safety of NMBDs. In general, transmission at the NMJ is abnormal in these disorders, and there are ultrastructural and biochemical changes in motor nerves, muscle, or both.
   A. **Burns and immobilization**
      1. **Thermal injury** affects fluid and electrolyte balance, cardiovascular and pulmonary function, drug metabolism, and musculoskeletal structure and function.
      2. **Burn patients** and many **immobilized patients** have a greatly exaggerated response to depolarizing agents, and a decreased responsiveness to nondepolarizing agents requiring higher doses. Burn patients exhibit ultrastructural and biochemical alterations in both muscle cells and neuromuscular contacts. These effects can be seen for more than 1 year after the initial thermal insult. Administration of SCh can cause fatal hyperkalemia. Similar problems have been reported in patients with major crush injuries or large areas of devitalized tissue.
   B. **Critical illness**
      1. **Myopathy of critical illness** is a collective group of disorders that can cause weakness in intensive care unit (ICU) patients. The prevalence is high (30% to 70%). The underlying pathology is quite heterogeneous, ranging from pure neuropathies and myopathies to mixed neuromuscular transmission disorders. Sepsis and multiorgan system failure are commonly associated with myopathy of critical illness.
      2. **Weakness** is the common manifestation of all these myopathic disorders, and they contribute to ventilator dependence and increased morbidity and mortality. Myopathy may also produce altered deep tendon reflexes, increased creatine kinase levels, and electrophysiologic alterations in nerves, muscles, or both.
      3. **Corticosteroids, NMBDs, and certain antibiotics** can contribute to or precipitate weakness in ICU patients. One subtype of myopathy of critical illness, acute necrotizing myopathy, has been linked to the repeated

administration of NMBDs, often in conjunction with high doses of corticosteroids.

C. Myasthenia gravis (MG)

1. MG is an **autoimmune disease** with a prevalence of 14 to 20 per 100,000 population in the United States. It is most common in young adult women.
2. **The loss of AChRs at motor endplates** in MG is induced by **antireceptor antibodies.** These antibodies are detectable in the serum of 90% of patients with MG, but antibody titers correlate poorly with clinical signs.
3. MG often presents with the gradual onset of **pharyngeal or ocular weakness.** All muscle groups may be affected. The hallmark of MG is weakness that becomes worse with exercise.
4. **Treatment** includes anticholinesterases (eg, pyridostigmine), corticosteroids, immunosuppressive drugs (eg, azathioprine and cyclophosphamide), plasmapheresis, and thymectomy. Remission of the disease is common after thymectomy.
5. Special attention needs to be given to patients with MG receiving either regional anesthesia or general anesthesia.
    a. **Anticholinesterase therapy** should not be discontinued before surgery.
    b. **Neuraxial regional anesthesia** is associated with skeletal muscle relaxation and some degree of diaphragmatic weakness. This normal effect of regional anesthesia often unmasks underlying weakness. These patients, therefore, may suffer from profound respiratory weakness and need careful respiratory monitoring throughout anesthesia and recovery.
    c. These patients are often **resistant to depolarizing agents** due to AChR loss, although clearance of SCh is inhibited by pyridostigmine. They are also **extremely sensitive to nondepolarizing agents.** Both longer-acting agents such as pancuronium and shorter-acting agents such as cisatracurium have been associated with prolonged blockade, refractoriness to neostigmine reversal, and profound postoperative weakness.
    d. **Monitoring of the degree of NMB is strongly recommended**, although complete recovery of the TOF does not ensure recovery of the muscles of the upper airway or adequate spontaneous ventilation.
    e. **Surgery and anesthesia may exacerbate the underlying illness.** Postoperative ventilatory support may be required even after minor surgical procedures.

D. Muscular dystrophies
are a heterogeneous group of inherited muscle disorders characterized by a progressive loss of skeletal muscle function. **Duchene muscular dystrophy** is the most common and the most severe of the disorders. The responsible gene encodes a membrane-associated protein known as dystrophin that is critical for the stability of the muscular membrane. The disorder is X-linked recessive and clinically evident in males. The clinical course is characterized by painless degeneration and atrophy of skeletal muscle, which manifests as weakness by the age of 5 years. By the preteen years, the patient often is confined to a wheelchair, and death usually occurs by the mid-20s secondary to congestive heart failure.

1. Cardiac (progressive systolic dysfunction and ventricular thinning) and smooth muscles (gastrointestinal hypomotility with delayed gastric emptying) are affected to various degrees. Although the diaphragm is spared, accessory muscle weakness produces a restrictive pattern on pulmonary function testing. Because coughing is impaired, pneumonia is a frequent complication.

2. **SCh** can cause massive rhabdomyolysis, hyperkalemia, and death. Because the intensity and duration of drug effect are hard to predict, short-acting NMBDs may be preferable. Although no longer commonly used, a **volatile inhalational agent,** halothane, can have exaggerated myocardial depressant effects. **MH** occurs with increased frequency. The delayed gastric emptying and ineffective cough place these patients at greater risk for regurgitation and aspiration. Postoperatively, these patients require aggressive pulmonary physiotherapy to ensure adequate secretion clearance. **Opioids**, which may further depress deep breathing and coughing, should be used cautiously.
E. **The myotonic syndromes** are a group of disorders characterized by a defect in skeletal muscle relaxation and persistent contraction of skeletal muscles after stimulation. The persistent contraction is a consequence of ineffective calcium removal from the cytoplasm to the sarcoplasmic reticulum. **Myotonic dystrophy** is the most common syndrome in this group of disorders.
    1. Patients with myotonic dystrophy have progressive involvement and deterioration of skeletal, cardiac, and smooth muscles throughout the body, with weakened respiratory effort, a restrictive pattern on pulmonary function testing, and diminished gastrointestinal motility. Other symptoms include cataracts, cardiac conduction abnormalities, baldness, and intellectual disability.
    2. **Regional anesthesia, neuromuscular-blocking agents, and increasing depth of general anesthesia do not relieve myotonic muscle rigidity.** Pregnancy exacerbates this condition, and cesarean section is often indicated because of uterine muscle dysfunction. These patients are exquisitely sensitive to the respiratory depressant effects of opioids, benzodiazepines, and inhalational agents. Neuraxial opiates that have minimal effect on respiratory function in normal persons can have a substantial effect in these patients. Similar to patients with Duchene muscular dystrophy, these patients have frequent cardiac arrhythmias and are at increased risk for cardiac arrest during general anesthesia.
    3. **SCh** should be avoided as it induces prolonged skeletal muscle contraction. **Nondepolarizing agents** can be used; however, the use of short-acting agents and careful titration of reversal agents are recommended.

ACKNOWLEDGMENT

We gratefully acknowledge the contributions of previous edition authors, Aditi Balakrishna and Matthew W. Vanneman, as portions of those chapters have been retained in this revision.

Suggested Readings

Ali HH, Savarese JJ. Monitoring of neuromuscular function. *Anesthesiology*. 1976;45:216–249.

Berg H, Roed J, Viby-Mogensen J, et al. Residual neuromuscular block is a risk factor for postoperative pulmonary complications. A prospective, randomised, and blinded study of postoperative pulmonary complications after atracurium, vecuronium and pancuronium. *Acta Anaesthesiol Scand*. 1997;41:1095–1103.

Blobner M, Hunter JM, Meistelman C, et al. Use of a train-of-four ratio of 0.95 versus 0.9 for tracheal extubation: an exploratory analysis of POPULAR data. *Br J Anaesth*. 2020; 124(1):63–72.

Briggs ED, Kirsch JR. Anesthetic implications of neuromuscular disease. *J Anesth*. 2003; 17:177–185.

Bruintjes MH, van Helden EV, Braat AE, et al. Deep neuromuscular block to optimize surgical space conditions during laparoscopic surgery: a systematic review and meta-analysis. *Br J Anaesth*. 2017;118(6):834–842.

Cheng CR, Sessler D, Apfel CC. Does neostigmine administration produce a clinically important increase in postoperative nausea and vomiting? *Anesth Analg.* 2005;101(5):1349–1355.

Eriksson LI. Residual neuromuscular blockade. Incidence and relevance. *Anaesthesist.* 2000;49:S18–S19.

Eriksson LI. The effects of residual neuromuscular blockade and volatile anesthetics on the control of ventilation. *Anesth Analg.* 1999;89:243–251.

Kirmeier E, Eriksson LI, Lewald H, et al; POPULAR Contributors. Post-anaesthesia pulmonary complications after use of muscle relaxants (POPULAR): a multicentre, prospective observational study. *Lancet Respir Med.* 2019;7(2):129–140.

Kopman AF, Yee PS, Neuman GG. Relationship of the train-of-four fade ratio to clinical signs and symptoms of residual paralysis in awake volunteers. *Anesthesiology.* 1997;86:765–771.

Lien C. Development and potential clinical impact of ultra-short acting neuromuscular blocking agents. *Br J Anaesth.* 2011;107:i60–i71.

Martyn JA, Richtsfeld M. Succinylcholine-induced hyperkalemia in acquired pathologic states: etiologic factors and molecular mechanisms. *Anesthesiology.* 2006;104:158–169.

Murphy GS, Szokol JW. Monitoring neuromuscular blockade. *Int Anesthesiol Clin.* 2004;42:25–40.

Murphy GS, Szokol JW, Marymont JH, Franklin M, Avram MJ, Vender JS. Residual paralysis at the time of tracheal extubation. *Anesth Analg.* 2005;100:1840–1845.

Pandit L, Agrawal A. Neuromuscular disorders in critical illness. *Clin Neurol Neurosurg.* 2006;108:621–627.

Plaud B, Meretoja O, Hofmockel R, et al. Reversal of rocuronium-induced neuromuscular blockade with sugammadex in pediatric and adult surgical patients. *Anesthesiology.* 2009;110:284–294.

Shear TD, Martyn JA. Physiology and biology of neuromuscular transmission in health and disease. *J Crit Care.* 2009;24:5–10.

Thilen SR, Hansen BE, Ramaiah R, et al. Intraoperative neuromuscular monitoring site and residual paralysis. *Anesthesiology.* 2012;117(5):964–972.

Thilen SR, Weigel WA, Todd MM, et al. 2023 American Society of Anesthesiologists practice guidelines for monitoring and antagonism of neuromuscular blockade: a report by the American Society of Anesthesiologists Task Force on neuromuscular blockade. *Anesthesiology.* 2023;138(1):13–41.

Monitoring
Julia M. Danford and Elisa C. Walsh

I. STANDARD MONITORING
The American Society of Anesthesiologists Standards for Basic Anesthetic Monitoring state that qualified anesthesia personnel should be present during all anesthetics (general, regional, monitored anesthesia care [MAC]), and that oxygenation, ventilation, circulation, and temperature should be continually evaluated.

A. Standard monitoring for general anesthesia
The minimal requirements for general anesthesia include an oxygen analyzer to confirm the administered FIO_2, pulse oximetry, expired carbon dioxide monitoring, an alarm to detect disconnection of components of the breathing system, electrocardiogram (ECG), blood pressure measurement, and the ability to assess temperature. Capnography (Chapter 11: Administration of General Anesthesia and Chapter 13: Airway Evaluation and Management) is mandatory for general anesthesia and recommended for MAC and regional anesthesia.

B. Additional monitoring
The patient's comorbidities and operative procedure may require additional monitors to measure invasive arterial and venous pressures, cardiac function (Chapter 3: Specific Considerations for Cardiac Disease and Chapter 29: Anesthesia for Cardiac Surgery), depth of sedation, neuromuscular blockade (Chapter 14: Neuromuscular Blockade), and central nervous system activity (Chapter 16: Monitoring Anesthetic Brain States and Chapter 23: Anesthesia for Neurosurgery).

II. CARDIOVASCULAR SYSTEM
Circulation may be assessed with clinical signs, ECG, noninvasive and invasive blood pressure monitoring, central venous pressure (CVP), pulmonary artery catheter (PAC) measurements, and echocardiography (transthoracic and transesophageal).

A. ECG.
The ECG is used to determine the heart rate and to detect and diagnose dysrhythmias, myocardial ischemia, pacemaker function, and electrolyte abnormalities. The presence of an ECG signal does not guarantee cardiac contraction and output.

1. Mechanism of monitoring
a. ECG leads. ECG leads are electrodes that measure a small electrical signal (about 1 mV). This makes the ECG prone to electrical interference from outside sources and requires proper electrode application to clean, dry skin.

b. Lead locations. To effectively detect dysrhythmias and ischemia, the leads must be placed in consistent locations on the body. Limb leads must be placed on or near their appropriate limbs and the precordial lead (V5) at the fifth intercostal space, anterior axillary line. With the standard five lead ECG, it is common practice to display leads II and V5 on the continual monitor. Lead II lies parallel to the

electrical axis of the atria and allows for the most sensitive detection of arrhythmias. Lead V5 is most sensitive for detecting anterior and lateral wall ischemia.
- **c. Modes and options**
  1. Monitors often have several choices for filtering of noise, commonly called "diagnostic" and "monitor" modes. The monitor mode filters out noise by using a narrowed bandpass (0.5 to 40 Hz), whereas the diagnostic mode filters less signal and noise by using a wider bandpass (0.05 to 100 Hz). The diagnostic mode should be used when monitoring for ischemia.
  2. Automatic trending of ST segment changes is useful monitoring for the development of ischemia over time.
- **2. Rhythm detection.** The relationship between the P and QRS waves allows for dysrhythmia diagnosis; the P wave is best seen in lead II.
- **3. Ischemia detection.** Monitoring leads II and V5 allows for detection of ischemia in 95% of patients since they represent activity in a large area of the myocardium. Lead II monitors the inferior portion of the heart, supplied by the right coronary artery. Lead V5 monitors the bulk of the left ventricle, supplied by the left anterior descending artery. Lead I may be monitored on patients in whom the left circumflex artery is at risk.
- **B. Arterial blood pressure.** Arterial blood pressure is a function of vascular resistance and blood flow. Blood supply to an organ may be low despite adequate blood pressure because of high vascular resistance. Therefore, arterial blood pressure should be interpreted as an indicator of organ perfusion, but not a direct measurement. Autoregulation in an individual organ may cause local changes in resistance to maintain a constant blood flow.
  1. Measuring blood pressure
     - **a. Mean arterial pressure** (MAP) is a time-weighted average of arterial blood pressure and may be measured directly or calculated (MAP = [systolic blood pressure + 2*(diastolic blood pressure)]/3)
  2. **Automated noninvasive blood pressure** is the most common noninvasive method of measuring blood pressure in the operating room. Most commonly, this method uses oscillometry to deduce blood pressure. The monitor electronically detects the pressures at which there is change in the amplitude of oscillations caused by arterial pulsations, and derives systolic, diastolic, and MAPs. **Manual blood pressure** directly measures the systolic and diastolic blood pressures by auscultation of Korotkoff sounds, palpation, or Doppler.
     - **a. Limitations**
       1. An appropriate cuff size is required for correct determination of blood pressure. A cuff that is too small may result in falsely high blood pressures, whereas a cuff that is too large may result in falsely low blood pressures. The cuff width should cover two-thirds of the upper arm or thigh.
       2. Dysrhythmias and motion artifact may result in erroneous values or may render an automated blood pressure cuff incapable of detecting a blood pressure, resulting in a delay in accurate measurements when using an automated cuff.
       3. Venous congestion and ischemia may result from frequent blood pressure measurements during rapid or large blood pressure fluctuations.
       4. Very low or high blood pressures may not correlate with intra-arterial measurements; noninvasive blood pressure measurement

often overestimates low blood pressure (systolic blood pressure below 80 mm Hg).
      5. Because of the effect of gravity, the level of sampling affects measurement of blood pressure. For example, the difference between pressure measured in the arm in seated or "beach chair" position versus the blood pressure in the head would equal the height of a column of water between the two sites multiplied by conversion factor (1 cm H_2O = 0.74 mm Hg). This difference is usually ~20 cm H_2O or 14.7 mm Hg.
 3. **Palpation may be used to estimate systolic blood pressure** based on whether the pulse may be palpated at key points: radial artery (≥80 mm Hg), femoral artery (≥60 mm Hg), or carotid artery (≥50 mm Hg). This method is inaccurate and is only an estimation when the blood pressure is very low.
 4. **Invasive blood pressure monitoring** uses an indwelling arterial catheter coupled to a pressure transducer via fluid-filled tubing. The transducer converts pressure into an electrical signal for display.
    a. **Indications**
       1. Need for precise blood pressure control (eg, induced hypertension or hypotension).
       2. Hemodynamically unstable patient.
       3. Frequent arterial blood sampling.
       4. Inability to utilize noninvasive blood pressure measurements (eg, during cardiopulmonary bypass when there is nonpulsatile flow).
       5. Access for mechanical circulatory support devices (eg, venoarterial extracorporeal membrane oxygenation).
    b. **Materials** include appropriately sized arterial catheter and transducer apparatus. Generally, the catheter size is 22 to 24 gauge for infants, 20 to 22 gauge for children, and 18 to 20 gauge for adults.
       1. The **transducer** is connected to fluid-filled tubing and a pressurized bag of saline. The pressurized saline enables a continuous infusion at 3 mL/h to prevent thrombosis.
       2. The **tubing** should be rigid and as short as possible, with no kinks or air bubbles.
       3. **Setup.** The transducer should be electronically zeroed while open to air and placed at the height of the coronary sinus for most patients (phlebostatic axis). Exceptions include placing the transducer at the level of the external auditory meatus (representing perfusion in the circle of Willis) during cerebral aneurysm surgery.
 5. **Procedure: Arterial cannulation**
    a. **Locations.** The radial artery is the most common site of insertion. Other locations include ulnar, brachial, axillary, femoral, posterior tibial, and dorsalis pedis arteries. As distance from the heart increases, systolic blood pressure increases, diastolic pressure decreases, pulse pressure increases, and MAP generally has little variation.
    b. **Procedure. Radial artery cannulation**
       1. Supinate and hyperextend the wrist and secure in place with an arm board or tape. Prep the skin and use local anesthetic if placing in an awake patient (**Figure 15.1**).
       2. Two approaches to insertion
          a. **Catheter-over-needle technique.** This technique is the same technique used for peripheral venous cannulation. For this

FIGURE 15.1 Radial artery cannulation using the transfixing technique. As shown in the upper drawing, the needle catheter is advanced through the artery. The lower drawing shows the needle withdrawn and the catheter removed until pulsatile flow is obtained. The catheter then is advanced into the artery with a guidewire using the Seldinger technique. (Reprinted with permission from Gerhardt MA, Walosik-Arenall KM. Monitoring the cardiac surgical patient. In: Hensley FA Jr, Gravlee GP, Martin DE, eds. *A Practical Approach to Cardiac Anesthesia*. 5th ed. Wolters Kluwer Health/Lippincott Williams & Wilkins; 2013:117–155.)

procedure, a standard intravenous catheter is used. Advance the needle until blood flow is observed and then advance the catheter over the needle into the vessel. Remove the needle and attach the transducing tubing.

b. **Transarterial Seldinger technique (Figure 15.1).** The artery is palpated with tips of index and middle fingers of the nondominant hand to determine both the trajectory of artery and point of maximum impulse. The fingers are then moved just distal or lateral to point of maximum impulse, and an angiocath is advanced until blood flow is observed ("flash" in angiocath chamber). It is then advanced further until it is through the back wall of the artery. The needle is then removed and the catheter is slowly withdrawn until there is pulsatile flow of arterial blood through the catheter. A guidewire is then advanced through the angiocath, and the angiocath is inserted into the vessel along the wire. Alternatively, the angiocath can be withdrawn and a longer catheter inserted over the wire. The arterial catheter is then connected to preflushed pressure tubing.

c. **Ultrasound-guided technique.** Ultrasound can be used to guide placement if there is any difficulty with above techniques, and can be considered for primary attempt in patients with severe peripheral vascular disease (and therefore difficult to palpate peripheral pulses) or who are systemically anticoagulated. The ultrasound probe is covered with a sterile sheath and is

used to locate the artery. Once an appropriate portion of vessel is chosen, real-time ultrasound guidance is used to guide the angiocath into the artery. The ultrasound may be used to obtain a cross-sectional image of the artery with an out-of-plane needle approach to the vessel. Alternatively, a long-axis view of the vessel may be obtained and the needle inserted in the plane of the ultrasound beam. Transfixing the artery is not necessary with this approach.
   c. **Considerations for placement**
      1. Femoral and axillary artery cannulations are best performed with 18- or 20-gauge catheters to enter the vessel followed by the insertion of a longer 6-inch catheter of corresponding gauge via the Seldinger technique.
      2. The **modified Allen test** may assess the relative contribution of the radial and ulnar arteries to the blood supply to the hand, but the results are variable. An abnormal test result should be followed up with ultrasonographic evaluation prior to arterial manipulation.
      3. Blood pressure and pulse should be assessed on both right and left sides, particularly in patients with known peripheral vascular disease. If disparity exists, the catheter should be placed on the side with the higher pressure as this may indicate subclavian stenosis or other pathologies on the side with the lower pressure.
      4. Prior cannulation may result in thrombosis or dissection. Proximal pulsation should be assessed before placement. Distal pulsation may simply indicate collateral flow.
   d. **Complications**
      1. **An overdamped waveform** will cause an artifactually low blood pressure measurement. This may result from arterial obstruction, catheter occlusion, excess tubing length, stopcocks, air bubbles, or kinking of the pressure tubing.
      2. **An underdamped waveform** will result in an artifactually elevated systolic blood pressure measurement. This may result from use of nonrigid tubing or hyperresonance caused by reverberation of pressure waves.
      3. Rare complications include arterial thrombosis, ischemia, infection, and fistula or pseudoaneurysm formation. Pulse oximetry on the same hand as the arterial catheter may help to monitor for impending vascular compromise. The catheter should be removed, and the opposite side used if new placement is indicated. The ipsilateral ulnar artery should not be cannulated in the event of radial artery complication due to potential compromise of collateral flow to the hand.

III. CVP AND CARDIAC OUTPUT
   A. **CVP. CVP** is measured by coupling a central venous catheter to a pressure transducer using fluid-filled tubing.
      1. Pressure is monitored at the level of the vena cava or the right atrium. The transducer apparatus is placed at the level of the coronary sinus.
         a. **Indications**
            1. Measurement of right heart filling pressures to assess intravascular volume and right heart function.
            2. Drug administration to the central circulation.
            3. Intravenous access for patients with poor peripheral access.
            4. Access for insertion of PAC via an introducer.

FIGURE 15.2 The normal central venous pressure (CVP) trace and electrocardiogram (ECG). (Reprinted from Mark JB. Central venous pressure monitoring: clinical insights beyond the numbers. *J Cardiothorac Vasc Anesth.* 1991;5(2):163–173. Copyright © 1991 Elsevier. With permission.)

5. Access for total parental nutrition or renal replacement therapy in the intensive care unit.
6. Access for mechanical circulatory support devices (eg, venovenous extracorporeal membrane oxygenation).

b. **Waveform.** The CVP tracing contains three positive deflections—the **a**, **c**, and **v** waves—and two negative slopes—the **x** and **y descents** (**Figure 15.2**). The waves correspond to atrial contraction, tricuspid valve excursion during ventricular contraction, and right atrial filling, respectively. The x descent corresponds to atrial relaxation during systole and the y descent corresponds to early ventricular filling and tricuspid valve opening during diastole.

c. **Analysis**
 1. **Range.** The CVP is read between the **a** and **c** waves at end expiration, thus minimizing the interaction of respiration. The **normal CVP is 2 to 6 mm Hg.**
 2. **Decreased CVP.** Interpretation of diminished CVP is made with respect to corresponding blood pressure. If CVP decreases with an associated increase in blood pressure (without changes to the systemic vascular resistance), there has been an increase in cardiac output. If CVP and blood pressure are both decreased, there has been a decrease in intravascular volume *or* venous return. Of note, however, the use of CVP for the evaluation of fluid responsiveness has been questioned. In general, CVP is a poor indicator of fluid responsiveness. Values of either low (<5 mm Hg) or high (>12 mm Hg) CVP may have some predictive value, but the predictive value is still poor.
 3. **Increased CVP.** When increased CVP is associated with increased blood pressure, without changes to the systemic vascular resistance, the cause of increased CVP is an increase in volume or venous return. With an associated decrease in blood pressure, the increased CVP is due to decreased cardiac output.

d. **Pathology and CVP**
 1. **Cannon a waves** are caused by the atrium contracting against a closed tricuspid valve, as during atrioventricular dissociation.

2. **Large v waves** are caused by regurgitant flow during ventricular contraction, as with tricuspid regurgitation.
   e. **Positive-pressure ventilation** affects both cardiac output and venous return. According to the Starling rule, the transmural pressure (the difference between the atrial pressure and extracardiac pressure) correlates with the cardiac output. At low levels of PEEP, the CVP increases with increased positive end-expiratory pressure (PEEP). At high levels of PEEP (over about 15 cm H_2O), CVP increases as the cardiac output is depressed because of impaired right ventricular output.
2. **Procedure: Central venous catheter placement**
   a. **Sites for central venous catheter placement** are the internal jugular (IJ), subclavian, and femoral veins.
   b. **Materials** include a saline bag under pressure, fluid-filled tubing, and transducer. The transducer is placed at the level of the coronary sinus.
      1. **Catheters may be single lumen or multilumen.** Multilumen catheters consist of a number of smaller caliber catheters which are enclosed in a single sheath allowing for the simultaneous infusion of fluids, nutrition, or medications. Multilumen catheters may also be used for CVP monitoring or periodic blood sampling. These catheters should not be used if anticipating rapid transfusion or infusion of large volumes of fluids. The outer diameter of the catheter ranges from 7- to 8.5-French (Fr) caliber and 16- to 20-cm length with individual lumen sizes of 20 to 16 gauge for catheters intended for use in adult patients.
      2. **Introducers** are larger caliber (9 to 14 Fr), short (7.5 to 11 cm), catheters that allow introduction of an additional device for diagnostic or therapeutic purposes such as a pulmonary arterial catheter, temporary pacing wire, or multilumen catheters specially designed for use with an introducer. The larger size may also allow rapid administration of fluid if the main lumen is not occupied with another device.
      3. **Ultrasound** should be used to guide and verify central venous catheter placement. After proper training and orientation, real-time ultrasound-guided line placement has been shown to be superior to landmark technique by improving overall and first attempt success rates, reducing time for line placement, and reducing the incidence of complications. Therefore, ultrasound-guided placement is considered the gold standard for central venous access.
      4. Depending on the site of catheter placement, **transthoracic** or **transesophageal echocardiography or fluoroscopy** may be used to confirm the intravenous location of the guidewire during catheter placement.
   c. Catheter insertion into the **right IJ vein** is preferred because the vessel runs a straight course to the right atrium.
      1. **Position and preparation.** The patient is positioned supine in slight Trendelenburg position with the head turned slightly toward the contralateral side of insertion. To reduce catheter-related infections, the neck should be prepped with chlorhexidine and sterile drapes should cover the patient from head to toe. The proceduralist should wear a sterile gown and gloves. A short, linear ultrasound probe should be covered with a sterile sheath and should be available in the field.

2. **Two approaches to insertion**
   a. **Landmark-based technique.** While ultrasound-guided central-line placement (described next) has become the gold standard, it is still prudent to be familiar with the landmark-based approach. A number of landmark-based approaches to the IJ have been described. The anterior triangle approach is outlined here. The needle insertion site is located roughly halfway between the angle of the mandible and the sternal notch, at the medial border of the sternocleidomastoid muscle (SCM). At this level, the index finger of the nondominant hand is used to identify the pulsation of the carotid artery and placed over it. An 18-gauge needle with a syringe attached is inserted lateral to the index finger but medial to the SCM and directed such that it travels under the SCM toward the ipsilateral nipple. The angle of insertion with respect to the skin should not exceed 30 degrees. The plunger of the syringe is retracted during needle advancement to apply constant negative pressure at the needle tip. When the vein is entered, blood will fill the syringe, the syringe is then removed and IV tubing is connected to needle to confirm CVP via manometry. Once confirmed, the tubing is removed and a guidewire is threaded through the needle into the IJ. This should thread freely without resistance. The needle is then removed over the wire. A small skin incision is made where the wire enters the skin, to allow for dilation over wire. Once dilated, the prepped central line (with all ports flushed and clamped except for distal-most port where wire will exit) is threaded over the wire and wire is removed. Each port is aspirated and flushed using a saline-filled syringe. Sterile dressing should be applied. A chest radiograph is required to confirm the position and exclude complications such as pneumothorax. The tip of the catheter should be at the junction of the superior vena cava (SVC) and right atrium.
   b. **Ultrasound-guided technique** is the gold standard for placement of central lines. Using a short, linear, high-frequency probe, the IJ is identified (**Figure 15.3**). Confirm the venous versus arterial vessels by applying gentle downward pressure with the ultrasound probe. The IJ vein should collapse, whereas the carotid artery should remain pulsatile. Doppler ultrasound can also be used. Check for vein patency and ensure there are no preexisting anatomical variants or clot burden.
      i. There are several views that can be used with the ultrasound for this procedure.
         (i) Short axis. Using the cross-sectional view seen when scanning the neck, find the desired location on the IJ vein. Position the probe such that the vein underlies the middle of the probe and is centered on the screen. The probe will serve as the surface landmark for the vein. The needle approach will be out of the plane of the ultrasound beam. Insert the needle at a 60° angle to the vertical at the midline of the ultrasound probe. Advance the needle as directed below.
         (ii) Long axis. Typically, a short-axis view is first obtained as previously described. Then rotate the probe 90 degrees in a clockwise fashion to obtain the long-axis

FIGURE 15.3 Ultrasound-guided internal jugular catheterization. The top picture demonstrates the two-dimensional examination showing the internal jugular vein (IJV) lateral to the carotid artery (CA). The bottom picture with the transducer-oriented caudad using color Doppler demonstrates the IJV with blue flow and CA with red flow. (Reprinted with permission from Barash PG, Cullen BF, Stoelting RK, et al. *Clinical Anesthesia*. 6th ed. Wolters Kluwer Health/Lippincott Williams & Wilkins; 2009.)

view. This method uses a needle in-plane technique. Insert the needle at 30-degree angle to the vertical at the proximal end of the ultrasound probe. Advance the needle as directed below.

(iii) Oblique axis. This axis is essentially a combination of the short- and long-axis views. First, obtain a short-axis view and then rotate the probe approximately 45 degrees in a clockwise fashion. Both the IJ and carotid arteries should be visualized simultaneously. This axis uses a needle in-plane technique. Insert the needle in a 30-degree angle to the vertical at the proximal end of the ultrasound probe. Advance the needle as directed below.

(iv) Placement. Use the ultrasound imaging to guide the angle and approach of the needle to the vein. Be mindful of the length of the needle that is required to reach the vein. No more than half of the length of the needle should be used to reach the vein, so that at least half of the catheter can be inserted into the vein reducing the risk of inadvertent decannulation. Aspirate while advancing the needle until venous blood is aspirated. If using a short-axis view, take care to ensure that the portion of the needle which is visualized is actually the tip. Generally, this requires fanning the ultrasound back and forth to track the bevel which will appear brighter than the shaft. If using the long or oblique axis, ensure that the bevel is clearly visualized throughout the entire course of the needle. Once the vein is cannulated, the syringe is removed and a guidewire is passed through the needle or catheter.

(v) Confirm intravenous placement of the catheter using manometry as well as ultrasound in both the short axis and long axis. Transthoracic or transesophageal echocardiography and fluoroscopy may be used to specifically confirm the presence of the wire or catheter at the junction of the SVC and right atrium in real time. The remainder of the procedure is the same as the landmark technique above.

d. The **subclavian vein** may be easily accessed as the vessel passes under the clavicle at the midclavicular line. It is one of the most common central venous line locations. Although the artery is not compressible in case of puncture, coagulopathy is not a contraindication to placement. The subclavian vein is often preferred for patient comfort, and the left SCV is often chosen because of the natural course of the brachiocephalic vein into the SVC.

1. **Landmarks** include the clavicle, suprasternal notch, and lateral border of the SCM as it inserts onto the clavicle. The insertion site is 2 to 3 cm inferior to the clavicle, just medial to the midclavicular line.
2. In the landmark-based technique, the thin-walled needle is placed at the insertion site and aimed at the suprasternal notch. The tip of the needle is used to identify the clavicle, and the tip is then "walked" posteriorly under the clavicle. The key to avoid a pneumothorax is to always keep the needle parallel to the floor during insertion. The rest of the procedure is similar to that described for the IJ cannulation.
3. Ultrasound guidance is less common for subclavian access as the position of the vein under the clavicle is not amenable to ultrasound visualization. However, recent meta-analyses and systematic reviews have demonstrated that use of dynamic ultrasound likely reduces mechanical complications of subclavian access.

This is because dynamic ultrasound can identify the position of the axillary vein (which becomes the subclavian under the clavicle) relative to the axillary artery and apex of the lung, thus helping the operator avoid an inadvertent arterial cannulation or pneumothorax.

e. The **femoral vein** is one of the most easily accessible central veins. Limitations include hip immobility, obesity, and increased infection and thrombosis rate. Ultrasound guidance is preferred but the procedure is often done using landmark techniques in emergency cases.
  1. **Landmarks** include the femoral artery, inguinal ligament, anterior superior iliac spine (ASIS), and pubic tubercle. The femoral vein is immediately medial to the femoral artery. A common mnemonic to remember the anatomic relationship of structure within the femoral triangle is "NAVeL" from lateral to medial indicating femoral nerve, artery, vein, and lymphatics. If the artery is not palpable, the vein is reliably located one-third of the distance from the pubic tubercle to the ASIS. In either case, the insertion point is just inferior to the inguinal ligament, 1 to 2 cm medial to the artery.
  2. **Ultrasound technique.** Establish the relationship of vessels to each other while using standard landmark findings to assist in choosing the ideal puncture site. As previously described, a short axis, long axis, or oblique axis can be used.

3. **Complications**
  a. **Dysrhythmias**, caused by the guidewire irritating the endocardium, typically resolve with withdrawal of the wire.
  b. **Arterial puncture** can cause significant vessel damage and bleeding if the dilator or catheter is placed into the artery. Before dilation, intravenous position should be verified by ultrasound, echocardiography, manometry, or fluoroscopy. Blood gas measurement may be used as well. If an artery is punctured before dilation, the needle should be removed and pressure applied for at least 5 minutes (10 minutes in the case of coagulopathy) and a new site chosen. If the catheter is placed in the artery, it should remain in place and vascular surgery should be consulted.
  c. **Venous damage** during placement may be minor or significant. Never forcibly advance the guidewire if resistance is encountered. When the dilator is passed over the guidewire, continually confirm the mobility of the guidewire as the dilator is advanced. The guidewire should not feel tethered as this may signify a bend or kink in the wire caused by the dilator.
  d. **Malpositioning** may be intra- or extravascular. Intravascular malpositioning includes azygos, axillary, and intercostal vein placement. Extravascular malpositioning has been described in numerous neighboring structures in the case literature and should be suspected if blood cannot be drawn from one or more lumens of the central line. Computed tomography (CT) scanning may be helpful to identify the location of an extravascular catheter and direct further interventions.
  e. **Pneumothorax, hemothorax, hydrothorax, chylothorax, or pericardial tamponade** are more serious complications of central venous cannulation that may lead to hemodynamic instability or cardiovascular collapse. They are in part ruled out with chest radiography but may also be assessed with point-of-care ultrasound. The risk of pneumothorax is the highest with subclavian vein insertion.

f. Infection may develop at any time during the period that the catheter is in place. The longer the catheter remains in place, the greater the risk of developing an infection. The risk of infection is higher with femoral and IJ venous placement compared to subclavian placement. Infections are best prevented through observance of strict sterile technique during catheter placement, antiseptic technique when accessing catheter ports, and expeditious removal of the catheter as soon as clinically appropriate.

g. **Air embolism** may occur at any time during catheter insertion, removal, or accessing. To reduce air entrainment at the neck and subclavian sites, placing the patient in Trendelenburg position is helpful. To reduce the chance of air embolism upon catheter removal, the site is occluded with the patient performing a Valsalva maneuver.

4. **PAC and pulmonary artery occlusion pressures (PAOPs).** The PAC gives information about ventricular function and vascular volume by measuring CVP, pulmonary artery pressure (PAP), PAOP or "wedge" pressure, mixed venous oxygen saturation sampling, and cardiac output. Studies have demonstrated no hospital mortality benefit with the use of PACs in the intensive care unit setting and their placement can lead to catheter-related complications. Although PACs provide useful clinical data, they are not recommended for routine critical care.

   a. **Mechanism.** The PAC is inserted through a central venous introducer catheter. It passes through the vena cava, right atrium, and right ventricle into the pulmonary artery. Transducers are connected to separate ports to allow CVP and PAP measurements. Inflating the balloon at the tip of the catheter allows measurement of PAOP, reflecting the left atrial pressure and left ventricular (LV) preload. To minimize the effect of alveolar pressure on PAOP, the tip should rest in West Zone III, where the pulmonary venous pressure is greater than the alveolar pressure.

   b. **Indications**
      1. Unexplained hypotension.
      2. Access for cardiac pacing.
      3. Surgical procedures with significant, rapid physiologic changes (eg, open aortic aneurysm repair and lung or liver transplant).
      4. Acute myocardial infarction with shock

   c. **PAP and PAOP**
      1. **Waveform.** The PAP waveform is similar in shape to the systemic arterial waveform. Because of the location, the waveform is smaller and precedes the systemic waveform. With the balloon inflated, the PAC will measure the PAOP recording, which is similar to the CVP waveform, with **a** and **v** waves. This waveform approximates the left atrial pressures and is slightly delayed because of the interposed lung.
      2. **Range.** The **normal PAP is 15 to 30 mm Hg systolic and 5 to 12 mm Hg diastolic.** The **normal range for PAOP is 5 to 12 mm Hg.** At end expiration, this approximates the left atrial pressure and correlates with the LV end-diastolic volume.

   d. **PAOP analysis** is used to assess the left-sided heart performance. A basic model of left-sided heart function is given by the relationship between the end-systolic pressure–volume curve and end-diastolic pressure–volume curve. Because the left ventricular end-diastolic pressure (LVEDP), which correlates with the LV end-diastolic volume, is known, the following deductions are possible (**Figure 15.4**).

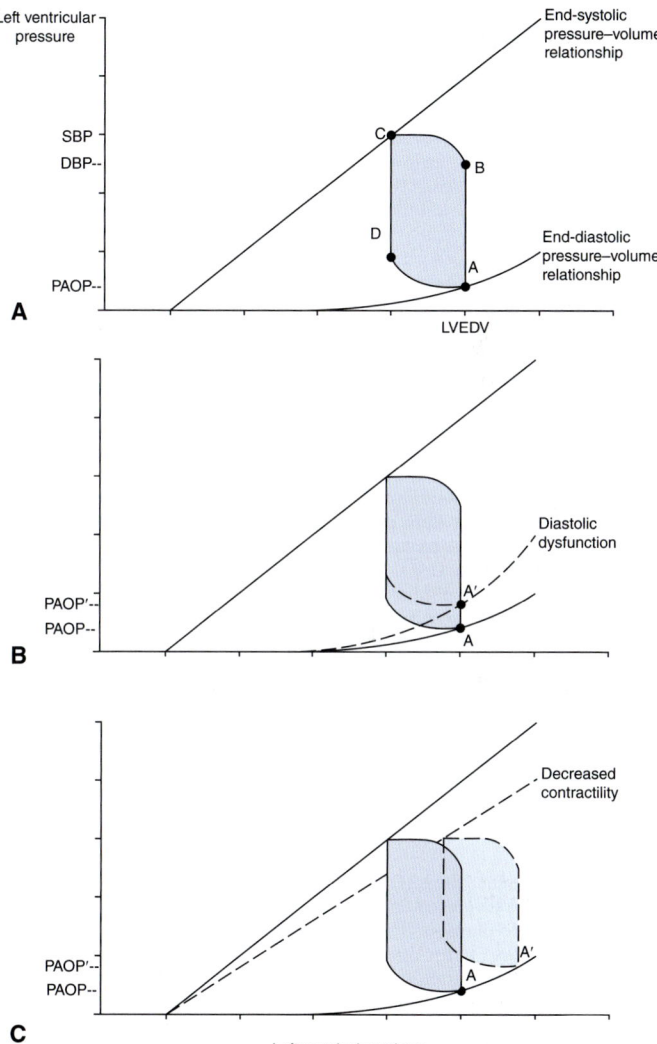

FIGURE 15.4 Left ventricular pressure–volume relationships. **A,** The cardiac cycle (A-B-C-D-A) is limited by the end-systolic pressure-volume relationship (describing the contractility) and the end-diastolic pressure-volume relationship. The PAOP approximates the LVEDP. An increase in PAOP may be ascribed to decreased diastolic compliance (**B**), an increase in left ventricular end-diastolic volume (LVEDV) (C), or a combination of both. An increase in LVEDV often results from decreased contractility in the setting of a properly performing right ventricle (**C**). DBP, diastolic blood pressure; SBP, systolic blood pressure.

1. **Increase in PAOP** can be due to an increase in LV end-diastolic volume, decrease in LV compliance, or both.
2. **Decrease in PAOP** can be due to a decrease in LV end-diastolic volume, increase in LV compliance, or both.

e. **Effects of pathology on waveform and PAOP**
   1. **Large a waves** may be due to either left ventricular hypertrophy (LVH) or atrioventricular dissociation. LVH will decrease the compliance of the left ventricle and will elevate the LVEDP. Thus, the PAOP should be measured at the peak of the **a** wave. During atrioventricular dissociation, pressure should be measured before the **a** wave.
   2. **Large v waves** are the result of mitral regurgitation.
   3. **Right-sided heart dilatation** can cause shifting of the interventricular septum into the left ventricle, effectively decreasing the LV end-diastolic compliance. Thus, LVEDP will be elevated.
   4. **Pulmonary embolism** may cause an elevation of the PAP without a concomitant elevation of the PAOP.

f. **Materials/catheter types.** Most catheters are available with or without bonded heparin. Types of PACs include the following:
   1. **Venous infusion** (VIP, VIP+) catheters provide extra ports for infusion and sampling.
   2. **Paceports** allow placement of cardiac pacing wires.
   3. **Continuous cardiac output** catheters perform frequent automated determinations of cardiac output by using frequent low-heat pulses to obtain a thermodilution curve; the values are usually an average over time.
   4. **Oximetric** catheters monitor mixed venous O_2 saturation.
   5. **Right ventricular ejection fraction** catheters use a rapid response thermistor to calculate the right ventricular ejection fraction in addition to cardiac output.

5. **Procedure: PAC placement**
   a. **Locations and preparation** are similar to those of the central venous catheter procedure described in Section IIIA2. The PAC is invariably placed through an introducer catheter. The operator typically dons a new pair of sterile gloves between the introducer and PAC placement.
   b. **Technique.** The PAC is prepared and examined as follows:
      1. **Sheath placement.** A sheath is placed over the catheter and locked into place at 70 cm. The sheath allows movement of the PAC to adjust to the optimum position while maintaining sterility.
      2. **Balloon** examination consists of inflating the balloon with 1.5 mL of air and inspecting prior to placement. The balloon should be symmetrical, inflate and deflate smoothly, and the tip of the PAC should not protrude past the balloon.
      3. All ports are flushed to ensure patency and are attached to calibrated pressure transducers. Raising and lowering the PAC distal end should produce changes in the PA pressure tracing and serve as a quick test of the system before insertion.
      4. **Placement (Figure 15.5).** The PAC is held so that it follows a natural curve through the heart during passage through the introducer. Once the 20-cm mark is reached, the balloon is inflated with 1.5 mL of air, and the CVP waveform is confirmed. As the catheter is advanced, the waveform will change to a right ventricular waveform and then to a pulmonary artery waveform characterized by

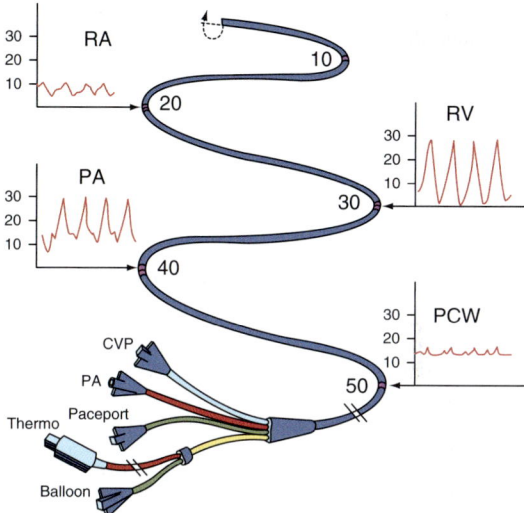

FIGURE 15.5 Pulmonary artery catheter (PAC) and pressure waveforms that will be encountered as it is inserted into the wedged position from the right internal jugular vein. Distances in centimeters on the catheter correspond to insertion distances read at the diaphragm of the introducer and are approximate. CVP, central venous pressure; PCW, pulmonary capillary wedge; RA, right atrium; RV, right ventricle; Thermo, thermistor connection for cardiac output determination. (Reprinted with permission from Gerhardt MA, Walosik-Arenall KM. Monitoring the cardiac surgical patient. In: Hensley FA Jr, Gravlee GP, Martin DE, eds. *A Practical Approach to Cardiac Anesthesia*. 5th ed. Wolters Kluwer; 2013:117–155.)

an increase in diastolic pressure and a change in the waveform during diastole from downsloping to upsloping. The PAC is advanced until a PAOP waveform is seen, and the balloon is then deflated. The waveform should return to a pulmonary artery tracing upon deflation. If it does not, then the PAC should be withdrawn about 5 cm with the balloon deflated, the balloon should be reinflated, and the PAC should be advanced until a PAOP tracing is encountered. The balloon should remain deflated normally.
5. **Securing** the sheath to the introducer proximally and at the 70-cm mark distally ensures the ability to manipulate the PAC aseptically. The introducer and PAC are secured to the patient, and an occlusive dressing is applied.
c. **Distances.** As a rough guide, distances from the right IJ vein to each chamber are "on the tens." Typically, the right atrium is encountered at around 20 cm, the right ventricle at around 30 cm, the pulmonary artery at around 40 cm, and the PAOP at around 50 cm. From the subclavian vein, subtract 5 cm from these distances; from the femoral vein, add 20 cm to these distances.
d. During PAC insertion, difficulty in passing the catheter into the right ventricle and pulmonary artery may be encountered because of balloon malfunction, valvular lesions, a low-flow state, or a dilated right ventricle. The monitoring equipment should be rechecked for calibration and scale. Inflating the balloon with a full 1.5 mL of air, rapid PAC

advancement (assuming no resistance), and large inspirations by the patient to augment venous return may be helpful. The PAC may have to be withdrawn to a depth of 20 to 30 cm, rotated slightly, and readvanced. Fluoroscopy can aid in the proper placement of the PAC.
  e. **Complications**
     1. **Dysrhythmias** may arise as the catheter tip comes into direct contact with the atrium, ventricle, and pulmonary outflow tract. They are usually transient and resolve spontaneously with continued passage or with withdrawal of the PAC. Complete heart block and ventricular tachycardia are possible (up to 0.3% of placements) and should be treated appropriately.
     2. **Right bundle branch block** is a specific risk in patients with either a left bundle branch block or a first-degree heart block, as this may result in complete heart block. In this event, the PAC should be withdrawn and temporary pacing initiated.
     3. **Pulmonary artery rupture** is possible from overinflation or prolonged inflation of the balloon or from direct pressure by the PAC. Thus, the balloon should be slowly inflated, and volume to achieve PAOP should be monitored. Furthermore, the PAP should always be monitored; if a persistent PAOP trace appears, the catheter should be pulled back immediately and repositioned.
     4. **Pacemakers** do not contraindicate PAC placement, although fluoroscopic guidance should be used if the pacemaker is less than 6 weeks old.
     5. **Balloon rupture** may occur with overinflation with more than the recommended 1.5 mL.
     6. **Valve damage, thrombus formation, and infection** can occur with PACs. Knotting of the catheter can happen when the catheter will not pass through the pulmonary valve and turns back on itself in the right ventricle.
6. **Cardiac output** is typically 4 to 8 L/min, whereas the cardiac index (CO/body surface area) is 2.4 to 4.0 L/min/m^2. CO is conventionally measured with a PAC using thermodilution. The risks of PAC placement have generated interest in alternative method for measuring CO.
   a. **Thermodilution with a PAC** is the gold standard for CO measurement. A known volume of cold saline is injected into the CVP port. The resulting temperature change in the PA is monitored by the thermistor located at the PAC tip. The area under the temperature–time curve correlates with cardiac output.
      1. **CO should be measured at end expiration.** Changes in intrathoracic pressure affect the CO measurement. Negative intrathoracic pressure during the inspiration phase of spontaneous breathing increases venous return and LV transmural pressure. Positive intrathoracic pressure during the inspiration phase of positive-pressure ventilation decreases venous return and LV transmural pressure.
      2. **Tricuspid regurgitation** often causes the CO and cardiac index to be underestimated by prolonging the time and increasing the area under the CO curve. Although underestimation is the most common error, values may be overestimated as well.
      3. **Errors in CO measurement** may also be caused by injectate spillage, very slow injection, use of the wrong catheter constant, concomitant infusion of fluids through central line, and intracardiac shunt.

b. **Pulse contour analysis** determines stroke volume and cardiac output by computer analysis of the arterial pulse pressure waveform. This method assumes that the aortic pulse pressure is proportional to stroke volume. The effects of vascular tone are included in the calculation as a conversion factor calculated from heart rate, MAP, and vessel compliance. The advantage is that central venous access is not needed. Available systems utilize patient demographics and physical characteristics for arterial impedance estimation (FloTrac System, Edwards Lifesciences, Irvine, CA) or injected indicators for calculation (see below). Limitations include:
   1. **Nonlinearity of aortic compliance changes.** The compliance of the aorta changes nonlinearly with pressure. This may limit the accuracy of stroke volume estimates.
   2. **Resonance and damping** may occur, as with use of any arterial catheter for invasive blood pressure monitoring.
   3. **Limited accuracy in tracking changes in stroke volume** after a volume challenge or the use of vasopressors.
   4. Need for **predefined optimal conditions** for testing. The literature supports increased accuracy with a control mode mechanical ventilation (no spontaneous breaths) on a patient with a closed chest, a fixed respiratory rate, TV ≥8 mL/kg, and generally a PEEP ≥5.
c. **Modified Fick techniques.** NICO (Philips Respironics, Pittsburgh, PA) uses sensors in the breathing circuit attached to an intubated patient to measure flow, airway pressure, and CO_2 concentration. During periods of rebreathing, CO_2 elimination is calculated from these measurements. The Fick principle is applied to calculate cardiac output, which is proportional to the change in CO_2 elimination divided by the change in end-tidal CO_2.
d. **Thoracic bioimpedance** uses skin electrodes placed along the neck and thorax to measure changes in voltage and impedance. Because blood is a stronger conductor than muscle, bone, and skin, changes in thoracic blood volume during the cardiac cycle result in impedance changes. Ohm's law is applied to use the change in impedance to determine CO. This method is completely noninvasive and the electrodes require minimal training to place. A large body habitus and fluid overload may result in inaccurate measurements.
e. **Thoracic bioreactance** (NICOM device, Cheetah Medical, Portland, OR) uses outer electrodes that apply an electric current of known frequency across the thorax and inner electrodes that record the signal after it interacts with the pulsatile blood flow within the thorax resulting in a time delay, or phase shift. The volume of pulsatile blood (stroke volume) that caused the specific time delay can be calculated and continually detected to create the NICOM signal. The continual, dynamic sensing results in less signal distortion than bioimpedance systems. Although further studies are needed, the CO as measured by bioreactance has been shown to be highly correlated with that measured by thermodilution.
7. **Echocardiography** (Chapter 2: Basics of Echocardiography and Lung Ultrasound)
   a. **Mechanism.** Echocardiography is performed with ultrasonic waves to create a two-dimensional image of the heart and surrounding structures. This may be done from a transthoracic or transesophageal approach, depending on the targeted structures, patient compliance, and conditions during placement. It provides independent

assessments of the same parameters that a PAC measures, but it also reveals cardiac valve function, ventricular contractility, diastolic function, and intracardiac structures.
- **b. Indications**
  1. **Hypotension of unknown cause**
  2. **Uninterpretable PAC values**
  3. **Suspected intracardiac masses or vegetations**
  4. **Valvular abnormalities**
  5. **Shunts**
  6. **Air embolism**
  7. **Pericardial disease**
  8. **Thoracic aneurysm/dissection**
- **c. Methods**
  1. **Transthoracic echocardiogram** can be performed with the patient awake and provides good visualization of right- and left-sided heart structures and qualitative estimates of contractile performance, although visualization intraoperatively may be limited depending on the location of surgery. The basic views are the parasternal short, parasternal long, subcostal, and apical four-chamber views.
  2. **Transesophageal echocardiogram** requires that the patient be topically, or generally anesthetized, but it may be performed intraoperatively and allows superior visualization of the left side of the heart. There are 20 standard views, but more may be incorporated for more intensive examinations or more subtle pathology.

IV. RESPIRATORY SYSTEM

The respiratory system is responsible for oxygen uptake and carbon dioxide removal and provides a conduit for delivery of anesthetic agents.

- **A. Mandatory respiratory monitors** during general anesthesia include pulse oximetry, capnography, inspired oxygen analyzer, and a disconnect alarm. Direct visualization of the chest and use of a stethoscope may provide additional information. During regional anesthesia, respiration may be monitored with direct visualization, oximetry, and capnography.
- **B. Oxygenation** is most easily measured by **pulse oximetry.** Other methods include qualitative assessment of skin color, transcutaneous oximetry, and arterial blood gas sampling.
  1. **Method.** Oxygenated and deoxygenated hemoglobin absorb light differently at most wavelengths, including 660 and 960 nm, the wavelengths examined by most devices. The Beer–Lambert law allows the concentration of each species to be calculated from the absorption of light at those wavelengths. The ratio of absorption is processed to give the oxygen saturation of hemoglobin. The sensor has at least two light-emitting diodes (960 and 660 nm) and a light detector. This may be applied to fingers, toes, earlobes, tongue, or, the nose.
  2. **Interpretation.** The normal range in a healthy adult is 96% to 99%, whereas values above 88% may be acceptable in patients with baseline lung disease. A high pulse oximeter reading (SpO_2) generally indicates that oxygen is available in the lungs, taken up in the blood, and delivered to distal tissues. A low SpO_2 may be due to a problem along the above pathway or due to an error in monitoring.
  3. **Limitations**
     a. Oximetry may be a late indicator of inadequate gas exchange.
     b. **Carboxyhemoglobin** absorbs light similarly to oxygenated hemoglobin at 660 nm and will provide falsely elevated readings, although it does not contribute to oxygenation.

c. **Methemoglobin** absorbs light at both 660 and 940 nm, resulting in a saturation of 85%, which does not correlate with the true saturation. Methemoglobinemia may be treated with methylene blue.
d. **Methylene blue, indocyanine green, indigo carmine,** and **isosulfan blue** injections transiently result in falsely low saturation readings.
e. SpO_2 tends to be falsely overestimated at low saturations (below 80%).
f. Low perfusion, motion, and nail polish (especially blue) may cause SpO_2 measurements to be uninterpretable or unreliable.

C. **Ventilation** is assessed by end-tidal carbon dioxide measurement via capnometry and spirometry. Capnometry and capnography are often used as synonyms, as both analyze and record carbon dioxide, with the latter including a waveform. Capnography not only evaluates respiration but also confirms of endotracheal intubation and is diagnostic of pathologic conditions.
  1. **Method.** The measurement of carbon dioxide is often based on infrared light absorption to determine concentration. Carbon dioxide may be measured either at the breathing circuit (mainstream capnograph) or via aspiration of gas samples by the capnograph (sidestream capnograph). Mainstream capnographs often cause traction on the endotracheal tube and can cause burns by radiant heat, whereas sidestream capnographs have a measurement delay based on sample volumes and may result in significant leaks from sampling. Sidestream capnography may also be used on a nonintubated patient to give a qualitative assessment of respiration.
  2. **Waveform.** The normal end-tidal carbon dioxide ($PetCO_2$) waveform (**Figure 15.6**) contains the expiratory portion (phases I, II, III, and occasionally IV) and inspiratory portion (phase 0). Two angles, the α angle (between phases II and III) and the β angle (between phases III and 0), also aide in interpretation.
      a. **Phase 0** is the inspiratory segment.
      b. **Phase I** is the carbon dioxide–free gas that is not involved in gas exchange (dead space).
      c. **Phase II** is the rapid upswing and includes both alveolar gas and dead space gas.
      d. **Phase III** is a plateau that involves alveolar gas and has a small positive slope. $PetCO_2$ is measured at the end of phase III.
      e. **Phase IV** is a terminal upswing seen in obese and pregnant patients with reduced thoracic compliance.
      f. The α **angle** is between phases II and III and is related to the ventilation: perfusion matching of the lung. The β **angle** is between phases III and 0 and usually is about 90 degrees, and it may be used to assess rebreathing.
  3. **Range and analysis**
      a. Normally, $PetCO_2$ is 2 to 5 mm Hg lower than arterial CO_2 pressure, so the typical range for end-tidal carbon dioxide during general anesthesia is 30 to 40 mm Hg.
      b. Owing to swallowed gas, **esophageal intubation** may initially result in carbon dioxide return similar to that of endotracheal intubation, except that $PetCO_2$ diminishes to zero with a few breaths.
      c. **An early sign of malignant hyperthermia** is a rapidly rising end-tidal carbon dioxide, especially if it is unresponsive to hyperventilation.
      d. Shock/low perfusion, embolism, auto-PEEP, airway obstruction, and system leaks will result in diminishing end-tidal carbon dioxide.
      e. Carbon dioxide absorption during laparoscopic procedures, reperfusion after releasing an arterial clamp or tourniquet, and absorbent

A

B

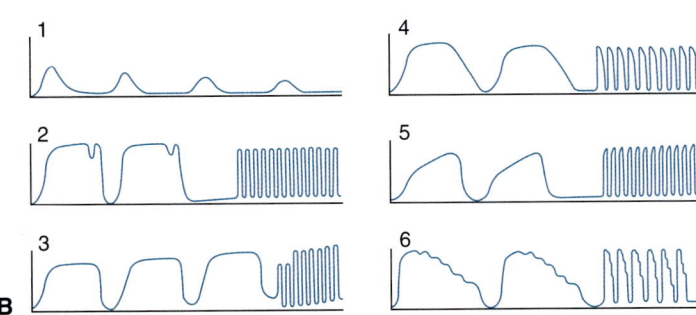

FIGURE 15.6 A, Normal capnograph. I, dead space expiration; II, mixed dead space and alveolar gas expiration; III, alveolar gas expiration and plateau; 0, inspiration. Phase IV is an upswing that occurs at the end of phase III. **B,** Capnographs that may be seen in practice. 1, rapidly extinguishing uncharacteristic waveform, compatible with esophageal intubation; 2, regular dips in end-expiratory plateau, seen in underventilated lungs or in patients recovering from neuromuscular blockade; 3, upward shift in baseline and plateau, seen with rebreathing of carbon dioxide, miscalibration, and so forth; 4, restrictive pulmonary disease; 5, obstructive pulmonary disease; 6, cardiogenic oscillations.

exhaustion or channeling will result in rising end-tidal carbon dioxide.
- f. Widening of the β angle with an elevation of both phases 0/I and III is a sign of **inspiratory valve failure.**
- g. Elevation of both phase 0/I and phase III is a sign of **expiratory valve failure** or **absorbent malfunction.**
4. **Esophageal manometry.** Using an esophageal pressure probe to obtain a surrogate for pleural pressures. Esophageal manometry is used to calculate transpulmonary pressures and to optimize PEEP to reduce the risk of trauma and improve oxygenation for the lungs. Optimizing these pressures allows for the reduction of lung overdistension, prevention of lung atelectasis and atelectrauma, and increase of functional lung volumes. Changes in esophageal pressures reflect changes in pleural pressures. To accurately obtain the esophageal pressure, the esophageal probe should be placed approximately 40 cm or when cardiac oscillations are seen on the pressure tracing.
5. **Airway pressures.** When a patient is sedated, paralyzed, and mechanically ventilated, the airway pressures (peak and plateau) are generally used to guide ventilator parameters since these are assumed to closely approximate the pressure in the lung parenchyma. This assumption

is reasonable in patients with normal chest wall elasticity and pleural pressure. As chest wall compliance decreases or pleural pressure increases, such as in conditions like ARDS, pleural effusion, ascites, or obesity, the portion of airway pressure that distends lungs decreases, resulting in atelectasis and overdistension in the nonatelectic lung.
  a. Calculations to consider:
    1. Plateau pressure = tidal volume/compliance and represents airway pressure due to endogenous alveolar compliance. It is measured at end inspiration when flow has ceased. In ARDS, it has been suggested to target plateau pressures below 30 cm H_2O.
    2. Peak pressure is the sum of alveolar and airway pressures. An isolated high peak pressure with normal plateau pressure represents an issue with airway resistance, including organic (eg, bronchospasm) and mechanical (eg, kinked endotracheal tube) problems.
    3. Driving pressure = Plateau pressure − PEEP. This represents the pressure delivered to the respiratory system (includes the chest wall and lung parenchyma). In ARDS, it has been suggested to target a driving pressure below 14 cm H_2O.
    4. Transpulmonary pressure = Plateau pressure − Pleural pressure. This represents the actual pressure to the lung parenchyma. Using esophageal manometry, the optimal PEEP may be identified by estimating the transpulmonary pressure. Optimal PEEP can prevent atelectasis and improve oxygenation as well as prevent barotrauma.

V. TEMPERATURE MONITORING
  A. **Mechanism.** Temperature may be measured intermittently or continuously. The limitation of more external methods of temperature determination is that they may not reflect changes in the core body temperature, especially in the presence of vasoconstriction.
  B. **Indications**
    1. **Need to control temperature** during induced hypothermia and rewarming (eg, during cardiopulmonary bypass or vascular neurosurgery).
    2. **Infants and small children** are prone to thermal lability owing to their high surface area-to-volume ratio.
    3. **Adults subjected to large evaporative losses or low ambient temperatures** (as occurs with exposed body cavity, large volume transfusion of unwarmed fluids, or burns) are prone to hypothermia.
    4. **Febrile patients** need to be monitored because of the risk of hyper- or hypothermia.
    5. Patients with **autonomic dysfunction** are unable to autoregulate their body temperature.
    6. **Malignant hyperthermia** is always a possible complication of general anesthesia, and temperature monitoring should always be available.
  C. **Monitoring sites**
    1. **Skin temperature**, as measured on the forehead, is normally 3 °F to 4 °F below the core temperature, and this gradient may increase with further cooling.
    2. **The axilla** is a common site for noninvasive temperature determination and is usually 1 °F below body **temperature.** The probe needs to be placed at the axillary artery with the arm adducted.
    3. **Tympanic membrane temperature** correlates well with the core temperature. Intervening cerumen may enlarge the gradient with respect to core temperature.

4. **Rectal temperature** changes lag behind those of the core body temperature. This phenomenon is often noted during rewarming after hypothermia and indicates the slower peripheral, or "shell," rewarming. The risk of rectal perforation is a rare complication.
5. **Nasopharyngeal temperature**, measured at the posterior nasopharynx, reflects the brain temperature. This measurement is performed by measuring the distance from the external meatus of the ear to the external naris and inserting the temperature probe to that distance. This method may be associated with epistaxis in coagulopathic or pregnant patients or may result in skin necrosis if the probe is allowed to press on the naris during longer procedures. This method is discouraged in patients with head trauma or cerebrospinal fluid rhinorrhea.
6. **Esophageal temperature** monitoring reflects the core temperature well. The probe should be located at the lower third of the esophagus and rarely may be misplaced in the airway.
7. **Blood temperature** measurements may be obtained with the thermistor of a PAC.

ACKNOWLEDGMENTS

We gratefully acknowledge the contributions of previous edition author(s), Christopher M. Aiudi and Kyan C. Safavi, as portions of those chapters have been retained in this revision.

Suggested Readings

Akoumianaki E, Maggiore SM, Valenza F, et al. The application of esophageal pressure measurement in patients with respiratory failure. *Am J Respir Crit Care Med.* 2014; 189(5):520–531.

Jacobsohn E, Chorn R, O'Connor M. The role of the vasculature in regulating venous return and cardiac output: historical and graphical approach. *Can J Anaesth.* 1997;44:849–867.

Kodali BS. *Capnography: A Comprehensive Educational Website.* Harvard Medical School; 2005. Accessed September 30, 2005. http://www.capnography.com

Lake CL, Hines RL, Blitt CD. *Clinical Monitoring: Practical Applications for Anesthesia & Critical Care.* 1st ed. WB Saunders; 2001.

Marik PE. Noninvasive cardiac output monitors: a state-of the-art review. *J Cardiothorac Vasc Anesth.* 2012;27(1):121–134.

Mark JB. *Atlas of Cardiovascular Monitoring.* Churchill Livingstone; 1998.

Pagel PS, Grossman W, Haering JM, Warltier DC. Left ventricular diastolic function in the normal and diseased heart (1). *Anesthesiology.* 1993;79:836–854.

Pagel PS, Grossman W, Haering JM, Warltier DC. Left ventricular diastolic function in the normal and diseased heart (2). *Anesthesiology.* 1993;79:1104–1120.

Perret C, Tagan D, Feihl F, Marini JJ. *The Pulmonary Artery Catheter in Critical Care.* Blackwell Science; 1996.

Safavi KC, Driscoll W, Wiener-Kronish JP. Remote surveillance technologies: realizing the aim of right patient, right data, right time. *Anesth Analg.* 2019;129(3):726–734.

Sagawa K, Maughan L, Suga H, et al. *Cardiac Contraction and the Pressure-Volume Relationship.* Oxford University Press; 1988.

Walsh EC, Fitzsimons MG. Preventing mechanical complications associated with central venous catheter placement. *BJA Educ.* 2023;23(6):229–237.

16 Monitoring Anesthetic Brain States
Christian Guay and Johanna Lee

I. GENERAL CONSIDERATIONS
General anesthesia is defined as a drug-induced reversible condition characterized by unconsciousness, amnesia, analgesia, immobility, and maintenance of physiologic stability. Monitoring brain and behavioral states under general anesthesia is challenging, and the brain states of patients under general anesthesia are often tracked using physiologic signs and, at times, electroencephalography (EEG)-based markers of anesthesia.

- **A.** During the maintenance of general anesthesia, anesthesia providers often use changes in the physiologic measures of heart rate, blood pressure, respiratory rate, and movement to track anesthetic states and guide the administration of anesthetic and analgesic medications.
- **B.** The changes in heart rate and blood pressure that anesthetized patients show in response to a nociceptive stimulus can be explained in terms of the **nociceptive–medullary–autonomic (NMA) circuit**, which is comprised of the spinoreticular tract, the brainstem arousal circuits, and the sympathetic and parasympathetic efferent pathways.
    1. The **ascending nociceptive (pain) pathway** begins with A-delta and C-fibers whose free nerve endings bring nociceptive (painful) information from the periphery to the spinal cord.
    2. In the spinal cord, these fibers synapse in the dorsal horn on projection neurons that travel through the anterolateral fasciculus and synapse at multiple sites in the brainstem, including the nucleus of the tractus solitarius in the medulla.
    3. The **autonomic response to a painful stimulus** is initiated within the nucleus of the tractus solitarius, which mediates sympathetic output through the rostral ventral lateral medulla and the caudal ventral lateral medulla to the heart and peripheral blood vessels through projections to the thoracolumbar sympathetic ganglia. The parasympathetic output from the nucleus of the tractus solitarius is mediated through the nucleus ambiguus, which projects through the vagus nerve to the sinoatrial node of the heart.
- **C.** A potentially nociceptive operative stimulus initiates an increase in sympathetic output and a decrease in parasympathetic output through the NMA circuit that rapidly results in an increase in heart rate and blood pressure. As such, these signs can be a rapid indicator of an inadequate level of analgesia.
- **D.** Apart from physiologic signs, intraoperative EEG can be used to track brain states induced by general anesthesia and sedation.

II. ELECTROENCEPHALOGRAM-BASED INDICES OF LEVEL OF UNCONSCIOUSNESS
- **A.** The EEG changes systematically in relation to the dose of anesthetic drug administered. As a consequence, the EEG signal tracing and various forms of processed EEG have been used to track the anesthetic state of patients receiving general anesthesia and sedation.

B. Basic biophysics of EEG
   1. The EEG detects postsynaptic potentials, or local field potentials, in the cerebral cortex. As neurons synapse in a region of the cortex, they produce macroscopic extracellular currents that can be detected as electrical potential differences by surface electrodes.
   2. Subcortical structures, like the thalamus, produce smaller field potentials because the strength of the electrical field diminishes with distance from the surface recording electrodes.
   3. However, cortical and subcortical structures are highly interconnected, and as a result, the EEG may reflect the dynamics of both cortical and subcortical structures.
   4. EEG signals comprise oscillations of varying frequencies and amplitudes (**Figures 16.1 and 16.2**).
C. Several **EEG-based index systems** have been studied and used in clinical practice, including the bispectral index (BIS), patient state index (PSI), Narcotrend, and Entropy. These systems process the EEG and provide an index value or set of values in near real time to track the level of unconsciousness. In general, the indices are designed to decrease with deepening levels of unconsciousness and increase as consciousness returns. The anesthesia provider can use these indices, along with physiologic signs such as changes in heart rate and blood pressure, to track the patient's state of unconsciousness and, to some degree, antinociception.
D. **BIS**
   1. The BIS uses a four-lead frontal EEG montage to record EEG signals for processing and analysis in near real time.
   2. The BIS uses a proprietary algorithm that measures specific features of the spectrogram, bispectrum, and level of burst suppression to compute an index between 0 and 100 that indicates the patient's level of unconsciousness. A value of 100 corresponds to being completely awake, whereas 0 corresponds to a profound state of coma or unconsciousness that is reflected by an isoelectric or flat EEG.
   3. **A patient is considered to be appropriately anesthetized when the BIS value is between 40 and 60.**
   4. Along with the index value, the BIS monitor also displays the EEG signal tracing, the spectrogram, the level of electromyographic (EMG) activity, and the degree of EEG suppression. The EMG indicator displays power in the frequency range of 70 to 110 Hz that is believed to be attributable to muscle activity.
E. **PSI**
   1. The PSI also uses a four-lead frontal EEG montage to record EEG signals for processing and analysis in near real time.
   2. Like the BIS, a proprietary algorithm is used to compute an index between 0 and 100, where 0 reflects unconsciousness and 100 reflects complete alertness.

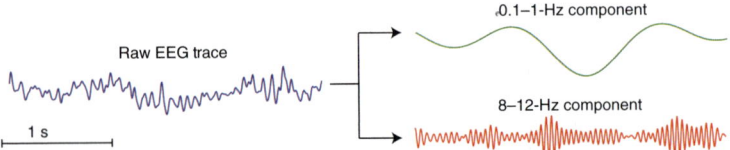

FIGURE 16.1 A typical electroencephalogram trace can be split into a slower oscillatory (0.1- to 1-Hz component **[top]**) with an overlying higher frequency (8- to 12-Hz component **[bottom]**).

FIGURE 16.2 Anesthetic states and electroencephalogram signatures. Slow (0.1- to 1-Hz), delta (1- to 4-Hz), and alpha (8- to 12-Hz) oscillations are typically seen during unconsciousness at surgical planes. Beta (12- to 25-Hz) oscillations are frequently associated with an arousable state of sedation. Gamma (25 to 40 Hz) is associated with an awake pattern with eyes open.

   3. **A patient is considered to be appropriately anesthetized when the PSI value is between 25 and 50.**
   4. Like the BIS, the PSI monitor also shows the EEG signal tracing in real time with its spectrogram from the left and right sides of the head, the level of EMG activity, an artifact index, and a suppression ratio that measures the amount of time the EEG is in burst suppression.

F. **Narcotrend**
   1. Like the BIS and PSI, the Narcotrend uses a proprietary algorithm that converts the EEG into different states, reporting both a Narcotrend Stage (A to F) and Narcotrend Index (0 to 100).
      a. Narcotrend stage A corresponds to patients who are awake, whereas stage F corresponds to general anesthesia with increasing burst suppression. Target stage D is meant to indicate an appropriate depth of anesthesia.
      b. Like the BIS and PSI indices, a Narcotrend Index of 100 correlates with the awake state, whereas an index of 0 correlates with a suppressed EEG.
   2. The monitor also displays the EEG times-series and its spectrogram.

G. Entropy

1. Entropy is a measure of disorder within a system, and this concept has been applied to EEG analysis to indicate the depth of anesthesia or level of unconsciousness. This measure relies on the observation that the EEG becomes highly structured and ordered under general anesthesia (ie, less disorder, and thus less entropy).
2. The Entropy monitor, which uses a publicly available algorithm, reports two values, **response entropy (RE)** and **state entropy (SE)**.
   a. RE (range, 0 to 100) is computed from EEG power in frequencies from 0.8 to 47 Hz.
   b. SE (range, 0 to 91) is computed from EEG power in frequencies from 0.8 to 32 Hz.
   c. In general, EMG artifact due to facial muscle activity will have a higher frequency and will thus be reflected in the RE. Therefore, in instances when RE is greater than SE, SE should be favored to reflect the underlying brain state because RE is reflecting EMG activity. As such, it has been proposed that the relative changes in RE and SE can be used to track brain states under anesthesia and distinguish recovery of consciousness from movement artifacts.
3. **Target RE or SE values for appropriate depth of anesthesia are from 40 to 60.**

H. Limitations of EEG-based indices

Although EEG-based indices have been available for nearly 20 years, there are several reasons why they are not part of standard practice in anesthesiology.

1. The use of EEG-based indices does not ensure that awareness under general anesthesia can be prevented.
2. Indices are considered less reliable in the elderly and pediatric populations.
3. Indices do not relate directly to the neurophysiology of how a specific anesthetic exerts its effects in the brain. Therefore, they cannot give an accurate picture of the brain's responses to the drugs. In particular, the EEG-based indices (in the previous sections) tend to be unreliable with the use of ketamine, nitrous oxide, and dexmedetomidine. See Section V for more information.
4. Indices assume that the same index value reflects the same level of unconsciousness for all anesthetics, across all patients.

III. END-TIDAL ANESTHETIC CONCENTRATION

A. The **median minimal alveolar concentration (MAC)** value (the MAC of inhaled anesthetic required for immobility, or more precisely lack of movement in response to a noxious stimuli, in 50% of patients) remains the gold standard for dosing inhaled anesthetics. However, MAC cannot be used to define or predict brain states in anesthetized patients. Animal experiments have demonstrated that there is no clear association between anesthetic-induced EEG patterns and that inhaled anesthetics produce immobility primarily by acting in the spinal cord, rather than in the brain.
B. Regardless, the end-tidal anesthetic concentration is widely used as a way to monitor the level of unconsciousness induced by inhaled anesthetics and guide anesthetic dosing.
   1. This use of MAC has been supported by the B-UNAWARE and BAG-RECALL trials that reported no significant difference in the incidence of intraoperative awareness with an anesthetic protocol that maintained the BIS between 40 and 60 compared with a protocol that maintained the end-tidal anesthetic between 0.7 and 1.3 MAC.

C. Unlike the BIS, PSI, Narcotrend, and Entropy, which provide EEG-based measures of brain activity, the end-tidal anesthetic concentration is indirectly related to brain activity through the concentration of anesthetic expired in the lungs.
D. Two additional concepts related to MAC are (1) MAC-aware, which is the MAC of inhaled anesthetic required for unconsciousness, which is approximately one-third of MAC; and (2) MAC-BAR (block of adrenergic response), which is the MAC of inhaled anesthetic required for the blunting of autonomic responses to nociception, and is approximately two times the MAC.
   1. The use of opioids can reduce MAC, MAC-aware, and, in particular, MAC-BAR, by decreasing nociception-induced arousal.
E. Another important drawback of MAC is that it cannot be used with total intravenous anesthesia. Analogous metrics have been developed for estimated plasma and effect site concentrations of propofol, though they exhibit much wider variance than what has been reported for inhaled anesthetics.

IV. THE SPECTRAL ANALYSIS OF THE EEG
A. The changes in brain states under sedation and general anesthesia are readily visible in the EEG signal tracing. However, it is challenging to interpret dynamic changes in frequencies and amplitudes in the real-time EEG signal, which is typically displayed in a 4-second sliding time window.
B. The **power spectrum** is a decomposition of a segment of EEG into its power (usually in dB) as a function of frequency. Because the spectrum captures only one instance in time, it has limited utility during a dynamic anesthetic state (**Figure 16.3**).

FIGURE 16.3 The plot of power (usually in decibels, dB) against the frequencies being analyzed is the power spectrum.

C. Taking the spectrum plots at several adjacent time intervals and stacking them together forms a **spectrogram**. The spectrogram is a plot of power by frequency as a function of time.

D. The 3D spectrogram (also called the compressed spectral array) can be flattened into a 2D plot (also called the density spectral array) with power mapped onto a color scale, which is displayed on monitors in the operating room (**Figure 16.4**). These 2D spectrograms give a visual representation of the EEG structure in a manner that facilitates analysis and tracking of the brain states under anesthesia over time.

V. EFFECTS OF DIFFERENT ANESTHETICS ON THE BRAIN
A. Propofol
1. Molecular mechanism
   a. Propofol is an agonist at postsynaptic gamma-aminobutyric acid type A ($GABA_A$) receptors, inducing an inward chloride current that hyperpolarizes postsynaptic neurons and enhances inhibition.
2. Neural circuit mechanism
   a. Propofol acts on $GABA_A$ receptors at multiple sites, including the cortex, thalamus, brainstem, and spinal cord.
   b. By enhancing GABAergic inhibition in the thalamus and brainstem, which are highly interconnected with the cortex, propofol decreases excitatory inputs and enhances the inhibition of cortical pyramidal neurons.
   c. The potentiation of GABAergic circuits is thought to produce the various features of anesthesia, including loss of consciousness, apnea, and atonia.
3. EEG signatures
   a. EEG signatures are markers of altered arousal states induced by each anesthetic.
   b. **Propofol-induced unconsciousness is characterized by slow–delta (0.1- to 4-Hz) and frontally coherent alpha (8- to 12-Hz) oscillations (Figure 16.5).**
   c. Slow–delta oscillations are thought to result from GABA-mediated inactivation of arousal circuits and appear to disrupt cortical integration by isolating local cortical networks and impairing intracortical communication. Specifically, slow–delta oscillations may be associated with neurons across the cortex being activated and inactivated at different times (up–down or on–off states). This fragments brain activity into asynchronous windows and impairs communication, which is also referred to as "cortical fragmentation" (**Figure 16.5**).
   d. Based on modeling studies, alpha oscillations are thought to reflect highly structured rhythms within thalamocortical circuits. During propofol-induced unconsciousness, these abnormally coherent or synchronous alpha oscillations are thought to interfere with communication between the thalamus and frontal cortex (**Figure 16.5**).
   e. High concentrations of propofol (and several other anesthetics) can lead to **burst suppression**, which is characterized by alternating periods of brief bursts of high-amplitude activity and isoelectricity (suppression). Intraoperative burst suppression is generally avoided for routine cases owing to concerns about potential adverse effects but can be at times targeted for specific indications like status epilepticus, intracranial hypertension, or deep hypothermic circulatory arrest.

FIGURE 16.4 Construction of the spectrogram: The power spectrum plot at several points in time can be stacked together to form a 3D spectrogram **(middle)**. The spectrogram still retains the frequency and power axes but has the helpful addition of a time axis. The 3D spectrogram flattened into a 2D plot **(bottom)** is what is displayed intraoperatively on brain function monitors. Of note, as indicated on the power scale, *red* indicates high power and *blue* indicates low power.

FIGURE 16.5 Spectrogram of propofol showing a pathologic alpha oscillation (8 to 12 Hz), which corresponds with prevention of communication between the thalamus and cortex, and slow wave (0.1- to 1-Hz) cortical fragmentation.

    f. Systematic changes in the amplitude of alpha and frequency of slow–delta oscillations can be used to track anesthetic depth prior to burst suppression. Specifically, as anesthetic concentrations increase, the amplitude of alpha oscillations tends to decrease, and the dominant frequency of slow–delta oscillations tend to increase. Monitoring these changes can help clinicians anticipate a deepening state of unconsciousness before the onset of burst suppression.
- **B. Ether-derived anesthetics** (sevoflurane, isoflurane, desflurane)
  - **1.** Molecular mechanism
    - **a.** Ether-derived anesthetics bind at multiple targets within the central nervous system, including GABA$_A$ receptors, N-methyl-d-aspartate (NMDA) receptors, potassium channels, and others.
  - **2.** Neural circuit mechanism
    - **a.** Although the neural circuit mechanisms of ether-derived anesthetics have not been fully characterized, the EEG signature under general anesthesia with inhaled anesthetics is very similar to propofol-induced anesthesia, suggesting that the primary mechanism is GABA$_A$-mediated inhibition of similar thalamocortical and corticocortical dynamics.
  - **3.** EEG signatures
    - **a.** Under sevoflurane general anesthesia, the EEG is characterized by prominent **alpha** and **slow–delta** oscillations, similar to propofol general anesthesia, with the addition of **theta** (4- to 8-Hz) oscillations, particularly at higher concentrations.
    - **b.** The addition of theta oscillations creates a "fill-in" effect between the slow and alpha oscillations (**Figure 16.6**).

FIGURE 16.6 Spectrogram of sevoflurane showing an alpha (8- to 12-Hz) and slow wave (0.1- to 1-Hz) oscillation at low concentration and the "fill-in" effect at high concentrations of anesthetic.

C. Dexmedetomidine (Precedex)
1. Molecular mechanism
   a. Dexmedetomidine is an agonist at presynaptic **α_2-adrenergic receptors** on neurons that project from the locus coeruleus.
   b. Binding of dexmedetomidine at the α_2 receptors hyperpolarizes the locus coeruleus neurons and decreases the release of norepinephrine.
   c. Dexmedetomidine may also directly bind to **α_2-adrenergic receptors** on neurons in the thalamus and basal forebrain.
2. Neural circuit mechanism
   a. The locus coeruleus synapses with multiple areas of the brain, including excitatory inputs to the cortex, preoptic area of the hypothalamus, basal forebrain, and intralaminar nucleus of the thalamus.
   b. Hyperpolarization of the locus coeruleus neurons leads to decreased norepinephrine release, resulting in the loss of inhibitory inputs to the preoptic area of the hypothalamus.
   c. The loss of inhibitory inputs results in activation of the GABAergic inhibitory pathways from the preoptic area to arousal centers, leading to sedation.
   d. This neural circuit mechanism is similar to the mechanism implicated in nonrapid eye movement (NREM) sleep.
3. EEG signatures
   a. At **clinically recommended doses used for light sedation**, the EEG is characterized by **spindles** (intermittent bursts of 9- to 15-Hz

FIGURE 16.7 Spectrogram of dexmedetomidine showing both spindles (9- to 15-Hz) and slow wave (0.1- to 1-Hz) oscillations at low doses and a predominance of slow-wave oscillations at high doses.

oscillations) and **slow–delta oscillations** that resemble NREM stage II sleep (**Figure 16.7**).
  b. The slow oscillations seen with dexmedetomidine likely result from decreased excitatory inputs to the cortex (owing to the disinhibition of inhibitory circuits, as described in the previous section).
  c. The spindles observed with dexmedetomidine, like sleep spindles and propofol-induced alpha oscillations, are thought to be generated by thalamocortical mechanisms. Of note, spindles are brief intermittent bursts of EEG activity, in contrast to propofol alpha oscillations, which are continuous.
  d. These slow oscillations and spindles are smaller in amplitude than the slow and alpha oscillations observed with propofol general anesthesia, likely reflective of a lower level of circuit inhibition and thus lighter levels of sedation.

D. Ketamine
  1. Molecular mechanism
     a. Ketamine is an **NMDA** receptor antagonist that binds to receptors within the brain and spinal cord. Ketamine also interacts with opioid, monoaminergic, cholinergic, nicotinic, and muscarinic receptors.
  2. Neural circuit mechanism
     a. At **low to moderate doses**, ketamine primarily **inhibits** excitatory glutamatergic inputs to inhibitory interneurons, thereby disinhibiting downstream excitatory neurons. This can lead to increased cerebral metabolism, as well as neuroexcitatory effects like hallucinations, dissociative states, and euphoria.

FIGURE 16.8 Spectrogram of ketamine showing notable 30-Hz gamma oscillations.

   b. At **high doses**, ketamine will also block the NMDA receptors on the excitatory glutamatergic neurons and lead to loss of consciousness.
   c. The antinociceptive effect of ketamine is likely due to its actions on NMDA receptors in the dorsal root ganglia and non-NMDA mechanisms (eg, monoaminergic) in supraspinal regions.
3. EEG signatures
   a. In patients receiving ketamine, the EEG is characterized by **beta–gamma oscillations**, ranging approximately between 20 and 30 Hz, in addition to the slow–delta oscillations characteristic of other anesthetics (**Figure 16.8**).
   b. For this reason, the numeric EEG-based index value associated with a ketamine anesthetic is often high, despite adequate anesthesia.

E. Nitrous oxide
1. Molecular mechanism
   a. The mechanism of nitrous oxide is not completely understood, as it acts on many receptors. However, its anesthetic effects seem to be primarily due to antagonism of **NMDA** receptors.
2. EEG signatures
   a. One common practice is to transition from an inhaled anesthetic (eg, sevoflurane, isoflurane) to high-concentration nitrous oxide (>50%) at the end of surgery to facilitate rapid emergence from anesthesia.
   b. During this transition to nitrous oxide, the EEG is characterized by transient, prominent slow–delta oscillations (lasting 3 to 12 minutes), followed by high-frequency beta–gamma (20- to 35-Hz) oscillations that are more commonly associated with nitrous oxide alone (**Figure 16.9**).
   c. The beta–gamma oscillations observed under nitrous oxide are thought to be induced by a similar mechanism to ketamine, owing to the shared mechanism of NMDA antagonism.
   d. The mechanism underlying the transient slow–delta oscillations is not fully understood.

F. Sevoflurane plus ketamine
1. Patients will often receive a combination of medications under anesthesia, such as an inhaled anesthetic like sevoflurane for unconsciousness and ketamine for analgesia.

FIGURE 16.9 Spectrogram of nitrous oxide during a transition from isoflurane as the anesthetic to nitrous oxide, as may occur clinically toward the end of surgery to facilitate emergence. The spectrogram of nitrous oxide profound slow–delta oscillations that transition to gamma oscillations.

2. When ketamine is added to sevoflurane general anesthesia, the alpha and delta oscillations typically observed with sevoflurane are reduced in power, whereas beta oscillations are increased in power. These observed changes may be due to ketamine causing an excitatory effect on neurons with lower intrinsic spiking frequencies to higher-frequency spiking.
3. Of note, the use of ketamine as an adjunct in a patient already receiving an inhaled anesthetic or propofol may lead to burst suppression.
4. Although not all combinations of anesthetics and their adjuncts have been studied at this time, understanding their mechanisms and the neural circuits involved can help provide insight into predicted or observed EEG patterns, as well as possible limitations with certain combinations of medications.

VI. AGE-RELATED CHANGES IN ANESTHETIC-INDUCED EEG SIGNATURES
A. The EEG signatures of patients under general anesthesia vary with age, most notably in children and in the elderly.

B. Children
1. In infants from 0 to approximately 3 months of age, the EEG under propofol- or sevoflurane-induced general anesthesia consists of slow–delta oscillations but not alpha oscillations.
2. In children greater than approximately 3 months of age, the EEG consists of both slow–delta and alpha oscillations. The alpha oscillations become frontally coherent by approximately 1 year of age, reflecting patterns that are more similar to the adult EEG under general anesthesia.
3. The alpha band in children and young adults tends to be broader, encompassing 8 to 15 Hz, compared with a narrower band of 8 to 12 Hz in older adults. Power in the alpha band is also greater in children and young adults.
4. **Figures 16.10 and 16.11** demonstrate age-related changes in the spectrogram in the pediatric population.
5. These age-related changes seen in the EEG under propofol or sevoflurane general anesthesia likely reflect the development and maturation of underlying brain circuits, such as the thalamocortical circuit.

FIGURE 16.10 Age-varying spectral changes in the frontal spectrogram during infancy to childhood, showing the absence of alpha oscillation power from 0 to 3 months of age, with a gradual increase in alpha oscillation power thereafter, becoming more prominent and sustained at approximately 6 months of age. (Reprinted from Cornelissen L, Kim SE, Lee JM, et al. Electroencephalographic markers of brain development during sevoflurane anaesthesia in children up to 3 years old. *Br J Anaesth*. 2018;120(6):1274–1286. Copyright © 2018 Elsevier. With permission.)

- **C.** Elderly
  1. The power and frontal coherence of the alpha oscillations decrease with age. This may reflect neurologic changes that occur with aging, including but not limited to cortical thinning, decline in synaptic density, and decline in neurotransmitter synthesis (**Figure 16.12**).
  2. The elderly appear to have a higher probability for burst suppression, characterized by alternating periods of isoelectricity and short bursts of high-amplitude activity, under general anesthesia compared with younger adults.
  3. There is an association between burst suppression and postoperative delirium. The ENGAGES randomized clinical trial, which randomized patients to EEG-guided anesthetic administration or usual anesthetic care, did not show that the use of the EEG to guide anesthesia decreased the incidence of postoperative delirium. More recent studies suggest that a small portion of the total effect of previously described postoperative delirium risk factors (eg, cognitive status, physical function) is mediated by burst suppression.
- **D.** There can be considerable interindividual differences in the EEG signature under general anesthesia. For example, some individuals may exhibit particular age-related changes, such as diminished alpha oscillations, at younger ages than others. These interindividual EEG differences may reflect underlying comorbidities.

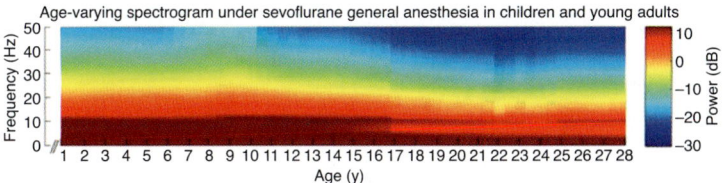

FIGURE 16.11 Age-varying spectral changes in the frontal spectrogram in children and young adults from 1 to 28 years of age, highlighting that, although the EEG structure is qualitatively preserved, the power of the oscillations changes as a function of age. (Reprinted from Akeju O, Pavone KJ, Thum JA, et al. Age-dependency of sevoflurane-induced electroencephalogram dynamics in children. *Br J Anaesth*. 2015;115(suppl 1):i66–i76. Copyright © 2015 Elsevier. With permission.)

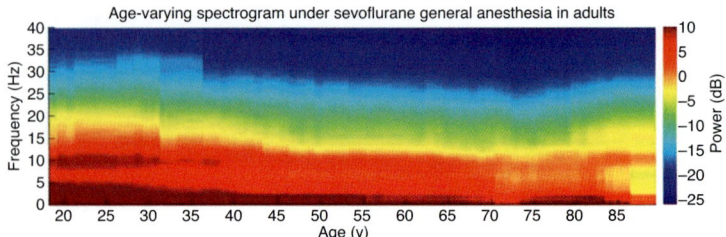

FIGURE 16.12 Age-varying spectral changes in the frontal spectrogram in adults ranging from 18 to 90 years of age, illustrating that alpha oscillation power decreases with age. (Reprinted from Purdon PL, Pavone KJ, Akeju O, et al. The Ageing Brain: age-dependent changes in the electroencephalogram during propofol and sevoflurane general anaesthesia. *Br J Anaesth.* 2015;115(suppl 1): i46–i57. Copyright © 2015 Elsevier. With permission.)

VII. CLINICAL MONITORING OF ANESTHETIC STATES
  A. The real-time EEG tracing and spectrogram can be used to track brain states in patients under sedation or general anesthesia. A foundational understanding of anesthetic neurophysiology and the associated anesthetic signatures on the EEG equips clinicians with the tools necessary to interpret and use perioperative EEG to guide clinical care. EEG education resources have been developed by the following institutions and can be found at the following websites:
  1. Massachusetts General Hospital in collaboration with the International Anesthesia Research Society (eegforanesthesia.iars.org)
  2. International Consortium for EEG Training of Anesthesia Practitioners, Washington University School of Medicine in St. Louis (www.icetap.org)

  B. A personalized approach to monitoring brain states and guiding anesthetic management in patients may improve anesthetic care. Specifically, using these strategies to target specific brain states under general anesthesia may help avoid potential complications associated with overdosing or underdosing of anesthetic drugs.

VIII. CONCLUSION
  A. Although real-time EEG tracings can be difficult to analyze during clinical care, the spectrograms make clear that each anesthetic has a distinct EEG signature. These signatures can be related to the mechanisms by which the drugs act at specific receptors in specific neural circuits to alter arousal and can be used to monitor the brain states of patients under anesthesia care.

ACKNOWLEDGMENTS

We gratefully acknowledge the contributions of previous edition authors, Johanna Lee and Oluwaseun Johnson-Akeju, as portions of those chapters have been retained in this revision.

Suggested Readings

Adam E, Kwon O, Montejo KA, Brown EN. Modulatory dynamics mark the transition between anesthetic states of unconsciousness. *Proc Natl Acad Sci U S A.* 2023;120(30): e2300058120.

Akeju O, Pavone KJ, Thum JA, et al. Age-dependency of sevoflurane-induced electroencephalogram dynamics in children. *Br J Anaes.* 2015;115(Suppl 1):i66–i76.

Akeju O, Pavone KJ, Westover MB, et al. A comparison of propofol- and dexmedetomidine-induced electroencephalogram dynamics using spectral and coherence analysis. *Anesthesiology.* 2014;121:978–989.

Akeju O, Westover MB, Pavone KJ, et al. Effects of sevoflurane and propofol on frontal electroencephalogram power and coherence. *Anesthesiology.* 2014;121:990–998.

Avidan MS, Jacobsohn E, Glick D, et al; BAG-RECALL Research Group. Prevention of intraoperative awareness in a high-risk surgical population. *N Engl J Med.* 2011;365:591–600.

Avidan MS, Zhang L, Burnside BA, et al. Anesthesia awareness and the bispectral index. *N Engl J Med.* 2008;358:1097–1108.

Brown EN, Lydic R, Schiff ND. General anesthesia, sleep and coma. *N Engl J Med.* 2010; 363:2638–2650.

Brown EN, Purdon PL, Akeju O, et al. Monitoring the state of the brain and central nervous system during general anesthesia and sedation. In: Gropper MA, Cohen NH, Eriksson LI, Fleisher LA, Leslie K, Wiener-Kronish JP, eds. *Miller's Anesthesia.* 9th ed. Elsevier, Inc.; 2020:1279–1297.

Brown EN, Purdon PL, Van Dort CJ. General anesthesia and altered states of arousal: a systems neuroscience analysis. *Annu Rev Neurosci.* 2011;34:601–628.

Cornelissen L, Kim SE, Lee JM, Brown EN, Purdon PL, Berde CB. Electroencephalographic markers of brain development during sevoflurane anaesthesia in children up to 3 years old. *Br J Anaes.* 2018;120(6):1274–1286.

Cornelissen L, Kim S-E, Purdon PL, Brown EN, Berde CB. Age-dependent electroencephalogram (EEG) patterns during sevoflurane general anesthesia in infants. *Elife.* 2015;4:e06513.

Egan TE. Are opioids indispensable for general anaesthesia? *Br J Anaesth.* 2019;122(6): e127–e135.

Fritz BA, King CR, Abdallah AB, et al; ENGAGES Research Group. Preoperative cognitive abnormality, intraoperative electroencephalogram suppression, and postoperative delirium: a mediation analysis. *Anesthesiology.* 2020;132(6):1458–1468.

Kim MC, Fricchione GL, Brown EN, Akeju O. Role of electroencephalogram oscillations and the spectrogram in monitoring anaesthesia. *BJA Educ.* 2020;20(5):166–172.

Lewis LD, Weiner VS, Mukamel EA, et al. Rapid fragmentation of neuronal networks at the onset of propofol-induced unconsciousness. *Proc Natl Acad Sci U S A.* 2012;109: E3377–E3386.

Pedemonte JC, Plummer GS, Chamadia S, et al. Electroencephalogram burst-suppression during cardiopulmonary bypass in elderly patients mediates postoperative delirium. *Anesthesiology.* 2020;133(2):280–292.

Purdon PL, Pavone KJ, Akeju O, et al. The ageing brain: age-dependent changes in the electroencephalogram during propofol and sevoflurane general anaesthesia. *Br J Anaesth.* 2015;115(Suppl 1):i46–i57.

Purdon PL, Pierce ET, Mukamel EA, et al. Electroencephalogram signatures of loss and recovery of consciousness from propofol. *Proc Natl Acad Sci U S A.* 2013;110:E1142–E1151.

Purdon PL, Sampson A, Pavone KJ, Brown EN. Clinical electroencephalography for anesthesiologists: part I: background and basic signatures. *Anesthesiology.* 2015;123(4):937–960.

Wildes TS, Mickle AM, Abdallah B, et al; ENGAGES Research Group. Effect of electroencephalography-guided anesthetic administration on postoperative delirium among older adults undergoing major surgery: the ENGAGES randomized clinical trial. *JAMA.* 2019;321(5):473–483.

Intra-anesthetic Problems

Zeyu Hu, Ying Hui Low, and Alexander Nagrebetsky

I. HYPOTENSION

Hypotension is a significant decrease of arterial blood pressure below the patient's usual range. It may be due to a decrease in cardiac function (contractility), systemic vascular resistance (SVR or afterload), venous return (preload), or the presence of dysrhythmias.

A. Contractility

1. Most anesthetic agents, including **inhalational agents, barbiturates, benzodiazepines**, and **etomidate** (see Chapter 12: Intravenous and Inhalation Anesthetics) cause dose-dependent direct myocardial depression. **Opiates** are not direct myocardial depressants in usual clinical doses, although clinically significant bradycardia and hypotension may be observed owing to decreased sympathetic outflow. Although **ketamine** can cause a dose-dependent increase in sympathetic nervous system discharge, its direct myocardial depressant effects may be unmasked in patients with depleted endogenous catecholamines, **myocardial depressants** such as β-adrenergic antagonists, calcium channel blockers, and lidocaine.

2. Acute myocardial dysfunction may occur with myocardial ischemia or myocardial infarction (MI), hypocalcemia (eg, after massive transfusion), severe acidosis or alkalosis, severe hypothermia, acute pulmonary hypertension (ie, embolism), and systemic toxicity from local anesthetics (particularly bupivacaine).

B. Decreased SVR

1. A decrease in SVR can be seen with many of the drugs administered during anesthesia.
   a. **Inhalational fluorinated anesthetics**, including **Isoflurane** and, to a lesser extent, sevoflurane and desflurane produce a dose-dependent decrease in SVR.
   b. **Opiates** and **propofol** produce loss of vascular tone by reducing sympathetic nervous system outflow.
   c. **GABAergic medications**, including benzodiazepines and barbiturates may decrease SVR, particularly when administered at high doses in conjunction with opiates.
   d. **Direct vasodilators** (eg, nitroprusside, nitroglycerin, and hydralazine).
   e. **$α_1$-Adrenergic blockers** (eg, droperidol, chlorpromazine, phentolamine, and labetalol, prazosin, doxazosin).
   f. **$α_2$-Adrenergic agonists** (eg, clonidine and dexmedetomidine).
   g. **Histamine-releasing medications** (eg, d-tubocurarine, mivacurium, and morphine).
   h. **Calcium channel blockers.**
   i. **Angiotensin-converting enzyme inhibitors** and **angiotensin receptor blockers.**
   j. **Inodilators** (eg, milrinone).
   k. Heparin administration in large doses.

2. **Sympathetic blockade** can occur during neuraxial anesthesia, particularly when sympathetic output derived from thoracolumbar level (T1–L2) nerve roots are blocked, leading to a reduction in SVR and/or preload secondary to vasodilation and venous pooling due to unopposed vagal tone.
3. **Sepsis** causes the release of vasoactive substances that mediate peripheral vasodilation.
4. **Vasoactive metabolites** are released during bowel manipulation, aortic cross-clamp release, or tourniquet release.
5. **Allergic reactions** (see Section XVIII).
6. **Profound hypoxia.**
7. **Adrenal insufficiency** (including iatrogenic causes).

C. **Inadequate venous return (preload)**
  1. **Hypovolemia** may be caused by blood loss, insensible evaporative losses, and preoperative deficits (eg, NPO (nothing by mouth) status, vomiting, diarrhea, nasogastric tube suction, enteric drains, and certain bowel preparations), or polyuria (eg, diuretic use, diabetes mellitus, diabetes insipidus, or postobstructive diuresis).
      a. *Positive pressure variation.* In patients undergoing positive-pressure ventilation, changes in cardiac output, and therefore the intra-arterial blood pressure trace, are correlated with volume responsiveness. Hypovolemia can be considered based on the delta-down component (the difference between the systolic blood pressure during apnea and the lowest systolic blood pressure after a positive pressure breath) on an intra-arterial tracing of a patient that is paralyzed, mechanically ventilated (ideally with tidal volumes >8 cc/kg for greatest sensitivity), and in sinus rhythm. A systolic pressure variation of greater than 12% difference in mm Hg predicts volume responsiveness in an otherwise hypotensive patient and therefore fluid resuscitation should be considered assuming no other contraindications.
  2. **Caval compression** may result from a gravid uterus, massive ascites, tumor, surgical maneuvers, or during laparoscopic insufflation of greater than 10 mm Hg leading to increased intra-abdominal or intra-thoracic pressure.
  3. **Increased venous capacitance** may occur with the following:
      a. Sympathetic blockade (eg, ganglionic blockers or regional anesthesia).
      b. Direct venodilators (eg, nitroglycerin).
      c. Histamine-releasing medications (eg, morphine, mivacurium).
      d. Medications that reduce sympathetic outflow (eg, propofol, inhalational agents, and opioids).
  4. **Increased intrathoracic pressure** will impair venous return. Possible causes include mechanical compression (eg, positioning, surgeon leaning on patient), mechanical ventilation with large tidal volumes, positive end expiratory pressure (PEEP), auto-PEEP (air trapping or dynamic hyperinflation), and continuous positive airway pressure (CPAP).
  5. **Acute primary increases in central venous pressure (CVP)** can cause a decrease in venous return as the increased CVP reduces the pressure gradient that drives blood from the periphery into the right heart.
      a. **Tension pneumothorax** leads to compression of the heart and great vessels. The resulting elevation in CVP decreases preload causing hypotension.

b. **Cardiac tamponade** is a collection of fluid or clot in the pericardial space causing compression of the heart, resulting in decreased filling due to elevated intrapericardial pressures.
c. **Pulmonary embolism (PE)** obstructs right ventricular ejection and in turn raises right atrial pressure, which can drastically reduce venous return.
d. **Intra-abdominal hypertension** causes increased intrathoracic pressure, which then compresses the heart and raises the CVP. Thus, the CVP can be elevated while the heart is severely underfilled.

D. **Dysrhythmias** (also see Section III)
1. **Tachydysrhythmias** often result in hypotension secondary to a decreased diastolic filling time.
2. **Atrial fibrillation, atrial flutter, and junctional rhythms** cause hypotension from loss of the atrial contribution to diastolic filling. This is particularly pronounced in patients with valvular heart disease or diastolic dysfunction, in whom atrial contraction may augment end-diastolic volume by more than 30%.
3. **Bradydysrhythmias** may cause hypotension if preload reserve is inadequate to maintain a compensatory increase in stroke volume.

E. **Treatment of hypotension** should be directed toward correcting the underlying cause. Depending on the etiology, appropriate maneuvers include:
1. **Decreasing anesthetic depth.**
2. **Volume expansion** (eg, administration of blood products, colloids, or crystalloids).
3. **Vasopressor support** to increase vascular resistance or decrease venous capacitance (eg, phenylephrine and vasopressin especially if acidemic) and increase stroke volume (eg, epinephrine).
4. **Correction of mechanical causes**, such as relief of pericardial tamponade, needle thoracostomy, and chest tube for pneumothorax, reducing or eliminating PEEP or CPAP, relieving obstruction of the vena cava (eg, left uterine displacement for a pregnant patient), surgically relieving intra-abdominal hypertension, or surgically removing a massive PE.
5. **Antidysrhythmics** (see Section III) may include β-blockers, calcium channel blockers, and amiodarone.
6. **Inotropic support** (eg, dobutamine, dopamine, norepinephrine, milrinone, and epinephrine).
7. **Anti-ischemic therapy** may include raising the systemic blood pressure with vasopressors and then treating the underlying ischemic myocardium (see Section XIV).
8. **In the case of refractory hypotension**, consider the use of additional noninvasive monitors (eg, transthoracic echocardiography [TTE] and noninvasive cardiac output devices) and the placement of invasive monitors (eg, arterial line, central venous catheter, pulmonary artery catheter, transesophageal echocardiography [TEE]) to facilitate the identification of decreased cardiac output or SVR. In ECMO-capable centers, consider venoarterial or venovenous cannulation for refractory hypotension due to obstructive shock (eg, massive PE) or severe hypoxemic shock. Intra-aortic balloon pumps and ventricular assist devices can also be considered when appropriate.

II. HYPERTENSION
A. **Etiologies**
1. **Catecholamine excess** may be seen with inadequate anesthesia, especially with increased sympathetic stimulation during laryngoscopy,

intubation, incision, emergence, patient anxiety, noxious stimulation/pain, hypoxia/hypercarbia, and prolonged tourniquet use.
2. **Preexisting disease** such as essential hypertension, secondary causes of hypertension such as pheochromocytoma, sleep apnea, or other endocrine, renal, or renovascular disorders.
3. **Increased intracranial pressure (ICP).** When ICP rises, systemic blood pressure increases to maintain cerebral perfusion pressure.
4. **Systemic absorption of vasoconstrictors** (eg, injection of local anesthetic with epinephrine).
5. **Aortic cross-clamping,** which leads to a significant increase in SVR.
6. **Rebound hypertension** from discontinuation of clonidine or β-adrenergic blockers.
7. **Drug interactions.** The administration of ephedrine to patients receiving **tricyclic antidepressants** (eg, amitriptyline, nortriptyline, doxepin) and **monoamine oxidase inhibitors** (eg, isoniazid, rasagiline, selegiline) may cause an exaggerated hypertensive response.
8. **Bladder distension.** Sympathetic response with bladder distension leads to increased blood pressure.
9. **Administration of indigo carmine dye** (via an α-adrenergic effect).

B. The treatment of hypertension is directed toward correcting the underlying cause. It may include the following:
1. Optimizing oxygenation and ventilation.
2. Increasing the depth of anesthesia (eg, volatile and IV anesthetics and analgesics).
3. Sedating an anxious patient or emptying a full bladder.
4. Medications (for further discussion, see Chapter 18: Perioperative Hemodynamic Control).
   a. ***Combined* α- and β-adrenergic blocking agents:** labetalol 5- to 10-mg increments IV.
   b. **β-Adrenergic blocking agents:** propranolol 0.5- to 1.0-mg increments IV; metoprolol 1.0 to 5.0 mg IV; or esmolol, 5- to 10-mg increments IV.
   c. **Vasodilators:** hydralazine 2.5- to 5-mg increments IV; nitroglycerin infusion, 30 to 50 μg/min IV and titrating to effect; nitroprusside infusion 30 to 50 μg/min IV and titrating to effect.
   d. **Calcium channel blockers:** verapamil 2.5 to 5 mg IV; diltiazem 5 to 10 mg IV, nicardipine infusion 2.5 to 15 mg/h IV, clevidipine infusion 1 to 15 mg/h IV.

III. DYSRHYTHMIAS
A. **Sinus bradycardia** is a sinus node–driven heart rate of less than 60 beats/min. Unless there is severe underlying heart disease, hemodynamic changes are minimal. With very slow rates, atrial and ventricular ectopic escape beats or rhythms may occur.
1. Etiologies
   a. **Hypoxia.**
   b. **Intrinsic cardiac disease** such as sick sinus syndrome or acute MI (particularly inferior wall MI).
   c. Medications such as **succinylcholine** (especially in young children via a direct cholinergic effect), **anticholinesterases**, **β-adrenergic blockers**, **calcium channel blockers**, **digoxin**, and synthetic **narcotics** (eg, fentanyl and remifentanil).
   d. **Increased vagal tone** can occur during laryngoscopy, traction on the peritoneum or spermatic cord; pressure on the globe via the oculocardiac reflex; pressure near the brainstem during craniotomies for

posterior fossa lesions; direct pressure on the vagus nerve or carotid sinus during neck or intrathoracic surgery; acute distension of the peritoneal cavity during laparoscopy; centrally mediated vagal response from anxiety or pain (vasovagal reaction); and Valsalva maneuvers.
- e. **Increased ICP (Cushing reflex).**
- f. **Reflex bradycardia.** From baroreceptor reflex (eg, with phenylephrine administration), atrial stretch, or cardiopulmonary reflex.

2. **Treatment of sinus bradycardia**
   a. Verify adequate oxygenation and ventilation.
   b. Bradycardia due to increased vagal tone requires discontinuation of the provocative stimulus. The vagal reflex may fatigue with repeat stimulus or be less pronounced with deeper anesthesia. Atropine 0.5 mg IV or low-dose epinephrine 10 to 50 μg IV may be needed if the patient is hypotensive. Glycopyrrolate 0.2 to 0.6 mg IV or ephedrine 5 to 10 mg IV may be given for hemodynamically stable bradycardia.
   c. In patients with intrinsic cardiac disease, treatment should proceed with atropine 0.5 mg IV, chronotropes (eg, ephedrine, dopamine), or cardiac pacing.

B. Sinus tachycardia is a sinus node–driven heart rate greater than 100 beats/min. The rate is regular and rarely exceeds 160 beats/min. Electrocardiogram (ECG) should demonstrate a P wave preceding each QRS complex with a fixed PR interval.

1. Etiologies. Catecholamine excess, inadequate anesthesia or analgesia, hypercarbia, hypoxia, hypotension, hypovolemia, medications (eg, pancuronium, desflurane, atropine, and ephedrine), fever, MI, PE, tamponade, tension pneumothorax, malignant hyperthermia, pheochromocytoma, and thyrotoxicosis.
2. Treatment should be directed toward correcting the underlying cause and may include the following:
   a. Correcting oxygenation and ventilation abnormalities.
   b. Increasing the depth of anesthesia and treating pain with analgesics.
   c. Correcting hypovolemia.
   d. Medications such as opioids and β-adrenergic blockers. Patients with active coronary artery disease and adequate blood pressure may benefit from treatment with β-adrenergic blockers to control the heart rate while the cause is being determined.

C. Heart block
1. **First-degree atrioventricular (AV) block** is characterized by a PR interval of 0.2 seconds or longer. In first-degree block, every atrial pulse is transmitted to the ventricle.
2. **Second-degree AV block** is divided into two types: Mobitz type 1 (Wenckebach) and Mobitz type 2.
   a. **Mobitz type 1** (Wenckebach) usually occurs when a conduction defect is in the AV node and is manifested by a progressive PR prolongation culminating in a nonconducted P wave. It is generally benign.
   b. **Mobitz type 2** is a conduction defect often distal to the AV node. It presents with a constant PR interval and frequent nonconducted P waves. It is more likely to progress to third-degree block.
3. **Third-degree AV block** (complete heart block) may be caused by intrinsic AV nodal or His Purkinje disease and occurs when there is a complete failure of any conduction from the atria to ventricles. It presents with AV dissociation (variable PR intervals) and either a junctional (narrow QRS) or ventricular (wide QRS) escape rhythm.

4. **Treatment of heart block**
    a. **First-degree AV block** does not usually require specific treatment; however, temporary pacing should be available in the case of first-degree heart block in combination with a bifascicular block (so-called trifascicular block).
    b. **Second-degree AV block**
        1. **Mobitz type 1** requires treatment only if the patient becomes symptomatic or hemodynamically unstable. Temporary transcutaneous or transvenous pacing may be necessary, particularly during an inferior MI, although the block may resolve following revascularization.
        2. **Mobitz type 2** may progress to complete heart block. Hemodynamically unstable patients should be urgently treated with atropine or epinephrine and often temporary cardiac pacing. Stable patients should be continuously monitored for progression to higher-grade conduction block warranting pacemaker placement while being evaluated for etiology.
    c. **Third-degree AV block** is treated in the short term with transcutaneous, transvenous, or epicardial pacing if the patient is acutely unstable, and in the long term with a permanent pacemaker.
D. **Supraventricular tachycardias (SVTs)** originate at or above the bundle of His. The resulting QRS complexes are narrow (<120 ms) except during aberrant conduction.
    1. **Atrial premature contractions (APCs or PACs)** occur when ectopic foci in the atria fire before the next expected impulse from the sinus node. The P wave of an APC characteristically looks different from preceding P waves, and the PR interval may vary from normal. APCs may cause aberrant QRS complexes. If the AV node is still in a refractory period, an APC will not elicit a ventricular response. APCs are common, usually benign, and typically require no treatment.
    2. **Junctional or AV nodal rhythms** are characterized by absent or abnormal P waves and normal QRS complexes. Although they may indicate ischemic cardiac disease, junctional rhythms are commonly seen in healthy individuals receiving inhalational anesthesia. In the patient whose cardiac output depends heavily on the contribution from atrial contraction, stroke volume, and blood pressure may decline precipitously. Treatment may include the following:
        a. Reduction of anesthetic depth.
        b. Increasing intravascular volume.
        c. Atropine in increments of 0.2 mg IV may convert a slow junctional rhythm to sinus rhythm, particularly if secondary to a vagal mechanism.
        d. Paradoxically, β-blockers may be used cautiously (eg, propranolol 0.5 mg IV and metoprolol 1 to 3 mg), especially with isorhythmic AV dissociation (independent atrial and ventricular rhythms that are similar in rate).
        e. If the dysrhythmia is associated with hypotension, increasing the blood pressure with vasopressors (eg, ephedrine or norepinephrine) may be required as a temporizing measure.
        f. If necessary, atrial pacing may be instituted to restore atrial contraction.
    3. **Atrial fibrillation** is an irregular rhythm with an atrial rate of 350 to 600 beats/min and a variable ventricular response. It may be seen with myocardial ischemia, mitral valvular disease, hyperthyroidism, PE, excessive sympathetic stimulation, and digitalis toxicity; after thoracic

surgery; or when the heart has been manipulated. Treatment is based on the hemodynamic status.
  a. **Rapid ventricular rate with stable hemodynamics** can be treated initially with β-adrenergic blockade, such as propranolol 0.5-mg increments IV, metoprolol 2.5- to 5-mg increments, esmolol 5- to 10-mg increments, or a calcium channel blocker such as verapamil 2.5- to 5-mg increments or diltiazem 10 to 20 mg IV (see Chapters 18: Perioperative Hemodynamic Control and Chapter 39: Adult, Pediatric, and Newborn Resuscitation). Amiodarone 150 mg IV can be used to promote conversion back to sinus rhythm (anticoagulation prior to cardioversion is recommended in patients with atrial fibrillation for longer than 24 hours).
  b. **Rapid ventricular rate with unstable hemodynamics** requires synchronized cardioversion (50 to 100 J if biphasic or 200 J if monophasic) (see Chapter 18: Perioperative Hemodynamic Control and Chapter 39: Adult, Pediatric, and Newborn Resuscitation).
4. **Atrial flutter** is usually a regular rhythm with an atrial rate of 250 to 350 beats/min and a characteristic sawtooth ECG configuration. It is often seen with underlying heart disease (ie, rheumatic heart disease and mitral stenosis). Conduction across the AV node is often 2:1 in patients not taking AV nodal blockers, but it may also be 1:1 or 4:1. A 2:1 block will result in a rapid ventricular rate (usually 150 beats/min). Treatment usually includes β-adrenergic, calcium channel blockade, or synchronized cardioversion (see Chapter 18: Perioperative Hemodynamic Control and Chapter 39: Adult, Pediatric, and Newborn Resuscitation).
5. **Paroxysmal SVT** is an abrupt-onset tachydysrhythmia (atrial and ventricular rates of 150 to 250 beats/min) with reentry usually through the AV node. This rhythm may be associated with **Wolff–Parkinson–White (WPW) syndrome**, thyrotoxicosis, or mitral valve prolapse. Patients without heart disease may develop this dysrhythmia owing to stress, caffeine, or excess catecholamines.
  a. Hemodynamically unstable patients with SVT should undergo synchronized cardioversion starting at 50 to 100 J. These patients are at high risk for ventricular fibrillation.
  b. For hemodynamically stable patients with SVT, treatment includes **adenosine** 6 to 18 mg IV, Valsalva maneuvers, carotid sinus massage, or propranolol 1 to 2 mg IV.
  c. Preexcitation syndromes refer to the presence of an accessory pathway. WPW syndrome is the most common. Conduction can be orthodromic (antegrade) or antidromic (retrograde).
    1. Orthodromic conduction means the ventricles are depolarized normally via the AV node and His–Purkinje system, consequently the QRS-complex on EKG will be narrow and regular. This is the most common form of WPW (>90% of cases). AV nodal blockers (including adenosine, calcium channel blockers, and β-blockers) are safe use in this population.
    2. Antidromic conduction means the ventricles are depolarized via the accessory pathway, which yields regular, wide-complex QRS (>0.12 s) on EKG. Nodal blockers are contraindicated in this population as unopposed conduction through the accessory pathway can induce ventricular fibrillation and cardiac arrest. The pharmacologic treatment of choice for antidromic conduction tachyarrhythmias is procainamide or ibutilide.

3. Preexcitation and atrial tachyarrhythmias including atrial fibrillation and flutter, can manifest as regular or irregular wide-complex tachycardia. Amiodarone may be considered in this case.
4. If uncertain about the diagnosis of an orthodromic preexcitation syndrome or if wide-complex QRS tracings are present on EKG, then nodal blockers should be prophylactically avoided and the arrhythmia should be approached as an undifferentiated wide-complex tachycardia. Refer to 2015 ACC/AHA/HRS Guideline on Management of Adult SVTs for a comprehensive summary of management.

E. Ventricular dysrhythmias
1. **Ventricular premature contractions (VPCs or PVCs)** occur when ectopic foci in the ventricle fire before the next expected impulse arrives. They are characterized by widened QRS (>120 ms) complexes. When these are coupled alternately with normal beats, ventricular bigeminy exists. VPCs are occasionally seen in healthy individuals but carry a worse prognosis in patients with underlying heart disease. Under anesthesia, they frequently occur during states of catecholamine excess, hypoxia, or hypercarbia. They may also signify myocardial ischemia or infarction, heart failure, digitalis toxicity, hypokalemia, or hypomagnesemia. **VPCs may require therapy when a patient becomes hemodynamically unstable. Other concerning features include sustained durations, increase in frequency (>10% of all ventricular depolarizations), or occurrence on or near the preceding T wave (R-on-T phenomenon);** these situations may precede the development of ventricular tachycardia, ventricular fibrillation, and cardiac arrest.
   a. Treatment in an otherwise hemodynamically stable patient should begin with ensuring adequate depth of anesthesia, oxygenation, and ventilation and assessing for electrolyte abnormalities (especially potassium and magnesium). Patients with coronary artery disease who continue to have ventricular irritability should have any ischemia treated. If the ectopy continues, then **amiodarone** (150 mg IV over 10 minutes followed by an infusion at 1 mg/min for 6 hours and then 0.5 mg/min thereafter) may be considered. Refractory ventricular ectopy may require further treatment (see Chapter 18: Perioperative Hemodynamic Control and Chapter 39: Adult, Pediatric, and Newborn Resuscitation).
2. **Ventricular tachycardia** is defined as three or more successive ventricular complexes. Nonsustained VT is three or more repetitive ventricular beats with a duration of <30 seconds. Sustained VT lasts for >30 seconds or is associated with hemodynamic impairment. Monomorphic VT is the repetition of the same basic QRS complex, whereas polymorphic VT refers to changing QRS morphology particularly if there is a change in axis. Polymorphic VT with a prolonged baseline QTc is called torsades de pointes.
   a. Hemodynamically unstable patients with a pulse should be treated as outlined in the advanced cardiac life support (ACLS) guidelines with cardiopulmonary resuscitation and cardioversion (120 to 200 J if biphasic, or 360 J if monophasic; if unresponsive, may increase energy in a stepwise fashion).
   b. For stable patients with sustained monomorphic VT, pharmacologic cardioversion can be attempted, but the patient should be monitored carefully as patients who are hemodynamically stable initially can rapidly become unstable. Underlying causes such as electrolyte disturbance, ischemia, and heart failure should also be treated.

c. Polymorphic VT is usually a hemodynamically unstable rhythm requiring urgent defibrillation.
d. In conscious, stable patients with torsades de points, intravenous magnesium sulfate is often an effective therapy.
3. **Ventricular fibrillation** is chaotic ventricular activity resulting in ineffective ventricular contractions. Prompt defibrillation is required with the same starting energy as above.
4. **Preexcited atrial fibrillation.** In patients with a wide-complex tachycardia who are hemodynamically stable, consider preexcited atrial fibrillation. Initial therapy with rhythm or rate control should be attempted (refer to WPW syndrome above).

IV. HYPOXEMIA

Hypoxemia occurs when oxygen delivery to the tissues is insufficient to meet metabolic demands.

A. Intraoperative etiologies

1. **Inadequate oxygen supply**
   a. Loss of the main pipeline supply with an empty reserve oxygen tank.
   b. An oxygen flowmeter that is not turned to a sufficient flow.
   c. Breathing system disconnection.
   d. Large leaks in the anesthesia machine, ventilator, carbon dioxide absorber, breathing circuit, or around the endotracheal tube or laryngeal mask airway. This condition may be managed acutely by increasing oxygen flow or using a self-inflating (Ambu) bag to deliver oxygen to the patient.
   e. Obstructed endotracheal tube (eg, kinked or mucous plug).
   f. Malpositioned endotracheal tubes (eg, esophageal or mainstem bronchial intubation).
   g. Upper airway obstruction.
   h. Laryngospasm in the unintubated patient (see Section X).
2. **Hypoventilation** (see Section V).
3. **Ventilation–perfusion inequalities or shunting**
   a. **Pulmonary shunt.** As seen with atelectasis, pneumonia, pulmonary edema, aspiration, pneumothorax, bronchospasm, mucous plugging, and other parenchymal pathologic states as well as with single lung ventilation. In some cases, these inequalities may be corrected by increasing mean airway pressure or applying PEEP.
   b. **Cardiac shunt.** Right-to-left cardiac shunt, as in ventricular septal defect (VSD), atrial septal defect (ASD), and tetralogy of Fallot.
4. **Reduction in oxygen-carrying capacity.** The oxygen-carrying capacity is reduced with anemia, carbon monoxide poisoning, and hemoglobinopathies, despite a normal oxygen saturation as measured by pulse oximetry. Methemoglobin reduces the oxygen-carrying capacity and at high levels will reduce oxygen saturation reading via pulse oximetry.
5. **A leftward shift of the hemoglobin-oxygen dissociation curve** results from hypothermia, decreased 2,3-diphosphoglycerate concentration, alkalosis, hypocarbia, and carbon monoxide poisoning.

B. Treatment of hypoxemia

1. If the patient is being mechanically ventilated, begin manual ventilation with 100% oxygen to assess pulmonary compliance. Evaluate breath sounds, check the surgical field for mechanical interference with ventilation, examine the endotracheal tube for obstruction or dislodgement, and confirm adequate movement of the chest wall or diaphragm. Elevated peak airway pressures may indicate bronchospasm,

pneumothorax, an obstructed endotracheal tube, or endobronchial intubation.
2. The breathing circuit, ventilator, and anesthesia machine should be checked for leaks. If a leak is present, ventilation should be started with high-flow 100% oxygen via an alternative source such as a self-inflating bag until the problem is rectified.
3. Adequate oxygen delivery to the patient should be confirmed with an inline oxygen analyzer.
4. Bronchoscopy may be valuable to help rule out obstructive causes, verify endotracheal tube placement, and remove mucus plugging.
5. Ultrasound or bedside chest x-ray may help evaluate for pneumothorax.
6. Further treatment is outlined in Chapter 13: Airway Evaluation and Management.

V. HYPERCARBIA

Hypercarbia is due either to inadequate ventilation or increased carbon dioxide production and can lead to respiratory acidosis, increased pulmonary artery pressure, and increased ICP.

A. Inadequate ventilation

1. **Central depression of the medullary respiratory center** can be caused by medications (eg, opioids, barbiturates, benzodiazepines, and volatile anesthetics) or primary central nervous system pathology (eg, tumor, ischemia, and edema). Controlled ventilation and the administration of reversal agents (eg, naloxone and flumazenil) may be required.
2. **Neuromuscular depression** may be seen with a high level of neuraxial anesthesia, phrenic nerve paralysis, and inadequate reversal of neuromuscular blockade.
3. **Inappropriate ventilator settings** may result in low-minute ventilation.
4. **Increased airway resistance** may occur with bronchospasm, upper airway obstruction, mainstem intubation, obstructed endotracheal tube, severe chronic obstructive lung disease, congestive heart failure, and hemothorax or pneumothorax.
5. **Rebreathing of exhaled gases** may occur owing to an exhausted carbon dioxide absorber, machine failure, inspiratory or expiratory valve failure, or inadequate fresh gas flow in nonrebreathing systems.
6. **One-lung ventilation** in patients with preexisting pulmonary pathology can lead to significant hypercarbia.

B. Increased carbon dioxide production
results from exogenous carbon dioxide (eg, reabsorption of carbon dioxide from insufflation or subcutaneous emphysema during laparoscopy), reperfusion of ischemic tissue, and hypermetabolic states (eg, hyperthermia, sepsis, burns, and malignant hyperthermia).

C. Treatment of hypercarbia
should be targeted to the cause. Depending on the etiology, treatment may include intubation, increasing minute ventilation, repositioning the endotracheal tube, suctioning, treatment of bronchospasm, diuresis, or placing a chest tube.

VI. ABNORMAL URINE OUTPUT

A. Oliguria
is defined as urine output less than 0.5 mL/kg/h. Prerenal, renal, and postrenal causes are described in Chapter 5: Specific Considerations With Renal Disease.
1. Treatment includes ruling out mechanical causes (eg, malpositioned, kinked, or obstructed Foley catheter) and renal dysfunction (can be accessed through renal ultrasound).

2. **Hypotension** should be corrected to ensure adequate renal perfusion pressure.
3. **Volume status should be assessed.** A fluid bolus may be given if hypovolemia is suspected. If oliguria persists, markers of end-organ perfusion, CVP measurement, or systolic variation in arterial tracing may help guide further fluid management. Patients with reduced ventricular function may benefit from placement of a pulmonary artery catheter for guiding inotropic support.
4. **If oliguria persists** despite an adequate volume status, urine output can be increased with the following drugs. Current evidence suggests that these medications do not affect renal function or outcome; however, they may aid in toxin elimination and reduce the formation of casts.
   a. Furosemide 2 to 20 mg IV.
   b. Dopamine infusion 1 to 3 µg/kg/min IV.
   c. Mannitol 12.5 to 25.0 g IV.
   d. Fenoldopam 0.1 to 0.4 µg/kg/min IV.
5. **Intraoperative diuretics** may be required to preserve urine output in patients on chronic diuretic therapy.
6. Syndrome of Inappropriate Antidiuretic Hormone (SIADH) is an uncommon complication after surgery and can also be caused by various medications such as SSRIs, diabetes medications, cyclophosphamide, and other chemotherapeutics. Patients may present with euvolemic hyponatremia and elevated urine osmolality.

B. **Anuria** is a rare occurrence in the perioperative period. Mechanical causes, including Foley catheter malfunction or ureteral obstruction, damage, or transection, must be excluded, and hemodynamic instability must be treated.

C. **High urine output** may occur in response to iatrogenic causes (eg, vigorous fluid administration, mannitol, and Lasix), but other causes must be considered, including hyperglycemia, cerebral salt wasting syndrome, and both neurogenic and nephrogenic diabetes insipidus (see Chapter 5: Specific Considerations With Renal Disease). A high urine output is not a problem unless associated with hypovolemia or electrolyte abnormalities. Treatment should be directed at the underlying cause, maintaining volume status, and correcting electrolyte abnormalities.

VII. HYPOTHERMIA

Hypothermia is a common problem in the perioperative period.

A. **Heat loss** during general anesthesia and surgery may occur from any or all of the following mechanisms:
   1. **Redistribution of heat from core areas** (eg, brain, heart) to peripheral tissues (eg, limbs, skin). Redistribution results in a reduction in the core temperature with maintenance of the mean body temperature.
   2. **Radiation.** Radiant heat loss depends on cutaneous blood flow and exposed body surface area.
   3. **Evaporation.** Energy is lost as liquid vaporizes from mucosal and serosal surfaces, skin, and lungs. Evaporative losses depend on the exposed surface area and the relative humidity of ambient gas.
   4. **Conduction,** which is heat transfer from a warm to a cool object. This heat loss is proportional to the area exposed, difference in temperature, and thermal conductivity.
   5. **Convection,** which is the loss of heat by conduction to a moving gas. High airflow rates in the operating rooms (10 to 15 room volume changes/h) may result in significant heat loss.

B. Pediatric patients are particularly susceptible to intraoperative hypothermia (see Chapter 33: Anesthesia for Pediatric Surgery and Care of the Neonate).

C. Geriatric patients are also more prone to hypothermia.

D. Anesthetic effects
1. Volatile anesthetics impair the thermoregulatory center located in the posterior hypothalamus and predispose the patient to heat redistribution and heat loss due to their vasodilatory properties.
2. Opioids will reduce the vasoconstriction mechanism for heat conservation because of their sympatholytic properties.
3. Muscle relaxants reduce muscle tone and prevent shivering.
4. Regional anesthesia produces sympathetic blockade, muscle relaxation, and sensory blockade of thermal receptors, which inhibit compensatory responses.

E. Severe hypothermia is associated with numerous physiologic changes.
1. **Cardiovascular.** Increased SVR, ventricular dysrhythmias, and myocardial depression may occur with severe hypothermia.
2. **Metabolic.** Decreased metabolic rate and decreased tissue perfusion (from catecholamine response) may occur.
3. **Hematologic.** Increased blood viscosity secondary to cold diuresis, leftward shift of the hemoglobin dissociation curve, impaired coagulation, and platelet dysfunction occur.
4. **Neurologic.** Decreased cerebral blood flow, increased cerebrovascular resistance, decreased minimum alveolar concentration, delayed emergence from anesthesia, drowsiness, and confusion may occur.
5. **Drug disposition.** Decreased hepatic blood flow and metabolism coupled with decreased renal blood flow and clearance result in decreased anesthetic requirement.
6. **Shivering** can increase heat production, oxygen consumption, and sympathetic tone. Shivering will stop once body temperature drops below 32 °C.

F. Prevention and treatment of hypothermia
1. **Maintain or increase ambient temperature.** Anesthetized patients frequently become hypothermic if the room temperature is below 21 °C.
2. **Cover exposed surfaces** to minimize conductive and convective losses. Forced-warmed air blankets placed under and over the patient can provide both insulation and active warming. Active warming should not be attempted on ischemic tissues such as those found distal to the level of an aortic cross-clamp.
3. **Warming transfused fluids and blood** is essential in cases with large fluid requirements or rapid infusion rates (see Chapter 35: Anesthesia for Trauma and Burns). Doing so will reduce heat loss by about 0.25 °C/L of crystalloid.
4. **Use of closed or low-flow semiclosed circuit anesthesia** will decrease evaporative losses and modestly reduce heat loss.
5. **Heated humidifiers** can be added to the anesthetic circuit when high gas flows are used. These will warm and humidify the inspired gas, minimizing evaporative loss from the lungs. The temperature of the inspired gas must be monitored and kept below 41 °C; otherwise, there is potential for airway burns. Alternatively, "artificial noses" (passive heat and moisture exchangers) can be placed between the endotracheal tube and the breathing circuit. These are hygroscopic membrane filters with large surface areas that trap the humidity of expired air.

6. **Warming blankets** placed beneath the patient can increase body temperature by conduction from warm water pumped through the blanket. This method is most effective in children weighing less than 10 kg. The temperature should be kept below 40 °C to avoid burns.
7. **Radiant warmers and heating lamps** warm the patients by infrared radiation and are useful only for infants. The warming lamps should be kept at least 70 cm from the patient to avoid burns.
8. **Warming irrigation solutions** prior to use.

VIII. HYPERTHERMIA

Hyperthermia is an increase in temperature of 2 °C/h or 0.5 °C/15 min. It is uncommon for a patient to become hyperthermic based solely on maneuvers to conserve body heat in the operating room. Therefore, any increase in temperature must be investigated. Hyperthermia and its accompanying hypermetabolic state produce an increase in oxygen consumption, cardiac work, glucose demand, and compensatory minute ventilation. Sweating and vasodilation may result in decreased intravascular volume and venous return.

A. Etiologies
1. **Malignant hyperthermia** must be considered during any perioperative temperature increase (see Section XVII).
2. **Inflammation, infection, and sepsis** with the release of inflammatory mediators may cause fever and hyperthermia.
3. **Hypermetabolic states** such as thyrotoxicosis may cause hyperthermia.
4. **Injury to the hypothalamic thermoregulatory center** from anoxia, edema, trauma, or tumor may affect temperature set points in the hypothalamus.
5. **Neuroleptic malignant syndrome** (NMS) triggered by neuroleptics such as phenothiazines (eg, haloperidol); it is a rare cause.
6. **Sympathomimetics**, such as monoamine oxidase inhibitors, amphetamines, cocaine, and tricyclic antidepressants, may produce a hypermetabolic state.
7. **Anticholinergics**, such as atropine, may suppress sweating.
8. **Iatrogenic** eg, Hyperthermic intraperitoneal chemotherapy (HIPEC) surgery

B. Treatment
1. **If malignant hyperthermia is suspected**, dantrolene treatment must be initiated (see Section XVII).
2. **Severe hyperthermia** can be treated by cooling exposed body surfaces (eg, skin) with ice, cooling blankets, and reduced ambient temperature or by performing internal lavage (eg, stomach, bladder, bowel, and peritoneum) with cold saline.
   a. Volatile liquids, such as alcohol, applied to the skin will promote evaporative heat loss.
   b. Conductive heat loss can be increased with vasodilators such as nitroprusside and nitroglycerin.
   c. Centrally active agents such as aspirin and acetaminophen can be given IV or by nasogastric tube or rectally.
   d. Shivering can be prevented by maintaining neuromuscular blockade.
   e. When hyperthermia is profound, **extracorporeal cooling** can be used. Cooling should be stopped when the body temperature reaches 38 °C to avoid hypothermia.

IX. DIAPHORESIS (SWEATING)

Diaphoresis (sweating) may occur in response to the sympathetic discharge caused by anxiety, pain, hypercarbia, or noxious stimuli in the presence of inadequate anesthesia. It may also be seen in conjunction with bradycardia, nausea, and hypotension as part of a generalized vagal reaction or as a thermoregulatory response to hyperthermia.

X. LARYNGOSPASM

A. Laryngospasm is most commonly caused by an irritative stimulus to the airway during a light plane of anesthesia. Common noxious airway stimuli that may elicit this reflex include secretions, vomitus, blood, inhalation of pungent volatile anesthetics, oropharyngeal or nasopharyngeal airway placement, laryngoscopy, painful peripheral stimuli, and peritoneal traction during light anesthesia. Laryngospasm can also result from sudden administration of high doses of synthetic narcotics (eg, fentanyl) during induction of anesthesia.

B. Reflex closure of the vocal cords, causing partial or total glottic obstruction, may be manifest in less severe cases by stridor and, when complete, by an obstructed pattern of breathing. In this situation, the abdominal wall rises with contraction of the diaphragm during inspiration, but because air entry is blocked the chest retracts or fails to expand. This can lead to the development of negative pressure pulmonary edema. During attempted expiration, the abdomen falls as the diaphragm relaxes and the chest returns to its original position. With complete obstruction, the anesthetist will not be able to ventilate the patient.

C. The hypoxia, hypercarbia, and acidosis that result from laryngospasm can cause hypertension and tachycardia, followed by hypotension, bradycardia, and ventricular dysrhythmias leading to cardiac arrest unless airway patency is restored. Children and pregnant women are particularly prone to these complications because of their small functional residual capacity and relatively high oxygen consumption.

D. Treatment

1. Deepening the anesthetic level and removing the stimulus (eg, by suction, withdrawal of an artificial airway, or stopping peripheral stimulation) while administering 100% oxygen may be adequate to relieve laryngospasm.
2. If laryngospasm is not relieved, **continuous positive pressure on the airway** with a jaw thrust may relieve the spasm; if not, a small dose of **succinylcholine** (eg, 10 to 20 mg IV in an adult) will relax the striated muscles of the larynx. In the pediatric population, 1.5 mg/kg of intravenous lidocaine prior to extubation has been shown to reduce the incidence of postextubation laryngospasm.
3. The lungs should be ventilated with 100% oxygen and the anesthetic level deepened before the noxious stimulation is resumed, or the patient may be allowed to awaken if laryngospasm has occurred during emergence.
4. Infrequently, laryngospasm may require reintubation.
5. Laryngospasm can result in negative-pressure pulmonary edema, which may need treatment after the laryngospasm resolves.

XI. BRONCHOSPASM

A. Reflex bronchiolar constriction may be centrally mediated or may be a local response to airway irritation. Bronchospasm is common in anaphylactoid or anaphylactic drug and blood transfusion reactions as well as in cigarette smokers and those with chronic bronchitis. Like laryngospasm, bronchospasm may be elicited by noxious stimuli such as secretions and endotracheal intubation.

B. Wheezing (usually more pronounced on expiration) characterizes bronchospasm and is associated with tachypnea and dyspnea in the awake patient. An anesthetized patient may be difficult to ventilate because of increased airway resistance. Decreased expiratory flow rates may produce air trapping and increase intrathoracic pressure, decreasing venous return, cardiac output, and blood pressure. End-tidal carbon dioxide curves often have an obstructive pattern (continual rise) during exhalation.

C. Histamine-releasing drugs (eg, morphine, mivacurium, vancomycin, and atracurium) may exacerbate bronchoconstriction.

D. Treatment
   1. The **endotracheal tube position** should be checked and, if carinal stimulation is the cause, withdrawn slightly.
   2. **Deepening the anesthetic level** will frequently reverse bronchospasm that is secondary to inadequate anesthesia. Deepening the level of anesthesia can usually be accomplished with an inhalational agent. An IV agent may be necessary when ventilation is significantly impaired. Propofol produces fewer symptoms of bronchoconstriction than barbiturates and is usually preferable. Ketamine has the advantage of causing bronchodilation by releasing endogenous catecholamines. The inspired oxygen concentration should be increased until adequate oxygenation is achieved.
   3. **Medical treatment** includes administering inhaled or intravenous β_2-adrenergic agonists. Inhaled bronchodilators have limited systemic absorption, which may minimize cardiovascular side effects. Nebulized forms may contain large particles, which deposit to a large extent in tubing and upper airways. The dosage of metered dose inhalers should be titrated to effect when administered into a breathing circuit. Large doses (10 to 20 puffs) may be necessary. If the condition is severe, low-dose ketamine 0.1 to 0.15 mg/kg/h based on case reports or low-dose IV epinephrine 0.02 to 0.05 µg/kg/min based on case reports should be started.
   4. **Adequate hydration and humidification** of inspired gases will minimize inspissation of secretions.

XII. ASPIRATION

General anesthesia causes depression of airway reflexes that predisposes patients to aspiration. Aspiration of gastric contents from vomiting or regurgitation may cause bronchospasm, hypoxemia, atelectasis, tachypnea, tachycardia, and hypotension. The severity of symptoms depends on the volume and pH of the gastric material aspirated. Conditions that predispose the patient to aspiration include gastric dysmotility, gastric outlet obstruction, gastroesophageal reflux, small bowel obstruction, symptomatic hiatal hernia, pregnancy, and recent food ingestion.

A. If vomiting or regurgitation occurs in an anesthetized patient whose airway is not protected by an endotracheal tube, the patient should be placed in the Trendelenburg position to minimize the passive flow of gastric contents into the trachea, the head should be turned to the side, the upper airway suctioned, and an endotracheal tube placed. Suctioning the endotracheal tube before instituting positive-pressure ventilation avoids forcing gastric contents into the distal airways. Evidence of significant aspiration includes wheezing, decreased lung compliance, and hypoxemia. A chest

radiograph should be obtained; however, radiographic evidence of infiltrates may be delayed. Bronchodilators may be useful.
- **B. Bronchoscopy** should be performed if a clinically significant aspiration is suspected. The airways should be suctioned clear, and foreign bodies such as teeth and food removed. Lavage with large volumes of saline is not helpful.
- **C. Aspiration of blood**, unless of large volume, is usually benign.
- **D. Administration of antibiotics** usually is not warranted unless the material aspirated contains a high bacterial load such as with bowel obstruction (see Chapter 8: Infectious Diseases and Infection Control in Anesthesia).
- **E. A sputum specimen** should be obtained for Gram stain and culture.
- **F. Steroids** are not useful for treating aspiration.
- **G. If significant aspiration has occurred**, close postoperative observation should be undertaken. This includes pulse oximetry and repeat chest radiography. Ventilatory support and supplemental oxygen may be necessary (see Chapter 37: The Post-Anesthesia Care Unit).

XIII. PNEUMOTHORAX

Pneumothorax is the accumulation of gas within the pleural space.
- **A. Etiologies**
    1. Spontaneous rupture of blebs and bullae.
    2. Blunt or penetrating chest trauma.
    3. Surgical entrance into the pleural space during thoracic, upper abdominal, or retroperitoneal surgery, tracheostomy, or surgery of the chest wall or neck.
    4. Iatrogenic complication of procedures such as subclavian or internal jugular vein catheter placement, thoracentesis, pericardiocentesis, or upper extremity nerve block.
    5. During positive-pressure ventilation using high pressures and volumes, causing barotrauma and alveolar rupture. Patients with chronic obstructive pulmonary disease are at particularly high risk.
    6. Malfunction of chest tubes.
- **B. Physiologic effects** of a pneumothorax are largely a function of the gas volume and the rate of expansion. A small pneumothorax may have no significant cardiopulmonary effect, whereas a larger one may result in significant lung collapse and hypoxemia. A tension pneumothorax occurs when there is a one-way leak into the pleural space, causing a significant increase in intrapleural pressure. This can result in decreased venous return, mediastinal shift, and compression of the heart. A small tension pneumothorax can cause hypotension, whereas a large tension pneumothorax can cause a cardiac arrest.
- **C.** The **diagnosis** of pneumothorax can be difficult.
    1. Signs of pneumothorax include decreased breath sounds on the affected side, a reduction in lung compliance, an increase in peak inspiratory pressure, and hypoxemia.
    2. Hypotension reflects the presence of a tension pneumothorax.
    3. A chest radiograph can usually reveal a pneumothorax as a hyperlucency between the chest wall, mediastinum, or diaphragm and lung parenchyma.
    4. Ultrasound imaging of the chest wall can provide a reliable and rapid diagnosis. Signs of a pneumothorax on ultrasound imaging will be the lack of parietal and visceral pleura sliding against each other during respirations. The "lung point," defined as the transition point from normal sliding lung to nonsliding lung due to collapse, if seen on ultrasound is diagnostic for pneumothorax.

D. Treatment. Nitrous oxide should be discontinued, and the patient should be ventilated with 100% oxygen. A tension pneumothorax requires immediate decompression. A large-bore catheter (14 to 16 gauge) can be inserted into the pleural space at the second intercostal space in the midclavicular line. A chest tube can then be placed at the fifth or sixth intercostal space in the midaxillary line.

XIV. MYOCARDIAL ISCHEMIA

A. Etiology. Myocardial ischemia is the result of an imbalance between myocardial oxygen supply and consumption and, if persistent, may lead to MI.

B. Clinical features

1. In the awake patient, myocardial ischemia may manifest as chest pain, dyspnea, nausea and vomiting, diaphoresis, or shoulder and jaw pain. **Asymptomatic ischemia is common** in the perioperative period, particularly in diabetic patients. In patients under general anesthesia, hemodynamic instability and ECG changes may occur with ischemia.

2. **ECG changes** such as **ST segment depression** greater than 1 mm or acute T-wave inversion may indicate subendocardial ischemia. **ST segment elevation** is usually seen with transmural myocardial ischemia. T-wave changes may also be seen with electrolyte abnormalities and thus are not particularly diagnostic of ischemia. Lead V_5 is the single most sensitive lead for detecting left ventricular ischemia (see Chapter 15: Monitoring).

3. **Other indicators of ischemia** include the following:
   a. Hypotension.
   b. Changes in central filling pressures or cardiac output.
   c. Regional wall motion abnormalities as detected with TEE.
   d. Dysrhythmias, particularly ventricular ectopy.

C. Treatment

1. **Hypoxemia and anemia should be** optimally managed to maximize myocardial oxygen delivery.

2. **β-Adrenergic antagonists** (eg, metoprolol in 1- to 3-mg increments IV or propranolol in 0.5- to 1.0-mg increments IV or esmolol in 5- to 10-mg increments IV) decrease myocardial oxygen consumption by decreasing heart rate and contractility. The initiation of β-blockers should be delayed in patients with active heart failure.

3. **Nitroglycerin** (starting at 25 to 50 µg/min IV or 0.15 mg sublingually) reduces ventricular diastolic pressure and volume through venodilation and thus decreases the myocardial oxygen demand. In addition, nitroglycerin may improve oxygen delivery by enhancing collateral coronary flow. Nitrates should be avoided if there is suspected or known right ventricular ischemia, severe hypotension, marked bradycardia, phosphodiesterase inhibitor use in the last 24 hours, hypertrophic cardiomyopathy, and severe aortic stenosis.

4. **Myocardial ischemia occurring in the setting of hypotension** may require a vasopressor such as phenylephrine (40 to 80 µg/min IV) or norepinephrine (2 to 20 µg/min IV) to improve myocardial perfusion pressure. Anesthetic depth may need to be decreased and intravascular volume optimized.

5. When myocardial ischemia results in a significant reduction in cardiac output and hypotension (cardiogenic shock), positive **inotropes** such as dopamine 5 to 20 µg/kg/min IV, dobutamine 5 to 20 µg/kg/min IV, milrinone 0.375 to 0.75 µg/kg/min (after loading dose of 50 µg/kg), and norepinephrine 2 to 20 µg/min IV are indicated.

Intra-aortic balloon counterpulsation or venoarterial ECMO may be lifesaving. A pulmonary artery catheter and transesophageal echocardiogram may be helpful in assessing ventricular function and response to therapy.
6. **Aspirin** should be administered.
7. **Heparin treatment, antiplatelet therapy, thrombolytic therapy, angioplasty, and coronary revascularization** may be considered in selected patients under the guidance of a cardiologist and cardiac surgeon.

XV. PULMONARY EMBOLISM

PE is the obstruction of pulmonary arterial blood flow by thrombus, air, fat, or amniotic fluid. Large emboli may lead to a sudden decrease in end-tidal carbon dioxide tension owing to an **acute increase in dead space**. Other signs include an increase in end-tidal nitrogen tension, as well as an increased CVP, hypoxemia, hypotension, tachyarrhythmias or bradyarrhythmias, and ventricular ectopy.

A. Thromboemboli most commonly arise from the deep venous system of the pelvis and lower extremities. Predisposing factors for the development of thrombi are stasis, hypercoagulability, and vascular wall abnormalities. Associated conditions include pregnancy, trauma, malignancy, prolonged bed rest, and vasculitis.

1. **Physical findings** are nonspecific and may include tachypnea and tachycardia, dyspnea, bronchospasm, and fever.
2. **Laboratory studies**
   a. The ECG reveals a nonspecific tachycardia unless embolization is severe, in which case right-axis deviation, right bundle branch block, and anterior T-wave changes may be seen. PE may cause atrial fibrillation.
   b. The chest radiograph may be unremarkable unless pulmonary infarction has occurred.
   c. Typically, hypotension and hypoxemia are present.
   d. In spontaneously breathing patients, hypocapnia and respiratory alkalosis may result from the increased respiratory rate.
   e. Definitive diagnosis requires a pulmonary angiogram or high-resolution computed tomography of the chest (spiral computed tomography).
3. **Intraoperative treatment** of a suspected PE is supportive. ACLS should be initiated if cardiac arrest occurs. Oxygenation may be increased with increased FIO_2 and hemodynamics should be optimized with inotropes and vasopressors as needed. For patients in profound cardiogenic shock, venoarterial ECMO may be considered as a bridge to catheter-directed thrombolysis or embolectomy, or surgical embolectomy with cardiopulmonary bypass. Intraoperative anticoagulation therapy, for example, heparin treatment or thrombolytic therapy can be considered and weighed against the risk of hemorrhage.

B. Air embolism occurs during entrainment of air into a vein or venous sinus. It occurs most commonly during intracranial surgery in the sitting position, where dural venous sinuses are stented open. Air embolism may also occur during central line placement or removal, liver transplantation, open cardiac procedures, and insufflation during laparoscopy.

1. **Additional signs indicating air embolism** include air seen by TEE or heard with a precordial Doppler. Possible vital sign changes include a sudden decrease in end-tidal CO_2, hypoxia, hypotension, or cardiovascular collapse.

2. **Treatment** begins with limiting the entrainment of additional air by flooding the surgical field with saline or repositioning the patient. Nitrous oxide should be discontinued to avoid enlarging air bubbles within the circulation. FIO_2 should be increased to facilitate the resorption of entrained air. Placing the patient in a head-down and left lateral decubitus position may help reduce air collection from blocking right ventricular filling and limit air entering the pulmonary artery. If a central venous catheter is in place, it may be aspirated in an attempt to remove air. Fluids, especially vasopressors (such as norepinephrine) and inotropes, are used to maintain blood pressure and support cardiac contractility. ACLS including chest compressions may be necessary.
3. **The use of PEEP** in the setting of air embolism is controversial. It will limit the entrainment of air by raising CVP but at the expense of reducing venous return and possibly cardiac output. **Hyperbaric oxygen** may be considered in cases where a large amount of gas has been entrained.

C. **Fat embolism** occurs after trauma or surgery involving the long bones, pelvis, or ribs.
  1. **Clinical features** are related to mechanical obstruction of the pulmonary circulation and are similar to those found with pulmonary thromboembolism. The release of free fatty acids may lead to diminished mental status, worsening hypoxemia, fat globules in the urine, disseminated intravascular coagulation, thrombocytopenia, and petechial hemorrhages.
  2. **Treatment is supportive**, with the administration of circulatory support plus supplemental oxygen and ventilation as necessary.

D. **Amniotic fluid emboli** (see Chapter 32: Anesthesia for Obstetrics and Gynecology).

XVI. CARDIAC TAMPONADE

Accumulation of fluid, clots, or loculations within the pericardial sac may prevent adequate ventricular filling and reduce cardiac output. When the accumulation is rapid, cardiovascular collapse may occur within minutes.

A. **Cardiac tamponade** may be associated with the following: chest trauma; cardiac or thoracic surgery; malignancy including lymphoma, leukemia, breast or lung cancer and radiation pericarditis; pericarditis (acute viral, pyogenic, uremic, or postradiation); myocardial perforation by a central venous or pulmonary artery catheter; and aortic dissection, acute MI, collagen vascular disease, and hypothyroidism with myxedema, or it may be idiopathic.

B. **Clinical features** include tachycardia, hypotension, jugular venous distention, muffled heart sounds, and a decrease in pulse pressure.
  1. An ECG may reveal **electrical alternans** (ECG finding of alternating QRS amplitude or axis) and diffusely low voltage.
  2. **Pulsus paradoxus** (a >10-mm Hg inspiratory decrease in systolic blood pressure) may be appreciated.
  3. There may be an **equalization of right- and left-sided heart pressures** as reflected in identical CVP, right ventricular end-diastolic pressure, pulmonary artery diastolic pressure, and pulmonary capillary wedge pressures.
  4. Radiographic findings may include an enlarged cardiac silhouette.
  5. An **echocardiogram** is usually diagnostic.

C. The **treatment** of a hemodynamically unstable patient with suspected cardiac tamponade is pericardiocentesis. Intravascular volume should be augmented, and vasopressors that maintain chronotropy and inotropy (ie, epinephrine) are administered to maintain blood pressure. A long needle is inserted between the xiphoid process and the left costal margin and directed toward the left shoulder. If the precordial lead of the ECG is attached to the needle, an injury current (ST segment elevation) will be observed when the needle contacts the epicardium. The needle should be withdrawn slightly and aspirated. Ultrasound-guided pericardiocentesis in the hands of a skilled operator can be accomplished by introducing a needle through the chest wall and aspirating the fluid accumulation where it is closest to the skin under continuous visualization. Positive-pressure ventilation should be avoided or used with caution as any increase in intrathoracic pressure could exacerbate tamponade physiology.

1. **Complications of pericardiocentesis** include pneumothorax, coronary artery laceration, and myocardial perforation. A surgical pericardial window is a more permanent approach to alleviating tamponade.

XVII. MALIGNANT HYPERTHERMIA

A. Etiology. Malignant hyperthermia is a hypermetabolic syndrome occurring in genetically susceptible patients after exposure to an anesthetic-triggering agent. **Triggering anesthetics** include all potent inhalational agents (eg, halothane, isoflurane, desflurane, and sevoflurane) and succinylcholine. Most cases are due to an inherited mutation in the ryanodine receptor, the calcium release channel in the sarcoplasmic reticulum. Abnormal function of this receptor causes a reduction in the reuptake of Ca^{2+} by the sarcoplasmic reticulum necessary for the termination of muscle contraction. Consequently, muscle contraction is sustained, resulting in signs of hypermetabolism, including tachycardia, acidosis, hypercarbia, muscle rigidity, tachypnea, hypoxemia, and hyperthermia. Malignant hyperthermia usually occurs in the operating room, but onset may be delayed until the patient reaches the postanesthesia care unit or even the postoperative floor.

B. Clinical features
1. Unexplained tachycardia.
2. Hypercarbia in the mechanically ventilated patient or tachypnea in the spontaneously breathing patient who is unresponsive to increased minute ventilation.
3. Metabolic acidosis.
4. Muscle rigidity even in the presence of neuromuscular blockade. Masseter spasm after giving succinylcholine is associated with malignant hyperthermia. However, not all patients who develop masseter spasm will develop malignant hyperthermia.
5. Hypoxemia.
6. Ventricular dysrhythmias.
7. Hyperkalemia.
8. Fever is often a late sign.
9. Myoglobinuria.

C. Treatment
1. **Summon help** as soon as malignant hyperthermia is suspected. Discontinue all triggering anesthetics and hyperventilate with 100% oxygen from a new source such as wall oxygen via an Ambu bag. Convert to a total intravenous anesthetic such as propofol. Surgery should be concluded as quickly as possible, and the anesthesia machine should be changed when feasible.
2. **Administer dantrolene or Ryanodex. Dantrolene** (Dantrium), 2.5 mg/kg IV is given initially and repeated to a total of 10 mg/kg or more if signs

of malignant hyperthermia persist. Dantrolene is the only known specific treatment for malignant hyperthermia. Its efficacy is due to its ability to inhibit Ca^{2+} release from the sarcoplasmic reticulum. Each ampule contains 20 mg of dantrolene and 3 g of mannitol and should be reconstituted with 50 mL of warm sterile water. **Ryanodex** is a newer formulation of dantrolene sodium with increased solubility. Each vial of Ryanodex contains 250 mg dantrolene sodium and 125 mg mannitol and should be reconstituted with 5 mL sterile water. Ryanodex dosing is the same as for the less soluble dantrolene.
3. **Sodium bicarbonate administration** should be guided by pH and partial pressure of carbon dioxide (PCO_2) measurements.
4. **Hyperkalemia** may be corrected with insulin, glucose, and an inhaled β-agonist (eg, albuterol). However, hypokalemia may occur as the hypermetabolic state is brought under control. Calcium administration should be avoided.
5. **Dysrhythmias** generally subside with the resolution of the hypermetabolic phase of malignant hyperthermia. Persistent dysrhythmias should be treated.
6. **Hyperthermia** is treated by a variety of methods (see Section VIII).
7. **Urine output** ideally should be maintained at 2 mL/kg/min to avoid renal tubular damage from myoglobin. A Foley catheter should be placed as soon as possible.
8. **Recrudescence, disseminated intravascular coagulation, and acute tubular necrosis** may occur after an acute episode of malignant hyperthermia. Therefore, dantrolene therapy (1 mg/kg IV or orally every 6 hours) and close observation should be continued for 48 to 72 hours after an episode of malignant hyperthermia.
9. Contact the malignant hyperthermia hotline if necessary, at 1-800-MH-HYPER (1-800-644-9737) from within the United States. Information can also be obtained at www.mhaus.org.

D. **Anesthesia for malignant hyperthermia–susceptible patients**
1. A **family history** of anesthetic problems suggesting susceptibility, such as unexplained fevers or death during anesthesia, should be sought in every patient.
2. **Malignant hyperthermia (MH)** may be triggered in susceptible patients who have had previous uneventful exposures to triggering agents.
3. **Pretreatment with dantrolene** is not recommended for malignant hyperthermia–susceptible patients. A malignant hyperthermia cart or other dantrolene supply, however, should be immediately available.
4. **The anesthesia machine** should be prepared by changing the carbon dioxide absorbent and fresh gas tubing, disconnecting the vaporizers, using a disposable breathing circuit with charcoal filters if available, and flushing the machine with oxygen at a rate of 10 L/min for at least 20 minutes. The preparation of modern anesthesia machines is variable. Some are more difficult to prepare and may require prolonged flushing times with maximal fresh gas flows, whereas others only require carbon filters in the inspiratory and expiratory limbs of the circuit.
5. **Local or regional anesthesia** should be considered, but general anesthesia with nontriggering agents is acceptable. **Safe drugs** for induction and maintenance of general anesthesia include barbiturates, propofol, benzodiazepines, opioids, and nitrous oxide. Nondepolarizing neuromuscular blockers may be used and safely reversed.
6. **Close monitoring** for early signs of malignant hyperthermia such as unexplained hypercarbia or tachycardia is crucial.

E. **Associated syndromes.** An increased risk of malignant hyperthermia has been reported in association with several disorders. In many of these cases, the association is not well established. However, patients with the following disorders should be treated as though they are susceptible to malignant hyperthermia:
   1. **King–Denborough syndrome,** characterized by dwarfism, mental retardation, and musculoskeletal abnormalities.
   2. **Central core disease,** a rare myopathy.
   3. **Multiminicore disease,** another rare myopathy.
   4. **Duchenne muscular dystrophy** and other **muscular dystrophies** are not associated with malignant hyperthermia but may be associated with hyperkalemia.
F. **Neuroleptic malignant syndrome (NMS)** is associated with the administration of neuroleptic drugs and shares many of the features of malignant hyperthermia.
   1. **Clinical features.** NMS typically develops over 24 to 72 hours and is clinically similar to malignant hyperthermia, presenting as a hypermetabolic episode consisting of hyperthermia, autonomic nervous system instability, pronounced muscle rigidity, and rhabdomyolysis. Creatine kinase and hepatic transaminases often are increased, and mortality approaches 30%.
   2. **Treatment** of NMS is with dantrolene, although benzodiazepines, dopamine antagonists such as bromocriptine, and nondepolarizing muscle relaxants will also decrease muscle rigidity.
   3. **Anesthetic implications.** The exact relationship between NMS and malignant hyperthermia is unclear. Some patients with a history of NMS may be at risk for malignant hyperthermia, and a conservative approach may be warranted (eg, avoidance of known triggering agents). Patients with NMS must be appropriately monitored for malignant hyperthermia during all anesthetics (eg, temperature and end-tidal carbon dioxide). They should not be pretreated with dantrolene.

XVIII. ANAPHYLACTIC AND ANAPHYLACTOID REACTIONS
A. **Anaphylaxis** is a life-threatening allergic reaction. It is initiated by antigen binding to preformed IgE antibodies on the surface of mast cells and basophils, which cause the release of vasoactive substances (eg, histamine, leukotrienes, prostaglandins, kinins, and platelet-activating factor). Anaphylaxis is characterized by an acute elevation in tryptase levels.
B. **Anaphylactoid reactions** are clinically similar to anaphylactic reactions, but they are not mediated by IgE and do not require prior sensitization to an antigen.
C. **Clinical features** of anaphylactic or anaphylactoid reactions may include the following:
   1. Urticaria and flushing.
   2. Bronchospasm or airway edema, which can produce respiratory failure.
   3. Hypotension and shock due to peripheral vasodilation and increased capillary permeability.
   4. Pulmonary edema.
D. **Treatment**
   1. **Discontinue anesthetic agents** if circulatory collapse is present.
   2. **Administer 100% oxygen.** Assess the need to intubate and support ventilation. Airway edema can persist beyond the acute event.
   3. **Begin intravascular volume expansion.**

4. **Treat hypotension by giving epinephrine** 50 to 100 μg IV. For overt cardiovascular collapse, epinephrine 0.5 to 1.0 mg IV is indicated, followed by an infusion if hypotension persists. Epinephrine is useful for treating hypotension and bronchospasm and for limiting mast cell degranulation. Other catecholamines such as norepinephrine may be added. Vasopressin should be added in refractory causes.
5. **Steroids** (eg, hydrocortisone 250 mg to 1.0 g IV, or methylprednisolone 1 to 2 g IV) may reduce the inflammatory response.
6. **Histamine antagonists** (eg, diphenhydramine 50 mg IV and ranitidine 50 mg IV in the adult) may be useful as second-line therapy.
7. **Consider** drawing a tryptase level after stabilization of the patient to aid in final diagnosis.

E. **Prophylaxis for drug hypersensitivity reactions**
1. **Histamine (H_1) antagonists.** Diphenhydramine 0.5 to 1.0 mg/kg or 50 mg IV in the adult the night before and morning of exposure.
2. **H_2 antagonists.** Ranitidine 50 mg IV or 150 mg orally in the adult the night before and the morning of exposure.
3. **Corticosteroids.** Prednisone 1 mg/kg or 50 mg for adults, four doses every 6 hours before exposure.

XIX. FIRE AND ELECTRICAL HAZARDS IN THE OPERATING ROOM

A. **Fire** in the operating room is a rare event that requires the presence of an ignition source, fuel, and an oxidizing agent.
1. **Lasers and electrocautery devices** are the most common ignition sources.
2. **Fuels** include alcohol, solvents, sheets, drapes, and plastic or rubber materials (including endotracheal tubes). Modern potent inhalation anesthetics are not fuels. During an electrical fire, it is important to unplug the electrical source.
3. **Oxygen** is by far the most common oxidizing agent, although nitrous oxide also supports combustion. Materials that are only marginally combustible in air can produce a massive flame in the presence of a high oxygen concentration. Supplemental oxygen can accumulate under surgical drapes and should be administered only when medically indicated.
4. **Fire extinguishers** should be readily available in all anesthetizing locations. Carbon dioxide and halon fire extinguishers offer the advantage of efficacy against a variety of fires without producing the particulate contamination associated with dry chemical extinguishers.

B. **Electrical safety**
1. **Macroshock** is an electrical injury caused when a large current passes through intact skin producing a thermal, neural, or muscular injury. It may disrupt normal physiologic function and cause cardiac or respiratory arrest. The level of injury varies with the source frequency and individuals, but, in general, the following guidelines can be applied for an alternating current of 60 cycles/s:
   a. **1 mA for 1 second.** Threshold of perception
   b. **5 mA for 1 second.** Accepted as maximum harmless current intensity. Level at which line isolation monitors alarm.
   c. **10 to 20 mA for 1 second.** Current that results in sustained muscular contraction, referred to as the "Let go current."
   d. **100 mA for 1 second.** Threshold for ventricular fibrillation.
2. **Microshock** occurs when small currents pass directly to the heart. This occurs intentionally when using cardiac pacemakers but can be harmful if it occurs inadvertently. Ventricular fibrillation can be produced

by as little as **100 μA** of current applied to the myocardium. This current is well below the 2- to 5-mA threshold of the line isolation monitor alarm; thus, line isolation monitors do not protect a patient from microshock. To minimize the likelihood of microshock, all equipment should be properly grounded with a three-prong plug and connections to the patient should be electrically isolated. Battery operation does not ensure electrical isolation.
3. **Line isolation monitors** are designed to alert the anesthesiologist when faulty ground connections place patients and operating room personnel at risk of potential exposure to large currents (2 to 5 mA). The line isolation monitor alarms when one of the two "hot" power lines becomes grounded, creating a first fault. This event signals that someone in the operating room may receive a macroshock if they touch any electrical equipment supplied by this circuit, as they now serve as the ground for the system, creating the second fault. If the line isolation monitor alarms, unplug the last appliance that was plugged in. Further investigation into the appliance or circuit will be necessary. Although line isolation monitors continue to be used in operating rooms, most electrical equipment used today have built-in electrical isolation, and many modern operating rooms contain ground fault interrupters on electrical outlets.
4. **Burns from electrosurgical units** may result from poor contact between the dispersive electrode (grounding pad) and the patient. Under such conditions, anything that is grounded may provide an alternative pathway for current, resulting in a burn at these sites. The risk of burns can be minimized by ensuring that the electrode gel is adequate, that the dispersive electrode is placed near the surgical site, and that the patient is insulated from possible alternative pathways for current flow.

XX. EQUIPMENT MALFUNCTIONS

For further information on monitoring, see Chapter 15: Monitoring. In the section that follows, common technical challenges that arise with monitoring equipment and suggestions for troubleshooting are discussed.

A. Cardiovascular system
1. **ECG**
   a. Electrocautery, motion, or inadequate pad contact with skin may interfere with ECG reading.
   b. Magnetic resonance imaging (MRI)-safe ECG pads may encounter interference when the MRI is actively scanning.
   c. Placement of ECG pads will affect the morphology of the waveform. Check that ECF electrodes are appropriately placed to detect dysrhythmias and ischemia.
2. **Noninvasive blood pressure monitoring**
   a. Check that the blood pressure cuff size is appropriate for the patient. A cuff that is too small may result in a falsely high reading. A cuff that is too large may result in a falsely low reading.
   b. External compression (eg, surgeon leaning on patient's arm) may cause reading errors.
3. **Arterial line**
   a. **An overdampened waveform** will cause an artificially low blood pressure measurement with a narrowed pulse pressure. This may be due to arterial obstruction, catheter occlusion, excess tubing, stopcocks, air bubbles, or pressure tubing kinks.
   b. **An underdampened waveform** will cause an artificially high blood pressure measurement with a wide pulse pressure. This may be due

to the use of nonrigid tubing or hyperresonance caused by the reverberation of pressure waves.
B. Respiratory system
1. Pulse oximeter
   a. Ensure proper placement of light-emitting diodes.
   b. Inadequate perfusion, motion, artificially colored or augmented fingernails, the presence of carboxyhemoglobin or methemoglobin, and injections of methylene blue, indocyanine green, indigo carmine, and isosulfan blue may cause saturation readings to be uninterpretable or unreadable.
2. **End-tidal CO_2**
   a. Sampling can be obscured by moisture in the sample line or water trap. Consider replacing clogged parts.
C. Neurologic system
1. EEG monitoring. Current methods of intraoperative electroencephalographic (EEG) recordings rely on surface electrodes placed on the frontal scalp.
   a. Ensure adequate contact between electrodes and the patient's skin.
   b. Adjust amplitude scale to maximize visualization of all frequencies.
   c. Use of electrocautery and patient movement may interfere with EEG monitoring.

ACKNOWLEDGMENT

We gratefully acknowledge the contributions of previous edition author, Frances K. W. Chen, as portions of those chapters have been retained in this revision.

Suggested Readings

Chacko T, Ledford D. Peri-anesthetic anaphylaxis. *Immunol Allergy Clin North Am.* 2007; 27(2):213–230.

Cottron N, Larcher C, Sommet A, et al. The sevoflurane washout profile of seven recent anesthesia workstations for malignant hyperthermia-susceptible adults and infants: A bench test study. *Anesth Analg.* 2014;119:67–75.

Ebo DG, Fisher MM, Hagendorens MM, Bridts CH, Stevens WJ. Anaphylaxis during anaesthesia: Diagnostic approach. *Allergy.* 2007;62:471–487.

Flood P, Rathmell JP, Shafer S. *Stoelting's Pharmacology and Physiology in Anesthetic Practice.* 5th ed. Wolters Kluwer; 2014.

Fuchshuber P, Jones S, Josens D, Feldman LS, Schwaitzberg S, Rozner MA. Ensuring safety in the operating room—the "fundamental use of surgical energy" (FUSE) program. *Int Anesthesiol Clin.* 2013;51:65–80.

Gaba DM, Fish KJ, Howard SN, et al. *Crisis Management in Anesthesiology.* 2nd ed. Churchill Livingstone; 2014.

Hines RL, Marschall KE. *Stoelting's Anesthesia and Co-existing Disease.* 6th ed. Saunders; 2012.

Kim TW, Nemergut ME. Preparation of modern anesthesia workstations for malignant hyperthermia-susceptible patients: A review of past and present practice. *Anesthesiology.* 2011;114:205–212.

Lobato EB, Gravenstein N, Kirby RR. *Complications in Anesthesiology.* Lippincott; 2007.

Marik PE. Aspiration pneumonitis and aspiration pneumonia. *N Engl J Med.* 2001;344: 665–671.

Marik PE, Cavallazzi R, Vasu T, Hirani A. Dynamic changes in arterial waveform derived variables and fluid responsiveness in mechanically ventilated patients: A systematic review of the literature. *Crit Care Med.* 2009;36:2642–2647.

Simons ER, Ardusso LR, Bilo MB, et al. International consensus on (ICON) anaphylaxis. *World Allergy Organ J.* 2014;7:1–19.

Zacharias M, Mugawar M, Herbison GP, et al. Interventions for protecting renal function in the perioperative period. *Cochrane Database Syst Rev.* 2013;9:CD003590.

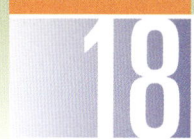

Perioperative Hemodynamic Control

Victoria Bass and William Benedetto

I. BLOOD PRESSURE

The aim of perioperative hemodynamic management strategies is to maintain adequate organ perfusion. Since organ perfusion itself is difficult to measure, systemic blood pressure is monitored as an indicator of blood flow and organ perfusion. The relationship between systemic blood pressure and systemic perfusion can be modeled by the mechanical analogue of Ohm law: $MAP - CVP = CO \times SVR$, where MAP represents mean arterial pressure, CVP represents central venous pressure, CO represents cardiac output, and SVR represents systemic vascular resistance. By solving the equation for CO, it becomes apparent that changes in MAP do not always reflect changes in CO.

A. CO is influenced by heart rate, preload, afterload, myocardial compliance, and contractility. These variables are intimately interdependent and regulated by the autonomic nervous system and humoral factors.

II. AUTOREGULATION

Autoregulation describes the ability of an organ to maintain adequate blood flow despite varying **perfusion pressure**, the pressure gradient across an organ's vascular bed. Organs vary in autoregulatory reserve or the ability to increase or decrease vascular resistance in order to couple organ blood flow with metabolic demand. Vasodilating anesthetic agents interfere with organ autoregulation mechanisms. Accordingly, organ perfusion under anesthesia becomes more dependent on systemic blood pressure.

III. ADRENERGIC RECEPTOR PHYSIOLOGY (TABLE 18.1)

Adrenergic receptors bind **catecholamines** to mediate many physiologic functions. The endogenous catecholamines include epinephrine, norepinephrine, and dopamine. Many drugs used to control blood pressure perioperatively act on adrenergic receptors. α-adrenergic receptors are activated by norepinephrine, epinephrine, and isoproterenol in descending order of responsiveness. β-adrenergic receptors demonstrate the inverse, with the greatest activity in response to isoproterenol, followed by epinephrine, and finally norepinephrine. Receptors that interact with dopamine are termed **dopaminergic**. Adrenergic receptors can be further subdivided based on their anatomic location and downstream effects:

A. α_1-receptors are located postsynaptically in vascular smooth muscle, the uterus, skin, intestinal mucosa, iris, splanchnic bed, and myocardium. Activation causes arteriolar and venous constriction, mydriasis, and relaxation of the intestinal tract. Activation of cardiac α_1-receptors results in a mild increase in inotropy.

B. α_2-receptors exist in multiple subtypes and are found throughout the central nervous system (CNS) and autonomic nervous system, playing roles in wakefulness, attention, nociception, and autonomic modulation.

   1. Presynaptic α_2-receptors at peripheral adrenergic nerve terminals are involved in feedback inhibition to decrease sympathetic transmission.

TABLE 18.1 Adrenergic Receptors and Their Effect Sites

Receptor	Site of Action	Effect	Agonists	Antagonists
α_1	Vascular smooth muscle Uterus Skin Intestinal mucosa Iris Splanchnic bed	Inotropy Vasoconstriction Mydriasis Uterine contraction Sphincter constriction Bronchoconstriction Inhibition of insulin secretion	Phenylephrine[a] Norepinephrine Epinephrine Methyldopa Clonidine Dexmedetomidine	Phenoxybenzamine Phentolamine Terazosin Prazosin Labetalol Carvedilol
α_2	Presynaptic: CNS Adrenergic nerve terminals Postsynaptic: Vascular smooth muscle Gastrointestinal tract Pancreatic β cells CNS	Inhibit neurotransmitter release (NE, ACh, DA, 5-HT) Hypnosis, sedation, analgesia ↓ sympathetic tone (bradycardia, vasodilation) Vasoconstriction ↓ insulin release ↓ salivation Hypnosis, sedation, analgesia ↓ sympathetic tone (bradycardia, vasodilation)	Dexmedetomidine Clonidine Tizanidine Epinephrine Norepinephrine Phenylephrine Methyldopa	Phenoxybenzamine Phentolamine Labetalol
β_1	Myocardium SA node Cardiac conduction system Kidneys Adipose tissue	Inotropy Chronotropy Renin release Lipolysis	Isoproterenol Epinephrine Dobutamine Norepinephrine Dopamine Ephedrine[b] Terbutaline	Atenolol[c] Esmolol[c] Metoprolol[c] Propranolol Labetalol

Receptor	Site of Action	Effect	Agonists	Antagonists
β_2	Vascular smooth muscle Bronchial smooth muscle Myocardium Uterus	Vasodilation Bronchodilation Uterine relaxation Inotropy Insulin release	Isoproterenol Terbutaline Epinephrine Ephedrine[b] Dopamine	Labetalol Propranolol
D_1	Renal smooth muscle Mesenteric smooth muscle	Vasodilation	Fenoldopam Dopamine Dopexamine	[d]
D_2	CNS	Inhibit norepinephrine release	Dopamine Dopexamine	[d]

[a] Agonists listed in descending order of effect.
[b] Primary mode of action for ephedrine is indirect stimulation of catecholamine release.
[c] Selective for β_1-receptors.
[d] Only hemodynamically significant drugs included in table.
5-HT, serotonin; ACh, acetylcholine; CNS, central nervous system; DA, dopamine; NE, norepinephrine; SA, sinoatrial.

Their activation reduces norepinephrine release and has an overall vasodilating effect. Activation of presynaptic α_2-receptors within the CNS also inhibits the release of norepinephrine and other neurotransmitters and is associated with sedation, analgesia, and reduced sympathetic outflow, which contributes to vasodilation and bradycardia.
2. **Postsynaptic α_2-receptors** are located within the CNS and peripherally in vascular smooth muscle, the gastrointestinal (GI) tract, and pancreatic β cells. Activation of peripheral postsynaptic α_2-receptors causes vasoconstriction, decreased salivation, and decreased insulin release. Activation of central postsynaptic α_2-receptors is also associated with sedation, analgesia, and reduced sympathetic outflow.
C. **β_1-receptors** are located in the myocardium, sinoatrial (SA) node, ventricular conduction system, adipose tissue, and renal tissue. Activation increases inotropy, chronotropy, myocardial conduction velocity, renin release, and lipolysis.
D. **β_2-receptors** are located in the myocardium and smooth muscle of the vasculature, bronchi, uterus, and GI tract. Stimulation leads to vasodilation, bronchodilation, uterine relaxation, and a mild increase in inotropy. β_2-receptor activation also promotes gluconeogenesis, insulin release, and potassium uptake by cells.
E. **β_3-receptors** are involved in lipolysis and regulation of metabolic rate.
F. **Dopamine receptors** are divided into five subtypes (D_1, D_2, D_3, D_4, and D_5). These are further classified into a D_1-like family, consisting of D_1 and D_5 receptors, and a D_2-like family, consisting of D_2, D_3, and D_4 receptors.
   1. **D_1-like family dopamine receptors** are mainly located postsynaptically in the peripheral nervous system and CNS. In the renal and mesenteric vascular smooth muscle cells, they directly mediate vasodilation.
   2. **D_2-like family dopamine receptors** are mainly located presynaptically in the peripheral nervous system and CNS. Stimulation of some peripheral D_2-like receptors inhibits norepinephrine release, indirectly causing vasodilation.
G. **Receptor regulation.** There is an inverse relationship between exposure to circulating adrenergic agonists and adrenergic receptor availability through a process of **receptor upregulation and downregulation**. For example, chronic β-blocker therapy leads to the upregulation of β-adrenergic receptors. As a result, the sudden cessation of β-blocker therapy may be associated with hypersensitivity to endogenous catecholamines, resulting in rebound hypertension and tachycardia with increased risk for developing myocardial ischemia.

IV. ADRENERGIC AGONISTS (TABLE 18.2)
A. **α-agonists**
   1. **Phenylephrine** is a direct-acting α_1-agonist at typical clinical doses of 40 to 200 µg/min. Phenylephrine causes both arterial and venous vasoconstriction. This dual action increases venous return and mean arterial blood pressure, frequently resulting in reflex bradycardia. Phenylephrine maintains CO in patients with normal myocardial function but may decrease cardiac performance in the presence of myocardial ischemia. Phenylephrine has a short duration of action, which makes it easily titratable.
   2. **Midodrine** is an orally administered α_1-agonist approved for the treatment of symptomatic orthostatic hypotension at doses of 2.5 to 10 mg TID. It is a prodrug that mediates its clinical effect through its active metabolite, desglymidodrine. Midodrine is increasingly used off-label

TABLE 18.2 Drug Dosages of Commonly Used Vasopressors and Inotropes

Drug Name (Trade Name)	IV Bolus	Mix[a]	IV Infusion Kinetics[b]	Dose	α₁	β₁	β₂	D₁	V₁
Arginine vasopressin (Pitressin)	NR	50 units/250 mL (0.2 units/mL)	O: <15 min D: 10–20 min	0.04 unit/min (range 0.01–0.1 unit/min)					+++
Dobutamine (Dobutrex)	NR	250 mg/250 mL (1000 μg/mL)	O: <10 min D: 5–10 min	2–20 μg/kg/min	+	+++	++		
Dopamine (Inotropin)	NR	200 mg/250 mL (800 μg/mL)	O: <5 min D: 5–10 min	1–5 μg/kg/min 5–10 μg/kg/min 10–20 μg/kg/min	+ ++ +++	+ ++ ++	+ +	+++ ++ +	
Ephedrine	5–10 mg	NR	O: <5 min D: 15–20 min[c]	NR	++	++			
Epinephrine (Adrenaline)	20–100 μg (hypotension) 0.5–1 mg (cardiac arrest)	1 mg/250 mL (4 μg/mL)	O: <1 min D: 1–2 min	0.01–0.03 μg/kg/min 0.03–0.1 μg/kg/min >0.1 μg/kg/min	+ +++	+++ +++ ++	+ +		
Isoproterenol (Isuprel)	NR	1 mg/250 mL (4 μg/mL)	O: <1 min D: 10–15 min	2–10 μg/min		+++	+++		
Milrinone	NR	20 mg/100 mL (200 μg/mL)	O: 5–15 min D: 3–5 h	0.375–0.75 μg/kg/min[d]					
Norepinephrine (Levophed)	2–8 μg	4 mg/250 mL (16 μg/mL)	O: <1 min D: 1–2 min	1–30 μg/min	+++	++			
Phenylephrine (Neosynephrine)	40–100 μg	10 mg/250 mL (40 μg/mL)	O: <1 min D: 5–10 min	10–150 μg/min	+++				

[a]Massachusetts General Hospital infusion mix in 5% dextrose in water.
[b]O, onset; D, duration of action.
[c]Times given for single IV bolus dose.
[d]Optional 50 μg/kg IV load over 10 min; dosage adjustments required for renally impaired patients.
D₁, dopamine-1 receptor; IV, intravenous; V, vasopressin receptor; NR, not recommended.

to prevent hemodialysis-related hypotension and to facilitate weaning of vasopressors in the ICU despite limited data on safety and efficacy. A recent meta-analysis demonstrated that the use of midodrine to wean off vasopressors was not associated with a significant decrease in ICU length of stay, hospital length of stay, mortality, or ICU readmissions.
3. **Clonidine** is a centrally acting antihypertensive with relative selectivity for α_2-adrenoreceptors. Its actions include reducing sympathetic tone, increasing parasympathetic tone, reducing anesthetic and analgesic requirements, causing sedation, and decreasing salivation. It may be administered intravenously, intramuscularly, orally, transcutaneously, epidurally, and intrathecally. Abrupt cessation of clonidine is associated with rebound hypertension, thus doses should be gradually tapered when discontinuing.
4. **Dexmedetomidine** is a selective α_2-adrenoreceptor agonist approved for intensive care unit sedation (intubated and mechanically ventilated patients) and procedural sedation (nonintubated patients) in adults. Its action on presynaptic receptors inhibits the release of norepinephrine, and its activation of postsynaptic α_2-receptors in the CNS inhibits sympathetic activity. These effects decrease blood pressure and heart rate. Dexmedetomidine offers potential advantages over other sedatives, including reduced respiratory depression, delirium, and hypotension.

B. β-agonists (please refer to Table 18.2 for recommended dose ranges)

1. **Isoproterenol** is a direct-acting, nonselective β-adrenergic agonist. It increases heart rate and contractility through its actions at β_1-receptors and reduces SVR through its actions on β_2-receptors. Its overall effect on CO is neutral. Other β_2-mediated effects of isoproterenol include bronchodilation and pulmonary vasodilation.
   a. **Indications**
      1. Hemodynamically significant, atropine-resistant bradycardia
      2. Atrioventricular (AV) nodal block, until temporary pacing can be instituted
      3. Maintenance of an elevated heart rate, such as in pediatric patients who have a fixed stroke volume and cardiac transplant recipients
      4. Status asthmaticus
      5. β-blocker overdose
   b. **Monitoring.** Continuous electrocardiographic monitoring is recommended with IV administration. Isoproterenol may be safely administered through a peripheral IV.
   c. **Adverse effects** include hypotension and tachydysrhythmias. Isoproterenol may contribute to an imbalance in myocardial oxygen supply and demand, leading to myocardial ischemia.

C. Mixed agonists

1. **Epinephrine** is a direct-acting α- and β-receptor agonist, produced by the adrenal medulla.
   a. **Indications**
      1. Cardiac arrest
      2. Anaphylaxis
      3. Bronchospasm
      4. Cardiogenic shock
      5. Symptomatic bradycardia or heart block
   b. **Clinical use.** The clinical effect of epinephrine is determined by its activation of both α- and β-receptors, with β effects predominating at lower doses. At very low doses (eg, 0.01 µg/kg/min), epinephrine

primarily causes bronchodilation. At usual clinical doses (0.03 to 0.1 µg/kg/min), epinephrine acts on α- and β-receptors to increase inotropy, chronotropy, and vasoconstriction. At even higher doses (>0.1 µg/kg/min), α effects predominate, and stroke volume may fall as SVR increases. Dose-limiting adverse effects include significant tachycardia, dysrhythmias, and myocardial ischemia. Volatile anesthetics can sensitize the myocardium to epinephrine, leading to potentially life-threatening dysrhythmias. Epinephrine should be administered through central venous access whenever possible as extravasation may lead to tissue necrosis.

2. **Norepinephrine** is released by postganglionic sympathetic neurons and binds adrenergic receptors at target organs. Biosynthetically, it is the precursor of epinephrine. Norepinephrine is a potent α_1- and β_1-receptor agonist, with α effects predominating at lower doses. Compared to epinephrine, norepinephrine has minimal effects on β_2-receptors. Norepinephrine increases blood pressure by increasing SVR. However, organ perfusion may suffer despite increases in MAP due to increased vascular resistance across organs. CO remains relatively unchanged. As with most vasoactive agents, intra-arterial blood pressure monitoring and continuous cardiac rhythm monitoring are recommended. In most cases, norepinephrine should be administered centrally, although dilute concentrations (eg, 16 µg/mL) may be safely administered through reliable peripheral access temporarily. Adverse effects include arrhythmias and worsening microvascular perfusion (eg, digital ischemia), particularly at higher doses.

3. **Dopamine,** the biosynthetic precursor of norepinephrine, produces a dose-related combination of α-, β-, and dopamine receptor effects. It also causes the release of norepinephrine from nerve terminals in the heart. At lower doses (<5 µg/kg/min), dopamine primarily activates renal and splanchnic vessel D_1 receptors, resulting in increased renal blood flow, glomerular filtration, and sodium excretion. Although dopamine administration often increases urine output, it has not been shown to improve mortality outcomes or the need for renal replacement therapy. At 5 to 10 µg/kg/min, β effects become more apparent, leading to increases in myocardial contractility, heart rate, and arterial blood pressure. At high doses (>10 µg/kg/min), α_1 effects predominate, leading to marked increases in arterial and venous blood pressure and decreases in renal blood flow. Dopamine is used in the management of cardiogenic shock, vasodilatory shock, heart failure, and refractory bradycardia. Adverse effects include tachycardia, ventricular arrhythmias, increased myocardial oxygen consumption, and profound vasoconstriction.

4. **Dobutamine** is a synthetic catecholamine available clinically as a racemic mixture of stereoisomers with the L(−)-isomer stimulating α_1-receptors and the D(+)-isomer stimulating β_1- and β_2-receptors. Through its effect on cardiac β_1-receptors, dobutamine increases myocardial contractility and chronotropy. In the peripheral vasculature, dobutamine generally has a vasodilatory effect owing to its more dominant β_2 action, despite its α_1 properties. Dobutamine is a useful agent for treating low CO states caused by acute myocardial infarction, cardiomyopathy, and myocardial depression after cardiac surgery. Dobutamine typically reduces or has a neutral effect on pulmonary vascular resistance (PVR), which may be beneficial for patients with right ventricular failure. Systemic hypotension, increased myocardial oxygen consumption, and tachydysrhythmias are the most common side effects.

5. **Ephedrine** is a noncatecholamine, indirect adrenergic agonist that causes the release of norepinephrine and other endogenous catecholamines stored within nerve terminals. It is used primarily in the management of anesthetic-related hypotension and bradycardia. Administration is limited to intermittent boluses as tachyphylaxis develops quickly.

V. NONADRENERGIC AGENTS
A. Nonadrenergic vasopressors
1. **Arginine vasopressin (AVP)** is a synthetic analogue of antidiuretic hormone. AVP causes vasoconstriction by direct stimulation of vascular smooth muscle V_1 receptors. It is frequently used as a second pressor in septic shock requiring high-dose norepinephrine, although a mortality benefit has not been demonstrated. Results of the Vasopressin and Septic Shock Trial (VASST) suggest a benefit when AVP is used in patients with less severe shock or in those at risk for renal failure. AVP may also be beneficial as a low-dose (0.04 unit/min) IV infusion in vasodilatory shock exacerbated by chronic angiotensin-converting enzyme (ACE) inhibitor therapy. AVP may be preferred in the setting of pulmonary hypertension as it preferentially constricts peripheral vasculature while sparing the pulmonary vasculature. AVP has a rapid onset with a duration of action of 10 to 20 minutes. Administration through a central venous catheter is recommended.
2. **Methylene blue** is used therapeutically as a redox agent in the treatment of methemoglobinemia (1 mg/kg IV over 5 minutes) and used diagnostically as an indicator dye in urologic surgery to assess the integrity of the urinary system. Methylene blue competitively inhibits guanylate cyclase, which decreases the production of cyclic guanosine monophosphate (cGMP), and renders the vascular endothelium less sensitive to cGMP-mediated vasodilators including **nitric oxide**. Methylene blue has been effective in the management of vasoplegia associated with cardiopulmonary bypass (eg, slow bolus of 2 mg/kg followed by an infusion of 0.5 mg/kg/h for 12 hours). As a reversible inhibitor of monoamine oxidase, methylene blue must be used with caution in patients on serotonergic medications including selective serotonin reuptake inhibitors, serotonin and norepinephrine reuptake inhibitors, and monoamine oxidase inhibitors, as fatal cases of serotonin syndrome have been reported. Other adverse effects include dysrhythmias, increased PVR, coronary vasoconstriction, and acute hemolytic anemia in patients with glucose-6-phosphate dehydrogenase deficiency. Administration of methylene blue may produce falsely low readings on pulse oximetry.

B. Nonadrenergic inotropes
1. **Cardiac glycosides** were the first inotropes to be used clinically. They are naturally occurring compounds found in plants (eg, foxgloves). Within this family of drugs, **digoxin** remains in clinical use today. The inotropic effect of digoxin derives from the inhibition of the sodium-potassium ATPase, secondarily promoting an influx of calcium into cardiac myocytes via the sodium-calcium exchanger. It additionally has a direct suppressive effect on the AV node. Therapeutically, digoxin is reserved for rate control refractory to β-blockers and for refractory chronic heart failure symptoms despite maximal medical management. Its use is limited by its narrow therapeutic window, many drug interactions, and lack of mortality benefit. Perioperatively, digoxin should be continued for patients on a stable regimen.

2. **Phosphodiesterase III inhibitors** act by inhibiting type III phosphodiesterase (PDE3), thereby increasing cyclic adenosine monophosphate, leading to increased contractility as well as pulmonary and peripheral vasodilation. PDE3 inhibitors are synergistic with adrenergic agents.
    a. **Milrinone** is used for cardiac support in patients with acute heart failure, pulmonary hypertension, chronic heart failure, and after cardiac surgery. Typical dosing involves a loading dose of 50 μg/kg administered over 10 minutes followed by an infusion of 0.375 to 0.75 μg/kg/min. Adverse effects include hypotension, ventricular arrhythmias, cardiac ischemia, and torsades de pointes. Its prolonged elimination half-life of 2 to 4 hours requires that it be introduced with caution in unstable patients. Coadministration with a vasopressor is often necessary to counter vasodilation.

VI. β-ADRENERGIC ANTAGONISTS (TABLE 18.3)

A. **β-blockers** are a mainstay of the perioperative management of sinus tachycardia, other tachyarrhythmias, hypertension, myocardial infarction, and heart failure. They can be distinguished by their adrenergic receptor selectivity and intrinsic sympathomimetic activity.
    1. According to the 2014 American College of Cardiology and American Heart Association guidelines on the management of patients undergoing noncardiac surgery, patients should continue chronic β-blocker perioperatively as abrupt β-blocker cessation may be associated with increased adverse cardiac events. Preoperative initiation of β-blocker therapy may also be considered in patients with three or more revised cardiac risk index risk factors, which include prior stroke (or transient ischemic attack), diabetes mellitus requiring insulin, serum creatinine ≥2 mg/dL, congestive heart failure, coronary artery disease, and high-risk surgery (thoracic, abdominal, or suprainguinal vascular surgery). Both of these guidelines are supported by level B evidence.
    2. β-blockers are contraindicated in patients with severe decompensated heart failure, symptomatic bradycardia in the absence of a pacemaker, and in patients with Wolff–Parkinson–White (WPW) syndrome in atrial fibrillation.
B. **Propranolol** is a nonselective β_1- and β_2-adrenergic receptor antagonist available in both IV and oral forms. Hemodynamic effects of propranolol and other β-adrenergic antagonists are secondary to the reduction of CO and suppression of the renin-angiotensin system. Owing to their β_2-blocking action, nonselective β-blockers may worsen obstructive pulmonary disease. Propranolol has been shown to significantly reduce FEV1 in patients with COPD and is not recommended for use in this population.
C. **Metoprolol** is a selective β_1-adrenergic receptor antagonist available in both oral and IV forms. It is used to treat supraventricular tachycardia (SVT), such as for rate control of atrial fibrillation. It is also effective in the treatment of angina pectoris, in reducing mortality from myocardial infarction and heart failure, and in treating mild hypertension.
D. **Esmolol** is a selective β_1-adrenergic receptor antagonist that is metabolized rapidly by esterases within red blood cells. These esterases are distinct from plasma pseudocholinesterase and are not affected by anticholinesterases. Esmolol has a rapid onset and short duration of action, achieving its peak effect in 5 minutes with an elimination half-life of 9 minutes. These favorable kinetics make it a commonly used drug perioperatively. Prolonged infusions of esmolol in propylene glycol may lead to propylene

TABLE 18.3 β-Adrenergic Antagonists

Drug Name (Trade Name)	β₁-Selective	α₁-Blockade	Bioavailability	Half-Life	Elimination	Oral Dose	IV Dose
Atenolol (Tenormin)	+	−	—	6–7 h	R (85%)	50–100 mg daily	5 mg q10min up to 10 mg total[a]
Esmolol (Brevibloc)	+	−	—	9 min	RBC esterase	—	1 mg/kg bolus; 50–200 μg/kg/min[b]
Metoprolol (Lopressor)	+	−	50%	3–4 h	H	25–100 mg q6h[c]	2.5–5 mg q5min up to 15 mg total
Carvedilol (Coreg)	−	+	30%	7–10 h	H	6.25–50 mg q12h	—
Labetalol (Trandate, Normodyne)	−	+	25%	3–8 h	H	100–800 mg q12h–q8h	5–20 mg initial bolus redosing 20–80 mg q10min up to 300 mg daily
Nadolol (Corgard)	−	−	30%	14–24 h	R (75%)	40–320 mg daily	—
Propranolol (Inderal)	−	−	30–50%	3–6 h	H	10–40 mg q12h–q8h	0.25- to 1-mg increments
Timolol (Blocadren)	−	−	75%	2–4 h	H (80%)	5–20 mg q12h	NA

[a]Not available in the United States.
[b]Optional 0.25 to 0.5 mg/kg load prior to infusion.
[c]Dosing for metoprolol tartrate.
H, hepatic elimination; IV, intravenous; R, renal elimination; RBC, red blood cell.

glycol toxicity marked by encephalopathy and osmolal gap with or without an anion gap metabolic acidosis.

E. **Labetalol** is a combined α- and β-adrenergic receptor antagonist with a β- to α-adrenergic receptor blockade ratio of 3:1 when administered orally and 7:1 when administered intravenously. Its combined effect on both α- and β-receptors leads to decreased blood pressure without reflex tachycardia. Labetalol also decreases PVR and minimally affects CO. Labetalol is useful in the treatment of acute perioperative hypertension due to its rapid onset within 2 to 5 minutes. It is effective in the management of hypertension related to pregnancy, pheochromocytoma, and clonidine withdrawal.

VII. VASODILATORS (TABLE 18.4)

A. **Calcium channel antagonists,** or **calcium channel blockers (CCBs)**, bind L-type calcium channels that regulate calcium entry into vascular smooth muscle, myocardial cells, and cardiac pacemaker cells. They decrease the vascular resistance of peripheral organs, cause coronary artery vasodilation, and are myocardial depressants. CCBs are distinguished by their relative affinities for cardiac versus vascular L-type calcium channels.

1. **Dihydropyridine (DHP)** CCBs are more selective for vascular smooth muscle and are used to treat hypertension. Their physiologic effect is largely arterial vasodilation with minimal effects on venous capacitance.

TABLE 18.4 Vasodilator Infusions

Drug Name (Trade Name)	Mix[a]	IV Infusion Kinetics[b]	Dose	Mechanism of Action
Clevidipine (Cleviprex)	25 mg/50 mL lipid emulsion (0.5 mg/mL)[c]	O: 2–4 min D: 5–10 min	Initial: 1–2 mg/h[d] Usual: 4–8 mg/h	CCB; arterial > venous vasodilation
Nicardipine (Cardene)	40 mg/200 mL (0.2 mg/mL)[c]	O: 5–10 min D: 0.5–8 h	Initial: 5 mg/h[e] Usual: 5–15 mg/h	CCB; arterial > venous vasodilation
Nitroglycerin	50 mg/250 mL (400 μg/mL)	O: 1 min D: 5 min	Initial: 50 μg/min[f] IV bolus: 50–100 μg	NO; venodilation
Nitroprusside (Nipride)	50 mg/250 mL (200 μg/mL)	O: 1–2 min D: 5–10 min	Initial: 0.5 μg/kg/min[f] Usual: 0.5–4 μg/kg/min	NO; arterial > venous vasodilation
Fenoldopam (Corlopam)	10 mg/250 mL (40 μg/mL)	O: 5–10 min D: 1–4 h	Initial: 0.05 μg/kg/min[g] Usual: 0.05–1.5 μg/kg/min	D_1-agonism; arteriodilation

[a]Infusion mix in 5% dextrose in water unless otherwise specified.
[b]O, onset; D, duration of action.
[c]Manufacturer preparation.
[d]Double dose every 90 seconds until approaching blood pressure goal, up to maximum 21 mg/h.
[e]Increase dose by 2.5 mg/h every 5 to 15 min, up to maximum 15 mg/h.
[f]Increase dose every 5 min based on patient responsiveness, up to maximum dose of 400 μg/min.
[g]Increase dose by 0.05 to 0.1 μg/kg/min every 15 minutes, up to a maximum dose of 1.5 μg/kg/min.
CCB, calcium channel blocker; D_1, dopamine-1 receptor; NO, nitric oxide; NR, not recommended.

a. **Clevidipine** is an ultrashort-acting antihypertensive administered by IV infusion ideal for perioperative use due to its rapid onset, titration, and elimination half-life of approximately 1 minute by serum esterases. After cessation, effects last 5 to 10 minutes, with a 90% return to baseline blood pressure by 7 minutes. Infusions are started at 1 to 2 mg/h and doubled every 90 seconds until blood pressure approaches target range. Usual doses are 4 to 8 mg/h. The maximum allowable dose is 21 mg/h.
b. **Nicardipine** is another short-acting antihypertensive administered in IV infusion perioperatively. Infusions are started at 5 mg/h, increased by 2.5 mg/h every 5 to 15 min until target blood pressure is reached, up to a maximum dose of 15 mg/h. Onset is within minutes. After cessation, effects may last up to 8 hours.
c. **Nifedipine** is limited to oral administration for the treatment of hypertension, including hypertension associated with pregnancy, at daily doses of 30 to 90 mg.
d. **Nimodipine** is an oral CCB approved for the prevention of vasospasm in subarachnoid hemorrhage at a dose of 60 mg q4h. Dose reductions are required in hepatic insufficiency.
e. **Amlodipine** is a common oral antihypertensive at daily doses of 5 to 10 mg.
2. **Non-DHP** CCBs are more selective for myocardial and pacemaker L-type calcium channels and are termed **cardioselective**. Verapamil and diltiazem are the two non-DHP CCBs in clinical use.
    a. **Indications**
        1. Antianginal therapy (by decreasing myocardial oxygen consumption and coronary vasospasm)
        2. Rate control (by depressing AV nodal conduction)
        3. Conversion of hemodynamically stable SVTs (by prolonging AV nodal repolarization, blocking reentry)
        4. Hypertension (by affecting vascular smooth muscle L-type calcium channels)
    b. **Contraindications** to CCBs are similar to those of β-blockers. CCBs are not appropriate antiarrhythmics for patients with WPW syndrome in atrial fibrillation/flutter, as they may allow for preferential conduction through the accessory pathway.
    c. **Verapamil** is initially dosed 2.5 to 5 mg IV over 2 minutes, with subsequent doses of 5 to 10 mg IV every 15 to 30 minutes.
    d. **Diltiazem** is initially dosed 10 to 20 mg IV over 2 minutes, which can be redosed up to 0.35 mg/kg after 15 minutes if needed. An infusion of 5 to 15 mg/h can be initiated in responders.
B. **Sodium nitroprusside** is a direct-acting vasodilator that acts on arterial and venous smooth muscle, reducing afterload through arteriolar dilation and reducing preload through venous dilation. Both SVR and PVR decrease.
    1. **Mechanism of action.** Nitroprusside degrades to release **nitric oxide**, an endogenous vasodilator that activates guanylate cyclase, which increases cGMP, and leads to smooth muscle relaxation.
    2. **Dosing.** Infusions may be started at 0.5 μg/kg/min and titrated upward based on blood pressure response every 5 minutes up to a maximum per-minute dose of 400 μg/min (note: not weight based).
    3. **Kinetics.** Nitroprusside is useful perioperatively because it has a fast onset within 2 minutes and its effects dissipate within 2 minutes of discontinuation.

4. **Adverse effects**
   a. **Reflex tachycardia.** Nitroprusside's reduction of preload and afterload typically causes a reflex increase in heart rate and myocardial contractility and an increase in CO.
   b. **Increased intracranial pressure (ICP).** Nitroprusside dilates cerebral blood vessels and should be used with caution in patients with elevated ICP.
   c. **Vascular steal phenomenon.** Global vasodilation may give rise to unintentional imbalances in blood flow. Under normal conditions, ischemic regions are vasodilated by metabolic factors in order to maximize blood supply. Vascular steal phenomenon results when blood supply to a vasodilated ischemic region gets shunted to newly dilated nonischemic regions. This is of particular importance in the coronary vasculature where regional ischemia may be exacerbated by vasodilator-related steal, even when afterload reduction reduces overall myocardial oxygen consumption.
   d. **Cyanide toxicity.** Nitroprusside reacts nonenzymatically with sulfhydryl groups in hemoglobin to release five cyanide radicals. Cyanide toxicity results when cyanide radicals bind cytochrome oxidase, disrupting the electron transport chain, leading to cellular hypoxia and death even in the presence of oxygen. Cyanide radicals can be converted by tissue and liver rhodanese to thiocyanate, which is excreted in the urine. Thiocyanate accumulation in renal insufficiency can cause **thiocyanate toxicity,** which is characterized by abdominal pain, vomiting, and altered mental status.
      1. **Clinical features.** Symptoms of cyanide toxicity include fatigue, nausea, muscle spasms, angina, and confusion. Cyanide toxicity typically occurs when more than 1 mg/kg sodium nitroprusside has been administered within 2.5 hours or when the blood concentration of cyanide reaches 100 µg/dL. Metabolic acidosis and elevated mixed venous oxygen tensions are early signs of cyanide toxicity.
      2. **Treatment.** Sodium thiosulfate is a sulfur donor in the rhodanese reaction that converts cyanide to thiocyanate. After discontinuing nitroprusside and administering 100% oxygen, 150 mg/kg **sodium thiosulfate** should be administered over 15 minutes. Severe cyanide toxicity (base deficit >10 mEq, hemodynamic instability) may require the additional administration of **amyl nitrate** (0.3 mL by inhalation) or 3% **sodium nitrite** (5 mg/kg IV over 5 minutes). These two compounds create methemoglobin, which binds cyanide ions to form inactive cyanmethemoglobin.
C. **Nitroglycerin,** also known as trinitroglycerin, is a potent venodilator that also relaxes arterial, pulmonary, ureteral, uterine, GI, and bronchial smooth muscles. It mediates its effect via conversion to nitric oxide. Nitroglycerin decreases MAP primarily by increasing venous capacitance.
   1. **Indications.** Nitroglycerin is useful for treating congestive heart failure and myocardial ischemia by increasing coronary flow and improving left ventricular performance. Nitroglycerin increases venous capacitance, decreases venous return, and consequently decreases ventricular end-diastolic volume. A decrease in end-diastolic volume is associated with a decrease in ventricular wall tension, which reduces myocardial oxygen consumption.
   2. **Dosing.** Nitroglycerin can be administered as an IV bolus of 50 to 100 µg. The effects of a single bolus disappear within 5 minutes. An initial test

dose of 50 µg or less is often useful to gauge patient responsiveness, which varies widely. Infusions may be started conservatively at 50 µg/min and titrated based on patient responsiveness every 5 minutes up to a maximum dose of 400 µg/min. Nitroglycerin is also available in oral, sublingual, and transdermal routes.
   3. **Reflex tachycardia** frequently occurs and must be treated with β-blockers to avoid increasing myocardial oxygen consumption.
   4. **Tachyphylaxis** often develops within 24 hours of continuous infusion.
   5. **Complications.** Nitroglycerin is metabolized by the liver and has no known toxicity in the clinical dose range. High doses (>250 µg/min) and prolonged continuous use may produce methemoglobinemia. Nitroglycerin produces cerebral vasodilation and should be used with caution in patients at risk for elevated ICP.
D. **Hydralazine** is a direct-acting vasodilator that reduces arteriolar tone in the coronary, cerebral, renal, uterine, and splanchnic beds. It is commonly used to treat hypertensive emergencies or to augment the effect of other hypotensive agents.
   1. **Reflex tachycardia.** The vasodilation induced by hydralazine triggers a reflex increase in heart rate and causes activation of the renin–angiotensin system. These effects can be attenuated by the concomitant use of a β-blocker.
   2. **Dosing.** Hydralazine can be administered as an IV bolus of 5 to 20 mg.
   3. **Kinetics and pitfalls.** Hydralazine's IV time to peak effect is 20 minutes, thus a reasonable initial bolus of 5 to 10 mg can be redosed in 20 minutes if blood pressure remains elevated. With its relatively longer elimination half-life of 3 to 7 hours, a single dose of hydralazine may act for up to 12 hours. Owing to its delayed onset, hydralazine can easily be dosed in excess of intention, resulting in hours of unwanted hypotension.
E. **Enalaprilat,** an active metabolite of enalapril, is currently the only ACE inhibitor available for IV use. It reduces systolic and diastolic blood pressure by inhibiting the conversion of angiotensin I to angiotensin II.
   1. **Kinetics.** It has an onset of action of approximately 15 minutes, peak effect of 1 to 4 hours, and overall duration of action of about 4 hours. Elimination is primarily renal.
   2. **Contraindications.** ACE inhibitors interfere with renal autoregulation and must be used with caution in patients with renal dysfunction.
F. **Fenoldopam** is a synthetic dopamine (D_1) receptor agonist that acts by selective dilation of arterial beds while maintaining renal perfusion.
   1. **Uses.** A continuous IV infusion may be used perioperatively for the management of severe hypertension in patients with impaired renal function.
   2. **Evidence.** Despite reducing the incidence of postoperative acute kidney injury (AKI), fenoldopam has not been shown to improve mortality or the need for renal replacement therapy.
   3. **Dosing.** "Renal dose" fenoldopam at 0.1 µg/kg/min has diuretic and natriuretic properties that increase renal blood flow without greatly effecting systemic blood pressure. For hypertension, it can be dosed up to 0.3 µg/kg/min.
   4. **Kinetics.** Onset is within 5 to 15 minutes, and the dose should be adjusted every 15 to 20 minutes until optimal blood pressure control is achieved.
   5. **Adverse effects** include dose-dependent tachycardia and occasional hypokalemia. Hypotension may occur with concomitant use of β-adrenergic receptor blockade.

Chapter 18 Perioperative Hemodynamic Control

G. Adenosine is a nucleoside that, in high doses, has inhibitory effects on cardiac impulse conduction through the AV node.
  1. **Clinical uses**
     a. Adenosine's ability to slow conduction through the AV node aids in diagnosing and treating SVT.
     b. The transient asystole and hypotension from an adenosine bolus facilitate clipping of cerebral aneurysms by decompressing the aneurysm and improving visualization.
     c. Adenosine dilates coronary arteries. Infusions of adenosine take advantage of coronary steal in pharmacologic stress testing to diagnose myocardial perfusion defects. Regadenoson (Lexiscan) is a more stable analogue of adenosine, which is commonly used for this purpose as a bolus dose of 0.4 mg.
  2. **Dosing.** Because of rapid degradation by the vascular endothelium, adenosine boluses must be rapidly delivered and followed by flushes. The starting dose is 6 mg, which may be followed by up to two 12 mg boluses, if ineffective.
  3. **Precautions.** Adenosine may induce acute myocardial ischemia, prolonged sinus pauses, and bradyarrhythmias, thus application of pads for transcutaneous pacing and defibrillation is recommended.
  4. **Contraindications.** Adenosine should be avoided in patients with WPW syndrome in atrial fibrillation/flutter as it may allow for preferential conduction through the accessory pathway.

H. α-adrenergic antagonists
  1. **Phentolamine** is a short-acting selective α-adrenergic receptor antagonist that causes predominantly arterial vasodilation.
     a. **Dosing.** It is used in 5 mg IV boluses to treat states of hypertension and catecholamine excess (eg, pheochromocytoma). It is additionally used for local infiltration to prevent tissue necrosis after extravasation of norepinephrine, phenylephrine, dopamine, or epinephrine (5 to 10 mg diluted in 10 mL of saline).
     b. **Kinetics.** Systemic doses have a rapid onset within 2 minutes and may last up to 30 minutes.
  2. **Phenoxybenzamine** is an irreversible, long-acting α-adrenergic receptor antagonist approved for the preoperative management of patients with pheochromocytoma. While it effectively prevents intraoperative hypertension in patients with pheochromocytoma, postoperative hypotension is common given its long duration of action of up to a few days.
  3. Selective α_1-adrenergic receptor antagonists including **tamsulosin, terazosin,** and **doxazosin** are used to induce prostatic smooth muscle relaxation in the management of benign prostatic hyperplasia. Orthostatic hypotension is an adverse effect common to this class of drugs.

I. Pulmonary vasodilators are used to treat pulmonary hypertension and right ventricular failure.
  1. **Prostaglandin E₁ (alprostadil)** is a stable metabolite of arachidonic acid that causes peripheral and pulmonary vasodilation (Appendix I).
  2. **Epoprostenol (Veletri, Flolan)** is a prostacyclin (PGI$_2$) analogue with pulmonary and peripheral vasodilating and antiplatelet effects (Appendix I).
     a. **Pharmacokinetics.** Epoprostenol must be given as a continuous infusion because of its short half-life (6 minutes in vivo.)
     b. **Dosing.** Infusion of VELETRI should be initiated at 2 ng/kg/min and increased in increments of 1 to 2 ng/kg/min every 15 minutes

or longer until a tolerance limit to the drug is reached or further increases in the infusion rate are not clinically warranted.

- c. **Adverse effects.** Chronic administration of epoprostenol most frequently leads to complications associated with the delivery system, such as catheter-related sepsis and thrombotic events. Epoprostenol has also been associated with thrombocytopenia.

3. **Inhaled nitric oxide** selectively delivers vasodilating nitric oxide to ventilated areas to improve V/Q matching, whereas systemic nitric oxide donors such as nitroprusside and nitroglycerin result in nonselective pulmonary vasodilation.
4. **Sildenafil** is a selective phosphodiesterase-5 inhibitor that decreases cGMP degradation, increasing pulmonary levels of nitric oxide. It is primarily used in its intravenous formulation to treat pulmonary hypertension. In this patient population, it has been shown to improve exercise capacity and hemodynamics.
5. **Bosentan** is an oral endothelin receptor antagonist that competitively blocks the binding of endothelin, a potent pulmonary vasoconstrictor. It is approved for pulmonary arterial hypertension.

VIII. INDUCED HYPOTENSION

Induced hypotension is a technique used to improve visualization of the surgical field in microsurgery (eg, middle ear, cerebral aneurysm clipping, and plastic surgery) or to reduce the need for transfusion in orthopedic and spinal surgery or in patients with rare blood groups or religious objections to transfusion.

- **A. Patient selection.** This technique is not appropriate for patients at risk for ischemia, including those with vascular insufficiency to vital organs, cardiac instability, uncontrolled hypertension, anemia, or hypovolemia. It should be utilized with caution as serious complications, while rare in healthy patients, include cerebral infarction, myocardial infarction, and AKI.
- **B. Hemodynamic goals.** It is acceptable to target a MAP goal of around 30% below a patient's baseline, given that it is no lower than 50 mm Hg in an otherwise healthy patient or lower than 80 mm Hg in an elderly patient.
- **C. Techniques.** Hypotension can be achieved using neuraxial blockade, high concentrations of volatile anesthetics, β-blockers, potent short-acting opioids (eg, remifentanil), peripheral vasodilators (eg, nitroprusside or nitroglycerin) and dexmedetomidine. A 2021 meta-analysis comparing agents to induce hypotension demonstrated the superiority of dexmedetomidine in reducing intraoperative bleeding as compared to β-blockers, opioids, and nitroglycerine.

IX. DRUG DOSAGE CALCULATIONS

Drug concentrations must frequently be converted between various units of measurement prior to administration.

A. A drug concentration expressed as $Z\%$ contains

$$Z \, \text{mg/dL} = Z \, \text{g}/100 \, \text{mL} = (10 \times Z) \, \text{g/L} = (10 \times Z) \, \text{mg/mL}$$

Example: A 2.5% solution of sodium thiopental is equivalent to 25 g/L or 25 mg/mL.

B. A drug concentration that is expressed as a ratio is converted as follows:
$1:1000 = 1 \, \text{g}/1000 \, \text{mL} = 1 \, \text{mg/mL}$
$1:10,000 = 1 \, \text{g}/10,000 \, \text{mL} = 0.1 \, \text{mg/mL}$
$1:100,000 = 1 \, \text{g}/100,000 \, \text{mL} = 0.01 \, \text{mg/mL}$

C. Continuous drug infusions in 250 mL can be calculated based on a simple formula:

Z mg/250 mL = Z μg/min at an infusion rate of 15 mL/h

Standard drug mixes in use at Massachusetts General Hospital are shown in **Table 18.1**. The desired rate of infusion for any drug is easily calculated as a fraction or multiple of 15 mL/h.

Example: An 80-kg patient needs dopamine at 5 μg/kg/min. What is the infusion rate in mL/h using the standard MGH mix?

Desired rate in μg/min: 5 μg/kg/min × 80 kg = 400 μg/min

Find Z: There is 200 mg dopamine in the 250 mL solution. Thus, 200 μg/min = 15 mL/h

Desired rate in mL/h: 400/200 × 15 mL/h = 30 mL/h

ACKNOWLEDGMENT

We gratefully acknowledge the contributions of previous edition author, Devan Cote, as portions of those chapters have been retained in this revision.

Suggested Readings

Al-Abdouh A, Haddadin S, Matta A, et al. Impact of adjuvant use of midodrine to intravenous vasopressors: a systematic review and meta-analysis. *Crit Care Res Pract.* 2021;2021:5588483.

Barak M, Yoav L, Abu el-Naaj I. Hypotensive anesthesia versus normotensive anesthesia during major maxillofacial surgery: a review of the literature. *Sci World J.* 2015;2015:1–7.

Cardenas-garcia J, Schaub KF, Belchikov YG, Narasimhan M, Koenig SJ, Mayo PH. Safety of peripheral intravenous administration of vasoactive medication. *J Hosp Med.* 2015;10(9):581–585.

De Backer D, Biston P, Devriendt J, et al. Comparison of dopamine and norepinephrine in the treatment of shock. *N Engl J Med.* 2010;362(9):779–789.

Dutton RP. Controlled hypotension for spinal surgery. 2004;13(Suppl 1):S66–S71.

Espinosa A, Ripollés-Melchor J, Casans-Francés R, et al; Evidence Anesthesia Review Group. Perioperative use of clevidipine: a systematic review and meta-analysis. *PLoS One.* 2016;11(3):e0150625.

Fleisher LA, Fleischmann KE, Auerbach AD, et al. 2014 ACC/AHA guideline on perioperative cardiovascular evaluation and management of patients undergoing noncardiac surgery. Executive summary: a report of the American College of Cardiology/American Heart Association Task Force on practice guidelines. *Circulation.* 2014;130(24):2215–2245.

Gulea C, Zakeri R, Alderman V, Morgan A, Ross J, Quint JK. Beta-blocker therapy in patients with COPD: a systematic literature review and meta-analysis with multiple treatment comparison. *Respir Res.* 2021;22(1):64.

Jadadzadeh M, Hosseini SH, Mostafavi Pour Manshadi SM, Naderi N, Emami Meybodi M. Effect of milrinone on short term outcome of patients with myocardial dysfunction undergoing off-pump coronary artery bypass graft: a randomized clinical trial. *Acta Med Iran.* 2013;51(10):681–686.

Kim DH, Lee J, Kim SW, Hwang SH. The efficacy of hypotensive agents on intraoperative bleeding and recovery following general anesthesia for nasal surgery: a network meta-analysis. *Clin Exp Otorhinolaryngol.* 2021;14(2):200–209.

Kingman M, Archer-Chicko C, Bartlett M, Beckmann J, Hohsfield R, Lombardi S. Management of prostacyclin side effects in adult patients with pulmonary arterial hypertension. *Pulm Circ.* 2017;7(3):598–608.

Lawson N, Meyer D. Autonomic nervous system: physiology and pharmacology. In: Barash PG, Cullen BF, Stoelting RK, eds. *Clinical Anesthesia.* 3rd ed. Lippincott-Raven Publishers; 1997:243–309.

Morozowich ST, Ramakrishna H. Pharmacologic agents for acute hemodynamic instability: recent advances in the management of perioperative shock – a systematic review. *Ann Card Anaesth.* 2015;18(4):543–554.

Onwochei DN, Ngan Kee WD, Fung L, Downey K, Ye XY, Carvalho JCA. Norepinephrine intermittent intravenous boluses to prevent hypotension during spinal anesthesia for cesarean delivery: a sequential allocation dose-finding study. *Anesth Analg.* 2017; 125(1):212–218.

Rhodes A, Evans LE, Alhazzani W, et al. Surviving sepsis campaign. international guidelines for management of sepsis and septic shock: 2016. *Intensive Care Med.* 2017;43(3): 304–377.

Rizvi MS, Trivedi V, Nasim F, et al. Trends in use of midodrine in the ICU: a single-center retrospective case series. *Crit Care Med.* 2018;46(7):e628–e633.

Rodriquez MA, Kumar SK, De Caro M. Hypertensive crisis. *Cardiol Rev.* 2010;18(2):102–107.

Russell JA, Walley KR, Singer J, et al; VASST Investigators. Vasopressin versus norepinephrine infusion in patients with septic shock. *N Engl J Med.* 2008;358(9):877–887.

Uhlig K, Efremov L, Tongers J, et al. Inotropic agents and vasodilator strategies for the treatment of cardiogenic shock or low cardiac output syndrome. *Cochrane Database Syst Rev.* 2020;11(11):CD009669.

Wachter SB, Gilbert EM. Beta-adrenergic receptors, from their discovery and characterization through their manipulation to beneficial clinical application. *Cardiology.* 2012;122(2):104–112.

Local Anesthetics

Lillye Anderson and Ken Solt

I. GENERAL PRINCIPLES

A. Introduction. Local anesthetics are a group of drugs which cause a reversible loss of sensation by blocking nerve conduction. This is accomplished through tissue infiltration, topical application, peripheral nerve blocks and neuraxial anesthesia techniques. The first local anesthetic used clinically was cocaine, isolated from the coca plant. Modern local anesthetics are **sodium channel blockers** derived from the cocaine molecule.

B. Chemistry. Local anesthetics are composed of a terminal amine attached to an aromatic ring via an ester or amide linkage. Local anesthetics are weak bases with both charged (protonated) and uncharged (unprotonated) forms at physiologic pH ~7.4. Only uncharged molecules can cross the lipid bilayer to block sodium channels intracellularly.

1. **Esters.** Benzocaine, cocaine, chloroprocaine, procaine, and tetracaine. Ester hydrolysis is catalyzed by pseudocholinesterase and the degradation product is *p*-aminobenzoic acid (PABA).
2. **Amides.** Bupivacaine, etidocaine, lidocaine, mepivacaine, prilocaine, and ropivacaine. The amide linkage is cleaved through initial *N*-dealkylation followed by hydrolysis, which occurs primarily in the liver. The elimination half-life for most amide local anesthetics is 2 to 3 hours.

C. Mechanism of action

1. **Local anesthetics inhibit voltage-gated Na^+ channels (NaV)** by binding to the intracellular pore of NaV. To enter the cell, the uncharged molecule must traverse the lipid bilayer through passive nonionic diffusion.
2. **Local anesthetics block nerve conduction** by inhibiting sodium influx and impairing the propagation of action potentials.
3. **Physiochemical properties** of the local anesthetics affect neural blockade.
    a. **Lipid solubility.** More lipophilic local anesthetics exhibit increased potency because they more easily permeate nerve membranes. Higher lipid solubility also leads to prolonged duration of action.
    b. **pK_a.** Agents with a lower pK_a will have faster onset since a greater fraction of the drug will exist in the uncharged form.
    c. **pH of the drug solution.** Higher pH will accelerate the onset by increasing the proportion of molecules in the uncharged form.
    d. **Drug concentration.** Higher concentrations will accelerate onset owing to mass effect.
4. **Differential blockade of nerve fibers**
    a. **Peripheral nerves** are classified according to size and function (**Table 19.1**). Local anesthetics block conduction based on the number of NaV channels, with thin, myelinated fibers more susceptible to blockade than thick, unmyelinated fibers.
    b. Local anesthetics block sensitivity to pain and temperature first, followed by fine touch. Finally, motor function is impaired. However, this differential blockade is imperfect (eg, it is nearly **impossible to produce a full sensory block without impairing motor function**).

Table 19.1 Classification of Nerve Fibers

Class	Myelin	Diameter (μm)	Local Anesthetic Sensitivity	Function
A-α	+++	12–20	++	Motor
A-β	+++	5–12	++	Touch/pressure
A-γ	++	1–4	+++	Proprioception/motor tone
A-δ	++	1–4	+++	Pain/temperature
B	+	1–3	++	Preganglionic autonomic
C	−	0.5–1	+	Pain/temperature

      c. **Sequence of block** progresses in the following order: Sympathetic ≥ pain and temperature ≥ proprioception ≥ fine touch and pressure ≥ motor.

  5. **Pathophysiologic factors affecting the neural block**

      a. **Decreased cardiac output** reduces the plasma and tissue clearance of local anesthetics, increasing plasma concentrations and the potential for toxicity.

      b. **Severe hepatic disease** may prolong the duration of action of amides.

      c. **Reduced cholinesterase activity.** Newborns, pregnant patients and patients with **atypical cholinesterase or cholinesterase deficiency** may have decreased clearance of ester-type anesthetics, but this is not usually associated with toxicity.

      d. **Fetal acidosis** may cause **ion-trapping** (eg, accumulation of ionized local anesthetic in the fetal circulation) potentially resulting in fetal toxicity. This is more likely with amides not cleared rapidly by maternal liver enzymes.

      e. **Sepsis, malignancy, and cardiac ischemia** can increase plasma levels of α_1-**acid glycoprotein,** an acute phase reactant with high affinity for amide local anesthetics, decreasing the plasma concentration of unbound local anesthetics.

D. **Commercial preparations.** In most commercial preparations, the pH is adjusted with hydrochloric acid or sodium hydroxide to a final value of 4 to 6. Solutions with epinephrine are adjusted to pH 3 to 4 to minimize the degradation of epinephrine.

  1. **Antimicrobial preservatives. Methylparaben** or other paraben derivatives are used as antiseptic agents for multidose vials. **Preservative-free solutions are used for neuraxial** anesthesia to avoid the neurotoxic effects of preservatives.

  2. **Epinephrine.** Epinephrine is often added to prolong the duration of nerve blocks and to act as a marker for intravascular injection (see Section II.B).

  3. **Antioxidants** (sodium metabisulfite, sodium ethylenediaminetetraacetic acid [EDTA]) are added to mixtures containing epinephrine **to slow oxidization.**

  4. **Liposomal bupivacaine.** Bupivacaine liposome injectable suspension, marketed under the trade name **Exparel** was designed for slow release of bupivacaine from liposomes to prolong its local anesthetic effects and reduce toxicity. It is approved by the US Food and Drug Administration

(FDA) for TAP block, interscalene block, adductor canal block and popliteal block as well as for local infiltration at the surgical site.

II. CLINICAL USES OF LOCAL ANESTHETICS
The choice of local anesthetic must account for the duration of surgery, regional technique used, surgical requirements, potential for toxicity, and metabolic constraints (**Tables 19.2** and **19.3**).
A. Combinations of local anesthetics
1. **Mixtures of local anesthetics** (eg, mepivacaine–bupivacaine) may accelerate onset. However, data suggest that mixtures do not speed onset but do reduce duration.
2. Mixture of **nonbupivacaine** local anesthetics with **liposomal bupivacaine** will perturb liposomes and alter the release of bupivacaine. A mixture of **bupivacaine** with liposomal bupivacaine alters the pharmacokinetics of release.
3. **Eutectic mixture of local anesthetics (EMLA)** cream is a mixture of 2.5% lidocaine and 2.5% prilocaine for use as a topical skin anesthetic. It must be applied to unbroken, healthy skin for at least 30 minutes to take effect.

B. Adjuncts for local anesthesia
1. **Epinephrine.** The most common additive after preservatives
   a. **Benefits** of epinephrine
      1. To assist in the **detection** of **intravascular injections**.
      2. To **decrease systemic toxicity** by decreasing the rate of absorption of the local anesthetic into the circulation.
      3. To **prolong the duration of anesthesia**. This varies with the anesthetic agent, concentration, and block performed.
   b. **Limitations** of epinephrine
      1. Epinephrine is neurotoxic in diabetic animal models. Systemic epinephrine is dangerous in patients with severe coronary artery disease, arrhythmias, uncontrolled hypertension, and hyperthyroidism; **it should be used with caution in susceptible patients**.
      2. Epinephrine should be **avoided** in peripheral nerve blocks for areas with **poor collateral blood flow** (eg, digits, penis, and nose) or in intravenous local anesthetic techniques (ie, Bier block).
   c. **Fresh epinephrine** can be added to make a 1:200,000 to 1:400,000 solution (2.5 to 5 µg/mL) prior to administration (while maintaining a high pH to achieve rapid onset of the nerve block). These doses balance the detection of intravascular injection while minimizing the cardiovascular risk of higher doses of epinephrine.
   d. The **maximum dose of epinephrine** should not exceed **10 µg/kg in pediatric** patients and **5 µg/kg in adults** to avoid ventricular arrhythmias.
2. **Opioids** including fentanyl, morphine, and hydromorphone are useful adjuncts for neuraxial anesthesia because they bind to opioid receptors in the spinal cord. They are less useful for peripheral nerve blocks.
   a. **Buprenorphine** can generate a 1.5- to 3-fold increase in the duration of peripheral blocks (0.15 to 0.3 mg or 3 µg/kg) but is associated with an increased risk of postoperative nausea and vomiting (PONV).
   b. **Meperidine.** Given its opioid and local anesthetic properties, meperidine is sometimes used as the sole anesthetic agent in spinal anesthesia. However, this practice is often avoided in the United States given the risk for toxicity from its metabolite, normeperidine.
3. **Sodium bicarbonate** raises the pH to increase the concentration of uncharged local anesthetic that can cross the cell membrane. This

TABLE 19.2 Clinical Uses of Local Anesthetics

Anesthetics	pK_a	Onset	Duration[a]	Relative Toxicity	Highest Recommended Dose (mg)[b]	Clinical Use/Comments
Esters						
Procaine (Novocaine)	8.9	Slow	Short	Low	500 (600)	Infiltration, spinal Allergic potential
Chloroprocaine (Nesacaine)	9.1	Fast	Short	Low	800 (1000)	All[d], rapid hydrolysis in plasma
Tetracaine (Pontocaine)	8.5	Slow	Long	High	10 (20)	Spinal, topical
Benzocaine	2.5	Moderate	Short	n/a[c]	n/a[c]	Topical only Methemoglobinemia
Amides						
Lidocaine (Xylocaine)	7.9	Fast	Medium	Medium	300 (500)	All[d]
Prilocaine (Citanest)	7.7	Fast	Medium	Medium	400 (600)	All[d], methemoglobinemia
Mepivacaine (Carbocaine)	7.6	Fast	Medium	Medium	400 (550)	All[d]
Bupivacaine (Marcaine, Sensorcaine)	8.1	Moderate	Long	High	175 (225)	All[d], differential block with low concentration
L-Bupivacaine (Chirocaine)	8.1	Moderate	Long	High	150 (n/a)	All[d] S-enantiomer of bupivacaine—less cardiotoxic
Ropivacaine (Naropin)	8.1	Moderate	Long	High	225 (n/a)	All[d]
Etidocaine (Duranest)	7.7	Moderate	Long	High	300 (400)	All[d] Motor greater than sensory blockade

[a]Duration of dose depends on the site of administration and proximity to vasculature.
[b]Dose in epinephrine-containing solution in parenthesis. Maximum dose may require clinical judgment based on other comorbidities.
[c]The 20% spray has been removed from practice owing to high risk of methemoglobinemia.
[d]"All" indicates that the drug can be used for any type of local anesthesia (infiltration, local, regional, neuraxial).

Table 19.3 Local Anesthetic Agents

Anesthetic Technique	Anesthetic	Concentration (%)	Duration (minutes)[a]	Usual Volume (mL; 70-kg Patient)[b]
Local infiltration	Procaine	1–2	20–30 (30–45)	
	Lidocaine	0.5–1	30–60 (120)	
	Mepivacaine	0.5–1	45–90 (120)	
	Bupivacaine	0.25–0.5	120–240 (180–240)	
	Ropivacaine	0.2–0.5	120–240 (180–240)	
Peripheral nerve blocks (drug with epinephrine 1:200,000)	Lidocaine	1–2	(120–240)	30–50
	Mepivacaine	1–1.5	(180–300)	30–50
	Bupivacaine	0.25–0.5	(360–720)	30–50
	Ropivacaine	0.2–0.5	(360–720)	30–50
Epidural (drug with epinephrine 1:200,000)	Chloroprocaine	2–3	(30–90)	15–30
	Lidocaine	1–2	(60–120)	15–30
	Mepivacaine	1–2	(60–180)	15–30
	Bupivacaine	0.25–0.5	(180–350)	15–30
	Levobupivacaine	0.25–0.75	(180–350)	15–30
	Ropivacaine	0.2–0.75	(180–350)	15–30
Spinal	Lidocaine + glucose (hyperbaric)	1.5, 5.0	30–60	1–2
	Bupivacaine (isobaric)	0.5	90–200	3–4
	Bupivacaine + glucose (hyperbaric)	0.75	90–200	2–3
	Tetracaine (hypobaric)	0.25	90–200	2–6
	Tetracaine (isobaric)	1.0	90–200	1–2
	Tetracaine + glucose (hyperbaric)	0.25–1.0	90–200	1–4

[a]Duration of epinephrine-containing solution in parenthesis.

[b]Doses should be reduced for patients with specific risk factors and when nonepinephrine–containing solutions are used.

accelerates the onset of neural blockade. Typically, 1 mL of 8.4% sodium bicarbonate is added to each 10 mL of lidocaine, chloroprocaine, or mepivacaine. Alkalinization can cause precipitation of bupivacaine and ropivacaine, so sodium bicarbonate is usually avoided for these anesthetics.
4. **Alpha-2 adrenergic agonists** bind to presynaptic receptors in the CNS to produce analgesia. Higher doses are associated with sedation and bradycardia.
   a. **Clonidine** prolongs the duration of neuraxial anesthesia (15 to 50 μg single dose) with less effect on peripheral nerve block duration (100 to 150 μg or 0.5 to 5 μg/kg).
   b. **Dexmedetomidine** prolongs the duration of both neuraxial anesthesia (intrathecal 5 to 10 μg, epidural 1 μg/kg) and peripheral nerve blocks (20 to 150 μg).
5. **Dexamethasone**, an anti-inflammatory steroid, extends the duration of regional blocks over intramuscular or intravenous injection (neuraxial 4 to 8 mg, peripheral nerve block 1 to 8 mg).

III. TOXICITY
A. Allergic reactions
1. True allergic reactions to local anesthetics are rare. Vasovagal episodes and responses to intravascular injection of local anesthetic/epinephrine are more common.
2. **Ester-type local anesthetics** may cause allergic reactions from the metabolite PABA. Patients allergic to PABA should avoid **methylparaben** owing to the structural similarity.
3. **Epinephrine-containing solutions with sulfa-based antioxidants** may cause allergic reactions in patients with sulfa allergies.
4. **Local hypersensitivity reactions** may produce local erythema, urticaria, edema, or dermatitis.
5. **Systemic hypersensitivity reactions** are rare and can present with generalized erythema, urticaria, edema, bronchoconstriction, hypotension, and cardiovascular collapse.
6. **Treatment** is supportive.

B. Local toxicity
1. **Tissue toxicity** is rare with short-term use.
2. **Post spinal pain syndrome** may occur after subarachnoid injection of local anesthetic with pain or dysesthesia in the buttocks or legs. The risk is higher with lidocaine than with bupivacaine, prilocaine, or procaine. Symptoms typically resolve spontaneously within 5 days.
3. Large volumes of intrathecal or epidural chloroprocaine may cause intense back pain, potentially due to spasms of the paraspinal muscles from EDTA.

C. Local anesthetic systemic toxicity (LAST) results from intravascular accumulation of local anesthetic due to inadvertent intravascular injection, absorption from a tissue depot, accumulation of metabolites, and/or intentional intravenous infusion.
1. **Clinical characteristics**
   a. In the setting of **landmark-based anesthesia**, LAST is primarily due to **inadvertent intravascular injection**. Intravascular injection can be reduced by:
      1. Aspirating before injection
      2. Using an intravascular marker (eg, **epinephrine**)
      3. **Incremental injection** to establish the block (eg, 5 mL per injection)
      4. **Ultrasound guidance**

b. **Ultrasound** has changed the clinical characteristics of LAST with increasing frequency of delayed toxicity from **depot absorption.**
   c. **Incidence** of systemic toxicity is ~1 to 2 per 1000 blocks with wide variation in published incidence.
   d. **Risk factors for toxicity** include total dose, vascularity of block site (penile > paravertebral > upper extremity block > lower extremity block), and prolonged infusions.
   e. **Patient risk factors** include low body mass index, hypoalbuminemia, renal disease, liver failure, heart failure, mitochondrial disease, carnitine deficiency, and acidosis (which causes intracellular ion trapping).
   f. **Perceived safety of local anesthesia** (particularly lidocaine) leads to overrepresentation of LAST in ASA I/II patients and **lidocaine as the causative agent.**
   g. A **nonanesthesiologist** is involved in administration of local anesthetic in up to 50% of cases of LAST.
2. **Presentation of toxicity.** LAST presents with **neurologic symptoms, cardiovascular symptoms,** or **both.** Early symptoms do not always precede late symptoms. The first observed symptom can be a seizure or cardiac arrest.
   a. **Central nervous system** toxicity can cause dizziness, lightheadedness, tinnitus, perioral numbness, metallic taste, and progress to muscle twitching, tremors, **seizures, and coma.**
   b. **Cardiovascular toxicity** will present with electrocardiographic changes (bradycardia, prolonged PR interval, widened QRS) and hemodynamic instability, and can progress to complete heart block and/or cardiac arrest.
      1. **Early cardiac toxicity** is due to sodium (and calcium) channel blockade with disruption of the conduction apparatus in the myocardium.
      2. **Vascular toxicity** will cause a **bimodal effect** of early (and often unobserved) hypertension with subsequent hypotension (due to smooth muscle inhibition).
      3. **Profound toxicity** is due to an **uncoupling of oxidative phosphorylation** in mitochondria.
   c. Toxicity is **associated with lipophilicity (LogP)** with bupivacaine > ropivacaine > lidocaine > chloroprocaine.
   d. **Pregnancy** increases sensitivity to cardiotoxicity.
   e. **Acidosis and hypoxia** markedly worsen cardiotoxicity and neurotoxicity, making airway management a priority.
3. Treatment of LAST
   a. **Secure** airway. **Ventilate with 100% O_2** and consider intubation to minimize respiratory and/or metabolic acidosis.
   b. **Lipid emulsion therapy.** If LAST is suspected, **lipid emulsion is the definitive treatment.** Administration should not be delayed, as benefits far outweigh risks.
      1. For a patient ≥ 70 kg, **bolus 100 mL 20% lipid emulsion** (eg, Intralipid) intravenously (or intraosseously) over 2 to 3 minutes followed by 0.25 mL/kg/min until 250 mL is infused.
      2. For a patient < 70 kg, **bolus 1.5 mL/kg** (lean body mass) followed by 0.25 mL/kg/min for at least 10 minutes after circulatory stability is achieved.
      3. The provider can **repeat the bolus** for persistent cardiovascular collapse and **double the infusion rate** (0.5 mL/kg/min) for persistent hypotension.

4. Continue lipid emulsion infusion for at least 15 minutes after the patient is hemodynamically stable.
5. **An upper limit of 12.5 mL/kg is** recommended by FDA guidelines.
   c. **Treat seizures** with **benzodiazepines.** If only propofol is available, use small incremental doses such as 10 to 20 mg, especially in patients with cardiovascular instability.
   d. If **cardiac arrest** occurs, start chest compressions immediately and provide advanced cardiac life support.
      1. **Epinephrine (<1 μg/kg)** can be used.
      2. **Avoid vasopressin, calcium channel blockers, β-blockers, or local anesthetics.**
      3. Treatment of arrhythmias with **amiodarone** is preferred.
   e. **Cardiopulmonary bypass (CPB).** If the patient fails to respond, CPB may be required. Given time required for CPB, notify CPB center ASAP if anticipated.
   f. Monitor for **4 to 6 hours** for cardiovascular symptoms given risk for recrudescence, or **2 hours** if symptoms are limited to the central nervous system and quickly resolve.
4. Emerging areas of concern for LAST: **local infiltration anesthesia** by surgeons, **intravenous lidocaine infusion** in unmonitored settings, prolonged **catheter infusions,** especially in patients with risk factors, and novel formulations (eg, **liposomal bupivacaine**) where mixing can lead to toxic dosing.
5. **Maximum allowable doses (Table 19.2)** of local anesthetics are estimates of toxicity but are not strictly evidence-based and can vary among publications. They should be taken into consideration, though systemic toxicity can still occur within these ranges. The lowest possible dose should be used to achieve the desired effect.

D. **Methemoglobinemia results from** the oxidation of heme groups within deoxyhemoglobin (Fe^{2+}) to form methemoglobin (Fe^{3+}), which cannot transport oxygen.
   1. **Causes: prilocaine** (in EMLA cream), which is metabolized to *o*-toluidine in the liver and oxidizes hemoglobin to methemoglobin; **benzocaine**, which is found in topical sprays.
   2. **Treatment** is with **methylene blue** (1 to 2 mg/kg intravenously over 5 minutes), which reduces methemoglobin to hemoglobin.

ACKNOWLEDGMENTS

We gratefully acknowledge the contributions of previous edition authors, Michael R. Fettiplace and Xiaodong Bao, as portions of those chapters have been retained in this revision.

Suggested Readings

Desai N, Kirkham KR, Albrecht E. Local anaesthetic adjuncts for peripheral regional anaesthesia: A narrative review. *Anaesthesia.* 2021;76:100–109.

Lirk P, Berde CB. Local anesthetics. In: Miller RE, ed. *Anesthesia.* 9th ed. Elsevier; 2020: 865–890.

Macfarlane, AJR, Gitman, M, Bornstein KJ, El-Boghdadly K, Weinberg G. Updates in our understanding of local anaesthetic systemic toxicity: A narrative review. *Anaesthesia.* 2021;76:27–39.

Neal JM, Barrington MJ, Fettiplace MR, et al. The Third American Society of Regional Anesthesia and Pain Medicine Practice Advisory on local anesthetic systemic toxicity: Executive summary 2017. *Reg Anesth Pain Med.* 2018;43(2):113–123.

Prabhakar A, Ward CT, Watson M, et al. Liposomal bupivacaine and novel local anesthetic formulations. *Best Pract Res Clin Anaesthesiol.* 2019;33(4):425–432.

Rosenberg PH, Veering BT, Urmey WF. Maximum recommended doses of local anesthetics: a multifactorial concept. *Reg Anesth Pain Med.* 2004;29(6):564–575.

Suresh S, Ecoffey C, Bosenberg A, et al. The European Society of Regional Anaesthesia and Pain Therapy/American Society of Regional Anesthesia and Pain Medicine recommendations on local anesthetics and adjuvants dosage in pediatric regional anesthesia. *Reg Anesth Pain Med.* 2018;43:211–216.

Spinal, Epidural, and Caudal Anesthesia

James S. Cho and Joseph L. McDowell

I. GENERAL CONSIDERATIONS

A. Preoperative assessment of the patient for **neuraxial and regional** anesthesia is similar to that for general anesthesia. The details of the procedure to be performed, including its anticipated length, patient position, and a complete review of any coexisting diseases, should be taken into account in determining the appropriateness of a regional technique.

B. Review of systems. A comprehensive review of cardiovascular and pulmonary systems should be performed. Preexisting neurologic abnormalities should be well documented. Any history of abnormal bleeding and a review of the patient's medications may indicate a need for additional coagulation studies.

C. Physical examination. Review of the patient's airway, cardiovascular, and pulmonary examinations should be performed. The area where the block is to be administered should be examined for potential pathology, such as abnormal anatomy (kyphoscoliosis) or evidence of overlying infection.

D. Informed consent should be obtained including a detailed explanation of the planned procedure, with procedure-specific risks and benefits—these include bleeding, infection, nerve damage, paresthesias, and dural puncture headache. Patients should be reassured that additional sedation and anesthesia can be given during the operation and that general anesthesia is an option if the block fails or the operation becomes more prolonged or extensive than originally thought; therefore, general anesthesia must also be on the consent form. In some instances, it is planned from the onset to have a combination of regional and general anesthesia.

E. Monitoring. As with general anesthesia, patients should receive appropriate monitoring (see Chapter 15: Monitoring) and have an intravenous (IV) line in place. Oxygen, equipment for intubation and positive-pressure ventilation, and drugs to provide hemodynamic support must be available.

II. SEGMENTAL LEVEL REQUIRED FOR SURGERY

A. Knowledge of the sensory, motor, and autonomic distributions of spinal nerves will help the anesthetist determine the correct segmental level required for a particular operation and anticipate the potential physiologic effects of producing a sensory block to that level. **Figure 20.1** illustrates the dermatomal distribution of the spinal nerves.

B. Afferent autonomic nerves innervate visceral sensation and viscerosomatic reflexes at spinal segmental levels much higher than would be predicted from skin dermatomes.

C. Minimal suggested levels for common surgical procedures are listed in **Table 20.1**.

III. CONTRAINDICATIONS TO NEURAXIAL ANESTHESIA

A. Absolute
1. Patient refusal
2. Localized infection at skin puncture site

FIGURE 20.1 Skin dermatomes corresponding to respective sensory innervation by spinal nerves.

3. Significant coagulopathy
4. Increased intracranial pressure

B. Relative
1. Septicemia or bacteremia
2. Hypovolemia
3. Central nervous system disease

IV. SPINAL ANESTHESIA

Spinal anesthesia involves administering local anesthetic into the subarachnoid space.

A. Anatomy
1. The **spinal canal** extends from the foramen magnum to the sacral hiatus. The boundaries of the bony canal are the vertebral body anteriorly,

TABLE 20.1 Suggested Minimum Cutaneous Levels for Spinal Anesthesia

Operative Site	Level
Lower extremities	T12
Hip	T10
Vagina, uterus	T10
Bladder, prostate	T10
Lower extremities with tourniquet	T8
Testis, ovaries	T8
Lower intra-abdominal	T6
Other intra-abdominal	T4

the pedicles laterally, and the spinous processes and laminae posteriorly (**Figure 20.2**).

2. Three **interlaminar ligaments** bind the vertebral processes together.
   a. Superficially, the **supraspinous ligament** connects the apices of the spinous processes.
   b. The **interspinous ligament** connects the spinous processes on their horizontal surface.

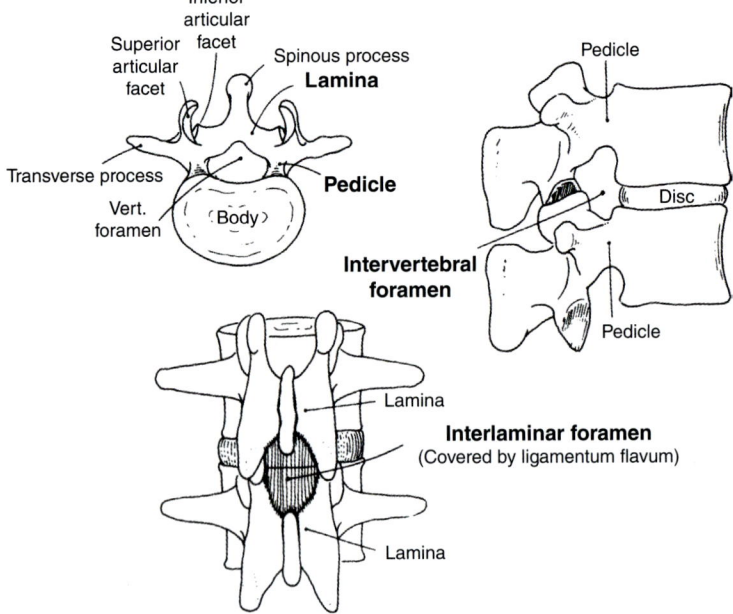

FIGURE 20.2 Vertebral anatomy.

c. The **ligamentum flavum** connects the caudal edge of the lamina above to the cephalad edge of the lamina below. This ligament is composed of elastic fibers and is usually recognized by its increased resistance to the passage of a needle.
3. The **spinal cord** extends the length of the vertebral canal during fetal life, ends at about L3 at birth, and is moved progressively to a cephalad position as the vertebral column grows to reach near the adult L1 level by 2 years of age. The conus medullaris, lumbar, sacral, and coccygeal nerve roots branch out distally to form the cauda equina. Spinal needles are placed in this area of the canal (below L2) because the mobility of the nerves reduces the danger of trauma from the needle.
4. The spinal cord is invested in three **meninges.**
    a. The pia mater **directly invests the spinal cord.**
    b. The **arachnoid mater,** which lies between the pia and the dura mater.
    c. The **dura mater,** which is a tough fibrous sheath running longitudinally along the length of the spinal cord and is tethered caudally at S2.
5. The **subarachnoid space** lies between the pia mater and the arachnoid mater and extends from the attachment of the dura at S2 to the cerebral ventricles above. The space contains the spinal cord, nerves, cerebrospinal fluid (CSF), and blood vessels that supply the spinal cord.
6. **CSF** is a clear colorless fluid that fills the subarachnoid space. The total volume of CSF is 100 to 150 mL, and the volume that exists in the spinal subarachnoid space is ~25 to 35 mL. CSF is continuously formed at a rate of 450 mL/d by secretion or ultrafiltration of plasma from the choroid arterial plexuses located in the lateral, third, and fourth ventricles. CSF is reabsorbed into the bloodstream through the arachnoid villi and granulations that protrude through the dura to lie in contact with the endothelium of the cerebral venous sinuses.

B. Physiologic changes
1. **Neural blockade. Differential blockade** refers to the varying sensitivity of different types of nerve fibers to the effects of local anesthetics. Smaller C fibers conveying autonomic impulses are more easily blocked than the larger sensory and motor fibers. As a result, the level of autonomic blockade extends above the level of the sensory blockade by two to six segments. Similarly, fibers conveying sensation are more sensitive to local anesthetics than the larger motor fibers, and as a result, the sensory blockade will extend above the level of the motor blockade. Causes of this phenomenon are multifactorial and include nerve fiber diameter and myelination.
2. **Cardiovascular. Hypotension** is directly proportional to the degree of **sympathetic blockade** produced. Sympathetic blockade results in dilatation of arteries and venous capacitance vessels, leading to decreased systemic vascular resistance and decreased venous return. If the block is below T4, increased baroreceptor activity produces an increase in activity to the cardiac sympathetic fibers and vasoconstriction of the upper extremities. Blockade above T4 interrupts cardiac accelerator sympathetic fibers, leading to bradycardia, decreased cardiac output, and a further decrease in blood pressure. These changes are more marked in patients who are hypovolemic or elderly or have obstruction to venous return (eg, pregnancy). Risk factors for bradycardia after spinal anesthesia include baseline bradycardia, the American Society of Anesthesiologists (ASA) physical status 1, use of β-blockers, age younger than 50 years, prolonged PR interval, and sensory level above T6.

3. **Respiratory.** Low spinal anesthesia has no effect on ventilation. With ascending height of the block into the thoracic area, there is progressive ascending intercostal muscle paralysis. This has little effect on ventilation in the supine surgical patient with intact diaphragmatic function mediated by the phrenic nerve (C3–C5), but patients may report a sensation of dyspnea due to decreased sensation of chest wall expansion. Conversely, ventilation in patients with poor respiratory reserve, such as the morbidly obese, may be profoundly impaired. Paralysis of both intercostal and abdominal muscles decreases the efficiency of coughing, which may be important in patients with chronic obstructive pulmonary disease. Usually, a spinal level of T4 does not result in impaired ventilation, but respiratory compromise may occur in patients with limited respiratory reserve or higher spinal levels.
4. **Visceral effects**
   a. **Bladder.** Sacral blockade (S2 to S4) results in an atonic bladder that can retain large volumes of urine. Blockade of sympathetic afferent and efferent innervation of the sphincter and detrusor muscle produces urinary retention.
   b. **Intestine.** Sympathetic blockade (T5 to L1) produced by spinal anesthesia leads to contraction of the small and large intestines because of a predominance of parasympathetic tone.
5. **Neuroendocrine.** Peridural block to T5 inhibits part of the neural component of the stress response through its blockade of sympathetic afferents to the adrenal medulla and blockade of sympathetic and somatic pathways mediating pain. Other components of the stress response and central release of humoral factors are unaffected. Vagal afferent fibers from the upper abdominal viscera are not blocked and can stimulate release of hypothalamic and pituitary hormones, such as antidiuretic hormone and adrenocorticotropic hormone. Glucose tolerance and insulin release are normal.
6. **Thermoregulation.** Hypothermia may occur due to several mechanisms. The predominant cause is redistribution of the central heat to the periphery secondary to vasodilatation, which makes forced air warming particularly effective at raising the patient's temperature. Core temperature may drop even though surface temperature is preserved and patients can feel warm despite a decrease in temperature. Thermoregulation is impaired given the loss of vasoconstriction to preserve heat below the level of sympathectomy. Shivering is common.
7. **Central nervous system effects.** Spinal anesthesia may have direct effects on suppressing consciousness, probably secondary to decreased afferent stimulation of the reticular activating system. During spinal or epidural anesthesia, doses of sedative agents may be decreased.

C. **Technique**
   1. **Spinal needle.** There are two main categories of spinal needles: those with a beveled tip that cut the dura ("cutting tip") and those with a conical tip ("pencil-point") with a lateral opening.
   2. **Sprotte** and **Whitacre** needles. Pencil-point needle; may reduce the incidence of postdural puncture headache (PDPH) (<1%) compared with traditional cutting-tip needles by splitting rather than cutting dural fibers during insertion. Twenty-four and 25-gauge needles are easily bent and are often inserted through a 19-gauge introducer needle.
   3. **Quincke needle.** Cutting tip. More prone to causing PDPH. The 22-gauge **Quincke** needle is more rigid and is easily directed when inserted. It can be useful in older patients in whom access may be more difficult and the incidence of PDPH is low.

4. **Patient position.** The lateral decubitus, prone, and sitting positions can be used for administration of spinal anesthesia.
   a. In the **lateral position**, the patient is placed with the affected side up if a hypobaric or isobaric technique is to be used and with the affected side down if a hyperbaric technique is to be used. The spine is horizontal and parallel to the edge of the table. The knees are drawn up toward the chest, and the chin is flexed downward onto the chest to obtain maximal flexion of the spine.
   b. The **sitting position** is useful for low spinal blocks required in certain gynecologic and urologic procedures and is commonly used in obese patients to assist in identification of the midline. It is often used in conjunction with hyperbaric anesthetics. The head and shoulders are flexed downward onto the trunk with the arms resting on a stand. An assistant should be available to stabilize the patient, and the patient should not be oversedated.
   c. The **prone position** is used in conjunction with hypobaric or isobaric anesthetics for procedures on the rectum, perineum, and anus. A prone jackknife position can be used for administration of spinal anesthesia and subsequent surgery.
5. **Procedure**
   a. With all regional anesthetic procedures, the patient should be monitored with standard ASA monitors including electrocardiogram (ECG), blood pressure, and oxygen saturation.
   b. The L2–L3, L3–L4, or L4–L5 interspaces are commonly used for spinal anesthesia. The spinous process of L4 is aligned with the upper borders of the superior iliac crests.
   c. Disinfect a large area of skin with an appropriate antiseptic solution. Care must be taken to avoid contamination of the spinal kit with antiseptic solution as the solution is potentially neurotoxic.
   d. Check the stylet for correct fit within the needle; this can be done by pulling the stylet back and then replacing it.
   e. Raise a skin wheal with 1% lidocaine and a 25-gauge needle at the spinal puncture site.
   f. **Approaches**
      1. **Midline.** Place the spinal needle (or introducer) through the skin wheal and into the interspinous ligament. The needle should be in the same plane as the spinous processes and angulated slightly cephalad toward the interlaminar space (**Figure 20.3**).
      2. **Paramedian.** This approach is useful in patients who cannot adequately flex their backs because of pain or whose interspinous ligaments may be ossified. Place the spinal needle approximately 1 cm lateral and 1 cm caudad to the center of the selected interspace. Aim the needle medially and slightly cephalad, passing lateral to the supraspinous ligament. If the lamina is contacted, redirect the needle and walk the tip off the lamina in a medial and cephalad direction.
      3. **Needle placement.** Always keep the stylet in place when advancing the needle so that the needle's lumen does not become occluded with tissue. If paresthesias occur during placement, immediately withdraw the needle. Allow the paresthesia to pass and reposition the needle before proceeding again. Advance the needle until increased resistance is felt as it passes through the ligamentum flavum. As the needle is advanced beyond this ligament, a sudden loss of resistance will occur as the needle "pops" through the dura.

FIGURE 20.3 Spinal needle insertion, lateral view. For the classic midline approach, the needle is introduced in the middle of the interspace and advanced with a slight cephalad angulation. If correctly angled (**A**), it will enter the interspinous ligament, ligamentum flavum, and epidural space. If bone is contacted, it may be the inferior spinous process (**B**), and cephalad redirection will identify the correct path. If angling cephalad causes contact with bone again at a shallower depth (**C**), it is probably the superior spinous process. If bone is encountered at the same depth after several attempts at redirection (not shown), the needle is most likely on the lamina lateral to the interspace, and the position of the true midline should be reassessed. (Reprinted with permission from Mulroy MF. *Regional Anesthesia: An Illustrated Procedural Guide*. 2nd ed. Little, Brown and Company; 1996:79.)

4. Remove the stylet and confirm correct placement by noting free flow of CSF into the hub of the needle. Rotate the needle in 90-degree increments if necessary to confirm or reestablish good flow of CSF.
5. **Administration of anesthetic.** Connect the syringe containing the predetermined dose of local anesthetic to the needle. Gently aspirate CSF into the syringe, which produces birefringence within dextrose-containing solutions and confirms free flow. Inject the drug slowly. Repeat aspiration of CSF at the end of the injection confirms that the needle point is still within the subarachnoid space. Remove the needle and place the patient gently into the desired position.

g. **Closely monitor** (every 60 to 90 seconds) blood pressure, pulse, and respiratory function for 10 to 15 minutes. Determine the ascending anesthetic level by noting the response to a gentle pinprick, alcohol swab, or bag of ice. Stabilization of the local anesthetic level takes approximately 20 minutes.

h. **Continuous spinal anesthesia** allows small aliquots of drug to be injected repeatedly to produce the desired level of sensory blockade. With this technique, a high or rapid sympathetic block can be avoided (of particular concern in patients who are sensitive to drastic changes in blood pressure, such as severe aortic stenosis). A 20-gauge catheter is inserted through a 17-gauge epidural needle. The catheter is advanced 2 to 4 cm into the subarachnoid space. Stimulation of nerve roots during catheter insertion necessitates repositioning of the catheter. **Neurotoxicity** from hyperbaric glucose-containing local anesthetic solutions injected through microbore spinal catheters (26 to 32 gauge) has been reported and may be due to the development of very high concentrations of local anesthetic around the nerves of the cauda equina. There are currently no such approved microbore catheters marketed in the United States.

D. Determinants of the level of spinal blockade
1. **Major**
   a. **Baricity of local anesthetic solution.** Local anesthetic solutions can be described as hyperbaric, hypobaric, or isobaric in relation to the specific gravity of CSF (1.004 to 1.007 g/mL).
      1. **Hyperbaric solutions** are typically prepared by mixing the drug with dextrose. They settle by gravity to the most dependent parts of the CSF column (**Figure 20.4**).
      2. **Hypobaric solutions** are prepared by mixing the drug with sterile water. They slowly rise to the highest part of the CSF column.
      3. **Isobaric solutions** may have the advantage of a predictable spread through the CSF that is less dependent on patient position. Increasing the dose of an isobaric anesthetic has more of an effect on the duration of anesthesia than on the dermatomal spread. Patient positioning can be altered to limit or increase the spread of these mixtures.
   b. **Drug dose.** The anesthetic level varies directly with the dose of the agent used (**Table 20.2**).
   c. **Drug volume.** The greater the volume of the injected drug, the further the drug will spread within the CSF. This is especially applicable to hyperbaric solutions.
   d. **Patient position.** This has a lesser effect on the spread of isobaric solutions.
2. **Minor**
   a. **Turbulence of CSF.** Turbulence created within the CSF during or after the injection will increase the spread of the drug and the level obtained. Turbulence is created by rapid injection, barbotage (the repeated aspiration and reinjection of small amounts of CSF mixed with drug), coughing, and excessive patient movement.

FIGURE 20.4 Spinal column curvatures that influence the spread of anesthetic solutions.

Table 20.2 Drugs and Dosages (in mg) for Spinal Anesthesia

Drug	Level T10	T8	T6	Duration (min)
Tetracaine[a]	10	12	14	90–120
Bupivacaine[a]	7.5	9.0	10.5	90–120
Mepivacaine	30	45	60	60–90

[a]Doses are based on a 66-inch patient. An additional 2 mg of tetracaine or 1.5 mg of bupivacaine should be added or subtracted for each 6 inches in height above or below 66 inches.

      b. **CSF volume.** Lumbosacral CSF volume is inversely correlated with the extent of the spread of local anesthetic.

      c. **Increased intra-abdominal pressure.** Pregnancy, obesity, ascites, and abdominal tumors increase pressure within the inferior vena cava. This pressure increases blood volume within the epidural venous plexus, concomitantly reducing the volume of CSF within the vertebral column, which permits greater spread of injected local anesthetic. In obese patients, this effect is potentiated further by increased fat within the epidural space.

      d. **Spinal curvature.** Lumbar lordosis and thoracic kyphosis influence the spread of hyperbaric solutions. Drug injected above the L3 level will tend to spread cephalad but will be limited by the thoracic curvature at T4 (**Figure 20.4**).

E. Determinants of the duration of the spinal blockade

    1. Drugs and dose. A characteristic duration is specific for each drug (see Chapter 19: Local Anesthetics). The addition of opioids to the injected solution can modify the character of the block (see also Chapter 38: Pain Management). **Hydrophilic opioids** (eg, morphine) offer analgesia that is slow in onset and long in duration. Undesired side effects are more common, and delayed respiratory depression may occur. If hydrophilic opioids are given intrathecally, patients should be closely observed for at least 24 hours. **Lipophilic opioids** (eg, fentanyl) have a lower risk of delayed respiratory depression. Onset is fast, and duration is moderate.

    2. Vasoconstrictors. The addition of epinephrine can prolong the duration of some spinal anesthetics by up to 50%. This effect has not been definitively demonstrated for bupivacaine, although there is evidence that epinephrine prolongs the analgesic effects of low-dose bupivacaine and fentanyl combinations used for labor analgesia. A typical concentration of epinephrine used in spinal anesthetics is 1:400,000 to 1:200,000 (2.5 to 5 µg/mL).

F. Complications and side effects

    1. Neurologic. Nerve injury is infrequent but can be a serious problem. Several types of nerve injury may occur.

      a. **Direct nerve injury related to needle or catheter placement.** Pain during insertion of the catheter or injection of the drug is a warning sign for potential nerve injury resulting from needle or catheter placement and requires repositioning of the needle or catheter. **Transient paresthesias reported by the patient** typically resolve immediately and are usually without any long-term sequelae.

b. **Transient neurologic syndrome (TNS)** is a spontaneous severe radicular pain that occurs after resolution of the spinal anesthetic and may last for 2 to 7 days. Symptoms include buttock and thigh pain described as achy or burning in quality. TNS is usually responsive to conservative measures, such as nonsteroidal anti-inflammatory drugs and warm compresses. The incidence is highest with lidocaine administration but has also been observed with other local anesthetics, including tetracaine, bupivacaine, and mepivacaine. Obesity, ambulatory surgery, knee arthroscopic surgery, and lithotomy position are additional risk factors.
c. **Back pain** following spinal anesthesia may be related to the relaxation of the ligaments that occurs with anesthesia. There is a similar incidence of back pain following general anesthesia, again likely related to the effects of anesthetic agents and muscle relaxants on the structures of the back. Reassurance should be provided.
d. **Bloody tap.** Puncture of an epidural vein during needle insertion may result in either blood or a mixture of blood and CSF emerging from the spinal needle. If the fluid does not rapidly clear, the needle should be withdrawn and reinserted in a different space.
e. **Spinal hematoma** is a surgical emergency. The overall incidence is around 1/150,000. The signs and symptoms of severe back pain and persistent neurologic deficit usually present within 48 hours. Risk is higher among patients who are coagulopathic or anticoagulated. Bloody taps are not generally thought to cause a spinal hematoma in patients with normal coagulation. A bloody tap may be a risk factor for spinal hematoma in patients who undergo subsequent anticoagulation, but there are no data to support the mandatory cancellation of a case under these circumstances. Instead, we advocate direct communication with the surgeon and that a specific risk–benefit decision about proceeding be made on an individual basis. **Close postoperative monitoring** for signs consistent with hematoma is warranted. Diagnosis is usually made with magnetic resonance imaging (MRI), and treatment is via emergent hematoma evacuation. Because catheter removal as well as needle placement may cause spinal hematoma, anesthesiologists need to check a patient's coagulation status and the use of anticoagulants not only at the time of needle placement but also at the time of catheter removal. The approach to the use of anticoagulants, antiplatelet agents, and nonsteroidal anti-inflammatory drugs at Massachusetts General Hospital is listed in **Table 20.3**.
f. **PDPH** usually develops within 3 days; 70% of headaches resolve within 7 days and 90% within 6 months. The classic "spinal headache" is frontal and occipital in distribution, although the temporal area can be affected as well. The headache is exacerbated by upright posture and relieved by lying supine. Other manifestations can include visual disturbances or hearing impairment. Risk factors include younger age, female gender, larger needle size, pregnancy, multiple dural punctures, and a history of previous PDPH. The incidence may be reduced by using smaller needles and noncutting needles (eg, pencil-point needles). Initial treatments of symptoms include rehydration, maintenance of supine position, pain medication including opioids, and caffeine. Maintenance of supine position as a prevention is neither proven nor recommended. Caffeine exerts its effect by vasoconstriction of cerebral vessels. The recommended

Table 20.3 Anticoagulation and Epidural Anesthesia/Analgesia Guidelines

Drug (Generic)	Common Trade Names	Time Interval for Catheter Placement or Neuraxial Procedure After Last Dose	Time Interval for Catheter Removal After Most Recent Dose	Time Interval to Restart Med After Neuraxial Procedure or Catheter Removal
Abciximab	ReoPro	48 h	48 h	24 h
Argatroban	Acova	At least 6 h; check for normal PTT or ACT	Check for normal PTT or ACT	2 h
Cilostazol[a]	Pletal	42 h	42 h	5 h
Clopidogrel[b]	Plavix	7 d	7 d if single 75 mg dose given	6 h
Eptifibatide	Integrilin	8 h	8 h	24 h
Fondaparinux[c]	Arixtra	7 d	4 d	6 h
Heparin subcutaneously (twice daily)	Heparin	4–6 h or assess AC status	4–6 h or assess AC status	Can be started immediately
Heparin IV	Heparin	IV: 4–6 h SC: 12 h and assess AC status	IV: 4–6 h SC: 12 h and assess AC status	1 h
Dalteparin (low dose)[d]	Fragmin (≤5000 U daily)	12 h	12 h	4 h
Dalteparin (high dose)[d]	Fragmin (5000 U twice daily or 120 U/kg twice daily or 175 U/kg daily)	24 h	24 h	4 h
Enoxaparin (low dose)[d]	Lovenox (<60 mg daily)	12 h	BID dosing: indwelling catheter should be removed before initiation Daily dosing: 12 h after last dose	4 h after catheter removal and >12 h after needle/catheter placement
Enoxaparin (high dose)[d]	Lovenox (>60 mg daily or 1 mg/kg twice daily)	24 h	Indwelling catheter should be removed before initiation	4 h after catheter removal and >24 h after needle/catheter placement

Anticoagulation and Epidural Anesthesia/Analgesia Guidelines (*continued*)

Drug (Generic)	Common Trade Names	Time Interval for Catheter Placement or Neuraxial Procedure After Last Dose	Time Interval for Catheter Removal After Most Recent Dose	Time Interval to Restart Med After Neuraxial Procedure or Catheter Removal
NSAID, ASA	Celebrex, Motrin, Naprosyn, Vioxx, etc.	No significant risk		
Thrombolytics: streptokinase, alteplase (tPA)	Streptase, Activase	10 d	10 d	10 d
Ticagrelor	Brilinta	5 d	5 d	6 h
Tirofiban	Aggrastat	8 h	8 h	24 h
Warfarin	Coumadin	3–5 d, INR ≤1.5	Check INR if treatment >24 h, INR ≤1.5	Same day

ACT, activated clotting time; ASA, aspirin; NSAID, nonsteroidal anti-inflammatory drug; PTT, partial thromboplastin time.

[a]If cilostazol (Pletal) is the only anticoagulant given, then an epidural catheter placement is most likely safe. If cilostazol (Pletal) is combined with other anticoagulant medicines (eg, aspirin), neuraxial procedure or catheter placement should be delayed for at least 48 h.

[b]Clopidogrel (Plavix) has a 24–48-h window to remove an epidural catheter once the medication is given. If it has been more than 48 h since dosing of clopidogrel, you must wait for 7 d.

[c]Fondaparinux should not be given if regional anesthesia is anticipated or has been used. If, however, fondaparinux 2.5 mg is given, we suggest the guidelines noted in this table. For larger doses (5–10 mg), neuraxial procedure should not be done for 7 d.

[d]Low–molecular-weight heparin: single-daily dosing may be started 6 to 8 h postoperatively. Twice-daily dosing should be started at least 24 h postoperatively. Epidural catheters should be removed before initiation of therapy.

dose of caffeine is 300 to 500 mg orally or IV. One cup of coffee contains 50 to 100 mg of caffeine. If initial therapy fails and severe symptoms persist more than 24 hours, an **epidural blood patch** can be done. Epidural needle insertion is done at the level of presumed dural puncture. Blood is drawn in a sterile fashion and injected into the epidural space. This procedure usually requires two providers. The typical blood volume is 20 to 30 mL or less if the patient complains of back discomfort during injection. The success rate ranges from 65% to 98%, and results are often immediate. A second blood patch can be tried with a success rate about the same as the first attempt. The use of a prophylactic epidural blood patch before the onset of headache symptoms is of controversial benefit, but is still performed by some anesthetists.

2. **Cardiovascular**
   a. **Hypotension.** The incidence of hypotension may be reduced by IV administration of 500 to 1000 mL of isotonic solution before

performing the block. Patients with decreased cardiac function require care in administering large volumes of IV fluid, because translocation of fluid from the peripheral to the central circulation during cessation of the block and return of systemic vascular tone could produce volume overload and pulmonary edema. Treatment of hypotension includes increasing venous return and treating severe bradycardia. Trendelenburg position, fluid administration, raising lower extremities to autotransfuse blood, or the use of vasopressors may be necessary.

  b. **Bradycardia.** Bradycardia can be a sign of a vagal response or could be indicative of a high spinal (less common). If present, bradycardia can be treated with atropine or glycopyrrolate. If bradycardia is severe and accompanied by hypotension, ephedrine or epinephrine may be used.

3. **Respiratory**
  a. **Dyspnea** is a common complaint with high spinal levels. It is caused by the proprioceptive blockade of afferent fibers from abdominal and chest wall muscles. Reassuring the patient may be all that is required, although adequate ventilation must be ensured. Supplemental O_2 can be provided for patient comfort.
  b. **Apnea** can be caused by reduced medullary blood flow accompanying severe hypotension or from direct blockade of C3–C5 ("total spinal"), inhibiting phrenic nerve output. Immediate ventilatory support is required in this scenario, so the provider should be prepared to mask ventilate and secure the airway if indicated.

4. **Visceral**
  a. **Urinary retention.** The mechanism of urinary retention is described in Section IV.B.4.a. Urinary retention may outlast the sensory and motor blockade. A urinary catheter should be placed if anesthesia or analgesia is maintained for a prolonged period.
  b. **Nausea and vomiting** are usually caused by hypotension or unopposed vagal stimulation. Treatment involves first restoring blood pressure, followed by administering oxygen, and IV atropine if needed.

5. **Infection** after spinal anesthesia is exceedingly rare. Nevertheless, meningitis, arachnoiditis, and epidural abscess can occur. Possible etiologies include chemical contamination and viral or bacterial infection due to lack of sterility. Consultation and prompt diagnosis and treatment are essential.

6. **Pruritus** commonly occurs with the use of neuraxial opioids and is more frequent with intrathecal administration as opposed to epidural. The exact mechanism is unclear. Pharmacologic treatments include nalbuphine (5 to 10 mg IV), naloxone (1 to 2 µg/kg/h), naltrexone (6 to 9 mg PO), diphenhydramine (25 to 50 mg IV/PO), ondansetron (4 to 8 mg IV), and propofol (10 to 20 mg IV bolus).

7. **Shivering** has a high incidence and may be treated with IV meperidine (25 mg IV). Clonidine (65 to 300 µg IV) has been shown to have a similar efficacy.

V. EPIDURAL ANESTHESIA

Epidural anesthesia is achieved by introducing local anesthetics into the epidural space.

  A. Anatomy. The epidural space is a potential space extending from the base of the skull to the sacrococcygeal membrane. Posteriorly, it is bounded by the ligamentum flavum, the anterior surfaces of the laminae, and the articular processes. Anteriorly, it is bounded by the posterior longitudinal ligament covering the vertebral bodies and intervertebral discs. Laterally, it is bounded by intervertebral foramina and the pedicles. It has direct communications with the paravertebral space. It contains fat and lymphatic tissue as well as epidural veins, which are most prominent in the lateral aspects of the space. The veins have no valves and directly communicate with the intracranial veins. The veins also communicate with the thoracic and abdominal veins through the intervertebral foramina and with the pelvic veins through the sacral venous plexus. The epidural space is widest in the midline and tapers off laterally. In the lumbar region, it is 5 to 6 mm wide in the midline; in the midthoracic region, the space is 3 to 5 mm wide.

B. **Physiology**
1. **Neural blockade.** Local anesthetic placed in the epidural space acts directly on the spinal nerve roots located in the lateral aspect of the space. These nerve roots are covered by the dural sheath. Local anesthetic gains access to the CSF by uptake through the dura. The onset of the block is slower than with spinal anesthesia, and the intensity of the sensory and motor block is less. Anesthesia develops in a segmental manner, and selective blockade can be achieved.
2. **Cardiovascular.** Physiologic changes from sympathetic blockade are similar to those described for spinal anesthesia (see Section IV.B.2), but usually, hemodynamic change is slower. Large doses of local anesthetic may be absorbed or inadvertently injected into the vasculature and could depress the myocardium. Epinephrine used to prolong the duration of the local anesthetics may also be absorbed or injected into the systemic circulation, producing tachycardia and hypertension.
3. **Respiratory.** Physiologic changes are similar to those described for spinal anesthesia. When we use postoperative epidural analgesia with dilute local anesthetics after major abdominal or thoracic surgery, the reduction in functional residual capacity and impairment of diaphragm function are minimized, which improves overall pulmonary outcome. With epidural anesthesia, the incidence of postoperative hypoxemia can be decreased by reducing the need for systemic opioids.
4. **Coagulation.** Epidural anesthesia has been reported to reduce venous thrombosis and subsequent pulmonary embolism. Proposed mechanisms include increased pelvic blood flow, decreased sympathetic response to surgery, and earlier mobility. Epidural anesthesia may reduce intraoperative blood loss during hip, pelvic, and lower abdominal surgeries.
5. **Gastrointestinal.** Epidural anesthesia can be administered for patients undergoing bowel resection with anastomosis. As with spinal anesthesia, the predominance of the parasympathetic system may cause contraction of the bowel. Patients often have earlier return of bowel function with the use of an epidural.
6. Other physiologic changes seen are similar to those described for spinal anesthesia (see Section IV.B).

C. **Technique**
1. **Epidural needles.** Most commonly, the 17-gauge **Tuohy** or **Weiss** needle is used for identification of the epidural space. These needles are stylletted, have a blunt leading edge with a lateral opening, and have a thin wall to allow passage of a 20-gauge catheter.
2. **Patient position.** Patients can be positioned for epidural anesthesia in either the sitting or the lateral position. The same considerations apply to spinal anesthesia (see Section IV.C.4).

3. **Monitoring.** The patient should be monitored with standard monitors including ECG, blood pressure, and oxygen saturation.
4. **Approaches.** Whether from a midline or paramedian approach, the needle should enter the epidural space in the midline, because the space is widest here and there is a decreased risk of puncturing epidural veins, spinal arteries, or spinal nerve roots, all of which lie predominantly in the lateral aspects of the epidural space. Palpation of landmarks, skin preparation, and draping are as described for spinal anesthesia (see Section IV.C.5) (**Figure 20.5**).
   a. **Lumbar.** Use a long 25-gauge needle for superficial and deep infiltration of local anesthetic into the supraspinous and interspinous ligaments. This needle also assists in defining the direction in which the epidural needle should be inserted. Advance the epidural needle through the supraspinous and interspinous ligaments in a slightly cephalad direction, until it comes to lie within the "rubbery" ligamentum flavum.
      1. **Loss-of-resistance techniques.** Remove the stylet and attach a glass or plastic loss-of-resistance syringe containing approximately 3 mL of air or saline to the needle hub. Apply constant pressure to the plunger of the syringe while slowly advancing the needle. When the bevel enters the epidural space, there is a marked "loss of resistance" to plunger displacement. Alternatively, an "intermittent" technique can be used, where the change in resistance

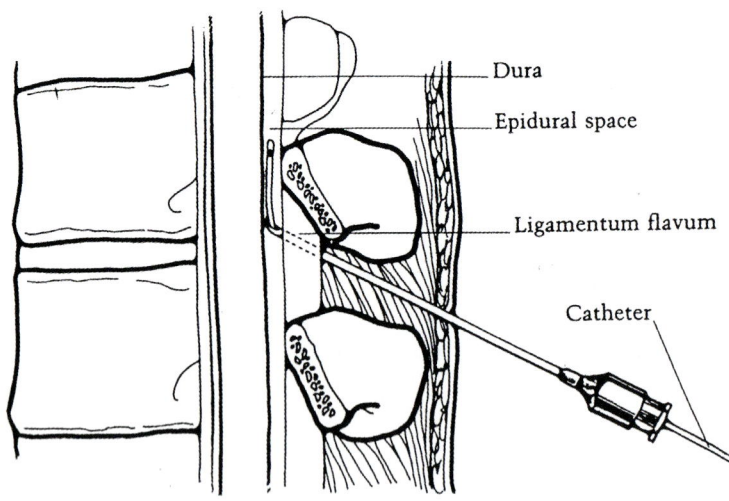

FIGURE 20.5 Insertion of an epidural catheter. The needle is secured by resting one hand on the back and grasping the hub firmly (not shown) while the other hand inserts the catheter into the hub and gently advances it beyond the tip of the needle. The bevel is usually directed cephalad, which produces the most reliable insertion; caudad orientation may allow the catheter to exit one of the intervertebral foramina. Ideally, the catheter is advanced 3 to 4 cm beyond the needle tip; further placement increases the potential for lateral misdirection or foraminal exit. (Reprinted with permission from Mulroy MF. *Regional Anesthesia: An Illustrated Procedural Guide.* 2nd ed. Little, Brown and Company; 1996:109.)

is tested repeatedly in between small careful advances of the epidural needle. When air is used for loss of resistance, the amount of air injected should be minimized. Patchy block, pneumocephalus, and air embolism have been reported with the loss of resistance with air technique.
2. The **hanging drop technique** relies on the principle that a drop of fluid placed on the hub of the epidural needle (once the ligamentum flavum has been entered) will retract into the needle as the tip of the needle is advanced into the epidural space. This negative pressure is provided by "tenting" of the dura by the needle tip but may be altered by transmitted changes in intra-abdominal and intrathoracic pressure (eg, pregnancy and obesity). Drop retraction occurs only about 80% of the time, so if a change in compliance is felt while advancing through the ligamentum flavum, it should be checked by loss of resistance to prevent unanticipated dural puncture.
3. In cases where landmarks are difficult to palpate, **ultrasound** can be used to identify the interspaces as well as midline. When placed perpendicular to the spinal cord (transverse approach), the spinous process can be identified as a hyperechoic signal close to the skin, continuing as a vertical acoustic shadow (can be triangular in shape), thus designating midline. The longitudinal paramedian approach involves placing the ultrasound probe parallel to the spinal cord just a few centimeters lateral and angled toward midline. This view allows visualization of the interspaces, as well as other structures including ligamentum flavum, vertebral body, and sacrum.

b. **Thoracic epidural anesthesia** provides upper abdominal and thoracic anesthesia with a smaller dose of local anesthetic. Postoperative analgesia can be produced without lower extremity blockade. Although the technique is the same as for lumbar placement, the thoracic vertebral spinous processes are much more sharply angulated downward so that the tip of the superior spinous process overlies the lamina of the vertebra below, and the epidural needle should be directed in a more acute cephalad direction. In addition, there is a risk of producing trauma to the underlying spinal cord if dural puncture occurs. In some patients, a paramedian approach is necessary.

c. **Technique for catheter placement.** An epidural catheter permits repeated injections of local anesthetic for prolonged procedures and provides a route for postoperative analgesia.
1. Thread a 20-gauge radiopaque catheter with 1-cm graduations through the epidural needle. If the catheter contains a wire stylet, the stylet should first be withdrawn 1 to 2 cm before insertion of the catheter to decrease the incidence of paresthesia and dural or venous puncture. Many individuals prefer to completely remove the stylet since it is stiff enough to allow placement into extraepidural tissue. If the catheter passes easily without the stylet, it is usually located in the epidural space. Polyvinyl chloride catheters are relatively stiff and resist kinking but can be associated with dural and venous puncture. Teflon catheters are very soft and flexible but may be more likely to kink and occlude. Newer catheters of nylon, polyamide, and polyvinyl offer compromises between flexibility and rigidity. Wire-reinforced

soft catheters do not kink and are much less prone to slipping out. When multipore catheters are used, the distance from the catheter tip to the most proximal lateral hole should be noted to ensure that all injected medication reaches the epidural space.
2. Make note of the depth at which loss of resistance occurred by counting the 1-cm markings on the Tuohy or Weiss needle that are exposed superficial to the patient's skin. A standard epidural needle measures 10 cm in length. By subtracting the number of 1-cm markings exposed superficial to the patient's skin from 10, an estimated distance between the skin and epidural space, or "depth" to the epidural space, can be obtained. Advance the catheter through the needle until the 15-cm marking on the catheter is within the shaft of the epidural needle to ensure that approximately 5 cm of catheter is exposed distal to the needle tip. The patient may experience an abrupt paresthesia, which is usually transient. If it is sustained, the catheter must be repositioned. If the catheter must be withdrawn, the catheter and needle should be removed together to avoid shearing the catheter tip.
3. Carefully withdraw the needle over the catheter making sure not to inadvertently withdraw the catheter as well. Make note of the marking on the catheter at the skin. Be sure to leave the catheter approximately 5 cm within the epidural space by securing the catheter at the skin 5 cm "deeper" than the "depth" to the epidural space (ie, if loss of resistance occurred at a "depth" of 6 cm, secure the catheter at the skin at a "depth" of 11 cm).
   d. After aspirating for CSF using a 3 mL syringe, administer a **test dose** of local anesthetic agent through the needle if a single-dose technique is used or through the catheter for continuous techniques. A test dose usually consists of 3 mL of 1.5% lidocaine with 1:200,000 epinephrine. This should have little effect on the epidural space. If the solution has been injected into the CSF, a spinal block will occur rapidly. If the solution has been injected into an epidural vein, a 20% to 30% increase in heart rate may be seen. Other symptoms of an intravascular injection include perioral numbness, a metallic taste, tinnitus, and palpitations. The patient should be instructed to report any of these sensations if they arise. A corresponding increase in blood pressure can also be seen if the patient's heart rate is controlled with β-blockers.
   e. **Injection of anesthetic.** Administer the anesthetic solution in 3- to 5-mL increments every 3 to 5 minutes until the desired total dose has been given. Aspirate the catheter or needle, checking for the appearance of blood or CSF, before each injection.
D. **Determinants of the level of the epidural blockade**
   1. **Volume of local anesthetic.** A maximum dose of 1.6 mL of local anesthetic per segment has been suggested for the induction of epidural blockade. This maximum can be exceeded if dilute mixtures of medications are used, as for postoperative or labor analgesia.
   2. **Age.** The volume of local anesthetic should be reduced by approximately 50% in the elderly and in neonates. Stenosis of intervertebral foramina in the elderly reduces the lateral paravertebral spread of the injected drug, allowing for a more cephalad spread.
   3. **Pregnancy.** A 30% reduction in dose is expected in pregnant women. Hormonal effects during pregnancy render nerves more sensitive to the effects of local anesthetic, and inferior vena cava compression increases

blood volume within the epidural venous plexus, reducing the potential volume of the epidural space.
4. **Speed of injection.** Rapid injection of drug into the epidural space may produce a less reliable block than a slow, steady injection at approximately 0.5 mL/s. Very rapid injection of large volumes of drug has the potentially hazardous effect of increasing pressure within the epidural space. Such a rise in pressure can produce headache, increased intracranial pressure, and possibly spinal cord ischemia by decreasing spinal cord blood flow.
5. **Position.** The position of the patient has a slight effect on the level of the epidural blockade. Patients sitting upright have greater caudad spread of blockade; patients in the lateral position have a higher level of block on the dependent side. This can be helpful if patients are reporting a "one-sided block," as the painful side can be positioned down during a bolus to overcome this.
6. **Spread of epidural blockade.** Onset of blockade occurs first and is most dense at the level of injection. Spread of the block usually occurs faster in a cephalad than in a caudad direction. This is likely because of the relative difference in size between the large lower lumbar and sacral nerve roots compared with the smaller thoracic nerve roots. L5–S1 are large nerve roots making them difficult to anesthetize and often leading to sparing of this area during epidural block.

E. Determinants of the onset and duration of the epidural blockade
1. **Selection of drug** (see Chapter 19: Local Anesthetics).
2. **Addition of epinephrine.** Epinephrine, added at a concentration of 1:200,000, decreases the systemic uptake and plasma levels of local anesthetic, and prolongs its duration of action (see Chapter 19: Local Anesthetics).
3. **Addition of opioid.** The addition of fentanyl, 50 to 100 µg, to the local anesthetic solution speeds the onset, increases the level, prolongs the duration, and improves the quality of the block. Fentanyl is thought to produce this effect by having a selective action at the substantia gelatinosa of the dorsal horn of the spinal cord to modulate pain transmission. This action appears to be synergistic with the actions of the local anesthetics.
4. **pH adjustment of solution.** The addition of sodium bicarbonate to the local anesthetic solution in a ratio of 1 mL of 8.4% sodium bicarbonate to each 10 mL of lidocaine (0.1 mL for each 10 mL of bupivacaine as excess bicarbonate will precipitate in bupivacaine) decreases the onset time for the blockade. It is thought that this effect is due to an increased amount of local anesthetic base, which increases the rate at which nonionized drug crosses axonal membranes.

F. Additional confirmation of epidural catheter placement
1. **Incidence of misplaced catheters.** The loss-of-resistance technique has low specificity, leading to frequent misplacement of epidural catheters. In teaching hospitals, the incidence of thoracic epidural analgesia failure due to misidentification of the epidural space may exceed 20%.
2. **Additional confirmatory methods.** Using additional confirmatory methods can reduce epidural failure rates and facilitate the early detection of misplaced epidural catheters.
    a. **Sensory testing.** Sensory testing with a pinprick or ice following a local anesthetic bolus is commonly used to confirm epidural placement. However, this method is limited by the slow onset of sensory blockade and its reliance on patient feedback.

b. **Waveform analysis.** Measuring pressure at the tip of a correctly placed epidural needle or catheter allows visualization of a characteristic waveform corresponding to arterial pulsations. An advantage of this method is that it can be used for patients under general anesthesia. However, waveform analysis cannot exclude intrathecal catheter placement, which also produces a similar waveform.

c. **Electrical stimulation.** Electrical stimulation via epidural catheters can produce myotomal contractions. The catheter tip can be repositioned to the desired level based on the myotomal response.

d. **Fluoroscopy.** Fluoroscopy allows visualization of the needle tip and catheter position, providing visual confirmation of catheter placement in the epidural space. The administration of contrast can provide further confirmation.

G. Complications

1. **Dural puncture** occurs in about 1% of epidural catheter placements. If dural puncture occurs during attempted epidural catheter insertion, the chance of PDPH is higher than with spinal anesthesia due to the larger size of the needle. Furthermore, it is important to minimize the amount of CSF leakage from the epidural needle by either covering the proximal hole of the needle with your finger or reinserting the stylet. Several management options are available after dural puncture. A conversion to spinal anesthesia can be made by injecting an appropriate amount of anesthetic into the CSF. Continuous spinal anesthesia can be performed by inserting an epidural catheter into the subarachnoid space through the epidural needle. If epidural anesthesia is required (eg, for postoperative analgesia), the catheter can be repositioned at a different interspace so that the tip of the epidural catheter lies well away from the site of dural puncture. The possibility of spinal anesthesia occurring with injection of the epidural catheter should be considered.

2. **Bloody tap.** If a bloody tap occurs during epidural needle placement, some practitioners advocate for epidural placement at a different interspace. Advantages include minimizing confounding effects of visualized blood on determination of correct catheter placement and potentially decreasing amounts of systemically absorbed local anesthetic that may be falsely interpreted as a positive test dose. In patients with normal coagulation, such bloody taps rarely lead to serious sequelae (eg, epidural hematoma). Bloody epidural taps may be risk factors for epidural hematoma in patients who undergo subsequent anticoagulation, but there are no data to support the mandatory cancellation of a case under these circumstances. Instead, we advocate direct communication with the surgeon and that a specific risk–benefit decision about proceeding be made on an individual basis. Close postoperative monitoring for signs consistent with hematoma is warranted.

3. **Catheter complications**

   a. **Inability to thread the epidural catheter** is relatively common. This problem can occur if the epidural needle is inserted into the lateral aspect of the epidural space rather than the midline or if the bevel of the needle is at too acute an angle to the epidural space for the catheter to emerge. It can also occur if the level of the needle is only partially through the ligamentum flavum when loss of resistance is found. In the latter case, slight (1 mm) advancement of the needle into the epidural space may facilitate catheter insertion.

   b. **The catheter can be inserted into an epidural vein.** Blood cannot always be aspirated back through the catheter. This may be noticed only when an initial test dose with epinephrine is administered, and tachycardia is noted. The catheter should be withdrawn until blood can no longer be aspirated, flushed with saline, and then retested. Withdrawal of the catheter more than 1 to 2 cm should prompt removal and reinsertion.

  c. **Catheters can break off or become knotted** within the epidural space. In the absence of infection, a retained catheter is no more reactive than a surgical suture. The patient should be informed of the problem and reassured. The complications of surgical exploration and removal of an asymptomatic catheter are greater than in conservative management.
  d. **Cannulation of the subdural space.** The subdural space is a potential space between the dura and the arachnoid membranes and may be entered with a needle or with a catheter. CSF is not aspirated but the effects of the local anesthetic are quite different from usual epidural anesthesia and are often quite variable. In the absence of myelography, it is a diagnosis of exclusion. It can result in dissociation of blocked modalities (eg, full sensory anesthesia without motor block or motor block with minimal sensory block). It should be suspected whenever an epidural dose produces a more extensive spread than expected. Subdural catheters should be removed and an epidural catheter should be placed.
4. **Unintentional subarachnoid injection.** The injection of a large volume of local anesthetic into the subarachnoid space can produce total spinal anesthesia. Treatment is similar to that described for spinal complications (see Section IV.F).
5. **Intravascular injection** of local anesthetic into an epidural vein causes central nervous system and cardiovascular toxicity and may result in convulsions and cardiopulmonary arrest. Resistant ventricular fibrillation with IV bupivacaine has been described. The treatment for intravascular injection includes IV lipid emulsion for local anesthetic-related cardiotoxicity. A bolus of Intralipid 20%, 1.5 mL/kg, over 2 to 3 minutes followed by a continuous infusion (0.25 mL/kg/min) with repeat bolus doses once or twice for a total maximum dose of 12 mL/kg is the treatment of choice. Cardiopulmonary bypass is an option if ventricular fibrillation or cardiac arrest is resistant to pharmacologic therapy (see Chapters 19: Local Anesthetics and 39: Adult, Pediatric, and Newborn Resuscitation).
6. **Local anesthetic overdose.** Systemic local anesthetic toxicity may occur due to the relatively large amounts of drug required for anesthesia. Inadvertent intravascular injection is the most common cause of local anesthetic overdose. Vasoconstrictors such as epinephrine decreases the incidence of toxicity by decreasing the rate of absorption of local anesthetic.
7. **Direct spinal cord injury** is more likely if the epidural injection is above L2. The onset of a unilateral paresthesia during needle insertion suggests lateral entry into the epidural space. Further injection or insertion of a catheter at this point may produce trauma to a nerve root. Small feeder arteries to the anterior spinal artery also run in this area as they pass through the intervertebral foramen. Trauma to these arteries potentially may result in anterior spinal cord ischemia or an epidural hematoma. Placement of epidural catheters after the induction of general anesthesia negates the ability to appreciate symptoms of paresthesia and is done only when such potential risk is deemed

necessary. Pediatric patients frequently have catheters placed after induction of general anesthesia, often at the caudal level.
8. **PDPH.** If the dura is punctured with a 17-gauge epidural needle, there is a greater than 75% chance of a young patient developing a PDPH. Management is the same as that described under spinal anesthesia (see Section IV.F.1.f.).
9. **Epidural abscess** is an extremely rare complication of epidural anesthesia. The source of infection usually is from hematogenous spread to the epidural space from an infection in another area. Infection can also arise from contamination during insertion, contamination of an indwelling catheter used for postoperative pain relief, or a cutaneous infection at the insertion site. The patient presents with fever, severe back pain, and localized back tenderness. Progression to nerve root pain and paralysis can occur. Initial laboratory investigations include evaluation for a leukocytosis and a lumbar puncture suggestive of a parameningeal infection. Definitive diagnosis is by MRI. Treatment includes antibiotics and sometimes urgent decompression laminectomy. Rapid diagnosis and treatment are associated with good neurologic recovery. Epidural catheter dressings should be inspected daily for signs of leakage and inflammation.
10. **Epidural hematoma** is an extremely rare complication of epidural anesthesia. An epidural hematoma is a surgical emergency. Trauma to epidural veins in the presence of a coagulopathy may result in a large epidural hematoma. The patient can present with severe back pain and persistent neurologic deficit after epidural anesthesia. Diagnosis is confirmed by MRI. A decompressive laminectomy within 8 hours from the onset of symptoms is required to preserve neurologic function.
11. **Horner syndrome** is seen in 1% to 4% of epidural anesthetics. The constellation of ptosis, miosis, anhidrosis, and enophthalmos occurs due to the sympathetic blockade of the upper thoracic spinal segments. Reassurance is provided to the patient as these symptoms resolve.

VI. COMBINED SPINAL–EPIDURAL ANESTHESIA
A. Spinal anesthesia offers the benefits of rapid onset. Placement of an epidural catheter at the same time offers the advantage of prolonged anesthesia and analgesia for longer procedures or postoperative pain management. This technique often is used in the labor and delivery setting (see Chapter 32: Anesthesia for Obstetrics and Gynecology).

B. Technique. Prepare the patient as for epidural placement (see Section V.C). After placing the epidural needle in the epidural space, advance a long spinal needle (Sprotte 24 gauge × 120 mm or Whitacre 25 gauge) through the epidural needle until the characteristic pop of dural penetration occurs. At this point, withdraw the stylet from the spinal needle and confirm free flow of CSF. Before withdrawing the stylet, it is recommended to grasp both the spinal needle and the epidural Tuohy needle at the same time to stabilize the position of the spinal needle. Inject medication into the subarachnoid space and withdraw the spinal needle. Thread an epidural catheter through the epidural needle in the standard fashion. If epidural anesthesia is used subsequently, a test dose is required (can be administered intraoperatively).

VII. CAUDAL ANESTHESIA
Caudal anesthesia is obtained by placing local anesthetic into the epidural space in the sacral region. This technique is often used for pediatric

anesthesia. The details in the section that follows are intended for the adult population.

A. Anatomy. The caudal space is an extension of the epidural space. The sacral hiatus is formed by the failure of the laminae of S5 to fuse. The hiatus is bounded laterally by the sacral cornua, which are the inferior articulating processes of S5. The **sacrococcygeal membrane** is a thin layer of fibrous tissue that covers the sacral hiatus. The caudal canal contains the sacral nerves, the sacral venous plexus, the filum terminale, and the dural sac, which usually ends at the lower border of S2. In neonates, the dural sac may extend to S4.

B. Physiology. The physiology of caudal anesthesia is similar to that described for epidural anesthesia (see Section V.B). It is indicated for surgical and obstetric procedures of the perineal and sacral areas.

C. Technique
   1. Caudal epidural anesthesia is performed with the patient in the lateral, prone, or jackknife position.
   2. Palpate the sacral cornua. If they are difficult to palpate directly, the location of the sacral hiatus in adults can be estimated by measuring 5 cm from the tip of the coccyx in the midline.
   3. Skin preparation and draping are as described for spinal anesthesia (see Section IV.C.5).
   4. Raise a skin wheal with 1% lidocaine between the sacral cornua.
   5. Insert a 22-gauge spinal needle at an angle of 70° to 80° to the skin. Advance the needle through the sacrococcygeal membrane, which is identified by a characteristic pop. Avoid attempting to thread the needle up the caudal canal because this increases the likelihood of puncturing an epidural vein (**Figure 20.6**).
   6. Withdraw the stylet and inspect the hub of the needle for passive CSF or blood flow. The needle can be aspirated as a further check. Reposition the needle if either blood or CSF appears.
   7. Administer a test dose of 3 mL of local anesthetic solution with epinephrine (1:200,000), similar to that used for lumbar epidural anesthesia (see Section V.C.4.d), observing the patient for signs of subarachnoid or IV injection. Because the caudal canal has a rich epidural venous plexus, IV injections are seen frequently and can occur even though blood cannot be aspirated from the needle.
   8. A caudal catheter can be placed in a manner analogous to that for lumbar epidural anesthesia with a 17-gauge Tuohy needle (see Section V.C.4.c). The catheter can be used for postoperative analgesia.
   9. The level, onset, and duration for caudal anesthesia follow the same principles outlined for epidural anesthesia (see Sections V.D and V.E). The extent of caudal block is less predictable than other epidural techniques because of the variability in content and volume of the caudal canal and the amount of local anesthetic solution that leaks out of the sacral foramina. To obtain sacral anesthesia, a volume of 12 to 15 mL should be sufficient.

D. Complications. The complications of caudal anesthesia are similar to those of epidural anesthesia (see Section V.G).

VII. ANTICOAGULATION AND NEURAXIAL BLOCKADE

Neuraxial blockade should be avoided in the presence of prophylactic or therapeutic anticoagulation because of the increased risk of epidural hematoma formation. Massachusetts General Hospital guidelines regarding neuraxial anesthesia in anticoagulated patients are listed in **Table 20.3**.

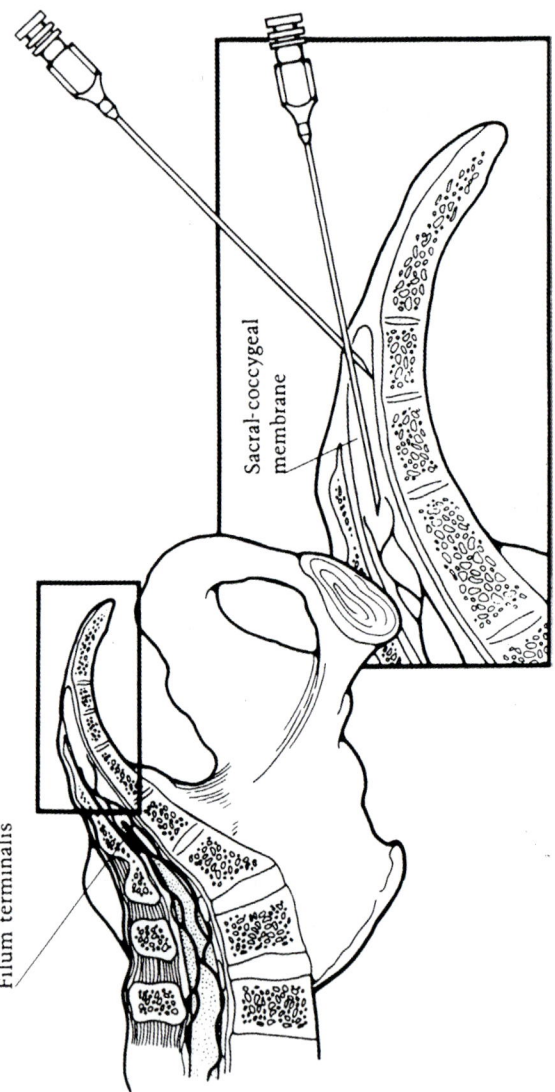

FIGURE 20.6 Sacral anatomy, lateral view. A needle directed through the sacral-coccygeal membrane at a 45-degree angle will usually "pop" through the ligament and contact the anterior bone of the sacral canal. The needle needs to be rotated so that the bevel does not scrape the periosteum of this layer, and the angle of advancement changed to allow passage directly 2 to 3 cm up the canal without contacting the bone again. This space is generously endowed with blood vessels, and the terminal point of the dural sac extends a variable distance in the sacral canal but usually lies at the S2 level. (Reprinted with permission from Mulroy MF. *Regional Anesthesia: An Illustrated Procedural Guide.* 2nd ed. Little, Brown and Company; 1996:124.)

A. **Oral anticoagulants.** In patients receiving low-dose oral anticoagulants (warfarin), regional techniques may be performed if the thromboprophylaxis was initiated less than 24 hours previously. If epidural or spinal anesthesia is planned, hold warfarin 3 to 5 days before the operation, and the patient's international normalized ratio (INR) should be checked before the operation. An INR less than or equal to 1.5 is generally acceptable for many anesthesiologists, but there is no definite cutoff value above which epidural or spinal anesthesia is specifically discouraged.
B. **Unfractionated heparin.** Twice-daily subcutaneous heparin prophylaxis is not a contraindication for the use of neuraxial techniques. There is an unknown risk with prophylactic subcutaneous heparin dosed three times per day. In these cases, a coagulation profile should be obtained. Caution should be used in debilitated patients, in whom the action of the drug may be prolonged and in whom neurologic monitoring may be difficult. IV heparin should be stopped 2 to 4 hours before the initiation of neuraxial blockade, and a repeat coagulation profile should be obtained if there is any question about the state of anticoagulation. Administration of heparin should be delayed for at least 2 hours after placement. Removal of a catheter should be treated with the same anticoagulation guidelines as the placement of a catheter.
C. **Low–molecular-weight heparin (LMWH).** Patients receiving LMWH for thromboembolism prophylaxis have altered coagulation parameters. Spinal or epidural needle placement should not be done for at least 12 hours after the last dose. Patients receiving higher doses of LMWH (enoxaparin 1 mg/kg twice daily) will require longer delays (24 hours). In patients requiring continuing LMWH administration, spinal or epidural catheters should be removed before administration of LMWH. The subsequent administration of LMWH should be delayed for 4 hours after catheter removal.
D. **Antiplatelet drugs.** Patients receiving aspirin or nonsteroidal anti-inflammatory drugs do not appear to be at higher risk for epidural hematoma formation. These drugs could contribute to an increased bleeding risk, however, if they are used concurrently with other anticoagulants. With regard to thienopyridine derivatives (ticlopidine and clopidogrel), the suggested time interval between discontinuation of medication and initiation of neuraxial block is 14 days for ticlopidine and 5 to 7 days for clopidogrel. Following platelet GPIIb/IIIa inhibitors, normal platelet function returns in 24 to 48 hours with abciximab and in 4 to 8 hours with eptifibatide and tirofiban.
E. **Fibrinolytic and thrombolytic agents.** Although the plasma half-life of thrombolytic drugs is only for hours, it takes several days before thrombolytic effects disappear. Surgery or puncture of noncompressible vessels within 10 days of thrombolytic therapy is contraindicated. There is no definitive guideline regarding the neuraxial anesthesia and thrombolytic therapy. Measurement of the fibrinogen level may be helpful in guiding the decision.
F. **Herbal medication** (see Chapters 1: Evaluating the Patient Before Anesthesia and 38: Pain Management). Herbal medications including garlic, ginkgo, and ginseng are all known to affect coagulation. Currently, there are no specific guidelines for timing the neuraxial block in relation to herbal medication use. Because it is not known at which doses potential coagulopathies occur, management decisions are often based more on a clinical history of abnormal bleeding. Herbal medications are thought to be more problematic when taken concurrently with other conventional anticoagulant medications.

ACKNOWLEDGMENT

We gratefully acknowledge the contributions of previous edition author, Erica L. Gee, as portions of those chapters have been retained in this revision.

Suggested Readings

Aida S, Taga K, Yamakura T, Endoh H, Shimoji K. Headache after attempted epidural block: the role of intrathecal air. *Anesthesiology.* 1998;88:76–81.

Horlocker TT, Wedel DJ, Rowlingson JC, et al. Regional anesthesia in the patient receiving antithrombotic or thrombolytic therapy: American Society of Regional Anesthesia and Pain Medicine Evidence-Based Guidelines (Third Edition). *Reg Anesth Pain Med.* 2010;35(1):64–101.

Moen V, Dahlgren N, Irestedt L. Severe neurological complications after central neuraxial blockades in Sweden 1990–1999. *Anesthesiology.* 2004;101:950–959.

Moraca RJ, Sheldon DG, Thirlby RC. The role of epidural anesthesia and analgesia in surgical practice. *Ann Surg.* 2003;238:663–673.

Tran Q, Booysen K, Botha HJ. Primary failure of thoracic epidural analgesia: revisited. *Reg Anesth Pain Med.* 2024;49(4):298–303.

Turnbull DK, Sheperd DB. Post-dural puncture headache: pathogenesis, prevention and treatment. *Br J Anaesth.* 2003;91(5):718–729.

Regional Anesthesia

David Rollins and A. Sassan Sabouri

ABBREVIATIONS

ASA—American Society of Anesthesiologists
ASIS—anterior superior iliac spine
BP—brachial plexus
CPB—cervical plexus block
CCB—costoclavicular block
EOM—external oblique muscle
ESM—erector spinae muscle
FIB—fascia iliaca block
GA—general anesthesia
IOM—internal oblique muscle
IP—in-plane
IPB—interpectoral plane block (IPP)
IV—intravenous
LA—local anesthetic
LAST—local anesthetic systemic toxicity
LFC—lateral femoral cutaneous
OOP—out-of-plane
PENG—pericapsular nerve group
PCNT—posterior cutaneous nerve of the thigh
PIP—parasternal intercostal plane
PNS—peripheral neurostimulation
PSP—pectoserratus plane block
QL—quadratus lumborum muscle
RA—regional anesthesia
SAP—serratus anterior plane block
SCM—sternocleidomastoid muscle
SCN—sciatic nerve
SCTL—superior costotransverse ligament
TAM—transversus abdominis muscle
TAP—transversus abdominis plane
TP—transverse process
TPVS—thoracic paravertebral space
UGRA—ultrasound-guided regional anesthesia

I. GENERAL CONSIDERATIONS

A. Peripheral nerve blockade can be an excellent addition or alternative to GA for many surgical procedures. RA may provide sensory and motor blockade without significantly disrupting systemic autonomic function. RA can also provide postoperative analgesia that may last for hours and days.

B. **Continuous peripheral nerve catheters** prolong the analgesia of RA techniques beyond the maximum duration of a single injection block. This can be especially useful for patients with chronic pain or opioid tolerance. A nerve block catheter is inserted percutaneously adjacent to the peripheral nerves or fascia plane, often with ultrasound guidance. LA is then infused through the catheter(s), providing analgesia while the catheter(s) are in place.

C. **The preoperative evaluation** includes a routine preoperative evaluation with particular focus on history of coagulopathy, and physical examination, with special attention to any preexisting neurologic deficits. ASA guidelines for perioperative care are similar between GA and RA.

D. **Surgical considerations** must be incorporated into the regional anesthetic plan. These intraoperative factors include projected surgical incision and extension, total surgical time, tourniquet placement, and postoperative factors, like anticipated level of pain and duration of recovery.

E. **Consent** for RA should include a thorough description of the risks, benefits, options, and common side effects. The need for supplemental LA, sedation, or potential for GA should be discussed. The laterality of the procedure and, thus, block placement must be confirmed with the patient, case booking, available preprocedure imaging or notes, and markings made by the surgical team on the day of surgery.

F. **Preoperative anxiolysis** may be appropriate as long as the patient remains alert and cooperative. RA is usually performed under conscious sedation to monitor the potential side effects or complications, like intraneural injection or LAST. Conscious sedation is usually achieved by using short-acting agents such as midazolam and/or fentanyl. RA can be performed under GA in pediatrics and selected patients.

G. **Standard ASA monitoring** of electrocardiogram, blood pressure measurement, and pulse oximetry with audible pitch tone must be used during the placement of all blocks. Resuscitation medications and equipment must be readily available (see Section IV.G).

H. A **time-out** must be conducted prior to starting regional block placement to confirm patient identity, the correct procedure site, and the regional anesthetic to be used.

I. **An aseptic technique must be employed during the** performance of all blocks. This includes removing jewelry, hand hygiene, wearing caps, masks, and sterile gloves, using individual packets of chlorhexidine solution (preferably alcohol based) for skin preparation and adequate drying time, using sterile equipment including sterile occlusive sheath on ultrasound probes, placing sterile occlusive dressings over catheter insertion sites, and limiting disconnection and reconnection of LA delivery systems.

J. **Postoperative follow-up** should include an assessment of block efficacy and duration, the presence of residual sensory or motor blockade, paresthesia or other side effects, and patient satisfaction.

II. GENERAL CONTRAINDICATIONS

Absolute contraindications to RA include lack of patient consent, local skin infection at the site of needle insertion, or when nerve blockade would hinder the surgery or desired postoperative neurologic examination. Relative contraindications include coagulopathy, neuropathy, systemic infection, excessive patient anxiety, cognitive deficits or movement disorders, and anatomic distortion. Peripheral nervous system disorders such as diabetic neuropathy and inflammatory neuropathies may be aggravated by peripheral nerve blockade.

III. COMPLICATIONS COMMON TO ALL NERVE BLOCKS
  A. **Complications of LAs** include intravascular injection, LAST (see Chapter 19: Local Anesthetics), and allergic reactions. Use of ultrasound, addition of epinephrine to LA solutions, and intermittent aspiration during injection may help identify intravascular injection.
  B. **Nerve damage is rare**, with long-term neurologic injury occurring in 0.02% to 0.04% of peripheral nerve blocks. Damage may result from needle trauma, nerve compression, stretch, or ischemia, or direct LA-induced neurotoxicity. Paresthesia with needle advancement or injection is not predictive of nerve injury. However, if pain or paresthesia is encountered, one must consider this complication and redirect the needle. A combination of monitoring techniques, such as peripheral nerve stimulation, injection pressure monitoring, and ultrasound can be used for prevention.
  C. **Hematomas** may result from vascular puncture but usually resolve without residual issue. When considering RA for an anticoagulated or coagulopathic patient, one should consider following neuraxial guidelines (see Chapter 20: Spinal, Epidural, and Caudal Anesthesia), particularly for deeper blocks (eg, infraclavicular, paravertebral) where vessel compression for bleeding control is challenging.
  D. **Infection** risk is reduced with the use of an aseptic technique (see Section I.I).
  E. **Failure or incomplete block** can be identified with a careful neurologic examination prior to the beginning of the surgical procedure.

IV. EQUIPMENT
  A. **Needles used for nerve blockade**
    1. **The needle gauge** should be optimized for patient comfort and block efficiency. A 22-gauge needle is most commonly used. **Short-beveled needles** (45 degrees) have become standard for peripheral nerve blocks. **Insulated** needles used in nerve stimulator-guided techniques have a small conductive area at the needle tip, allowing for more accurate nerve stimulation at lower amplitudes of current. Ideal **needle length** varies by block. Upper- and lower-extremity blocks are best performed with a 50- to 150-mm needle depending on nerve depth. **Echogenic needles** designed for use in UGRA have modifications such as special coating, scoring of the needle's surface, and reflector placement to enhance the reflection of ultrasound waves and improve needle visualization.
  B. Connecting a large-volume (20-mL) **syringe** to the block needle with sterile extension tubing ensures stable needle position during aspiration and injection.
  C. A variety of **continuous catheter kits** and infusion pumps for continuous nerve blockade are commercially available.
  D. **Nerve stimulators (Figure 21.1)** designed for RA can deliver a current of 0.1 to 10.0 mA at a frequency of 0.5 to 4 Hz with a stimulus duration of 0.05 to 1.0 ms.
  E. **Ultrasound machines** that are portable and utilize transducers of various shapes, sizes, and frequencies facilitate imaging of relevant anatomy and serve as an alternative/adjuvant to nerve stimulator approaches. Sterile transducer covers and gel allow for real-time imaging within a sterile field.
  F. **The selection of LA** for a block depends upon the desired speed of onset and duration (see Chapter 19: Local Anesthetics).
  G. **Resuscitation drugs** must be immediately accessible for any provider performing RA. These medications include lipid emulsion with dosing guidelines and resuscitation medications, including epinephrine. **Emergency**

FIGURE 21.1 Nerve stimulator attached to the regional block needle. The negative (*black*) lead is attached to the exploring needle, whereas the positive (*red*) is connected to a reference electrocardiogram pad used as a "ground." (Reprinted with permission from Mulroy MF, Bernards CM, McDonald SB, et al. *A Practical Approach to Regional Anesthesia*. 4th ed. Wolters Kluwer Health/Lippincott Williams & Wilkins; 2009.)

equipment includes an oxygen supply, airway management devices, suction, and defibrillators.

H. To provide for the safe and effective practice of RA, a designated and centralized **regional anesthesia bay** with equipment and nurses who are familiar and experienced with RA techniques is recommended (**Figure 21.2**).

V. NERVE LOCALIZATION TECHNIQUES

The classic approach uses anatomical landmarks, tactile feedback from fascial "clicks," elicited paresthesias, and transarterial approaches to guide

FIGURE 21.2 Regional anesthesia bay and team. **A,** A well-maintained and equipped regional anesthesia bay is essential to the safe practice of regional anesthesia techniques. **B,** A "block nurse" (N) who is familiar with regional anesthesia techniques is an important member of the team (physician [P], fellow [F], and resident [R]).

needle advancement and LA injection. This technique has largely been replaced by PNS and/or UGRA. **PNS techniques** allow the operator to estimate the distance of the needle tip from the target nerve based on the magnitude of current required to elicit the desired motor response. Although it does not require direct nerve contact, nerve stimulation can cause patient discomfort and may be affected by variations in tissue impedance or peripheral neuropathy. In contrast, UGRA techniques enable realtime visualization of the target anatomy, needle tip position, trajectory, and local anesthetic spread. These techniques have seen widespread adoption in recent years. Studies have shown ultrasound may reduce the time to perform a block, number of needle passes, volume of LA required for successful block, and may also reduce the incidence of vascular puncture. Nevertheless, complications such as intravascular and intraneural injection have occurred even with the use of ultrasound, and visualization of some structures like the lumbar plexus and smaller and deeper nerves may be limited.

A. PNS elicits a motor response without causing significant pain. Proficiency in surface anatomy and understanding the potential location(s) of the nerve is crucial for effective use of PNS.
   1. Ground the positive lead of the stimulator to the patient and attach the negative terminal of the stimulator to the needle (**Figure 21.1**).
   2. Set the nerve stimulator to an initial current of 0.5 to 1.0 mA and move the needle toward the nerve until a motor response in the desired muscle group occurs. Stimulation of the target nerve at a current of 0.5 mA suggests accurate needle placement for LA administration. Motor response at less than 0.5 mA is suggestive of intraneural placement, and the needle should be withdrawn slightly.
B. **UGRA** may supplement or replace the above techniques.
   1. **Ultrasound** uses high-frequency sound waves (>20 kHz) to visualize structures and tissues in real time without ionizing radiation. Within the ultrasound transducer, an electric current is applied to a piezoelectric crystal array, which vibrates at a high frequency to generate sound waves. As these waves travel through the tissue being imaged, some are reflected to the transducer. The intensity and delay of the reflected sound waves are used to construct a 2D gray-scale image. Denser structures such as bone reflect more sound waves and appear brighter or

hyperechoic. Less dense substances such as air or fluid reflect less and appear darker or **hypoechoic.**
2. **Knobology.** Commercially available ultrasound machines allow the operator to adjust several parameters to optimize visualization. **Depth** should be set to the minimum that allows visualization of target structures. **The focus** of the ultrasound waves should be placed just beyond the depth of the target structures. **Gain** determines the overall brightness of the image and may be increased or decreased as needed. **Frequency** affects both image resolution and depth of penetration. Higher frequencies increase the resolution at the expense of penetration. Conversely, lower frequencies increase the depth of penetration at the expense of resolution. Most nerve blocks are performed at an intermediate depth and thus utilize intermediate frequencies. **Color Doppler** is useful to identify blood flow in vasculature.
3. **The block's performance depends on optimal visualization of target structures, proper needle positioning, and adequate LA spread** around the nerve(s).
   a. The initial positioning of the ultrasound transducer is determined by surface landmarks and refined by scanning to obtain the optimal view of the desired anatomy. The left-right orientation of the transducer in relation to the display should be confirmed prior to scanning. Basic scanning maneuvers include sliding the transducer in the horizontal plane, tilting its vertical axis to various angles in relation to the skin surface, rotating around its vertical axis, and applying more or less vertical pressure. Anatomic structures may be viewed in sagittal, transverse, or oblique planes.
   b. There are two options for needle visualization. In the OOP approach, the needle is inserted immediately above or below the midline of the transducer and advanced perpendicularly to the plane of the ultrasound beam. This provides a cross-sectional view of the needle tip as a hyperechoic dot. In the IP approach, the needle is inserted a few centimeters lateral to the transducer and advanced in the plane of the ultrasound beam, allowing continuous visualization of the length of the needle as a hyperechoic line.
   c. **The needle insertion angle** influences the visibility of the needle tip. When the needle is nearly parallel to the ultrasound probe, the tip is easier to identify. However, at steeper angles of entry, needle tip visibility can be more difficult. An echogenic needle can help improve visualization in those cases.
   d. The needle tip should be positioned near the target nerve. Injection of 0.5 to 1 mL of dextrose water or normal saline can help localize the needle tip (**hydrolocalization**). Spread of LA should be observed both for evidence of intraneural injection, which may result in nerve injury and should prompt adjustment of needle position, and for adequacy of spread. The circumferential spread of LA around the target nerve suggests injection in the proper fascial plane. For some blocks, multiple injection sites may be needed to achieve the desired distribution of LA.

VI. REGIONAL ANESTHESIA OF THE NECK
A. CPB
1. **Anatomy.** The cervical plexus lies in the paravertebral region of the upper four cervical vertebrae, formed from the anterior rami of the C1–C4 spinal nerve roots. The plexus is situated between the prevertebral muscle anteromedially and the muscles attached to the posterior tubercles

of the cervical TP posterolaterally. The plexus has cutaneous, muscular, and communicating branches. The **superficial cutaneous branches**, which include the lesser occipital, greater auricular, transverse cervical, and supraclavicular nerves, pierce the prevertebral fascia anteriorly, just deep to the SCM at the level of the C5 TP. They innervate the skin and fascia of the back of the head, lateral neck, top of the shoulder and chest, and the clavicle (**Figure 21.3**). The **deep muscular branches** are

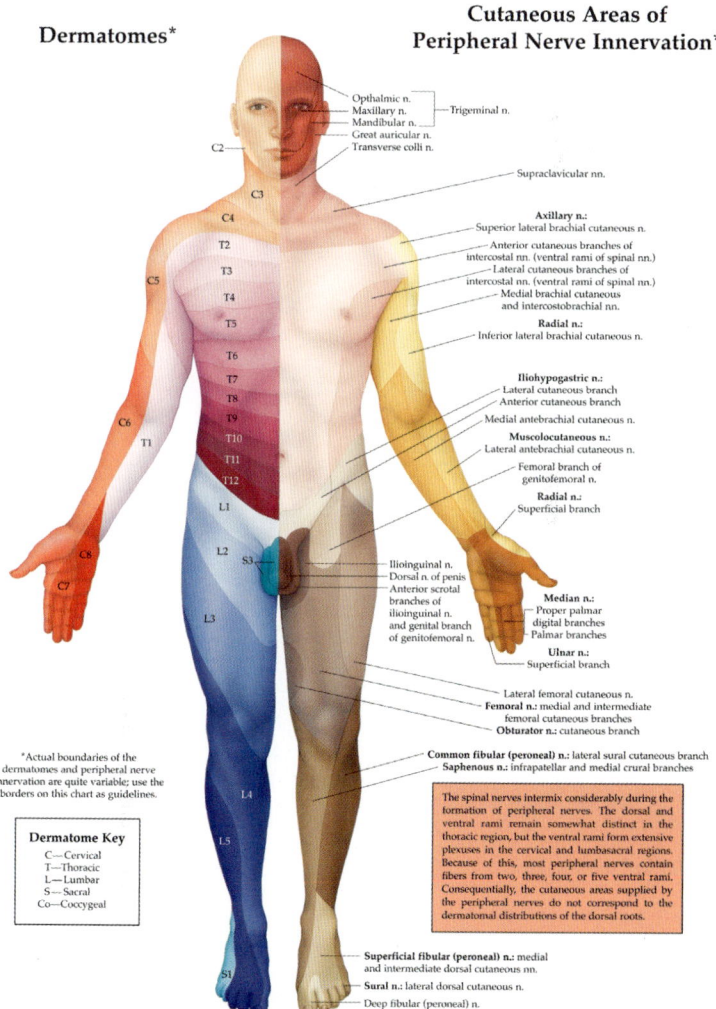

FIGURE 21.3 A map of the dermatomes. (Adapted from Anatomical Chart Company. Dermatomes Anatomical Chart. *Classic Anthology of Anatomical Charts*. 8th ed. Wolters Kluwer; 2014 and Jaffe RA, Schmiesing CA, Golianu B, eds. *Anesthesiologist's Manual of Surgical Procedures*. 6th ed. Wolters Kluwer; 2020.) *(continued)*

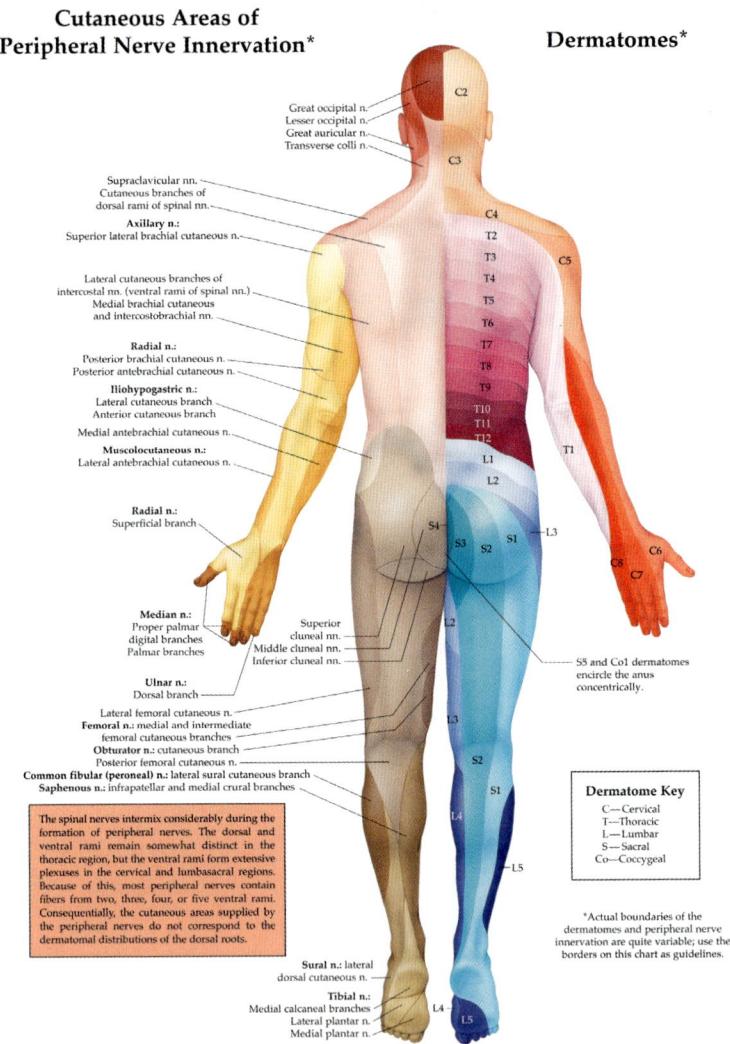

FIGURE 21.3 *(Continued)*

deep to the prevertebral fascia and supply the muscles and deep structures of the neck and form the phrenic nerve.

2. **Indications. Superficial CPB** (C2–C4) produces cutaneous anesthesia and is useful for superficial procedures on the neck and shoulder. It has been shown that superficial CPB is as effective as **paravertebral cervical root block**, known previously as **deep CPB**, for carotid endarterectomy with fewer complications.

3. **Superficial CPB using UGRA** (see **Figure 21.5**). Position the patient supine with the neck slightly extended and the head turned toward the opposite side. Place the ultrasound probe transversely over the SCM at the level of the cricoid cartilage and scan posteriorly until the posterior edge of the SCM is visualized in the center of the screen. The SCP may be visualized as two to three small hypoechoic structures between the SCM and scalene muscles. Using an IP approach, insert a 23- to 25-gauge 50-mm needle lateral to the probe and advance until the needle tip is beneath the posterior border of the SCM and adjacent to the plexus. After negative aspiration, inject 10 mL of LA in a fan-like fashion along the posterior border of the SCM, 2 to 3 cm above and below the needle insertion site. LA should spread between the SCM and the underlying prevertebral fascia.
4. **Complications. Vagus nerve block** and **recurrent laryngeal nerve block** can occur if LA spreads too medially, causing hoarseness and vocal cord dysfunction.

VII. REGIONAL ANESTHESIA OF THE UPPER EXTREMITY
A. Anatomy (Figures 21.3 and 21.4)
1. The shoulder, axilla, and upper extremity are innervated by the BP. The skin of the medial aspect of the upper arm is innervated by the **intercostobrachial nerve** formed by T2 and the **medial cutaneous nerve of the arm**. The **supraclavicular nerve**, which is formed by C3–C4, innervates the skin of the top of the shoulder (see Section VI.A.1).
2. The BP is formed from the ventral rami of the spinal nerves from C5 to C8 and T1, with frequent contributions from C4 and T2. It is traditionally divided into five parts: roots, trunks, divisions, cords, and branches.
3. Each **root** or ventral ramus exits posterior to the vertebral artery and travels laterally in the trough of its cervical TP, in between the fascial sheaths of the anterior and middle scalene muscles.
4. The **trunks** (superior, middle, and inferior) pass over the first rib through the space between the anterior and middle scalene muscles in

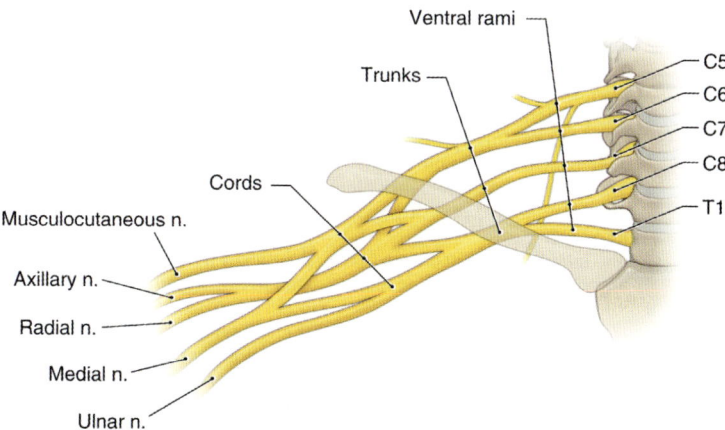

FIGURE 21.4 Diagram of the brachial plexus and its terminal branches. (From Horn JL, Nasiri M. Regional blocks—A brief overview. In: Jaffe RA, Schmiesing CA, Golianu B, eds. *Anesthesiologist's Manual of Surgical Procedures*. 6th ed. Wolters Kluwer; 2020:1763–1799.)

association with the subclavian artery, which shares the same fascial sheath.
5. As the trunks pass over the first rib and under the clavicle, they split into the anterior (flexor) and posterior (extensor) **divisions**, which then reorganize to form the three **cords** (lateral, medial, and posterior, named for their usual positions relative to the axillary artery) of the plexus.
6. Branches of the lateral and medial cords form the **median nerve**. The lateral cord also gives off a branch that forms the **musculocutaneous nerve**. The medial cord also forms the **ulnar, medial antebrachial cutaneous**, and **medial brachial cutaneous nerves**. The posterior cord becomes the **axillary and radial nerves (Figure 21.4)**. In the axilla, the median nerve classically lies lateral to the axillary artery, the radial nerve posterior and over the conjoint tendon (of the teres major and latissimus dorsi muscles), and the ulnar nerve medial, but variation in these relative positions occurs. The musculocutaneous and axillary nerves exit the sheath high up in the axilla. The musculocutaneous nerve travels through the coracobrachialis muscle before becoming subcutaneous below the elbow, and the axillary nerve travels through the quadrilateral space (bordered by the humeral shaft, long head of the triceps, and teres major and minor muscles) before dividing into its terminal branches.
7. **Figure 21.3** summarizes the dermatomal distribution of the body's nerves. Cutaneous innervation does not necessarily correlate with deep structures, including the bones; therefore, knowledge of the osteotomes is useful in predicting the ultimate success of any regional technique.
8. The **major motor functions** of the five nerves are as follows: **axillary (circumflex nerve)**: shoulder abduction; **musculocutaneous**: elbow flexion; **radial**: wrist and finger extension; **median**: forearm pronation, wrist and finger flexion, thumb flexion and opposition; and **ulnar**: wrist flexion and adduction, thumb adduction.

B. Indications
1. The **interscalene approach** blocks the BP at the level of the roots to the upper trunks. This approach is most useful for surgeries of the shoulder and proximal humerus. As the inferior trunk (C8–T1) and, therefore, the ulnar nerve are usually spared, it is less useful for forearm and hand operations.
2. **Superior truck block** is used as an alternative to the interscalene block, offering a lower risk of phrenic nerve palsy and better preservation of respiratory parameters.
3. The **supraclavicular approach** blocks the plexus at the level of the trunks to divisions. This approach allows for reliable anesthesia of the entire arm distal to the shoulder.
4. The **costoclavicular approach** blocks the plexus at the level of the cords. This new approach will provide analgesia or anesthesia to the arm and hand.
5. The **infraclavicular approach** blocks the plexus at the level of the cords and provides coverage for surgery distal to the midhumerus.
6. The **axillary approach** blocks the terminal branches of the BP. The block is combined with the blockade of the **musculocutaneous nerve** and is used for surgical procedures involving the forearm and hand.
7. For procedures involving the medial arm or using a proximal humeral tourniquet, the **intercostobrachial nerve** must be blocked in addition to the BP.
8. **Suprascapular and axillary nerve blocks** provide shoulder analgesia similar to that of an interscalene block but avoid complications like phrenic nerve paralysis.

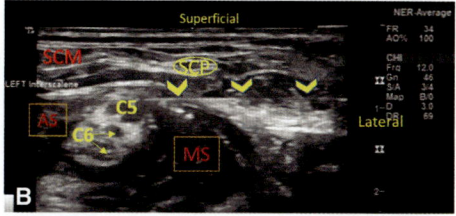

FIGURE 21.5 Superficial cervical plexus/interscalene block using ultrasound (US) guidance. **A,** US probe and needle position for performing the block. **B,** US image of brachial plexus (C5 and C6) at the level of interscalene. The *yellow arrows* delineate the path of the needle toward the plexus. *Please note, in actual practice, the ultrasound probe must have a sterile covering. In this figure, the covering is omitted to better demonstrate correct probe orientation and needle insertion point.* AS, anterior scalene muscle; MS, middle scalene muscle; SCM, sternocleidomastoid; SCP, superficial cervical plexus.

    9. **Blockade of an individual peripheral nerve** may be useful when limited anesthesia is required, or a BP block is incomplete and requires a rescue block.
- **C. Techniques and complications**
  1. **Interscalene block using UGRA (Figure 21.5; ⊙ Video 21.1).** Position the patient supine and semireclined or lateral decubitus with the arms at the side and head turned away from the side to be blocked. Place the probe over the SCM at the level of the cricoid cartilage (C6) and identify the internal carotid artery and internal jugular vein. Move the probe laterally and identify the anterior and middle scalene muscles. At this time, the roots and trunks, usually C5 and two branches of C6, will come into view as hypoechoic nodular structures often stacked in a "stoplight" configuration between the anterior and middle scalene. After centering the nerves on the screen, infiltrate skin with LA, insert a 22-gauge 50-mm needle just lateral to the probe site, and advance with IP approach toward the target nerves in a lateral-to-medial direction. **Stimulation of the BP using PNS** will result in a muscle twitch in the deltoid, biceps, triceps, or pectoralis major muscles. After negative aspiration, deposit 15 to 20 mL LA solution between the two scalene muscles.
     - a. **Complications. Phrenic nerve palsy** and hemidiaphragm paralysis almost always occur. The **cervical sympathetic nerve block** can produce an ipsilateral Horner syndrome.
  2. **Superior truck block using UGRA.** The position for this block is similar to interscalene block. For this block, after identifying the roots and scalene muscles, the probe is moved distally until the suprascapular nerve branches off from the superior trunk are visible. Insert a 22-gauge 50-mm needle just lateral to the probe and advance IP until it reaches the superior truck. After negative aspiration, slowly administer 15 to 20 mL of LA solution.
  3. **Supraclavicular block using UGRA (Figure 21.6; ⊙ Video 21.2).** Position the patient similar to that for the interscalene block. In some cases, a blanket roll or pillow behind the shoulder may facilitate visualization by extending the head and neck to increase space around the clavicle. Place the probe in the transverse plane with caudal tilt in the supraclavicular fossa. The BP will be visualized as a hypoechoic group of nerves ("cluster of grapes") located laterally and posterior to the subclavian artery. Deep to the artery, the hyperechoic first rib and part of the

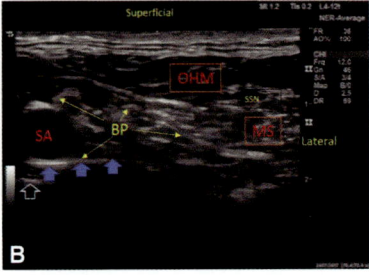

FIGURE 21.6 **A,** Supraclavicular block using ultrasound guidance. US probe and needle position for performing the block. **B,** The BP is at the posterolateral border of the SA and superior to the first rib (*blue arrows*). The pleura can be seen as a hyperechoic line deep to the first rib (*white arrow*). *Please note, in actual practice the ultrasound probe must have a sterile covering. In this figure, the covering is omitted to better demonstrate correct probe orientation and needle insertion point.* BP, brachial plexus; MS, middle scalene muscle; OHM, omohyoid muscle; SA, subclavian artery. SSN, Suprascapular nerve.

pleura are typically seen, with the portions of the pleura often obscured by the rib's acoustic shadow. Insert a 22-gauge 50-mm needle just lateral to the probe and advance IP in a lateral-to-medial direction until it reaches the BP. **Stimulation of the BP using PNS** is manifested by finger flexion or extension. After negative aspiration, slowly administer 15 to 20 mL of LA solution. LA should spread throughout the BP, between the middle scalene and subclavian artery, just above the first rib.
  a. **Complications** include pneumothorax (0.04% with UGRA), phrenic nerve block, and Horner syndrome.
4. **Costoclavicular block using UGRA (Figure 21.7, ⊚ Video 21.3).** Position the patient similarly to the supraclavicular approach, supine with the ipsilateral arm abducted and the head turned slightly to the opposite side of the BP block. Place the ultrasound probe transversely on the midclavicular and infraclavicular fossa. Optimize the ultrasound image until all three cords of the BP are clearly visualized laterally to the axillary artery. The axillary/cephalic vein and pleura should also be visible.

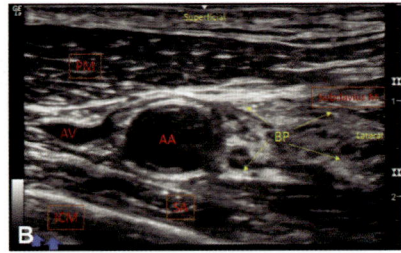

FIGURE 21.7 Costoclavicular block using ultrasound guidance. **A,** US probe and needle position for performing US-guided costoclavicular block. **B,** BP stays at the lateral border of the axillary artery and vein. *Please note, in actual practice, the ultrasound probe must have a sterile covering. In this figure, the covering is omitted to better demonstrate correct probe orientation and needle insertion point.* PM, pectoralis major; AV, axillary vein; AA, axillary artery; BP, brachial plexus; SA, serratus anterior muscle; ICM, intercostal.

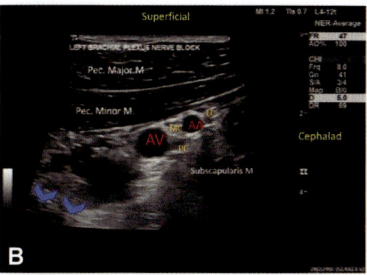

FIGURE 21.8 Infraclavicular block using ultrasound guidance. **A,** US probe and needle position for performing the block. **B,** The LC, MC, and PC are located around the AA. The PC can be obscured by the acoustic enhancement of the artery. The *blue arrows* designate the pleura. *Please note, in actual practice the ultrasound probe must have a sterile covering. In this figure, the covering is omitted to better demonstrate correct probe orientation and needle insertion point.* AA, axillary artery; AV, axillary vein; LC, lateral cord; MC, medial cord; PC, posterior cord.

Insert a 22-gauge 50-mm needle just lateral to the probe and advance it in a lateral-to-medial direction until it reaches the BP. **PNS stimulation** of the posterior cord will produce extension at the wrist and/or finger (radial nerve), and stimulation of the medial cord produces flexor carpi ulnaris movement with some flexion of the wrist and/or fingers (median and ulnar nerves); stimulation of the posterior cord generally results in a higher success rate. Deposit 20 to 30 mL of LA solution around the cords, which may require needle repositioning.

5. **Infraclavicular block using UGRA (Figure 21.8, Video 21.4).** Position the patient supine with the arm supinated and abducted 90 degrees at the shoulder, with the forearm supinated. Place the probe sagittally in the infraclavicular fossa (at the deltopectoral groove) and under the coracoid process. Identify the axillary artery and vein with hyperechoic lateral, posterior, and medial cords lying in a U-shape configuration around the artery. A needle-insertion site is identified approximately 1 cm superior to the probe, just inferior to the clavicle. A 22-gauge 100- to 150-mm needle is appropriate. Insert the needle and advance caudally at a steep angle to the skin in an IP approach until the tip is positioned posterior to the axillary artery (ie, in the 6 o'clock position). PNS stimulation is similar to the costoclavicular block (see above). After negative aspiration, deposit 20 to 30 mL of LA solution with a goal of a U-shaped spread around the axillary artery. This may require repositioning the needle to achieve the desired spread and coverage of the medial and lateral cords.

    a. **Complications** include pneumothorax in addition to those mentioned in Section III.

6. **Axillary block using UGRA (Figure 21.9; Video 21.5).** Position the patient supine with the arm abducted 90 degrees at the shoulder, externally rotated, and flexed at the elbow. Place the transducer transversally over the axillary artery, perpendicular to the axis of the arm, and position the artery in the center of the screen. The hyperechoic median, ulnar, and radial nerves can be appreciated in the perivascular area. Special care should be taken to identify veins, as pressure from the transducer may easily compress and obscure them from view. Insert a 22-gauge 25- to 50-mm needle superior to the transducer and advance toward the nerves with an IP approach. **PNS stimulation** of each nerve will result

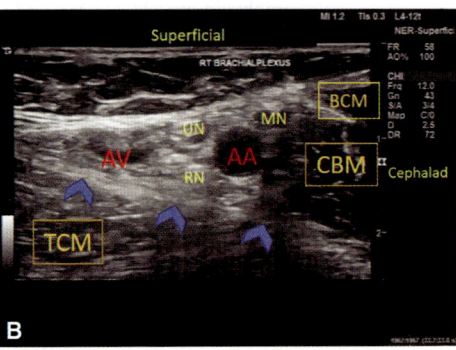

FIGURE 21.9 Axillary block using ultrasound guidance. **A,** US probe and needle position for performing the block. **B,** The axillary approach to the terminal branches of the brachial plexus is achieved by placement of the US probe over the axillary artery. The *blue arrows* trace the conjoined tendon of the latissimus dorsi and teres major muscle. *Please note, in actual practice the ultrasound probe must have a sterile covering. In this figure, the covering is omitted to better demonstrate correct probe orientation and needle insertion point.* AA, axillary artery; AV, axillary vein; BCM, biceps muscle; CBM, coracobrachialis muscle; MN, median nerve; RN, radial nerve; TCM, triceps muscle; UN, ulnar nerve.

in different motor stimulation (see Section VII.A.8). After negative aspiration, inject a total of 20 to 30 mL of LA near each terminal nerve. The goal is to cover each of the terminal nerves, which may be achieved by a single injection of 5 to 7 mL of LA around the median, radial, and ulnar nerves. Next, identify the **musculocutaneous nerve** as a hyperechoic oval or triangular structure between the coracobrachialis and biceps muscles or within one of the muscles. Without changing the needle entry site, redirect the needle adjacent to the nerve and inject 5 to 7 mL of LA solution. **PNS stimulation** of the musculocutaneous nerve leads to flexion of the elbow.

  a. **Complications** include LAST secondary to injection into the axillary artery or vein in addition to those mentioned in Section III.

7. **Intercostobrachial nerve block.** Insert a 25-gauge needle inferior to the axillary artery at the level of the axillary fossa. Subcutaneously infiltrate 5 mL of LA superiorly and inferiorly along the axillary crease. Using high frequency and high-resolution ultrasound, this nerve can be found between the axillary fascia and skin on the medial side of the axilla.

8. **Suprascapular and axillary nerve block.** A suprascapular nerve block, with or without an axillary nerve block, is considered a phrenic nerve-sparing regional anesthesia technique for shoulder surgery.

  a. **Suprascapular nerve block using UGRA.** With the **posterior approach**, position the patient in the lateral position with the shoulder fully adducted. Place the ultrasound probe transversely over the supraspinous fossa and trace it from the medial end of the spine of the scapula to the greater suprascapular notch laterally. Insert a 22-gauge needle and advance with an IP approach to the lateral aspect of the supraspinous fossa beneath the supraspinatus muscle. After negative aspiration, inject 10 to 12 mL of LA. With the **anterior approach**, position the patient and the probe as for the supraclavicular block. Identify the omohyoid muscle on the top of the BP. Follow

the omohyoid muscle laterally and posteriorly. Locate the suprascapular nerve as it separates from the upper trunk (**Figure 21.6**). Insert a 22-gauge needle and advance with an IP approach under the inferior belly of the omohyoid muscle. Inject 10 to 12 mL of LA adjacent to the nerve.
   b. **Axillary nerve block using UGRA.** Position the patient in the lateral position. Locate the humeral head and neck on the posterolateral aspect of the arm. Identify the humeral circumflex artery and visualize the axillary nerve located superior to the artery. Advance a 22-gauge needle IP through the deltoid muscle, and after negative aspiration, deposit 10 mL of LA solution around the axillary nerve. LA should fill the potential space between the deltoid and the posterior surface of the humerus.
   c. **Complications** include concurrent radial nerve block due to the spread of the LA proximally to the posterior cord in addition to those in Section III. The suprascapular and axillary nerve block does not anesthetize all-terminal nerves of C5 and C6, supplemental analgesic is frequently necessary.
9. **Blockade of an individual terminal nerve of the BP**
   a. **Ulnar nerve block using UGRA. At the forearm,** the ulnar nerve is just lateral to the flexor carpi ulnaris and medial to the ulnar collateral artery, lying over the flexor digitorum profundus. Place the ultrasound probe transversally over the midforearm, and using an IP approach, inject 3 to 6 mL of LA around the nerve.
   b. **Median nerve block using UGRA. At the elbow,** the median nerve is just medial to the brachial artery and on the top of the brachialis muscle at the level of the epicondyles. Using the same approach as above for the ulnar nerve, inject 3 to 5 mL of LA around the median nerve, avoiding penetration of the brachial artery. **At the wrist,** the median nerve lies between the palmaris longus tendon and the flexor carpi radialis tendon. At this level, isolating the nerve from the tendons can be difficult with ultrasound. Sliding the probe alongside the forearm will help to visually separate tendons from the nerve, as tendons become muscles and their appearance will change while the nerve will stay the same. The approach is the same as above at the elbow.
   c. **Radial nerve block using UGRA. At the elbow,** the radial nerve lies lateral to the biceps tendon and medial to the brachioradialis muscle at the level of the lateral epicondyle of the humerus. Place the ultrasound probe transversally about 3 to 4 cm above the lateral epicondyle to locate the radial nerve. Follow the radial nerve until it reaches the lateral margin of the humerus to confirm the nerve. Use an IP approach to reach the nerve and inject 3 to 5 mL of LA around it.
   d. **Lateral cutaneous nerve of the forearm block using UGRA.** This is the primary cutaneous branch of the musculocutaneous nerve. It may be blocked **in the axilla**, as described in Section VII.C.4, or **at the elbow**, where it is usually located on the lateral side of the forearm and can be seen between the biceps tendon and the brachioradialis muscle, usually accompanying the cephalic vein. The block technique is the same as above but with 5 to 10 mL of LA.
D. **IV RA (Bier block).** IV administration of LA distal to a tourniquet is a simple way to anesthetize an extremity for short procedures (60 minutes or less).
   1. Place a 20- to 22-gauge IV catheter as distally as possible in the extremity to be blocked. Apply a pneumatic double tourniquet proximally and

exsanguinate the extremity by elevating it and wrapping it distally to proximally with an Esmarch bandage.
2. Inflate the proximal cuff to 150 mm Hg greater than systolic pressure. The absence of pulses after inflation ensures arterial occlusion. Remove the Esmarch bandage and slowly inject the anesthetic into the previously placed IV catheter. Average drug doses are 50 mL of 0.5% lidocaine for an arm. Although Bier block has been described for the leg, it is generally not utilized as it is difficult to achieve complete vascular occlusion of the leg with a tourniquet, and the volume of LA required increases the risk of systemic toxicity.
3. Anesthesia occurs within 5 minutes of LA injection. Tourniquet pain generally becomes unbearable after 1 hour and is the limiting factor for the success of this technique. When the patient complains of pain, the distal tourniquet that overlies the anesthetized skin should be inflated, and the proximal tourniquet should be released.
4. The major **complication** associated with IV RA is LA toxicity. It may occur during injection if the tourniquet fails or after tourniquet deflation, particularly with a short inflation time.

VIII. REGIONAL ANESTHESIA OF THE LOWER EXTREMITY
A. Anatomy. Two major plexuses innervate the lower extremity: the lumbar plexus and the sacral plexus.
1. The **lumbar plexus** (**Figure 21.10A**) is formed within the psoas muscle from the anterior rami of the L1–L4 spinal nerves, with contribution from the 12th thoracic nerve (subcostal nerve). The most cephalad nerves of the plexus are the **iliohypogastric**, **ilioinguinal**, and **genitofemoral**. These nerves pierce the abdominal musculature anteriorly before supplying the skin of the hip, groin, and genital regions. The three caudal nerves of the lumber plexus are the **LFC**, **femoral**, and **obturator**.
   a. The **LFC nerve** passes under the lateral end of the inguinal ligament, supplying sensory innervation to the lateral thigh and buttock.
   b. The **femoral nerve** passes under the inguinal ligament just lateral to the femoral artery and vein, under the fascia iliaca, on the surface of the iliacus muscle. It supplies the muscles and skin of the anterior thigh as well as the knee and hip joints. From there, it courses with the femoral artery and vein through the **adductor canal**, an anatomic tunnel bounded by the fascial planes of the sartorius, the vastus medialis, and the adductor longus and magnus muscles. The nerve and vessels exit the canal at the adductor hiatus just above the medial femoral condyle. The **saphenous nerve** is the cutaneous termination of the nerve, supplying the skin of the medial leg and foot. It is the only nerve of the lumbar plexus that innervates below the knee (**Figure 21.3**).
   c. The **obturator nerve** exits from the pelvis through the obturator canal of the ischium, innervating the adductor muscles of the thigh, the hip and knee joints, and a portion of the skin of the medial thigh.
2. The **sacral plexus** (**Figure 21.10B**) is formed from the anterior rami of the L4–L5 nerves and the S1–S3 nerves (lumbosacral trunk). The two major nerves of the sacral plexus are the **SCN** and the **PCNT**. Other branches of the sacral plexus are the pudendal, superior, and inferior gluteal nerves.
   a. The **PCNT** travels with the SCN to its proximal extent and supplies the skin of the posterior thigh, extending at times to the posterior calf.
   b. The **SCN** passes out of the pelvis through the greater sciatic foramen, becomes superficial at the lower border of the gluteus maximus,

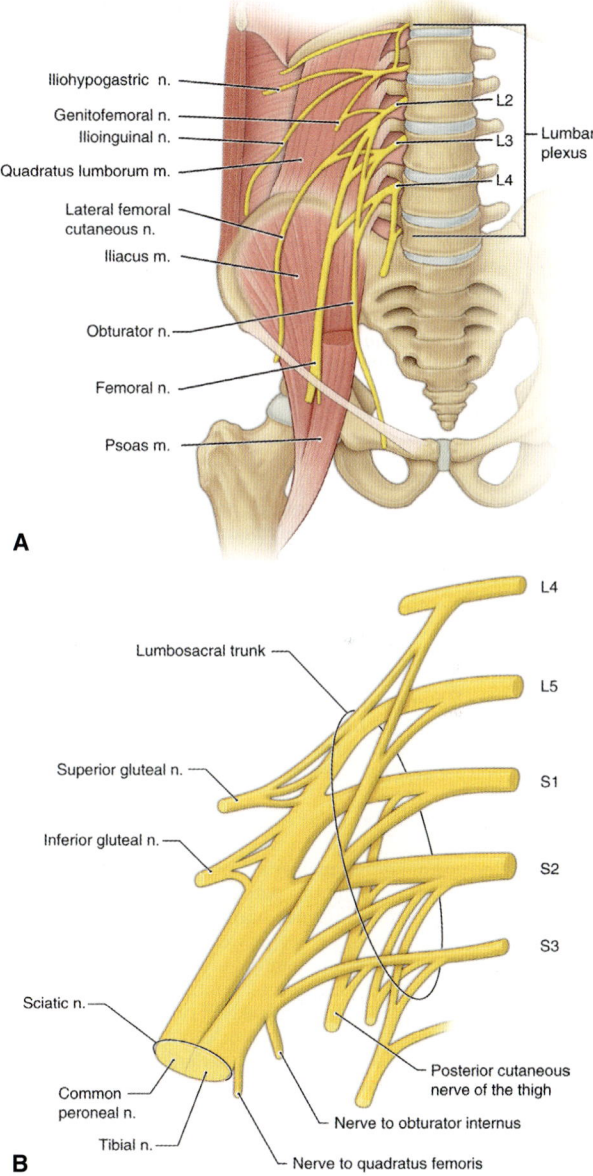

FIGURE 21.10 Diagram of the lumbar (**A**) and sacral plexus (**B**). (From Horn JL, Nasiri M. Regional blocks—A brief overview. In: Jaffe RA, Schmiesing CA, Golianu B, eds. *Anesthesiologist's Manual of Surgical Procedures*. 6th ed. 2020:1763–1799.)

descends along the medial aspect of the femur supplying branches to the hamstrings, and becomes superficial again at the popliteal fossa, where it lies between the semimembranosus and semitendinosus muscles medially and biceps femoris muscle laterally. There, it divides into the tibial nerve and the common peroneal nerve.
   1. The **tibial nerve** travels down the posterior calf and passes under the medial malleolus before dividing into its terminal branches. It supplies the skin of the medial and plantar foot and causes plantar flexion (**Figure 21.3**).
   2. The **common peroneal nerve** winds around the head of the fibula before dividing into the superficial and deep peroneal nerves.
      a. The **superficial peroneal nerve** is a sensory nerve that passes down the lateral calf, dividing into its terminal branches just medial to the lateral malleolus, supplying the dorsal aspect of the foot (**Figure 21.3**).
      b. The **deep peroneal nerve** enters the foot just lateral to the anterior tibial artery, lying at the superior border of the malleolus, in between the anterior tibialis tendon and the extensor hallucis longus tendon. Although primarily a motor nerve causing dorsiflexion of the foot, it also sends a sensory branch to the web space between the first and second toes (**Figure 21.3**).
      c. The **sural nerve** is a sensory nerve formed from branches of the common peroneal and tibial nerves. It passes under the lateral malleolus, supplying the lateral foot (**Figure 21.3**).
B. Indications. Anesthetizing the entire lower extremity requires blocking components of both the lumbar and sacral plexuses.
   1. Innervation of the **hip joint** includes many nerves from both lumbar and sacral plexuses, including genitofemoral, LFC, femoral, obturator, sciatic, superior cluneal, and superior gluteal nerves, and the nerve to the quadratus femoris muscle. This complex innervation makes it difficult to find one single RA technique for hip surgeries. However, the **lumbar plexus block**, **femoral nerve block** (including **fascia iliaca block**), **SCN block**, and **periarticular injection techniques** have been used for post–hip surgery pain control.
   2. An **LFC nerve block** provides excellent analgesia for skin graft donor sites on the anterior thigh. An isolated **femoral nerve block** is useful for providing postoperative analgesia for femoral shaft fractures as well as quadricepsplasty or repair of a patellar fracture.
   3. **Knee joint** innervation includes branches of the LFC, tibial, common peroneal, and obturator nerves, as well as the nerves to the vastus lateralis and intermedius, and femoral branches like the saphenous and medial femoral cutaneous nerves, contribute to knee joint innervation. This complex innervation makes it difficult to find one single RA technique for open knee surgery. Blocks of the lumbar plexus, femoral nerve, SCN, and **adductor canal** and **periarticular injection between the popliteal artery and posterior capsule of the knee (IPACK)** have been used for postoperative analgesia for open knee surgeries.
   4. **Operations distal to the knee** can be performed under **sciatic and saphenous nerve blocks**.
C. Complications specific to lower extremity blocks are common to all nerve blocks (see Section III).
D. Techniques
   1. **Lumbar plexus (psoas) block using UGRA (Figure 21.11).** Place the patient in the lateral position with hips flexed, and surgical side up. Place a curved

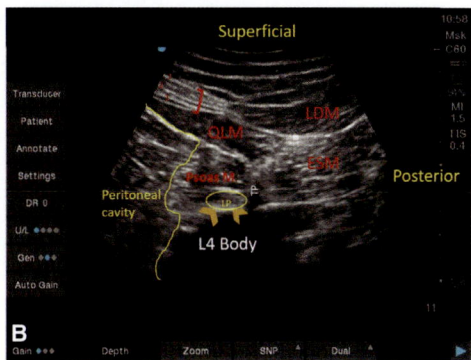

FIGURE 21.11 Lumbar plexus (psoas)/quadratus lumborum block using ultrasound guidance. **A,** The ultrasound probe and needle are placed between the iliac crest and costal margin. **B,** The red bracket delineates the three abdominal muscle layers (1: external oblique, 2: internal oblique, 3: transversus abdominis). The TP of the lumbar vertebra separates the psoas muscle from the ESM. The LP is embedded within the psoas muscle. *Please note, in actual practice the ultrasound probe must have a sterile covering. In this figure, the covering is omitted to better demonstrate correct probe orientation and needle insertion point.* ESM, erector spinae muscle; LDM, latissimus dorsi muscle; LP, lumbar plexus; QLM, quadratus lumborum muscle; TP, transverse process.

array transducer in the transverse plane along the posterior axillary line above the iliac crest at the level of L2–L4. Scan from medial to lateral and identify the TP, ESM superficial to the TP, psoas muscle (deep to the TP), and peritoneum, noting the depth of all structures. Identify the posterior one-third of the psoas muscle, where the lumbar plexus is located. The plexus itself may not be visualized inside the psoas muscle. Insert a 22-gauge 150-mm needle medial to the transducer and advance IP from medial to lateral until the needle tip lies in the posterior one-third of the psoas muscle. PNS is helpful for localization and will cause quadriceps contraction. After negative aspiration, inject 25 to 30 mL of LA. **Complications** specific to this block include epidural blockade with potential sympathectomy, vascular injury, perforated viscus, and renal injury.

2. **LFC nerve**
   a. **LFC nerve block using landmark.** Insert a 22-gauge 25-mm needle 1 to 2 cm caudal and medial to the ASIS. Direct the needle in a slightly lateral and cephalad direction, striking the iliac bone medially just below the ASIS, and inject 5 to 10 mL of LA.
   b. **LFC nerve block using UGRA.** Place the probe inferior to the ASIS, parallel to the inguinal ligament. The LFC nerve is localized on the "fat pad" between the tensor fasciae lata and sartorius muscles. Insert a 22-gauge 25-mm needle with an IP approach and inject 5 to 10 mL of LA around the nerve. Note that the nerve may pass through the sartorius muscle in up to 22% of the population.
3. **Femoral nerve block using UGRA** (**Figure 21.12**, ◉ **Video 21.6**). With the patient supine, place the probe over the femoral artery at the level of the femoral crease and move approximately 1 cm laterally to align the artery at the medial edge of the image. Two separate fascial layers can be visualized overlying the iliopsoas muscle: the superficial fascia lata and the deeper fascia iliaca. The nerve can be visualized just deep to

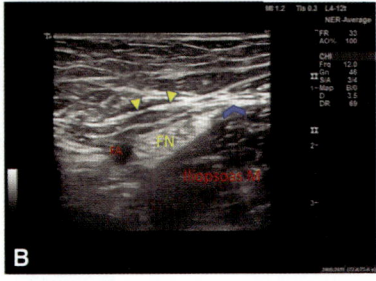

FIGURE 21.12 Femoral nerve/fascia iliaca compartment block (infrainguinal) using ultrasound guidance. **A,** The US probe and the block needle are placed parallel and caudad to the inguinal ligament. **B,** The FN is located deep to the fascia lata (*yellow arrows*) and fascia iliaca (*blue arrow*) and lateral to the FA. *Please note, in actual practice the ultrasound probe must have a sterile covering. In this figure, the covering is omitted to better demonstrate correct probe orientation and needle insertion point.* ASIS, anterior superior iliac spine; FA, femoral artery; FN, femoral nerve.

the fascia iliaca and lateral to the artery. Insert a 22-gauge needle at least 50 mm in length and advance medially at a 60-degree angle to the skin using an IP approach. As the needle is advanced, two distinct "pops" are felt and seen as the two fascial layers are traversed. At this point, the needle tip should lie between the fascia iliaca and the iliopsoas muscle on the lateral side of the nerve. If the needle is in the proper plane, with **PNS,** a quadriceps twitch (patella dance) is elicited, and a 20 cc LA spread is seen mostly in the horizontal direction, easily reaching the femoral nerve.

4. **Fascia iliaca compartment block (FICB) using UGRA.** FICB can block the LFC and femoral nerves and provide analgesia for hip and femur surgeries.
   a. **Infrainguinal approach (Figure 21.12).** This approach mirrors the femoral nerve block. Approximately 35 to 40 mL of diluted LA is injected at the lateral edge under the fascia iliaca and should spread medially toward the femoral nerve.
   b. **Suprainguinal approach (Figure 21.13 and Video 21.7).** In this technique, in a supine position, an ultrasound probe is placed sagittally

 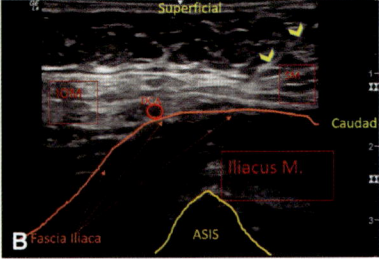

FIGURE 21.13 Suprainguinal fascia iliaca compartment block using ultrasound guidance. **A,** The US probe is placed sagittal to the inguinal ligament. The blue line represents the iliac crest. **B,** The block needle (*yellow arrows*) is directed toward fascia iliaca. *Please note, in actual practice the ultrasound probe must have a sterile covering. In this figure, the covering is omitted to better demonstrate correct probe orientation and needle insertion point.* DCA, deep circumflex artery; ASIS, anterior superior iliac spine; SM, sartorius muscle; IOM, internal oblique muscle.

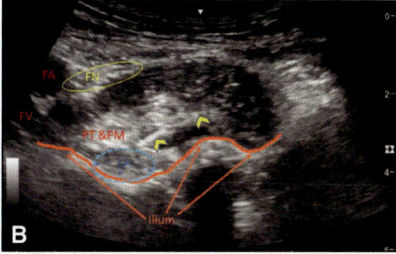

FIGURE 21.14 Pericapsular nerve group (PENG) block using ultrasound guidance. **A,** Direction of the US probe and the block needle. **B,** The ultrasonographic image of PENG block. The *yellow arrows* outline the block needle. *Please note, in actual practice the ultrasound probe must have a sterile covering. In this figure, the covering is omitted to better demonstrate correct probe orientation and needle insertion point.* FN, femoral nerve; FA, femoral artery; FV, femoral vein; PT, psoas tendon; PM, psoas muscle; LA, local anesthetic.

to obtain an image of the ilium and iliacus muscle. Move the probe inferiorly and medially along the inguinal ligament to visualize the femoral artery. The probe is then shifted laterally and superiorly along the inguinal ligament toward the ASIS. The deep circumflex artery is identified as superficial to the fascia iliaca and 1 to 2 cm cephalad to the inguinal ligament. The needle is inserted 2 to 4 cm caudad to the inguinal ligament, beneath the fascia iliaca cephalad to the inguinal ligament. The spread of 30 to 35 cc of dilute LA should be seen between the fascia iliaca and iliacus muscle, extending into the iliac fossa.

5. **PENG block using UGRA (Figure 21.14, ⊙ Video 21.8).** In this block, LA is deposited between the psoas tendon and the ilium, targeting part of the articular branches of the hip arising from the femoral and accessory obturator nerves. This novel block is used for hip surgeries. After prepping and draping, a curvilinear low-frequency ultrasound probe is placed in an oblique plane over the anterior inferior iliac spine and aligned with the pubic ramus. In this view, the femoral vessels, iliopubic eminence, and iliopsoas muscle/tendon are identified. The needle is inserted lateral to medial IP until the needle tip is between the psoas tendon and ilium. Hydrolocalization ensures the injectate is placed in the fascial plane rather than intramuscularly. Following this, 20 mL of LA is administered.

6. **Adductor canal block using UGRA (Figure 21.15; ⊙ Video 21.9).** This block anesthetizes the terminal branches of the femoral nerve (saphenous nerve and nerve to the vastus medialis) and the branches of the obturator nerve at the level of the midthigh as they course through the adductor canal. Blocking the femoral nerve terminal branches here as opposed to at the inguinal crease has been shown to result in equivalent knee analgesia with potentially less motor blockade of the quadriceps. Place the patient in the supine position, with the operative leg externally rotated and slightly flexed at the knee. Scan with the ultrasound probe to identify the femoral artery deep into the sartorius at the medial aspect of the midthigh. The nerve bundles can be visualized as echo-dense structures lateral to the femoral artery. Insert a 22-gauge 80- to 100-mm needle lateral to the probe and advance toward the target structures. After negative aspiration, deposit a total of 15 to 20 mL of LA on each side of the femoral artery.

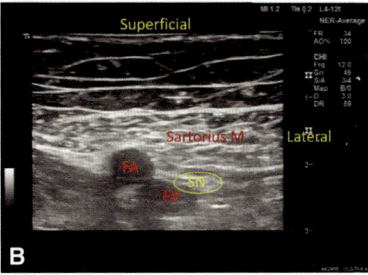

FIGURE 21.15 Adductor canal block using ultrasound guidance. **A,** US probe and needle position for performing the block. **B,** The FA and FV are located beneath the sartorius muscle, with the SN usually located lateral to the artery. *Please note, in actual practice the ultrasound probe must have a sterile covering. In this figure, the covering is omitted to better demonstrate correct probe orientation and needle insertion point.* FA, femoral artery; FV, femoral vein; SN, saphenous nerve.

7. **Periarticular IPACK** (Video 21.10). This block provides knee analgesia by targeting the posterior articular branches of the knee joint. It can be performed in a prone or supine position with the leg flexed at the level of the knee and rotated laterally (frog leg position). The probe is placed transversely at or just above the popliteal crease to visualize the femoral condyles and the popliteal artery in cross-section. The femoral condyles appear as curved hyperechoic lines, while the popliteal artery is seen as a pulsating anechoic structure in the center. By adjusting the tilt of the transducer, the tibial nerve (superficial to the popliteal artery) and the common peroneal nerve (at the lateral edge) can be visualized. The needle is inserted IP from medial to lateral. Typically, 20 mL (range 15 to 25 mL) of local anesthetic is infiltrated into the tissue plane, reaching the lateral border of the popliteal artery.
8. **Saphenous nerve block using UGRA.** The adductor canal approach is used for saphenous nerve block at the level of the midthigh. For the saphenous nerve block below the knee, position the patient supine with the leg straight. Place the probe at the level of the tibial tuberosity. Visualize the saphenous vein and fascia lata and inject LA around the saphenous nerve close to the saphenous vein. Using a tourniquet above the knee may help to engorge the saphenous vein.
9. **Obturator nerve block using UGRA.** Position the patient supine. Place the transducer on the medial thigh just below the inguinal crease. Identify the anterior branch of the obturator nerve in the fascial plane between the adductor longus and brevis muscles. Identify the posterior branch in the fascial plane between the adductor brevis and magnus muscles. Advance a 22-gauge 80-mm needle with the IP or OOP approach until the tip lies in the appropriate fascial plane. **PNS** of the obturator nerve will elicit an adductor twitch. Inject 5 to 10 mL of LA around each branch (total of 10 to 20 mL).
10. **SCN block**
    a. **Gluteal/subgluteal approach using UGRA (Figure 21.16; Video 21.11).** Place the patient in the Sims position, a lateral decubitus position with the leg to be blocked uppermost and flexed at the hip and knee. Place a curved transducer between the greater trochanter and ischial tuberosity. Visualize the hyperechoic SCN in the transverse plane at the level of the ischial spine, deep to the gluteus maximus

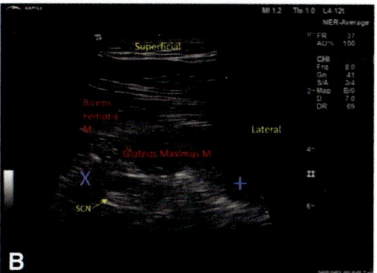

FIGURE 21.16 Sciatic nerve block with subgluteal approach using ultrasound guidance. **A,** US probe and needle position for performing the block. It is placed between the ischial tuberosity (X) and the greater trochanter (+). **B,** The nerve (*yellow arrow*) is located deep to the gluteus maximus muscle. *Please note, in actual practice the ultrasound probe must have a sterile covering. In this figure, the covering is omitted to better demonstrate correct probe orientation and needle insertion point.* SCN, sciatic nerve.

muscle and superficial to the quadratus femoris muscle. Insert a 22-gauge 80- to 100-mm needle lateral to the transducer and advance in the plane until the needle tip is in proximity to the nerve. **PNS** elicits a motor response in the SCN distribution (contraction of hamstring or gastrocnemius, foot dorsiflexion, or plantar flexion) or paresthesia in the leg or foot. After negative aspiration, inject 15 to 25 mL of LA with the goal of circumferential spread around the nerve. In the **subgluteal approach** (the needle is inserted a few centimeters more distally where the gluteus maximus is thinner, and the SCN is more superficial.

b. **Popliteal approach using UGRA (Figure 21.17; ⊙ Video 21.12).** This may be performed posteriorly with the patient in the prone, lateral, or supine position with the leg elevated. The linear or curved probe is placed at the level of the popliteal crease, and the popliteal artery should be seen in cross-section. The artery is then followed cephalad 5 to 7 cm.

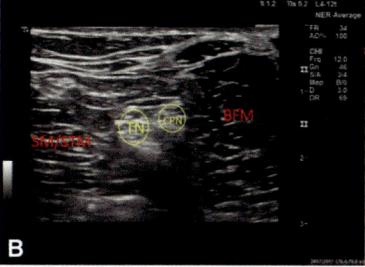

FIGURE 21.17 Sciatic nerve block with popliteal fossa approach using ultrasound guidance. **A,** US probe and needle position for performing the block. **B,** The SM/STM is seen medially, and the BFM is seen lateral to the sciatic nerve, which is composed of the TN and CPN. *Please note, in actual practice the ultrasound probe must have a sterile covering. In this figure, the covering is omitted to better demonstrate correct probe orientation and needle insertion point.* BFM, biceps femoris muscle; CPN, common peroneal nerve; SM, semimembranosus muscle; STM, semitendinosus muscle; TN, tibial nerve.

The popliteal vein classically lies superficial and lateral to the artery, and the SCN lies even more superficial and lateral to the vein. The semimembranosus muscle is seen medially and the biceps femoris laterally to the nerve. The nerve should be traced to identify the site of bifurcation into the tibial and common peroneal nerves. With the SCN centered in the image and taking an IP approach, a needle insertion site is chosen approximately 1 cm lateral to the probe. Insert a 22-gauge 80-mm needle and advance the needle tip adjacent to the nerve at the point of bifurcation and between common peroneal and tibial nerves. A distinct pop is felt with entry into the perineural sheath. **PNS** causes foot dorsiflexion or plantar flexion and/or paresthesia in the leg or foot. After negative aspiration, inject 20 to 30 mL of LA to achieve circumferential spread around the nerve.

11. **Ankle block**
    a. The five nerves supplying the foot can be blocked at the ankle. These include two deep nerves (tibial and deep peroneal) and three superficial nerves (superficial peroneal, sural, saphenous) (**Figure 21.18**). The ankle block can be performed with the landmark technique or UGRA with a small linear high-frequency probe.
        1. At the superior border of the malleoli, the **deep peroneal nerve (◉ Video 21.13)** is situated between the anterior tibialis tendon and

FIGURE 21.18 Cross-section of anatomic structures at the level of the ankle. The deep peroneal nerve is located lateral to the extensor hallucis longus tendon and dorsalis pedis artery. The posterior tibial nerve is posterior to the distal medial malleolus and posterior tibial artery. (From Horn JL, Nasiri M. Regional blocks—A brief overview. In: Jaffe RA, Schmiesing CA, Golianu B, eds. *Anesthesiologist's Manual of Surgical Procedures*. 6th ed. 2020:1763–1799. Figure 16.41.)

the extensor hallucis longus tendon, which are easily palpable with dorsiflexion of the foot and extension of the great toe. Place the transducer transversely at the level of the extensor retinaculum on the anterior ankle and identify the nerve lateral to the anterior tibial artery. Insert a 25-mm needle just lateral to the anterior tibial artery while depositing 5 to 10 mL of LA close to the nerve.

2. Block the **superficial peroneal nerve** (⊙ **Video 21.13**) by placing the transducer transversely 5 to 10 cm proximal and anterior to the lateral malleolus. Identify the nerve in the subcutaneous tissue and between the peroneus longus and extensor digitorum longus muscles superficial to the fascia. Alternatively, inject 10 mL of LA subcutaneously across the anterior surface of the tibia, from malleolus to malleolus. The latter approach will block the **superficial peroneal nerve** laterally and the **saphenous nerve** medially.
3. To block the **tibial nerve** (⊙ **Video 21.13**), place the transducer transversely at the level of the medial malleolus and visualize the nerve posterior to the posterior tibial artery under the flexor retinaculum of the ankle. Insert a needle OOP or IP posterior to the medial malleolus, directed toward the posterior tibial nerve, and inject 5 to 10 mL of LA in a fan-shaped area.
4. Block the **sural nerve** (⊙ **Video 21.13**) by placing the probe lateral and proximal to the lateral malleolus. Find the small saphenous vein, identify the nerve superficial to the deep fascia and adjacent to the saphenous vein, and inject 5 mL of LA.

IX. REGIONAL ANESTHESIA OF THE TRUNK
A. Anatomy
1. The **thoracic spinal nerves** exit from the intervertebral foramina and divide into dorsal and ventral rami. The **ventral rami** become the **intercostal nerves**, which travel within the intercostal spaces below the inferior border of the superior rib and innervate the thoracic and abdominal walls. All intercostal nerves except for T1 give off a lateral cutaneous branch, which innervates the lateral chest. The anterior cutaneous branches of intercostal nerves T2–5 provide sensory innervation to the **medial breast**, and the lateral cutaneous branches innervate the **lateral breast**, while the supraclavicular nerve innervates the **superior pole of the breast**. Other nerves that contribute to breast innervation are lateral and medial pectoral, long thoracic, intercostobrachial (which innervates the axilla and axillary tail of the breast), and thoracodorsal nerves (**Figure 21.3**).
2. The **TPVS** is a wedge-shaped space that exists on both sides of the thoracic vertebra and is limited anterolaterally by the pleura, medially by vertebra, and posteriorly by the SCTL. It contains the ventral and dorsal rami, sympathetic chain, and intercostal vessels.
3. The intercostal nerves arising from T6 to T11 ultimately terminate in the **anterolateral abdominal wall** and are known as the **thoracoabdominal nerves**. The ventral ramus of T12 is known as the subcostal nerve and travels entirely in the abdominal wall. The anterior abdominal wall receives sensory innervation from the ventral rami of the T6–L1 spinal nerves. The terminal branches of these nerves travel through the lateral abdominal wall within the TAP, the fascial plane between the IOM and the TAM, and generate a plexus. The upper T6–T9 segmental nerves exit the intercostal space and enter the TAP lateral to the linea

alba. The anterior cutaneous branches of the thoracoabdominal nerves enter the rectus muscle and sheath lateral to the linea semilunaris and form a plexus with each other. The presence of both TAP and rectus sheath plexuses explains why the precise dermatomal map maybe inaccurate. The L1 nerve divides into iliohypogastric and ilioinguinal nerves (see Section VIII.A.1).

B. RA of the thorax using UGRA

1. **Indications.** Thoracic wall blocks provide analgesia for the chest and upper abdomen, including patients with rib fractures or those undergoing thoracotomy, breast surgery, gastrostomy, cholecystectomy, and herniorrhaphy.
2. **Complications** specific to thoracic wall blocks include pneumothorax and intrathecal or epidural injection for paravertebral blocks.
3. **Techniques**
   a. **Thoracic paravertebral block.** The TPVS can be accessed to provide unilateral somatic and sympathetic sensory loss. The block may be performed with a **sagittal paramedian approach.** With the patient prone, place the probe parasagittally, lateral to the spinous processes, and scan medially until the TP and TPVS are visualized, as well as the pleura and the SCTL. Insert a 22-gauge 80-mm needle and advance OOP until the SCTL is pierced. A depression of the pleura with LA injection should be visualized if the SCTL has been traversed. Alternatively, a **transverse approach (Figure 21.19; Video 21.14)** may be used to allow continuous visualization of the needle. Place the probe transversely, lateral to the spinous processes. The rib is visualized as a shallow hyperechoic structure with acoustic shadowing below it. Move the probe slightly cranially or caudally off the rib into the intercostal space and visualize the hyperechoic pleura and the shadow of the TP. The TPVS appears as a hypoechoic triangle bounded by the pleura below, the hyperechoic innermost intercostal membrane above, and the TP medially. Insert a 22-gauge 80- to 100-mm needle lateral to the probe and advance IP medially toward the TPVS. Continuous visualization of the needle tip is essential to avoid pleural puncture. Hydrolocalization may be used to help find the needle tip. After negative aspiration, 3 to 5 mL of LA may be injected at multiple

 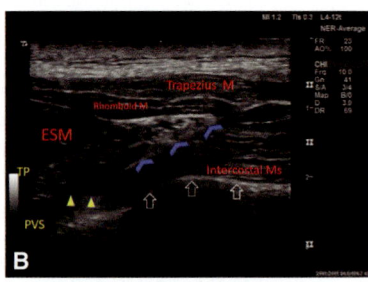

FIGURE 21.19 Thoracic paravertebral block with transverse approach using ultrasound guidance. **A,** US probe and needle position for performing the block. **B,** The PVS is located ventral to the superior costotransverse ligament (*yellow arrows*) and posterior to the TP. The *blue arrows* show the needle approaching the PVS, and the *white hollow arrows* designate the pleura. *Please note, in actual practice the ultrasound probe must have a sterile covering. In this figure, the covering is omitted to better demonstrate correct probe orientation and needle insertion point.* ESM, erector spinae muscle; PVS, paravertebral space; TP, transverse process. (Courtesy of Dr. Heitor Jose Medeiros.)

single levels, or a larger volume (up to 20 mL) may be injected at a single midpoint level. A catheter may be placed to provide continuous analgesia. Depression of the pleura is observed with injection of LA and spread can be traced cranially and caudally.

b. **Thoracic interfascial plane blocks** are newer UGRA techniques that rely on the spread of LA on the target fascial plane and were developed initially as safer alternatives to epidural, thoracic paravertebral, and intercostal blocks.

 1. **Pectoral nerve block (Pecs).** The pectoral nerves innervate the pectoral major and minor muscles, providing analgesia for postoperative pectoral muscle spasms and myofascial pain. The interpectoral plane block or the **Pecs I block** (◉ **Video 21.15**), involves LA injection between the pectoralis major and minor muscles to block the lateral and medial pectoral nerves. Position the patient supine with the arm next to the chest or abducted to 90 degrees. Place the probe parasagittally, similar to the infraclavicular approach above. Rotate the transducer slightly from medial to lateral to help locate the pectoral branch of the thoracoacromial artery and allow for an IP approach. Hydrodissection is used to confirm the correct fascial plane. After negative aspiration, inject 10 mL of LA. The pectoserratus plane block or **Pecs II block** (◉ **Video 21.16**) involves two separate LA injections along two fascial planes and is essentially a combination of the Pecs I and injection between the serratus anterior muscle and pectoralis minor muscle. Both injections can be performed with a single needle pass. Positioning is the same as for Pecs I. The first injection is made in the same manner as Pecs I. The transducer is then moved laterally to identify the pectoralis minor and serratus anterior, and the second injection is made between these two muscles at the anterior axillary line at the level of the fourth rib. This will block the lateral cutaneous branches of T2–4 and the intercostobrachial nerves.

 2. **Erector spinae block (Figure 21.20;** ◉ **Video 21.17).** This block has been used for rib fractures and procedures requiring truncal analgesia. LA is injected in the fascial plane deep to the ESM and superficial to the tips of the TP. The block relies on the spread of LA to the paravertebral and epidural spaces. Place the probe parasagittally over the tip of the TP. Insert a 22-gauge 80-mm needle using an IP approach until the needle tip is in contact with the TP. A single injection of 20 mL provides coverage to 6 to 10 levels in the intercostal area.

 3. **PIP block (Figure 21.21).** The PIP blocks are described as surficial and deep; targeting anterior cutaneous branches of T2–T6, which provide sensory innervation to the anterior chest wall and sternum. The superficial PIP block targets the plane superficial to the internal intercostal muscles and ribs and deep to the pectoralis major muscle lateral to the sternum. The deep PIP block targets the plane between the internal intercostal muscle and transversus thoracis muscles and has also been known as the transversus thoracis muscle plane block.

 4. **Serratus anterior plane block (Figure 21.22).** This block targets the lateral cutaneous branches of the intercostal nerves and thoracic and thoracodorsal nerves, extending from T2 to T7, and is used for breast analgesia and thoracotomy. It is performed in the axillary region between the 2nd and 7th ribs, in a more lateral and posterior position than the Pecs blocks. To perform this block, place the

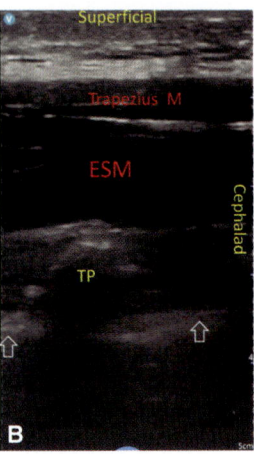

FIGURE 21.20 Erector spinae block using ultrasound guidance. **A,** US probe and needle position for performing the block. **B,** Erector spinae muscle (ESM) located dorsal to the transverse process (TP). While *hollow arrows* show the pleura. *Please note, in actual practice the ultrasound probe must have a sterile covering. In this figure, the covering is omitted to better demonstrate correct probe orientation and needle insertion point.* (Courtesy of Dr. Heitor Jose Medeiros.)

 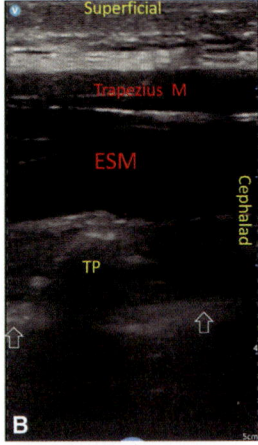

FIGURE 21.21 Parasternal Intercostal Plane (PIP) Blocks using ultrasound guidance. **A,** US probe and needle position for performing the block. **B,** US image of PIP. Superficial PIP is the fascia plane between pectoralis major and intercostal muscles. The deep PIP is the fascia plane between intercostal and transversus thoracis muscles. While *hollow arrows* show the pleura. *Please note, in actual practice the ultrasound probe must have a sterile covering. In this figure, the covering is omitted to better demonstrate correct probe orientation and needle insertion point.* (Courtesy of Dr. Heitor Jose Medeiros.)

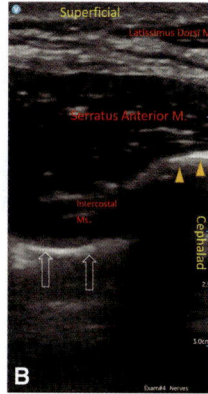

FIGURE 21.22 Serratus anterior plane (SAP) blocks using ultrasound guidance. **A,** US probe and needle position for performing the block. **B,** US image of SAP. Interfascial injection is usually performed between the latissimus dorsi muscle and serratus anterior muscle or between the serratus anterior muscle and intercostal muscle. While *hollow arrows* show the pleura. *Yellow arrowheads* show the rib. *Please note, in actual practice the ultrasound probe must have a sterile covering. In this figure, the covering is omitted to better demonstrate correct probe orientation and needle insertion point.* (Courtesy of Dr. Heitor Jose Medeiros.)

probe between the fourth and fifth ribs to locate the latissimus dorsi. Identify the thoracodorsal artery, which runs in the fascial plane between the serratus anterior and latissimus dorsi. LA may be injected superficially or deep to the serratus anterior.

5. **Retrolaminar block.** This block has been used for TP fractures and truncal analgesia, and although similar to the erector spinae block, it targets the vertebral laminae rather than TP. Place the probe closer to the midline to visualize the lamina. A single injection of 20 mL provides coverage to 2 to 4 sensory levels in the paravertebral and epidural spaces.

c. **Intercostal nerve block.** This block involves LA injection in the proximal intercostal space between the internal intercostal membrane and endothoracic fascial/parietal pleura. It can be performed with the patient in prone, sitting, or lateral decubitus positions. Place the probe in a paramedian, sagittal orientation and identify the tip of the TP, then laterally to visualize the rib. Insert a 22-gauge 25- to 50-mm needle using an IP approach until the tip of the needle is below the internal intercostal membrane and above the pleura. After negative aspiration, a 3- to 5-mL injection of LA will spread laterally and in a single intercostal level. Multiple injections may be needed to provide extensive analgesia.

C. **RA of the abdomen using UGRA**
1. **Indications.** Abdominal wall blocks provide analgesia for periumbilical abdominal incisions, including laparoscopy, laparotomy for colorectal surgery, appendectomy, retropubic prostatectomy, abdominal hysterectomy, Cesarean section, and hernia repair. Bilateral blocks are required for midline incisions.
2. **Complications** specific to these blocks include perforated viscus, intravascular injection into epigastric arteries, and LAST given the large amount of LA injection required.

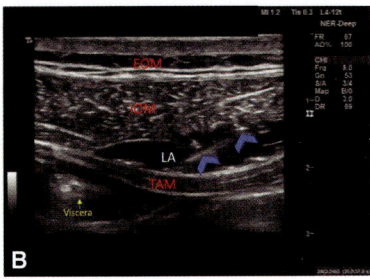

FIGURE 21.23 Transverse abdominis block with lateral approach using ultrasound guidance. **A,** US probe and needle position for performing the block. **B,** LA is deposited by the block needle (*blue arrows*) between the IOM and TAM. *Please note, in actual practice the ultrasound probe must have a sterile covering. In this figure, the covering is omitted to better demonstrate correct probe orientation and needle insertion point.* EOM, external oblique muscle; IOM, internal oblique muscle; LA, local anesthetic; TAM, transversus abdominis muscle. (Courtesy of Dr. Heitor Jose Medeiros.)

3. **Techniques**
   a. **TAP block**. The TAP block provides analgesia of the anterior abdominal wall, including the skin, muscles, and parietal peritoneum. Theoretically, the T7–L1 block can be achieved; however, the extent of this block is variable clinically. There are two approaches to the TAP block.
      1. **Lateral (Figure 21.23; ⊙ Video 21.18)**. This approach targets the lateral abdominal wall between the mid- and anterior axillary lines. Position the patient supine with the abdomen exposed from the costal margin to the iliac crest. Place the probe along the midaxillary line between the subcostal margin and the iliac crest. Identify the three muscular layers of the abdominal wall: the EOM, IOM, and TAM. The parietal peritoneum can be visualized deep to the TAM with loops of bowel sliding beneath it. Insert a 22-gauge 80- to 100-mm blunt-tipped needle 2 cm medial to the probe at a 30-degree angle to the skin. Advance the needle IP until the needle tip is in the fascial plane between the IOM and TAM. After negative aspiration, inject 20 to 30 mL of LA per side or thread a catheter for continuous analgesia. The spread can be traced superiorly and inferiorly.
      2. **Subcostal.** The subcostal approach targets the anterior abdominal wall from the xiphoid process to the ASIS and is typically used for upper abdominal sensory block (T6–10). Positioning is the same as above. Place the probe along the subcostal margin. Identify the rectus abdominis muscle and posterior rectus sheath. Deep to the rectus sheath is the TAM. Insert the needle until the tip is between the posterior rectus sheath and the TAM, and inject LA and follow it laterally toward the ASIS.
   b. **Rectus sheath block (Figure 21.24, ⊙ Video 21.19)**. The rectus sheath block is useful for analgesia after umbilical hernia repair and other midline abdominal incisions. The rectus abdominis muscle is located beneath the superficial fascia of the abdomen. Position the patient supine with the abdomen exposed. Place the probe transversely just lateral to the umbilicus. Insert a 22-gauge 80- to 100-mm needle medial to the probe and advance IP in a medial-to-lateral direction through the anterior rectus sheath and rectus abdominis muscle until the tip rests against the posterior rectus sheath. Avoid

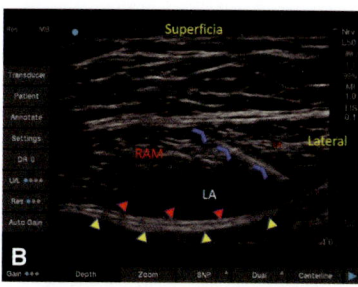

FIGURE 21.24 Rectus sheath block using ultrasound guidance. **A,** US probe and needle position for performing the block. **B,** LA is injected by the block needle (*blue arrows*) between the RAM and the rectus sheath (*red arrows*). The *yellow arrows* show the endoabdominal fascia. *Please note, in actual practice the ultrasound probe must have a sterile covering. In this figure, the covering is omitted to better demonstrate correct probe orientation and needle insertion point.* EA, epigastric artery; LA, local anesthetic; RAM, rectus abdominis muscle. (Courtesy of Dr. Heitor Jose Medeiros.)

the inferior epigastric vein and artery. After negative aspiration, inject 10 to 20 mL of LA per side.

c. **Iliohypogastric/ilioinguinal block.** This block provides excellent analgesia for groin operations (eg, hernia repair). Place the transducer medial to the ASIS along a line connecting the ASIS and the umbilicus. Identify the nerves as hyperechoic structures in the fascial plane between the IOM and TAM. The superficial iliac circumflex vein and artery may present in the same plane and can be used to identify the plane. Insert a 22-gauge 25-mm needle medial to the probe and advance IP in a medial-to-lateral direction until the needle tip is within the previously described fascial plane. After negative aspiration, inject 10 mL of LA.

d. **QL block.** This block involves LA injection adjacent to the QL and covers T7–L1. There are several different variations of the block that are named based on the location of the needle tip and deposition of LA relative to the muscle. The patient may be positioned supine, lateral, sitting, or prone for any type.

   1. **QL type 1 (lateral).** Using a linear transducer, place the probe in the midaxillary line and move it laterally until the aponeurosis of the TAM is visualized. Using an IP approach, insert a 22-gauge 80- to 150-mm needle lateral to the probe with an anterior–posterior needle trajectory. Advance the needle tip until it crosses the transversus abdominis aponeurosis but is superficial to the transversalis fascia. LA is injected at the lateral border of the QL.
   2. **QL type 2 (posterior).** The approach is similar to type 1 with probe positioning and needle insertion. The difference is that LA is injected on the posterior surface of the QL, at the fascial layer separating the QL and ESM.
   3. **Transmuscular QL (anterior)** (**Figure 21.11**; ⊙ **Video 21.20**): Using a curved array transducer, place the probe just cranial to the iliac crest. Visualize the "shamrock sign," which contains the TP of L4 as the stem, QL laterally, ESM posteriorly, and psoas major anteriorly. Insert the needle using an IP approach in a posterior-to-anterior fashion. Inject the LA in the fascial plane between the QL and psoas major muscle and visualize the spread of LA to the paravertebral space.

ACKNOWLEDGMENTS

We gratefully acknowledge the contributions of previous edition author(s), Lucy T. Li and Shika Card, as portions of those chapters have been retained in this revision.

We also would like to extend their gratitude to Dr. Heitor Jose Medeiros for his contributions to video editing and graphic visualization of the anatomical structures related to each nerve block technique.

Suggested Readings

Amaral S, Lombardi RA, Medeiros H, Nogueira A, Gadsden J. Superior trunk block is an effective phrenic-sparing alternative to interscalene block for shoulder arthroscopy: a systematic review and meta-analysis. *Cureus*. 2023;15(11):e48217.

ASA House of Delegates. *Standards for Basic Anesthetic Monitoring*. 2015:1–4.

American Society Anesthesiologists Task Force on Infectious Complications Associated With Neuraxial Techniques. Practice advisory for the prevention, diagnosis, and management of infectious complications associated with neuraxial techniques. *Anesthesiology*. 2010;112:530–545.

Bigeleisen PE, Moayeri N, Groen GJ. Extraneural versus intraneural stimulation thresholds during ultrasound-guided supraclavicular block. *Anesthesiology*. 2009;110:1235–1243.

Chin KJ. Thoracic wall blocks: From paravertebral to retrolaminar to serratus to erector spinae and back again – A review of evidence. *Best Pract Res Clin Anaesthesiol*. 2019;33(1):67–77.

Chin KJ, McDonnell JG, Carvalho B, Sharkey A, Pawa A, Gadsden J. Essentials of our current understanding: abdominal wall blocks. *Reg Anesth Pain Med*. 2017;42(2):133–183.

Chin KJ, Pawa A, Forero M, Adhikary S. Ultrasound-guided fascial plane blocks of the thorax: pectoral I and II, serratus anterior plane, and erector spinae plane blocks. *Adv Anesth*. 2019;37:187–205.

Desmet M, Vermeylen K, Van Herreweghe I, et al. A longitudinal supra-inguinal fascia iliaca compartment block reduces morphine consumption after total hip arthroplasty. *Reg Anesth Pain Med*. 2017;42(3):327–333.

El-Boghdadly K, Albrecht E, Wolmarans M, et al. Standardizing nomenclature in regional anesthesia: an ASRA-ESRA Delphi consensus study of upper and lower limb nerve blocks. *Reg Anesth Pain Med*. 2024;49(11):782–792.

El-Boghdadly K, Wolmarans M, Stengel AD, et al. Standardizing nomenclature in regional anesthesia: an ASRA-ESRA Delphi consensus study of abdominal wall, paraspinal, and chest wall blocks. *Reg Anesth Pain Med*. 2021;46(7):571–580.

Elsharkawy H, El-Boghdadly K, Barrington M. Quadratus lumborum block: anatomical concepts, mechanisms, and techniques. *Anesthesiology*. 2019;130(2):322–335.

Elsharkawy H, Pawa A, Mariano E. Interfascial plane blocks: back to basics. *Reg Anesth Pain Med*. 2018;43(4):341–346.

Feigl GC, Litz RJ, Marhofer P. Anatomy of the brachial plexus and its implications for daily clinical practice: regional anesthesia is applied anatomy. *Reg Anesth Pain Med*. 2020;45(8):620–627.

Greengrass RA, Narouze S, Bendtsen TF, Hadzic A. Cervical plexus and greater occipital nerve blocks: controversies and technique update. *Reg Anesth Pain Med*. 2019;44:623–626.

Halaszynski TM. Ultrasound brachial plexus anesthesia and analgesia for upper extremity surgery: essentials of our current understanding, 2011. *Curr Opin Anaesthesiol*. 2011;24(5):581–591.

Helander EM, Webb MP, Kendrick J, et al. PECS, serratus plane, erector spinae, and paravertebral blocks: a comprehensive review. *Best Pract Res Clin Anaesthesiol*. 2019;33(4):573–581.

Horlocker TT, Vandermeulen E, Kopp SL, Gogarten W, Leffert LR, Benzon HT. Regional anesthesia in the patient receiving antithrombotic or thrombolytic therapy: American Society of Regional Anesthesia and Pain Medicine evidence-based guidelines (fourth edition). *Reg Anesth Pain Med*. 2018;43:263–309.

Hussain N, Golder G, Ragina N, Banfield L, Laffey JG, Abdallah FW. Suprascapular and interscalene nerve block for shoulder surgery: a systematic review and meta-analysis. *Anesthesiology*. 2017;127(6):998–1013.

Ilfeld BM. Continuous peripheral nerve blocks: a review of the published evidence. *Anesth Analg*. 2011;113:904–925.

Jones MR, Novitch MB, Sen S, et al. Upper extremity regional anesthesia techniques: a comprehensive review for clinical anesthesiologists. *Best Pract Res Clin Anaesthesiol.* 2020;34(1):e13–e29.

Kandarian B, Indelli PF, Sinha S, et al. Implementation of the IPACK (Infiltration between the Popliteal Artery and Capsule of the Knee) block into a multimodal analgesic pathway for total knee replacement. *Korean J Anesthesiol.* 2019;72(3):238–244.

Kang R, Jeong JS, Chin KJ, et al. Superior trunk block provides noninferior analgesia compared with interscalene brachial plexus block in arthroscopic shoulder surgery. *Anesthesiology.* 2019;131(6):1316–1326.

Li JW, Songthamwat B, Samy W, Sala-Blanch X, Karmakar MK. Ultrasound-guided costoclavicular brachial plexus block: sonoanatomy, technique, and block dynamics. *Reg Anesth Pain Med.* 2017;42(2):233–240.

Lin X, Liu CW, Goh QY, et al. Pericapsular nerve group (PENG) block for early pain management of elderly patients with hip fracture: a single-center double-blind randomized controlled trial. *Reg Anesth Pain Med.* 2023;48(11):535–539.

Mian A, Chaudhry I, Huang R, Rizk E, Tubbs RS, Loukas M. Brachial plexus anesthesia: a review of the relevant anatomy, complications, and anatomical variations. *Clin Anat.* 2014;27(2):210–221.

Neal JM, Bernards CM, Hadzic A, et al. ASRA practice advisory on neurologic complications in regional anesthesia and pain medicine. *Reg Anesth Pain Med.* 2008;33:404–415.

Neal JM, Gerancher JC, Hebl JR, et al. Upper extremity regional anesthesia. *Reg Anesth Pain Med.* 2009;34:134–170.

Ochroch J, Qi V, Badiola I, et al. Analgesic efficacy of adding the IPACK block to a multimodal analgesia protocol for primary total knee arthroplasty. *Reg Anesth Pain Med.* 2020;45(10):799–804.

O'Reilly N, Desmet M, Kearns R. Fascia iliaca compartment block. *BJA Educ.* 2019;19(6):191–197.

Sabouri AS, Crawford L, Bick SK, Nozari A, Anderson TA. Is a retrolaminar approach to the thoracic paravertebral space possible? A human cadaveric study. *Reg Anesth Pain Med.* 2018;43(8):864–868.

Sala-Blanch X, Reina MA, Pangthipampai P, Karmakar MK. Anatomic basis for brachial plexus block at the costoclavicular space: a cadaver anatomic study. *Reg Anesth Pain Med.* 2016;41(3):387–391.

Singelyn FJ, Lhotel L, Fabre B. Pain relief after arthroscopic shoulder surgery: a comparison of intraarticular analgesia, suprascapular nerve block, and interscalene brachial plexus block. *Anesth Analg.* 2004;99:589–592.

Sinha SK, Suter S. New blocks for the same old joints. *Curr Opin Anaesthesiol.* 2018;31(5):630–635.

Sites BD, Taenzer AH, Herrick MD, et al. Incidence of local anesthetic systemic toxicity and postoperative neurologic symptoms associated with 12,668 ultrasound-guided nerve blocks: an analysis from a prospective clinical registry. *Reg Anesth Pain Med.* 2012;37(5):478–482.

Tagariello V. Sciatic nerve blocks: approaches, techniques, local anaesthetics and manipulations. *Anaesthesia.* 1998;53(Suppl 2):15–17.

Tran DQ, Bravo D, Leurcharusmee P, Neal J. Transversus abdominis plane block: a narrative review. *Anesthesiology.* 2019;131(5):1166–1190.

Tran DQ, Salinas F, Benzon HT, Neal JM. Lower extremity regional anesthesia: essentials of our current understanding. *Reg Anesth Pain Med.* 2019;44:143–180.

Woodworth GE, Ivie RMJ, Nelson S, Walker CM, Maniker RB. Perioperative breast analgesia: a qualitative review of anatomy and regional techniques. *Reg Anesth Pain Med.* 2017;42(5):609–631.

Xing T, Ge L. Ultrasound-guided brachial plexus block by costoclavicular space approach: a narrative review. *Med Sci Monit.* 2023;29:e939920.

Yurgil JL, Hulsopple CD, Leggit JC. Nerve blocks: Part I. Upper extremity. *Am Fam Physician.* 2020;101(11):654–664.

Yurgil JL, Hulsopple CD, Leggit JC. Nerve blocks: Part II. Lower extremity. *Am Fam Physician.* 2020;101(11):669–679.

Anesthesia for Orthopedic Surgery
Megan Abbott and Amy Du

I. GENERAL CONSIDERATION
There are multiple features of orthopedic surgery that mandate special consideration. Orthopedic anesthesia requires mastery of a wide range of anesthetic approaches: general, neuraxial, and regional anesthesia. It is critical to know the indications, limitations, and potential complications for each type of anesthesia and surgery. The anesthetist also must be comfortable caring for patients who may range from young and completely healthy to those nearing the end of life with multiple medical comorbidities. These patients may require simple elective, major reconstructive, or palliative surgeries.

II. ANESTHESIA FOR TOTAL HIP AND KNEE ARTHROPLASTY
Total hip and total knee arthroplasties are two of the most common surgical procedures performed in the United States. An aging population has increased the prevalence of degenerative and traumatic diseases in both healthy and frail patients. Modern medicine now offers the hope of maintaining a reasonable quality of life even for those patients who previously may have been deemed nonoperative candidates. Robotic-assisted techniques for these operations have gained more popularity over the years. These methods allow for integration with joint imaging to improve implant fit and positioning. Other benefits include haptic interfaces and burring tool technologies to prevent operating outside established parameters.

A. Neuraxial anesthesia is a staple of anesthetic practice in orthopedic surgery, especially for total hip arthroplasty (THA) and total knee arthroplasty (TKA). Neuraxial anesthesia is described in Chapter 20: Spinal, Epidural, and Caudal Anesthesia, and its use for specific orthopedic operations is explained here. Isobaric, preservative-free 0.5% bupivacaine is the most common drug used for hip and knee arthroplasties at the Massachusetts General Hospital (MGH); the dose is adjusted for the patient's height, weight, complexity of case, and estimated surgical time. We strive to provide neuraxial anesthesia sufficient for the entire operation. This can usually be achieved with doses of 1.6 to 1.8 mL for THA and 1.2 to 1.4 mL for TKA. These lower-dose ranges allow for early recovery of motor function. Higher doses may be considered for more complex operations, including revision arthroplasties and robotic-assisted cases. Neuraxial anesthesia allows for adequate relaxation during surgery; if neuraxial anesthesia is not completed, then surgeons may request muscle paralysis for the operation. Considerations should be given to provide appropriate intravascular volume repletion in the setting of vasodilation and subsequent hypotension seen with neuraxial anesthesia. In ambulatory surgical centers, there has been a trend toward using mepivacaine, instead of bupivacaine, as the spinal anesthesia for THA and TKA. A 2022 meta-analysis comparing mepivacaine and bupivacaine showed that patients undergoing total joint arthroplasties who received mepivacaine spinals demonstrated quicker

return of motor function and shorter length of stay as compared to bupivacaine spinals, without a difference in pain scores.
B. **Regional anesthesia** is often provided prior to TKA. The most common nerve block performed is the adductor canal block, which aims to anesthetize the saphenous nerve proximal to the knee. While blocking the saphenous nerve only anesthetizes the anteroinferior and medial aspects of the knee, this block can help with postoperative pain control. Moreover, the adductor canal block is preferable because the saphenous nerve is purely sensory, so patients can participate in physical therapy soon after surgery while still benefiting from pain relief. However, the nerve to the vastus medialis can be affected, resulting in some motor weakness.
C. **Pneumatic tourniquets** are often used in TKA and produce optimal surgical conditions by creating a bloodless field. Despite common use of this tool in the operating room, the optimal pressure to which to inflate the tourniquet is unclear. Generally, surgeons may request pressures of 250 to 350 mm Hg in adults. Intravenous antibiotics and tranexamic acid should be administered prior to tourniquet inflation to ensure adequate plasma concentration at the surgical site.
  1. Significant "tourniquet pain" despite profound neuraxial anesthesia can occur. It may manifest as a sympathetic nervous system response, which reportedly may be mitigated by short-acting beta-adrenergic inhibitors, ketamine, dexmedetomidine, clonidine, magnesium sulfate, or remifentanil. Rarely, this necessitates conversion to general anesthesia. Usually, this response is seen when the tourniquet time is greater than 60 minutes. Multiple expert opinions have suggested deflating the tourniquet for 10 minutes and then reinflating the tourniquet in this situation. Severe postoperative neuropraxias may occur if the inflation time exceeds 120 minutes.
  2. Deflation of the pneumatic tourniquet at any time during the procedure can cause multiple physiologic changes; the anesthetist should be prepared to manage these events. Tourniquet release will lower central venous pressure and mean arterial pressure as the extremity is perfused. The washout of metabolic products from the extremity will increase $PaCO_2$, $EtCO_2$, and potassium and lactate levels; and will decrease pH and body temperature. These changes can cause an increase in minute ventilation in the spontaneously breathing patient. Rarely, cardiac arrhythmias, ST segment changes, and T wave changes can occur.
D. **Tranexamic acid (TXA)** is an antifibrinolytic drug often used to reduce perioperative blood loss and minimize transfusion requirements in orthopedic surgery. Its use has been studied widely in joint arthroplasty, spine surgery, and trauma surgery. At MGH, we routinely use TXA over aminocaproic acid, although the mechanism of action and outcomes are similar.
  1. Mechanism of action: TXA is a synthetic analogue of lysine. It binds the lysine receptor sites on plasminogen and plasmin and thereby inhibits conversion of plasminogen to plasmin and direct action of plasmin on fibrin, respectively.
  2. Dosing: recent evidence shows that a single 1-g dose of TXA provides similar results to two doses in reducing perioperative transfusions, blood loss, and hospital length of stay after THA and TKA. At MGH, the dosing regimen is dependent on patient risk factors and should be discussed with the surgeon. Generally, one dose is given as a 1-g intravenous infusion over 10 minutes, ideally administered 20 minutes before incision. If a second dose is requested, it is given 15 minutes before closure.

3. Contraindications: (1) active or a history of arterial or venous thromboembolic disease; (2) recent cardiac stent placement (within 6 months); (3) allergy to TXA; (4) recent cerebrovascular accident (within 6 months) or intracranial hemorrhage; (5) color vision defect or retinal disease. Dose reduction is recommended in patients with renal impairment.
E. **Multimodal analgesia mixture** is often injected by the surgical team prior to closure of the incision. The doses per mL consist of ropivacaine 2.46 mg, ketorolac 0.3 mg, epinephrine 0.005 mg, and clonidine 0.0008 mg. Usually, 100 mL of the mixture is injected into the periarticular space, with considerations for dose adjustment in patients with extreme weights and those who received high doses of local anesthetics for preoperative peripheral nerve blocks.
F. **Bone cement implantation syndrome** is a feared complication of joint arthroplasty. "Cement" is polymethyl methacrylate, a synthetic resin. It is prepared on the surgical field by mixing a liquid with a powder, which results in the polymerization of methyl methacrylate. This exothermic reaction creates a paste, which is placed in the femoral canal and on the femoral and tibial prosthesis components during THA and TKA, respectively. Placement can cause intramedullary hypertension, which can then cause embolization of cement, bone marrow, or fat. The primary pathophysiology is an increase in pulmonary vascular resistance. Hence, patients with preexisting right-sided heart dysfunction or pulmonary hypertension are especially vulnerable.
  1. **Clinical presentation** includes hypotension, hypoxia, and arrhythmias.
  2. To avoid these complications, our practice is to increase the FiO_2 and intravascular volume status prior to cement placement. Clear communication between the surgical and anesthesia teams is paramount; if the patient is unstable, then cement placement should be delayed. A discussion about the suitability of cement should occur before surgery in patients with complex conditions who require hemiarthroplasty or THA for repair of a hip fracture. The team should consider an uncemented prosthesis in patients with known pulmonary hypertension or right-sided heart failure, in patients with a dire prognosis, and when palliative surgery is necessary to allow transfer to home or hospice care.
G. **Bilateral THA or TKA**, defined as same-day bilateral hip or knee arthroplasty, is less frequently performed. Several studies have reviewed outcomes of bilateral arthroplasty surgery. The benefits of decreased rehabilitation time and patient convenience must be weighed against the potentially increased risk of perioperative complications of bilateral procedures (including higher risk of mortality, cardiac events, and thrombotic events) when compared with their staged, unilateral counterparts.
  1. A consensus statement by the Consensus Conference on Bilateral Total Knee Arthroplasty Group in 2013 recommended the use of the following exclusion criteria for patients considering bilateral arthroplasty: (1) age over 75 years; (2) ASA physical status class III or higher; (3) presence of certain comorbidities, especially morbid obesity and a history of cardiopulmonary disease.

III. ANESTHESIA FOR SHOULDER SURGERY

Shoulder surgery can be performed with general anesthesia, regional anesthesia, or both. These operations include total shoulder arthroplasty, anterior acromioplasty, rotator cuff repair, repair of humeral or clavicular fractures, and scapulothoracic arthrodesis (STA). Surgery may be performed via an arthroscopic or open approach. Elderly, frail, and high-risk patients

FIGURE 22.1 Beach chair positioning, shown on the T-MAX table by Smith & Nephew. (Courtesy of Smith & Nephew, Inc.)

especially may benefit from regional anesthesia, when administered solely or as an adjunct to general anesthesia.

A. Positioning is a critical consideration in shoulder surgery. The sitting or "beach chair" position has become more popular than the traditional lateral position (**Figure 22.1**). The sitting position has implications for airway management and hemodynamic stability. The patient's head is supported on a mobile headrest, and then the operating table is turned 45 degrees. It is essential to protect the patient's head and eyes throughout surgery. Periodic inspection of the patient may help to prevent injury.

B. Blood pressure measurement in the upright position: Recall that actual blood pressure will change by 7.4 mm Hg for every 10-cm difference in vertical height. For example, if the blood pressure measurement for a cuff placed at the level of the heart is 120/80 mm Hg, and the circle of Willis is now at a 25 cm elevation above the heart, the pressure for cerebral perfusion will be 102/62 mm Hg. Aiming for higher blood pressure to offset this change in vertical height is a strategy we employ. The surgeon may request permissive hypotension for improved hemostasis, but this request must be considered carefully in patients with cerebrovascular disease. Invasive measurement of arterial pressure may be necessary to manage hemodynamics in a patient with complex conditions or sepsis.

C. The Bezold–Jarisch reflex can complicate up to 20% of sitting cases in patients who receive preoperative regional anesthesia prior to shoulder surgery, resulting in a combination of bradycardia and hypotension. The sudden onset of these hemodynamic alterations begins about 60 minutes after block placement. It is likely the result of a hyperdynamic heart and may be associated with epinephrine used in the block or due to anxiety in a conscious patient. This heart vigorously contracts against a volume-depleted ventricle owing to decreased preload in the sitting position. These conditions combine to activate receptors in the ventricular wall, and reflexive bradycardia occurs. One might consider volume repletion prior to cases requiring a sitting position to mitigate the effects of this reflex.

- **D. Airway management** usually necessitates the use of an endotracheal tube in these patients, as the upright position and operative field can make it difficult to reposition a malfunctioning laryngeal mask airway.
- **E. Interscalene nerve block** is often ideal when considering regional anesthesia, as most of the deep shoulder is innervated by the C5–C7 nerve roots. A catheter also can be inserted for prolonged postoperative analgesia. Occasionally, an intercostobrachial nerve block can help augment anesthesia in the medial or posterior shoulder and for anterior arthroscopic port placement.
- **F. Intense muscle relaxation** is often needed in total shoulder arthroplasty and repair of dislocated humeral fractures; this provides optimal conditions for proper realignment and fixation. Regional anesthesia has the benefit of offering excellent muscle relaxation without the necessity for dense neuromuscular blockade.
- **G. Scapulothoracic arthrodesis (STA)** is generally done in the prone position. Double-lumen endotracheal tube or bronchial blocker should be utilized when lung isolation is anticipated during these cases. Complete coverage using regional anesthesia may be challenging for STA. Truncal (paravertebral or erector spinae plane) nerve block catheters, interscalene nerve block catheters, or both purportedly can help decrease postoperative opioid requirement in select patients.

IV. ANESTHESIA FOR LOWER EXTREMITY SURGERY

These operations include fusions, tendon transfers, fracture repairs, arthroscopies, and amputations. The decision between general and regional anesthesia with sedation as the choice of primary anesthetic is based on the type of procedure, operative plan, length of surgery, and patient factors. Peripheral nerve blocks should be considered for all patients while being mindful of specific contraindications, as discussed in Subsection F that follows. Both regional and neuraxial anesthesia may be used to achieve excellent intraoperative anesthesia in lower extremity surgeries.

- **A.** The intraoperative use of a thigh tourniquet may often necessitate general anesthesia, because the pain from the applied pressure is not covered by many lower extremity nerve blocks.
- **B.** Knee arthroscopies usually do not require muscle relaxation. Thus, general anesthesia using laryngeal mask airway may be considered in patients without contraindications.
- **C.** Positioning plays a role in anesthetic choice. Most foot and ankle surgeries can be performed in the supine or lateral position. Achilles tendon surgery and calcaneal fractures are often performed in the prone position. Regional anesthesia may be appropriate if airway management is safe and comfortable for the patient. However, general anesthesia with controlled airway management may be necessary.
- **D.** The surgeon may need to evaluate the neurovascular integrity of the distal extremity after the operation; this concern may influence the choice of primary anesthesia. The aging of our patient population, commonly presenting with advanced cardiovascular and pulmonary diseases, may shift our anesthetic practices toward regional anesthesia. However, it has not been shown that use of regional anesthesia with sedation decreases incidence and severity of postoperative delirium or shortens rehabilitation time, as compared to general anesthesia.
- **E.** Nerve blocks to consider:
    1. Sciatic or popliteal nerve block is one of the most common blocks used in foot and ankle surgeries. Anesthetizing the sciatic nerve in the

popliteal fossa proximal to its bifurcation into the tibial and common peroneal nerves provides complete sensory loss below the knee, except the *medial* aspects of the leg and foot.
2. The saphenous nerve innervates the medial leg and foot and can be anesthetized most commonly in the adductor canal. Other recognized locations for saphenous nerve block are at the tibial tuberosity and just superior to the medial malleolus.
3. Ankle block can be utilized for foot surgeries when sensory loss above the ankle is not needed. Five nerves innervate the foot and can be blocked with a circumferential ring at the level of the malleolus. These include the saphenous, sural, tibial, and superficial and deep peroneal nerves.

F. Contraindications to regional anesthesia include the following: (1) infection at the site of injection; (2) allergy to local anesthetic; (3) risk for compartment syndrome; (4) acute neurologic deficit; (5) block near noncompressible blood vessels in an anticoagulated patient; (6) patient refusal.

V. ANESTHESIA FOR ELBOW, ARM, AND HAND SURGERY

These operations include fracture repair, tendon manipulation and transfer, hardware removal, and carpal tunnel release. Regional anesthesia, alone or as an adjunct to general anesthesia, should be considered for upper extremity surgery. The same discussion surrounding patient position, tourniquet use, length of surgery, and need for muscle relaxation influences the anesthetic approach (see Section IV).

A. Elbow and upper arm surgeries can often be performed with an interscalene (see Section III.E.) or lower brachial plexus nerve block. The former does have a higher incidence of incomplete blockade of the inferior trunk of the brachial plexus and can result in inadequate blockade within the ulnar nerve distribution.
1. Axillary block, often with separate musculocutaneous nerve block, will provide reliable anesthesia of the upper extremity from the mid-arm down to the hand. The area superficial to the deltoid is not anesthetized because the axillary nerve leaves the posterior cord more proximally in the axilla.
2. Of note, intercostobrachial and medial cutaneous nerve blocks may be used to augment an axillary block if medial incision of the upper arm is expected. This is performed by injecting local anesthetic into the subcutaneous tissue superiorly and inferiorly along the axillary crease.
3. Contraindications are similar for all regional techniques; axillary lymphadenopathy is a relative contraindication to regional anesthesia at this location.
4. For a complete description of regional anesthesia techniques, drugs, and doses please see Chapter 21: Regional Anesthesia. The New York Society of Regional Anesthesia (NYSORA) website, listed in *Suggested Readings*, has detailed descriptions of many techniques.

B. Forearm and hand surgeries can often be performed with regional anesthesia and sedation. Tourniquet use and its location will influence the specific block.
1. Lower brachial plexus blocks (supraclavicular, infraclavicular, and axillary) can be used for operations of the hand, forearm, and elbow.
2. Traditionally, an additional block of the intercostobrachial nerve, which innervates the medial aspect of the upper arm and is not covered by the brachial plexus block (see Section V.A.2.), is used to cover upper arm tourniquet pain. However, recent evidence suggests that this may not be necessary.

3. Peripheral nerve blocks at the wrist are often used for minor procedures that do not require a forearm or upper arm tourniquet. The median, ulnar, and radial nerves are easily accessible.
4. Intravenous regional anesthesia or the Bier block can be used for minor surgical procedures of the wrist and hand, including carpal tunnel release. A smaller volume of local anesthetic drug can be used if a forearm, rather than an upper arm, tourniquet is used.

VI. ANESTHESIA FOR ORTHOPEDIC ONCOLOGY

Orthopedic malignancies include primary tumors—osteosarcoma, chondrosarcoma, and Ewing sarcoma—and metastatic tumors, which are usually breast, prostate, and lung cancers. Bone, cartilage, and soft tissue malignancies can occur in every age group. Over the past 3 decades, aggressive surgical treatment and creative reconstructive techniques have revolutionized care, and limb salvage is a reality for many patients. Significant preoperative, intraoperative, and postoperative concerns must be considered in this patient population.

A. Preoperative concerns
1. Chemotherapy is a critical concern; patients may have had extensive treatment prior to surgery. Myelosuppression, anemia, thrombocytopenia, leukopenia, and end-organ chemotherapy side effects may be present. Preoperative erythropoietin and red blood cell or platelet transfusion may be necessary.
2. The specific chemotherapy regimen should be reviewed; doxorubicin is an anthracycline drug and is frequently administered preoperatively to patients with bone tumors. Its cardiac side effects are dose related and include arrhythmias, electrocardiographic changes such as ST segment and T wave abnormalities, congestive heart failure, and cardiomyopathy. The incidence of cardiomyopathy is related to dose, extremes of age, concomitant use of other cardiotoxic antitumor medications, and mediastinal radiation therapy. Echocardiography is performed before initiating doxorubicin therapy; serial cardiac examinations are part of the regimen.
3. Radiation is an equally important consideration, as previous radiation of a tumor can result in scar tissue, which poses the risk of large intraoperative hemorrhage.
4. Highly vascularized tumors pose an additional risk of large blood loss. Preoperative embolization of the tumor should be considered. Multidisciplinary management of complex tumors is now our standard approach; for example, in addition to an orthopedic oncology surgeon or a spine surgeon, a general surgeon may isolate the bowel, a urologic surgeon may place ureteral stents, a vascular surgeon may identify blood vessels, a thoracic surgeon may assist in resection of chest tumors, and a plastic and reconstructive surgeon may create a "free flap" for coverage of an extensive wound.

B. Intraoperative considerations include precise identification of the tumor, the anticipated length of surgery, the potential for staged surgery, patient positioning, and the possible need for neurophysiologic monitoring such as somatosensory and motor evoked potentials. For cross-reference, please see Chapter 24: Anesthesia for Spine Surgery.
1. Anesthetic approach will depend on tumor location and burden. Often, isolated tumors of distal extremities lend themselves to excision with regional anesthesia unless an intraoperative or immediate postoperative neurovascular examination is planned. The postoperative plan for

thromboprophylaxis must be discussed prior to choosing an anesthetic approach that may limit options for antithrombotic therapy, such as neuraxial anesthesia or certain peripheral nerve blocks.
2. Massive blood loss should be anticipated from highly vascularized tumors; major peripheral and central venous access, ability for rapid blood product transfusion, blood component availability, arterial access, and additional anesthesia staff are essential. These patients may have significant airway edema and vasopressor requirements; thoughtful discussion with the surgical team about postoperative transfer to an intensive care unit is recommended.
C. Postoperative pain control may be difficult and usually involves a multimodal analgesic approach. Oncology patients often have significant pain prior to surgery and may be taking high doses of opioid, tricyclic antidepressants, and anticonvulsant (eg, gabapentin) medications. The anesthetist should understand the patient's tolerance and preoperative requirements, as this regimen likely will need to be escalated in the postoperative period. Early consultation of the acute pain service may be useful to help the patient achieve an acceptable level of pain control after surgery.

VII. ANESTHESIA FOR ORTHOPEDIC TRAUMA

Orthopedic trauma is often one component of a polytrauma, and all standard procedures should be followed for triage and patient preoperative evaluation. If possible, investigation of underlying comorbidities, current medications, allergies, and previous surgeries should be attempted. Patients may have concomitant cervical spine injuries, which necessitate careful positioning and airway management. Along with standards of trauma care, including appropriate intravenous access, control of the airway, and management of comorbid diseases and implanted devices, some unique considerations are described.

A. Emergent and urgent orthopedic procedures are those that should be started immediately and within 4 hours, respectively. Emergent cases include those that threaten loss of limb or life and include vascular injuries, traumatic amputations, pelvic fractures accompanied by major blood loss, and compartment syndrome. Urgent cases are those at risk for complications without prompt fixation or repair; these include open fractures with the potential for soft tissue or bone infection and joint injuries that may lead to avascular necrosis.

B. Monitoring. The potential for hemodynamic instability, blood loss, and frequent laboratory tests will dictate the need for arterial and central venous access. Transesophageal or transthoracic echocardiography and, occasionally, a pulmonary artery catheter, can be considered for detailed information on cardiac function and volume status. Radiographic and ultrasound examination of the heart, chest, and lungs can be quite useful if pneumothorax, hemothorax, and lung or cardiac contusions are suspected. In polytrauma cases with traumatic brain injuries, intracranial pressure may also be monitored by external ventricular drains.

C. Hip fracture is one of the most common orthopedic trauma injuries in the United States. This injury can have devastating consequences for the elderly. Death is rare after orthopedic surgery; however, a 2022 retrospective cohort study found that 1-year mortality rates after hip fracture ranged from 6.5 to 19.6%, which was higher than all other lower extremity fractures. Significant preoperative risk factors for death include chronic renal failure, congestive heart failure, chronic obstructive pulmonary disease, and age greater than 70 years.

1. The care of the patient with a hip fracture can range from reasonably simple to profoundly complex. Although the surgery may be straightforward, the patient's comorbidities often present challenges to the anesthesia team. At MGH, the geriatric service is often consulted prior to operative repair to help optimize medical management of the elderly patient with a traumatic hip fracture. In addition, the type of repair planned by the orthopedic team will have implications for anesthetic management; these can include fixation of a femoral neck fracture with cannulated screws, fixation of a hip fracture with a sliding hip screw (SHS), a cephalomedullary nail such as the trochanteric femoral nail (TFN) or Gamma Nail, and hip hemiarthroplasty or THA. An SHS or TFN repair requires traction, and the patient must be positioned on an appropriate fracture table (**Figure 22.2**). Hemiarthroplasty or THA is performed while the patient is in the lateral position. Extensive manipulation and intraoperative fluoroscopy can extend surgical time, which influences the choice of a regional or general anesthetic approach.
2. One might wonder whether the type of anesthesia—general or regional—influences acute and long-term morbidity, mortality, and other outcomes. Early retrospective reviews suggested that regional anesthesia was associated with lower odds of inpatient mortality and pulmonary complications among patients with hip fracture when compared with general anesthesia. However, more recent studies have supported similar outcomes in general and neuraxial anesthesia approaches. For example, the REGAIN trial, a multicenter randomized controlled trial across 46 North American hospitals, demonstrated there were similar outcomes after 60 days (including survival and recovery of ambulation) between those who received general and spinal anesthesia for hip fractures. Secondary analysis of these data showed these results were consistent at 1-year postsurgery. See *Suggested Readings* for detailed reviews of this topic.
3. The timing of hip fracture repair may also affect outcomes. Currently, the American Academy of Orthopedic Surgeons recommends repair of hip fractures within 24 to 48 hours of injury. At MGH, we strive to

FIGURE 22.2 An example of fracture table positioning on the Hana orthopedic table by Misuho OSI. (Courtesy of Mizuho OSI, Union City, CA.)

repair frailty fractures within 48 hours of injury. Surgery may be delayed if the patient has the following conditions: acute myocardial infarction with increasing troponin levels, acute congestive heart failure, acute pneumonia with worsening oxygen saturation levels, acute metabolic derangements, and acute mental status changes necessitating evaluation and imaging. Other factors that may contribute to delaying surgery include transfer from a referral hospital, resource availability, and patient and family wishes.

D. There are several complications relevant to orthopedic trauma.
  1. Fat embolism syndrome (FES) is a rare but potentially fatal condition affecting orthopedic trauma patients. Care should be taken for prevention, early diagnosis, and treatment.
     a. Pathophysiology of FES is usually considered to be either mechanical or biochemical in origin. In the *mechanical* theory, large fat droplets are released into the venous system during injury and circulate through pulmonary capillaries and arteriovenous shunts into the cerebral circulation. The microvascular lodging of these fat droplets then produces inflammation and local ischemia. In the *biochemical* theory, the inciting event, such as an injury, causes the release of fatty acids into the circulation. Fatty acids and resultant inflammation combine to damage the capillary beds of the lungs and other organs.
     b. Clinical presentation usually occurs 12 hours to 3 days after long bone or pelvic trauma. The characteristic triad of respiratory distress, neurologic dysfunction, and skin petechiae may be present in varying degrees.
     c. Diagnosis is clinical in nature and can be aided by using diagnostic tools, such as Gurd's Diagnostic Criteria or the Schonfeld FES Index (**Table 22.1**).

Fat Embolism Syndrome Diagnostic Tools: Gurd's Diagnostic Criteria and Schonfeld FES Index

Scoring System	Criteria
Gurd Diagnostic Criteria: Must have 2 major OR 1 major and 4 minor criteria	*Major criteria* • Respiratory insufficiency with bilateral radiographic changes • Cerebral depression unrelated to hypoxemia or head injury • Petechial rash *Minor criteria* • Tachycardia >110 bpm • Fever >38.5 °C • Jaundice • Emboli present in retina on fundoscopy • Anuria or oliguria • Fat macroglobulinemia • Thrombocytopenia • Elevated erythrocyte sedimentation rate • Anemia
Schonfeld Fat Embolism Syndrome Index: Must have ≥5 points	• 5 points: Petechial rash • 4 points: Diffuse alveolar infiltrates • 3 points: Hypoxemia (PaO$_2$ <70 mm Hg with FiO$_2$ 100%) • 1 point each: Confusion, fever, tachycardia >120 bpm

d. Prevention likely consists of early operative fixation of long bone fractures. If internal fixation must be delayed, then external fixation for pelvic and long bone fractures should be considered.
   e. Treatment focuses on supportive measures, which will depend on the severity of lung and other end-organ dysfunction. Steroids, heparin, and vena cava filters have been proposed, but prospective, randomized, controlled studies are currently inconclusive. Patients with sickle cell disease who develop FES require urgent red blood cell exchange, because FES can cause acute chest syndrome and multiorgan failure in these patients.
2. Acute compartment syndrome (ACS) is a true orthopedic emergency. Regional anesthesia may potentially delay diagnosis, and therefore, anesthetists must be aware of its presentation and management when selecting an anesthetic approach. ACS develops most commonly in the forearm and lower leg, although it can occur in the upper arm and upper leg.
   a. Early clinical signs are variable, although pain out of proportion to injury is an important symptom. The other classic "P's" of pulselessness, pallor, and paresthesia have been found to be nonspecific in predicting compartment syndrome.
   b. At MGH, the threshold for diagnosing ACS (indicating the need for a fasciotomy) is a delta pressure (ie, the difference between the diastolic blood pressure and the compartment pressure) of 30 mm Hg. Notably, the patient's blood pressure should not be pharmacologically elevated or reduced (such as by vasopressors or anesthetics, respectively) at the time of measurement.
   c. Definitive treatment of ACS is emergent fasciotomy, which confers a good chance of complete recovery.
3. Crush injury and muscle compression can cause rhabdomyolysis. These injuries can lead to acute renal failure, which has a significant mortality rate.
   a. Serum creatinine kinase levels correlate with the degree of muscle damage and are useful for diagnosis and monitoring.
   b. Potassium is released from injured and necrotic muscle tissue, which can lead to rapid hyperkalemia and ventricular arrhythmias. Hemodialysis may be necessary to prevent serious sequelae.
   c. Therapy includes measures to avoid myoglobin precipitation in the renal tubules. Aggressive treatment of hypovolemia and diuresis are often employed.
4. The treatment of intraoperative hypotension and shock and the process of massive transfusion is discussed in Chapter 35: Anesthesia for Trauma and Burns.

VIII. ANESTHESIA FOR SPINE SURGERY
This topic is covered separately in Chapter 24: Anesthesia for Spine Surgery.

ACKNOWLEDGMENT

We gratefully acknowledge the contributions of previous edition author(s), Susan A. Vassallo, Philipp Gerner, and Shauna Williams, as portions of those chapters have been retained in this revision.

Suggested Readings

American Academy of Orthopaedic Surgeons. *Management of Hip Fractures in Older Adults. Evidence-Based Clinical Practice Guideline.* Published December 3, 2021. https://www.aaos.org/hipfxcpg

Anderson MR, Jeng CL, Wittig JC, Rosenblatt MA. Anesthesia for patients undergoing orthopedic oncologic surgeries. *J Clin Anesth*. 2010;22(7):565–572.

Dimet-Wiley A, Golovko G, Watowich SJ. One-year postfracture mortality rate in older adults with hip fractures relative to other lower extremity fractures: Retrospective cohort study. *JMIR Aging*. 2022;5(1):e32683.

Fenelon C, Murphy EP, Pomeroy E, Murphy RP, Curtin W, Murphy CG. Perioperative mortality after cemented or uncemented hemiarthroplasty for displaced femoral neck fractures – a systematic review and meta-analysis. *J Arthroplasty*. 2021;36:777–787.

Griffiths R, Babu S, Dixon P, et al. Guideline for the management of hip fractures 2020: Guideline by the Association of Anaesthetists. *Anaesthesia*. 2021;76(2):225–237.

Kumar K, Railton C, Tawfic Q. Tourniquet application during anesthesia: "What we need to know?" *J Anaesthesiol Clin Pharmacol*. 2016;32:424–430.

Luff D, Hewson DW. Fat embolism syndrome. *BJA Educ*. 2021;21(9):322–328.

Memtsoudis SG, Hargett M, Russell LA, et al; Consensus Conference on Bilateral Total Knee Arthroplasty Group. Consensus statement from the consensus conference on bilateral total knee arthroplasty group. *Clin Orthop Relat Res*. 2013;471(8):2649–2657.

Murphy GS, Greenberg SB, Szokol JW. Safety of beach chair position shoulder surgery: A review of the current literature. *Anesth Analg*. 2019;129(1):101–118.

Neuman MD, Feng R, Carson JL, et al; REGAIN Investigators. Spinal anesthesia or general anesthesia for hip surgery in older adults. *NEJM*. 2021;385:2025–2035.

New York Society of Regional Anesthesia. https://www.nysora.com/filter-techniques/

Rojas J, Familiari F, Bitzer A, Srikumaran U, Papalia R, McFarland EG. Patient positioning in shoulder arthroscopy: which is best? *Joints*. 2019;7(2):46–55.

Siddiqi A, Mahmoud Y, Secic M, et al. Mepivacaine versus bupivacaine spinal anesthesia for primary total joint arthroplasty: a systematic review and meta-analysis. *J Arthroplasty*. 2022;37:1396–1404.

Vail EA, Feng R, Sieber F, et al; REGAIN (Regional versus General Anesthesia for Promoting Independence after Hip Fracture) Investigators. Long-term outcomes with spinal versus general anesthesia for hip fracture surgery: a randomized trial. *Anesthesiology*. 2024;140:375–386.

von Keudell AG, Weaver MJ, Appleton PT, et al. Diagnosis and treatment of acute extremity compartment syndrome. *Lancet*. 2015;386(10000):1299–1310.

Warltier DC, Campagna JA, Carter C. Clinical relevance of the Bezold–Jarisch reflex. *Anesthesiology*. 2003;98(5):1250–1260.

Yang YZ, Cheng QH, Zhang AR, et al. Efficacy and safety of single- and double-dose intravenous tranexamic acid in hip and knee arthroplasty: a systematic review and meta-analysis. *J Orthop Surg Res*. 2023;18(1):593.

Anesthesia for Neurosurgery
Daniel Ankeny and Gabrielle White-Dzuro

I. PHYSIOLOGY
A. Cerebral blood flow (CBF) is equal to cerebral perfusion pressure (CPP) divided by the cerebral vascular resistance. **CPP is defined as the difference between the mean arterial pressure (MAP) and intracranial pressure (ICP) or central venous pressure, whichever is higher.** CBF averages 50 mL/100 g of brain tissue per minute in the normal brain and is affected by blood pressure, metabolic demands, $Paco_2$, Pao_2, blood viscosity, vasoactive agents, and neurogenic regulation. The brain receives approximately 15% of the cardiac output.

1. **CBF** is maintained at a constant level by constriction and dilation of arterioles (autoregulation) (**Figure 23.1**) when the MAP is between 50 and 150 mm Hg. This concept is known as **cerebral autoregulation.** When MAP is outside these limits, CBF varies directly with the MAP. Chronic hypertension shifts the autoregulatory curve to the right, rendering hypertensive patients susceptible to cerebral ischemia at blood pressures considered normal in healthy individuals. Chronic antihypertensive therapy likely normalizes the autoregulatory range. Cerebral ischemia, trauma, hypoxia, hypercarbia, edema, mass effect, and volatile anesthetics attenuate or abolish autoregulation and may make blood flow to the affected area dependent on MAP.

2. **$Paco_2$** has profound effects on CBF by its effect on the pH of the brain extracellular fluid (ECF). CBF increases linearly with increasing $Paco_2$ in the range from 20 to 80 mm Hg, with an absolute change of 1 to 2 mL/100 g/min for each mm Hg change in $Paco_2$. The effect of $Paco_2$ on CBF decreases over 6 to 24 hours because of slow adaptive changes in the brain ECF bicarbonate concentration. Sustained hyperventilation causes cerebrospinal fluid (CSF) bicarbonate production to decrease, allowing CSF pH to gradually normalize. Rapid normalization of $Paco_2$ after a period of hyperventilation results in a significant CSF acidosis with vasodilation and increased ICP.

3. **Pao_2.** Hypoxia is a potent cerebral vasodilator. CBF increases markedly below a Pao_2 of 60 mm Hg. Pao_2 above 60 mm Hg has little influence on CBF. However, hyperoxia may be deleterious under conditions of neuropathology, via promotion of oxidative injury.

4. **Neurogenic regulation.** The cerebral vasculature receives extensive cholinergic, adrenergic, serotonergic, and VIPergic innervation, though the exact role these systems play in regulation of CBF is not clear. Evidence suggests, however, that increased sympathetic tone in hemorrhagic shock shifts the lower end of the autoregulatory curve to the right and results in lower CBF at a given MAP.

5. **Viscosity.** Normal hematocrit (33% to 45%) in a healthy brain has little influence on CBF.

B. Cerebral metabolic rate ($CMRO_2$) and CBF are tightly coupled because the brain requires a constant supply of energy to meet its high metabolic

FIGURE 23.1 Autoregulation maintains a constant level of cerebral blood flow (CBF) over a wide range of carotid artery mean blood pressures. Independent of this effect, CBF is elevated by hypercarbia ($PaCO_2$) and hypoxemia (PaO_2); hypocarbia diminishes CBF.

demands. Regional or global increases in $CMRO_2$ elicit a corresponding increase in CBF, probably mediated by signaling molecules such as nitric oxide. Other factors that modulate $CMRO_2$ (and CBF through this mechanism) include the following:
1. **Anesthetics.** Variable effect (Sections II.A and B).
2. **Temperature.** Hypothermia decreases $CMRO_2$ by 7% per 1 °C below 37 °C, while hyperthermia increases $CMRO_2$.
3. **Seizures.** Increases $CMRO_2$.
4. **Pain or arousal.** Increases $CMRO_2$.

C. **ICP** reflects the relationship between the volume of the intracranial contents (brain, blood, and CSF) and the fixed container of the cranial vault. **Normal ICP varies between 5 and 15 mm Hg.** A sustained elevation of ICP greater than 22 mm Hg in the setting of intracranial pathology is considered abnormal.
1. **The cranial vault is rigid**, and its capacity to accommodate increases in intracranial volume is limited. A developing intracranial mass (eg, tumor, edema, hematoma, or hydrocephalus) initially displaces blood and CSF, and ICP remains relatively normal (**Figure 23.2**). As intracranial volume increases further, intracranial compliance decreases, and ICP rises rapidly (**Figure 23.2**). Thus, patients with decreased compliance may develop marked increases in ICP even with small increases in intracranial volume (eg, cerebral vasodilation due to anesthesia, hypertension, or carbon dioxide retention) (**Figure 23.2**).
2. **Clinical features of elevated ICP.** ICP elevation usually decreases CPP and may cause ischemia in regions of the brain where autoregulation is defective and CBF depends on CPP. Early signs and symptoms of increased ICP include headache, nausea, vomiting, blurred vision, papilledema, and decreased levels of consciousness. As ICP increases, brain herniation may occur causing mechanical injury and/or ischemia to

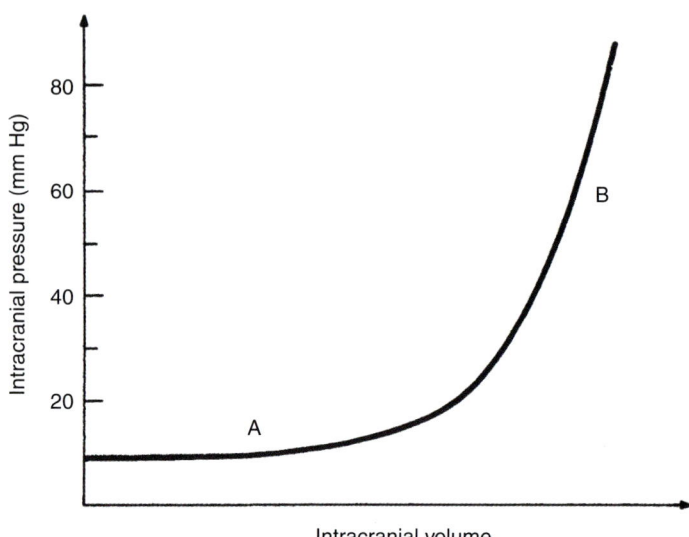

FIGURE 23.2 The intracranial compliance curve. In the normal intracranial pressure (ICP) range (*A*), increases in intracranial volume produce minimal changes in ICP. Further, small increases in ICP after the "elbow" of the curve can produce abrupt increases in ICP (*B*).

the brainstem and cranial nerves. This may result in hypertension with bradycardia or tachydysrhythmia, irregular respiration, oculomotor (third cranial nerve) palsy leading to ipsilateral pupillary dilation with absent light reflex, abducens (sixth cranial nerve) palsy, contralateral hemiparesis or hemiplegia, and ultimately, coma and respiratory arrest.

3. **Treatment of elevated ICP** involves strategies aimed at decreasing the volume of the intracranial components, as outlined below:
   a. **Hyperventilation to a Paco$_2$ of 25 to 30 mm Hg produces cerebral vasoconstriction and may be used as a temporizing measure in the management of acutely increased ICP.** Hyperventilation is potentially deleterious, however, and can cause ischemia in injured brain and penumbra where CBF is low. Therefore, hyperventilation should be withdrawn when effective, definite therapy is established. Moreover, the effect of hyperventilation on ICP decreases over time as CSF pH normalizes. Conversely, **hypoxia and hypercarbia cause cerebral vasodilation** and should be avoided.
   b. **Decrease jugular venous pressure.** Elevating the head at least 30° from supine promotes venous drainage and decreases intracranial venous blood volume, thereby lowering ICP. Avoid excessive flexion or rotation of the neck and prevent increases in the intrathoracic pressure (eg, coughing, straining, and elevated intrathoracic pressure), since each of these may decrease jugular outflow.
   c. **Control CMRO$_2$.** Propofol decreases cerebral blood volume while decreasing CMRO$_2$. Prevent increases in CMOR$_2$ due to arousal/seizures with adequate sedation and seizure prophylaxis where indicated.
   d. **Maintaining high serum osmolality** (305 to 320 mOsm/kg) may reduce cerebral edema and decrease brain volume via promotion of

favorable fluid gradients (hydrostatic and oncotic pressures). Fluid management is designed to achieve this goal (Section V.D). In addition, **mannitol** (0.5 to 1.0 g/kg intravenous [IV]) and **hypertonic saline** produce a hyperosmolar state and are effective in the acute reduction of ICP.

e. **CSF volume can be reduced by** draining the CSF through ventriculostomy catheter. This can be placed preoperatively when ICP is dangerously elevated.

f. Surgical removal of tumor or hematoma reduces intracranial volume and ICP.

g. Decompressive craniectomy is an option to decrease ICP by increasing the volume of the cranial vault. It results in lower mortality but higher disability at 6 months when compared with maximal medical therapy.

h. Steroids may reduce cerebral edema associated with tumors, though this is a gradual process and likely does not contribute to acute ICP management.

II. PHARMACOLOGY

Agents used in anesthesia may affect $CMRO_2$ and CBF.

A. Inhalation anesthetics

1. **Nitrous oxide** (N_2O) can increase $CMRO_2$, CBF, and ICP. These effects are variably reported to be enhanced, attenuated, or abolished when N_2O is administered in conjunction with IV anesthetic agents. Nitrous oxide should be avoided when intracranial airspaces (eg, pneumocephalus) exist because it diffuses more rapidly into these spaces than nitrogen diffuses out and may thereby produce an acute increase in ICP.

2. Volatile agents increase CBF due to their direct vasodilatory actions. Autoregulation can be attenuated or abolished by increasing the concentrations of these drugs (1.5 × minimum alveolar concentration), but cerebrovascular responsiveness to carbon dioxide is preserved (**Table 23.1**). The vasodilatory effect of inhalational agents is clinically insignificant in patients with normal intracranial compliance. These agents should be used with caution in patients with compromised intracranial compliance (eg, large intracranial mass lesion and acute intracranial hematoma).

3. Volatile anesthetics produce dose-dependent reductions in metabolism ($CMRO_2$), probably by depressing neuronal electrical activity.

Cerebral Physiologic Effects of Inhalational Anesthetics

	Nitrous Oxide	Desflurane	Sevoflurane	Isoflurane
CBF	↑	↑↑	↑	↑↑
CPP	↓	↓↓	↓	↓↓
ICP	↔/↑	↔/↑	↔/↑	↔/↑
Metabolic demands	↑	↓	↓	↓
CO_2 reactivity	↔	↔	↔	↔
Seizure threshold	↓	↓	↓	↓

CBF, cerebral blood flow; CPP, cerebral perfusion pressure; ICP, intracranial pressure.

Isoflurane is the most potent in this respect and is the only volatile agent that induces an isoelectric electroencephalogram (EEG) at clinically relevant concentrations (2 × minimum alveolar concentration).
- B. **IV anesthetics** generally cause coupled reduction in CBF and $CMRO_2$ in a dose-dependent manner. **Barbiturates, etomidate,** and **propofol** markedly decrease CBF and $CMRO_2$ and can produce isoelectric EEGs. Etomidate has been associated with seizures and is best avoided in seizure-prone patients. **Lidocaine** in therapeutic doses decreases both CBF and $CMRO_2$. **Ketamine,** by contrast, increases CBF and $CMRO_2$ and is used infrequently in neuroanesthesia. **Opioids** and **benzodiazepines** produce minimal changes in CBF and $CMRO_2$. Autoregulation and carbon dioxide responsiveness appear to be preserved with IV agents.
- C. **Muscle relaxants** have no direct effect on CBF and $CMRO_2$.
- D. **Vasoactive drugs**
    1. **Adrenergic agonists.** α-Adrenergic agonists and low-dose β-adrenergic agonists have little influence on CBF if MAP is within the limits of autoregulation.
    2. **Vasodilators.** Sodium nitroprusside, nitroglycerin, hydralazine, nimodipine, and nicardipine can increase CBF and ICP by direct cerebral vasodilation if MAP is maintained. β-Adrenergic–blocking agents probably have minimal effects. Despite these profiles, all these agents have been used safely during neuroanesthesia, particularly if CPP is maintained.
- E. **Cerebral protection**
    1. **Focal versus global cerebral ischemia**
        - a. **Focal ischemia** is characterized by an area of densely ischemic tissue that is surrounded by nonischemic brain, which may provide collateral flow to the penumbral margins. This blood flow may allow neurons to survive for varied periods of time (eg, thrombolysis within 3 hours after stroke onset may prevent a full infarct due to reperfusion).
        - b. **Complete global ischemia** is characterized by absent CBF (eg, cardiac arrest). Tolerance for surviving global ischemia is on the order of minutes. Targeted temperature management (see section on Hypothermia that follows) after cardiac arrest may improve survival and decrease neural dysfunction.
    2. **Agents**
        - a. **IV anesthetic agents.** High-dose **barbiturates** may slightly improve neurologic recovery from focal ischemia, possibly by decreasing metabolic rate or more likely by a direct pharmacologic effect. **Propofol** may also reduce focal ischemic cerebral injury, although it is not as extensively studied as barbiturates. Etomidate aggravates ischemic brain injury.
        - b. **Volatile anesthetic agents** may provide some cerebral protection, but data are conflicting, and it is unclear whether this neuroprotection is sustained.
        - c. The 1,4-dihydropyridine calcium channel blocker **nimodipine** has beneficial effects on cerebral vasospasm after subarachnoid hemorrhage (SAH). These effects are well established and are likely mediated through neuronal rather than vascular effects. Clinical trials failed to detect a beneficial effect for patients with acute stroke.
        - d. **Steroids** have not been found to be beneficial after stroke or severe head injury. Their effects on recovery after traumatic spinal cord injury are also controversial.

e. **Hypothermia** reduces metabolism for both neuronal and cellular functions and therefore may be beneficial in the setting of decreased cerebral perfusion. Induced mild hypothermia (maintaining core temperature at 33 °C compared with 36 °C for 28 to 36 hours) has been studied extensively and has not shown to be effective in improving survival, functional outcomes, or quality-of-life measures in patients who sustain cardiac arrest. Similarly, two clinical studies did not demonstrate improved outcomes when induced mild hypothermia was used in patients after significant head injury or intraoperatively for aneurysm surgery.

f. **Hyperthermia** profoundly worsens outcome from focal cerebral ischemia and should be avoided.

g. Moderate **hyperglycemia** (>180 mg/dL) exacerbates neurologic injury after an ischemic insult. There are human data suggesting that normalizing blood glucose improves outcome in patients with stroke.

h. **Other physiologic variables.** In addition to the aforementioned variables of temperature and glucose, meticulous management of perfusion pressure, P_{CO_2}, P_{O_2}, pH normalization, and seizure prophylaxis contributes significantly to improved neurologic outcomes in the setting of cerebral ischemia. Maintenance of a high-normal CPP can augment collateral CBF. By contrast, hypotension reduces CBF and exacerbates the injury. Normocapnia should be maintained. Seizures, which can increase CBF and ICP and decrease CPP, should be prevented and rapidly treated.

3. There is preliminary evidence that female sex hormones may confer some neuroprotection after traumatic brain injury or spinal cord injury.

III. ELECTROPHYSIOLOGIC MONITORING

A. Electroencephalography (EEG) measures the electrical activity of neurons in the cerebral cortex and is thus used as a threshold marker for detecting ischemia due to inadequate CBF. EEG is used frequently during procedures that jeopardize cerebral perfusion, such as carotid endarterectomy, or to ensure electrical silence before circulatory arrest.

1. Normal CBF in gray and white matter averages 50 mL/100 g/min. With most anesthetic techniques, the EEG becomes abnormal when CBF decreases to 20 mL/100 g/min. Cellular survival is endangered when CBF decreases to 12 mL/100 g/min. Thus, EEG changes can warn of ischemia before CBF becomes insufficient to maintain tissue viability. Prompt detection of EEG changes may be treated with increases in perfusion pressure or shunting to restore CBF, thereby preventing infarction.

2. The EEG may exhibit changes intraoperatively with no demonstrable neurologic deficit during postoperative examination. Cerebral ischemia can produce electrical dysfunction without causing neuronal cell damage because the blood flow threshold for electrical failure is higher than that needed to maintain cellular integrity.

3. Factors other than anesthetics that may affect the EEG include hypothermia (which may limit the usefulness of EEG during cardiopulmonary bypass), hypotension, hypoglycemia, hypoxia, tumors, vascular abnormalities, and epilepsy. An abnormal EEG in patients with preexisting neurologic deficits, an evolving stroke, or recent reversible ischemic neurologic deficits can also make it difficult to interpret new changes.

4. **Anesthetic effects on the EEG** are generally global, which often helps distinguish them from the focal changes of ischemia. A predominance of slow activity is seen as the anesthetic depth increases. "Deep"

anesthesia may cause marked EEG slowing, making detection of superimposed ischemic changes during critical periods difficult to interpret. Maintaining a constant level of anesthesia during critical periods (eg, carotid clamping) facilitates EEG interpretation.

B. Evoked potential monitoring

1. **Sensory-evoked potentials** are electrical potentials generated within the neuraxis in response to stimulation of a peripheral or cranial nerve. As they travel from the periphery to the brain, these potentials can be recorded by electrodes placed over the scalp and along the transmission pathway. Evoked potentials (EPs) have lower voltage than background EEG activity, but summation of hundreds using neurophysiologic recording devices allows the neurophysiologist to visualize them by averaging and subtracting out the random background EEG. A normal response implies that the conduction pathway is intact. **Damage to the pathway generally decreases the amplitude and/or prolongs latency** (ie, the time from peripheral stimulus to the arrival of potentials at the recording site) of the electrical waveform peaks. EPs are classified according to the nerve tract being evaluated.

    a. **Somatosensory-evoked potentials (SSEPs)** are obtained by stimulating a peripheral nerve (eg, median nerve at the wrist or posterior tibial nerve at the ankle or in the popliteal fossa) and recording the elicited signals over the spinal cord (spinal SSEPs) or cerebral cortex (cortical SSEPs). SSEPs are used most commonly to monitor spinal cord function during spinal cord or vertebral column surgery (eg, major spine surgery with instrumentation) and may be used during peripheral nerve, brachial plexus, or thoracic aortic surgery (to detect spinal ischemia during aortic cross-clamping). Because SSEPs are conducted primarily by the spinal cord dorsal column, there are concerns about the reliability of SSEP monitoring for detecting threatened motor function (ie, anterior spinal cord ischemia). For this reason, the "wake-up test" is used in some centers (Section VII.B.2), and the neurophysiologist can also perform motor-evoked potential (MEP) monitoring.

    b. **Brainstem auditory–evoked potentials (BAEPs)** are recorded by delivering an auditory stimulus to one ear through an ear-insert headphone. BAEPs reflect the transmission of electrical impulses along the auditory pathway and are monitored during posterior fossa surgery in an attempt to avoid brainstem or auditory (eighth cranial) nerve damage.

    c. **Visual-evoked potentials (VEPs)** are specialized potentials of the visual pathway recorded from the visual cortex after flash stimulation of the retina through closed eyelids. Utility has not been established, and VEPs are highly susceptible to effects from general anesthetics.

2. **MEPs.** Monitoring the integrity of the motor tracts within the spinal cord may be more reliable than SSEP monitoring during spinal surgery, as indicated above. The ventral motor columns of the spinal cord may be more susceptible to ischemia than the posterior proprioceptive fibers. Motor impulses can be generated by transcranial electrical stimulation. The evoked responses are measured as a potential over the spinal cord below the surgical field and in the muscle of interest. Anesthetics substantially modify transcranial-induced potentials but less so if the stimulus is measured in the spinal cord below the surgical field.

3. **Electromyography** (EMG) records muscle responses to the stimulation of peripheral motor nerves. EMG is used frequently when there is a risk

of facial nerve injury during cerebellopontine angle surgery (eg, posterior fossa surgery for meningioma). Because the EMG records motor responses to stimulation, neuromuscular-blocking agents are avoided during the periods of electrical stimulation and monitoring.
4. **Confounding factors.** Interpretation of EP changes is confounded by factors similar to those that affect the EEG (eg, anesthetics, temperature, hypotension, hypoxia, anemia, preexisting neurologic lesions). Volatile anesthetics can depress SSEPs by reducing the amplitude or prolonging the latency of the SSEPs and can abolish the far more sensitive MEPs. BAEPs are more resistant to the depressive effects of anesthetics than cortical SSEPs. IV anesthetics, including propofol and remifentanil, have smaller effects than volatile anesthetics and are compatible with effective monitoring of cortical SSEPs and MEPs.
5. **False positives.** Changes in EPs occur frequently and often are not associated with postoperative neurologic complications. Further work is required to establish the nature, magnitude, and duration of EP changes associated with irreversible damage.

IV. PREOPERATIVE CONSIDERATIONS FOR NEUROSURGICAL PROCEDURES

A. **Intracranial compliance** may be decreased by intracranial mass lesions (eg, tumor, hematoma, or abscess). Surrounding normal brain tissue may be compressed, leading to blood–brain barrier compromise, cerebral edema, loss of cerebral autoregulation, and local ischemia. Signs and symptoms of increased ICP are discussed in Section I.C.2.

B. **A computed tomography (CT) or magnetic resonance imaging scan** should be reviewed. Midline shift, basal cistern obliteration, loss of cortical sulci, and ventricular effacement suggest the presence of increased ICP. The degree of brain edema surrounding the mass and the site of the lesion in relation to major intracranial vessels and structures should be noted. Lesions near the dural venous sinuses risk exposure of the sinuses to the atmosphere and may be associated with elevated risk of venous air embolism (Section VI.C.3).

C. **The pathology of the mass** is important in anticipating possible perioperative problems. Vascular lesions (eg, meningiomas and some metastatic brain tumors) may bleed profusely, prompting alterations in the anesthetic plan. Infiltrating malignant tumors may render the patient particularly prone to postoperative cerebral edema.

D. **Preoperative fluid and electrolyte imbalances and glucose intolerance may be present due to poor oral intake, use of diuretics and steroids, and centrally mediated endocrine abnormalities.**

E. **Anticonvulsants** may be required to control seizures. **Corticosteroids** may be necessary to treat edema. These drugs should be continued perioperatively.

F. **Premedication** with anxiolytics such as benzodiazepines and opioids should be prescribed cautiously because patients with intracranial disease may be sensitive to the effects of central nervous system (CNS) depressants. Frequently, no premedication is given. If sedation is needed, midazolam (1 to 2 mg) can be used. Additional sedation can be given once the patient arrives in the operating room. If the patient has impaired intracranial compliance and/or a high ICP, opioids should be avoided because of their respiratory-depressant effects and the increases in CBF that occur with hypercarbia.

G. In addition to standard anesthetic monitoring (Chapter 15: Monitoring), arterial catheters are used in most patients undergoing craniotomy. Capnography is particularly useful when reducing ICP by hyperventilation.

A urinary catheter is placed to aid fluid management and diuretic therapy. Invasive monitoring (eg, pulmonary artery catheter or transesophageal echocardiography [TEE]) may be indicated for patients with severe cardiac, renal, or pulmonary disease in the context of marked diuretic-induced fluid shifts. A second IV catheter for drug administration is often useful.

V. INTRAOPERATIVE MANAGEMENT

Anesthetic goals for intracranial procedures include hypnosis, amnesia, immobility, control of ICP and CPP, and a "relaxed brain" (ie, optimal surgical conditions). Whenever possible, promptly following the procedure, the anesthetist should endeavor to provide an awake and interactive, extubated patient who can be evaluated neurologically by the neurosurgical team.

A. Induction of anesthesia must be accomplished without increasing ICP or compromising CBF. Hypertension, hypotension, hypoxia, and hypercarbia should be avoided.

1. While propofol (1.0 to 2.5 mg/kg), midazolam (0.2 to 0.4 mg/kg), and etomidate (0.3 to 0.4 mg/kg) are all reasonable IV induction agents, the hemodynamic effects caused by these agents should be carefully considered.

2. **An adequate mask airway** is essential to prevent hypoventilation and increased $PaCO_2$. After induction, hyperventilation by mask can be started with 100% oxygen.

3. An intubating dose of muscle relaxant is given. Nondepolarizing agents are commonly chosen, if there are no neuromonitoring considerations. Adequate relaxation should be obtained before laryngoscopy and intubation to avoid coughing and straining.

4. **Opioids** cause minimal changes in cerebral hemodynamics and are useful in blunting responses to intubation and craniotomy. Because intubation, placement of head pins, and craniotomy (skin incision and manipulation of the periosteum) are the most physiologically stimulating periods during intracranial procedures, generous doses of narcotics are given before these manipulations. Fentanyl and remifentanil are most commonly used because both have rapid onset and high potency. Lidocaine (1 mg/kg IV) or esmolol (~0.5 mg/kg IV) can also be used to attenuate the cardiovascular and ICP responses to intubation.

5. After intubation, the eyes are covered with watertight patches to prevent irritation from surgical preparation solutions, and the head is carefully checked after final positioning to ensure good venous return. Because **access to the airway is limited during neurosurgical procedures**, breath sounds and ventilation should be checked after final positioning to ensure proper placement of the endotracheal tube, the tube should be adequately secured, and all connections in the breathing circuit should be securely tightened.

B. Maintenance

1. **Adequate brain relaxation** is necessary before opening the dura. This is achieved by ensuring adequate oxygenation, venous return, muscle relaxation, anesthetic depth, a $PaCO_2$ of 33 to 35 mm Hg (hyperventilation if dictated by surgical field), and often the administration of furosemide (10 to 20 mg IV), mannitol (0.5 to 1.5 g/kg IV), and dexamethasone before the craniotomy is completed. The surgeon can then assess the need for further brain relaxation by checking the tension of the dura. If necessary and possible, CSF can be drained through a previously placed lumbar subarachnoid catheter or external ventricular drain.

2. **Anesthetic requirements** are substantially lower after craniotomy and dural opening because the brain parenchyma is devoid of sensation. If supplemental narcotics are needed, small doses of morphine or fentanyl can be given. A continuous infusion of propofol (50 to 150 μg/kg/min) and/or remifentanil (0.05 to 0.1 μg/kg/min) produces a stable level of anesthesia and allows for a rapid emergence. Large doses of **long-acting narcotics and sedatives are usually avoided during the last 1 to 2 hours of the procedure** to facilitate neurologic examination at the end of surgery and avoid potential drowsiness and hypoventilation.
3. **Muscle relaxants** are frequently continued throughout the procedure to prevent movement. Patients receiving anticonvulsants (e g, phenytoin) may require more frequent administration of muscle relaxants.

C. **Emergence** should occur promptly without straining or coughing. IV lidocaine may be administered to suppress the cough reflex but may delay emergence. Toward the end of the procedure, $Paco_2$ is normalized gradually if hyperventilation is employed. Hypertension should be controlled to minimize bleeding; rapidly acting IV agents such as labetalol, esmolol, sodium nitroprusside, and nitroglycerin are often used. Muscle relaxation is usually maintained until the head dressing is completed and then reversal agents are administered. Before leaving the operating room, the patient should be awake and responsive so that a brief neurologic examination can be performed. The differential diagnosis of persisting unconsciousness after discontinuation of all anesthetics should include residual anesthesia, narcosis, hypothermia, hypoxia, hypercapnia, residual neuromuscular blockade, metabolic causes, and surgically induced increases in ICP (bleeding, edema, and hydrocephalus). Naloxone (0.04 to 0.4 mg IV) may help antagonize pharmacologically induced CNS depression. The presence of new localized or generalized neurologic deficits should be immediately addressed and may be evaluated by CT and/or surgical reexploration.

D. **Perioperative fluid management** is designed to decrease brain water content, thereby reducing ICP and providing adequate brain relaxation, while maintaining hemodynamic stability and CPP.
1. **The blood–brain barrier is selectively permeable.** Gradients for osmotically active substances ultimately determine the distribution of fluids between the brain and intravascular spaces.
    a. **Water freely passes through the blood–brain barrier.** Intravascular infusion of free water may increase brain water content and elevate ICP. Isoosmotic glucose solutions (eg, 5% dextrose in water) have the same effect because the glucose is metabolized, and free water remains. As such, these are usually avoided during neurosurgery.
    b. **The blood–brain barrier is impermeable to most ions** including Na^+. Unlike the peripheral vasculature, total osmolality, rather than colloid oncotic pressure, determines the osmotic pressure gradient across the blood–brain barrier. Consequently, maintenance of high-normal serum osmolality can decrease brain water content, while administration of a large amount of hypoosmolar crystalloid solution may increase brain fluid content.
    c. **Large, polar substances cross the blood–brain barrier poorly.** Albumin has little effect on brain ECF because the colloid oncotic pressure contributes to only a small portion of total plasma osmolality (approximately 1 mOsm/L).
    d. If the blood–brain barrier is disrupted (eg, by ischemia, head trauma, or tumor), permeability to mannitol, albumin, and saline increases

so that these molecules have equal access to brain ECF. Under such circumstances, isoosmolar colloid and crystalloid solutions seem to have similar effects on edema formation and ICP.
2. **Severe fluid restriction** can produce marked hypovolemia, leading to hypotension, reduced CBF, and ischemia of the brain and other organs, while only modestly decreasing brain water content. **Excessive hypervolemia** may cause hypertension and cerebral edema.
3. **Specific treatment recommendations are outlined in the section that follows.** The overarching goal is to maintain normal intravascular volume and to produce a hyperosmolar state.
   a. **Fluid losses.** The fluid deficit incurred by an overnight fast is usually not replaced. Physiologic maintenance fluids are given. Third spacing of fluids during intracranial surgery is minimal and usually does not warrant replacement. Two-thirds of total intraoperative urine output is replaced with crystalloid. If signs of hypovolemia develop, additional fluid is administered.
   b. **Assessment of blood loss** may be difficult during intracranial procedures because significant amounts can be hidden under the drapes. Also, irrigating solutions are used generously by the neurosurgeon. As such, the anesthetist should keep track of total irrigation fluids used during the procedure.
   c. **The serum osmolality** is increased to between 305 and 320 mOsm/kg. If large fluid requirements are anticipated, isoosmolar crystalloid solutions such as 0.9% normal saline (309 mOsm/kg) may be preferable to hypoosmolar solutions such as lactated Ringer (272 mOsm/kg). However, large volumes of 0.9% normal saline may cause a metabolic acidosis that can be deleterious to end-organ function. Therefore, it is prudent to follow the arterial blood gases and change to lactated Ringer if indicated. Mannitol (0.5 to 2.0 g/kg IV) and/or furosemide (5 to 20 mg IV) are also often administered. The marked diuresis produced by these agents demands close monitoring of intravascular volume and electrolytes.
   d. **Hypokalemia** may develop from the use of steroids or potassium-wasting diuretics and is exacerbated by hyperventilation. Nevertheless, intraoperative administration of potassium is rarely necessary.
   e. **Hyponatremia** may be produced by diuretics or syndrome of inappropriate antidiuretic hormone (SIADH) secretion.
   f. **Hyperglycemia** may worsen neurologic outcome after ischemia (Section II.E.2.g). Glucose-containing solutions are avoided in patients at risk for CNS ischemia.
E. **Immediate postoperative care.** Patients are observed closely in an intensive care setting after most intracranial neurosurgical procedures.
   1. **The head of the bed** should be elevated 30° to promote venous drainage.
   2. **Neurologic function**, including the level of consciousness, orientation, pupillary size, and motor strength, should be assessed frequently. Deterioration of any of these may indicate development of cerebral edema, hematoma, hydrocephalus, or herniation.
   3. **Adequate ventilation and oxygenation** are essential in patients with reduced consciousness.
   4. **Continuous monitoring of ICP** may be indicated if intracranial hypertension exists at the time of dural closure or is anticipated in the postoperative period.
   5. **Serum electrolytes and osmolarity** should be checked and corrected as appropriate.

6. **SIADH** can be diagnosed by hyponatremia and low serum osmolality with high urine osmolality. It is treated by restricting free water intake.
7. **Cerebral salt-wasting syndrome** can occur in the setting of brain tumors or injury to the brain. It is characterized by hyponatremia and polyuria. Polydipsia, extreme salt cravings, and dehydration may also be seen. It is a diagnosis of exclusion and can be difficult to distinguish from SIADH, with the main difference being volume status (hypovolemia in cerebral salt wasting syndrome and normal to hypervolemia in SIADH).
8. **Diabetes insipidus** may occur after any intracranial procedure, but is most common after pituitary surgery. **Polyuria** is associated with hypernatremia, serum hyperosmolality, and low urine osmolality. Conscious patients can compensate by increasing their fluid intake; otherwise, adequate IV replacement is mandatory. **Aqueous vasopressin** (5 to 10 USP units subcutaneously or 3 units/h by IV infusion) may be given. Larger doses may cause hypertension. Alternatively, **desmopressin** (1 to 2 mg IV or subcutaneously every 6 to 12 hours) can be used and is associated with a lower incidence of hypertension than vasopressin.
9. **Seizures** may indicate the presence of an expanding intracranial hematoma or cerebral edema. If a seizure occurs, airway patency, oxygenation, and ventilation must be ensured. The patient should be protected from injury and the IV secured. For acute therapy, midazolam (2 to 4 mg IV), or lorazepam (2 mg) may be used. Fosphenytoin (15 to 20 mg/kg IV, 100 to 150 mg/min) can be administered to prevent recurrence.
10. **Tension pneumocephalus** may occur and should be suspected after failure to awaken from anesthesia. Skull radiographs or head CT scans confirm the diagnosis; treatment consists of opening the dura to release the air.

VI. SPECIFIC NEUROSURGICAL PROCEDURES

A. Patients with **intracranial aneurysms** present for surgery electively or emergently following **SAH**.
   1. Preoperative evaluation of patients with SAH should include all components of a routine anesthetic preoperative evaluation (Chapter 1: Evaluating the Patient Before Anesthesia), with attention to known associated physiologic perturbations. These include the **neurologic grade** (**Table 23.2**), presence of **vasospasm** (and the hemodynamic parameters that have been effective in relieving clinical symptoms),

	Classification of Patients With Subarachnoid Hemorrhage According to Surgical Risk (Hunt and Hess Classification)
Grade	**Characteristics**
I	Asymptomatic or minimal headache and slight nuchal rigidity
II	Moderate to severe headache, nuchal rigidity, no neurologic deficit other than cranial nerve palsy
III	Drowsiness, confusion, mild focal deficit
IV	Stupor, moderate to severe hemiparesis, possibly early decerebrate rigidity, vegetative disturbances
V	Deep coma, decerebrate rigidity, moribund

degree of hydrocephalus, ICP elevation, and concurrent drug therapy such as calcium channel blockade with nimodipine, which may moderately lower systemic blood pressures intraoperatively.

Electrocardiographic changes are common after SAH and include arrhythmias and fluctuating ST-segment, QT-interval, and T-wave changes. These are probably caused by subendocardial injury following the autonomic discharge that occurs in association with the initial SAH. Provided these are not associated with cardiac dysfunction, no modification of patient management is necessary, although recent data suggest that a heart rate of either less than 60 or greater than 80 or the presence of nonspecific ST/T wave abnormalities are independently associated with increased mortality in patients with SAH receiving aneurysm clipping. Cardiac biomarkers may be increased as well.

2. Current practice is to intervene early during the first 24 to 48 hours after SAH for patients with neurologic grades I to III, which decreases the risk of rebleeding and facilitates the hypertensive management of vasospasm.
3. **Specific anesthetic considerations** include the following:
    a. **Avoidance of hypertension**, which may increase the risk of aneurysm rupture before aneurysm clipping. Prophylactic use of agents such as IV nicardipine, fentanyl, β-adrenergic blockers, lidocaine, or additional doses of propofol will often attenuate the blood pressure response to noxious stimuli such as laryngoscopy and intubation.
    b. **Avoidance of hypotension** to maintain adequate CPP in the setting of altered autoregulation.
    c. **Providing adequate brain relaxation** to optimize surgical exposure. Rapid reductions in ICP may affect transmural pressure and increase the risk of aneurysm rupture. This should be done cautiously before opening the dura.
    d. **Induced hypertension** may be requested during temporary clipping to improve collateral blood flow to regions that were perfused by the clipped arteries. Often, IV phenylephrine is used for this purpose. It is critical that hypertension be induced only **after** the temporary clip has been placed, otherwise the risk of aneurysm rupture is markedly increased.
    e. **Intraoperative aneurysm rupture** can produce rapid and **massive blood loss** requiring large-bore IV access for volume resuscitation. Accurate estimation of blood loss is essential to guide volume repletion. Induced hypotension, adenosine-mediated cardiac standstill, or, occasionally, manual pressure on the ipsilateral carotid artery may be helpful during the desperate situation of a large and uncontrolled premature rupture.
    f. **Mild hypothermia** (34 °C) has previously been used as a protective strategy for the brain during periods of cerebral ischemia. **Data from the Intraoperative Hypothermia for Aneurysm Surgery Trial, suggests that hypothermia does not improve either neurologic or neuropsychologic outcome in patients with good-grade (grade I to III) surgical SAH.** Given the results of this trial, targeted temperature management during aneurysm surgery is now the standard of care.
    g. Once the permanent clips have been placed on the aneurysm, prevention of postoperative vasospasm becomes important. Blood pressure is increased moderately.
    h. When appropriate, the anesthetic should be designed for a prompt emergence from anesthesia to enable an immediate neurologic

examination to ensure that clip placement does not compromise the parent vessel.
- B. **An arteriovenous malformation** (AVM) is a direct communication between cerebral arteries and veins without an intervening capillary bed. Because an AVM is a high-flow, low-resistance system, surrounding brain regions may be hypoperfused by the diversion of blood through the AVM (steal phenomenon). The most common presentations of an AVM are SAH, seizures, headaches, and, rarely, progressive neurologic deficits due to steal phenomenon.
  1. Patients with AVMs may require anesthetic care for embolization procedures or surgical resection.
     a. **Embolizations** are usually done to decrease blood flow to the AVM prior to surgical resection. Embolization may decrease the risk of intraoperative bleeding and postoperative reperfusion hyperemia.
     b. Embolizations can be done under general anesthesia or monitored anesthesia care, which has the advantage of permitting continuous neurologic evaluation.
     c. The anesthetist should be prepared for adverse reactions to the contrast dye (eg, anaphylaxis and osmotic load that may cause congestive heart failure), vessel perforation (sudden and rapid blood loss requiring immediate craniotomy), and neurologic changes.
  2. **Anesthetic management for surgical resection** of an AVM is similar to that for cerebral aneurysms.
     a. The primary focus is on tight blood pressure control because hypotension can lead to ischemia of hypoperfused regions. Hypertension can exacerbate perfusion pressure breakthrough, a poorly understood phenomenon that is thought to be caused by abrupt diversion of the AVM's blood flow to adjacent, previously marginally perfused brain, which produces sudden cerebral engorgement and hemorrhage. Should perfusion pressure breakthrough and brain swelling occur, they are commonly treated with propofol and modest lowering of blood pressure.
     b. Potential for large blood loss occurs in cases in which the AVM is large and has arterial feeders from more than one part of the cerebral arterial vasculature or when the preoperative embolization has been unsuccessful.
     c. **Postoperative angiography** to confirm complete AVM resection is usually done immediately after surgery. Should any residual AVM be detected, further resection is indicated.
- C. **Posterior fossa surgery**
  1. **Posterior fossa tumors** may cause cranial nerve palsies, cerebellar dysfunction, and hydrocephalus due to obstruction of the fourth ventricle. Tumors or surgery around the glossopharyngeal and vagus nerves may impair the gag reflex and increase the risk of postoperative aspiration. Tumor resection that results in edema in the floor of the fourth ventricle may damage respiratory centers and necessitate postoperative mechanical ventilation.
  2. **Cardiovascular instability** resulting from surgical manipulation is common. Sudden severe bradycardia and hypertension or hypotension occur if the trigeminal nerve is stimulated. Bradycardia, asystole, or hypotension may follow stimulation of the glossopharyngeal or vagus nerve. In such cases, the surgeon should be notified immediately because the instability usually resolves with cessation of the stimulus. Pharmacologic treatment (eg, atropine, glycopyrrolate, ephedrine) is rarely necessary.

3. **A sitting position** is occasionally used for posterior fossa surgery. The advantages include better surgical exposure, improved venous and CSF drainage, and diminished bleeding due to lower venous pressures. The sitting position is also associated with a higher incidence of venous air embolism and cardiovascular instability. Modified supine, prone, and three-quarter prone positioning may be substituted for the sitting position because of these concerns.
    a. **Venous air embolism** is a risk whenever the operative site is above the level of the heart and there is an open vein. Under these circumstances, an open venous sinus can entrain air and produce hypoxia, hypercarbia, bronchoconstriction, hypotension, and ultimately, cardiovascular collapse. Systemic arterial air embolism is a risk whenever right-to-left shunts exist and can cause myocardial and cerebral ischemia. Monitoring devices for the detection of air embolism and central venous catheters for aspiration of air are often placed when there is risk for venous air embolism.
    b. **Methods used to monitor for venous air embolism** include Doppler ultrasound (which reveals a characteristic "mill wheel" murmur when air is entrained), capnography (which may reveal a sudden decrease in end-tidal CO_2), and TEE. Of these, TEE is the most sensitive of the invasive monitors, and Doppler ultrasound the most sensitive of noninvasive monitors.
    c. **If air is detected**, the focus is to prevent further air entrainment and treatment of the adverse consequences. First, the surgeons are notified so they can eliminate the source of air (close the dural opening, place bone wax, or flood the surgical field), and the air is aspirated from the central venous pressure catheter. If possible, patient positioning should be modified to place the surgical site below the level of the heart to reverse the pressure gradient facilitating air entry. If the patient remains stable, the prevention of further air entry may be all that is needed. If hypotension develops, Trendelenburg positioning, fluid administration, and inotropic support may be required. If being used, nitrous oxide should be discontinued.
4. At the end of surgery, the adequacy of the airway and respiration should be verified before extubation. Surgical manipulation may damage the cranial nerves or respiratory centers in the brainstem with resulting pharyngeal or respiratory dysfunction. Postoperative infarction, edema, or hematoma formation in the posterior fossa can cause rapid clinical deterioration. Close observation and prompt support including intubation, mechanical ventilation, and circulatory management may be required.

D. Awake craniotomy
1. Recommended for removal of tumors involving or adjacent to speech centers and for epileptogenic focus resection. Intraoperative cortical mapping allows maximal resection with minimal postoperative neurologic dysfunction.
2. The goals are to provide adequate analgesia and sedation as well as to ensure hemodynamic stability, a patent airway, and patient cooperation with neurologic testing during cortical stimulation. Adequate local anesthesia is required. Conscious sedation with propofol, dexmedetomidine, remifentanil, or other agents may be used. Alternatively, an "asleep-awake-asleep" technique may be used as long as the patient is fully cooperative during testing. A laryngeal mask airway (LMA) may be necessary for airway patency during the "asleep" portions of the case.

3. Be prepared to treat a **cortical stimulation–induced seizure.** If one occurs, ask the neurosurgeons to irrigate the cortex with iced saline. Next, the seizure may be aborted with either midazolam or propofol. Small doses may stop the seizure and not overly sedate the patient so that testing may continue. It is important that the IV catheter is not placed across a joint, which may be flexed and ineffective during a grand mal seizure. Before the procedure, the patient's anticonvulsant level should be checked to ensure that it is therapeutic.
4. **Allow adequate access to the patient's airway.** This should include sufficient room to provide mask ventilation and LMA insertion should the circumstances require these interventions.

E. **Transsphenoidal resection of the pituitary gland** is performed through a nasal, transsphenoidal approach.
1. Although nonfunctioning **pituitary adenomas** are the most common tumor type, some patients have endocrine deficiencies due to hypothalamopituitary compression. Various hyperpituitarism syndromes may accompany functioning adenomas, including Cushing syndrome, acromegaly (with associated airway difficulties), and amenorrhea–galactorrhea.
2. ICP is not a concern as these tumors are usually small and unlikely to compromise intracranial compliance.
3. **Uncontrollable bleeding** is rare but can be massive and catastrophic due to lack of exposure. Frontal craniotomy ultimately may be required to achieve hemostasis.
4. **Monitoring.** The endotracheal tube must be firmly secured to the lower lip to keep it out of the surgical field. Continuous monitoring of ventilation is essential. Arterial monitors are usually not indicated unless indicated by other medical comorbidities.
5. **Throat packs** will prevent blood from accumulating in the stomach and may reduce postoperative vomiting. The throat pack must be removed before extubation.
6. At the conclusion of surgery, nasal breathing will be obstructed by packs. Patients should be prepared for this preoperatively.
7. **Diabetes insipidus** may occur after transsphenoidal hypophysectomy (usually 4 to 12 hours postoperatively). Treatment with IV fluids or desmopressin may be necessary (Section V.E.8). Some patients may develop postoperative adrenal insufficiency and require corticosteroids postoperatively.

F. **Stereotactic surgery** is usually performed through a burr hole, using a three-dimensional reference grid attached to the head with pins placed in the outer table of the skull. This approach allows localization of a discrete area of brain for biopsy or ablation. In most cases, the procedure is done under general anesthesia. However, when intraoperative testing is required, the procedure can be done under monitored anesthetic care. Because the stereotactic apparatus precludes full access to the airway, sedation must be given with caution. The stereotactic frame can be removed in an emergency; newer models can be quickly removed to provide more rapid access to the airway.

G. **Deep brain stimulators** are inserted in patients with movement disorders (mostly Parkinson disease) who have failed medical therapy. Microelectrodes are inserted through burr holes to a precise location in the subthalamic nuclei, globus pallidum, or thalamus. A stereotactic headframe with image-guided navigation is required to identify and locate the electrode target.

1. Patients often do not receive their morning dose of either dopaminergic or anticholinergic medications to improve electrode recordings that guide electrode placement to a specific cell layer.
2. Patients are awake and often not sedated during the electrode placement, since most sedatives can alter the electrode recordings. Once the electrodes are secure, appropriate sedation is implemented.

H. Epilepsy surgery is performed in patients with epilepsy of focal origin who are refractory to medical therapy or intolerant of the side effects of anticonvulsants.

1. **Excision of a seizure focus.** Electrophysiologic mapping of the epileptic focus and other cortical areas (eg, language, memory, sensorimotor) is often performed to maximize the resection of the epileptogenic lesion while minimizing the neurologic deficits. This procedure is often done with general anesthesia and electrocorticography. It offers the advantages of patient comfort, immobility, a secure airway, and the ability to control $PaCO_2$ and other variables. The anesthetic technique is chosen for its ability to augment (eg, methohexital, etomidate, ketamine) or attenuate (eg, benzodiazepines, isoflurane) the seizure focus and its compatibility with intraoperative monitoring (Section III). Because there is often an initial increase in seizure activity postoperatively, anticonvulsants should be resumed promptly.
2. **Vagal nerve stimulators** (VNS) may be placed for medically refractory epilepsy. The electrodes are typically placed through an incision in the left neck and then tunneled to a generator located above the left pectoralis fascia. VNS are typically placed under general anesthesia with endotracheal intubation. Patients frequently are taking multiple antiepileptic drugs, which may cause resistance to neuromuscular-blocking drugs. Additionally, medications that may trigger seizure activity (e.g., ketamine) should be avoided. Postoperatively, monitoring for peritracheal hematoma and vocal cord paralysis should be performed.

I. Head trauma. Anesthetic management of the patient with head trauma is complicated by the challenging combination of a "tight" head, full stomach, and potentially unstable cervical spine. While following the "ABCs" of resuscitation, the anesthesiologist should ascertain the mechanism and extent of injury. **Cervical spinal cord injury** must be suspected, and the neck stabilized until cervical injury is excluded.

1. Patients who are responsive and ventilating adequately should receive supplemental oxygen and be observed closely for evidence of neurologic deterioration.
2. Comatose patients require immediate endotracheal intubation for airway protection and to avoid hypercarbia and hypoxia, which can exacerbate increases in ICP and contribute to secondary brain injury.
3. **Endotracheal intubation** should be accomplished rapidly, with blood pressure stability and without coughing or straining.
    a. **A rapid sequence induction** is usually performed. If a cervical spine injury has not been excluded, the neck should be immobilized with manual in-line stabilization (MILS). The anterior part of the cervical collar may be removed to apply gentle cricoid pressure (excessive pressure may displace a fracture) and obtain sufficient mouth opening. A short-acting induction agent such as propofol or etomidate is used to induce anesthesia, which is immediately followed by an intubating dose of muscle relaxant. Succinylcholine can be used safely unless contraindicated for other reasons (Section II.C and Chapter 14: Neuromuscular Blockade). Nondepolarizing relaxants also may

be used. When MILS is used, the laryngoscopist should anticipate an increased likelihood of poor glottic visualization during direct laryngoscopy due to limited extension of the occiput, C1, and C2.

  b. **Awake intubation** may be advocated because of full-stomach considerations, the potential for worsening neck injuries during manipulation of the airway, and anticipation of a difficult airway due to associated facial injuries. Awake approaches are often impractical or unwise in head-injured patients because of lack of cooperation, airway bleeding, and increases in ICP that can be induced by hypertension, coughing, and straining.

  c. **Nasal intubation and nasogastric tube placement** are contraindicated in the presence of a basilar skull fracture (eg, CSF rhinorrhea, otorrhea, Le Fort III facial fracture).

4. **Hypertension** in head-injured patients may be the body's compensatory effort to maintain CPP in the face of increased ICP. CPP should be maintained at 60 mm Hg. **Hypotension can be detrimental** in patients with elevated ICP and, when combined with tachycardia, should lead one to suspect bleeding from other injuries. Interventions to stop bleeding and restore intravascular volume should occur in concert with surgical treatment of the head injury.

5. **Hypoxia should be aggressively treated** as its presence dramatically worsens neurologic outcome in head-injured patients.

6. **Hyperglycemia should be treated** to improve neurologic outcome.

7. **ICP monitoring** can be performed if severe or progressive intracranial hypertension is suspected.

8. **Seizures** may accompany direct cerebral injury or signal the expansion of an intracranial hematoma.

9. **Brain contusion** is the most common type of head injury. Surgery is usually reserved for acute epidural hematomas and acute subdural hematomas. Subdural hematomas are much more common than epidural hematomas and carry a worse prognosis. Intracranial hypertension is frequently seen even after evacuation of hematomas because of severe brain swelling.

10. **Penetrating brain injuries** require early debridement of injured tissue, removal of bone fragments, and evacuation of hematoma. Skull fractures may require debridement, cranioplasty, and repair of dural lacerations.

11. **Anesthetic management** follows the general rules of maintaining CPP and ICP, and reducing cerebral edema. Postoperative intubation and ventilatory support are frequently required for ICP control and airway protection in patients with prolonged loss of consciousness or an inadequate gag reflex. Preoperative alteration in the level of consciousness is helpful in predicting the need for postoperative intubation.

12. **Disseminated intravascular coagulation** is a frequent complication of an acute head injury, particularly those associated with a subdural hematoma. Frequent monitoring of the patient's coagulation status is recommended throughout the procedure and early postoperative period.

13. **Corticosteroids are not indicated for head trauma** and may increase morbidity and mortality.

J. **CSF shunts** are inserted in patients with hydrocephalus. A ventriculoperitoneal (VP) shunt is the most common treatment for hydrocephalus. A ventricular catheter is placed through a frontal burr hole and is attached to a valve. These are then attached to the draining catheter that is tunneled subcutaneously to the upper abdomen, where laparoscopy is performed to insert the catheter under direct visualization.

1. The anesthetic management of these patients is determined primarily by the acuity of their disease. Acute hydrocephalus is a neurosurgical emergency where rapidly rising ICP could cause ischemic neurologic damage. Management should focus on measures that will reduce the patient's ICP, maintain a CPP of at least 60 mm Hg, and enable rapid neurosurgical decompression. Anesthetic management of elective VP shunt insertion or revision employs a standard, well-managed, and safe anesthetic where factors that cause extreme ICP elevation are avoided.

VII. SURGERY ON THE SPINE AND SPINAL CORD

Surgery on the spine and spinal cord is undertaken for a variety of conditions, including intervertebral disk disease, spondylosis, stenosis, neoplasm, scoliosis, and trauma. The physiology of the spinal cord and brain is similar, even though absolute rates of blood flow and metabolism are lower in the spinal cord. Maintaining spinal cord perfusion pressure (which equals MAP minus intraspinal pressure) and reducing cord compression are clinical management objectives.

  A. **The prone position** is frequently used. Most patients can be anesthetized on a stretcher and "logrolled" onto the operating room table after endotracheal intubation. Awake intubation should be considered for patients with tenuous neurologic conditions that may be worsened by laryngoscopy/intubation or positioning (eg, patients with unstable cervical or thoracic spine injuries). Under these circumstances, an abbreviated neurologic examination should be performed after intubation and transfer to ensure that injury has not occurred. The anesthetist should ensure that all pressure points are padded; neck and extremities are in neutral positions; eyes, ears, nose, breasts, and genitalia are free from pressure; and all monitors and lines are secured in place and functioning. Special attention should be paid to the endotracheal tube, since it can move or kink in the process of positioning. **Ischemic optic neuropathy is a potential complication** of prone cases associated with length of procedure (usually >5 hours), blood loss (usually >2 L), hypotension, medical comorbidities, and fluid resuscitation. Increased facial swelling may alter venous hemodynamics in the globe, leading to optic nerve ischemia and postoperative visual deficits. There are no standard preventive guidelines, but maintenance of systemic blood pressure near baseline values, frequent eye checks to assess for direct pressure on the globe, and maintenance of adequate perfusion are likely beneficial.

  B. **Surgery to correct scoliosis** can be accompanied by significant blood loss. Various techniques can be used to reduce homologous blood transfusion, including preoperative autologous donation, use of intraoperative blood-scavenging techniques, and meticulous patient positioning to prevent increased abdominal and intrathoracic pressures that can increase venous bleeding. Because of concern of neurologic sequelae, induced hypotension may not be advantageous in this procedure. Scoliosis surgery is accompanied by a 1% to 4% incidence of serious postoperative neurologic complications. Spinal instrumentation and distraction can cause spinal cord ischemia and result in paraplegia. Intraoperative monitoring of spinal cord function is used routinely.

  1. **SSEP and MEP monitoring** provide continuous evaluation of spinal cord function (Section III.B).
  2. **The selective wake-up test.** Intraoperatively, if there is uncertainty about the neurophysiologic monitoring, the presence of neuromuscular function is assured when patients are awakened briefly and asked to move

their legs. If there is no leg movement, the spine distraction is released until movement is observed. Patients should be prepared for this event preoperatively. Wake-up tests can be performed in older children and adults.
   3. **Total IV anesthesia** with propofol and remifentanil is often selected because it is less likely to interfere with neurophysiologic monitoring than volatile anesthetics. Communication of anesthetic interventions with the clinical neurophysiologist or technician is important.
C. **After acute spinal cord injury**, surgery may be required to decompress and stabilize the spinal cord. The primary goal in the initial management of acute spinal cord injury is to prevent secondary damage to the injured cord. This is accomplished by stabilizing the spine and correcting circulatory and ventilatory abnormalities that can exacerbate the primary injury. The presence of cervical cord injury should lead one to suspect associated head, face, or tracheal trauma; thoracic and lumbar spine injuries often are associated with chest or intra-abdominal trauma.
   1. **Spinal shock** is characterized by systemic vasodilation and hypotension from impaired activation of the sympathetic nervous system. If the lesion involves the sympathetic cardiac accelerator nerves (T1–T4), bradycardia, bradyarrhythmias, atrioventricular block, and cardiac arrest can occur due to unopposed vagal activity. Spinal shock occurs because of functional transection of sympathetic innervation below the level of the injury and may persist for days to weeks. Bradycardia can be treated with atropine. Hypotension can be treated by fluid, vasopressors, or both. Patients with high spinal cord injury may be unusually sensitive to the cardiovascular depressant effects of anesthetics because of an inability to increase sympathetic tone.
   2. **Lesions above C3–C4 necessitate intubation and mechanical ventilatory support** because of loss of innervation to the diaphragm (C3–C5). Lesions below C5–C6 may still cause as much as 70% reduction in vital capacity and FEV_1 with impaired ventilation and oxygenation.
   3. **Atony of the gastrointestinal tract and urinary bladder** necessitates a nasogastric tube and an indwelling urinary catheter, respectively. These patients are also **prone to heat loss** because of inability to vasoconstrict.
   4. **Methylprednisolone** (30 mg/kg IV loading dose, followed by an infusion of 5.4 mg/kg/h for 23 hours) may improve the functional recovery of patients with acute spinal cord injuries if treatment is begun within the first 3 hours after injury. There is considerable controversy surrounding this therapy for spinal cord injury, and some centers do not follow this protocol.
   5. **Chronic spinal cord injuries** are discussed in Chapter 24: Anesthesia for Spine Surgery.
   6. **Airway management** of patients with cervical spine injury is discussed in Section VI.I.
D. Neuroradiologic procedures are performed in suites often remote from the main operating room. For a detailed discussion of anesthetic issues pertaining to the patient having a magnetic resonance imaging or interventional radiologic procedures, see Sections IV and V in Chapter 34: Non-Operating Room Anesthesia.

ACKNOWLEDGMENT

We gratefully acknowledge the contributions of previous edition author, Eleanor M. Mullen, as portions of those chapters have been retained in this revision.

Suggested Readings

Cottrell JE, Young WL, eds. *Cottrell and Young's Neuroanesthesia*. 5th ed. Mosby; 2010.

Dankiewicz J, Cronberg T, Lilja G, et al; TTM2 Trial Investigators. Hypothermia versus Normothermia after out-of-hospital cardiac arrest. *N Engl J Med*. 2021;384(24):2283-2294.

Drummond JC, Patel PM. Neurosurgical anesthesia. In: Miller RD, ed. *Miller's Anesthesia*. 7th ed. Churchill Livingstone; 2010:2045-2088.

Koht A, Sloan TB, Toleikis JR, eds. *Monitoring the Nervous System for Anesthesiologists and Other Health Care Professionals*. Springer; 2012.

Mashour GA, Farag E. *Case Studies in Neuroanesthesia and Neurocritical Care*. Cambridge; 2011.

Newfield P, Cottrell JE. *Handbook of Neuroanesthesia*. 5th ed. Lippincott; 2012.

Nielsen N, Wetterslev J, Cronberg T, et al; TTM Trial Investigators. Targeted temperature management at 33°C versus 36°C after cardiac arrest. *N Engl J Med*. 2013;369(23):2197-2206.

Patel PM, Drummond JC. Cerebral physiology and the effects of anesthetic drugs. In: Miller RD, ed. *Miller's Anesthesia*. Churchill Livingstone; 2010:305-339.

Seubert CN, Mahla ME. Neurologic monitoring. In: Miller RD, ed. *Miller's Anesthesia*. Churchill Livingstone; 2010:1477-1514.

Anesthesia for Spine Surgery

John J. A. Marota and Zachary Achen

I. GENERAL CONSIDERATIONS

Pathologic conditions of the spine treated with surgical intervention include intervertebral disk disease, spinal stenosis, scoliosis, spondylosis, spondylolisthesis, kyphosis and lordosis, tumors, and trauma. In the United States, the demand for these procedures has increased dramatically, owing to the widespread prevalence of low back pain, an aging demographic, and advancements in minimally invasive methods of surgical intervention. It is important that anesthetists be familiar with the challenges associated with these procedures including the prone position, fluid shifts, prolonged surgeries, and manipulations adjacent to nerves and major blood vessels. While general anesthesia is the predominant choice for anesthetic management of these procedures, both regional and local anesthesia are potential options for lumbar microdiscectomy or laminectomy.

A. Spinal cord injury

1. Acute spinal cord injury may present with neurogenic shock, more commonly with lesions above T6. Presentation is hemodynamic instability due to sympathectomy with resultant arterial and venous vasodilation; hypotension and increased heat loss are common. Weeks to months after the acute phase of spinal shock, autonomic dysreflexia may develop, characterized by hypertension and bradycardia in response to stimulation below the level of loss of sensation; hypertension may result in myocardial ischemia, retinal/cerebral hemorrhage, and seizures. While a variety of physical stimulations can trigger this autonomic hyperresponse, the majority are associated with the most caudal root levels below the region of injury. Bladder distention is responsible for up to 75% to 82% of episodes of autonomic dysreflexia.

2. Cervical spine injury is commonly associated with head trauma. Injury to the spinal cord at C5 presents with weakness of the deltoid, biceps brachialis, brachioradialis, and partial diaphragmatic paralysis. Cervical cord injury above C6 can compromise ventilatory function with either partial or total loss of ventilation. Approximately 55% of all spinal cord injuries occur in the cervical region; the most common cervical spine fracture occurs at C2 and accounts for ≈24% of injuries.

3. Prolonged immobility secondary to paraplegia/quadriplegia leads to increased proliferation of extrajunctional acetylcholine receptors at the neuromuscular junction. Accordingly, succinylcholine is contraindicated starting at 48 hours after spinal cord injury due to risk of resultant hyperkalemia.

B. Airway

1. In addition to standard concerns for securing the airway, additional caution is required for patients with cervical spine injuries to prevent or not worsen damage to the spinal cord. Hard cervical collars permit 72% to 73% of normal extension and flexion of the cervical spine. Movement

of the cervical spine during direct laryngoscopy predominantly occurs at the occipital/C1 and C1/C2 levels with much less potential for movement at lower levels.
2. Video laryngoscopy has emerged as a useful technique for intubation of patients with cervical spine injury because it requires less cervical spinal motion during laryngoscopy.
3. Awake fiberoptic intubation followed by awake positioning for surgery should be considered for any patients with severe cervical spine instability after injury; directed neurologic examination is performed immediately before and after intubation to confirm that no change has occurred with manipulation. This approach should be discussed in advance with the surgical team as well as the sequence of events should be explained to the patient before proceeding with awake intubation; this approach requires a cooperative patient. Intubation is achieved with minimal or no sedation and adequate topicalization of the upper and lower airway with local anesthetic, after which the brief neurologic examination is repeated. The patient can be positioned on the operating (OR) table awake and then general anesthesia induced after confirming postposition neurologic examination.
4. Manual inline stabilization of the cervical spine can be performed to limit cervical motion. With the patient supine, a second provider stands by the top of the head and provides traction on the head to maintain alignment and immobility relative to the shoulders; this limits motion of the neck during intubation and positioning. The laryngoscopist usually stands at the patient's side by the left shoulder. Although this technique has gained wide acceptance and is a component of Advanced Trauma Life Support, its effectiveness has been questioned due to potential increase in craniocervical motion and worsening view during laryngoscopy. This technique can be performed with or without cervical collar in place and with direct laryngoscopy, video laryngoscopy, or fiberoptic intubation.
5. In emergency situations where there is no evidence of facial/basal skull fractures, blind nasotracheal intubation is an acceptable option.

C. Prone position

1. For patients undergoing posterior procedures, induction of general anesthesia and intubation is performed supine, typically on a stretcher or hospital bed, and then the patient is rolled prone onto OR table. Before turning prone, eyes are protected with tape or clear plastic adhesive; bite blocks, orogastric tube, and temperature probe are placed. Nasogastric or nasal temperature probes are discouraged because of the potential for bleeding when prone; the nasal approach is not recommended in cases with basal skull fracture or evidence of CSF leak from the nose.
2. There are several options to support the head in the prone position. It can be placed on a commercially available foam head and/or face rest in which there are cut-out spaces for eyes and nose to remain free from compression; endotracheal tubes may be positioned either straight down through a hole in the rest or accessed to the side. Alternatively, the head can be supported by sharp pins screwed into the outer table of skull; Gardner–Wells tongs have two-pin fixation; Mayfield skull clamp system has a three-pin fixation. Gardner–Wells tongs system provides continuous traction; Mayfield skull clamp system holds the head rigidly in place, attached to the OR table. Alternatively, the halo of a halo vest immobilizer can be used either with traction, fixed to the OR table, or with the vest fixation.

3. The physiologic changes associated with prone positioning may include depressed cardiac index from reduced filling pressures, inferior vena cava obstruction with decreased venous return to the heart, peripheral pooling of blood volume, increase in airway ventilation pressure with increase in intrathoracic pressure, increased functional residual capacity, and redistribution of pulmonary blood flow and lung ventilation to dependent areas. The prone position predisposes to atelectasis; PEEP may be necessary to maintain oxygenation.
4. Care should be taken so that the eyes, abdomen, genitalia, and breasts are free from compression; the stomach can be decompressed with an orogastric tube and bladder with a urinary catheter. Improper positioning of arms can result in vascular compromise or brachial plexus injury, as well as increased pressure within the cubital tunnel with elbow flexion greater than 130 degrees. Complications such as shoulder dislocation, facial and laryngeal edema, eye injuries, and peripheral nerve palsy have been reported as well as hip dislocation with rolling into position. Bite injuries can occur during motor-evoked potential (MEP) monitoring due to jaw muscle contractions; bilateral molar bite blocks will decrease the likelihood of forceful apposition of the teeth. Turning from supine to prone presents the greatest risk for injury to the spinal cord with or without instability; care should be taken to maintain good alignment of the spine across the area of instability.

D. Monitoring

1. Intraoperative monitoring of spinal cord functional integrity involves electrophysiologic monitoring of the sensory and/or motor transmission pathways; changes in functional activity could result from transection, direct compression, or ischemia produced by compromise or distortion of blood vessels. Different techniques to monitor integrity of spinal cord function include somatosensory-evoked potentials (SSEPs), MEPs, epidural electrodes, direct stimulation of spinal roots, F-responses, H-reflexes, testing specific reflexes, electromyography, transcranial electrical stimulation with screw electrodes, neuromuscular junction monitoring, and electrical impedance testing. Combining multiple methods increases sensitivity when the risk of spinal cord, nerve root, or peripheral nerve damage is high. Use of intraoperative monitoring has been shown to reduce postoperative neurologic morbidity and may identify functional compromise caused by surgical manipulation (eg, retractor or pedicle screw placement) so as to permit immediate correction of a reversible deficit.
2. SSEPs and MEPs are the two most commonly utilized modalities for monitoring integrity of the spinal cord and peripheral nervous system; amplitude and latency of the electrophysiologic complex wave generated by depolarization of either nerve or muscle, respectively, are detected from multiple electrodes placed on the patient. Peripheral nerves at sites distal to the surgical site are stimulated repetitively to obtain SSEPs; interruption of the blood supply of the posterior spinal arteries or nerve compression causes loss of these signals. Transcranial electrical stimulation of the motor cortex or direct stimulation of the spinal cord or nerve roots generates MEPs detected as action potentials within specific muscles; spinal cord motor pathways are supplied by the single anterior spinal artery.
3. Intraoperative "wake-up test" can be used to assess motor function. Patients are coached about testing before induction of general anesthesia. At the appropriate time, typically immediately after distraction

of the spinal cord, the anesthetic is reduced sufficiently to permit the patient response to command to move the hands and feet; the anesthetic is deepened after confirming adequate neurologic function. The procedure requires adequate analgesia and reversal of muscle relaxation before the "wake-up." The test carries the potential complications of coughing, displacement or loss of the endotracheal tube, venous air embolism (VAE), and awareness.

4. All general anesthetics decrease the effectiveness of neuromonitoring in a dose-dependent manner by increasing latency and/or decreasing amplitude of the electrophysiologic signal detected from neuronal depolarization; these same changes are suggestive also of ischemia. Hypothermia and cortical burst suppression on EEG will suppress both detection of SSEPs and evoked neuronal depolarization necessary for MEPs; hypothermia and neuromuscular blockers suppress MEP detection. Low concentrations of isoflurane, desflurane, and N_2O do permit intraoperative monitoring but with reduced signal. The goal of anesthetic management is to maintain patient immobility for surgery; both inhalational agents as well as intravenous anesthetics including propofol and dexmedetomidine at sufficient dose can suppress EEG activity and decrease effectiveness of SEP and MEP to detect integrity of function. Opioids have a minor impact on evoked potentials. Total intravenous anesthetic with propofol and opioid infusions is a widely used technique with the caveat that the dose of propofol is adjusted to maintain adequate EEG activity. Ketamine increases EEG activity and may mask suppression of activity produced by propofol that obscures detection of SSEP and MEP; alternatively, etomidate increases SSEP signal amplitude, but variations in dose can lead to alterations in signal inappropriately interpreted as decrement of function. Nonetheless, the combination of propofol infusion, opioids (including remifentanil), ketamine, lidocaine, and dexmedetomidine can provide adequate patient immobility for surgery and permit adequate signal detection for monitoring evoked potentials. Bolus doses of anesthetic agents and sudden increases in inhaled agent concentration should be avoided when possible to minimize the deleterious impact on the detection of evoked potential signal changes.

II. BLOOD LOSS

Epidural vessel bleeding and decortication of bone during instrumentation and fusion of the vertebral column account for significant blood loss during spinal surgery. Factors predicting blood loss requiring transfusion include type of surgery (fusion, laminectomy, pedicle subtraction osteotomy, osteotomy), degree of osteoporosis, low preoperative hemoglobin, tumor surgery, number of spine levels involved, and underlying cardiopulmonary disease. Factors likely to decrease blood loss include use of the Jackson table, hypotensive techniques, and use of tranexamic acid or aminocaproic acid. In nontumor surgery, use of a "cell saver" to capture blood cells for reinfusion decreases requirement for the use of allogenic blood transfusion. Monitoring for development of intraoperative coagulopathy includes testing prothrombin time/international normalized ratio, partial thromboplastin time, platelet count, and fibrinogen level. Thrombocytopenia should be treated with platelet transfusion. Cryoprecipitate transfusion is sometimes necessary to correct acquired bleeding disorders. Use of DDAVP, 0.3 mcg/kg bolus dose, has been advocated to reduce blood loss during spine surgery when significant blood loss is anticipated.

III. SPINAL CORD PERFUSION

Spinal cord perfusion may be compromised by the initial trauma, surgical manipulation, hematoma formation, and reductions in blood pressure and cardiac output. Similar to cerebral perfusion pressure, spinal cord perfusion pressure (SCPP) is determined by mean arterial pressure (MAP) and intraspinal pressure (ISP) (or central venous pressure [CVP] if CVP > ISP): SCPP = MAP − ISP. Blood vessel injury (decreased local blood flow), systemic hypotension (decreased MAP), and obstruction to blood flow (either segmental or elevated ISP) will decrease SCPP. Methods to maximize SCPP include elevating MAP to maximize perfusion, monitoring cerebrospinal fluid (CSF) pressure within the thecal sac, and CSF drainage.

A. Complications

1. Spinal surgery carries significant risks with complication rates that are higher than many other procedures; major complications occur in 11% of cases and minor complications in 24%. The lowest complication rates were among adolescents undergoing idiopathic scoliosis surgery and highest among patients with neuromuscular scoliosis. Surgeries that combine anterior/posterior approach carry greater complication rate than staged procedures. Age older than 60 years increases the complication rate.

2. VAE can be fatal during spinal surgery. Risk is elevated because of the large surface area of exposed and decorticated bone and the surgical site elevated above the heart. Routine monitoring is accomplished with capnography and/or precordial Doppler. Transesophageal echocardiography is the most sensitive monitor for detection. If VAE is suspected, treatment includes irrigating the wound with saline, discontinuing N_2O, vasopressors to treat hypotension, turning from prone to supine (difficult with an open surgical exposure), institution of advanced life support, and potentially initiating cardiopulmonary bypass in cases refractory to resuscitation attempts.

3. Bone cement embolism is a rare complication of vertebroplasty or kyphoplasty treatment of vertebral compression fractures; cement emboli migrate to the pulmonary vasculature from leakage of bone cement into the low-pressure venous drainage system of vertebrae. Most emboli are incidental findings, <1% present with symptoms, typically dyspnea. Diagnosis is made with imaging demonstrating cement in a vascular distribution with chest x-ray or CT; treatment is typically conservative monitoring but may require systemic anticoagulation and surgical embolectomy based on the severity of symptoms.

4. Postoperative visual loss occurs in approximately 0.2% of cases and has been postulated to involve optic nerve ischemia by venous engorgement, decreased arterial perfusion pressure from hypotension, hemodilution, or increased intraocular pressure in the prone position. Risk factors include vascular disease, preoperative anemia, prolonged procedure time, substantial blood loss, obesity, and tobacco use. The American Society of Anesthesiologists recommends continuous blood pressure monitoring, use of colloids or crystalloids to treat substantial blood loss, periodic monitoring of hemoglobin/hematocrit, and case-by-case consideration for use of deliberate hypotension, CVP monitoring, and staging surgical procedures in high-risk patients.

5. Peripheral nerve injury. Ulnar nerve injury is the most common peripheral nerve injury during spine surgery. Elbow flexion greater than 130 degrees results in increased pressure within the cubital tunnel, which may compress the ulnar nerve. Brachial plexus injury can occur from

TABLE 24.1 Major Blood Vessels at Risk of Injury During Common Surgical Spine Procedures

Surgical Procedure	Vessel(s)
Anterior screw fixation of the odontoid fracture	Vertebral artery Internal carotid artery
Anterior cervical spine surgery	Vertebral artery
Posterior C1–C2 arthrodesis	Vertebral artery
Posterior cervical spine surgery	Vertebral artery
Anterolateral approach for thoracolumbar spine fracture	Aorta Inferior vena cava
Posterior thoracic spine surgery	Thoracic aorta
Scoliosis surgery	Superior mesenteric artery
Anterior lumbar interbody fusion	Inferior vena cava Iliac veins and arteries (L > R)
Lumbar disk surgery	Inferior vena cava Iliac veins
Posterior lumbar spine surgery	Epidural venous bleeding

arm positioning that places traction on the plexus or compression from the clavicle.

6. Spinal cord injury can result in postoperative paraplegia and may occur despite monitoring of SSEPs and MEPs. Cervical traction has been demonstrated as an effective method to decrease motion at the occipitocervical junction to prevent cervical spine injury. Minimizing cervical manipulation during positioning/turning and fiber-optic technique for orotracheal intubation reduces cervical motion.
7. Vascular injury can occur in major vasculature structures adjacent to and within the spine. The major vessels at risk are summarized in **Table 24.1**.

IV. DISPOSITION

Immediate postsurgical care is dependent upon procedure and patient comorbidities. For all patients, frequent checks of neurologic function in the postsurgical time period are advocated to assess for the development of edema, compressive hematomas, or vascular compromise that can compromise function. Factors determining disposition to an ICU include extensive surgery, significant blood loss, significant facial and airway edema, and requirement for postoperative ventilation and endotracheal intubation to maintain airway patency.

V. POSTOPERATIVE PAIN MANAGEMENT

A. Postoperative pain management may be a significant issue for patients with chronic pain, specifically back pain, who present with history of long-term high-dose opioid therapy prior to surgical intervention.
B. Intraoperative administration of methadone has been reported to reduce pain scores and analgesic requirements with acceptable side effects after complex spine surgery; most likely this is due to the long effective half-life of

the drug. Continuous infusions of short-acting opioids during surgery, such as fentanyl or remifentanil, have been demonstrated to provide adequate intraoperative analgesia and may facilitate an intraoperative "wake-up test." Postoperative pain is typically managed initially with intravenous opioids, either by patient-controlled analgesia or continuous infusion as necessary.

C. Adjuncts with demonstrated efficacy to reduce postprocedure analgesic requirements in the immediate postoperative period include preoperative acetaminophen, celecoxib, and either gabapentin or pregabalin as well intraoperative administration of dexamethasone and ketamine infusion. Ketamine 0.15 mg/kg bolus before surgical stimulus followed by infusion of 0.015 to 0.02 mg/kg/min has been shown to reduce opioid requirements. Infiltration of the surgical field with long-acting local anesthetic at incision and/or at closure and intravenous acetaminophen may be helpful for immediate postprocedure pain control. Intravenous administration of the nonsteroidal anti-inflammatory ketorolac can also aid in postsurgical analgesia; some surgeons prefer to avoid this medication because of concern for bleeding and possible impact on bone fusion.

D. Multimodal approach to pain management is gaining in popularity as an option for treatment of postsurgical pain. While some individual adjuncts themselves have been demonstrated neither to improve pain scores nor reduce opioid use, there may be an "additive effect" on analgesia when given in conjunction with other medications that have different mechanisms of action.

ACKNOWLEDGMENTS

We gratefully acknowledge the contributions of previous edition authors, Raissa Quezado da Nobrega and John Marota, as portions of those chapters have been retained in this revision.

Suggested Readings

Alboog A, Bae S, Chui J. Anesthetic management of complex spine surgery in adult patients: a review based on outcome evidence. *Curr Opin Anaesthesiol.* 2019;32(5):600–608

American College of Surgeons. *Best Practices Guidelines: Spine Surgery*; 2022.

American Society of Anesthesiology. Practice advisory for perioperative visual loss associated with spine surgery: an updated report by the American Society of Anesthesiologists Task Force on Perioperative Visual Loss. *Anesthesiology.* 2012;116(2):274–285.

Bae S, Alboog A, Esquivel KS, et al. Efficacy of perioperative pharmacological and regional pain interventions in adult spine surgery: a network meta-analysis and systematic review of randomised controlled trials. *Br J Anaesth.* 2022;128(1):98–117.

Banoub M, Tetzlaff JE, Schubert A. Pharmacologic and physiologic influences affecting sensory evoked potentials. *Anesthesiology.* 2003;99(3):716–737.

Edgcombe H, Carter K, Yarrow S. Anaesthesia in the prone position. *Br J Anaesth.* 2008; 100(2):165–183.

Farag E. Airway management for cervical spine surgery. *Best Pract Res Clin Anaesthesiol.* 2016;30(1):13–25.

Hambly PR, Martin B. Anaesthesia for chronic spinal cord lesions. *Anaesthesia.* 1998;53(3): 273–289.

Henry SM. *ATLS Advanced Trauma Life Support 10th Edition Student Course Manual*, 10e; 2018.

Inamasu J, Guiot BH. Vascular injury and complication in neurosurgical spine surgery. *Acta Neurochir (Wien).* 2006;148(4):375–387.

Kawaguchi M, Iida H, Tanaka S, et al; The MEP Monitoring Guideline Working Group of the Safety Committee of the Japanese Society of Anesthesiologists (JSA). A practical guide for anesthetic management during intraoperative motor evoked potential monitoring. *J Anesth.* 2020;34(1):5–28.

Klatt JWB, Mickelson J, Hung M, Durcan S, Miller M, Smith JT. A randomized prospective evaluation of 3 techniques of postoperative pain management after posterior spinal instrumentation and fusion. *Spine (Phila Pa 1976)*. 2013;38(19):1626–1631.

Kong CY, Hosseini AM, Belanger LM, et al. A prospective evaluation of hemodynamic management in acute spinal cord injury patients. *Spinal Cord*. 2013;51:466–471.

Legatt AD, Emerson RG, Epstein CM, et al. ACNS Guideline: transcranial electrical stimulation motor evoked potential monitoring. *J Clin Neurophysiol*. 2016;33(1):42–50.

Lennarson PJ, Smith DW, Sawin PD, Todd MM, Sato Y, Traynelis VC. Cervical spinal motion during intubation: efficacy of stabilization maneuvers in the setting of complete segmental instability. *J Neurosurg*. 2001;94(2):265–270.

Li G, Sun TW, Luo G, Zhang C. Efficacy of antifibrinolytic agents on surgical bleeding and transfusion requirements in spine surgery: a meta-analysis. *Eur Spine J*. 2017;26(1):140–154.

McCahon RA, Evans DA, Kerslake RW, McClelland MH, Hardman JG, Norris AM. Cadaveric study of movement of an unstable atlanto-axial (C1/C2) Cervical segment during laryngoscopy and intubation using the Airtraq®, Macintosh and McCoy laryngoscopes. *Anaesthesia*. 2015;70(4):452–461.

McDonnell MF, Glassman SD, Dimar JR, Puno RM, Johnson JR. Perioperative complications of anterior procedures on the spine. *J Bone Joint Surg Am*. 1996;78(6):839–847.

Murphy GS, Avram MJ, Greenberg SB, et al. Postoperative pain and analgesic requirements in the first year after intraoperative methadone for complex spine and cardiac surgery. *Anesthesiology*. 2020;132(2):330–342.

Murphy GS, Szokol JW, Avram MJ, et al. Clinical effectiveness and safety of intraoperative methadone in patients undergoing posterior spinal fusion surgery: a randomized, double-blinded, controlled trial. *Anesthesiology*. 2017;126(5):822–833.

Nuttall GA, Horlocker TT, Santrach PJ, Oliver WC Jr, Dekutoski MB, Bryant S. Predictors of blood transfusions in spinal instrumentation and fusion surgery. *Spine (Phila Pa 1976)*. 2000;25(5):596–601.

Raw DA, Beattie JK, Hunter JM. Anaesthesia for spinal surgery in adults. *Br J Anaesth*. 2003;91(6):886–904.

Riddell JM, Trummel JM, Onakpoya IJ. Low-dose ketamine in painful orthopaedic surgery: a systematic review and meta-analysis. *Br J Anaesth*. 2019;123(3):325–334.

Werndle M, Saadoun S, Phang I, et al. Monitoring of spinal cord perfusion pressure in acute spinal cord injury: initial findings of the injured spinal cord pressure evaluation study. *Crit Care Med*. 2014;42(3):646–655.

Wiles MD. Manual in-line stabilisation during tracheal intubation: effective protection or harmful dogma? *Anaesthesia*. 2021;76(6):850–853.

Anesthesia for Transplant Surgery

Lauren Alderette and James Taylor Lloyd

I. HISTORY AND ETHICAL CONSIDERATIONS

A. The first successful human organ transplant (kidney) was performed in 1954. Since that time, the **heart, lungs, liver, pancreas, intestine, stomach, testis, penis, hand, thymus**, and **uterus** have all been successfully transplanted. It is not uncommon today to have a patient undergo a transplant of two organs in the same surgery (eg, heart–liver, heart–kidney, pancreas–kidney, etc.).

B. From the mid-1950s to the early 1970s, individual hospitals and organ procurement organizations independently managed most aspects of organ donation and transplantation. In 1984, the **United Network for Organ Sharing (UNOS)** was established to coordinate the allocation of organs and systematically collect data regarding donors, transplant candidates, and recipients across the United States. Since then, UNOS has played a central role in overseeing the national organ procurement and transplantation network. Recently, however, legislative and regulatory efforts have emerged aimed at diversifying, modernizing, and potentially restructuring the framework governing organ procurement and transplantation in the United States.

C. Although demand continues to exceed supply, modifications of the organ allocation system, expansion of criteria for acceptable donor organs, and advances in organ preservation techniques have increased the availability of organs and improved allograft survival.

   1. The LifePort Kidney Transporter is a perfusion preservation machine for donor kidneys that works by pumping the renal vasculature continuously with a cold perfusate, reducing the odds of delay in kidney function and improving first-year posttransplant success compared with static storage.

   2. US Food and Drug Administration–approved transport systems have been developed for donor lungs (eg, TransMedics' OCS Lung, a "lung-in-a-box" device). This machine maintains normothermia, breathing, and perfusion throughout transport, allowing expanded retrieval ranges and successful use of organs that had been rejected by transplant centers using cold storage.

   3. Similar devices are now under investigation for donor hearts and livers. Recently, there have been significant advancements in organ preservation and procurement technologies designed to enhance transplant outcomes and expand the donor organ pool. Two prominent normothermic machine perfusion platforms—the OrganOx metra device and the TransMedics Organ Care System (OCS)—are increasingly utilized in clinical practice. These devices maintain donor organs, such as livers, at physiologic temperatures while providing oxygenation, nutrients, and the ability to monitor organ function prior to transplantation. This approach contrasts with traditional static cold storage, potentially allowing for prolonged preservation, improved organ assessment, and utilization of marginal organs. In addition, normothermic regional perfusion (NRP) is an emerging technique in which circulation is reestablished in the donor following circulatory death, enabling organs to be assessed and recovered under physiologically optimal conditions. Similar perfusion devices and methods are currently under investigation for heart transplantation, reflecting an evolving landscape toward broader use of normothermic perfusion technologies to improve transplant outcomes and expand access to transplantation.

D. The success of solid organ transplantation critically depends on the careful selection of transplant recipients. The suitability of candidates is typically determined by a multidisciplinary committee and based on national criteria.
  1. Patients require a thorough **history and physical examination** as well as **psychosocial evaluation** to identify any behavioral, social, or financial issues that may preclude adherence to immunosuppressive therapy and medical follow-up after transplantation.
  2. In addition to **standard laboratory tests**, **serologic tests** for varicella, measles, mumps, rubella, HIV, hepatitis, tuberculosis, syphilis, cytomegalovirus, Ebstein–Barr virus; **drug screening**; **ABO-Rh blood typing**; **age-appropriate screening**; and **electrocardiography (ECG)** are required.
  3. Lifesaving transplants, defined by liver, lungs, heart) are per the decision of the primary team and OR team.
  4. The need for additional cardiac and pulmonary testing is dependent on patient comorbidities as well as the type of transplant to be performed.
  5. **Absolute contraindications** include active infection, active malignancy, substance abuse not in stable remission, uncontrolled psychiatric disease, life expectancy less than 1 year, and ongoing nonadherence to medical or psychiatric treatment.
  6. **Ethical issues** in transplantation are numerous and include how death and brain death are defined, financial incentives, organ trafficking, and coerced donation. A full discussion is beyond the scope of this chapter.

II. ANESTHESIA FOR KIDNEY TRANSPLANTATION
A. In 2022, 26,309 kidney transplants were performed in the United States from 20,511 deceased donors and 5798 living donors. The 5-year survival is estimated to be 81.4% and 90.0% for recipients of cadaveric and living grafts, respectively. Xenotransplantation, such as pig kidney transplantation, remains experimental and is currently under FDA investigation. While innovative combined approaches—such as kidney and hematopoietic stem-cell transplants—represent important areas of research, inclusion in isolation may prompt consideration of other advanced transplant techniques. These include more common variations like simultaneous liver-kidney (SLK) transplants, zero-HLA-mismatch (perfect match) kidney transplants, simultaneous islet-kidney transplants, living donor liver transplants, and ABO-incompatible (A2 to O) liver transplants, each of which also carries significant clinical implications. Therefore, careful consideration is warranted when determining which advanced transplantation strategies merit dedicated sections in the context of anesthesia management.

B. **Indications and recipient selection**
  1. A kidney transplant may be indicated for patients with **end-stage renal disease (ESRD)** from any cause.
  2. Patients are generally referred to a transplantation center when the **estimated glomerular filtration rate is under 30 mL/min/1.73 m²** in order to

TABLE 25.1 UNOS Guidelines for Maximum Cold Ischemic Times for Commonly Transplanted Organs

Organ	Cold Ischemic Time (Hours)
Kidney	24–36
Pancreas	12–18
Liver	8–12
Heart/Lung	4–6

ensure timely completion of evaluation and any interventions required to address candidacy for transplantation.

3. The scheduling of a deceased donor kidney transplantation should take into consideration the limited viability of the donated kidney (**Table 25.1**). Transplantation from a living donor is generally elective, although in some instances transplants are conducted as part of a donor chain and thus timing is more critical.

C. Preanesthetic considerations

1. Preoperative evaluation for the patient with ESRD is discussed in **Chapter 5**: Specific Considerations With Renal Disease.
2. Patients presenting for kidney transplantation will have already undergone a thorough preoperative evaluation prior to listing. In the patient presenting for surgery, we recommend a tailored evaluation of at least the following:
   a. **Volume status** can be assessed through a number of modalities, including physical examination, comparison with estimated dry weight, and chest radiographs.
   b. **Electrolyte imbalances** including hyponatremia, hyperkalemia, hypocalcemia, hyperphosphatemia, and metabolic acidosis can be diagnosed with a comprehensive metabolic panel and arterial blood gas.
   c. **Anemia** can be assessed with a complete blood count. **Coagulopathy** arising from uremic platelet dysfunction is difficult to predict or quantify but should be anticipated.
   d. **Relevant medications** (at least of diuretics, antihypertensives, nephrotoxins, and any other renally cleared medication) and **dialysis type and schedule** should be confirmed.
   e. **Comorbid cardiovascular disease** may be assessed through history, physical examination, and electrocardiogram with additional testing (eg, echocardiography) as indicated.

D. Monitoring

1. **Standard monitors** (see **Chapter 15: Monitoring**) including continuous ECG display of leads II and V5 with ST segment analysis and temperature monitoring are required.
2. For patients with significant cardiac history, **intra-arterial, invasive blood pressure monitoring** may be necessary.
3. Intraoperative fluid management remains a challenge. Urine output will not be a reliable measurement of volume status intraoperatively. Traditionally, **central venous pressure** (CVP) or **pulmonary arterial pressure (PAP) monitoring** has been used. The use of **transesophageal echocardiography, arterial pulse waveform analysis,** and **thoracic electrical bioimpedance** has also been described. If a central line were not necessary nor

utilized and a CVP was desired to assess fluid status, one could transduce from a dedicated peripheral intravenous catheter (PIV), with only minor margin of error from the CVP (be sure to use a PIV that is not being used for infusions or drug access).

E. Preoperative management
1. **Peripheral venous access** should be established with two intravenous catheters in separate venous systems. One PIV catheter will be reserved for the administration of rabbit antithymocyte globulin with a filter.
2. For patients undergoing regular dialysis, it is important to confirm their most recent session as well as the method of dialysis (hemodialysis or peritoneal dialysis), and to assess their volume status. If a patient is deemed to be hypovolemic, **volume expansion** may be necessary prior to anesthetic induction with 250 to 500 mL of nonpotassium-containing isotonic fluid. A patient who is floridly hypervolemic may require **immediate, preoperative dialysis.**
3. It is essential to confirm that the patient has received **oral immunosuppressant** (usually mycophenate mofetil) prior to arrival to the operating room.
4. If there are no contraindications, patients should be consented for a **transversus abdominis plane block (TAP block)** that can be done at the conclusion of surgery or postoperatively for postoperative pain management. Neuraxial techniques are typically avoided owing to concern for uremic platelet dysfunction that will persist postoperatively.

F. Intraoperative management
1. **Rapid sequence induction** is indicated for patients receiving peritoneal dialysis, patients with a diagnosis of autonomic neuropathy, and should be considered, given the patient has taken oral immunosuppressant preoperatively. It may also be considered for patients taking glucagon-like peptide-1 receptor agonists (GLP1-RA) which may, if not stopped preoperatively, increase their risk of aspiration. Those with comorbidities such as gastroesophageal reflux disease (GERD), obesity, diabetes, or any disorder that may predispose to delayed gastric emptying.
2. For immunosuppression, **methylprednisolone** 125 to 250 mg is administered as a bolus after intubation followed by **rabbit antithymocyte globulin** 1.5 mg/kg over 6 hours via dedicated intravenous catheter with a filter. Lower-risk patients may receive basiliximab instead of thymoglobulin.
   a. Rabbit antithymocyte globulin can produce a cytokine release syndrome due to activation of T cells, manifesting in fevers, hypotension, and rigors, and more rarely, noncardiogenic pulmonary edema, acute respiratory distress syndrome, or other untoward complications. **Diphenhydramine** 50 mg is often given to reduce these risks.
3. **Maintenance anesthesia** can be established with either **volatile anesthetic** or **propofol**. **Processed electroencephalography** can be used to appropriately titrate the anesthetic.
4. **Analgesia** can be maintained with intermittent doses of nonrenally cleared opioids such as **fentanyl** or **hydromorphone**. Morphine and meperidine are contraindicated owing to the accumulation of active, renally cleared metabolites (morphine-6-glucuronide and normeperidine, respectively) (see Chapter 5: Specific Considerations With Renal Disease).
5. **Neuromuscular blockade** is best accomplished with **cisatracurium** owing to its organ-independent elimination.
6. The surgery typically takes **3 to 5 hours.** The procedure begins with a vertical curvilinear incision extending from the pubis symphysis to above

the anterior superior iliac spine. During incision and dissection, there is increased surgical stimulation and potentially exaggerated hemodynamic response. Analgesics, anesthetics, and relaxants should be used and titrated accordingly.
7. After exposure and mobilization, the external iliac vein is clamped and anastomosed to the donor renal vein. The external iliac artery is then clamped and anastomosed to the donor renal artery.
    a. In order to increase renal blood flow and promote allograft function, the mean arterial pressure (MAP) should be maintained in the range of **70 to 90 mm Hg or within 15% to 20% of the patient's preoperative baseline.**
8. **Intraoperative volume expansion** with isotonic crystalloid or albumin 5% and **titration of anesthetic agents** is favored over the administration of vasopressors owing to theoretical concern for graft malperfusion with alpha agonists.
    a. **Mannitol** (12.5 g) is often administered after the vascular anastomoses and prior to reperfusion to decrease the incidence of acute tubular necrosis in the allograft. A 0.2- to 5-micron filter is necessary before infusing mannitol to reduce the administration of the typically existing crystals in mannitol vials. **Furosemide** (60 to 100 mg) is also often administered at this time to promote diuresis after reperfusion.
    b. Rarely, removal of the vascular clamps is associated with significant blood loss requiring resuscitation and transfusion.
9. The donor ureter is then implanted into the recipient bladder, which is filled with antibiotic saline irrigation solution. The surgeon will request that the Foley be clamped prior to retrograde infusion of a methylene blue solution into the bladder to check for leaks.
10. It is **essential that neuromuscular blockade is maintained** until surgical closure of the abdominal fascial layer owing to the risk of damage to the vascular anastomoses with coughing or other unexpected movement.
11. The majority of patients are **extubated** in the operating room and taken to a typical postanesthesia care unit for recovery.

G. Postoperative management
1. **Urine output is strictly monitored.** Suspected hypovolemia is managed with volume resuscitation. Ureteral obstruction, vascular thrombosis, and hemorrhage are managed with early surgical re-exploration.
2. **Delayed graft function**, defined as a need for dialysis within 7 days of transplant, is a common complication with a rising incidence due to the increasing use of marginal donor organs. In addition to urine output monitoring, patients should have a basic metabolic panel postoperatively to check for electrolyte imbalances that may require immediate dialysis.
3. Analgesia can be achieved with oral or IV analgesic medications. If inadequate, **patient-controlled analgesia** with intravenous fentanyl or hydromorphone can be administered. Morphine and meperidine are still avoided owing to the accumulation of renally excreted toxic metabolites. Nonsteroidal anti-inflammatory drugs are also avoided owing to nephrotoxicity. **TAP blocks,** mentioned earlier, if consent was obtained preoperatively, may reduce postoperative opioid requirements.

III. ANESTHESIA FOR PANCREAS TRANSPLANTATION
A. Indications and recipient selection
1. The goal of pancreas transplantation is to **restore euglycemia and halt the progression of diabetic complications** in patients who are unable to produce insulin owing to dysfunction of the beta cells of the pancreas.

2. Pancreas transplantation is most commonly performed as a **simultaneous kidney–pancreas transplant** or **pancreas after kidney transplant** for patients with ESRD and type 1 diabetes mellitus. Select patients with insulin-dependent type 2 diabetes mellitus may also be candidates for pancreas transplantation.
3. **Pancreas transplant alone** is generally reserved for patients with severe complications of type 1 diabetes mellitus including a history of frequent severe metabolic complications (eg, diabetic ketoacidosis) and failure of exogenous insulin therapy to prevent these complications.
4. **Islet cell transplantation** is an experimental therapy wherein islet cells from a deceased donor pancreas are harvested and then injected percutaneously into the portal vein.
5. In 2023, 62 pancreas transplants and 810 kidney–pancreas transplants were performed in the United States. The 5-year survival rates are estimated at greater than 91.9% and 87.3% for type I and type II diabetes, respectively.

B. Preanesthetic considerations
1. Preoperative evaluation for the patient with pancreatic disease is discussed in **Chapter 7:** Specific Considerations With Endocrine Disease.
2. For patients presenting for pancreatic transplant, we recommend a tailored evaluation including at least the following:
    a. **Macro- and microvascular complications of diabetes** should be confirmed by history and physical examination. Special attention should be paid to cardiac, neurologic, and renal comorbidities. Patients with **comorbid ESRD** presenting for dual kidney–pancreas transplant should be evaluated as described in the prior section in addition.
3. **Acute metabolic abnormalities** such as diabetic ketoacidosis or hypoglycemia can be identified with a basic metabolic panel and frequent blood glucose measurements.
4. **Recent insulin administration and baseline insulin requirements** should be assessed and documented. If the patient has an insulin pump, especially a patient with type 1 diabetes mellitus, the surgical, anesthesia, and often endocrinology teams should discuss if the pump will remain in situ and on during surgery or when to disconnect the pump intraoperatively during explantation and transplantation.

C. Monitoring
1. **Standard monitors** (see Chapter 15: Monitoring) including continuous ECG display of leads II and V5 with ST segment analysis and temperature monitoring are recommended.
2. For patients with a significant cardiac history, **intra-arterial, invasive blood pressure monitoring** may be necessary.
3. Owing to the necessity of frequent intraoperative glucose monitoring, a **glucometer** or an intra-arterial catheter must be available.

D. Preoperative management
1. **Peripheral venous access** should be established with two intravenous catheters in two separate venous systems. One catheter should be reserved for the administration of an immunosuppression induction agent, most often rabbit antithymocyte globulin, to be infused with a filter.
2. It is essential to confirm that the patient has received oral immunosuppressant prior to arrival in the operating room.
3. Patients may benefit from the preoperative placement of a **thoracic epidural** at the T5–T8 level if there are no contraindications. In patients with significant comorbid renal disease or who are undergoing a kidney–pancreas transplant, neuraxial anesthesia may be deferred

owing to concern for uremic platelet dysfunction. A postoperative **TAP block** is a reasonable alternative and preoperative consent should be obtained.

E. Intraoperative management

1. **Rapid sequence induction** is recommended owing to the expected risk of gastroparesis from long-standing diabetes, the increasing frequency at which longstanding diabetic patients are receiving GLP1-RAs, increasing aspiration risk, and the administration of an oral immunosuppressant preoperatively.
2. Immediately after intubation, **methylprednisolone** 125 to 250 mg is administered as a bolus, followed by **rabbit antithymocyte globulin** 1.5 mg/kg over 6 hours via dedicated PIV with a filter.
3. **Maintenance anesthesia** can be maintained with either volatile anesthetic or propofol infusion.
4. **Analgesia** is usually accomplished with intermittent opioid dosing or epidural anesthesia/analgesia.
5. **Neuromuscular blockade** is best accomplished with cisatracurium or rocuronium depending on their renal function.
6. **Insulin and dextrose (D5W or D10W) infusions** should be titrated to maintain blood glucose levels of **110 to 180 mg/dL** to prevent hyperglycemia-induced islet cell dysfunction intraoperatively.
7. Case length is typically **3 hours** for a pancreas transplant and **up to 6 hours** for a combined kidney–pancreas transplant. A midline surgical incision is used for both procedures during this surgery. After dissection and mobilization, three anastomoses for the donor pancreas must be performed: (1) **arterial**, typically from the recipient iliac artery; (2) **venous**, typically to the recipient iliac vein; and (3) **exocrine**, most commonly to the intestine or bladder.
   a. Following allograft perfusion, pancreatic beta cells begin secreting insulin within 5 minutes. **Blood glucose levels** should be assessed **every 15 minutes** for the first hour after reperfusion, then **every 30 minutes** thereafter.
   b. To promote graft perfusion after reperfusion, **intraoperative volume expansion** with isotonic crystalloid or albumin 5% and **titration of anesthetic agents** is favored over the administration of vasopressors owing to theoretical concern for graft malperfusion with alpha agonists.
   c. Rarely, there is significant blood loss associated with the vascular anastomoses requiring resuscitation and transfusion.
8. It is essential that **neuromuscular blockade is maintained** until the abdominal fascial layer is closed owing to the risk of damage to the vascular anastomoses with coughing or other unexpected movement.
9. The majority of patients **are extubated** in the operating room and taken to a typical postanesthesia care unit for recovery.

F. Postoperative management

1. **Blood glucose and electrolytes are strictly monitored.** Exogenous insulin is administered as necessary for delayed graft function, defined as hyperglycemia exceeding 180 to 200 mg/dL.
2. Technical failures such as pancreatic thrombosis, leaks, and bleeding may require imaging or early reoperation.
3. In the absence of a working thoracic epidural, pain control is generally achieved with **patient-controlled analgesia** with intravenous hydromorphone or morphine (dependent on their renal function, and not if they underwent a kidney–pancreas transplant), or the aforementioned TAP blocks if consented preoperatively.

IV. ANESTHESIA FOR LIVER TRANSPLANTATION
A. Introduction
1. In 2022, 9527 liver transplants were performed in the United States from 8924 deceased donors and 603 from living donors. There were also 800 liver–kidney transplants performed in 2022.
2. The 5-year survival is estimated at approximately 80% and over 80% for recipients of cadaveric and living grafts, respectively.

B. Indications for liver transplantation include, but are not limited to:
1. Acute fulminant hepatic failure (highest priority).
2. Cirrhosis with evidence of portal hypertension and markers of serious decompensation including variceal hemorrhage, ascites, hepatic encephalopathy, hepatorenal syndrome, portopulmonary hypertension, and hepatopulmonary syndrome. Etiologies include chronic hepatitis B or C, alcoholic liver disease, biliary cirrhosis, cryptogenic cirrhosis, autoimmune hepatitis, hemochromatosis, nonalcoholic steatohepatitis.
3. Hepatocellular carcinoma (HCC), stage I or II.
4. Budd–Chiari syndrome (hepatic vein thrombosis).
5. Sclerosing cholangitis.
6. Biliary atresia and inborn errors of metabolism.

C. Recipient selection
1. Priority on the liver transplant waitlist is based on a patient's **Model for End-Stage Liver Disease (MELD)** score, an objective and accurate predictor of short-term survival in patients with cirrhosis. The MELD score is derived from the patient's **serum bilirubin, serum creatinine, and international normalized ratio.** For patients who are on hemodialysis, the score is calculated using a serum creatinine value of 4 mg/dL. For patients with a MELD score greater than 11, the serum sodium concentration is also factored in to yield the **MELD-Na score**, which reflects the vasodilatory state in cirrhosis and predicts mortality independent of the MELD score.
2. Exception points
   a. Certain conditions are associated with a higher mortality than reflected in the MELD score. Patients with **stage I or II HCC, hepatopulmonary syndrome, portopulmonary hypertension**, and **hereditary hemorrhagic telangiectasia** receive **exception points** in addition to their calculated MELD score that lead to higher prioritization on the waitlist.
   b. Patients with other complicating medical conditions related to their liver disease but not qualifying for standard MELD exception points may **petition** for additional points.

D. Preanesthetic considerations
1. Preoperative evaluation for the patient with liver disease is discussed in **Chapter 6:** Specific Considerations With Liver Disease.
2. Preoperative testing is typically initiated at a MELD score of **10 to 15 points.** The goals of this assessment are to determine the extent of **hepatic dysfunction**, to screen for cardiac, pulmonary, and renal **comorbidities** unique to cirrhotic patients, and to evaluate for potential **posttransplantation survival.** The decision to list a patient is based on the review of the test results by a **multidisciplinary committee** that includes liver transplant anesthesiologists.
3. For cardiac clearance, each patient is screened for **structural heart disease, coronary artery disease**, and **portopulmonary hypertension.**
   a. Our institution's approach for patients under age 50 years is to acquire a **transthoracic echocardiogram**, with special attention paid

to the estimated right ventricular systolic pressure (RVSP), right ventricular function, and right ventricular size. Contrast-enhanced echocardiography may be employed to identify intrapulmonary shunting. **Right heart catheterization** is necessary for any patient with elevated RVSP to ascertain the mean pulmonary arterial pressure (mPAP) and pulmonary vascular resistance (PVR). The RVSP cutoff varies by institution but is usually either **40 or 50 mm Hg.**
- b. **Portopulmonary hypertension** is defined by an mPAP greater than 25 mm Hg, pulmonary capillary wedge pressure (PCWP) less than 15 mm Hg, and a PVR greater than 240 dynes/s/cm^5.
- c. Patients with an **mPAP greater than 35 mm Hg or a PVR greater than 250 dynes/s/cm^5** have a 36% mortality rate within 18 days of transplantation.
- d. Patients over age 50 years or with significant cardiac risk factors undergo **dobutamine stress echocardiography** to assess cardiac function in response to an elevated heart rate. For patients on a beta-blocker who are unable to mount a heart rate response, we obtain a **nuclear stress test** with a coronary vasodilator. **Cirrhotic cardiomyopathy** is a syndrome defined by increased cardiac output and contractility at rest with a blunted contractile response and/or diastolic dysfunction with stress.
4. For preoperative pulmonary assessment, we acquire **pulse oximetry, pulmonary function testing,** and **arterial blood gas testing** for age-adjusted alveolar–arterial gradient.
- a. **Hepatopulmonary syndrome** is defined by a triad of portal hypertension with or without cirrhosis, arterial hypoxemia (Pao$_2$ less than 60 to 80 mm Hg with room air at rest in a sitting position), and the presence of intrapulmonary shunts. These patients can also demonstrate severe platypnea and orthodeoxia on physical exam. The degree of hypoxemia is directly related to perioperative mortality.
5. **Chest** and **abdominal imaging** is generally required to rule out the presence of occult malignancy and to assess the presence of any anatomic barriers to transplantation. **Multiphase contrast-induced computed tomography or contrast-enhanced magnetic resonance imaging** is preferred to assess hepatic vasculature and stage HCC, if present.
6. **Upper endoscopy** is performed to assess for the presence of significant esophageal varices or if prior varices were treated, that those are stable, and there are no new varices requiring treatment.

E. Monitoring
1. **Standard monitors** (see **Chapter 15: Monitoring**) including continuous ECG display of leads II and V5 with ST segment analysis and temperature monitoring, are required.
2. **Intra-arterial, invasive blood pressure monitoring** is essential both for hemodynamic management and frequent laboratory draws intraoperatively.
3. **Pulmonary arterial catheter monitoring** is frequently used to assess PAP and cardiac output intraoperatively.
4. **Transesophageal echocardiography** is increasingly used to assess intraoperative cardiac output and chamber function, particularly in the presence of cirrhotic cardiomyopathy or other preexisting cardiac disease. It is necessary to first exclude significant esophageal variceal disease. If it is safe to proceed and varices are not limiting the use of transesophageal echocardiography, consent the patient preoperatively.

F. Preoperative management
1. At least one **large-bore PIV** should be established. Insertion of a short 7.5-French catheter may be considered for rapid infusion within that PIV site. The left arm is preferred for placement as the right arm is often tucked. The largest catheter should be attached to a rapid transfusion system capable of delivering resuscitative fluids or blood products at up to 1.0 to 1.5 L/min at 38 °C.
2. An intra-**arterial catheter** is placed on the left arm. We suggest the ultrasound-guided single-puncture technique to avoid the through-and-through technique in the setting of cirrhosis-associated coagulopathy. Emphasis on successfully obtaining intra-arterial access on the first attempt is highlighted by the high probability that the patient's other arm may be tucked and inaccessible or a patient may have a fistula if concurrent ESRD, limiting the options for intra-arterial access. Brachial–arterial access can be done in the setting of cirrhosis-associated coagulopathy, but is not recommended unless the anesthesiologist is experienced in both the placement of these lines (institution and anesthesiologist dependent), the risks associated with brachial arterial access, and its risk of hematoma if the catheter is not removed correctly in this patient population.
3. **Blood products** should be ordered prior to induction in anticipation of significant bleeding during the initial stages of surgery. Blood loss during a liver transplant is highly variable, ranging from 500 mL to several patient blood volumes. A number of variables have been associated with increased transfusion during liver transplantation, including (but not limited to) the **severity of liver disease, history of prior abdominal procedures**, and **cold ischemic time** of the donor organ. Knowledge of the patient blood antibody status and the ability to cross-match large volumes of blood are critical. We suggest starting with the following:
   a. **5 to 10 units of packed red blood cells** in the room and **10 units crossed and available when needed.**
   b. **5 to 10 units of fresh frozen plasma** in the room and **10 units crossed and available when needed.**
   c. **Five aliquots of 5% albumin** (250 mL each). If 5% albumin in 250 mL bags is not available, one could dilute 25% albumin and give an equivalent dose.
4. It is essential to confirm that the patient has received oral immunosuppressant (usually mycophenate mofetil) prior to arrival in the operating room.

G. Intraoperative management
1. **Induction. Rapid-sequence induction** is advised owing to the preoperative administration of oral immunosuppressants and the presence of ascites.
2. **Maintenance anesthetic** is most often established with a balanced technique including a volatile anesthetic and opioid administration. In the setting of even mild hepatic encephalopathy, a lower concentration of anesthetic is often sufficient and can be titrated using processed electroencephalography.
3. **Central venous access** with a central venous catheter (CVC) should be established for drug administration as well as monitoring of CVP. Depending on the adequacy of peripheral volume access and expected blood loss, a single- or double-lumen 9-French cannula may be inserted. Our institution utilizes venovenous bypass (VVBP) for liver transplants; if a need for VVBP is anticipated, a 15-French VVBP inflow cannula can

be inserted ideally in the right internal jugular vein (RIJV), even accompanying a RIJV CVC.
4. The ideal agent for **neuromuscular blockade** is cisatracurium owing to its organ-independent elimination and the often underappreciated proportion of rocuronium metabolism that relies on the biliary system, which is often deficient in liver failure patients. However, rocuronium may be used with careful train-of-four monitoring. Liver failure produces a large volume of distribution that may lead to delayed onset and recovery from neuromuscular blockade.
5. **Preanhepatic stage**
   a. The total case length is typically **6 to 8 hours.**
   b. The preanhepatic stage begins with the **bisubcostal (Chevron) incision** and ends with **cross-clamping of the portal vein.** The diseased liver is dissected and mobilized.
   c. If **VVBP** is being used, the surgical team will place outflow cannulas in the femoral and portal veins. Bypass is initiated prior to the anhepatic phase.
   d. During the preanhepatic stage, the most common problem encountered is **hypotension.**
   e. **Drainage of large-volume abdominal ascites** can be managed with anticipatory administration of colloid-containing fluid to minimize changes in preload.
   f. **Bleeding** is related to the degree of preexisting coagulopathy, presence and severity of portal hypertension, and duration and complexity of surgical procedure (eg, severe adhesions).
   g. **Compression of the inferior vena cava** with the manipulation of the liver during dissection can lead to hypotension owing to a reduction in venous return.
   h. Along with hemodynamic monitoring, the patient's hemoglobin and metabolic status should be assessed at regular and frequent intervals.
   i. **Methylprednisolone 250 mg** is given for immunosuppression when the recipient's liver is removed.
6. **Anhepatic stage**
   a. The anhepatic stage begins with **portal vein cross-clamp** and ends with **graft reperfusion.** The recipient liver and a portion of the inferior vena cava is removed, and the donor liver is inserted with caval and portal anastomoses.
   b. Approaches (**Figure 25.1**)
      1. In the **bicaval or "classic" technique,** the suprahepatic and infrahepatic cava are clamped prior to removal of the liver. To preserve venous return, **VVBP** allows diversion of blood flow from the recipient's inferior vena cava and portal vein to the axillary vein and attenuates the decrease in preload. However, the use of VVBP incurs risks including postoperative acute renal failure, air embolism, thromboembolism, and inadvertent decannulation.
      2. If the VVBP technique is utilized, after initiation, if the patient becomes hypotensive with caval cross-clamping, the VVBP flows should be increased to maintain adequate venous return. If the flows cannot be increased ("line chatter"), additional volume should be administered to the patient.
      3. Instead, if the **"piggyback" technique is utilized,** a side-biting clamp is placed across the base of the hepatic vein, preserving caval flow and venous return. The suprahepatic cava of the donor liver is then anastomosed to the base of the hepatic vein.

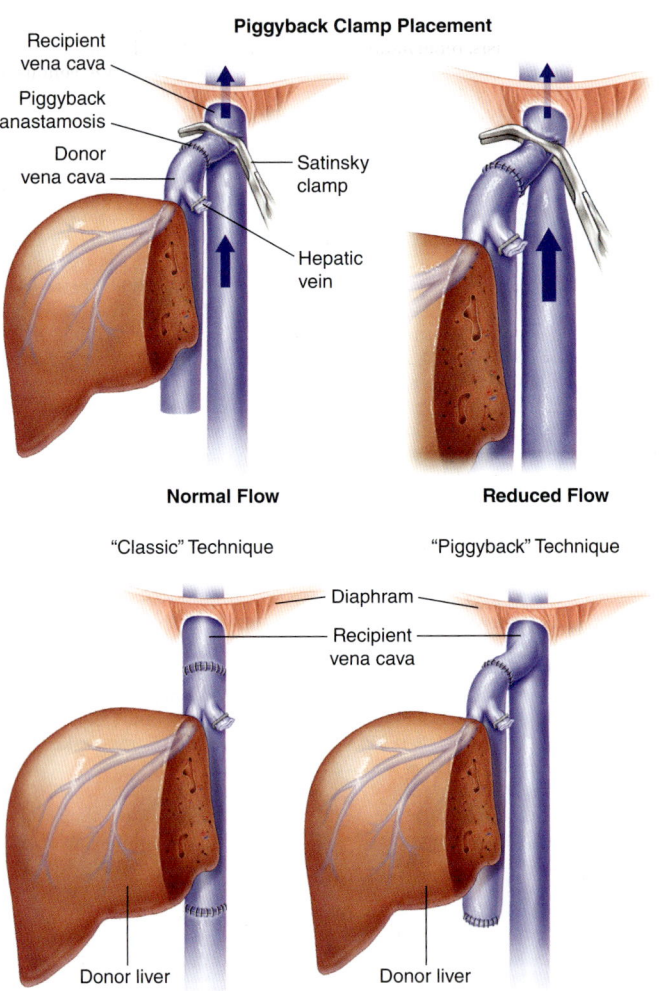

FIGURE 25.1 "Classic" versus piggyback technique for donor liver implantation.

This technique preserves the recipient's inferior vena cava and avoids the VVBP.
4. **Fibrinolysis** may occur during the anhepatic stage owing to the unopposed action of tissue plasminogen activator in circulation.
5. Hypocalcemia may occur as citrate, a component of blood product transfusion, is not metabolized with the complete absence of hepatic function. Citrate chelates with calcium reducing its serum concentration. Serum ionized calcium less than 1.0 mg/dL is typically treated with 100 to 200 mg of calcium chloride given slowly as bolus or infusion.

6. Metabolic acidosis may develop in patients with preexisting acidosis, renal failure, or a prolonged anhepatic phase.
7. **Reperfusion** is defined as the release of portal venous clamp following completion of caval anastomosis and portal venous anastomosis.
8. Prior to completion of the anastomosis and graft reperfusion, the donor liver is flushed into the field to wash out the preservative solution. It may be flushed with a colloid/crystalloid solution or with blood through the portal vein.
9. Reperfusion is associated with hypotension, hyperkalemia, acidemia, and arrhythmias. **Postreperfusion syndrome** is defined as a >30% decrease in MAP lasting over 1 minute and occurring within 5 minutes of reperfusion. It is estimated to occur in 15% to 30% of patients. Typical management includes the administration of vasopressors and volume.
10. **Hyperkalemia** with reperfusion should be managed with calcium chloride, insulin (and a glucose source), hyperventilation, furosemide, and albuterol dependent on patient comorbidities.

7. **Neohepatic stage**
   a. This stage begins following **graft reperfusion** and ends with **abdominal closure**. The primary considerations for anesthetic management are the treatment of coagulopathy and fibrinolysis and the maintenance of low CVP.
   b. **Fibrinolysis**, caused by rising tissue plasminogen activator from graft endothelial cells, is often managed with the administration of fresh frozen plasma, cryoprecipitate, and platelets as guided by **frequent laboratory testing, thromboelastography, or thromboelastometry**. In cases of profound coagulopathy, infusion of antifibrinolytic agents such as aminocaproic acid or tranexamic acid may be necessary.
   c. **Volume resuscitation** is carried out in a judicious manner to target a **CVP <10 mm Hg** to prevent hepatic congestion and graft dysfunction.

H. **Postoperative management**
   1. Patients are transported to the **intensive care unit (ICU)** upon completion of surgery. If clinically stable and fluid shifts or blood loss permit, patients may be extubated in the operating room prior to transport.
   2. Immediate complications of liver transplantation include **postoperative bleeding, biliary leaks, graft dysfunction**, and **vascular thromboses (hepatic artery or portal vein)** that may require emergent reoperation in the postoperative period.

V. ANESTHESIA FOR ORGAN PROCUREMENT
A. **Types of donors**
   1. **Donation after brain death (DBD)** donors are patients who have had a terminal neurologic insult and have been declared brain dead in accordance with the American Academy of Neurology guidelines and any institutional policies.
   2. **Donation after cardiac death** (DCD) donors are patients who have had a terminal neurologic insult but do not meet criteria for brain death. Death is declared based on cardiopulmonary criteria after life support is withdrawn. A period of 5 minutes is allowed to elapse prior to procurement to ensure no autoresuscitation.
   3. **Living donors** are patients who willingly donate an organ, most often a kidney. Living liver donation can occur with left lateral segment or lobe donation to a pediatric recipient or a right lobe to an adult recipient.

a. Living organ donation boasts improved survival rates, reduced wait times to transplant, and opportunity to electively schedule and plan for surgery. However, it presents a significant **ethical challenge** as it is the only surgery from which a patient derives no benefit for the risk they take.
   b. Living liver donations should involve a liver transplant anesthesiologist who is familiar with the anesthetic considerations for dissection and mobilization of the hepatic segment, which can present significant risk to the donor.
 B. Preanesthetic considerations for DBD procurement
   1. For the purposes of our discussion, we will focus on the **DBD donor** presenting for organ procurement as these cases directly involve the anesthesiology team and present unique challenges.
   2. Brain death precipitates a number of **profound physiologic changes** affecting nearly every organ system, as summarized in **Table 25.2**.
 C. Preoperative management for DBD organ procurement
   1. PIV access should be established with at least two large-bore PIV catheters in each arm.
   2. Intra-arterial, invasive pressure monitoring is preferred owing to the high chance of hemodynamic instability and the potential need for laboratory draws during the dissection and procurement.
   3. CVC access should be established for dynamic measurement of CVP and vasopressor administration.
   4. Pulmonary arterial catheter monitoring may be indicated.
 D. Intraoperative management for DBD procurement
   1. Neuromuscular blockade is necessary to inhibit spinal motor reflexes.
   2. Analgesia via intravenous opioids and a low to moderate dose of volatile anesthetic is often employed to minimize hemodynamic response to incision.
   3. A **lung-protective ventilator strategy** with tidal volumes of 6 to 8 mL/kg of ideal body weight, positive end-pulmonary pressure of <10 mm Hg (depending on patient factors), and peak inspiratory pressures below 35 cm H_2O is recommended. There may be more involved lung

	Pathologic Changes in Donation After Brain Death Donors by Organ System

Organ System	Pathology
Pulmonary	• Increased pulmonary capillary permeability • Pulmonary edema
Cardiovascular	• Profound vasoplegia • Myocardial injury • Hypovolemia • Autonomic storming
Hematologic	• Coagulopathy progressing to disseminated intravascular coagulation
Endocrine	• Pituitary infarction leading to diabetes insipidus, adrenal insufficiency, and hypothyroidism • Insulin resistance leading to hyperglycemia

Adapted by permission from Springer: Anderson TA, Bekker P, Vagefi PA. Anesthetic considerations in organ procurement surgery: a narrative review. *Can J Anaesth*. 2015;62(5):529–539. Copyright © 2015 Springer Nature.

4. **Hemodynamic goals** of systolic blood pressure greater than 100 mm Hg and <180 mm Hg, CVP of 4 to 8 mm Hg, MAP greater than 70 mm Hg, and heart rate of 60 to 120 bpm are accomplished with the use of **continuous vasopressor infusions, vasodilator infusions, and boluses** as needed. Vasopressin is the vasopressor of choice as it both raises systemic vascular resistance and treats diabetes insipidus, which is often seen after brain death.
5. In the presence of significant diabetes insipidus, **intravascular volume replacement** is necessary with administration of colloids such as albumin 5% or packed red blood cells (for a hemoglobin goal of greater than >7 g/dL) preferred over balanced crystalloids. Synthetic colloids are avoided entirely. **Desmopressin (ddAVP)** (1 to 4 μg every 6 hours intravenously) may also be employed for diabetes insipidus treatment.
6. **Heparin** is delivered immediately prior to **thoracic and abdominal aortic cross-clamping.** After this, the organs are cooled and removed in the following order: heart, lung, liver, pancreas, and kidneys.
7. After aortic cross-clamping, the anesthesiologist closes the intraoperative record and turns off the ventilator as well as all ongoing infusions.

ACKNOWLEDGMENTS

We gratefully acknowledge the contributions of previous edition author(s), Elisa C. Walsh and Hovig V. Chitilian, as portions of those chapters have been retained in this revision.

Suggested Readings

Anderson TA, Bekker P, Vagefi PA. Anesthetic considerations in organ procurement surgery: a narrative review. *Can J Anesth.* 2015;62:529–539.

Aniskevich S, Perry D. Anesthesia for pancreas transplantation. *Pancreatic Dis Ther.* 2013;3:1–3.

Carton EG, Plevak DJ, Kranner PW, Rettke SR, Geiger HJ, Coursin DB. Perioperative care of the liver transplant patient. Part I and II. *Anesth Analg.* 1994;78(2):382–399.

Deshpande R, Chadha RM. Tutorial 377. Anaesthesia for orthotopic liver transplantation. In: Doane MA, Poon C, eds. *Anesthesia Tutorial of the Week.* 2018. Accessed March 29, 2020. https://resources.wfsahq.org/wp-content/uploads/377_english.pdf

Gruessner RWG, Gruessner AC. The current state of pancreas transplantation. *Nat Rev Endocrinol.* 2013;9:555–562.

Krowka M, Wiesner RH, Heimbach JK. Pulmonary contraindications, indications, and MELD exceptions for liver transplantation: a contemporary view and look forward. *J Hepatol.* 2013;59(2):367–374.

Moers C, Pirenne J, Paul A, Ploeg RJ; Machine Preservation Trial Study Group. Machine perfusion or cold storage in deceased-donor kidney transplantation. *N Engl J Med.* 2009;360:7–19.

Organ Procurement and Transplantation Network (OPTN). U.S. Department of Health and Human Services. Last updated March 29, 2020. Accessed March 29, 2020. https://resources.wfsahq.org/wp-content/uploads/377_english.pdf

Schmid S, Jungwirth B. Anesthesia for renal transplant surgery: an update. *Eur J Anaesthesiol.* 2012;29:552–558.

Steadman RH. Anesthesia for liver transplant surgery. *Anesthesiol Clin North Am.* 2004;22:687–711.

Steadman RH, Wray CL. Anesthesia for abdominal organ transplantation. In: Miller RD, ed. *Miller's Anesthesia.* 8th ed. Elsevier; 2015:2262–2289.

TransMedicsOCS: Science That Mirrors life. TransMedics; 2020. Accessed April 5, 2020. https://www.transmedics.com/ocs-hcp/

United Network for Organ Sharing (UNOS). 2020. Accessed April 1, 2020. https://unos.org/

Xia V, Steadman RH. Anesthesia for organ procurement. In: Miller RD, ed. *Miller's Anesthesia*, 8th ed. Elsevier; 2015:2262–2289.

Anesthesia for Abdominal Surgery
Scott Cao and J. Paul Fleming

I. PREANESTHETIC CONSIDERATIONS

Patients undergoing abdominal surgery necessitate a complete history and physical examination as outlined in Chapter 1: Evaluating the Patient Before Anesthesia. Additional concerns germane to abdominal surgery should be considered including:

A. Volume status. Surgery in the abdomen has the potential to cause severe derangements in volume status and fluid homeostasis. These derangements causes are multifactorial, and their assessment can be difficult.

1. Assessment of volume status

a. Orthostasis, inferior vena cava (IVC) ultrasound assessment and clinical signs including dry mucous membranes, decreased skin turgor or mottling, and delayed capillary refill may suggest hypovolemia or dehydration. Jugular venous distention, and lower extremity swelling can indicate hypervolemic states.

b. Laboratory analysis of base excess or deficit, hematocrit, serum osmolality, BUN (blood urea nitrogen) to creatinine ratio, serum and urine electrolyte concentrations, and urine output may be helpful in estimating volume deficits.

c. Dynamic hemodynamic monitoring may also be considered to guide assessment of intravascular volume status. Under positive pressure mechanical ventilation, pulse pressure variation (PPV) and systolic pressure variation (SPV) obtained from an arterial catheter waveform may aid in estimating volume responsiveness. Generally, a delta-down component of 5 mm Hg for SPV or PPV greater than 13% is indicative of volume responsiveness. Traditional assessments of volume status including central venous pressure (CVP) and pulmonary artery occlusion pressures may provide additional context to guide intraoperative fluid management.

2. Etiologies of hypovolemia

a. Preoperative fasting, reduced oral intake, malabsorption, gastrointestinal tract dysmotility, active bleeding, and bowel preparation may predispose a patient to hypovolemia or dehydration in the perioperative period.

b. Emesis, gastric drainage, or diarrhea may produce significant fluid and electrolyte derangements. Monitoring the quantity, quality, and frequency of output is recommended.

c. Distributive shock common can result from severe intra-abdominal pathologies including sepsis and pancreatitis. Volume resuscitation is the recommended first-line treatment of distributive shock.

d. Bleeding from the gastrointestinal tract may be occult and include sources like ulcers, neoplasms, esophageal varices, diverticula, angiodysplasia, and hemorrhoids.

e. Sequestration of fluid may occur either into the bowel lumen from ileus or into the interstitium from peritonitis.

f. Fever increases insensible fluid loss.

B. **Metabolic derangements** occur frequently in patients requiring emergency abdominal surgery. Hypokalemic, hypochloremic metabolic alkalosis is common in patients with large gastric losses (emesis or nasogastric [NG] tube drainage). Severe diarrhea, hypovolemia, or septicemia may cause profound metabolic acidosis.

C. **Length of surgery** is influenced by the history of previous abdominal surgery, intra-abdominal infection, radiation therapy, steroid use, surgical technique, and surgeon experience.

D. **All patients for emergency abdominal procedures should be considered as high risk for aspiration and induced as a "full stomach."** A rapid sequence induction (RSI) is indicated with the goal of minimizing aspiration risk. Cricoid pressure is an area of active controversy with respect to its role and efficacy in minimizing aspiration. Premedication with histamine (H_2) antagonists and oral nonparticulate antacids may decrease gastric acidity.

II. ANESTHETIC TECHNIQUES

A. **General anesthesia (GA)** is the most commonly employed technique.
  1. Advantages particularly relevant to abdominal surgery include airway protection, control of ventilation parameters, and use of neuromuscular blockade to relax abdominal wall musculature.
  2. Disadvantages include loss of airway reflexes necessitating advanced airway management, which increases the risk of aspiration upon induction and emergence, and potential hemodynamic instability.

B. **Monitored anesthesia care (MAC)** describes a spectrum of anesthesia that ranges from anxiolysis to deep sedation without the need for advanced airway management. For abdominal surgeries, MAC is often employed with other analgesic modalities such as surgeon-administered local anesthetics. For example, various hernia repairs can be accomplished under this technique (local anesthetic with sedation).

C. **Regional anesthetic techniques** for abdominal surgery include neuraxial anesthetics and peripheral nerve blocks performed on the trunk. The abdominal wall is innervated via the anterior divisions of the thoracolumbar nerves (T6–L1). The abdominal viscera innervation arises from cervical, thoracic, lumbar, and sacral spinal levels. Regional techniques can be used as a primary anesthetic or as a complementary technique such as when an epidural or a nerve block is used as an adjuvant to GA. For example, umbilical and inguinal hernia repairs can be performed under neuraxial anesthesia with no additional sedation. Significant intraoperative and postoperative analgesia can be achieved by decreasing the need for opioids.
  1. **Neuraxial anesthesia** involves the administration of local anesthetics and adjuvant medications into the epidural or intrathecal spaces via single injection or catheter placement for continuous infusion. These blocks have the benefit of providing muscle relaxation and profound analgesia to the abdominal wall and viscera. Neuraxial techniques are contraindicated due to concerns for infection, anticoagulation or coagulopathy, severe spinal stenosis, severe peripheral nerve disease, intracranial hypertension, expected hemodynamic instability after loss of sympathetic tone or patient refusal.
     a. Spinal anesthesia is usually performed with a single, lumbar, intrathecal injection. Block coverage and duration is determined by the choice of local anesthetic and adjuvants (see Chapter 20: Spinal, Epidural, and Caudal Anesthesia).
     b. Epidural anesthesia is usually performed with a continuous catheter technique.

c. Paravertebral blocks are performed most commonly in the thoracic spine by injection into the paravertebral space to provide unilateral anesthesia to the dorsal and ventral rami of the spinal nerve and the sympathetic chain. Multiple unilateral and/or bilateral injections may be required.
d. Caudal anesthesia is performed via single-dose injection or catheter placement through the sacral hiatus into the epidural space most commonly in infants. This technique provides analgesia for infraumbilical procedures.
2. **Peripheral Nerve blocks** primarily provide anesthesia to the abdominal wall and are most commonly used as adjuvant techniques for postoperative analgesia. They may be performed awake, or more commonly just prior to emergence (postprocedure) from GA. The nerve blocks can provide significant intraoperative and postoperative analgesia, creating an opioid-sparing technique. Peripheral nerve blocks can often be employed when neuraxial techniques are contraindicated due to bleeding, hemodynamic, or infectious concerns.
   a. **Types**
      1. **TAP blocks** can be used for most lower abdominal procedures, often as an alternative for epidural anesthesia. A regional needle is placed in the anterior axillary line, between the costal margin and the iliac crest. The local anesthetic spreads between the transversus abdominis and internal oblique muscle planes. Catheters are often used for TAP blocks to provide postoperative analgesia, providing a significant opioid-sparing effect.
      2. **Rectus sheath blocks** are appropriate for midline procedures, particularly periumbilical procedures. Local anesthetic is deposited via a regional needle between the rectus muscle and posterior rectus sheath.
      3. **Erector spinae plane (ESP) block** is a paraspinal fascial plane block where local anesthetic is deposited between the erector spinae muscle and thoracic transverse process to anesthetize the dorsal and ventral rami of the spinal nerve providing somatic and visceral coverage. Local anesthetic spread of up to four spinal levels above and below the block location inside this facial plane can result in a unilateral, multidermatomal sensory blockade of the thoracic and abdominal walls.
   b. **Advantages**
      1. If awake for the procedure, patients maintain the ability to communicate symptoms (eg, chest pain).
      2. Airway reflexes are maintained.
      3. Profound muscle relaxation after neuraxial anesthesia optimizes surgical exposure.
      4. Sympathectomy after neuraxial anesthesia increases blood flow to the bowel.
      5. Continuous catheter techniques provide a ready means for postoperative analgesia.
      6. Regional techniques are opioid sparing.
      7. There is some evidence to support earlier return of bowel function in patients with prolonged postoperative ileus when epidural catheters are used for postoperative analgesia.
   c. **Disadvantages**
      1. Local anesthetic toxicity from inadvertent IV injection or rapid absorption.
      2. Patient cooperation is necessary for the institution of block and positioning during surgery.

3. Primary block failure necessitates intraoperative conversion to GA.
4. Regional nerve blockade may be contraindicated in patients with abnormal bleeding profile or localized infection at the site of injection.
5. Sympathectomy with neuraxial techniques may lead to vaso/venodilation and bradycardia that can precipitate profound hypotension, especially in patients who are hypovolemic. Unopposed parasympathetic activity causes the bowel to contract and may make construction of bowel anastomoses more difficult; this can be reversed with glycopyrrolate, 0.2 to 0.4 mg IV, or 1 mg glucagon.
6. Blockade of upper thoracic nerves may compromise pulmonary function in patients reliant on accessory muscles.
7. Awake patients often require frequent communication and reassurance; this may distract the anesthesiologist during complicated cases.
8. Upper abdominal procedures (above the umbilicus at T10) are unlikely to be well tolerated under regional anesthesia alone. Spinal or epidural anesthesia for upper abdominal procedures may necessitate a sensory level of T2–T4. Although minute ventilation is maintained, paralysis of intercostal muscles from a high thoracic level impairs deep breathing, often resulting in an intolerable sensation of dyspnea. Intraperitoneal air or upper abdominal exploration commonly generates a dull pain referred to the C5 dermatomal distribution (usually over the shoulders) requiring supplemental intravenous (IV) analgesics.

D. A combined technique makes use of a regional technique along with a general anesthetic or MAC. This technique is often employed for extensive abdominal surgeries when an epidural and general anesthetic are used, or to avoid the need for GA such as an ESP or paravertebral block combined with MAC for a liver nodule microwave ablation. In either case, utilization of a regional technique will decrease intraoperative anesthetic requirements and postoperative pain.

III. MANAGEMENT OF ANESTHESIA
A. Standard monitors are used as described in Chapter 15: Monitoring.
B. Induction of anesthesia
   1. Restoration of volume deficits prior to induction should be considered.
   2. RSI or awake intubation is indicated for all patients considered to have full stomachs. This includes conditions in which gastric emptying is delayed, intra-abdominal pressure is increased, or lower esophageal tone is compromised. Examples include trauma, bowel obstruction or ileus, hiatal hernia, gastroesophageal reflux disease, pregnancy beyond the first trimester, significant obesity, ascites, and diabetes with gastroparesis and autonomic dysfunction. Preinduction NG tube placement should be considered in such cases.

C. Intraoperative management
   1. Fluid replacement is guided by clinical judgment and may be aided by invasive monitoring. Traditionally, extended operative cases with significant bowel exposure and preoperative hypovolemia have necessitated fluid replacement of up to 10 to 15 mL/kg/h. Emerging evidence, though, suggests that a more restrictive approach to fluid resuscitation may be associated with faster recovery and fewer complications.
   2. A "protocol-based" strategy for fluid administration is claimed to reduce impairment of bowel motility, cardiopulmonary complications, and bowel edema. It may also improve anastomosis healing and reduce

hospital length of stay (LOS). Currently, no clear consensus exists on definitions or protocols for fluid-restrictive strategies. Literature has been published measuring multiple parameters including volume of fluid, perioperative weight, and hemodynamic responsiveness. A deliberate and planned strategy for intraoperative fluid administration on a case-by-case basis seems to be the most prudent approach.
- a. Bleeding may be estimated both by direct observation of the surgical field and suction traps and by weighing sponges. Blood loss may be concealed (eg, beneath drapes or within the patient) and labs should be checked as clinically indicated.
- b. Insensible losses may range from 0.5 to 1 mL/kg/h for larger abdominal cases.
- c. In spite of an overnight NPO period, blood volume is possibly near normal in many patients, and perceived fluid deficits may not necessitate IV fluid repletion. Clinical judgment will guide the need for resuscitation prior to starting the case.
- d. Abrupt drainage of ascitic fluid with surgical entry into the peritoneum has the potential to cause acute hypotension from a sudden decrease of intra-abdominal pressure and pooling of blood in mesenteric vessels, reducing venous return to the right heart. Postoperative reaccumulation of ascitic fluid may produce significant intravascular fluid losses.
- e. NG and other enteric drainage should be quantified and replaced appropriately.

3. Fluid losses should be replaced with crystalloids, colloids, or blood products.
   - a. Initially, fluid should be replaced by administration of an isotonic salt solution. When an isotonic crystalloid solution is used to replace blood loss, goal-directed therapy and fluid responsiveness is likely more optimal than traditional 3:1 replacement. Evidence suggests that aggressive normal saline resuscitation may cause non–anion gap metabolic acidosis.
   - b. Colloids are fluids with particles large enough to exert oncotic pressure with the theory of remaining in the intravascular space longer than crystalloids. Multiple studies comparing fluid resuscitation with crystalloids to colloids have reported no benefit with colloids. Colloid solutions are more expensive than crystalloids, and routine use may not be justified. Albumin may be superior to crystalloid in certain patients including significant burns, hepatorenal disease, or acute lung injury. Hydroxyethyl starch solutions (eg, Hextend or Hespan) are non–blood-derived colloids that are rarely used methods of volume expansion due to their deleterious effects on renal function, coagulation, and potentially all-cause mortality.

4. Muscle relaxation is required for all but the most superficial abdominal procedures. Sufficient relaxation is critical for abdominal closure as bowel distention, edema, and organ transplantation may increase the volume of abdominal contents.
   - a. Titrating relaxants to obtain a single twitch by train-of-four monitoring is generally sufficient for surgical closure and allows for reversal of muscle relaxants for extubation.
   - b. Potent inhalational agents are synergistic with muscle relaxants in blocking neuromuscular conduction.
   - c. Flexing the operating table may decrease tension on transverse abdominal and subcostal incisions and facilitate surgical closure

without the need for profound muscular relaxation as may be requested by the surgeons.
5. Use of nitrous oxide (N_2O) may cause bowel distention as N_2O diffuses into the bowel lumen. The amount of distention depends on the concentration of N_2O delivered, blood flow to the bowel, and duration of N_2O administration. Under normal conditions, the initial volume of bowel gas is small; doubling or tripling of this volume does not pose a significant problem. Studies have shown that N_2O may be used in lower fractions and shorter (<3 hours) open and laparoscopic surgeries, without causing clinically significant bowel distention. Use of N_2O is relatively contraindicated in bowel obstruction because the initial volume of bowel gas may be large. Abdominal surgical procedures are associated with an increased risk of postoperative nausea and vomiting (PONV). N_2O is associated with increased risk of PONV, correlating with concentration and duration of administration.
6. NG tubes are frequently placed in the perioperative period.
    a. Preoperative placement is indicated for decompression of the stomach, especially in trauma victims and patients with bowel obstructions. Although suction via a large-bore NG tube may reduce the volume of gastric contents, they should not be assumed to completely evacuate the stomach. Alternatively, they may facilitate aspiration by stenting open the lower esophageal sphincter and compromise mask fit.
    b. Intraoperative placement is required to drain gastric fluid and air during abdominal surgery. During laparoscopic surgery, stomach decompression is necessary to avoid injury during trocar placement. NG and orogastric tubes should never be inserted with excessive force. Lubrication and head flexion facilitate insertion. Tubes can be directed into the esophagus by using a finger within the oropharynx or using Magill forceps under direct visualization with a laryngoscope.
    c. Complications of NG tube insertion include bleeding, submucosal dissection of the retropharynx, and placement in the trachea. Intracranial placement has been described in patients with basilar skull fracture. The NG tube should be secured carefully to avoid excessive pressure on the nasal septum or nares, as this may cause ischemic necrosis.
    d. As discussed in the previous section, the need for a gastric tube should be discussed with the surgeon, as placement for elective procedures is not recommended in many cases.

D. Enhanced recovery after surgery (ERAS)
ERAS is a concept of multimodal evidence-based care designed to enhance postoperative recovery and optimize patients for discharge. Core tenets center on a continuum of preoperative, intraoperative, and postoperative pathway strategies.

Current literature suggests that ERAS protocols may be associated with reduced hospital LOS, faster recovery, reduced overall morbidity and nonsurgical complications, and similar rates of readmission compared to traditional care. As most ERAS pathways are instituted as a "bundle" there is a paucity of evidence as to which elements of a specific bundle are more or less meaningful than others.

E. Notable highlights of ERAS protocols for elective colorectal surgery are discussed in the section that follows. Specific components continue to be increasingly mapped to ERAS protocols for other surgeries.

1. Minimization of preoperative fasting. Clear liquids and carbohydrate drinks are encouraged up to 2 hours before surgery. Modifications may be based on disease state (eg, bowel obstruction).
2. Avoidance of routine preoperative sedative premedications due to the potential impairment of postoperative psychomotor function and ability to mobilize and begin PO intake.
3. Avoidance of routine mechanical bowel preparation due to adverse physiologic effects related to dehydration and association with prolonged ileus and spillage of bowel contents.
4. Avoidance of routine postoperative NG tubes to minimize patient discomfort and delay in time to oral intake. NG tubes placed intraoperatively should be removed prior to emergence.
5. Intraoperative maintenance of normothermia.
6. Intraoperative fluid management strategy continues to be an area of active research and debate. Goal-directed fluid management guided by administration of fluid to a physiologic objective is a cornerstone of ERAS protocols but the specific goals continue to be ill-defined. Noninvasive methods of measuring cardiac output, stroke volume, and stroke volume variation may be employed, with no evidence currently suggesting any method as being superior or better than rational management by clinical judgment.
7. Minimization of postoperative fluids to maintain normovolemia and minimize fluid overload.
8. Use of multimodal analgesia to reduce opioids thus facilitating early postoperative ambulation and rehabilitation. This includes regional techniques and utilization of preoperative oral medications such as acetaminophen and celecoxib.
9. Administration of multiple medications for prophylaxis against PONV in accordance with patient risk factors.

IV. ANESTHETIC CONSIDERATIONS FOR SPECIFIC ABDOMINAL TECHNIQUES AND PROCEDURES

A. **Laparoscopic surgery.** Laparoscopic approaches are utilized for a wide variety of surgical procedures including appendectomy, cholecystectomy, hernia repair, hysterectomy, fundoplication, nephrectomy, bariatric surgery, liver resection, and bowel resection. Benefits of laparoscopic surgery include smaller incisions, reduced postoperative pain, decreased postoperative ileus, early ambulation, and shorter hospital LOS.
  1. GA is usually required for laparoscopy. Creation of pneumoperitoneum and steep Trendelenburg positioning may compromise ventilatory function and are generally not tolerated in an awake patient under neuraxial anesthesia.
  2. Operative technique involves intraperitoneal insufflation of CO_2 through a needle or trocar inserted into the abdomen via a small incision. Insufflation typically increases intra-abdominal pressure to 12 to 15 mm Hg. Pneumoperitoneum creation has multiple anesthetic considerations.
     a. Hemodynamic changes occur in response to volume and pressure of insufflated CO_2. Mean arterial pressure and systemic vascular resistance generally increases with the creation of pneumoperitoneum due to catecholamine release and activation of the renin–angiotensin system. Alternatively, peritoneal stretching can trigger a vagally mediated bradycardic response. Increased intra-abdominal pressure can cause compression of the vena cava and other venous structures

decreasing cardiac preload. Hypovolemic patients or those with coexisting cardiac disease may be susceptible to the physiologic effects of pneumoperitoneum and manifest with decreased cardiac output and hypotension.
   b. Absorption of CO_2 across the peritoneal surface typically causes hypercarbia and acidosis, thus increasing sympathetic nervous system stimulation and decreasing cardiac contractility.
   c. Reduction in functional residual capacity (FRC) associated with GA is compounded by the creation of pneumoperitoneum, and FRC may be further compromised by the Trendelenburg position and patient body habitus. Frequent recruitment and titration of positive end-expiratory pressure (PEEP) may be necessary to mitigate against alveolar collapse.
   d. Embryonic channels between the peritoneal and pleural or pericardial cavities may open with increased intraperitoneal pressure, resulting in pneumomediastinum, pneumopericardium, and pneumothorax. Diffusion of gas cephalad from the mediastinum may lead to subcutaneous emphysema of the face and neck.
   e. Vascular or other internal organ injuries due to incorrect introduction of the needle or trocar may produce sudden blood loss and necessitate conversion to an open procedure and vascular repair to control bleeding.
   f. Clinically significant venous gas embolism is rare but may occur on induction of pneumoperitoneum if the needle or trocar is placed into a vessel or abdominal organ, or if gas is trapped in the portal circulation. The high capacity of blood to absorb CO_2 and rapid elimination in the lungs increases the margin of safety in cases of accidental IV injection of CO_2. Insufflation of gas under high pressure can lead to an "air lock" in the vena cava and right atrium; this will decrease venous return and cardiac output and produce circulatory collapse. Embolization of gas into the pulmonary circulation leads to increased dead space, ventilation–perfusion mismatch, and hypoxemia. Systemic gas embolization (with occasionally devastating effects on cerebral and coronary circulation) may occur with massive gas entrainment or via a patent foramen ovale. Treatment is supportive and includes immediate cessation of gas insufflation, increasing FiO_2 to minimize hypoxemia, positioning the patient in steep head-down left-lateral decubitus to displace gas from the right ventricular outflow tract (see Chapter 17: Intra-anesthetic Problems), and inotropic right ventricular support.
3. Trendelenburg or reverse Trendelenburg positioning is often necessary to facilitate operative exposure.
   a. Attention to cardiovascular function with positioning in steep Trendelenburg or reverse Trendelenburg is essential due to change in venous return. Carbon dioxide pneumoperitoneum may have synergistic deleterious cardiovascular and respiratory effects.
   b. In Trendelenburg positioning, abdominal contents are translocated cephalad with a corresponding reduction of FRC and lung compliance. Patients may be prone to ventilation–perfusion mismatch, increased peak airway pressures, and atelectasis.
   c. CVP, pulmonary artery pressure, and pulmonary capillary wedge pressure are increased and correspond to the degree of head-down tilt. Arterial vasculature compression increases systemic and pulmonary vascular resistance.

d. Swelling of the face and upper airway may be seen with the steep and prolonged positioning. A restrictive fluid management strategy may be beneficial. A small period of reverse Trendelenburg at the end of the case may allow venous drainage of airway structures and may be particularly helpful in patients with difficult airways on induction.
   4. IV and radial artery access may be limited by draping and position of the patient. Pelvic procedures are generally performed with the arms tucked as the surgeons stand at the patient's shoulders while foregut procedures can be performed with the shoulders abducted.
B. **Robotic surgery** is utilized as a telemanipulator technique in surgical specialties with the goal of affording the surgeon a higher degree of precision and control with purported benefits of decreased hospital LOS and improved postoperative recovery.
   1. Advantages of the robotic systems include true three-dimensional depth perception and magnification of the operative field. In addition, the system filters natural hand tremors and scales movements for precision work. Compared to laparoscopic surgery, the surgeon is afforded a cumulative six degrees of freedom of movement.
   2. Anesthetic considerations and management
      a. Robotic surgery often entails steep Trendelenburg or reverse Trendelenburg positioning and intraperitoneal insufflation, which has the potential for serious physiologic derangements as discussed above. Patients with coexisting cardiovascular, respiratory, intraocular, or central nervous system pathology may be considered for alternative approaches.
      b. Any lines, monitors, or patient-protective devices must be placed and secured beforehand as access to the patient is limited after robot positioning and engagement. Depending on the robotic model and equipment, the position of the operating table may need to be maintained stationary throughout the procedure.
      c. Deep neuromuscular blockade must be maintained until the robot is undocked at the end of the procedure. A continuous infusion of a nondepolarizing neuromuscular blocking agent may be indicated. The robotic arms have minimal flexibility, and any movement has the potential for serious morbidity to organs and vasculature. Sugammadex may be indicated to reverse deep neuromuscular blockade in a timely fashion.
      d. Vigilant assessment of patient positioning and padding is imperative as the patient is often in a steep position for several hours.
      e. Shoulder supports and other patient-protective devices for securing the patient on the operating table during steep positioning may create suboptimal conditions for airway access on induction.
C. **Esophageal surgery** for gastroesophageal reflux disease can be performed via either an abdominal approach (see below) or a thoracic approach.
   1. Fundoplication surgery is a common treatment for reflux disease. It involves wrapping the fundus of the stomach around the lower part of the esophagus. This creates a collar in which intragastric pressure serves to constrict the wrapped esophagus rather than push the gastric contents into the esophagus. Hiatal hernias, if present, are repaired at the time of surgery. This procedure is often performed using laparoscopic techniques to decrease the duration of postsurgical hospitalization.
      a. Anesthetic considerations. This procedure is performed most commonly with GA or combined GA-epidural (for open procedures).

Patients who come to surgery often have been treated medically with proton pump inhibitors, H_2-receptor antagonists, or prokinetic agents. These should be continued until the day of surgery. An RSI is likely indicated because of the high risk of gastroesophageal reflux and the potential for aspiration.

    b. An esophageal bougie may be placed to calibrate fundoplication; this ensures an adequate esophageal lumen to minimize postoperative dysphagia. The stomach or esophagus may be perforated by passage of the bougie or NG tube. Correct angulation of the esophagus or stomach during this maneuver is extremely important in preventing injury. The dilator or NG tube should be passed slowly and should be directly visualized. Particular attention should be paid to patients with esophageal strictures.

D. Gastric surgery for gastric cancer, lymphoma, and uncontrolled bleeding is usually performed with combined GA epidural. The high likelihood of aspiration in these patients necessitates rapid-sequence intubation.

  1. Gastrectomy or hemigastrectomy with gastroduodenostomy (Billroth I) or gastrojejunostomy (Billroth II) is usually performed for gastric adenocarcinoma, lymphoma, or intractable bleeding from gastric or duodenal ulcers. Rarely, it is necessary in Zollinger–Ellison syndrome.

  2. Gastrostomy tube placement can be performed through a small upper abdominal incision or percutaneously with an endoscope. Local anesthesia with sedation is often adequate in the debilitated elderly patient, although some require GA.

E. Intestinal and peritoneal surgery. Indications for small bowel resection include infection, penetrating trauma, Crohn disease, obstructing adhesions, Meckel diverticulum, carcinoma, and infarction (from volvulus, intussusception, or thromboemboli). Patients are often hypovolemic and are considered to have a full stomach.

  1. Appendectomy is performed through a small lower abdominal incision or via laparoscopy. IV hydration before induction is indicated because fever, poor oral intake, and vomiting may produce hypovolemia. GA with rapid-sequence intubation is generally indicated. TAP blocks may be opioid sparing and can be considered as an adjuvant for this procedure.

  2. Colectomy or hemicolectomy is used to treat colon cancer, diverticular disease, Crohn disease, ulcerative colitis, trauma, ischemic colitis, and abscess. Emergency colectomy on unprepared bowel carries a risk of peritonitis from fecal contamination. Some emergencies involving the colon are treated with an initial diverting colostomy, followed later by bowel preparation and elective colectomy. Patients must be evaluated for hypovolemia, anemia, and sepsis. All emergency colectomies and colostomies should be treated as if at risk for aspiration. Combination general/regional anesthetics are common, although epidural analgesia use is decreasing with laparoscopic techniques and the intraoperative use of adjuvants.

  3. Perirectal abscess drainage, hemorrhoidectomy, and pilonidal cystectomy are relatively noninvasive and brief procedures. Pilonidal cysts are excised with patients positioned prone; abscess drainage and hemorrhoidectomy can be performed in either a prone or a lithotomy position. If GA is used, deep planes of anesthesia or the use of muscle relaxants may be necessary to achieve adequate sphincter relaxation. Hyperbaric spinal anesthesia can be used for procedures in the lithotomy position, whereas a hypobaric technique is useful for the flexed

prone (jackknife) or knee–chest position. A caudal block may be performed for either position.
  4. Inguinal, femoral, or ventral herniorrhaphies can be performed under local anesthesia, regional anesthesia (spinal, epidural, caudal, or nerve block), MAC, GA, or a combination of these techniques. Maximum stimulation and profound vagal responses may occur during spermatic cord or peritoneal retraction. Communication with surgeons is important, as they may need to reduce traction if necessary. Techniques to minimize coughing on emergence that can strain the repair are indicated, and deep extubation can be considered in patients where it is not contraindicated (ie, difficult mask airway, difficult intubation, high risk of aspiration, etc.).
  5. **Hyperthermic intraperitoneal chemotherapy (HIPEC)** is an intraoperative adjuvant therapy after cytoreduction surgery to treat peritoneal carcinomatosis. Surgical resection is accomplished via a large midline laparotomy. Subsequently, high temperature chemotherapy agents are instilled into a closed abdominal cavity and continuously circulated over 1 to 2 hours via an extracorporeal system. During treatment, careful attention must be paid to the patient body temperature, metabolic derangements, and fluid losses. The patient must be actively cooled with forced cool air, ice packs, and cooled fluids. Arterial access should be established to allow frequent blood sampling for electrolyte monitoring. Finally, fluid shifts and losses are common after HIPEC. Patients will require aggressive resuscitation continuing into the postoperative setting.

F. Hepatic surgery
  1. Partial hepatectomy is performed for hepatoma, unilobar metastasis of a carcinoma, arteriovenous malformation, or echinococcal cysts. Extensive hemorrhage should be anticipated and standard monitors are supplemented with placement of arterial and large-bore IV access and/or central venous catheters. Blood loss during hepatic parenchymal division can be reduced by temporary occlusion of portal venous and arterial inflow at the level of the hepatic pedicle (Pringle maneuver). Low CVP techniques have been shown to reduce blood loss during the case and improve survival. The CVP is generally kept in the range of 2 to 5 mm Hg. CVP essentially represents the back pressure which causes bleeding during the resection, since there are no valves between the right atrium and the liver. Fluids should be restricted with a goal of maintaining a nonzero urine output and an acceptable blood pressure (variable depending on the patient). If fluid restriction is not adequate, nitrates and opioids can be used as well. Resuscitation of the patient occurs after the resection is completed and hemostasis has been achieved. This can be guided by signs of hypovolemia such as the respiratory variation of arterial systolic pressure, arterial PPV, cardiac output, CVP, and stroke volume variation. The normal liver has considerable reserve, and extensive resection is required before clinical impairment of drug metabolism is evident. The effects of liver disease on anesthetic management are discussed in Chapter 6: Specific Considerations With Liver Disease. Epidural or paravertebral catheters can be placed in patients with normal coagulation status.
  2. Transjugular intrahepatic portosystemic shunts (TIPS) procedure has replaced portacaval or splenorenal shunt procedures for patients with portal hypertension because of superior outcomes. The procedure entails access of internal jugular vein (most on the right side). A shunt between portal vein and hepatic vein will be created after verifying the

position with both contrast and pressure measurement. TIPS procedure can be performed under MAC, but is usually performed under GA. Although the anesthetic for a TIPS is simple, a high-level vigilance is required because of potential bleeding.

G. Biliary tract procedures
1. Cholecystectomy is a common procedure performed via either open laparotomy or laparoscopic techniques. GA is favored for either technique. During laparoscopic cholecystectomy, the patient is placed in a steep reverse Trendelenburg position, and the gallbladder is dissected from the liver bed by using either cautery or laser. The amount of hemorrhage is difficult to assess because of the limited field of view and high magnification of the laparoscope; heavy bleeding from the cystic or hepatic arteries may occur.
2. Biliary drainage procedures include transduodenal sphincteroplasty for extensive choledocholithiasis; cholecystojejunostomy for distal common bile duct obstruction from pancreatic cancer; and choledochojejunostomy for chronic pancreatitis, stone disease, and benign strictures of the distal bile duct. Endoscopic and transhepatic techniques are increasingly common, but open surgical drainage is occasionally required.

H. Pancreatic surgery
1. Although the initial treatment of acute pancreatitis is supportive, surgical intervention may be necessary for complications of pancreatitis. Surgical management is indicated for infected pancreatic necrosis and hemorrhagic pancreatitis unresponsive to resuscitation with blood products and correction of coagulopathy. Pancreatic pseudocysts may require drainage either surgically or via endoscopy. The cyst may be anastomosed to a Roux-en-Y limb of jejunum, the posterior wall of the stomach, or duodenum. Surgical intervention can produce significant bleeding and third-space fluid losses. In severe acute pancreatitis, activation of inflammatory mediators can produce sepsis and multiple organ dysfunction that require fluid resuscitation, mechanical ventilation, and vasopressor support.
2. Pancreaticojejunostomy with gastrojejunostomy and choledochojejunostomy (Whipple procedure) is typically performed for resection of adenocarcinoma of the pancreas, malignant cystadenoma, or refractory pancreatitis confined to the head of the pancreas. These procedures have a high potential for hemorrhage and fluid loss often necessitating arterial line and large-bore IV access placement. Epidural catheters and other regional techniques such as paravertebral blocks are generally helpful for postoperative pain control in the absence of contraindications. Intraoperative neurolytic celiac plexus blocks can be used in unresectable cases where significant postoperative pain is expected.

I. Splenectomy
may be performed emergently after blunt or penetrating trauma or electively for the treatment of idiopathic thrombocytopenic purpura or Hodgkin lymphoma. GA and muscle relaxation are required. Large-bore IV access is necessary because major blood loss requiring transfusion can be encountered. A combined epidural and general anesthetic technique is appropriate with the caveat that a sympathectomy may significantly potentiate hypotension from hemorrhage. Occasionally, a transthoracic approach to gain control of the hilar vessels of a very large spleen may be necessary. Splenectomy patients should receive polyvalent pneumococcal vaccine in the postoperative period.

J. Intraoperative radiation therapy for pancreatic, colonic, or other carcinomas may be performed during laparotomy for primary resection or tumor debulking. Specially designed operating rooms have been constructed to facilitate intraoperative radiotherapy. The patients must be hemodynamically stable and have a stable ventilatory status as they are monitored by remote television outside the radiation area. Aortic or IVC compression may occur when the sterile cone of the radiation therapy device is positioned in the abdominal wound. Ventilation with 100% oxygen can maximize the sensitivity of the tumor to radiation therapy. Treatments usually last just a few minutes and can be interrupted in the event of problems with hemodynamics or ventilation. Wound closure is performed after the radiation therapy is complete, and any necessary anastomoses are made.

K. Surgery for the obese patient. As the prevalence of obesity in the US population continues to rise, the perioperative management of the obese patient is increasingly relevant. Obesity is defined by the body mass index (BMI) and is calculated as follows: BMI = body weight (kg)/height (m^2). Patients are typically defined as obese if BMI exceeds 30 kg/m^2.

1. **Preanesthetic considerations**
   a. Obese patients have increased circulating blood volume and cardiac output to meet increased oxygen consumption. Depressed left ventricular function related to left ventricular hypertrophy may be seen even in young asymptomatic patients and is often correlated to the duration of obesity.
   b. Obese individuals have an increased risk for cardiovascular disease and may require additional cardiac evaluation or consultation to optimize management in the perioperative period.
   c. Respiratory system compliance is decreased in obesity due to reduced chest wall compliance. FRC and expiratory reserve capacity are also likely to be reduced. In the supine position, FRC may be less than the closing volume, leading to ventilation–perfusion mismatch and hypoxemia. The higher metabolic demand of the obese person results in increased oxygen consumption and CO_2 production, necessitates an increase in minute ventilation to maintain normocapnia.
   d. Increased submucosal fat in the pharynx increases collapse of the hypopharynx with normal sleep, thus predisposing to obstructive sleep apnea. Long-standing hypoxemia may result in pulmonary hypertension and right heart failure. Obstructive sleep apnea increases the risk of perioperative complications and screening may be accomplished with validated tools including the STOP-Bang questionnaire.
   e. Increased gastric emptying time resulting in high residual gastric contents despite appropriate preprocedure NPO time is common. This is exacerbated by GLP-1 agonists such as semaglutide and tirzepatide, commonly prescribed for diabetes management and weight loss. Gastric ultrasound can be used to assess the volume of gastric contents.
   f. Elevated intra-abdominal pressure and volume predisposes to a higher incidence of symptomatic gastroesophageal reflux.
   g. Type 2 diabetes with hyperglycemia, hyperinsulinemia, and insulin resistance is common in obesity. Because perfusion of adipose tissue is variable, IV insulin infusions may be necessary to control hyperglycemia. Guidelines for the management of glucose and insulin are covered in Chapter 7: Specific Considerations With Endocrine Disease.

h. Airway management is a challenge in obesity including difficulty with intubation and mask ventilation. Careful assessment of neck and jaw mobility, inspection of the oropharynx, and examination of dental status are required. If intubation is expected to be difficult, an airway management strategy should be discussed and advanced airway management techniques should be considered.

i. Positioning of the upper body with the external auditory meatus in line with the sternal notch has been shown to provide a better view for direct laryngoscopy. This is often accomplished by making a "ramp" of blankets under the thorax, which facilitates alignment of the thorax with the trachea. In addition, a reverse Trendelenburg position should be used in morbidly obese patients to increase FRC and utilize gravity to displace soft tissue away from the neck and airway.

2. Surgical techniques. Bariatric surgery is currently the most effective treatment of morbid obesity. Patients with a BMI ≥40 kg/m^2 or with a BMI ≥35 kg/m^2 with obesity-related comorbidities may be candidates for surgery. Currently, two basic types of bariatric surgery are performed.

a. Vertical banded gastroplasty (gastric sleeve) produces a small gastric pouch that restricts the volume of food that can be ingested. Long-term weight loss may be limited by maladaptive eating patterns (liquids with high caloric content) or by staple line disruption. Gastroplasty procedures, particularly the laparoscopic sleeve gastrectomy, are popular due to lower complications than formal bypass procedures.

b. Roux-en-Y gastric bypass surgery consists of formation of a small gastric pouch and anastomosis of the pouch to the proximal jejunum. Weight loss occurs due to both a restrictive anatomy as well as decreased absorption of calories because of the bypassed small intestine. Patients who undergo this surgery may experience a "dumping" syndrome in which ingestion of high–energy-density food leads to nausea, abdominal cramping, and diarrhea. The Roux-en-Y gastric bypass is often performed laparoscopically.

3. Anesthetic management

a. Standard operating tables are often unable to accommodate the size and weight of the obese patient; tables specifically designed for obese patients should be used. Extra padding and skin protection are necessary even for short procedures.

b. Standard noninvasive monitoring is acceptable in obese patients without significant comorbidities. An appropriately sized blood pressure cuff is critical; a regular-sized cuff placed on the forearm may be more effective than an oversized cuff on the upper arm.

c. Obtaining IV access can be challenging due to the structure depth, making it difficult to see or palpate a target vein. IV catheters are more likely to infiltrate due to increased vein depth resulting in less angiocatheter within the vein and tissue mobility.

d. Regional and neuraxial anesthetic techniques may be challenging due to less defined anatomic landmarks. For neuraxial techniques, the midline of the spine may be more readily apparent in the sitting position than in lateral decubitus, thus facilitating catheter placement. Long epidural needles (5 inches) may be necessary. The volume of local anesthetic volume injected may need to be decreased in obese patients as they have reduced epidural space resulting from

adipose infiltration and increased blood volume in the epidural venous system.
  e. The combination of increased metabolic demand and decreased FRC leads to rapid desaturation with apnea. This is exacerbated in the supine position. Preoxygenation for a minimum of 3 to 5 minutes and targeting an end-tidal concentration of O_2 greater than 90% is recommended. Preoxygenation may be augmented by reverse Trendelenburg positioning and PEEP. Mask ventilation may be challenging and adequate gas exchange is often limited. Use of an oral or nasopharyngeal airway or two-person bag-mask technique is frequently required.
  f. Morbidly obese patients have greater reductions in lung volumes than nonobese patients on induction of GA. Physiologically, this manifests as increasing atelectasis, airway closure, and hypoxemia. Titration of PEEP may be necessary to counteract this.
  g. Drug dosing is a challenge and subject of controversy in the obese patient. Obese patients have increased total body weight (TBW) and lean body weight (LBW). However, the ratio of LBW to TBW decreases with increases in TBW. Physiologically, obese patients have increased cardiac output, total body volume, glomerular filtration rate (GFR), and regional alterations in blood flow that alter pharmacokinetics and pharmacodynamics. Generally, lipid-soluble drugs have an increased volume of distribution, but exceptions exist.
     1. In obese patients, LBW is highly correlated with cardiac output, which determines early distribution kinetics, and drug clearance. Most anesthetic drugs should be dosed by LBW.
     2. LBW is determined by individual's height and weight and is best determined in obese patients by a modified LBW equation: $LBW_{men} = [9 \times 103 \times body\ weight/7 \times 103 + (216 \times BMI)]$; $LBW_{women} = [9 \times 103 \times body\ weight/9 \times 103 + (244 \times BMI)]$.
     3. Induction doses of propofol should be based on LBW, and maintenance dosing should be based on TBW.
     4. Doses of opioids, including remifentanil, should be based on LBW.
     5. With increased amount of pseudocholinesterase and extracellular fluid, succinylcholine administration should be based on TBW.
     6. Nondepolarizing muscle relaxants should be dosed on ideal body weight.
  h. The patient should be extubated in the operating room when awake, with adequate cough reflexes, and after confirmation of adequate reversal of muscle relaxation. Because the supine position decreases FRC, obese patients should be placed in a sitting position as soon as possible. Patients requiring continuous positive airway pressure for sleep apnea can resume this treatment as soon as necessary.
  i. Postoperative intensive care or step-down unit should be considered for patients with severe coronary artery disease, poorly controlled diabetes, and severe sleep apnea. Studies have shown that patients who are male, older (>50 years), heavier (BMI > 60 kg/m^2), and who have complications requiring reoperation are more likely to need intensive care.

L. Recovery of organs for transplantation
  1. A significant gap exists between the supply of suitable donated organs and the demand for these organs to treat end-stage disease. To increase the donor pool, strict exclusion criteria (age and coexisting illnesses)

are no longer used. In addition, some centers use aggressive care regimens for potential donors to prevent common perturbations in homeostasis that accompany brain death. An alternative is the non–heart-beating donor, who does not meet brain death criteria but has such a poor prognosis that the family might consider withdrawing life support. A transplant coordinator from an organ procurement organization must screen all potential donors.

2. Organs may be deemed unsuitable based on donor age, organ injury, disease, or gross abnormalities.

3. Hormonal therapy using methylprednisolone, arginine vasopressin, and triiodothyronine can increase the number of successfully implanted organs and reduce graft dysfunction when administered to brain-dead donors who demonstrate resistance to conventional resuscitation as manifested by low cardiac output, inadequate organ perfusion, or worsening lactic acidosis.

4. Anesthetic management for harvesting organs should focus on optimizing organ perfusion and oxygenation. Volatile anesthetics may help to blunt spinal reflex, reduce the adrenergic storm, and provide some ischemic preconditioning to the vital organs, although studies have not been done to confirm clinical significance. Opioids will also help with reduction in response to stimulation.

   a. Dissection of organs usually occurs in the following order: heart (30 minutes), lungs (1 to 1.5 hours), liver (1 to 1.5 hours), pancreas (1 to 1.5 hours), and kidneys (30 minutes to 1 hour).

   b. Once all organs are mobilized, heparin (20,000 to 30,000 units IV in adult donors) is administered and the aorta is cross-clamped. The distal aorta and IVC are cannulated, and the harvested organs are perfused in situ, topically cooled, and exsanguinated via the IVC.

   c. Ventilatory support is discontinued after the aorta is cross-clamped, and the anesthesiologist's role is completed with the discontinuation of all monitoring and supportive care, except during heart and lung procurement.

   d. Non–heart-beating organ donation, also referred to as donation after cardiac death (DCD), is reserved for patients who are not declared brain dead but whose family has chosen to remove them from life support because their condition is considered "hopeless." Life-sustaining treatment (mechanical ventilation and vasopressors) is discontinued after the patient is prepared for surgery to remove the organs. Five minutes after asystole occurs, a physician who is not part of the transplant team declares death. The body is rapidly cooled with preservative solution via an aortic cannula, and the abdomen entered and organs removed expeditiously. This technique has the disadvantage of significant warm ischemia time before organ procurement begins. In addition, there are ethical debates about the appropriateness of interventions (heparin treatment) aimed at improving grafts before the donor's death. Usually, anesthesiologists are not involved in DCD. However, if the lungs are donated, an anesthesiologist may be asked to intubate the deceased and briefly ventilate.

5. Specific management problems

   a. Hypoxemia may be caused by atelectasis, pulmonary edema, aspiration, or pneumonia. The FiO_2 and minute ventilation should be adjusted to maintain a $PaO_2 \leq 100$ mm Hg and $PaCO_2 = 35$ to 45 mm Hg with pH 7.35 to 7.45. Arterial blood gases should be determined every

30 to 60 minutes. High levels of PEEP should be avoided to preserve cardiac output and avoid barotrauma. High FiO_2 should be avoided in potential lung donors to minimize possible oxygen toxicity.
   b. Poikilothermia is common, and early aggressive measures should be taken to minimize heat loss.
   c. Hypertension often transiently accompanies brain death and can be dramatic. Reflex hypertensive responses to surgical stimulation may occur. Short-acting agents such as nitroprusside or esmolol should be used, anticipating hypertension that is often more challenging to control during organ procurement.
   d. Hypotension is common and is due to a combination of hypovolemia and neurogenic derangement of vasomotor control. Central venous or pulmonary artery catheterization may be necessary to optimize filling pressures. Hypovolemia can be treated with crystalloid, colloid solutions, and blood products as necessary. Hematocrit should be maintained greater than 30%. After restoration of intravascular volume, a vasopressor such as dopamine, epinephrine, or norepinephrine may be necessary.
   e. Dysrhythmias occur frequently, especially in the setting of electrolyte imbalance, hypothermia, increased intracranial pressure, hypoxemia and acidosis, and derangement of brainstem cardiovascular control centers. Standard therapy is indicated. Bradycardia is often resistant to atropine and may require pacing therapy.
   f. Polyuria may be secondary to volume overload, osmotic diuresis, or the diabetes insipidus resulting from derangement of the hypothalamic–pituitary axis. An IV infusion of vasopressin or desmopressin may be titrated to treat severe diabetes insipidus (see Chapter 7: Specific Considerations With Endocrine Disease) and should be done in consultation with the surgical team. If used, it is prudent to discontinue these infusions 1 hour before aortic cross-clamping to minimize the risk of uneven distribution or ischemic injury with the infusion of preservative solution.
   g. Oliguria should be treated by ensuring adequate intravascular volume. Dopamine is preferred for the initial treatment of hypotension. A brisk diuresis is preferred when the kidneys are to be harvested. If volume repletion and vasopressors are not effective in restoring adequate urine output, mannitol and/or furosemide may be administered.

ACKNOWLEDGMENTS

We gratefully acknowledge the contributions of previous edition authors, David Hao and Triffin J. Psyhojos, as portions of those chapters have been retained in this revision.

Suggested Readings

Ahmad S, Nagle A, McCarthy RJ, Fitzgerald PC, Sullivan JT, Prystowsky J. Postoperative hypoxemia in morbidly obese patients with and without obstructive sleep apnea undergoing laparoscopic bariatric surgery. *Anesth Analg.* 2008;107(1):138–143.

Akca O, Lenhardt R, Fleischmann E, et al. Nitrous oxide increases the incidence of bowel distention in patients undergoing elective colon resection. *Acta Aanesthesiol Scand.* 2004;48:894–898.

Ballantyne JC, Carr DB, deFerranti S, et al. The comparative effects of postoperative analgesic therapies on pulmonary outcome: Cumulative meta-analyses of randomized, controlled trials. *Anesth Analg.* 1998;86:598–612.

Boldt J, Haisch G, Suttner S, Kumle B, Schellhaass A. Effects of a new modified, balanced hydroxyethyl starch preparation (Hextend) on measures of coagulation. *Br J Anaesth.* 2002;89:722–728.

Brodsky JB, Lemmens HJ, Brock-Utne JG, Vierra M, Saidman LJ. Morbid obesity and tracheal intubation. *Anesth Analg.* 2002;94(3):732–736.

Brodsky JB, Lemmens HJ, Collins JS, Morton JM, Curet MJ, Brock-Utne JG. Nitrous oxide and laparoscopic bariatric surgery. *Obes Surg.* 2005;15:494–496.

Chappell D, Jacob M, Hofmann-Kiefer K, Conzen P, Rehm M. A rational approach to perioperative fluid management. *Anesthesiology.* 2008;109(4):723–740.

Choi PT, Yip G, Quinonez LG, Cook DJ. Crystalloids vs. colloids in fluid resuscitation: a systematic review. *Crit Care Med.* 1999;27:200–210.

Corcoran T, Rhodes J, Clarke S, Myles PS, Ho KM. Perioperative fluid management strategies in major surgery: a stratified meta-analysis. *Anesth Analg.* 2012;114(3):640–651.

Doherty M, Buggy DJ. Intraoperative fluids: how much is too much? *Br J Anaesth.* 2012;109(1):69–79.

Ebert TJ, Shankar H, Haake RM. Perioperative considerations for patients with morbid obesity. *Anesthesiol Clin.* 2006;24(3):621–636.

Gridelli B, Remuzzi G. Strategies for making more organs available for transplantation. *N Engl J Med.* 2000;343:404–410.

Gustafsson UO, Scott MJ, Schwenk W, et al; Enhanced Recovery After Surgery (ERAS) Society, for Perioperative Care; European Society for Clinical Nutrition and Metabolism (ESPEN); International Association for Surgical Metabolism and Nutrition (IASMEN). Enhanced recovery after surgery society. Guidelines for perioperative care in elective colonic surgery: enhanced Recovery After Surgery (ERAS(®)) Society recommendations. *World J Surg.* 2013;37(2):259–284.

Hartog CS, Bauer M, Reinhart K. The efficacy and safety of colloid resuscitation in the critically ill. *Anesth Analg.* 2011;112:156–164.

Hebbard PD, Barrington MJ, Vasey C. Ultrasound-guided continuous oblique subcostal transversus abdominis plane blockade: description of anatomy and clinical technique. *Reg Anesth Pain Med.* 2010;35(5):436–441.

Huntington JT, Royall NA, Schmidt CR. Minimizing blood loss during hepatectomy: a literature review. *J Surg Oncol.* 2014;109:81–88.

Ingrande J, Lemmens HJ. Dose adjustment of the anaesthetics in the morbidly obese. *Br J Anaesth.* 2010;105(suppl 1):i16–i23.

Lobo SM, Ronchi LS, Oliveira NE, et al. Restrictive strategy of intraoperative fluid maintenance during optimization of oxygen delivery decreases major complications after high-risk surgery. *Crit Care.* 2011;15(5):R226.

Lowham AS, Filipi CJ, Hinder RA, et al. Mechanisms and avoidance of esophageal perforation by anesthesia personnel during laparoscopic foregut surgery. *Surg Endosc.* 1996;10:979–982.

McKeown DW, Bonser RS, Kellum JA. Management of the heart beating brain-dead organ donor. *Br J Anaesth.* 2012;108(suppl 1):i96–i107.

Molenaar IQ, Warnaar N, Groen H, Tenvergert EM, Slooff MJ, Porte RJ. Efficacy and safety of antifibrinolytic drugs in liver transplantation: a systematic review and meta-analysis. *Am J Transplant.* 2007;7:185–194.

Myles PS, Leslie K, Chan MT, et al; ANZCA Trials Group for the ENIGMA-II Investigators. The safety of addition of nitrous oxide to general anesthesia in at-risk patients having major non-cardiac surgery (ENIGMA II): a randomised, single blind trial. *Lancet.* 2014;384(9952):1446–1454.

Neligan PJ, Porter S, Max B, et al. Obstructive sleep apnea is not a risk factor for difficult intubation in morbidly obese patients. *Anesth Analg.* 2009;109(4):1182–1186.

Ogunnaike BO, Jones SB, Jones DB, Provost D, Whitten CW. Anesthetic considerations for bariatric surgery. *Anesth Analg.* 2002;95(6):1793–1805.

Patel T. Surgery in the patient with liver disease. *Mayo Clin Proc.* 1999;74:593–599.

Pelosi P, Ravagnan I, Giurati G, et al. Positive end-expiratory pressure improves respiratory function in obese but not in normal subjects during anesthesia and paralysis. *Anesthesiology.* 1999;91:1221–1231.

Qadan M, Akca O, Mahid SS, Hornung CA, Polk HC Jr. Perioperative supplemental oxygen therapy and surgical site infection: a meta-analysis of randomized controlled trials. *Arch Surg.* 2009;144:359–366.

Robertson KM, Cook DR. Perioperative management of the multiorgan donor. *Anesth Analg.* 1990;70:546–556.

Shenkman Z, Shir Y, Brodsky JB. Perioperative management of the obese patient. *Br J Anaesth.* 1993;70:349–359.

Sinha AC. Some anesthetic aspects of morbid obesity. *Curr Opin Anaesthesiol.* 2009;22(3): 442–446.

Spanjersberg WR, Reurings J, Keus F, van Laarhoven CJ. Fast track surgery versus conventional recovery strategies for colorectal surgery. *Cochrane Database Syst Rev.* 2011;(2):CD007635.

Strunden MS, Heckel K, Goetz AE, Reuter DA. Perioperative fluid and volume management: physiological basis, tools and strategies. *Ann Intensive Care.* 2011;1(1):2.

Tympa A, Theodoraki K, Tsaroucha A, Arkadopoulos N, Vassiliou I, Smyrniotis V. Anesthetic considerations in hepatectomies under hepatic vascular control. *HPB Surg.* 2012;2012: 720–754.

White PF. The changing role of non-opioid analgesic techniques in the management of postoperative pain. *Anesth Analg.* 2005;101(5 suppl):S5–S22.

Zhuang CL, Ye XZ, Zhang XD, Chen BC, Yu Z. Enhanced recovery after surgery programs versus traditional care for colorectal surgery: a meta-analysis of randomized controlled trials. *Dis Colon Rectum.* 2013;56(5):667–678.

Anesthesia for Thoracic Surgery

Henry K. Su and Xiaodong Bao

I. PREOPERATIVE EVALUATION AND PREPARATION

A. Patients scheduled for thoracic surgery should undergo the standard preoperative assessment as detailed in Chapter 1: Evaluating the Patient Before Anesthesia.
  1. Any patient undergoing elective thoracic surgery should be carefully screened for underlying bronchitis or pneumonia and treated appropriately before surgery.
  2. Patients with tracheal stenosis or mediastinal masses should be evaluated for signs or symptoms of positional dyspnea, static or dynamic airway collapse, and evidence of hypoxemia. The history may also suggest the probable location of the lesion.

B. An arterial blood gas (ABG) may help clarify the severity of underlying pulmonary disease but is not routinely necessary.

C. Pulmonary function tests (PFTs) are useful for assessing the pulmonary risk of lung resection.
  1. Preoperative PFTs should include spirometry and the diffusing capacity of the lungs for carbon monoxide (DLCO). Both the forced expiratory volume in 1 second (FEV1) and DLCO are independent predictors of outcomes after lung resection.
  2. If either of these values is less than 80% of the predicted, the patient's predicted postoperative FEV1 (ppoFEV1) and predicted postoperative DLCO (ppoDLCO) should be calculated.
  3. If both ppoFEV1 and ppoDLCO are ≥60%, then the patient is considered to be of low risk for surgery.
  4. If either is <60% but both are ≥30%, then the patient should undergo a stair-climbing test (SCT) or a shuttle walk test (SWT). If SCT is ≥22 m or SWT ≥25 shuttles, the patient is considered to be of low risk.
  5. If either ppoFEV1 and ppoDLCO are <30%, or performance on the SCT or SWT is not satisfactory, cardiopulmonary exercise test to calculate maximum oxygen consumption (Vo_2 max) is needed. Vo_2 max >20 mL/kg/min or >75% indicates low-risk, while Vo_2 max of <10 mL/kg/min or <35% is high-risk group, and surgery is not recommended. Vo_2 max 10 to 20 mL/kg/min or 35% to 75% indicates moderate-risk and Vo_2 max <10 mL/kg/min or <35% indicates high-risk group and surgery is not recommended.
  6. Quantitative ventilation/perfusion (V/Q) scan can also be used to calculate ppoFEV1 in patients scheduled to undergo pneumonectomy.

D. Cardiac screening should be conducted in accordance with the ACC/AHA guidelines for noncardiac surgery (see Chapter 3: Specific Considerations for Patients With Cardiac Disease). **Cardiac function** should be assessed if there is a question about the relative contribution of cardiac and pulmonary diseases to the patient's functional impairment.
  1. Echocardiography can be used to assess right ventricular function. Echocardiographic estimation of right ventricular systolic pressure

can be used as a screening tool for pulmonary hypertension, although right heart catheterization is required for definitive diagnosis. This is especially important for procedures requiring clamping of a pulmonary artery (eg, pneumonectomy).
- E. **Chest imaging**, such as chest radiography, computed tomography (CT), and magnetic resonance imaging (MRI), are useful to determine the presence and extent of tracheobronchial, pulmonary, and mediastinal pathology.
  1. Imaging studies can also reveal the nature and degree of involvement of other thoracic structures in the disease process. Three-dimensional CT reconstruction can be used to define the anatomy of a stenotic airway.
  2. Imaging studies can also be helpful in planning for lung isolation if required.
- F. **Preoperative sedation** should be given carefully to patients with tracheal or pulmonary disease.
  1. Heavy sedation may impair postoperative deep breathing, coughing, and airway protection. Patients with poor pulmonary function will be more prone to hypoxemia when their respiratory drive is suppressed. When sedating these patients, it is prudent to monitor oxygenation and administer supplemental oxygen.
  2. In the presence of airway obstruction, oversedation may profoundly suppress ventilation, but an anxious patient may make exaggerated respiratory efforts. In this case, the increased turbulence may impair effective ventilation, leading to increased anxiety. Benzodiazepines, reassuring words, careful monitoring, and an expeditious start to the procedure are the best approaches.
  3. In patients with airway stenosis, administration of a mixture of 80% helium and 20% oxygen (Heliox) may reduce airway resistance, albeit at the cost of a lower fraction of inspired oxygen (FiO_2).
  4. Glycopyrrolate may be given to decrease oral secretions.

II. LUNG ISOLATION
- A. **A variety of devices designed for lung isolation** are available and are used to facilitate surgical exposure. They are also indicated for avoiding ventilation of an anatomic defect like a bronchopleural fistula or lung protection in the setting of hemorrhage or infection.
- B. **Double-lumen endobronchial tubes (DLTs)** are used for the majority of thoracic surgeries requiring lung isolation.
  1. Selection
     - a. Right- and left-sided DLTs are available and are designed to conform to either the right or the left mainstem bronchus. Each tube has two separate channels: one for ventilation of the bronchus and the other for the trachea and nonintubated bronchus. Right-sided tubes have a separate opening (Murphy eye) in the bronchial lumen to permit ventilation of the right upper lobe.
     - b. The choice of a left- or right-sided tube depends on the type and side of the operation. If a mainstem bronchus is absent, stenotic, disrupted, or obstructed, the DLT must be placed on the opposite side, preferably under direct fiberoptic guidance.
     - c. In most cases, the choice of left- versus right-sided tube is not absolute. Most surgical procedures can be performed with a left-sided DLT.
     - d. At MGH, we typically selectively intubate the nonoperative bronchus. This ensures that the DLT will not interfere with resection of the mainstem bronchus if this is necessary. An additional concern is if the operative bronchus is intubated, ventilation of the

nonoperative lung through the tracheal lumen may be compromised by mediastinal pressure pushing the tube against the tracheal wall and creating a "ball-valve" obstruction.
2. Size
   a. DLTs range in size from 26 to 41 French.
   b. For adult patients, a simplified approach is to choose the size based on the patient's sex and height. Many approaches exist; two sample approaches are offered below:

   Approach 1
   1. Female < 5′ 3″ = 35 Fr
   2. Female > 5′ 3″ = 37 Fr
   3. Male < 5′ 7″ = 39 Fr
   4. Male > 5′ 7″ = 41 Fr

   Approach 2
   1. Male > 6′ 0″ = 41 Fr
   2. Male 5′ 7″ to 6′ 0″ = 39 Fr
   3. Male 5′ 0″ to 5′ 6″ = 37 Fr
   4. Male < 5′ 0″ = 35 Fr
   5. Female: for equivalent heights, down-size by 2 Fr

3. Insertion
   a. The DLT, including both cuffs and all necessary connectors, should be carefully checked before placement. The tube is lubricated, and a stylet is placed in the bronchial lumen.
   b. After laryngoscopy, the DLT should be inserted initially with the distal curve facing anteriorly. Once the DLT passes the vocal cords, the stylet should be removed and the tube rotated to direct the bronchial lumen toward the appropriate side. The tube is then advanced to an average depth of 29 cm at the incisors for males and 28 cm at the incisors for females.
   c. Alternatively, a fiberoptic bronchoscope can be passed down the bronchial lumen as soon as the tube is in the trachea and then used to guide the tube into the correct mainstem bronchus.
   d. Once the tube has been inserted and connected to the anesthesia circuit, the tracheal cuff is inflated, and mechanical ventilation is initiated.
   e. Bronchoscopy should routinely be used to confirm tube position. When passed down the tracheal lumen, the bronchoscope should reveal the carina with the proximal edge of the bronchial cuff just visible in the mainstem bronchus. Passing the bronchoscope down the bronchial lumen should reveal either the left mainstem bronchus or the bronchus intermedius, depending on whether a left- or right-sided tube has been placed. The orifice of the right upper lobe should be visible through the side lumen of a right-sided tube. A bronchoscope should be kept available throughout the case.
   f. The bronchial cuff is inflated to a point just sufficient to eliminate air leak. Lung isolation can be monitored continuously if the anesthesia machine is able to measure inspiratory and expiratory volumes independently and display the leak.
   g. The procedure for passing a DLT through an existing tracheostomy stoma is identical. Bronchoscopy will help to determine how far the tube should be advanced once it is in the trachea.

4. Management
   a. DLT malposition commonly has a few patterns.
      1. The tube is placed too far into the bronchus so that the distal lumen ventilates a single lobe.

2. The tube is too shallow such that the bronchial balloon obstructs the entire tracheal lumen.
3. A left-sided tube is misplaced into the right mainstem bronchus, with the right upper lobe mistakenly thought to be the entire right bronchus. This malposition can be corrected under bronchoscopic guidance via the bronchial lumen, withdrawing the tube to the trachea and directing toward the left mainstem bronchus.

5. Removal
  a. Prior to extubation or any significant manipulation of the DLT, the bronchial cuff should be deflated.

C. Bronchial blockers

1. Bronchial blockers may be used routinely, but especially in situations in which it is not possible to place a DLT, including in pediatric patients, in those with difficult airway anatomy, where satisfactory lung isolation cannot be achieved by other means, or if it is anticipated that the patient will remain intubated postoperatively.
2. Vascular occlusion catheters, such as the Fogarty, have been traditionally used as bronchial blockers. An appropriately sized Fogarty catheter (8- to 14-French venous occlusion catheter with a 10-mL balloon) is selected and placed into the trachea before endotracheal intubation. After intubation, the balloon tip is positioned with a fiberoptic bronchoscope into the appropriate mainstem bronchus and inflated. Lung collapse occurs slowly, via absorption of gases. There is no ability to suction or perform maneuvers such as continuous positive airway pressure (CPAP) to the nonventilated lung.
3. The Arndt blocker (Cook Medical, Bloomington, Indiana) is a bronchial blocker especially designed for lung isolation. Placement is facilitated by a distal loop that can be snared with a bronchoscope. The airway connector is well designed, with separate access ports for the blocker, bronchoscope, and ventilation circuit. Like the Univent tube, the blocker has a small central lumen that can be used for lung collapse or CPAP.
4. The Y-shaped EZ-blocker is designed to simplify positioning. Like the Arndt blocker, it includes an airway connector that allows simultaneous ventilation, bronchoscopic visualization, and blocker placement. This blocker terminates at a Y shape that mimics the carinal division into the mainstem bronchi, terminating with a cuff on each extension. The blocker is placed such that the Y sits at the carina with the extensions in each mainstem bronchus. Each cuff can be inflated by its corresponding balloon. Like the other blockers, each extension has a small central lumen.
5. Univent tubes are large-caliber endotracheal tubes (ETTs) encompassing a small integrated channel for a built-in bronchial blocker. The Univent tube is inserted into the trachea in the usual fashion and is rotated toward the operative lung. After inflation of the tracheal cuff, the bronchial blocker is advanced into the operative mainstem bronchus under fiberoptic guidance. After appropriate positioning, the cuff of the bronchial blocker is inflated. Because the Univent tube is made of Silastic rather than polyvinyl chloride, thorough lubrication of the bronchoscope is required. Collapse of the operative lung occurs through both exhalation via the small distal opening in the blocker and progressive absorption of oxygen from the lung, which will produce alveolar collapse. This is a slow process but may be hastened by deflating the blocker and disconnecting the anesthesia circuit while observing the lung. Once collapse has occurred, the blocker can be reinflated and the circuit reconnected.

Chapter 27 Anesthesia for Thoracic Surgery   **469**

III. ONE-LUNG VENTILATION

A. Ventilation and perfusion are altered by general anesthesia, muscle relaxation, the lateral position, an open chest, surgical manipulations, and one-lung ventilation in ways that may lead to hypoxemia and hypoventilation.

B. Oxygenation
1. Perfusion of the nonventilated lung, also known as pulmonary shunt, is the fundamental reason for hypoxemia during OLV.
2. Perfusion of the nonventilated lung is reduced by hypoxic pulmonary vasoconstriction (HPV). HPV is the pulmonary vascular mechanism that diverts blood flow away from poorly ventilated areas of the lung, minimizing ventilation/perfusion mismatch.
3. Diseased lungs often have reduced perfusion secondary to vascular occlusion or vasoconstriction. This may limit shunting of blood through the nonventilated operative lung during one-lung ventilation.
4. Positive end-expiratory pressure (PEEP) has variable effect on the pulmonary vascular resistance, and PEEP has not been definitively shown to improve oxygenation during one-lung ventilation, but it is used as part of lung-protective strategies.
5. The lateral position (as opposed to supine) reduces pulmonary shunting, because gravity decreases blood flowing to the nondependent lung.

C. Ventilation
1. Controlled ventilation is generally required during open-chest operations. In select patients, these procedures can be performed with the patient breathing spontaneously.
2. Tidal volume should be maintained in the 4 to 6 mL/kg range for protective one-lung ventilation.
3. Arterial carbon dioxide tension is generally maintained at the same level as one would during two lung ventilation by increasing the respiratory rate. This should not be pursued at the expense of overdistending the ventilated lung or causing air trapping.
4. Plateau (or end-inspiratory) airway pressure should generally be maintained below 25 cm H_2O to avoid overdistention of the lung. The occurrence of high airway pressure is usually due to malpositioning of the DLT or the presence of secretions and deserves immediate attention.
5. When resuming two-lung ventilation at the conclusion of the operation, a few manual breaths with a prolonged inspiratory hold will help to reexpand collapsed alveoli.

D. Management of hypoxemia during one-lung ventilation
1. Difficulties with oxygenation during one-lung ventilation may be treated with a variety of maneuvers directed at increasing oxygen delivery to the ventilated lung, decreasing blood flow to the nonventilated lung (decreasing shunt fraction), minimizing atelectasis in the ventilated lung, or providing additional oxygen to the operative lung.
    a. Tube position should be reassessed by fiberoptic bronchoscopy and repositioned if necessary. In addition, the bronchial lumen should be suctioned to clear secretions and ensure patency.
    b. The FiO_2 should be increased. Tidal volumes could be enhanced to improve oxygen delivery.
    c. Recruitment maneuvers to overcome atelectasis have been shown to be effective.
    d. PEEP may be increased to the ventilated lung to treat atelectasis, but this may lower arterial oxygen saturation if a greater proportion of blood flow is forced into the unventilated lung as a result.

e. CPAP can be applied to the nonventilated lung with a separate circuit. Under direct visualization, the collapsed lung is inflated and then allowed to deflate to a volume that will not interfere with surgical exposure (usually 2 to 5 cm H_2O CPAP).
   f. Apneic oxygenation may be provided to the nonventilated lung by partially inflating it with 100% oxygen and then capping the exhalation port. In this way, a motionless partially collapsed lung is maintained. Reinstillation of oxygen will be necessary every 10 to 20 minutes.
   g. If hypoxemia persists, the surgeon can minimize shunt by compressing or clamping the pulmonary artery of the surgical lung or any of its available lobes.
   h. In the event of persistent hypoxemia that is uncorrectable by combinations of the aforementioned therapies or a sudden precipitous desaturation, the surgeon must be notified and the operative lung reinflated. Two-lung ventilation should be maintained until the situation has stabilized, after which the operative lung can be allowed to collapse again. Periodic reinflation or manual two-lung ventilation may be required to maintain adequate arterial oxygen saturation throughout some procedures. Consideration should also be given to nonpulmonary etiology of the shunt (ie, patent foramen ovale with right to left shunt) in the setting of elevated right-sided pressures during OLV.
   i. Extracorporeal life support (ECLS) can be instituted in extreme situations.
   j. Total intravenous anesthesia (TIVA) with propofol has not been shown to decrease shunt.

IV. DIAGNOSTIC PROCEDURES
   A. Flexible bronchoscopy permits visualization from the larynx to the segmental bronchi.
   1. A "working lumen" is used for suctioning, administering drugs, and passing wire instruments.
   2. Ventilation must occur around the flexible bronchoscope. Bronchoscopes range in external diameter from approximately 5 mm (standard adult size) to 2 mm (neonatal bronchoscopes that lack a working lumen). Larger "therapeutic" bronchoscopes and ultrasound-equipped scopes have diameters ranging to 7 mm.
   3. Topical anesthesia is a common anesthetic approach.
      a. The patient should meet the American Society of Anesthesiologists preoperative fasting guidelines.
      b. Lidocaine (various formulations from 1% to 4%) is applied to the oropharynx or nasopharynx, larynx, and vocal cords. The trachea can be sprayed with anesthetic through the bronchoscope or by transtracheal injection. If good topicalization of the airway is achieved, no further anesthesia is required.
      c. Care should be taken with the total dose of local anesthetic due to high systemic absorption from the orotracheal mucosa.
      d. Premedication with atropine or glycopyrrolate will limit salivary dilution of the anesthetic and may improve the onset and efficacy of the anesthetic.
      e. Nerve blocks may be used to supplement airway anesthesia (see Chapter 13: Airway Evaluation and Management).
      f. The patient should have nothing by mouth until tracheal and laryngeal reflexes return, 2 to 3 hours following administration, to prevent aspiration.

4. General anesthesia may be indicated in anxious or uncooperative patients; in more extensive bronchoscopic procedures; or if bronchoscopy is part of a larger surgical procedure.
   a. Bronchoscopy is very stimulating but does not cause significant postoperative pain, so a potent short-acting anesthetic is preferable.
   b. Muscle relaxation or topical anesthesia to the trachea is generally needed to prevent coughing during the procedure.
   c. The ETT used should be sufficiently large (7-mm inner diameter for a standard scope, 8.5 or 9 mm if ultrasound will be used) to permit ventilation in the annular space around the scope.
   d. If there are no contraindications to its use, a laryngeal mask airway (LMA) offers the advantages of a large lumen and the ability to visualize the vocal cords and proximal trachea.

B. **Endobronchial ultrasound** involves the use of ultrasound during bronchoscopy to visualize structures within the lungs, airway, and mediastinum. It is used to guide the biopsy needle for structures that are close to the airway (such as enlarged mediastinal lymph nodes).
   1. Although topical anesthesia with mild sedation can be used, the procedure is typically done under general anesthesia using a large ETT or LMA.
   2. Whichever anesthetic technique is used, it is imperative to prevent coughing and movement as this can increase the risk of injury of major vessels within the thorax during the procedure.

C. **Rigid bronchoscopy** permits visualization of the airway from the larynx to the mainstem bronchi.
   1. A rigid bronchoscope has better optics and a larger working channel than a flexible bronchoscope. It can be used to establish an airway, visualize the trachea, and treat tracheal pathologies such as obstruction, stenosis, and hemorrhage.
   2. Ventilation is accomplished through the lumen of the scope, allowing better control of a marginal airway. Rigid scopes are not cuffed, so a variable leak will occur depending on the size of the scope, lumen of the airway, and depth of insertion.
   3. General anesthesia is required for rigid bronchoscopy. It is important to prevent coughing or movement to avoid tracheal disruption. Either deep inhalation anesthesia or muscle relaxation is required to prevent movement and coughing.
   4. Conventional ventilation can be used, with the anesthesia circuit attached to a side arm of the rigid bronchoscope. The proximal end of the rigid bronchoscope is closed by a clear lens or by a gasket through which telescopes may be passed.
      a. The potentially large leak requires an anesthesia machine capable of delivering high oxygen flows.
      b. An intravenous anesthetic technique is preferred. It can be difficult to maintain adequate anesthesia with an inhalational technique due to leak and interruption of ventilation. There will also be considerable operating room contamination with volatile anesthetics.
      c. Close coordination between the surgeon and anesthetist is needed because ventilation may need to be interrupted for surgery, and surgery in turn may be interrupted by the need to ventilate.
   5. If spontaneous breathing is desired because of a severely compromised airway (eg, severe airway stenosis or airway disruption), a deep stage of anesthesia must be achieved prior to instrumenting the airway.
   6. Ventilating gas usually leaks out around the bronchoscope so that measurements of end-tidal carbon dioxide may be inaccurate. Adequacy of

ventilation should be assessed by observation of chest excursion, pulse oximetry, and, if necessary, blood gas analysis.
7. Rigid bronchoscopes are available that are designed for jet ventilation through a special small side lumen.
   a. The central lumen remains open. Severe barotrauma and pneumothorax may occur if gas is not allowed to escape. Observation of chest movement during the expiratory phase is critical. Conversely, ventilation may be ineffective with noncompliant lungs.
   b. An intravenous anesthetic technique (see Chapter 11: Administration of General Anesthesia) must be used. Muscle relaxation is required for the jet to inflate the lungs adequately.
   c. The inspired oxygen concentration is uncertain because the amount of room air entrained cannot be controlled.
   d. During laser surgery, the fractional inspired oxygen concentration should be reduced to below 0.3, either by jetting air or by using a gas blender for the jet intake.
   e. The advantage of the jet technique is that ventilation is not interrupted by suctioning or surgical manipulations because the proximal end of the bronchoscope is always open. This makes the bronchoscope suitable for use during laser surgery of the larynx, vocal cords, or proximal trachea.
   f. Automated jet ventilators carry the added safety feature of automatic hold when the expiratory airway pressure rises above a set threshold. This prevents breath stacking and subsequent barotrauma.
   g. Complications of bronchoscopy include dental and laryngeal damage from intubation, injuries to the eyes or lips, airway rupture, pneumothorax, air embolism, and hemorrhage. Airway obstruction may be caused by laryngospasm, bronchospasm, hemorrhage, a foreign body, or a dislodged mass.

D. Mediastinoscopy is conducted to evaluate the extrapulmonary spread of pulmonary tumors and to investigate mediastinal masses.
   1. Mediastinoscopy is performed through an incision just superior to the manubrium. A rigid endoscope is then introduced beneath the sternum, and the anterior surfaces of the trachea and the hilum are examined. The patient is supine with the neck extended.
   2. Any general anesthetic technique may be used, provided the patient remains immobile. Although the procedure is not very painful, intermittent stimulation of the trachea, carina, and mainstem bronchi occurs.
   3. Complications include pneumothorax, rupture of the great vessels, and damage to the airways.
   4. Large-bore IV access is required, and having blood cross-matched in the case of hemorrhage could be considered. IV access should be placed in the right upper extremity as the left innominate vein may be compressed during mediastinoscopy. If there is concern for trauma to the superior vena cava (SVC) intraoperatively, lower extremity IV access should be established.
   5. There is a risk of stroke from right innominate artery occlusion by compression between the mediastinoscope and the posterior surface of the sternum. Blood flow to the right arm should be monitored by pulse oximetry. Blood pressure monitoring in the left arm is essential to accurately monitor systemic blood pressure in the event of innominate arterial compression. Should innominate arterial compression occur and the surgeon be incapable of relieving the pressure (ie, while managing hemorrhage through the mediastinoscope), the mean systemic pressure

must be increased to encourage collateral flow to the right cerebral hemisphere.
   6. The trachea may be intermittently compressed by the mediastinoscope, and the position of the patient and surgeon increases the chance of accidental disconnection of the breathing circuit.
E. **Parasternal mediastinoscopy, also known as the Chamberlain procedure,** uses an anterior parasternal incision to obtain lung or anterior mediastinal tissue for diagnostic purposes or to drain abscesses. The incision is typically in the left second intercostal interspace.
   1. The procedure is performed with the patient in the supine position.
   2. One-lung ventilation is not required for lung biopsy, but manual ventilation in cooperation with the surgeon can facilitate the procedure.
   3. If no ribs are resected, the procedure is usually not very painful. Infiltration of the incision with local anesthetic or administration of small doses of IV analgesics is usually sufficient.
   4. If the pleural space is evacuated as it is closed, a chest tube generally is not required postoperatively, although the patient should be monitored carefully for any signs of pneumothorax.

V. PULMONARY RESECTION
A. **Lung resections** may be classified as anatomic or nonanatomic.
   1. Anatomic resections include segmentectomy, lobectomy, and pneumonectomy.
   2. Nonanatomic resections are typically described as wedge resections.
B. **Surgical techniques**
   1. The traditional approach to lung resection is via a thoracotomy. A posterolateral thoracotomy is the most common technique. The incision centers over the fourth to sixth interspaces and requires division of the latissimus dorsi and sometimes the trapezius muscles. An axillary or "muscle-sparing" thoracotomy is an alternative technique that avoids division of major chest wall muscles.
   2. Minimally invasive thoracic surgery (MITS) includes both video-assisted thoracoscopic surgery (VATS) and robotic-assisted thoracoscopic surgery (RATS) and has become the standard approach to lung resection.
      a. Instruments are inserted via one to four small incisions.
      b. Surgical exposure for RATS and some VATS procedures is facilitated by insufflation with low-pressure CO_2.
      c. Lung isolation is required for adequate visualization of the surgical field.
      d. RATS is a growing technique that is theoretically superior to VATS in that the accuracy of the robotic arm facilitates lymph node resection with the conservation of nerves and improved cure rates.
      e. It has been previously stated that once the robot is docked, the surgical bed must not be moved at all. However, newer robotic system allows the robot and the surgical bed to be moved as one unit, decreasing the risk of patient injury when the bed position is changed.
      f. It is important to ensure that adequate muscle relation during RATS as patient coughing or movement during surgery can be dangerous.
C. **Anesthetic techniques**
   1. General anesthesia, often in combination with epidural or regional anesthesia, is the typical approach.
   2. Lung isolation is typically employed to provide optimal surgical exposure. This is ideally achieved with a double-lumen endobronchial tube. A protective one-lung ventilation strategy is crucial.

3. Maintenance with either inhaled or intravenous anesthetics is appropriate. Compared to propofol, inhaled anesthetics are thought to cause greater inhibition of HPV; this is not usually clinically relevant.
4. Muscle relaxation is a useful adjunct but is not required to facilitate surgical exposure. Still, movement and coughing carry some risks and are especially undesirable during RATS.
5. Epidural anesthesia can provide excellent analgesia intraoperatively and is considered the gold standard for postoperative pain management after thoracotomy. Intercostal and paravertebral blocks provide adequate analgesia for MITS.
6. With careful patient selection and a combination of sedation and regional anesthesia, some minimally invasive thoracic surgeries can be performed on a spontaneously breathing patient.

D. Positioning

1. Operations for lung resection are most commonly performed in the lateral decubitus position with the bed sharply flexed. The goal is to maximally distract the ribs, lower the profile of the hip, and have the operative chest wall parallel to the floor.
2. Careful attention to positioning of the neck, arms, torso, and legs is essential to prevent patient injury.
   a. The neck should remain in a neutral position. Constant support of the head during the movement of the bed into the flexed position is required. The dependent eye and ear should be carefully checked to ensure that they are free from direct pressure.
   b. The arms are usually extended in front of the patient.
      1. Neither arm should be abducted or flexed more than 90 degrees at the shoulder to avoid traction on the brachial plexus.
      2. The axilla should be free of compression.
      3. The arms must be carefully padded to avoid compression of the radial and ulnar nerves.
      4. Venous and arterial cannulae may be obstructed by arm positioning. This can usually be avoided by placing lines in the dependent arm.
   c. The torso and hips must be supported anteriorly and posteriorly to prevent rotation. The point of lateral flexion should lie under the iliac crest, not the flank or ribcage.
   d. The lower extremities should be padded with attention to bony prominences. In male patients, the scrotum should be free of compression.
3. During the positioning process, vital signs should be closely observed. Pooling of blood in the dependent extremities may cause hypotension.
4. Positioning can move the endotracheal tube, affect respiratory system compliance, and change V/Q relationships. Respiratory parameters and lung isolation should be reassessed after any change in position.

E. Emergence

1. Chest tubes are inserted to drain the pleural cavity and maintain reexpansion of the operative lung. Postoperatively, chest tubes may be allowed to drain passively ("water seal") or actively with up to 20 cm H_2O of suction. Management of a chest tube after pneumonectomy is a notable exception; suction should never be applied and this could precipitate mediastinal shift, airway obstruction, and cardiovascular collapse.
2. Before closing the chest, the operative lung is inflated with 20 to 30 cm H_2O of pressure for 15 to 30 seconds. This serves both as a recruitment maneuver and as a method of identifying air leaks.

3. A smooth extubation avoids the potentially disruptive effects of endotracheal intubation and positive-pressure ventilation on fresh suture lines. If postoperative intubation and mechanical ventilation are required, the DLT should be exchanged for a conventional single-lumen ETT, and inspiratory pressures should be kept as low as possible.

F. Postoperative analgesia
1. A posterolateral thoracotomy is a painful incision, involving multiple muscle layers, rib resection, and continuous motion as the patient breathes. Posterolateral thoracotomy incisions typically center over the fourth to sixth interspaces. Chest tubes are typically placed below the incision, around the seventh and eighth interspaces.
2. Regional techniques
   a. Epidural analgesia is considered the gold standard for postoperative pain management after thoracotomy, but is not routinely employed for MITS.
   b. The paravertebral block is an effective alternative to epidural analgesia.
   c. Intercostal nerve blocks are easily placed under direct vision by the surgeon, and provide effective analgesia for 4 to 8 hours.
   d. The role of other regional techniques, such as the serratus anterior plane block and the erector spinae plane block, has yet to be established.
3. Opioids are useful but should be administered judiciously to avoid respiratory depression.
4. Ipsilateral shoulder pain after lung resection is common and thought to represent a combination of musculoskeletal pain and referred pain from phrenic nerve irritation. It is not covered by epidural analgesia but can be effectively managed with nonsteroidal anti-inflammatory drugs (NSAIDs) and acetaminophen.

VI. MEDIASTINAL MASS RESECTION
A. Patients with mediastinal masses may present a number of unique challenges.
1. Mediastinal masses may exert mass effect on adjacent structures. Anterior mediastinal masses are of particular concern because of the potential for compression of the heart, great vessels, and tracheobronchial tree. The anesthetic plan must account for the possibility of hemodynamic and airway compromise upon administration of sedation or induction of general anesthesia.
2. Signs and symptoms of associated syndromes should be identified, including myasthenia gravis and SVC syndrome. Anesthetic considerations for the patient with myasthenia gravis are detailed in Chapter 14: Neuromuscular Blockade.
   a. A thorough preoperative assessment and discussion with the surgeon about operative plan, possible perioperative complications and the intended management cardiovascular or airway compression are essential.

B. Preoperative evaluation
1. The patient's symptoms and imaging findings are the most important predictors of the risk for hemodynamic or respiratory compromise with induction of general anesthesia.
2. A focused history should elicit positional symptoms and the patient's ability to lie flat. The patients' most comfortable position should be assessed as it can be used as a "rescue position" in the event of airway obstruction.

3. Preoperative PFTs are not routinely obtained unless otherwise indicated. In addition, studies have shown that flow–volume loops are not useful clinically because of poor correlation with airway obstruction.
4. Venous and arterial compromise may affect the plan for vascular access. Lower extremity access may be considered.
5. If epidural analgesia is planned for postoperative pain control, it can be placed preoperatively; however, caution should be used in activating it prior to induction and mass removal. If there is a high probability of complete airway obstruction or cardiovascular collapse during induction process, femoral sheaths can be inserted to facilitate the rapid initiation of ECLS. ECLS can also be initiated prophylactically prior to induction.

C. Induction
1. The choice of induction technique and airway management strategy depends upon the findings of the preoperative evaluation. The surgeon should be present during this time and appropriate rescue airway equipment should be immediately available.
2. The patient should be placed in semi-Fowler position (or whichever position is most comfortable for them) until the airway is secured.
3. In patients with no symptoms or no evidence of airway or cardiovascular compression, routine IV induction can be performed carefully.
4. Although maintaining spontaneous ventilation until the airway is secured and potentially during the procedure has been advocated as the safest approach, studies in adult patients with large anterior mediastinal masses have shown that central airway collapse typically does not occur with institution of positive-pressure ventilation and neuromuscular blockade. An intravenous induction with muscle relaxation may provide better conditions for airway management.
5. Reinforced ETT is preferred if tracheal compression is present. It is important to have an array of ETTs including microlaryngoscopy tubes, DLTs, and bronchial blockers if one-lung ventilation might be required. It is important that the ETT should also be placed distal to obstruction.
6. If airway obstruction or hemodynamic collapse occurs after induction and ventilation is not possible, steps to take include position change or rigid bronchoscopy. The surgeon should also be prepared for emergency sternotomy to lift the mass and alleviate compression.

D. Monitoring and additional considerations
1. Invasive arterial blood pressure monitoring is mandatory.
2. Transesophageal echocardiogram (TEE) can be used to assess cardiovascular performance intraoperatively. The presence of associated esophageal pathology should be determined prior to insertion of the TEE probe.

VII. ESOPHAGEAL SURGERY
A. Esophagogastroduodenoscopy (EGD)
1. EGD may be performed under local anesthesia as described for flexible bronchoscopy or after the induction of general anesthesia and endotracheal intubation. Use of a smaller-caliber ETT will allow the surgeon more room to work in the pharynx and proximal esophagus.
2. Rigid esophagoscopy is commonly performed under general anesthesia with muscle relaxation. As with flexible esophagoscopy, a smaller ETT is used.

B. Esophageal surgery
includes procedures for resecting esophageal neoplasms, for treating reflux, and for repairing traumatic or congenital lesions.

C. General considerations

1. Patients may be chronically malnourished both from systemic illness (carcinoma) and anatomic interference with swallowing. Enteral or parenteral nutrition may have been initiated preoperatively.
2. Both esophageal carcinoma and traumatic disruption of the distal esophagus are associated with alcohol abuse; patients may have impaired liver function, elevated portal pressures, anemia, cardiomyopathy, and bleeding disorders.
3. Patients who have difficulty swallowing may be significantly hypovolemic. Cardiovascular compromise may be further exacerbated by preoperative chemotherapy with cardiotoxins.
4. Most patients presenting for esophageal procedures will be at risk for aspiration. Rapid sequence induction or awake intubation should be planned.
5. An arterial line and a urinary catheter are required for complex esophageal surgery.
6. Temperature conservation measures should be aggressively pursued. The use of a forced air blanket over the lower body is routine.

D. Operative approaches and anesthesia

1. An upper esophageal diverticulum (Zenker diverticulum) is typically approached through a lateral cervical incision, similar to carotid surgery. This incision may also be used for upper esophageal myotomies for swallowing disorders. A transoral endoscopic approach can also be adopted, which would require nasal intubation.
   a. The patient is positioned supine with the neck extended and the head turned to the contralateral side.
   b. Postoperative pain and fluid shifts are usually minimal with a cervical incision, and patients may be safely extubated at the conclusion of the procedure. The surgeons may or may not elect to leave a nasogastric tube in place.
2. **Carcinoma**
   a. General considerations
      1. Intraoperative repositioning and lung isolation are required for most of the surgical approaches that involve entering the thorax.
      2. Large-volume blood loss is uncommon. However, large-bore intravenous access and a preoperative type and screen should be acquired.
      3. Immediate postoperative extubation can be considered in healthier patients after uncomplicated procedures, and should be performed only when the patient is fully awake and can protect their airway.
      4. Epidural analgesia is commonly used in the postoperative period both for analgesia from large incisions and to avoid any risk of aspiration from somnolence secondary to parenteral narcotics. Epidural analgesia has been shown to improve esophageal blood flow, as long as hypotension and hypovolemia are treated.
      5. In rare instances, if postoperative intubation is deemed necessary, it is typical to exchange the DLT for a single-lumen ETT. Tissue edema may significantly narrow the airway, rendering reintubation difficult.
   b. Multiple surgical approaches exist which utilize a variety of incisions in the neck, chest and abdomen to access the esophagus.
   c. Lesions of the upper esophagus are approached by a "three-hole" approach, which includes a transverse cervical incision, a

laparotomy, and a right thoracotomy. Sometimes the lesion is high enough to be removed with a transhiatal approach, including only the anterior cervical incision and the laparotomy, avoiding the thoracotomy. The laparotomy (and sometimes the right thoracotomy) is required to mobilize the stomach and lower esophagus. A cervical incision allows for anastomosis of the proximal esophagus and distal stomach.

   d. Lesions of the middle esophagus are commonly approached with a laparotomy followed by a right-sided thoracotomy. This procedure is known as an Ivor Lewis esophagectomy. Mobilization of the stomach or jejunum is accomplished through a midline abdominal incision. The right thoracotomy allows for a proximal anastomosis above the level of the aortic arch. There are also minimally invasive versions of this procedure that use laparoscopic and thoracoscopic equipment for the abdominal and thoracic portions of the procedure, respectively.

   e. Lower esophageal lesions are approached through an extended left thoracoabdominal incision. After resection, the surgeon will perform a primary anastomosis of the esophagus and stomach. Occasionally, the stomach does not provide an adequate distal anastomosis, and the surgeon instead brings up a Roux-en-Y loop of jejunum.

3. Trauma to the entire esophagus, as with lye ingestion, may necessitate a total esophagectomy with subsequent interposition of a segment of the colon or jejunum to serve as a conduit between the pharynx and stomach.

   a. Surgical exposure may require two or three incisions, as described above.

   b. These patients may have a prolonged postoperative course with significant fluid shifts and nutritional depletion and are at risk for aspiration pneumonia. The trachea may remain intubated at the conclusion of the surgery, if a complex procedure has been done.

4. Gastrointestinal motility disorders may benefit from surgical repair. Fundoplication (eg, Belsey Mark IV, Hill, or Nissen) is performed to relieve gastroesophageal reflux. Heller myotomy is performed for severe achalasia.

   a. The surgical approach is transabdominal for the Hill and Nissen procedures, and transthoracic for the Belsey. Collapse of the left lung is required for the latter procedure.

   b. Rapid sequence induction is necessary due to the increased risk of aspiration, especially in patients with achalasia.

   c. Iatrogenic intraoperative pneumothorax is a possible complication, although it is usually well tolerated with appropriate adjustment in ventilation.

   d. Fluid shifts are usually less than after other esophageal surgeries.

VIII. TRACHEAL SURGERY
A. General considerations
   1. Surgery of the trachea and mainstem bronchi involves significant anesthetic risks, including interruption of airway continuity and the potential for total obstruction of an already stenotic airway.

   2. The surgical approach depends on the location and extent of the lesion. Lesions of the cervical trachea are approached through a transverse neck incision. Lower lesions necessitate an upper sternotomy. Lesions

of the distal trachea and carina may require a median sternotomy or a right thoracotomy.
3. The anesthetic technique must include a plan for preserving airway patency and adequacy of oxygenation and ventilation. Depending on the severity and nature of the lesion, this may include rigid bronchoscopy or ECLS.

B. Induction and initial examination
1. For most patients without significant tracheal obstruction, a routine intravenous induction and immediate transition to positive-pressure ventilation is safe.
2. Following induction of anesthesia, bronchoscopy is usually performed to define the anatomy and resectability of the tracheal lesion. For appropriate candidates, an LMA facilitates an initial flexible bronchoscopic exam. Traditionally, the standard approach was to perform rigid bronchoscopy for this purpose.
3. The patient is then intubated with the largest possible ETT. If the stenotic segment is too narrow or friable to allow intubation, ventilation through the LMA or rigid bronchoscope is continued until the trachea distal to the lesion can be accessed surgically. Alternatives include having the surgeon "core out" the tracheal lesion with the rigid bronchoscope, placing a tracheostomy distal to the stenotic segment, intubating the trachea above the lesion, or using a jet ventilation system to ventilate the patient from above the lesion.
4. For patients with critically stenotic lesions, the induction plan must be carefully considered and backup plans must be in place in case difficulty with maintaining airway patency is encountered. Emergency equipment and a skilled rigid bronchoscopic surgeon must be immediately available during induction.
5. Patients with preexisting, mature tracheostomies may be intubated through the stoma with a flexible, armored ETT. The surgical field is prepared around the ETT, which is later removed and replaced with a sterile one by the surgeon.

C. Intraoperative management
1. Anesthetic management is complicated by periodic interruption of airway continuity by the surgical procedure.
2. When the trachea is surgically divided, the orotracheal ETT is retracted proximal to the division. A suture may be placed in the distal end of the orotracheal tube before pulling it back into the pharynx to facilitate replacing it in the trachea at the end of the procedure. A sterile armored ETT is then placed into the distal trachea by the surgeon; this is used to perform cross-field ventilation. The ETT is frequently removed and reinserted by the surgeons as they work around it. Close coordination during this portion of the procedure will help avoid leakage of gas from the circuit.
3. Once the stenotic segment has been removed and the posterior tracheal anastomosis is complete, the transtracheal ETT is removed and the orotracheal ETT is readvanced from above. The distal trachea should be suctioned to remove accumulated blood and secretions. The patient's neck is then flexed forward, reducing tension on the trachea, and the anterior portion of the anastomosis is completed.
4. For lower tracheal or carinal resections, a long ETT with a flexible armored wall can be used. This allows the surgeon to position the tip in the trachea or either mainstem bronchus and to operate around it without interrupting ventilation.

5. Jet ventilation through a catheter held by one of the surgeons may be required during carinal resection if the distal airways are too small to accommodate an ETT. Jet ventilation rate and pressure should be carefully titrated by direct observation of the surgical field. Obstruction of exhalation will lead to "stacking" of breaths, increased airway pressure, and barotrauma.
6. In general, it is difficult to administer volatile anesthetic agents in a consistent manner intraoperatively. An intravenous maintenance agent should be chosen.

D. Emergence and extubation
1. At the conclusion of the procedure, a single large suture is placed from the chin to the anterior chest to preserve neck flexion and thereby minimize tension on the tracheal suture line. Several blankets under the head will help maintain flexion. Close attention to neck position during emergence, extubation, and transfer is essential.
2. Spontaneous ventilation should be resumed as soon as possible after the procedure to minimize trauma to the tracheal suture line.
3. Extubation at the conclusion of the surgical procedure is desirable, so as to avoid trauma to the tracheal anastomosis from an ETT.
4. The patient should be awake enough to maintain spontaneous ventilation and avoid aspiration but should be extubated before excessive head movement can damage the surgical repair. Remifentanil is a useful adjunct to facilitate a smooth emergence.
5. Fiberoptic examination of the surgical repair via LMA may be planned for the conclusion of the case, or done if there is suspicion of obstruction after extubation.
6. Only relatively small amounts of intravenous opioids are usually needed to treat the mild pain from the neck incision. Analgesia usually is administered after the patient is wide awake and responsive and with close monitoring for undesirable respiratory depression.
7. Most patients may be safely extubated, but in those for whom difficult anatomy or copious secretions make this undesirable, a small tracheostomy may be placed below the tracheal repair.
8. If tracheal collapse, airway edema, or secretions cause persistent respiratory distress after extubation, the patient should be reintubated fiberoptically with a small uncuffed ETT, preferably with the head maintained in forward flexion.
9. Frequent bronchoscopies at the bedside under local anesthesia may be required to remove secretions from the lungs in the postoperative period.

IX. LARYNGEAL SURGERY
A. Suspension microlaryngoscopy
1. Suspension of the laryngoscope allows for stable and hands-free access to the larynx and vocal cords. The laryngoscope may be suspended using either a device that rests the patient's chest or one attached to a table.
2. Laryngeal surgeries may also be performed via rigid bronchoscopy.
3. Operations on anterior glottic lesions may be performed with an ETT in place, but for posterior glottic lesions an ETT will obstruct the surgical field.
4. If an ETT is not used and the airway is open, TIVA is useful for maintaining a consistent depth of anesthesia and preventing pollution of the operating suite environment with anesthetic gasses. Jet ventilation may be necessary. Alternatively, shorter procedures may be safely

performed using apneic oxygenation techniques such as transnasal humidified rapid-insufflation ventilatory exchange (THRIVE) using high-flow nasal cannula. Other strategies include intermittent mask ventilation and maintenance of spontaneous ventilation.
   5. Intraoperative stimulation can be intense, but postoperative pain is minimal. Muscle relaxation is essential to avoid movement and coughing.
   6. Laryngeal suspension may trigger a vagal response and severe bradycardia. The surgeon can be asked to take the laryngoscope out of suspension until the bradycardia resolves. Glycopyrrolate or atropine may be required.
B. Medialization laryngoplasty
   1. Voice restoration operations are typically performed under sedation to allow for the patient to phonate intraoperatively.
   2. Local anesthesia with small doses of rapidly reversible hypnotic agents and analgesics are typically adequate to produce adequate operating conditions.

X. INTERVENTIONAL PULMONARY PROCEDURES
A. The application of minimally invasive techniques to diagnose and treat diseases of the airway, lungs and pleura is a growing field, especially for patients who are otherwise not considered surgical candidates.
B. Therapeutic bronchoscopy
   1. Many therapeutic procedures may be performed using either a flexible or rigid bronchoscope. A common indication is central airway obstruction.
   2. Airway obstructions may be relieved with bronchoplasty, in which a balloon is inflated under pressure to dilate a stenotic airway, or the placement of airway stents to help preserve airway patency.
   3. A variety of ablative therapies may be applied, often in combination. Three common therapies are laser, argon plasma coagulation (APC), and cryosurgery. APC refers to a technique in which argon gas is ignited in order to cauterize tissue. Cryosurgery uses the application of a cooling agent to destroy tissue. Lasers are useful because they both cut and coagulate. The specific properties depend on the type of laser used.
   4. All of the above therapies come with risks of air embolism and airway bleeding, edema, and perforation. Laser and APC use comes with the additional risk of airway fire; communication with the proceduralist and maintenance of an FiO_2 less than 0.3 when the laser is in use is essential.
C. Lung volume reduction
   1. For select patients with chronic obstructive pulmonary disease (COPD), lung volume reduction is an option to improve function by decreasing lung hyperinflation.
   2. Lung volume reduction surgery essentially involves multiple wedge resections of the affected lung. This is also referred to as reduction pneumoplasty.
   3. A bronchoscopic approach with placement of endobronchial valves avoids the need for surgery. One-way endobronchial valves allow for air and mucus to exit the treated area, but do not allow air to reenter. This results in atelectasis of the treated lobe.
   4. The procedure begins with an assessment of collateral ventilation between the target lobe and neighboring lung tissue. Lack of fissure integrity and the presence of collateral airflow will result in failure. The lobe is blocked with a specialized balloon catheter and an assessment of airflow distal to the balloon is made. If an appropriate target is

identified, the endobronchial valve is deployed under direct bronchoscopic visualization.
   5. General anesthesia is preferred, although sedation has been described. A large endotracheal tube is required to allow for ventilation around the bronchoscope. A narcotic-heavy emergence may be helpful to prevent coughing and dislodgement of the valve.
D. Medical thoracoscopy/pleuroscopy
   1. Medical thoracoscopy is similar to VATS but is typically performed by pulmonologists for more limited diagnostic and therapeutic interventions, hence the term "medical" thoracoscopy.
   2. Usually, only a single port is placed to access the chest cavity.
   3. Common applications include the diagnosis of pleural diseases, drainage of pleural fluid and chemical pleurodesis.
   4. These procedures are often performed under local anesthesia and sedation, but general anesthesia with or without lung isolation can also be considered.
E. Whole lung lavage
   1. Whole lung lavage is used to treat pulmonary alveolar proteinosis by removing accumulated lipoproteinaceous material from the lungs. The procedure involves instillation and then drainage of large volumes of normal saline into one or both diseased lungs.
   2. The procedure typically requires lung isolation by DLT to provide adequate irrigation and drainage. Excellent lung isolation must be achieved before the procedure starts to minimize the risk of cross-contamination.
   3. Core body temperature should be closely monitored as hypothermia may result from large-volume saline lavage.
   4. Hypoxemia develops due to removal of surfactant and resultant atelectasis. Patients may require noninvasive positive-pressure ventilation postoperatively or high-flow nasal cannula oxygen to treat persistent hypoxemia, or rarely may need to remain intubated and recover in the intensive care unit.

XI. SPECIAL CIRCUMSTANCES
A. Intrapulmonary hemorrhage
   1. Massive hemoptysis may be caused by thoracic trauma, pulmonary artery rupture secondary to catheterization, or erosion into a vessel by a tracheostomy, abscess, or airway tumor.
   2. The trachea must be immediately intubated and the lungs ventilated with 100% oxygen.
   3. An attempt should be made to suction the airway clear, ideally by rigid bronchoscopy.
   4. If a unilateral source is identified, lung isolation may be undertaken to protect the uninvolved lung and facilitate corrective surgery.
      a. Lung isolation may be achieved by placing an endobronchial blocker or a double-lumen endobronchial tube. Choice of technique depends on experience, equipment at hand, and the extent of active bleeding. Active bleeding may obscure airway visualization during flexible bronchoscopy. Obstruction of the ETT is an ever-present danger, and frequent suctioning may be necessary.
      b. In an emergency, the existing ETT can be advanced into the mainstem bronchus of the uninvolved lung and the cuff inflated.
      c. Fiberoptic bronchoscopy is essential for suctioning blood and confirming isolation.

5. Frequently, the source of bleeding is from the bronchial circulation. **Embolization** in the radiology suite is often attempted if the patient is stable.
6. Definitive treatment may require a thoracotomy and surgical repair.

B. Bronchopleural fistula
1. Bronchopleural fistula is a connection between a bronchial stump and the surrounding pleura. Symptoms include dyspnea, subcutaneous emphysema, persistent air leak, and purulent discharge from the chest tube.
2. General considerations
   a. Small fistulas may close spontaneously; a persistent leak indicates involvement of a larger bronchus.
   b. Treatment of subsequent sepsis involves antibiotics and chest tube drainage.
   c. Surgical approach varies, ranging from application of fibrin glue via bronchoscopy to thoracoplasty with a pedicled muscle flap.
3. Anesthetic management
   a. Positive-pressure ventilation may be inadequate if most ventilation escapes through the fistula. A functional chest tube must be in place before induction and positive-pressure ventilation.
   b. Patients often undergo inhalation induction with spontaneous ventilation and lung isolation via endobronchial intubation to minimize the amount of time spent ventilating the fistula.
   c. High-frequency jet ventilation (HFJV) has been used as an alternative to lung isolation to successfully decrease gas leak through the fistula by providing lower peak and mean airway pressures than with traditional positive-pressure ventilation. HFJV is not as effective in patients with noncompliant lungs such as those with acute respiratory distress syndrome. If mechanical ventilation via a standard ETT is to be used, flow redistribution may not be used to signal the end of a breath: The fistula will allow for gas flow at a constant velocity, causing the mechanical breath to continue indefinitely.

C. Tracheal injury
1. Tracheal disruption may be caused by airway instrumentation or thoracic trauma and may present with hypoxia, dyspnea, subcutaneous emphysema, pneumomediastinum, or pneumothorax.
2. Injury may occur at the cricoid, midtrachea, carina, or either mainstem bronchus. Several mechanisms of injury have been proposed, including high airway pressures, lateral stretch of the thoracic cavity, and deceleration injury.
3. Positive-pressure ventilation will exacerbate the air leak and rapidly worsen symptoms from pneumothorax or pneumomediastinum. If possible, the patient should be allowed to breathe spontaneously, following the protocol for the patient with critical tracheal stenosis.
4. Tracheal damage in the already anesthetized patient may be treated initially by advancement of a small ETT past the point of injury. In the case of a difficult airway in which the tube causes the injury, an immediate surgical tracheostomy must be performed and access to the distal trachea secured.
5. Once a tube has been placed across or distal to the site of tracheal disruption, controlled positive-pressure ventilation can begin. Further management is as for the patient undergoing elective airway surgery.

XII. INTRAOPERATIVE EXTRACORPOREAL LIFE SUPPORT
A. The term ECLS broadly describes a variety of applications of mechanical cardiopulmonary support, including extracorporeal membrane

oxygenation (ECMO) and cardiopulmonary bypass (CPB), which can provide hemodynamic and ventilatory support during thoracic surgery.
- **B.** The choice and specific configuration of ECMO and CPB is determined by the specific needs of the patient and the procedure. A full discussion of these modalities and their intraoperative management is beyond the scope of this chapter.
- **C.** The following are situations in which ECLS may find application:
    1. Airway surgery
        a. VV-ECMO may be used to support patients with airway obstruction or anticipated airway obstruction in whom oxygenation and ventilation may be difficult or impossible. For example, ECMO may be considered to support patients undergoing complex tracheal resection and reconstruction in which cross-field ventilation or jet ventilation fails to provide adequate oxygenation and ventilation.
        b. VA-ECMO or CPB can be utilized if airway reconstruction requires decompression of the heart.
    2. Difficult one-lung ventilation
        a. Patients with limited pulmonary reserve who may not tolerate intraoperative one-lung ventilation.
        b. Patients in whom lung isolation may be technically challenging.
    3. Mediastinal masses
        a. Patients with large anterior mediastinal masses who may not tolerate induction of general anesthesia and/or intraoperative positioning due to compression of the great vessels or the right side of the heart.
    4. Lesions requiring concomitant cardiac surgery
    5. Intraoperative iatrogenic large vessel injury
        a. CPB is generally favored in cases of severe, acute bleeding from an iatrogenic vascular injury. Reduction of blood flow facilitates surgical repair.

ACKNOWLEDGMENTS

We gratefully acknowledge the contributions of previous edition author(s), Peter O. Ochieng and Ryan J. Horvath, as portions of those chapters have been retained in this revision.

Suggested Readings

Ahmad S, Taneja A, Kurman J, Dagar G, Kumar G. National trends in lung volume reduction surgery in the United States: 2000 to 2010. *Chest.* 2014;146(6):e228–e229.

Ahuja S, Cohen B, Hinkelbein J, Diemunsch P, Ruetzler K. Practical anesthetic considerations in patients undergoing tracheobronchial surgeries: a clinical review of current literature. *J Thorac Dis.* 2016;8(11):3431–3441.

Brunelli A, Kim AW, Berger KI, Addrizzo-Harris DJ. Physiologic evaluation of the patient with lung cancer being considered for resectional surgery: diagnosis and management of lung cancer, 3rd ed: American College of Chest Physicians evidence-based clinical practice guidelines. *Chest.* 2013;143(5 suppl):e166S–e190S. Published correction appears in *Chest.* 2014;145(2):437.

Castillo M, Slinger P. Myths of anterior mediastinal masses. *South Afr J Anaesth Analg.* 2013;19(1):38–40.

Chenesseau J, Fourdrain A, Pastene B, et al. Effectiveness of surgeon-performed paravertebral block analgesia for minimally invasive thoracic surgery: a randomized clinical trial. *JAMA Surg.* 2023;158(12):1255–1263.

Detterbeck FC, Lewis SZ, Diekemper R, Addrizzo-Harris D, Alberts WM. Executive summary: diagnosis and management of lung cancer, 3rd ed: American College of Chest Physicians evidence-based clinical practice guidelines. *Chest.* 2013;143(5 suppl):7S–37S.

Duthie DJ. Anesthetic agents for thoracic surgery: what's best? *Curr Opin Anaesthesiol.* 2013;25:53–57.

Erdös G, Tzanova I. Perioperative anaesthetic management of mediastinal mass in adults, *Eur J Anaesthesiol.* 2009;26(8):627–632.

Hartigan PM, Karamnov S, Gill RR, et al. Mediastinal masses, anesthetic interventions, and airway compression in adults: a prospective observational study. *Anesthesiology.* 2022;136(1):104–114.

Hobai IA, Chhangani SV, Alfille PH. Anesthesia for tracheal resection and reconstruction. *Anesthesiol Clin.* 2012;30:709–730.

Ku CM. Anesthesia for patients with mediastinal masses. In: Slinger P, eds. *Principles and Practice of Anesthesia for Thoracic Surgery.* Springer; 2011.

Lederman D, Easwar J, Feldman J, Shapiro V. Anesthetic considerations for lung resection: preoperative assessment, intraoperative challenges and postoperative analgesia. *Ann Transl Med.* 2019;7(15):356.

Lennox PH, Umedaly HS, Grant RP, White SA, Fitzmaurice BG, Evans KG. A pulsatile pressure waveform is a sensitive marker for confirming the location of the thoracic epidural space. *J Cardiothorac Vasc Anesth.* 2006;20(5):659–663.

Pauli H, Eladawy M, Park J. Anesthesia for robotic thoracic surgery. *Ann Cardiothorac Surg.* 2019;8(2):263–268.

Pawlowski J. Anesthetic considerations for interventional pulmonary procedures. *Curr Opin Anaesthesiol.* 2013;25:6–12.

Roy PM. Preoperative pulmonary evaluation for lung resection. *J Anaesthesiol Clin Pharmacol.* 2018;34(3):296–300.

Subramanyam P, Sundaram PS. Which is better – a standalone ventilation or perfusion scan or combined imaging to predict postoperative FEV1 in one seconds in patients posted for lung surgeries with borderline pulmonary reserve. *Indian J Nucl Med.* 2018;33(2):105–111.

Vidal Melo MF, Musch G, Kaczka DW. Pulmonary pathophysiology and lung mechanics in anesthesiology: a cased-based overview. *Anesthesiol Clin.* 2012;30:759–784.

Yoo ID, Im JJ, Chung YA, Choi EK, Oh JK, Lee SH. Prediction of postoperative lung function in lung cancer patients using perfusion scintigraphy. *Acta Radiol.* 2019;60(4):488–495.

Wittenstein J, Scharffenberg M, Fröhlich J, et al. Effects of positive end-expiratory pressure on pulmonary perfusion distribution and intrapulmonary shunt during one-lung ventilation in pigs: a randomized crossover study. *Anesthesiology.* 2024;141:44–55.

28. Anesthesia for Vascular Surgery
Ann Norris and James Taylor Lloyd

I. PREOPERATIVE ASSESSMENT AND MANAGEMENT
Patients undergoing vascular surgery frequently have multiple comorbid conditions that should be optimized prior to surgery.

A. Cardiovascular system. Major adverse cardiac events (MACE) such as stroke, myocardial infarction (MI), cardiac arrest, and death are the leading cause of morbidity and mortality in patients undergoing vascular surgery. MI accounts for about one-half of early postoperative deaths. Accurate risk stratification based on preoperative patient characteristics remains a significant challenge in vascular surgery. Commonly used risk calculators such as the Revised Cardiac Risk Index (RCRI) and Gupta Myocardial Infarction or Cardiac Arrest have reduced performances in vascular surgery. Alternate scoring systems such as the Geriatric-Sensitive Perioperative Risk Calculator, Vascular Surgery Group of New England Cardiac Risk Index, and Vascular Quality Initiative Cardiac Risk Index tools have been proposed to address these shortcomings, but have their own limitations. Below are some specific considerations with regard to vascular surgical patients.

1. **Cardiac stress testing.** For nonemergent cases, in patients estimated to be at elevated risk (>1% risk of perioperative MACE) with poor functional capacity (<4 METS), noninvasive cardiac stress testing should be carried out if the results will impact patient care. Dobutamine stress echocardiography or myocardial perfusion imaging will be necessary for patients with physical limitations such as claudication or disability from prior stroke. The need for coronary artery catheterization is determined based on the results of the stress test.

2. **Echocardiography** may be indicated if the patient has a new murmur, dyspnea of unknown etiology, valvular heart disease, or heart failure with new or worsening symptomatology.

3. **Cardiac Biomarkers** such as beta-natriuretic peptide (BNP) to aid in preoperative risk stratification are not currently part of the American College of Cardiology guidelines but have been integrated into society guidelines in Europe and Canada. Several studies have shown an association between elevated preoperative BNP and adverse cardiovascular events in noncardiac surgery, though optimal cutoff levels or a precise algorithm for how to respond to elevated levels have not been well defined. Cardiac biomarkers represent a potential emerging area to further improve preoperative risk stratification, particularly in vascular surgery patients where the RCRI has not been shown to be as predictive.

4. **Blood pressures** should be measured in both arms to determine whether there is a difference. Due to the systemic nature of atherosclerosis, patients may have subclavian or axillary arterial stenoses. Blood pressure should be monitored in the extremity with the higher reading.

5. **Coronary revascularization** should be carried out only if medically indicated. According to the Coronary Artery Revascularization Prophylaxis trial, coronary revascularization in advance of major vascular surgery has not been shown to improve outcome when compared with medical management. This trial excluded patients with left main coronary artery disease, ejection fraction less than 20%, and severe aortic stenosis.
6. **β-Blocker therapy** should be maintained in patients already on chronic therapy. Initiation of β-blocker therapy is reasonable in patients with three or more RCRI risk factors or in patients with reversible ischemia on preoperative testing. However, improper timing and dose titration may increase risk of stroke and mortality. β-Blocker therapy should be started at least 2 days prior to surgery; 7 days is preferred. Therapy should be started at a low dose and titrated slowly to achieve target heart rate of 60 to 80 bpm and should be held for hypotension.
7. **Antiplatelet therapy.** Aspirin therapy should be continued in patients with coronary stents, cerebrovascular disease, or high-risk coronary artery disease. Continuation should be considered in all vascular surgical procedures in discussion with the surgical team. Aspirin therapy is associated with an increased risk of bleeding. POISE-2, a randomized, controlled trial of 10,000 patients undergoing noncardiac surgery, did not show a benefit of aspirin initiation or continuation with respect to MACE or death. However, it excluded patients who had recently received coronary stents and those undergoing carotid endarterectomy (CEA). Furthermore, only a small proportion of the study population underwent vascular surgery. Continuation of **clopidogrel** therapy depends on patient factors (eg, presence and type of coronary stents and when they were placed) as well as surgical factors.
8. **Statins** should be continued perioperatively. The initiation of statin therapy is reasonable in patients undergoing vascular surgery. The statin should ideally be started 1 week to 30 days prior to the surgical procedure. There is evidence that statins decrease coronary inflammation regardless of low-density lipoprotein level. Withdrawal prior to surgery has been associated with increased cardiac events.
9. **Warfarin,** depending upon the indication and in consultation with the surgical team and prescribing provider, should be discontinued at least 3 to 5 days before surgery, and heparin therapy initiated.
10. If **regional anesthesia** is planned, anticoagulant and antiplatelet agents should be held according to the most recent American Society of Regional Anesthesia (ASRA) guidelines and in consultation with the surgeon and cardiologist.

B. **Respiratory system.** Many vascular patients have histories of significant tobacco use and may have compromised pulmonary function (see Chapter 4: Specific Considerations With Pulmonary Disease). Routine pulmonary function testing is not indicated. Aortic cross-clamping and associated ischemia-reperfusion can produce a systemic inflammatory response that may contribute to postoperative lung injury.

C. **Renal system.** Preexisting renal dysfunction is common. It is related to atherosclerosis, hypertension, diabetes, and advanced age and may exist even in the absence of an abnormal serum creatinine value. These patients have a reduced capacity to autoregulate renal perfusion in the setting of hypotension and are often intolerant to perioperative insults such as ischemia-reperfusion, atheroembolism, and nephrotoxins like contrast dye. Patients with chronically elevated serum creatinine levels (>2 mg/dL) have substantially greater morbidity and mortality following vascular surgery. Open aortic and renal arterial surgeries carry the highest risk for postoperative renal dysfunction. Patients undergoing endovascular procedures are at risk for **contrast-induced acute kidney injury (CI-AKI)**. **CI-AKI** is diagnosed by an increase in serum creatinine beginning 24 to 48 hours following contrast exposure in a patient with no other reason for AKI. In otherwise healthy patients, the risk of CI-AKI is low and its clinical relevance is debated. The risk of CI-AKI is increased in patients with chronic kidney disease, diabetes, anemia, heart failure, and hemodynamic instability. Procedures using high-osmolar contrast or high volumes of contrast are higher risk. In patients at risk, crystalloid administration and the use of low volumes of iso-osmolar or low-osmolar contrast agents are recommended. Treatment with sodium bicarbonate and N-acetylcysteine (NAC) has also been used to prevent CI-AKI. However, results of the PRESERVE trial demonstrated neither a benefit of sodium bicarbonate over saline nor a benefit of NAC over placebo in preventing AKI.

D. **Central nervous system.** Patients should be examined for carotid bruits and questioned for a history of transient ischemic attacks (TIAs) and cerebrovascular accidents. Symptomatic carotid disease may warrant revascularization prior to other elective procedures.

E. **Endocrine system.** In addition to accelerated atherosclerosis, patients with long-standing diabetes may have extensive microvascular disease resulting in autonomic dysfunction, silent myocardial ischemia, and nephropathy. In consultation with the patient's endocrinologist, **metformin** should be discontinued prior to procedures that involve intravenous (IV) contrast dye or renal or hepatic ischemia due to the potential for the development of severe lactic acidosis. It should also be held in patients with preexisting renal dysfunction or heart failure.

Glucagon-like–peptide 1 (GLP-1) agonists are increasingly being prescribed for type 2 diabetes, cardiovascular risk reduction, and weight loss. These medications are associated with delayed gastric emptying and have been linked to cases of aspiration. Current American Society of Anesthesiologist (ASA) recommendations are to hold these medications on the day of surgery for patients taking GLP-1 agonists daily and the week prior to surgery for patients taking them weekly. Patients requiring surgery who have not held this medication appropriately should be managed as having a full stomach.

Sodium glucose co-transporter 2 (SGLT-2) inhibitors are another emerging medication with indications for diabetes, heart failure, and renal failure. SGLT-2 inhibitors are associated with euglycemic diabetic ketoacidosis (DKA), a process of ketosis characterized by normal or mildly elevated blood glucose and an anion-gap metabolic acidosis. Surgical stress can exacerbate the risk of euglycemic DKA and thus it is recommended to discontinue SGLT-2 inhibitors 3 to 4 days prior to surgery. Laboratory values (pH, bicarbonate, anion gap, beta-hydroxybutyrate) should be closely monitored in patients who haven't appropriately discontinued these medications preoperatively or in patients who develop otherwise unexplained metabolic acidosis during the intraoperative or postoperative period.

F. **Hematologic system.** The vascular surgical patient is at particularly high risk to develop **heparin-induced thrombocytopenia (HIT)** due to the need for repeated and occasionally prolonged exposure to heparin (see Chapter 24: Anesthesia for Spine Surgery). This syndrome is characterized by thrombocytopenia and/or thrombosis in the setting of heparin exposure and is due to the formation of antibodies to the heparin–platelet factor 4 (PF4) complex. The 4T score helps determine the pretest probability of a HIT diagnosis and should guide clinical management (eg, suspension of heparin administration if the probability is intermediate or high). The **acute management** of the patient with HIT includes discontinuation of all heparins, suspension of warfarin, avoidance of platelet transfusions, and the initiation of alternative, nonheparin anticoagulant therapy.

In patients with active HIT alternative anticoagulation with direct thrombin inhibitors such as argatroban and bivalirudin can be used. These medications are only FDA approved for use as an anticoagulant during percutaneous coronary intervention but bivalirudin has also been studied for use during cardiopulmonary bypass. Argatroban's effect can be monitored intraoperatively using activated clotting time (ACT). There is no currently approved method to monitor the effect of bivalirudin but ACT and activated partial thromboplastin time (aPTT) have been used. These alternative anticoagulants carry an increased risk of bleeding due to the lack of a reversal agent. In addition, bivalirudin is renally cleared and its elimination can be delayed in patients with renal dysfunction. Argatroban is hepatically cleared and similarly can have decreased elimination in patients with hepatic dysfunction.

II. PERIPHERAL ARTERIAL SURGERY

A. General considerations. Peripheral arterial procedures include the bypass or stenting of stenotic arteries; embolectomy or catheter directed thrombolysis of occluded arteries, and the repair of peripheral arterial aneurysms. Endovascular approaches are employed whenever possible and are typically performed in the operating room, angiography suites, or hybrid operating rooms. Special considerations for the provision of anesthesia outside of the operating room are discussed in Chapter 34: Non-Operating Room Anesthesia.

B. Percutaneous balloon angioplasty and stenting. Limb patency and amputation-free survival rates are similar to open bypass surgery. Patients must have a target lesion amenable to the endovascular approach: typically a focal short-segment occlusion with patent vessels distal to the treated lesion (ie, "good runoff"). Advantages of percutaneous therapy include faster patient recovery, shorter hospital stay, smaller wounds with lower complication rates, and potential cost savings. Procedures on the upper and lower extremities are typically performed in the operating room angiography suites and are frequently done under local anesthesia with sedation.

1. **Surgical approach** may be percutaneous or through a cutdown to the artery. Brachial artery access may be required, necessitating IV placement and blood pressure monitoring on the contralateral arm.
2. **Large amounts of IV contrast dye** may be administered and may require prophylaxis for CI-AKI (see Section I.C).
3. **Anesthetic technique** frequently involves monitored anesthesia care with standard monitors. Local anesthesia typically provides sufficient analgesia. Provisions should be made to allow for conversion to general anesthesia in the case of an unplanned conversion to open repair.
4. **IV unfractionated heparin** is often used as an adjunct and is given prior to arterial cannulation. A **vasodilator** may be administered intra-arterially by the surgeon to treat catheter- or wire-induced vasospasm. Treatment of systemic effects may be required.
5. **Distal embolization** is a potential serious complication with aggressive endovascular instrumentation.

C. Lower-extremity bypass grafting. In the presence of multisegment disease or poor distal runoff, open **surgical bypass** of the lower extremity is preferred over the endovascular approach. An autologous saphenous vein graft is the most commonly used conduit. If this is not available, or is of unacceptable quality, an upper extremity vein from the patient or cryopreserved cadaveric vein may be used. Preparation of the vein and subsequent anastomoses to the arterial circulation may be time consuming but rarely place significant hemodynamic stress on the patient. The use of synthetic grafts in selected patients may reduce the length of these procedures; however, long-term patency rates with prosthetic grafts are generally reduced relative to autologous vein grafts. **Blood loss is usually minimal**, but may be significant with revision of a previous bypass. **Routine monitoring** is usually sufficient. Patient comorbidities or surgical complexity may warrant placement of invasive monitors. **No significant differences in morbidity or mortality have been demonstrated between regional anesthesia and general anesthesia** for lower limb revascularization.
  1. **General anesthesia.** Any technique is appropriate provided hemodynamic stability is maintained.
  2. **Neuraxial and regional anesthesia.** Potential advantages may include sympathetic blockade, improved pain control, lack of airway instrumentation, improved ability to detect symptoms of myocardial ischemia in an awake patient, and reduced incidence of pneumonia. However, long procedures under regional anesthesia can pose a challenge for patients who may become uncomfortable and restless.
     a. A continuous **lumbar epidural catheter** may be used. It provides excellent analgesia and muscle relaxation as well as the ability to administer postoperative analgesia. Spinal anesthesia may be used if the length of the procedure is appropriate. For **femoral–popliteal** and distal lower extremity bypass limited to a single limb, combined lumbar plexus and sciatic nerve block may be used as an alternative to neuraxial anesthesia. For **iliofemoral bypass**, a spinal or epidural will require a higher level (ie, T8–T10) because of proximal extension of the incision and peritoneal retraction for exposure of the iliac artery. **Femoral–femoral bypass grafting** is used to treat symptomatic unilateral iliac occlusive disease.
     b. **An α-adrenergic agent** (eg, phenylephrine) should be available to treat the hypotension associated with sympathetic blockade.
D. Peripheral embolectomy and catheter-directed thrombolysis (CDT)
Embolectomy can be performed using either an open or a percutaneous technique. Due to its more rapid revascularization, embolectomy can be associated with more systemic effects of reperfusion than thrombolysis. CDT using tissue plasminogen activator (tPA) can be considered as a revascularization strategy in acute limb ischemia but is more appropriate in patients where there is no immediate threat to limb due to its slower timeframe of revascularization. Patients who have contraindications to thrombolytic therapy are not eligible for CDT. Patients must be monitored closely for bleeding complications or progression of ischemia. CDT is done percutaneously and can be done with local or general anesthesia. Regional or neuraxial anesthesia is usually contraindicated as many patients with acute limb ischemia have received systemic anticoagulation.
E. Femoral pseudoaneurysm. Femoral pseudoaneurysms are most often iatrogenic, occurring in the setting of femoral artery catheterization (eg, for coronary angiography or intra-aortic balloon pump placement). As such, these patients often have unstable cardiovascular disease (eg, recent MI

with stent placement). Some are anticoagulated or have recently received thrombolytic agents, thus precluding regional anesthesia. Field blocks with local anesthesia may be most appropriate in the setting of cardiovascular instability.

F. **Peripheral aneurysms.** Peripheral arterial aneurysms, such as popliteal artery aneurysms, rarely rupture but are associated with a high rate of thrombosis and embolism. Either general or neuraxial anesthesia may be used to manage their repair.

G. **Axillofemoral bypass grafting.** An axillofemoral bypass graft restores arterial blood flow to the lower extremities in patients with occluded aortoiliac vessels who are not candidates for aortic reconstruction for various reasons including high anesthetic risk, significant intra-abdominal adhesions due to prior abdominal surgeries, active abdominal infection, or an infected aortic prosthesis. A prosthetic graft is tunneled under the pectoralis muscle and positioned in the subcutaneous layer of the thorax and abdomen and anastomosed distally to the femoral artery. General anesthesia is most appropriate.

H. **Vascular surgery of the upper extremity.** Vascular surgery of the upper extremity usually includes distal embolectomy and repair of traumatic injuries. The surgery is localized, but there may be a need to harvest a vein graft at a site distant from the vascular repair. Possible anesthetic techniques include field block and regional or general anesthesia.

III. CAROTID REVASCULARIZATION

A. **General considerations.** Carotid revascularization is performed in patients with significant stenosis of the internal carotid artery, often manifesting clinically as carotid bruits or neurologic symptoms such as transient ischemic attacks (TIAs) or strokes. According to the 2021 American Heart Association/American Stroke Association guidelines, carotid endarterectomy (CEA) is strongly recommended for symptomatic patients (TIA or nondisabling stroke within the previous 6 months) with carotid stenosis of 70% to 99%, provided their life expectancy is at least 5 years and the surgeon's perioperative stroke and death rate is less than 6%. In addition, for symptomatic patients with moderate stenosis (50% to 69%), CEA can be beneficial depending on factors such as age, sex, comorbidities, and perioperative risk. For asymptomatic patients with carotid stenosis of 60% to 99%, CEA may be considered if the patient has a life expectancy exceeding 5 years and a surgeon's perioperative risk of stroke and death below 3%. Currently, the evidence supporting CEA for asymptomatic women remains less definitive. For patients not meeting surgical criteria, comprehensive medical therapy including high-intensity statins, antiplatelet agents, smoking cessation, blood pressure control, and diabetes management is essential.

CEA remains the preferred approach for carotid artery stenosis in suitable surgical candidates. The role of carotid artery stenting (CAS) is evolving, with evidence indicating similar long-term outcomes compared to CEA, but a generally higher periprocedural stroke and death rate, especially in older patients (>70 years). CAS is specifically recommended in select scenarios where anatomic or medical factors significantly elevate the surgical risk such as in patients with severe medical comorbidities or those who present anatomic challenges due to prior neck surgery or radiation.

B. **Carotid artery stenting**
  1. **Indications.** CAS may be preferred over CEA in patients with neck anatomy that is unfavorable for open surgery, such as with prior neck

surgery or radiation, or in patients with higher operative risk due to severe cardiac or pulmonary disease. Due to the potential for CI-AKI, CAS is generally avoided in patients with renal dysfunction.

2. **Monitoring.** An arterial catheter is indicated for continuous hemodynamic monitoring and facilitates frequent blood draws for monitoring of ACT. Close observation of the patient's **mental status** is necessary to detect new-onset stroke resulting from plaque embolization.
3. **Anesthetic management** usually consists of monitored anesthesia care combined with local anesthesia at the vascular access site. Care should be taken to maintain the patient's level of alertness to facilitate intraoperative neurologic monitoring. The femoral artery is typically accessed percutaneously. The awake patient may feel pain during balloon angioplasty and arterial dilation that resolves immediately with balloon deflation.
4. **IV contrast dye** and fluoroscopy are used intermittently throughout the procedure.
5. **Heparin** is administered prior to arteriotomy.
6. Vagally mediated **bradycardia** can occur following stent deployment. Pretreatment with glycopyrrolate is helpful.
7. **Complications** include stroke, vascular access site injuries, device malfunction, restenosis, and CI-AKI. Microembolic injuries are more frequent after CAS compared with CEA; embolic protection devices can reduce neurologic injuries if the operator is experienced with the apparatus.
8. Transcarotid artery revascularization (TCAR) is a system for carotid artery stenting which relies on blood flow reversal through a temporary carotid to femoral venous shunt to prevent distal embolization during stent deployment. It involves surgical dissection and exposure of the carotid artery as well as percutaneous insertion of a femoral venous sheath. Anesthetic considerations are similar to CAS. The procedure can be performed under general anesthesia or using a MAC with a field block for neck dissection. The Society for Vascular Surgery guidelines notes that TCAR outcomes are at least equivalent to CEA.

C. Carotid endarterectomy
1. **Monitoring.**
    a. **Intra-arterial blood pressure monitoring is necessary.**
    b. **Central nervous system (CNS) monitoring** is necessary, especially during carotid artery clamping to evaluate the adequacy of cerebral perfusion and to identify patients who may require **shunting**. The awake patient is the gold standard for intraoperative CNS monitoring. If the procedure is being conducted under general anesthesia, the CNS can be monitored using **electroencephalography** (EEG), transcranial Doppler ultrasound, or arterial stump pressure measurement. CEA can also be conducted with routine shunting without continuous CNS monitoring. There are no data to support the use of routine versus selective shunting. No particular method of CNS monitoring in selective shunting has been shown to produce better outcomes.
2. **Anesthetic technique.** The superiority of general versus regional anesthesia has been debated. Retrospective observational studies have suggested a benefit to regional techniques, including in a meta-analysis. However, pooled analysis of available randomized trials did not find a difference between the techniques. If a clinical difference exists, it is likely small and anesthetic technique is usually based on the preferences of the surgeon and the patient.

a. **Regional anesthesia**
   1. Regional anesthesia may be performed with a combined **superficial** and **deep cervical plexus block** or with a superficial plexus block that is supplemented in the field by the surgeon (see Chapter 18: Perioperative Hemodynamic Control). Both have potential complications.
   2. CEA under regional anesthesia **requires an alert, cooperative patient** who is able to tolerate lying still, with the head rotated to the side, under the drapes.
   3. **Access to the airway** may be necessary at any time, and the patient should be positioned and draped with this in mind. An appropriately sized laryngeal mask airway should be readily available.
   4. **Continuous neurologic** assessment is possible in the awake patient.
b. **General anesthesia**
   1. **Prior to induction, neuromonitoring baselines** are established.
   2. **Blood pressure** should be maintained at the patient's **high-normal** range that may require a vasopressor.
   3. **A hemodynamically stable induction** is desired to preserve cerebral perfusion.
   4. Minute ventilation should be adjusted to avoid hypocapnic cerebral vasoconstriction. Hypercarbia has no clinical benefit.
   5. When employing intraoperative EEG monitoring, communication with the neuromonitoring team is essential. Goals include a stable anesthetic plane to facilitate EEG interpretation and the avoidance of burst suppression. **Neuromuscular blockade** minimizes muscle artifact that can interfere with EEG interpretation and with inadvertent patient movement during delicate portions of the procedure.
   6. The goals during emergence are twofold: to minimize straining, which poses a risk to the arteriotomy closure, and to facilitate a **prompt neurologic examination** in case of new neurologic or cranial nerve deficit. This is best summarized as a crisp, smooth emergence.

3. **Carotid cross-clamping**
   a. **Systemic heparin** (100 IU/kg) is administered before cross-clamping with a target ACT of greater than or equal to 200 seconds.
   b. Prior to cross-clamp, **blood pressure** is typically increased by the use of a vasopressor, with the intention of maintaining ipsilateral cerebral perfusion through the Circle of Willis from the contralateral carotid.
   c. **Surgical manipulation of the carotid sinus** may cause intense vagal stimulation, leading to hypotension and bradycardia. Release of traction or infiltration with local anesthetic will typically abolish the response. Administration of anticholinergics is seldom required. Prophylactic infiltration of local anesthetic infiltration should be considered for patients with significant preoperative cardiac conduction delay, critical aortic stenosis, and significant coronary disease.
   d. **Routine shunting, selective shunting, or no shunting.** Shunting involves the placement of a temporary arterial graft to span the arteriotomy and preserve ipsilateral, antegrade cerebral perfusion during carotid artery cross-clamping. The approach to shunting is based on surgical preference. A number of case series have shown similar stroke risk with the three approaches. Selective shunting describes the practice of shunt placement upon EEG evidence of cerebral ischemia following carotid cross-clamping.

    e. **Unclamping** may produce reflex vasodilation and bradycardia. Vasopressors may be required as the baroreceptors adapt, which may continue into the postoperative period.
 D. **Postoperative considerations**
    1. Immediate postoperative complications include **neurologic deficits, blood pressure lability, and airway obstruction.**
    2. **Neurologic deficits** are typically due to emboli related to the surgical procedure. They should be managed aggressively with increased blood pressure and consultation with the surgeon and a stroke specialist.
    3. **Labile blood pressures** may be observed secondary to alterations in the carotid baroreceptor response brought about by the endarterectomy. Hypertension requiring administration of vasodilator (labetalol or hydralazine boluses or escalating to nitroglycerin or nicardipine as an IV infusion) may be a result of surgical denervation of the carotid sinus. Hypotension requiring a vasopressor (phenylephrine) may be a result of baroreceptor hypersensitivity and typically does not reflect hypovolemia.
    4. **Postextubation airway compromise** can be secondary to dehiscence at the arteriotomy suture line leading expanding hematoma. The immediate release of the superficial sutures with evacuation of the hematoma is necessary to prevent airway compromise.
    5. Other etiologies for postextubation airway compromise include **injury to the recurrent laryngeal, superior laryngeal, or hypoglossal nerves.** Unilateral recurrent laryngeal nerve injury manifests with a hoarse voice. Bilateral recurrent laryngeal nerve injury is rare but must be considered in patients who have undergone previous contralateral CEA or neck surgery.
    6. **Cerebral hyperperfusion syndrome** typically occurs several days postoperatively and may manifest as ipsilateral headache, seizure, focal neurologic signs, or intracranial hemorrhage. It is related to an abrupt increase in blood flow with loss of autoregulation in the surgically reperfused brain. Based on the pathophysiology of the syndrome, **it is reasonable to target postoperative blood pressures in the normal to slightly subnormal range** (often systolic blood pressure [SBP] <140 mm Hg).

IV. ABDOMINAL AORTIC REPAIR

Abdominal aortic repair may be required for atherosclerotic occlusive disease or aneurysmal dilation of the aorta. Aorto-occlusive disease usually presents as claudication. An abdominal aortic aneurysm (AAA) may be found incidentally. Alternatively, it may present with back pain or, if ruptured, severe shock. Ninety-five percent of all AAAs occur below the level of the renal arteries. Indications for repair are largest diameter greater than 5.5 cm; rate of expansion exceeding 1 cm/y; or symptoms secondary to the AAA. In females, repair of asymptomatic AAA may be indicated at a lower diameter threshold due to a higher rate of rupture, although females may also be at a higher perioperative risk. The annual risk of rupture of an expanding 5-cm aneurysm is about 4%. The operative mortality for elective AAA repair is less than 2%, while the overall mortality of aneurysm rupture is 70% to 80%.

A. **Endovascular abdominal aortic repair (EVAR)**
    1. **Overview.** The majority of infrarenal AAA are treated by EVAR. The procedure involves the endovascular placement of an expandable stent graft spanning the aneurysm under fluoroscopic guidance. The stent graft excludes the aneurysm from the circulation, preventing its further expansion and rupture. The application of an aortic **cross clamp is not required** consequently. **EVAR leads to greater intraoperative hemodynamic stability.** There is a lower incidence of postoperative pulmonary,

cardiovascular, and renal morbidity and significantly reduced 30-day operative mortality for EVAR compared to open surgery. The early survival benefit is lost over time. At about 2 years postprocedure, mortality rates are the same as those for patients who have undergone open aneurysm resection. Patients with endovascular repair also require regular follow-up imaging and may require additional EVAR-related interventions.

2. **Patient suitability** for EVAR depends on the size and morphology of the AAA. Most infrarenal AAAs with favorable neck anatomy are repaired endovascularly. EVAR has lower short-term, perioperative mortality, but higher incidence of leak and other long-term complications, and requires a lifetime of imaging surveillance. Younger patients with better risk profile may be more suited for open repair.

3. **Monitoring and access.** Intra-arterial blood pressure monitoring is required in addition to standard monitors. Large bore peripheral access (16 gauge or 14 gauge) is desirable. Central venous access is rarely required.

4. **Surgical considerations.** Systemic **heparinization** is required. If the aneurysm involves the renal or mesenteric arteries, a more complex endovascular stent graft with branches or fenestrations can be used. For infrarenal aneurysms, **surgical access is usually via bilateral common femoral arteries.** Exposure of the arteries followed by arteriotomies is typically performed with surgical repair afterward. Percutaneous access with subsequent closure using a specialized device is possible for select patients in the absence of femoral artery disease or stenosis. There is significant **radiation exposure** with **fluoroscopy** and a **contrast** dye load. **Ensuring the patient does not move** during digital subtraction angiography will reduce the patient's exposure by minimizing the need for repeated studies. Following stent graft deployment, an intra-aortic balloon is inflated to expand the stent graft and anchor it in place. Balloon inflation leads to temporary aortic occlusion. The occlusion is short lived, typically lasting 3 to 4 heartbeats. Hypertension may be observed during the period of balloon occlusion; however, it usually does not last long enough to warrant therapy. **Controlled hypotension** may be requested by the surgeon during stent graft deployment to prevent proximal hypertension and stent graft displacement.

5. **Types of grafts used in EVAR.** Advances and improvements in graft technology have expanded the pool of patients who are eligible for endovascular repair. Fenestrated grafts have radiopaque markers at fenestrations in the graft designed for aortic side branches and are typically used for juxtarenal aneurysms. Because these fenestrations need to be precisely placed according to a patient's anatomy, these grafts require customization and preoperative planning. Branched grafts are another type of customized endograft which have branches arising from the main body for insertion into the visceral arteries. For patients who are not able to wait for custom grafts, chimney stent grafts can be used. In this technique covered stents are deployed first into the visceral and renal arteries and then a conventional graft is deployed alongside these stents.

6. **Anesthetic technique.** EVAR may be performed under **local, regional,** or **general anesthesia.** Factors such as anticoagulant use, patient comfort, surgeon preference, and anticipated length of surgery will influence the choice of anesthetic. There are no randomized controlled trials which evaluate the optimal anesthetic approach. Retrospective studies have shown an association between local or regional anesthesia and reduced mortality, lengths of stay, and ICU admissions. Bilateral ilioinguinal or

iliohypogastric nerve blocks are alternatives along with local infiltration. Of note, in contrast to neuraxial anesthesia, local anesthesia will not alleviate the ischemia pain associated with femoral artery occlusion, and supplementation with systemic analgesics may be required.

7. **Conversion to open repair is rare (<1%).** It may be necessary in the setting of difficult arterial access (eg, with severely atherosclerotic arteries); vessel dissection at the arterial access site; tortuous iliac arteries that prevent passage of the deployment system; stent malposition or migration; and aneurysm rupture. Resuscitation equipment such as a red blood cell salvage device and a rapid infusion device should be available in centers performing EVAR.
8. **Bleeding** may occur around the femoral sheaths and is often difficult to quantify or track. Massive hemorrhage is rare.
9. **Complications of EVAR** include failure to exclude the AAA from the arterial system (endoleak), embolism, arterial injury, graft kinking, groin access injury, limb ischemia, and infection. AKI can result from contrast administration and embolization of debris dislodged by catheters and wires (see Section I.C).
    a. **Endoleak (Figure 28.1)** is the persistence of blood flow into the aneurysm sac despite leading to expansion. It occurs in 20% to 25% of EVARs. Types I and III endoleaks are considered at high risk for aneurysm sac pressurization and rupture and should be treated as soon as diagnosed. Type II endoleaks may spontaneously resolve and are followed closely with serial imaging. If they persist, they may require a subsequent procedure to embolize the responsible vessel. Treatment is not recommended for type IV endoleaks.

B. **Open abdominal aortic surgery**

Patient selection. Open surgical repair is indicated for patients whose aortic anatomy does not meet the specified minimum requirements for standard, commercially available endografts; for patients in whom delaying repair to wait for a custom-made endograft may result in significant risk of rupture; and for patients unlikely to comply with long-term imaging surveillance protocols following EVAR.

1. **Surgical approach.** The abdominal aorta is accessed through either a transabdominal or retroperitoneal (RP) approach. Compared with a **transabdominal** approach, the **RP** approach may result in a lower incidence of postoperative ileus, pulmonary complications, cardiovascular complications, and fluid shifts. The RP approach is technically advantageous in morbidly obese patients and in those who have had previous abdominal procedures.
2. **Monitoring.** A large peripheral IV, arterial line, central venous catheter, and Foley catheter are indicated. Procedures that require a supraceliac cross-clamp entail greater hemodynamic perturbations and blood loss. Enhanced intraoperative monitoring of cardiac function with TEE or PA catheter may be beneficial. Vasopressors and vasodilators must be available.
3. **Anesthetic technique.** Most patients receive combined general and epidural anesthesia using a low-thoracic to midthoracic epidural catheter. Although general anesthesia alone is acceptable, a combined technique reduces anesthetic requirements, facilitates earlier extubation, and provides effective postoperative analgesia. Retrospective data suggests a mortality benefit with epidural use in elective AAA repair.
4. The hemodynamic goal of **induction** is to **avoid hypertension**. It is helpful to establish a sensory level with the epidural catheter prior to the induction of general anesthesia.

Chapter 28 Anesthesia for Vascular Surgery 497

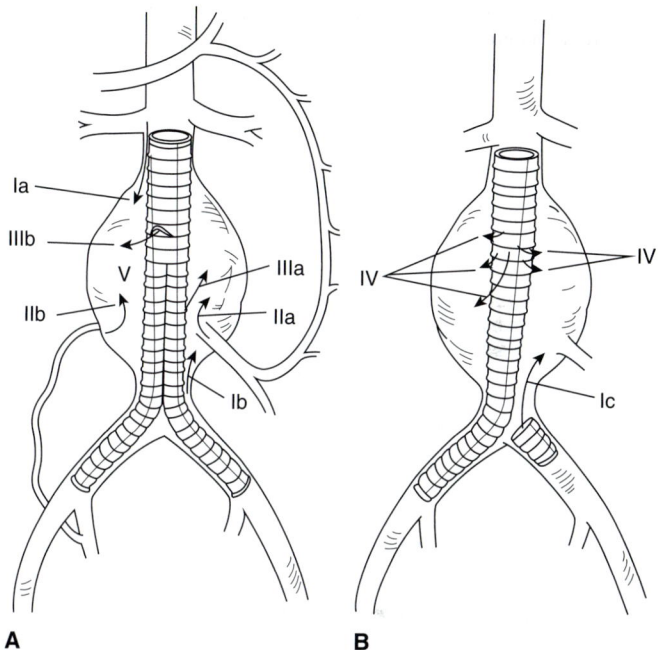

FIGURE 28.1 A, B, Schematic demonstrating the different types of endoleak after endovascular aneurysm repair. Type I endoleaks occur because of inadequate graft seal resulting in perigraft flow and include (*Ia*) perigraft flow occurring proximally, (*Ib*) perigraft flow occurring distally, and (*Ic*) perigraft flow around an iliac artery occlusion device. Type II endoleaks occur when branch arteries backbleed because of collateral flow. These endoleaks include (*IIa*) backbleeding inferior mesenteric artery and (*IIb*) backbleeding lumbar artery. Type III endoleaks occur when flow persists between the segments of a modular graft and include (*IIIa*) leaks between iliac limbs or an iliac limb and main body component and (*IIIb*) leaks between main body components. Type IV endoleaks (*IV*) occur when flow is present through endograft material (graft porosity). Type V endoleak, or, "endotension" (*V*), occurs when persistent or recurrent pressurization of the aortic aneurysm exists in the absence of demonstrable endoleak. (Drawings prepared by H. Fischer, MFA.)

5. **Heat conservation.** Heat loss during aortic procedures may be considerable. Strategies for heat conservation are discussed in Chapter 19: Local Anesthetics. Forced air warmers should **never** be used **below the level of the aortic cross-clamp.** Severe burns may develop during cross-clamping due to the absence of heat redistribution by normal blood flow.
6. **Bowel manipulation** is necessary to gain access to the aorta during the transabdominal approach and may be accompanied by skin flushing, decreased systemic vascular resistance, and profound hypotension. These changes may be caused by the release of prostaglandins and vasoactive peptides from the bowel and last for 20 to 30 minutes. Treatment consists of vasopressor administration and volume expansion.
7. **Fluid management.** There is the potential for significant intravascular volume depletion due to hemorrhage; insensible losses into the bowel and peritoneal cavity; and evaporative losses associated with the laparotomy. Volume resuscitation is guided by the patient's hemodynamics.

Aortic cross-clamp application will give rise to renal insufficiency, even with an infrarenal cross-clamp.
8. **Blood product administration** should be guided by the patient's laboratory values.
9. **Aortic cross-clamping**
    a. **Systemic heparin** is administered several minutes prior to the application of the aortic cross-clamp.
    b. **Hypertension** will occur with aortic cross-clamping. The degree of hypertension is a function of the cross-clamp location. A more proximal cross-clamp is associated with a greater increase in blood pressure. Consideration can be given to inducing mild hypotension prior to the application of the cross-clamp. The **increased afterload** is well tolerated by patients with normal cardiac function, but those with compromised left ventricular function may develop myocardial ischemia and hypotension. Hypotension with the application of the aortic cross-clamp may indicate left ventricular failure secondary to increased afterload or retrograde dissection into the coronary arteries. Cardiac function must be evaluated and supported.
    c. Avoidance of excessive hypertension is important during aortic cross-clamp to minimize the **risk of retrograde aortic dissection.**
    d. Following proximal clamping, **vascular control distal to the aneurysm** is established. The surgical plan is driven by anatomic considerations. If distal cross-clamping is not technically feasible because sufficient disease-free artery cannot be exposed to sew the distal anastomoses, then a balloon-tipped catheter is advanced antegrade through the arteriotomy to prevent retrograde blood flow. Once the aneurysm sac is opened, a balloon-tipped catheter is advanced distal to the aneurysm. Balloon inflation occludes the vessel to establish distal control and prevent retrograde hemorrhage into the field, establishing distal control. Significant retrograde hemorrhage may occur during this maneuver.
    e. There is no compelling evidence to support the use of renal protective adjuncts such as **mannitol and fenoldopam.** The application of an aortic cross-clamp at any level may lead to decreased renal cortical blood flow and urine output. With suprarenal clamping, renal perfusion is at even greater risk due to longer cross-clamp times and potential for cholesterol embolization. The maintenance of adequate hydration and urine output is paramount.
10. **Aortic unclamping**
    a. Unclamping will produce immediate **hypotension** due to a fall in systemic vascular resistance.
    b. The degree of hypotension is a function of clamp duration and the proximal location of the clamp.
    c. Prior to release of the aortic cross-clamp, steps should be taken to optimize the patient's intravascular **volume status** and **increase vascular tone.** Inspired oxygen concentration should be increased to 100%. **Minute ventilation** may also be increased to induce a mild respiratory alkalosis.
    d. Following unclamping, reperfusion of the ischemic organs and tissues leads to acidemia and systemic vasodilation. The magnitude of these disturbances is a function of the duration of the aortic cross-clamp and the metabolic activity of the organs that were ischemic. **Cross-clamping above the celiac or superior mesenteric artery can produce profound visceral ischemia and acidosis. Sodium bicarbonate** may

be administered at unclamping to mitigate the effects of acidosis. In the setting of profound hypotension that is unresponsive to fluids or vasopressors, the aortic cross-clamp may be reapplied to maintain adequate perfusion pressure while additional volume and vasopressors are administered.

11. **Emergence.** Most patients with working epidurals and infrarenal or juxtarenal cross-clamps can be extubated at the end of the procedure. Patients with hemodynamic instability, persistent hemorrhage, persistent acidosis, or severe hypothermia (<33 °C) are left intubated. Hypertension, tachycardia, pain, and shivering should be anticipated and treated.

C. **Emergent repair of a ruptured AAA.** Patients may be **hemodynamically stable or unstable** depending on the degree to which the rupture is contained. Rupture can occur into the peritoneal cavity or the RP space. Some measure of tamponade will temporarily reduce the volume of blood loss.

1. The priority for anesthetic management is the establishment of adequate **IV access** for large volume resuscitation.
2. **Blood products** should be ordered immediately. If type-specific blood and FFP are unavailable, universal donor-type blood (type O negative for women of childbearing age and type O positive for all others) and FFP (type AB) should be obtained, and a **blood bank sample** should be sent immediately to the lab for cross-matching. **Colloid solutions** should be ordered. A red blood cell salvage system as well as a rapid transfuser should be immediately available.
3. **Standard monitors** should initially be applied if the patient is unstable, so as not to delay definitive surgical control. The immediate priority is to control bleeding surgically by cross-clamping the aorta through a laparotomy or thoracotomy. Alternatively, the aorta may be occluded endovascularly using a balloon-tipped catheter. Invasive monitors (arterial line, central line, PA catheter) may be placed as time and hemodynamics permit. **Clear communication with the surgical team** regarding the surgical and anesthetic plans is essential. If the patient's hemodynamics permit, placement of a central venous catheter is often performed while the patient is awake.
4. **Hypotensive resuscitation** that involves restricting intravascular volume administration to maintain SBP in the 70 to 100 mm Hg range has been recommended. Evidence for this management strategy is borrowed from the trauma literature, and this strategy has not been studied in ruptured aortic syndromes. The physiologic rationale behind this strategy is to limit hypothermic and dilutional coagulopathy while avoiding clot disruption caused by increases in SBP.
5. Based on the clinical circumstances, the surgical plan, and the available equipment, it may be preferable to insert an occlusive balloon-tipped catheter into the aorta above the level of the aneurysm prior to the induction of general anesthesia. Such a catheter may be inserted percutaneously using local anesthesia. It can then be used to occlude the aorta in the event of circulatory collapse following anesthetic induction.
6. **Surgical technique: endovascular versus open**
   a. **Open repair**
      1. **Induction.** In moribund patients, endotracheal intubation should be performed immediately. Hypotensive patients should be preoxygenated and induced expeditiously. Hemodynamics may allow for only small doses of scopolamine, etomidate, ketamine, and a benzodiazepine. **Severe hypotension on induction may occur** as a result of vasodilation, loss of sympathetic drive, and loss

of peritoneal tamponade with abdominal wall relaxation. The patient should be prepped and draped prior to induction and the surgeon ready to make incision if needed.
2. Care must be taken to **avoid hypertension** during induction.
3. Once the aorta has been clamped and hemodynamic stability achieved, incremental doses of opioids and supplemental anesthetics may be given as tolerated.
4. Blood component therapy should be guided by the laboratory values. In the event of massive hemorrhage, packed red blood cells and FFP should be administered in a ratio of at least 2:1.
5. **Hypothermia** contributes to acidosis, coagulopathy, and myocardial dysfunction and should be treated.
6. **Renal protective strategies** such as aggressive hydration and the maintenance of appropriate perfusion pressure should be instituted. The administration of mannitol and fenoldopam may be considered, although there is no compelling evidence to support their use. Mortality in patients developing renal failure following a ruptured AAA is high.

b. **Endovascular repair** can be considered as an alternative to open repair provided anatomy is suitable, the center is appropriately equipped, and the team is appropriately experienced. The procedure may be performed under local anesthesia. Recent randomized controlled trials and meta-analyses have provided mixed results regarding survival outcomes for patients undergoing endovascular aneurysm repair (EVAR) compared with open repair for ruptured AAAs. While retrospective studies previously suggested a survival benefit favoring EVAR, contemporary evidence from prospective randomized trials indicates comparable short-term survival outcomes, with EVAR offering potential advantages in perioperative morbidity and shorter hospital stays. The overall survival benefit of EVAR compared to open repair remains uncertain, particularly in the long term, necessitating individualized patient selection based on clinical condition, anatomical suitability, and institutional expertise.

7. **Complications and prognosis.** Under the best of circumstances, there is a 40% to 50% mortality rate. The incidence of MI, acute renal failure, respiratory failure, and coagulopathy is high.

V. THORACOABDOMINAL AORTIC ANEURYSM REPAIR

A. **Etiology of thoracic aortic disease.** Causes of thoracic aortic disease include atherosclerosis, degenerative disorders of connective tissue (eg, Marfan and Ehlers–Danlos syndromes and cystic necrosis), infection (eg, syphilis), congenital defects (eg, coarctation and congenital aneurysms of the sinus of Valsalva), trauma (eg, penetrating and deceleration injuries), and inflammatory processes (eg, Takayasu aortitis). The most common problem affecting the thoracic aorta is **atherosclerotic aneurysm** of the descending portion, accounting for about 20% of all aortic aneurysms. When such aneurysms dissect proximally, they may involve the aortic valve or coronary ostia. Distal dissection may involve the abdominal aorta with renal or mesenteric involvement. The next most frequent problem is **traumatic disruption** of the thoracic aorta. Adventitial false aneurysms may form distal to the left subclavian artery at the insertion of the ligamentum arteriosum, because of penetrating or deceleration injuries. These false aneurysms may dissect proximally and involve the arch and its major branches.

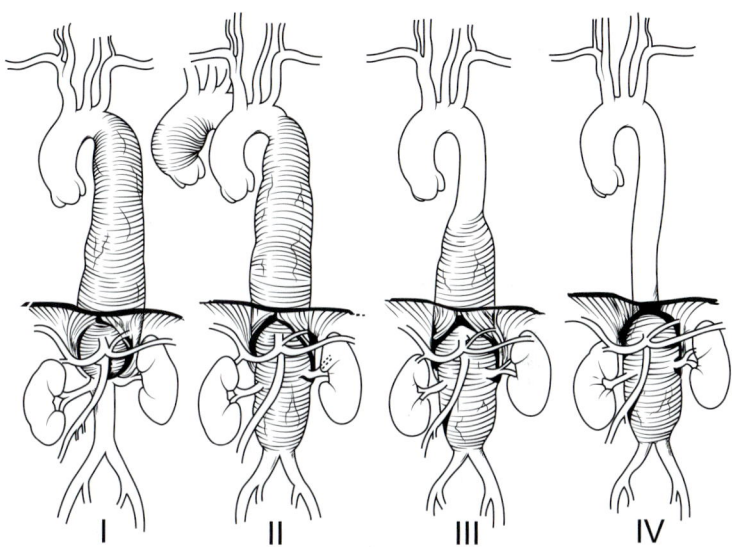

FIGURE 28.2 Crawford classification of thoracic and thoracoabdominal aortic aneurysms. (Reprinted from Crawford ES, Crawford JL, Safi HJ, et al. Thoracoabdominal aortic aneurysms preoperative and intraoperative factors determining immediate and long-term results of operations in 605 patients. *J Vasc Surg.* 1986;3:389–404, with permission from Elsevier.)

- **B. Crawford classification** of thoracoabdominal aneurysms (**Figure 28.2**).
    1. **Type I.** Aneurysm of the descending thoracic aorta distal to the subclavian artery, ending at or above the origin of the visceral vessels.
    2. **Type II.** Aneurysm from the origin of the subclavian artery to the distal abdominal aorta. This is the highest risk type in terms of paralysis, renal failure, and mortality.
    3. **Type III.** Aneurysm from the mid-descending thoracic aorta to the distal abdominal aorta.
    4. **Type IV.** Aneurysm from the diaphragm down to the distal aorta.
- **C. Associated findings**
    1. **Airway deviation or compression**, particularly of the left mainstem bronchus, producing atelectasis.
    2. **Tracheal displacement or disruption**, producing difficulties with endotracheal intubation and ventilation. Long-standing aneurysms may give rise to recurrent laryngeal nerve damage, resulting in vocal cord paralysis and hoarseness.
    3. **Hemoptysis**, due to the erosion of the aneurysm into an adjacent bronchus.
    4. **Esophageal compression** with dysphagia and an increased risk of aspiration.
    5. **Distortion and compression of the central venous and arterial anatomy**, producing markedly asymmetric pulses and difficult internal jugular vein cannulation.
    6. **Hemothorax and mediastinal shift** from rupture or leakage, producing respiratory and circulatory compromise.
    7. **Reduced distal perfusion** secondary to aortic branch vessel occlusion, producing renal, mesenteric, spinal cord, or extremity ischemia.

D. Open thoracic aortic aneurysm repair

1. **Surgical technique.** The patient is positioned in the right lateral decubitus position. The left arm is placed overhead on an armrest to avoid brachial plexus stretch, and care is taken to pad pressure points thoroughly. To the extent possible, the pelvis is rotated supine. This position allows access from the posterior thorax through the retroperitoneum to the distal abdominal aorta. The affected aortic segment is isolated, and an interposition graft is inserted. During aortic cross-clamping, visceral organ ischemic time can be reduced using distal aortic perfusion with atrial-femoral bypass (AFB). The **inclusion technique** involves using the portion of native aorta containing the celiac, superior mesenteric, and renal ostia as a component of the bypass graft.

2. **Spinal cord protection**
   a. **Anatomy**
      1. The anterior spinal artery arises from the vertebral arteries at the base of the skull. Its blood supply in the thoracic and lumbar regions is maintained through segmental arteries.
      2. The most dominant of the aortic radicular arteries is the **artery of Adamkiewicz**, which usually originates between T8 and T12.
      3. Cross-clamping of the thoracic aorta may compromise flow through these vessels and result in anterior spinal cord ischemia giving rise to anterior spinal artery syndrome.
   b. **Anterior spinal artery syndrome.** Manifestations include paraplegia, rectal and urinary incontinence, and loss of pain and temperature sensation. Vibratory and proprioceptive sensations are maintained. Paraplegia occurs in 2% to 4% of descending thoracic aortic aneurysm repairs and 3% to 10% of thoracoabdominal aortic aneurysm repairs. **Risk factors** include the location of proximal and distal cross-clamps; the duration of the cross-clamp; increased body temperature; the degree of collateralization of the spinal cord circulation; and previous abdominal aneurysm surgery.
   c. **Mechanism of spinal cord ischemia.** Spinal cord ischemia during aortic surgeries is multifactorial and likely results both from an initial insult causing decreased perfusion as well as the subsequent inflammatory response caused by reperfusion. Ischemia was traditionally thought to be directly related to interruption of flow in the artery of Adamkiewicz but more recent study has focused on the existence of an extensive collateral network with contributions from the lumbar segmental arteries, subclavian artery, internal thoracic artery, and hypogastric artery. Poor flow in this collateral circulation is thought to contribute to the development of spinal cord ischemia. Allowing for the development of an increased collateral network forms the basis for elective staged repairs of more extensive aortic aneurysms. Staged repairs can be done open, endovascularly, or as a hybrid approach.
   d. **Spinal cord protection strategies**
      1. **Cerebrospinal fluid (CSF) drainage** lowers the CSF pressure (CSFP) and promotes spinal cord perfusion. It has been shown to reduce the incidence of anterior spinal artery syndrome and is a class I recommendation for patients undergoing open thoracoabdominal aortic aneurysm repair who are at high risk for spinal cord ischemia in the 2022 ACC/AHA guidelines. The CSF drainage catheter is inserted at the L4–L5 level and advanced 8 to 12 cm into the subarachnoid space. Much of placement is guided by institutional practice. Drains can be placed in the sitting or lateral decubitus position. Fluoroscopy can be used to aid in

placement. Careful consideration should be given to spinal curvature, epidural scarring, or prior surgeries, as these may necessitate adjustments in approach. Thorough imaging evaluation is essential to inform the approach to subarachnoid catheter placement. Prior lumbar MRIs, if available, should be reviewed to determine the level of the conus medullaris and assess for spinal stenosis that may complicate catheter placement. Plain radiographs, already present as a part of the surgical planning, help evaluate for vertebral degeneration and rotational deformities that may influence needle trajectory or access. In addition, 3D reconstructions from cross-sectional CT imaging can be used for detailed procedural planning, particularly in patients with complex spinal anatomy or prior instrumentation. No specific recommendations exist on how to proceed in the event of a bloody puncture as there are no guidelines on optimal duration of delay prior to systemic anticoagulation in the event of a traumatic puncture. Some institutions admit patients to place lumbar CSF drains 24 hours prior to surgery to allow for delay should a traumatic puncture occur. CSFP is monitored throughout the procedure and CSF drained to a goal pressure of less than 10 mm Hg. Spinal drains should be zeroed at the level of the right atrium. The pressure transducer must not be attached to a pressurized bag of fluid. Complications include spinal headache, intracranial hypotension, subdural hemorrhage, epidural or spinal hematoma, meningitis, and persistent CSF leak. CSF can be drained intermittently or continuously, though if drained continuously it must be closely monitored as excessive drainage will increase the risk of subdural hemorrhage. It is typically recommended to drain no more than 10 to 15 mL/h though this can be increased to 20 mL/h in the event of active symptoms.
2. **Postoperative paraplegia** must be addressed immediately by increasing drainage. If no prophylactic drain is in place, emergent placement of a spinal drain should be considered. It is also recommended to target higher mean arterial pressure (MAP) and hemoglobin levels to improve spinal cord perfusion. Spinal cord hematoma is an important differential to consider in a patient with a spinal drain who develops motor weakness as it may require emergent surgical intervention.
3. **Maintaining an MAP greater than 80 mm Hg** is recommended. Spinal cord perfusion pressure (SCPP) is the difference between MAP and CSFP (or CVP if it is greater). The target SCPP is greater than 70 mm Hg. This goal can be achieved by maintaining a MAP greater than 80 mm Hg, CSFP less than 10 mm Hg, and CVP less than 10 mm Hg.
4. **Moderate systemic hypothermia** is reasonable for spinal cord protection.
5. **Distal aortic perfusion** using AFB may be used to minimize ischemic time to the spinal cord and visceral organs. Sequential aortic clamping has also been used to minimize ischemic time.
6. **Intraoperative motor-evoked potential (MEP) monitoring** and/or somatosensory-evoked potentials (SSEPs) monitoring can be used to detect spinal cord ischemia. In response to the degradation of MEPs or SSEPs, MAP can be raised to encourage collateral perfusion to the spinal cord. Furthermore, the surgeon may reimplant intercostal arteries into the graft.

3. **Renal protection.** Lasix, mannitol, and dopamine have not been demonstrated to reduce the incidence of renal insufficiency. Distal aortic perfusion when the distal clamp is proximal to the renal arteries reduces renal ischemic time. Perfusion of a cold crystalloid (sometimes including mannitol or methylprednisolone and cooled to 4 °C, "renal cold") directly into the renal arteries can reduce the incidence of renal injury.
4. **Monitoring** includes a right upper extremity intra-arterial cannula as application of the aortic cross-clamp proximal to the left subclavian artery is occasionally necessary. A femoral intra-arterial catheter connected to a pressure transducer is used to monitor distal aortic perfusion pressures during AFB. CSFP transducer is necessary. TEE or PA catheter may be used to monitor cardiac function. Care must be exercised with insertion of the TEE probe as the aneurysm may compress the esophagus.
5. **Anesthetic technique**
    a. **Vasopressors** (phenylephrine and norepinephrine) and **vasodilators** (nitroglycerin and nitroprusside) should be available prior to induction.
    b. **General anesthesia** is induced as detailed in Section IV.B. When MEPs are used for spinal cord monitoring, paralytics, and volatile anesthetics must be avoided. Total intravenous anesthesia (TIVA) is required.
    c. **Lung isolation** is achieved to facilitate surgical access and protect the left lung from trauma during left thoracotomy. Lung isolation can be accomplished using a double-lumen tube (DLT) or an endobronchial blocker (see Chapter 27: Anesthesia for Thoracic Surgery). A right-sided DLT is preferred in case where the aneurysm distorts the left bronchial anatomy. The advantage of using a bronchial blocker is that it avoids the need to change from a DLT to a single-lumen endotracheal tube (ETT) at the conclusion of the procedure.
    d. **Positioning.** The patient is turned to the right lateral decubitus position with the pelvis at a small degree of tilt to facilitate femoral access. Bite blocks are placed between the molars bilaterally with the tongue free to prevent injury during MEP monitoring.
6. **Maintenance**
    a. **TIVA** with propofol and opioid (and avoidance of neuromuscular blockade) is used for these cases because volatile anesthetics can interfere with spinal cord monitoring.
    b. **Fluid management** is based on the patient's hemodynamics. Fluid administration is limited to FFP, red blood cells, platelets, and colloids in an attempt to limit the development of a coagulopathy and edema brought about by excessive crystalloid administration. A red blood cell salvage system and a rapid infuser should be used.
7. **Aortic cross-clamping**
    a. Prior to cross-clamping, a target CSFP of 6 to 10 mm Hg is maintained.
    b. **Marked hypertension** is universal with proximal aortic cross-clamp application and can be treated with clevidipine or nitroprusside. If AFB has been instituted, the flow rate can be increased to help mitigate the pressure rise.
    c. **Renal ischemia is minimized** by the infusion of cold crystalloid directly into the renal arteries.
8. **Use of shunts**
    a. Perfusion of the mesentery can be maintained by inserting either an accessory limb from the AFB circuit into the origin of the celiac artery or by inserting a side-arm from the graft (Gott shunt) into the origin of the celiac artery once the proximal anastomosis is complete.
    b. Distal aortic perfusion through AFB maintains blood flow to organs distal to the distal aortic clamp. The adequacy of perfusion is

Table 28.1 Management of Flow Through the Atrial-to-Left-Femoral-Artery Bypass Shunt

Radial Artery Pressure	Femoral Artery Pressure	Intervention
↑	↓	Increase pump flow
↓	↑	Decrease pump flow
↓	↓	Administer volume or vasopressor
↑	↑	Administer vasodilator

monitored using a femoral arterial line. **Table 28.1** summarizes the management consideration for AFB.

9. **Aortic unclamping** produces hypotension by the mechanism discussed in Section IV.B.10. Volume administration before and during unclamping, slow release of the cross-clamp, and use of vasopressors are continued until myocardial function and vascular tone have returned to baseline.
10. **Systemic acidosis** is universal after the release of the aortic cross-clamp. The degree of acidosis depends on the ischemic time to the organs. An infusion of bicarbonate during the cross-clamping period may minimize the acidemia and preserve the function of the myocardium and vasopressor agents.
11. At the conclusion of the procedure, the patient is kept intubated and sedated. If a double-lumen ETT was employed for lung isolation, consider exchange to a single-lumen ETT if it is safe to do so. Due to the duration of the case and dependent positioning of the head, the oropharynx is often edematous. An ETT exchange catheter and videolaryngoscope can be used to facilitate intubation. An elevated MAP should be maintained to maximize collateral perfusion to the spinal cord.

E. **Endovascular thoracic/thoracoabdominal aortic aneurysm repair (TEVAR)**
   1. **Benefits and patient selection.** Endovascular thoracic aortic aneurysm repair leads to significantly lower morbidity than open repair. Patients with significant comorbidities who would be poor candidates for open surgical repair may particularly benefit from endovascular repair. Patients must have suitable aortic anatomy to accommodate a stent graft as well as suitable vascular access sites free from significant atherosclerotic disease to allow large-bore sheath insertion.
   2. **Spinal cord and bowel preservation.** Studies have not shown a demonstrable difference in rates of spinal cord ischemia between open and endovascular repair. The greatest factor associated with spinal cord ischemia risk is the extent of the aneurysm, with extent II thoracic aortic aneurysms being the highest risk. Risk factors for paraplegia after TEVAR include previous AAA surgery, occlusion of the left subclavian, hypogastric occlusive disease, and more extensive graft coverage. To minimize risk of spinal cord ischemia and paraplegia, **CSF monitoring and drainage** are recommended for all thoracic aortic procedures (see Section V.D.2.c.). For thoracoabdominal aortic aneurysm repairs, preservation of mesenteric perfusion may be achieved through the construction of extra-anatomic bypass grafts prior to endograft implantation. Creation of these extra-anatomic grafts via open surgical techniques, performed in combination with endovascular aortic stent grafting, is referred to as **hybrid repair.**

3. **Monitoring** includes an arterial line and central venous or PA catheter, based on patient indications. **TEE** is reasonable for cardiac monitoring as well as for procedural guidance.
4. **Surgical considerations** for TEVAR are similar to those for EVAR (Section IV.A.4).
5. **Anesthetic technique.** TEVAR is almost exclusively performed under general anesthesia. Neuraxial anesthesia may interfere with postoperative motor examination and neurologic monitoring.
6. Following the deployment of the stent graft, an elevated MAP should be maintained to encourage collateral perfusion to the spinal cord.
7. **Complications of TEVAR** include **paraplegia** as well as those discussed in Sections IV.A.6 to 9 for EVAR: injury to the vascular access site and thromboemboli to the lower extremities, kidneys, or mesentery. Endoleaks occur in 10% to 20% of patients. Six percent to 7% of patients require reintervention. Hypotension in the postoperative period increases the risk of delayed-onset paraplegia and should be avoided.

VI. AMPUTATIONS

A. **General considerations.** Amputations can be performed under general or regional anesthesia. There is no mortality difference between regional and general anesthesia. Regardless, insertion of an epidural catheter or perineural block is typically recommended for postoperative pain control. Postoperative stump pain is effectively treated with either continuous perineural infusion of bupivacaine or epidural infusion of bupivacaine combined with an opioid.

B. **Phantom limb pain (PLP)** has been reported to occur in 60% to 70% of patients undergoing amputation. It is controversial whether the use of perioperative neuraxial anesthesia decreases the risk of development of chronic PLP. The literature suggests that good perioperative pain control, starting in the preoperative period and extending postoperatively, may be associated with a reduced incidence of PLP. Further studies are needed.

VII. REGIONAL ANESTHESIA UNDER ANTICOAGULATION

Many patients presenting for vascular procedures are on systemic anticoagulation or antiplatelet agents. ASRA has guidelines for the recommended interval for discontinuation of these agents prior to neuraxial placement and removal. They also make recommendations for appropriate intervals for resuming these agents while an epidural catheter is in place. ASRA recommends a 1-hour interval between needle placement and intraoperative heparinization.

There is less evidence on bleeding complications in patients receiving plexus or peripheral nerve blocks. The current ASRA recommendation is for patients undergoing perineuraxial, deep plexus, or deep peripheral nerve blocks to be managed according to neuraxial guidelines. They recommend that other blocks be managed according to site compressibility, vascularity, and impact if bleeding did occur. ASRA does not specifically define what is considered a superficial versus deep peripheral block but the European Society of Regional Anesthesia (ESRA) categorizes common blocks as superficial or deep. Arteriovenous fistula creation and lower limb amputation are common vascular procedures that receive peripheral nerve blocks. For upper extremity nerve blocks, the ESRA classifies the infraclavicular block as a deep nerve block. For lower extremity blocks, proximal sciatic blocks such as transgluteal are considered deep nerve blocks.

VIII. GROIN ACCESS COMPLICATIONS

Femoral arterial access remains a critical entry site for vascular procedures and has several well recognized risks. Complications of femoral access include hematoma, pseudoaneurysm, arteriovenous fistula, vessel occlusion, and branch injury. Risk factors for complications include female sex, high or low body mass index (BMI), previous access, and high femoral artery bifurcation.

Manual compression was traditionally the recommended method for achieving hemostasis after femoral access. As percutaneous vascular procedures have increased in frequency, so has the use of vascular closure devices (VCD). VCD aim to close the arteriotomy to achieve hemostasis and are primarily organized into the method by which this is achieved, either with a collagen-based plug, sutures, or a staple-/clip-based. VCD have been shown to improve time to hemostasis, time to ambulation and patient satisfaction. Importantly, VCDs have not shown evidence of reduced vascular complications when compared to manual compression.

ACKNOWLEDGMENT

We gratefully acknowledge the contributions of previous edition author, Christopher J. Mariani, as portions of those chapters have been retained in this revision.

Suggested Readings

American College of Cardiology Foundation/American Heart Association Task Force on Practice Guidelines; American Society of Echocardiography; American Society of Nuclear Cardiology; Heart Rhythm Society; Society of Cardiovascular Anesthesiologists; Society for Cardiovascular Angiography and Interventions; Society for Vascular Medicine; Society for Vascular Surgery; Fleisher LA, Beckman JA, Brown KA, et al. 2009 ACCF/AHA focused update on perioperative beta blockade incorporated into the ACC/AHA 2007 guidelines on perioperative cardiovascular evaluation and care for noncardiac surgery. *J Am Coll Cardiol.* 2009;54(22):e13–e118.

Bardia A, Sood A, Mahmood F, et al. Combined epidural-general anesthesia vs general anesthesia alone for elective abdominal aortic aneurysm repair. *JAMA Surg.* 2016;151(12):1116–1123.

Brott TG, Halperin JL, Abbara S, et al. 2011 ASA/ACCF/AHA/AANN/AANS/ACRA/ASNR/CNS/SAIP/SCAI/SIR/SNIA/SVM/SVS guideline on the management of patients with extracranial carotid and vertebral artery disease: executive summary. *J Am Coll Cardiol.* 2011;57(8):1002–1044.

Carroll AM, King RW, Ghincea CV, Aftab M, Reece TB. Spinal cord protection for thoracoabdominal aortic aneurysm repair: from bench to bedside. *Ann Cardiothorac Surg.* 2023;12(5):438–449.

Chaikof EL, Brewster DC, Dalman RL, et al. Society for Vascular Surgery practice guidelines for the care of patients with an abdominal aortic aneurysm: executive summary. *J Vasc Surg.* 2009;50(4):880–896.

Chery J, Semaan E, Darji S, Briggs WT, Yarmush J, D'Ayala M. Impact of regional versus general anesthesia on the clinical outcomes of patients undergoing major lower extremity amputation. *Ann Vasc Surg.* 2014;28(5):1149–1156.

Coselli JS, LeMaire SA, Orozco-Sevilla V, et al. Current approaches to spinal cord protection during open thoracoabdominal aortic aneurysm repair. *Ann Cardiothorac Surg.* 2023;12:429–437.

Crowley K, Scanaill PÓ, Hermanides J, Buggy DJ. Current practice in the perioperative management of patients with diabetes mellitus: a narrative review. *Br J Anaesth.* 2023;131(2):242–252.

De Bruin JL, Baas AF, Buth J, et al; DREAM Study Group. Long-term outcome of open or endovascular repair abdominal aortic aneurysm. *N Engl J Med.* 2010;362(20):1881–1889.

Duncan D, Wijeysundera D. Preoperative cardiac evaluation and management of the patient undergoing major vascular surgery. *Int Anesthesiol Clin.* 2016;54(2):1–32.

Erickson KM, Cole DJ. Carotid artery disease: stenting vs. endarterectomy. *Br J Anaesth.* 2010;105:i34–i49.

Fedorow CA, Moon MC, Mutch AC, Grocott HP. Lumbar cerebrospinal fluid drainage for thoracoabdominal aortic surgery: rationale and practical considerations for management. *Anesth Analg.* 2010;111(1):46–58.

Fleisher LA, Fleischmann KE, Auerbach AD, et al. 2014 ACC/AHA guideline on perioperative cardiovascular evaluation and management of patients undergoing noncardiac surgery: executive summary: a report of the American College of Cardiology/American Heart Association Task Force on Practice Guidelines. *J Am Coll Cardiol.* 2014;130(24):2215–2245.

GALA Trial Collaborative Group; Lewis SC, Warlow CP, Bodenham AR, et al. General anaesthesia versus local anaesthesia for carotid surgery (GALA): a multicentre, randomised controlled trial. *Lancet.* 2008;372(9656):2132–2142.

Gaudino M, Khan FM, Rahouma M, et al. Spinal cord injury after open and endovascular repair of descending thoracic and thoracoabdominal aortic aneurysms: A meta-analysis. *J Thorac Cardiovasc Surg.* 2022;163(2):552–564.

Gelman S. The pathophysiology of aortic cross-clamping and unclamping. *Anesthesiology.* 1995;82(4):1026–1060.

Greenberg RK, Lu Q, Roselli EE, et al. Contemporary analysis of descending thoracic and thoracoabdominal aneurysm repair: a comparison of endovascular and open techniques. *Circulation.* 2008;118(8):808–817.

Guarracino F. Cerebral monitoring during cardiovascular surgery. *Curr Opin Anaesthesiol.* 2008;21(1):50–54.

Gutsche JT, Szeto W, Cheung AT. Endovascular stenting of thoracic aortic aneurysm. *Anesthesiol Clin.* 2008;26(3):481–499.

Hajibandeh S, Anoniou SA, Torella F, Antoniou GA. Meta-analysis and trial sequential analysis of local vs. general anaesthesia for carotid endarterectomy. *Anaesthesia.* 2018;73(10):1280–1289.

Hiratzka LF, Bakris GL, Beckman JA, et al. 2010 ACCF/AHA/AATS/ACR/ASA/SCA/SCAI/SIR/STS/SVM guidelines for the diagnosis and management of patients with thoracic aortic disease. *Circulation.* 2010;121(13):e266–e369.

Horlocker TT, Vandermeuelen E, Kopp SL, Gogarten W, Leffert LR, Benzon HT. Regional anesthesia in the patient receiving antithrombotic or thrombolytic therapy. *Reg Anesth Pain Med.* 2018;43(3):263–309.

IMPROVE Trial Investigators. Endovascular or open repair strategy for ruptured abdominal aortic aneurysm: 30 day outcomes from IMPROVE randomised trial. *Br Med J.* 2014;348:f7661.

Kansagra K, Kang J, Taon MC, et al. Advanced endografting techniques: snorkels, chimneys, periscopes, fenestrations, and branched endografts. *Cardiovasc Diagn Ther.* 2018;8(S1): S175–S183.

Kasipandian V, Pichel AC. Complex endovascular aortic aneurysm repair. *BJA Education.* 2012;12(6):312–316.

Kent KC. Abdominal aortic aneurysms. *N Engl J Med.* 2014;371(22):2101–2108.

Kietaibl S, Ferrandis R, Godier A, et al. Regional anaesthesia in patients on antithrombotic drugs: Joint ESAIC/ESRA guidelines. *Eur J Anaesthesiol.* 2022;39(2):100–132.

Koster A, Faraoni D, Levy JH. Argatroban and bivalirudin for perioperative anticoagulation in cardiac surgery. *Anesthesiology.* 2018;128(2):390–400.

LaMuraglia GM, Houbballah R, Laposata M. The identification and management of heparin induced thrombocytopenia in the vascular patient. *J Vasc Surg.* 2012;55(2):562–570.

Madhok J, Vanneman MW. SGLT-2 inhibitors: proliferating indications and perioperative pitfalls. *J Cardiothorac Vasc Anesth.* 2022;36(7):1815–1819

McFalls EO, Ward HB, Moritz TE, et al. Coronary artery revascularization before elective major vascular surgery. *N Engl J Med.* 2004;351(27):2795–2804.

Mehran R, Dangas GD, Weisbord SD. Contrast-associated acute kidney injury. *N Engl J Med.* 2019;380(22):2146–2155.

Moll FL, Powell JT, Fraedrich G, et al. Management of abdominal aortic aneurysms clinical practice guidelines of the European Society for Vascular Surgery. *Eur J Vasc Endovasc Surg.* 2011;41(suppl 1):S1–S58.

Moreno DH, Cacione DG, Baptista-Silva JC. Controlled hypotension versus normotensive resuscitation strategy for people with ruptured abdominal aortic aneurysm. *Cochrane Database Syst Rev.* 2018;6(6):CD011664.

Morrison H III. Catheter-directed thrombolysis for acute limb ischemia. *Semin Intervent Radiol.* 2006;23(3):258–269.

Motyl CM, Beck AW. Strategies for prevention and treatment of spinal cord ischemia during F/BEVAR. *Semin Vasc Surg.* 2022;35(3):297–305.

Nicolaou G, Ismail M, Cheng D. Thoracic endovascular aortic repair: update on indications and guidelines. *Anesthesiol Clin.* 2013;31(2):451–478.

Noori VJ, Eldrup-Jørgensen J. A systematic review of vascular closure devices for femoral artery puncture sites. *J Vasc Surg.* 2018;68(3):887–899.

Ohira S, Lansman SL, Spielvogel D. Collateral network concept and spinal cord protection. *ASVIDE.* 2023;10:152–152.

Pishko AM, Cuker A. Heparin-induced thrombocytopenia and cardiovascular surgery. *Hematology Am Soc Hematol Educ Program.* 2021;2021(1):536–544.

Reddy U, Smith M. Anesthetic management of endovascular procedures for cerebrovascular atherosclerosis. *Curr Opin Anaesthesiol.* 2012;25(4):486–492.

Ruzycki SM, Prystajecky M, Driedger MR, Kachra R. Peri-operative cardiac biomarker screening: a narrative review. *Anaesthesia.* 2020;75(S1):e165–e173.

Smaka TJ, Cobas M, Velazquez OC, Lubarsky DA. Perioperative management of endovascular abdominal aortic aneurysm repair: update 2010. *J Cardiothorac Vasc Anesth.* 2011;25(1):166–176.

Stone PA, Campbell JE. Complications related to femoral artery access for transcatheter procedures. *Vasc Endovascular Surg.* 2012;46(8):617–623.

Telford RJ. Anaesthesia for vascular surgery on the extremities. *Anaesth Intensive Care.* 2016;17(5):230–234.

United Kingdom EVAR Trial Investigators. Endovascular repair of aortic aneurysm in patients physically ineligible for open repair. *N Engl J Med.* 2010;362(20):1872–1880.

United Kingdom EVAR Trial Investigators. Endovascular versus open repair of abdominal aortic aneurysm. *N Engl J Med.* 2010;362(20):1863–1871.

Ushakumari DS, Sladen RN. ASA Consensus-based guidance on preoperative management of patients on glucagon-like peptide-1 receptor agonists. *Anesthesiology.* 2023;140(2):346–348.

Vaniyapong T, Chongruksut W, Rerkasem K. Local versus general anaesthesia for carotid endarterectomy. *Cochrane Database Syst Rev.* 2013;12:CD000126.

Vaughn SB, LeMaire SA, Collard CD. Case scenario: anesthetic considerations for thoracoabdominal aortic aneurysm repair. *Anesthesiology.* 2011;115(5):1093–1102.

Weisbord SD, Gallagher M, Jneid H, Garcia S. Outcomes after angiography with sodium bicarbonate and acetylcysteine. *N Engl J Med.* 2018;378(7):603–614.

Wesner L, Marone LK, Dennehy KC. Anesthesia for lower extremity bypass. *Int Anesthesiol Clin.* 2005;43(1):93–110.

Zarinsefat A, Henke P. Update in preoperative risk assessment in vascular surgery patients. *J Vasc Surg.* 2015;62(2):499–509.

Anesthesia for Cardiac Surgery
Brian J. Kinsman and Jason Zhensheng Qu

I. CARDIOPULMONARY BYPASS
Cardiopulmonary bypass (CPB) is used to temporarily perform the functions of the heart (circulation of blood) and lungs (gas exchange) during surgical procedures on the heart and great vessels. It involves a pump and oxygenator connected through an extracorporeal circuit that provides oxygenated blood flow to the systemic circulation, bypassing the heart and lungs.

A. Components of circuit
1. Venous blood is drained from the venous cannula (inserted into the right atrium) to a **venous reservoir.** Maintaining an adequate fluid level in the venous reservoir is critical to prevent air entrainment.
2. A **pump** (roller or centrifugal) propels the venous blood forward. Unlike roller pumps, centrifugal pumps are afterload sensitive and will decrease flow if resistance increases (eg, with outflow obstruction). Centrifugal pumps are less traumatic to blood and do not pump air.
3. Venous blood enters a **heat exchanger** and an **oxygenator** that adds oxygen and removes carbon dioxide by adjusting the FiO_2 and sweep rate. A volatile anesthetic (eg, isoflurane) is added to the oxygenator gas mixture. The arterialized blood enters the systemic circulation via an aortic cannula, which is usually inserted in the ascending aorta. The femoral artery is sometimes used for aortic cannulation for emergency or redo sternotomy situations.
4. **Cardioplegic solution** containing high potassium is infused into the coronary circulation to induce and maintain cardiac arrest. Cardioplegia can be infused via the aortic root or coronary ostia (antegrade) or through the coronary sinus (retrograde).
5. **Left ventricular (LV) vent** removes blood that accumulates in the LV to decrease wall tension by suctioning on the same catheter placed for antegrade cardioplegia or one inserted into the LV via the right pulmonary vein across the mitral valve (MV).

B. CPB pathophysiology.
Contact of blood with the CPB circuit can lead to an intense systemic inflammatory response via the complement, kallikrein, and coagulation cascades. A prolonged CPB time is associated with multisystem compromise including neurologic dysfunction, acute respiratory distress syndrome, coagulopathy, hepatic insufficiency, and acute kidney injury. A number of approaches have been tested to decrease inflammation in CPB including leukocyte depletion, hemofiltration, administration of monoclonal antibodies against inflammatory mediators, and the coating of circuitry with heparin. None have shown definitive clinical benefits in humans.

C. CPB effects on pharmacokinetics.
CPB results in increased volume of distribution and decreased protein binding. Acid–base shifts can affect the ionized and unionized concentrations of drugs. Decreased perfusion pressures during CPB can lead to reduced hepatic and renal clearance. Hypothermia further decreases hepatic enzyme function.

II. PREOPERATIVE ASSESSMENT FOR CARDIAC SURGERY

A. Issues **pertinent to the cardiac procedure** and the physiologic impact of CPB and circulatory arrest include the following:
1. **Prior surgery in the chest**, which technically complicates surgery.
2. **Evidence of aortic and cerebrovascular disease**—symptomatic or documented carotid arterial disease may warrant endarterectomy. Aortic disease can affect cannulation strategies for bypass and may sometimes require concomitant repair with the cardiac operation.
3. **History of bleeding, anticoagulation regimens, and prothrombotic** tendencies may reveal a condition responsive to perioperative therapy.
4. A history of **heparin-induced thrombocytopenia (HIT)** alerts the potential for the development of life-threatening thrombotic complications when exposed to heparin. HIT is discussed later in the chapter.
5. **Renal insufficiency** may indicate the need for intraoperative renal protective measures.
6. Patients with **pulmonary disease** can develop severe **post-CPB pulmonary dysfunction** and may benefit from preoperative antibiotics, bronchodilators, steroids, or chest physical therapy.
7. **Liver dysfunction** (eg, cardiac cirrhosis) may indicate derangements in coagulation and platelet function and the need for transfusion of coagulation factors, platelets, and fibrinogen.

B. **Cardiac evaluation** determines the major anatomic and physiologic characteristics of the cardiovascular system, to predict intraoperative ischemia and functional reserve of the heart.
1. **Radionuclide imaging** may demonstrate the regions and extent of myocardium at risk for ischemia. Radionuclide ventriculography characterizes cardiac chamber volume, ejection fraction, and right-to-left stroke volume ratios.
2. **Viability studies** in patients with severe LV dysfunction can help distinguish areas of myocardial necrosis from hibernation; the latter may recover after revascularization. Current modalities include nuclear imaging (SPECT or PET), dobutamine stress echocardiography, and magnetic resonance imaging (MRI).
3. **Echocardiography** provides an assessment of ventricular function and valve function. Regional wall motion abnormalities (WMAs) may reflect ischemia or prior myocardial infarction.
4. **CT scan and f-MRI** are noninvasive modalities to assess for coronary vascular disease. They can be useful in patients who are not candidates for cardiac catheterization.
5. **Cardiac catheterization** remains the gold standard diagnostic test for most forms of cardiac disease.
   a. **Anatomic data.** Coronary angiography reveals the location and extent of coronary stenoses, distal runoff, collateral flow, and coronary dominance. Significant **stenosis** implies a greater than 70% reduction in luminal diameter. **The dominant coronary artery** supplies the atrioventricular node and the posterior descending coronary artery.
   b. **Functional data.** Ventriculography may demonstrate WMA, mitral regurgitation (MR), and intracardiac shunts. LV ejection fraction is normally greater than 0.6. Impaired ventricular performance is a useful predictor of increased surgical risk.
   c. **Hemodynamic data** are compiled from both right and left heart catheterization. Intracardiac and pulmonary vascular pressures reflect volume status, valvular function, and the presence of pulmonary vascular disease (normal values are presented in **Table 29.1**). An

TABLE 29.1 Normal Intracardiac Pressure and Oxygen Saturation

	Pressure (mm Hg)	O₂ Saturation (%)
Superior vena cava	—	71
Inferior vena cava	—	77
Right atrium (mean)	1–8	75
RV (systolic/diastolic)	15–30/0–8	75
PA (systolic/diastolic)	15–30/4–12	75
PA occlusion pressure (mean)	2–12	—
Left atrium (mean)	2–12	98
LV (systolic/diastolic/end diastolic)	100–140/0–8/2–12	98
Aorta (systolic/diastolic)	100–140/60–90	98

LV, left ventricle; PA, pulmonary artery; RV, right ventricle.

elevated LV end-diastolic pressure (LVEDP) may be due to ventricular failure and dilation, volume overload (mitral or aortic insufficiency [AI]), poor compliance from ischemia or hypertrophy, or a constrictive process. The LVEDP may rise substantially in patients with coronary artery disease (CAD) after dye injection for ventriculography or coronary angiography, despite otherwise normal hemodynamic values.

    d. **Left-to-right intracardiac shunts** are demonstrated by an arterial oxygen saturation (SaO_2) "step up" in the right heart.

    e. **Cardiac output** is determined by thermodilution and can be used to derive the hemodynamic indices (**Table 29.2**).

C. Other studies

1. **Routine labs** for patients undergoing a cardiac operation usually include a CBC, prothrombin time, activated partial thromboplastin time (aPTT), platelet count, electrolytes, blood urea nitrogen, creatinine, glucose, liver function tests, and thyroid-stimulating hormone level. A heparin-platelet factor 4 antibody detection assay should be considered for patients with a low or rapidly falling platelet count associated with heparin, as these patients are at risk for developing HIT.
2. **Chest radiograph and a 12-lead ECG** with a rhythm strip.
3. **Pulmonary function tests** may be appropriate in patients with underlying lung disease.
4. **Vascular studies** such as carotid duplex and vein mapping.
5. Frailty assessments may aid preoperative evaluation and risk stratification of geriatric patients to identify surgical candidates with adequate physical and cognitive reserve who are likely to benefit and recover from proposed interventions.

D. Cardiac Medications

1. **β-Adrenergic antagonists, calcium channel blockers, antiarrhythmics, and nitrates,** including intravenous (IV) nitroglycerin, are routinely continued on schedule until the patient's arrival in the operating room (OR).
2. **Angiotensin-converting enzyme (ACE) inhibitors,** angiotensin receptor blockers, and **diuretics** are usually held before surgery. Patients with

TABLE 29.2 Ventricular Function Indices

Formula	Units	Normal Value
$SV = \dfrac{CO}{HR} \times 1000$	mL/beat	60–90
$SI = \dfrac{SV}{BSA}$	mL/beat/m^2	40–60
$LVSWI = \dfrac{1.36(MAP - PCWP)}{100} \times SI$	g-m/m^2/beat	45–60
$RVSWI = \dfrac{1.36(PAP - CVP)}{100} \times SI$	g-m/m^2/beat	5–10
$SVR = \dfrac{(MAP - CVP)}{CO} \times 80$	dyne-s/cm^5	900–1500
$PVR = \dfrac{(PAP - PCWP)}{CO} \times 80$	dyne-s/cm^5	50–150

BSA, body surface area; CO, cardiac output; CVP, mean central venous pressure; HR, heart rate; LVSWI, left ventricular stroke work index; MAP, mean arterial pressure; PAP, mean pulmonary artery pressure; PCWP, pulmonary capillary wedge pressure; PVR, pulmonary vascular resistance; RVSWI, right ventricular stroke work index; SI, stroke index; SV, stroke volume; SVR, systemic vascular resistance.

significant LV dysfunction are prone to vasodilatory shock when they receive an ACE inhibitor preoperatively.

3. **Aspirin** has a positive effect on graft patency and should be continued in most patients who have significant CAD. Bleeding related solely to aspirin therapy can be overcome with platelet transfusion provided the drug has been cleared from the circulation. Patients receiving multiple antiplatelet agents may or may not be rapidly reversible (**Table 29.3**).
4. **P2Y$_{12}$ inhibitors** such as oral clopidogrel and prasugrel are stopped 5 to 7 days prior to surgery. If a bare-metal stent was placed within the past month or a drug-eluting stent within the last year, clopidogrel is often continued up until the time of surgery. Conversely, cangrelor, a reversible P2Y$_{12}$ inhibitor, may be used for bridging in patients with recent coronary stent placement. It should be stopped 6 hours preoperatively.
5. **Direct oral anticoagulants (DOACs)** such as factor Xa inhibitors apixaban, rivaroxaban and edoxaban, and thrombin inhibitor dabigatran should be stopped 3 to 5 days before cardiac surgery. Andexanet Alfa is approved for emergency reversal of rivaroxaban and apixaban. Idarucizumab is approved for emergency reversal of dabigatran. Use of these DOAC reversal agents must be weighed against the risk of thrombotic events in consultation with Hematology. Off-label use of prothrombin complex concentrates may also be considered for refractory hemorrhage during cardiac surgery for patients on a DOAC.
6. **Warfarin** is held 3 to 5 days preoperatively to allow normalization of the international normalization ratio. IV vitamin K (5 to 10 mg) or

TABLE 29.3 Antiplatelet Agents

Drug	Inhibits	Half-Life	Duration	Reversible	Methods to Restore Function
Aspirin	Cyclooxygenase	15–20 min	7 d	No	Platelet transfusion
Abciximab (Reopro)	Glycoprotein IIb/IIIa receptor	30 min	48 h	Partially	Platelet transfusion
Eptifibatide (Integrilin)	Glycoprotein IIb/IIIa receptor	2.5 h	4–8 h	Yes	Delay surgery 8 h after stopping drug
Tirofiban (Aggrastat)	Glycoprotein IIb/IIIa receptor	1.5–3 h	4–8 h	Yes	Discontinue drug 8 h before surgery
Clopidogrel (Plavix)	Adenosine diphosphate receptor	8 h	7 d	No	Platelet transfusion
Prasugrel (Effient)	Adenosine diphosphate receptor	2–15 h	7 d	No	Platelet transfusion
Cangrelor	Adenosine diphosphate receptor	2–5 min	1 h	Yes	Platelet transfusion or wait 6 h before surgery
Ticagrelor (Brilinta)	Adenosine diphosphate receptor	6–9 h	5 d	No	Platelet transfusion
Ticlopidine (Ticlid)	Adenosine diphosphate receptor	12 h–5 d with repeated dosing	7 d	No	Platelet transfusion
Dipyridamole[a] (Persantine)	Adenosine uptake; phosphodiesterase	9–13 h	4–10 h	Yes	Platelet transfusion
Cilostazol (Pletal)	Phosphodiesterase III	11–13 h	48 h	Yes	Platelet transfusion
Herbal therapies[b]	Platelet aggregation	Variable	Variable	Variable	Limited data available

[a]Dipyridamole is available in a formulation with aspirin (Aggrenox).
[b]Includes garlic, ginkgo, ginseng, ginger, feverfew, fish oil, and dong quai.

fresh–frozen plasma (FFP) may be used emergently to correct coagulopathy. However, FFP will only transiently correct a warfarin-induced coagulopathy due to the relatively longer half-life of warfarin compared with the vitamin K–dependent cofactors (factors II, VII, IX, and X), thus putting the patient at risk for rebound coagulopathy. Emergent reversal requires the administration of four-component prothrombin complex concentrates.

7. **Heparin** infusions initiated for unstable angina or left main CAD are continued preoperatively. The anticoagulant effects of unfractionated heparin are reversible with IV protamine administration. In contrast, the anticoagulant effects of low–molecular-weight heparin (LMWH) preparations are not fully reversible with protamine. LMWH has been associated with increased perioperative hemorrhage in cardiac surgical patients.

III. ANESTHETIC MANAGEMENT
A. Monitoring
1. **Standard monitors**
   a. Continuous **ECG display of both leads II and V_5** with ST segment trend analysis.
   b. **Temperature monitoring** includes that of the oral or nasopharynx (core temperature), the blood temperature (measured from pulmonary artery [PA] catheter), and bladder or rectal temperature, which represents the average body temperature.
2. **Central venous and PA pressures**
   a. **Patients with normal ventricular function** can be effectively managed with either central venous pressure (CVP) monitoring with or without transesophageal echocardiography (TEE) or a PA catheter.
   b. A **PA catheter** provides helpful data in managing hemodynamics of patients with poor ventricular function, and valvular and redo surgeries. **Mixed venous oxygen saturation** ($SmvO_2$) monitoring is available continuously with PA catheters specially equipped with a fiberoptic-linked oximeter. A decrease in $SmvO_2$ is the result of decreased cardiac output, decreased hemoglobin, increased oxygen consumption, or decreased SaO_2.
3. **Intraoperative TEE** can help surgical and anesthetic decision making. The Society of Cardiovascular Anesthesiologists/American Society of Echocardiography TEE guidelines recommend the use of intraoperative TEE in all open heart (eg, valvular procedure) and thoracic aortic surgical procedures and to be considered in coronary artery bypass grafting (CABG) surgery. TEE provides guidance during catheter-based intracardiac procedures, and minimally invasive and robotic surgeries.
   a. The routine examination consists of **20 standard views.** The probe is advanced into the esophagus for upper and midesophageal views and then into the stomach for transgastric views.
   b. **Application** of intraoperative TEE includes confirmation of the placement of guidewire or cannula, assessment of global and regional ventricular function, chamber sizes, and valvular anatomy and function. TEE is very sensitive for detecting ischemia. It is also used to assess ventricular function, the presence of intracardiac air, and the presence of paravalvular leaks.
   c. **Absolute contraindications** to TEE:
      1. Esophageal stricture
      2. Tracheoesophageal fistula
      3. History of recent esophageal surgery and esophageal trauma.

4. TEE must be used cautiously in patients with esophageal varices and altered anatomy (eg, from gastric bypass surgery) and in those who have had radiation therapy to the neck and mediastinum. The incidence of severe complications such as esophageal perforation is on the order of 0.1%.
   d. **3-Dimensional TEE** can provide detailed images of valves, other structures, and ventricular function.
   e. **Tissue Doppler Imaging** measurement of myocardial velocities can be used to assess global and regional myocardial systolic and diastolic function with diagnostic and prognostic utility in many cardiac conditions.
4. **Neurologic monitors** such as transcranial Doppler, multichannel electroencephalography (EEG), and near-infrared spectroscopy may improve neurologic outcome by alerting the clinician of cerebral ischemia. Processed EEG (Bispectral index or Sedline) monitor is a useful guide to predict the depth of anesthesia.

B. Preinduction
1. **Peripheral venous access** is established with one large-bore (14- or 16-gauge) IV catheter. If excessive bleeding is expected (eg, a redo operation, transplant, or a patient with a preexisting coagulopathy), a second volume line will facilitate blood product administration.
2. **Sedation and analgesia:** Benzodiazepines should only be given to extremely anxious patients. Patients with severe aortic stenosis (AS), mitral stenosis (MS), pulmonary hypertension, or left main CAD may not tolerate even small degrees of hypotension and respiratory depression; minimal or no premedication is administered until the patient arrives in the OR.
3. **Arterial cannulation** is performed with a 20-gauge catheter inserted into the right radial artery.
   a. Left radial or femoral artery cannulation is used for systemic blood pressure monitoring when right axillary artery cannulation is planned for antegrade cerebral protection during deep hypothermic circulatory arrest (DHCA).
   b. Cannulation distal to a previous brachial artery cutdown site should be avoided.
   c. If blood pressure measurements are asymmetric, the arterial catheter should be placed on the side with the higher value.
   d. Be certain to note whether the surgeon will use the radial artery for CABG surgery.
   e. Femoral artery cannulation is a safe and reliable alternative to radial artery cannulation. Preoperative femoral artery cannulation can also be accessed for emergency CPB and intra-aortic balloon pump (IABP) insertion in patients with redo, severe CAD, and poor LV function. Brachial and axillary artery cannulations are third and fourth choices.
   f. Intra-aortic balloon central lumen pressure can be transduced as a monitor of central arterial pressure.
4. **Central venous access** may be established before or after induction.
5. **A defibrillator and an external pacemaker generator** must be available. Permanent pacemaker or implantable cardioverter defibrillator (ICD) should be interrogated, and a magnet should be available.
6. **Typed and cross-matched packed red blood cells** (2 to 4 units) should be immediately available.
7. **Baseline hemodynamics values**, including cardiac output or cardiac index, are recorded.

8. **Available medications** should include heparin, calcium chloride, lidocaine, amiodarone, inotropes, vasopressors, vasodilators, and nitroglycerin. Protamine should never be drawn up until the patient is safely separated from CPB.

IV. INDUCTION

A. **During induction**, a surgeon should be available, and the CPB pump should be ready in the event of severe hemodynamic instability during induction. A systematic and gradual induction involves minimizing the degree of cardiovascular depression while maintaining an adequate anesthetic depth.
  1. **Induction agents**
     a. **IV opioids** produce various degrees of vasodilation and bradycardia without significant myocardial depression. Opioids are commonly administered in conjunction with other central nervous system depressants as part of a balanced anesthetic technique, which has supplanted primary opioid anesthetics for adult cardiac surgery. Bolus dose fentanyl (1 to 5 mcg/kg) or sufentanil (0.5 to 2 mcg/kg) may be administered at induction to blunt laryngeal reflexes. Hydromorphone IV (0.01 to 0.02 mg/kg) is often administered for long-acting analgesia approaching sternotomy.
     b. **Sedative hypnotics and amnestics**, including propofol, etomidate, and dexmedetomidine are useful coinduction agents. Of these drugs, etomidate causes the least myocardial depression.
     c. **Volatile inhalation anesthetics** are useful supplementary and maintenance agents.
     d. **Muscle relaxants** with minimal cardiovascular effects are commonly chosen (eg, rocuronium, cisatracurium, and vecuronium). Pretreatment with a "priming dose" and early relaxant administration help to counteract chest wall rigidity often encountered during opioid-based inductions.
  2. **Specific considerations for valvular heart disease** (see also Chapter 2: Basics of Echocardiography and Lung Ultrasound).
     a. **Aortic stenosis (AS)**. Physiologic goals include the maintenance of adequate intravascular volume, sinus rhythm, contractility, and systemic vascular resistance (SVR), and the avoidance of tachycardia. Patients with AS typically have a hypertrophied and noncompliant ventricle and require higher filling pressures (LVEDP of 20 to 30 mm Hg). Anesthetic agents that reduce vascular tone or myocardial contractility should be avoided. An infusion of phenylephrine can be started 1 to 2 minutes before induction to decrease the risk of developing significant hypotension associated with induction. Dysrhythmias must be treated aggressively.
     b. **Aortic regurgitation (AR)**. Physiologic goals include maintenance of adequate intravascular volume and adequate contractility. Bradycardia and increases in SVR must be avoided. Patients with AR are often highly dependent on endogenous sympathetic tone. Patients with coexisting CAD may decompensate with significant bradycardia due to very low diastolic perfusion pressure. A means for rapid pacing should be available.
     c. **Mitral stenosis (MS)**. Hemodynamic goals mandate the maintenance of a slow rhythm, preferably sinus, and adequate intravascular volume, contractility, and SVR. Patients with severe MS and elevated pulmonary vascular resistance (PVR) are challenging to induce. Elevated PVR, often secondary to hypoventilation or positive

end-expiratory pressure (PEEP), must be avoided. Atrial fibrillation with rapid ventricular response must be treated aggressively, such as with immediate cardioversion.
- d. **Mitral regurgitation (MR).** Physiologic goals include the maintenance of adequate intravascular volume, myocardial contractility, a normal or elevated heart rate, and a reduction of systemic vascular tone. Increased SVR should be avoided. Anesthesia-induced decreases in SVR are usually well tolerated.
- e. **Mixed valvular lesions,** the most hemodynamically significant lesion, dominate the management goals. The addition of CAD to mixed valvular lesions makes planning even more complex (eg, AS with AR and CAD). In all situations, determine the most likely problems that could occur during induction and plan the management for each.

3. **Specific considerations for emergent inductions**
    - a. **Pulmonary embolus.** Induction of general anesthesia and the institution of positive-pressure ventilation can precipitate cardiovascular collapse. It is prudent to prepare and drape the unstable patient prior to induction. In patients with compromised RV function, cannulation of the femoral vessels under local anesthesia should be performed prior to induction to allow for the emergent institution of CPB if needed.
    - b. **Pericardial tamponade.** Similar concerns are present for patients with pericardial tamponade. Adequate volume administration is essential. Starting an inotropic agent and a vasopressor before induction may be helpful. A rapid sternotomy may be required if hemodynamic collapse occurs with anesthesia induction. If possible, the pericardial effusion should be drained under local anesthesia prior to induction.
    - c. **Aortic dissection.** Hypertension can precipitate aortic rupture. Packed red blood cells must be available in the OR before induction. Proximal extension of the dissection into the coronary arteries can occur, leading to myocardial ischemia or tamponade.
    - d. **Ventricular septal defect (VSD) and papillary muscle rupture after myocardial infarction.** Patients may present with extreme hypotension. Rapid initiation of CPB is essential. Preinduction initiation of intra-aortic balloon counterpulsation therapy is indicated in many of these patients.
    - e. **CABG.** Manage concomitant hemodynamic sequelae of STEMI or Non-ST-elevation myocardial infarction with inotropes, vasoconstrictors, and fluids as indicated. Nitroglycerin infusion should be continued. Patients may have undergone emergent percutaneous coronary intervention preceding operation necessitating administration of cangrelor and/or receiving a form of mechanical circulatory support (MCS).
    - f. **Mechanical circulatory support procedures**
        1. **VA-ECMO c**annulation may be performed in OR or non-OR settings. These patients are often in extremis requiring active resuscitation with blood products, inotropes, and vasoconstrictors. TEE is often indicated to assess cardiac function and potentially assist with aortic cannulation. A right radial or brachial arterial line is indicated to assess for differential hypoxemia.
        2. **Impella.** Similar to VA-ECMO, patients with an indication for Impella are often in decompensated LV failure (Impella 5.5) or RV failure (Impella RP); however, Impella placement may also serve to vent the LV when overdistended on VA-ECMO. TEE is usually needed to appropriately position the device.

B. **The prebypass period** is characterized by variable levels of stimulation during the preparation for CPB initiation. Stimulating periods include incision, sternotomy, sternal retraction, and pericardiotomy.
  1. **Baseline** Pao_2, $Paco_2$, pH, hematocrit (Hct), and activated clotting time (ACT) should be obtained.
  2. **Consider acute normovolemic hemodilution (ANH)** in patients with a starting Hct of 35% or greater. One to 2 units of whole blood may be removed with maintenance of normovolemia using crystalloid and/or colloid replacement fluid. The blood is later transfused into the patient following conclusion of CPB and heparin reversal.
  3. **The lungs are deflated during sternotomy.** Physical alterations of the chest wall can produce ECG changes (especially T-wave changes), which should be noted to avoid confusion with ischemia.
  4. **Left internal mammary artery dissection** may cause ipsilateral hemothorax and negatively affect pulmonary mechanics in patients with reduced pulmonary reserve.
  5. **Anticoagulation for cannulation and bypass**
     a. **Prior to the induction of anesthesia**, bolus dose of heparin should be drawn up and kept readily available in case the emergent initiation of CPB is necessary. The dose may be calculated by heparin dose-responsive formula or body weight (300 to 500 units/kg). The heparin should be administered through a centrally placed catheter.
     b. **Hypotension** often follows the heparin bolus and should be anticipated.
     c. The **ACT** is used to monitor the degree of anticoagulation and measured approximately 3 minutes after administering full-dose heparin. Baseline values are 80 to 150 seconds. Heparin treatment sufficient to prevent microthrombus formation during CPB correlates with an ACT of more than 400 seconds (at higher than 35 °C). Antithrombin concentrate (500 to 1000 units) or 2 to 4 units of FFP administration may be necessary to achieve ACT target in patients with antithrombin III deficiency.
     d. **Patients with a diagnosis of HIT type 2 (also known as HIT with thrombotic syndrome [HITTS])** require alternative anticoagulation management during CPB. The classification of HIT is determined by immune involvement. HIT type 1 is a nonimmunologic reaction of heparin with platelets that causes a mild thrombocytopenia. HIT type 2 is an immune-mediated phenomenon that activates platelets, resulting in platelet aggregation. Biochemical mediators from activated platelets can induce the generation of thrombin, leading to diffuse arterial and venous clotting. The diagnosis requires serologic and clinical evidence. Patients with a positive functional assay (serotonin release assay or platelet aggregation study), greater than 50% reduction in platelets (irrespective of starting platelet count), drop in platelet count less than 150,000, or history of a thrombotic event associated with heparin use are more likely to have an adverse outcome when reexposed to heparin. Patients with a positive ELISA test in the absence of a positive functional assay or clinical symptoms have a lower likelihood of having an adverse reaction to heparin.
     e. For patients with HIT type 2 or HITTS, **alternatives to standard heparin treatment** exist (**Table 29.4**); each has significant limitations that should be discussed with the surgeon and a hematologist before use.
        1. All forms of heparin are removed preoperatively. Saline is used to flush pressure transducers, and citrated saline is used to wash salvaged blood during the centrifugation process.

Table 29.4 Alternative CPB Anticoagulation in Patients With HIT

Drug	Mechanism	Half-Life	Lab Monitor	Reversible?
Bivalirudin (Angiomax)	Direct thrombin inhibitor	25 min (normal renal function)	ACT	No
Argatroban	Direct thrombin inhibitor	40–50 min (prolonged in hepatic insufficiency)	ACT	No
Tirofiban (Aggrastat) + unfractionated heparin[a]	Glycoprotein IIb/IIIa receptor inhibitor prevents platelet aggregation in HIT	1.5–3 h	ACT (platelets and D-dimer if heparin-induced thrombosis is suspected)	No

[a]Additional training is required to safely use this anticoagulation technique for patients requiring CPB.

ACT, activated clotting time; CPB, cardiopulmonary bypass; HIT, heparin-induced thrombocytopenia.

2. A heparin-free PA catheter is used.
3. Alternative anticoagulant regimens may be used. These include bivalirudin or unfractionated heparin in combination with an antiplatelet agent (see **Table 29.4**).
4. If unfractionated heparin is used, then a bypass dose of porcine heparin is administered before aortic cannulation (to minimize the likelihood of a repeat dose of heparin).
5. Aspirin is administered early in the postoperative period, and initiation of systemic anticoagulation with a direct thrombin inhibitor and warfarin may be indicated to prevent both early and late postoperative thromboembolic complications.
6. **Antifibrinolytic drugs** such as ε-aminocaproic acid (Amicar) are usually given as a bolus 7.5 g followed by an infusion 1.25 g/h during all on-pump procedures, with the intention of inhibiting excessive fibrinolysis (ie, plasmin activity and D-dimer formation) and possibly preserving platelet function. Tranexamic acid can be used as a substitute for Amicar with a different dose.
7. **Aortic cannulation** is conducted in the ascending aorta. **Epiaortic scanning** can be used to sonographically direct the cannulation site in patients with atherosclerotic disease. Maintaining a slightly low systolic blood pressure (90 to 100 mm Hg) during aortic cannulation decreases the risk of dissection.
8. **Venous return cannulas** are inserted via the right atrium. A single cavoatrial catheter is placed in the right atrial appendage, with the tip in the inferior vena cava (IVC) and fenestrations in the midatrium. For open-chamber procedures (ie, mitral and tricuspid valve surgeries), bicaval cannulation, consisting of separate superior vena cava (SVC) and IVC cannulas, is conducted.
9. **Retrograde autologous priming (RAP)** can be used to reduce the hemodilution from the crystalloid priming solutions of the bypass circuit. During

RAP, the patient's blood pushes the crystalloid prime out of the circuit, often necessitating use of α-agonist agents to maintain vascular tone and prevent hypotension.
C. Cardiopulmonary Bypass
1. **Initiation of CPB.** After an ACT greater than or equal to 400 seconds is obtained, the clamp on the venous line is released and CPB is initiated. The pump flow progressively increases to 2.0 to 2.4 L/min/m^2 with target mean arterial pressure (MAP) of 60 to 80 mm Hg. Ventilation is discontinued. Anesthesia is maintained using IV agents or inhalational agents administered through a vaporizer in the fresh gas line of CPB circuit. It is advisable to withdraw the PA catheter 2 to 5 cm to prevent the catheter tip from migrating into a wedge position during CPB. If two venous return lines are used and tourniquets are applied to achieve complete CPB, the CVP measured above the tourniquet is the SVC pressure. High CVP may indicate obstruction of SVC cannula. A vent cannula may be inserted via right pulmonary vein to drain the LV.
2. **Maintenance of CPB**
   a. **Myocardial protection** during the cross-clamp period is achieved primarily by reducing myocardial oxygen consumption through hypothermia, hyperkalemic arrest, or both.
      1. **Intermittent cold cardioplegia** is a commonly used technique. Cold (4 °C to 6 °C) hyperkalemic solution with or without blood is delivered to the coronary circulation approximately every 20 minutes as needed. Systemic cooling of the patient and topical cooling of the heart augment myocardial protection.
      2. The **warm cardioplegia technique** delivers a warm (32 °C to 37 °C) hyperkalemic solution mixed with blood at approximately 1:5 ratio. The solution is delivered continuously during the cross-clamp period with a few interruptions to allow visualization of the anastomotic sites. Mild systemic cooling to 32 °C to 34 °C is frequently performed. Blood glucose levels should be monitored and controlled between 80 and 180 mg/L with IV insulin bolus and infusion as needed.
   b. **Hypothermia (20 °C to 34 °C)** is commonly used during CPB. Oxygen consumption and blood flow requirements are reduced while blood viscosity is increased, thus counteracting prime-induced hypoviscosity. Adverse effects of hypothermia include impaired autoregulatory, enzymatic, and cellular membrane function; decreased oxygen delivery (leftward shift of the hemoglobin oxygen dissociation curve); and potentiation of coagulopathy. Metabolic requirements decrease by about 7% for every degree Celsius reduction in body temperature below 37 °C.
   c. **Hemodynamic monitoring**
      1. **Hypotension** during the initiation of CPB is usually due to hemodilution, hypoviscosity, and cardioplegia administration. Other causes include inadequate pump flow, vasodilation, aortic dissection, and aortic cannula mispositioning. A phenylephrine infusion may be required to treat transient hypotension. During CPB, a pressure gradient (as high as 40 mm Hg) may develop between the radial artery and the aorta. The lower radial artery pressure could lead to unnecessary administration of vasopressors if the discrepancy is not recognized. In the presence of carotid stenosis, MAP should be maintained at a higher level than usual (eg, 70 to 80 mm Hg), and hypocarbia should be avoided.

2. **Hypertension** (MAP >90 mm Hg) may be due to excessive flow rates or increased vascular resistance, which may be treated with vasodilators or anesthetics.
3. **Elevated PA pressures** indicate left heart distention, which may be due to inadequate venting, AI, or inadequate isolation of venous return. Severe distention may result in myocardial injury.

d. **Acid–base management.** In the setting of hypothermia, gas solubility increases and the dissociation constant for water decreases, resulting in a lower [H^+] and [OH^-] and a higher pH. While total CO_2 content remains constant, the partial pressure of CO_2 decreases.
  1. **pH-stat** corrects the patient's blood gas for temperature and strives to maintain a neutral pH of 7.4 and CO_2 near 40 mm Hg by adding CO_2 to the CPB circuit. This strategy potentially results in cerebral vasodilatation and more uniform cerebral cooling during DHCA; however, at an increased risk of cerebral microembolism.
  2. **Alpha-stat** involves the use of uncorrected gas tensions during hypothermia. No CO_2 is added to the oxygenator. The basis of the approach is that the total CO_2 content of blood and the intracellular electroneutrality (as primarily governed by the imidazole rings of histidine residues) are unchanged during hypothermia. Cerebral blood flow is autoregulated and coupled to cerebral oxygen demand.
  3. Most studies fail to reveal any significant difference in patient outcomes between the two methods. Generally, alpha-stat is used in adults and pH-stat in children when circulatory arrest is used.

e. **Metabolic acidosis and oliguria** may suggest inadequate systemic perfusion. Additional volume (blood or crystalloid depending on Hct) may be required to achieve increased flow. Brisk urine output should be established within the first 10 minutes of CPB.
  1. **Oliguria** (<1 mL/kg/h) may be treated with a trial of increased perfusion pressure and/or flow, mannitol (0.25 to 0.5 g/kg). Patients on chronic furosemide therapy may require their usual dose during CPB to sustain diuresis.
  2. **Hemolysis** during CPB is usually due to mechanical trauma to red blood cells from the bypass machine and the pump suction. Released pigments may cause acute renal failure postoperatively. For hemoglobinuria, diuresis is maintained using IV fluids with mannitol or furosemide. In severe cases, the urine is alkalinized by administering sodium bicarbonate at 0.5 to 1.0 mEq/kg.

f. **Additional heparin** bolus and/or infusion may be needed for prolonged CPB. The duration of heparin anticoagulation may be shorter in patients on chronic heparin therapy or during cases in which systemic hypothermia is not used. The ACT does not correlate well with plasma heparin levels when the patient is on CPB, but many centers routinely monitor the ACT during hypothermic (25 °C to 34 °C) CPB.

g. **Blood glucose** should be controlled between 80 and 180 mg/dL during bypass. Hyperglycemia may be associated with an increased risk of neurologic injury. Diabetic patients following a warm cardioplegia technique will typically require an insulin infusion.

h. **Table 29.5** lists some of the **problems** that can be encountered during CPB.

D. **Discontinuing CPB** implies transferring cardiopulmonary function from the bypass system back to the patient. In preparation for this transition, the anesthesiologist must examine and optimize the patient's metabolic, anesthetic, and cardiopulmonary conditions.

TABLE 29.5 Potential Problems During CPB

Problem	Possible Cause
Inadequate systemic pressures	Vasoplegia, inadequate flow, hemodilution
Poor gas exchange	Oxygenator failure, hypoxic gas mixture, inadequate coagulation, poor perfusion
High arterial line pressure	Mechanical obstruction, malpositioned aortic cannula, aortic dissection, inadequate anticoagulation, or cold agglutination
Distension of heart	Poor venous drainage, inadequate venting, increased regurgitation, or shunting
High coronary sinus pressure (during retrograde cardioplegia)	Small coronary sinus, malpositioning of catheter

CPB, cardiopulmonary bypass.

1. **Preparation for discontinuing CPB begins during rewarming.** The arterial blood is warmed but does not exceed 37 °C before discontinuation from CPB.
   a. **Laboratory data** to be acquired during rewarming include PaO_2, $PaCO_2$, pH, potassium, calcium, glucose, Hgb, and ACT. Clinical decisions concerning pH are usually made according to the values measured at 37 °C (alpha-stat management).
   b. **Adequate anticoagulation** during rewarming and separation from CPB is ensured with additional heparin if necessary.
   c. **Metabolic acidosis** should be treated with sodium bicarbonate, and the perfusionist may elect to increase the sweep rate to remove CO_2. **Hyperkalemia** frequently corrects spontaneously by redistribution and diuresis. If not, the administration of IV insulin/glucose with sodium bicarbonate will lower serum potassium.
   d. Usually, a **Hct >21%** should be achieved before separation, either by transfusion or by hemoconcentration, as indicated by the CPB reservoir volume.
   e. **FFP** and **platelets** should also be readily available to correct coagulopathy.
2. **Separation from CPB**
   a. **Deairing maneuvers** under TEE guidance are used to prevent air embolism to the cerebral or coronary circulations. Air in the left ventricle can be liberated and suctioned out via aortic root vent by manipulation of the heart and ventricular filling.
   b. **Aortic cross-clamp removal** reestablishes coronary perfusion.
   c. **Defibrillation** may be spontaneous; ventricular fibrillation is treated with internal paddles delivering 5 to 10 J of energy with a biphasic waveform defibrillator. Failure may indicate inadequate warming, graft problems, a metabolic disturbance, or inadequate myocardial protection. Additional lidocaine, magnesium (1-g IV slowly), or amiodarone (150-mg IV bolus followed by infusion at 1 mg/min for 6 hours, then 0.5 mg/min) may be required.
   d. **Rhythm is assessed.** With bradycardia, atrial pacing is established through epicardial wires. Ventricular pacing is added if there are

atrioventricular conduction abnormalities. Hypothermia as well as hypocalcemia, hyperkalemia, and hypermagnesemia caused by cardioplegia solutions may contribute to a high incidence of reversible heart block immediately after CPB. Other atrial dysrhythmias may be treated with overdrive pacing, cardioversion, and antiarrhythmics (eg, esmolol, propranolol, amiodarone, verapamil, or rarely digoxin).
- e. **The ECG should be inspected** for evidence of ischemia possibly related to intracoronary air or inadequate revascularization.
- f. During separation from CPB, volume administration may be guided by monitoring LV filling using TEE, mean PA, or wedge pressure. RV filling is indicated by the CVP or direct RV visualization. Patients without LVH will most likely need a mean PA pressure of 20 mm Hg or an LA pressure of 10 mm Hg. A patient with severe LVH and inadequate revascularization may need a mean PA pressure of 30 mm Hg or an LA pressure of 20 mm Hg.
- g. **If a gradient** between central (aortic) and peripheral (radial) arterial pressures is present, a femoral arterial line can be placed.
- h. **Compliance and resistance of the lungs** are tested with a few trial breaths. Ventilation should be reestablished when LV ejection begins even if the patient is still on CPB. To facilitate reexpansion of the lungs, the pleural cavities are drained if they have been opened previously or fluid is detected by TEE. If the lungs are difficult to ventilate, tracheobronchial suctioning and the administration of bronchodilators may be indicated.
- i. **Visual inspection of the heart** confirms atrioventricular synchrony. Contractility is assessed both by gross appearance and by systolic performance, as estimated by peak systolic and pulse pressure (taking into account pump flow and LA and PA pressures). If poor myocardial performance is demonstrated or anticipated (eg, impaired preoperative function or intraoperative ischemia), initiation of inotropic support before separation from CPB may be indicated. Pump flow rate is checked and compared with the patient's preoperative cardiac output. Significantly higher flows indicate the need to increase vascular tone.
- j. **Ionized Ca^{2+}** may be corrected slowly after the heart is reperfused. Rapid Ca^{2+} administration, especially in the presence of myocardial ischemia, is associated with Ca^{2+}-induced myocardial injury. Calcium will increase both contractility and SVR.

E. **At the time of separation from CPB**, venous lines to the pump are slowly clamped, allowing the heart to gradually fill and eject with each contraction. Prolonged partial venous line occlusion allows for "partial bypass," during which time cardiopulmonary function is shared and hemodynamics are assessed. After complete venous line occlusion, once adequate filling pressures are achieved, perfusion through the aortic cannula is stopped, and the heart alone provides systemic perfusion.
  1. **Pressure maintenance.** Transfusion from the CPB reservoir maintains an optimal filling condition assessed by MAP, PA, CVP, and TEE. Care is taken not to overdistend the heart. Should overdistention occur, the surgeon may "empty" the heart by transiently unclamping a venous line. Alternatively, the patient may be temporarily placed in reverse Trendelenburg position to decrease venous return to the overdistended heart.
  2. **At termination of bypass, it is important to assess** the ECG, systemic blood pressure, filling of the ventricles, and the cardiac output. These values

Table 29.6 Hemodynamic Changes and Management After CPB

Clinical Scenarios	SBP	CO	PAP	CVP	Management Options
Hypovolemia	↓	↓	↓	↓	Volume administration
LV failure	↓	↓	↑	↑	Inotropes, IABP, CPB, and LVAD
RV failure	↓	↓	↓	↑	Inotropes, increase MAP, decrease PVR, CPB, and RVAD
Biventricular failure	↓	↓	↑	↑	Treatment for LV and RV failure
Low SVR	↓	↑	Normal	Normal	Vasopressors; decrease anesthetic
High SVR	↑	↓	Normal	Normal	Vasodilators; deepen anesthetic
pHTN	↓	↓	↑	↑	Inotropes with pulmonary dilating properties (eg, milrinone), nitrous oxide; reinstitute CPB

CO, cardiac output; CPB, cardiopulmonary bypass; CVP, central venous pressure; IABP, intra-aortic balloon pump; LV, left ventricle; LVAD, left ventricular assist device; MAP, mean arterial pressure; PAP, pulmonary artery pressure; pHTN, pulmonary hypertension; PVR, pulmonary vascular resistance; RV, right ventricle; RVAD, right ventricular assist device; SVR, systemic vascular resistance.

are compared with target values for the patient. If the patient is unstable, correct any pacing problems, have the surgeon assess the patency of the grafts, and use TEE to assess the valve replacement or repair. Assuming there is no surgical cause for hemodynamic instability, the unstable patient will usually fall into one of the categories listed in **Table 29.6**. **If a return to CPB is necessary**, adequate anticoagulation must be ensured. A **full dose** of heparin is indicated if protamine has been administered.

F. Postbypass Period

1. **Hemodynamic stability** is the primary goal. CPB gives rise to myocardial functional impairment and a systemic inflammatory response. Maintain adequate volume status, perfusion pressure, and appropriate rate and rhythm. Continuously monitor and reassess the surgical field.
2. **Hemostasis.** Once cardiovascular stability has been achieved and surgical bleeding is controlled, **protamine** administration begins. Initially, 25 to 50 mg is given over 2 to 3 minutes, and the hemodynamic response is observed. Protamine often causes systemic vasodilation (type I reaction) that can be avoided by slow administration over 10 to 15 minutes with or without α-agonist support. Rarely, an anaphylactic or anaphylactoid reaction (type II reaction) resulting in hypotension, bronchospasm, and pulmonary edema is encountered. Type II reactions are more likely observed in diabetic patients taking subcutaneous injections of protamine-containing insulin preparations (ie, neutral protamine hagedorn insulin) and men who have had a vasectomy. Finally,

catastrophic pulmonary hypertension (type III reaction) can occur, manifested by elevated PA pressures, right ventricular dilatation, systemic hypotension, and myocardial depression. Upon severe reaction, protamine is immediately discontinued, appropriate resuscitative measures are used, and, if necessary, the patient is retreated with heparin (with a full loading dose), and CPB is reinitiated. If forward flow is compromised, ask the surgeon to inject the heparin into the right atrium.
- **a.** The protamine dose is calculated based on the patient's whole blood heparin level. Automated heparin-protamine titration assays calculate the protamine dose for complete heparin neutralization; this method is associated with reduced protamine requirement. Alternatively, 1 to 1.3 mg of protamine is administered for every 100 units of heparin administered throughout the procedure.
- **b.** ACT monitoring is useful for titrating protamine after initial dose. Thromboelastography may be used to provide information about coagulation factor activity, platelet function, and degree of fibrinolysis during and after CPB.
- **c.** Normothermia reduces post-CPB coagulopathy
3. **Pulmonary dysfunction may follow CPB.** Aggressive treatment of bronchospasm before sternal closure is imperative.
4. **Pulmonary hypertension** may arise during the post-CPB period. See **Table 29.6** for approaches to management.
5. **Sternal closure** may precipitate acute cardiovascular decompensation. **Cardiac tamponade** may develop from compression of the heart and great vessels in the mediastinum. Severe hemodynamic compromise may necessitate transport to ICU with open sternum.
- **a.** Volatile anesthetics and other negative inotropes are reduced in anticipation of sternal closure. Intravascular volume should be optimized.
- **b.** Immediately after sternal closure, the filling pressures and cardiac output are compared with preclosure values, and appropriate adjustments in volume or drug infusions are made.
- **c.** Mediastinal and pleural tubes are placed on suction to prevent tamponade and quantify blood loss.
- **d.** Epicardial pacing is rechecked to assure reliable capture and optimal pacing setting.

G. Transfer to the ICU
- **a.** Patients should always be hemodynamically stable before transport. Transport with full monitors and defibrillator.
- **b.** Upon arrival to the ICU, mediastinal and pleural drainage tubes are attached to suction. Detailed sign out should be given before transfer care to the ICU team.

V. POSTOPERATIVE CARE
A. Warming. Most cardiac surgical patients will be hypothermic upon arrival to the ICU, and their initial course is notable for warming and vasodilation. Adequate sedation will prevent unwanted waking and shivering during this period.

B. Complications
1. **Dysrhythmias and myocardial ischemia** are common in the immediate postoperative period. Diagnosis and management are discussed in Chapter 36: Transfusion Therapy.
2. **Unexplained profound hypotension**, unresponsive to volume and pharmacologic resuscitation, is an indication for immediate reopening of

the chest in the ICU. The OR should be notified, and blood products requisitioned.
3. **Cardiac tamponade** may occur insidiously. Most often, an accumulation of blood in the mediastinum and inadequate chest tube drainage secondary to clot are responsible. Placing mediastinal tubes on suction as soon as the sternum is closed will help to prevent the development of tamponade. Reopening the sternum may be lifesaving. The diagnosis is considered with hypotension or low-output state. TEE is very helpful in making quick diagnoses.

VI. ENHANCED RECOVERY AFTER SURGERY (ERAS) FOR CARDIAC SURGERY
A. ERAS programs apply best practices across phases of perioperative care to enhance patient outcomes. Based on these recommendations, MGH adopted an ERAS protocol for nonurgent, on-pump CABGs incorporating integrating consensus recommendations for perioperative care in cardiac surgery with institutional values.
B. **Preoperative Strategies** include Hgb A1C and albumin measurement for risk stratification, correction of nutritional deficiency when feasible, preoperative carbohydrate loading and clear liquid consumption, patient engagement tools, alcohol and tobacco cessation 4 weeks before surgery, and prehabilitation when feasible.
C. **Intraoperative Strategies** include implementation of a surgical site infection prevention bundle, avoidance of hyperthermia during CPB rewarming, rigid sternal fixation, and antifibrinolytic therapy for on-pump cardiac surgeries. MGH-specific practices include limiting use of PA catheters, use of radial artery derived cardiac output monitoring, early termination of NMB infusion, initiation of insulin therapy at blood glucose >170 mg/dL, and temperature >35.5 °C prior to transport to ICU.
D. **Postoperative Strategies** include perioperative glycemic control with insulin infusion for glucose >160 to 180 mg/dL, multimodal opioid-sparing pain management, delirium screening at least once per shift, early extubation within 6 hours postop, maintenance of chest tube patency without breaking the sterile field, initiation of chemical thromboprophylaxis by postop day 1, biomarker monitoring for acute kidney injury, and goal-directed fluid therapy.

VII. PEDIATRIC CARDIAC ANESTHESIA
A. **Transition from fetal to adult circulation.** The transition from fetal to adult circulation is a transformation from a parallel to a series circulation. In utero, there is right-to-left shunting of blood across the ductus arteriosus. After birth, as the lungs are expanded and alveolar oxygen tension rises, the PVR decreases. Simultaneously, the SVR increases in association with the loss of the low-resistance placental circulation. The net effect of the PVR falling below the SVR is a reversal of ductus flow. The ductus arteriosus will contract and functionally close in the first 10 to 15 hours of life. This is caused by a loss of placental-produced prostaglandins and an increase in neonatal blood oxygen tension. Accompanying the decrease in PVR is an increase in pulmonary blood flow, an improvement in RV compliance, and a decrease in right-sided pressures relative to the left. This drop in right atrial pressure results in the closure of the foramen ovale. With the closure of the ductus arteriosus and the foramen ovale, the circulation assumes an adult configuration. These changes in the neonatal period are tentative; however, reversion to fetal circulation can occur during periods of abnormal physiologic stress. Persistence of elements of fetal circulation is

common in many cases of congenital heart disease (CHD) and can occasionally be lifesaving.
- **B. Differences between neonatal and adult cardiac physiology**
  1. In infants, there is **parasympathetic nervous system dominance** that reflects the relative immaturity of the sympathetic nervous system. Infant hearts are more responsive to circulating catecholamines than to sympathetic nervous stimulation.
  2. Neonatal hearts have more inelastic membrane mass than elastic contractile mass. Consequently, infant hearts have less myocardial reserve, a greater sensitivity to myocardial depressants, and a greater sensitivity to volume overload. The relatively noncompliant ventricles make stroke volume less responsive to increases in preload or demand. As such, **increases in cardiac output largely depend on increases in heart rate.**
  3. The RV and LV are equal in muscle mass at birth. A left-to-right muscle mass ratio of 2:1 is not achieved until the age of 4 to 5 months.
- **C. Congenital heart disease (CHD).** The clinical presentation depends on both the anatomy and the physiologic changes secondary to intracardiac shunts and obstructive lesions. In general, there are three categories of lesions: shunt, mixing lesion, and flow obstruction.
  1. **Shunt.** A shunt is an abnormal communication between the systemic and pulmonary circulations. Examples are atrial septal defect (ASD), VSD, and patent ductus arteriosus (PDA). The direction of blood flow is dependent on the pressures on either side of the shunt and the size of the shunt orifice.
     a. **Left-to-right shunt**—occurs when the PVR is lower than the SVR, resulting in increased pulmonary blood flow. This can cause pulmonary circulation congestion, volume overload, and increased work for the LV. Prolonged exposure to increased pulmonary blood flow results in progressive elevations in PVR, eventually leading to pulmonary vascular obstructive disease.
     b. **Right-to-left shunt**—occurs when PVR or RV outflow tract resistance exceeds SVR, thereby reducing pulmonary blood flow and manifesting as hypoxemia and cyanosis. Pure right-to-left shunting due to high PVR is seen in Eisenmenger syndrome and persistent pulmonary hypertension of the newborn with atrial and ductal shunting.
     c. **Simple versus complex shunts: Simple shunts** are not associated with anatomic obstruction to ventricular outflow. Pulmonary and systemic blood flow is determined by both the size of the shunt and the relative PVR/SVR ratio. **Most left-to-right shunts are simple shunts**. In contrast, **most right-to-left shunts are complex shunts**. These shunts are accompanied by an anatomic obstruction to blood flow. Shunt flow depends less on the PVR/SVR ratio and more on the resistance of the obstructive lesion. For example, tetralogy of Fallot is a complex right-to-left shunt since shunting occurs through the VSD because of pulmonary outflow obstruction while PVR remains low.
     d. **Shunt flow calculation.** Measuring the Q_p/Q_s (ratio of pulmonary to systemic blood flow) quantifies the direction and degree of shunting.

     $Q_p/Q_s = (SaO_2 - SmvO_2)/(SpvO_2 - SpaO_2)$

     $Q_p/Q_2 > 1$ indicates left-to-right shunt

     (1–1.5 small shunt; 1.5–2.0 moderate shunt; >2.0 large shunt).

     $Q_p/Q_s < 1$ indicates right-to-left shunt

where Q_p is pulmonary blood flow, $SmvO_2$ is mixed venous oxygen saturation, Q_s is systemic blood flow, $SpvO_2$ is pulmonary venous oxygen saturation, SaO_2 is systemic arterial oxygen saturation, and $SpaO_2$ is PA oxygen saturation. When calculating the ratio, oxygen saturation can be conveniently used instead of oxygen content. To simplify the calculation, if systemic blood is fully saturated, one can approximate that there is no significant right-to-left shunting and that pulmonary venous oxygen saturation is equal to systemic oxygen saturation ($SpvO_2 = SaO_2$).
2. **Mixing lesions.** In these lesions, there is large mixing between the pulmonary and systemic circulation as if they act as a common chamber. The Q_p/Q_s is independent of the shunt size and entirely dependent on relative vascular resistance or outflow obstruction. In cases of LV outflow obstruction, the pulmonary blood flow may be excessive enough to impair systemic perfusion. Examples of mixing lesions include truncus arteriosus, single ventricle, and total anomalous pulmonary venous return.
3. **Obstructive lesions.** These include AS, pulmonic stenosis, coarctation of the aorta, and asymmetrical septal hypertrophy. These lesions have ductal-dependent circulations. For example, in left-sided obstructive defects, systemic perfusion is dependent on blood flow from the RV via the PDA. In right-sided obstructive lesions, pulmonary blood flow is supplied from the aorta via the PDA.

D. **Anesthetic management**
 1. **Preoperative evaluation**
    a. The **history** should provide an assessment of the extent of cardiopulmonary impairment. Documentation should be made of the presence of cyanosis or congestive heart failure (CHF), exercise tolerance, cyanotic spells, activity level, feeding and growth patterns, associated syndromes, and anatomic abnormalities.
    b. **Physical examination** should make note of skin color, activity level, respiratory pattern and frequency, heart and lung sounds, and appropriateness of development for given age. Peripheral pulses should be palpated, and blood pressure measurements obtained in both arms as well as the lower extremities to rule out coarctation.
    c. The **chest radiograph** should be examined for evidence of cardiomegaly, CHF, abnormalities in heart position, and the presence of any thoracic cage abnormalities.
    d. The **ECG** may be normal; however, abnormalities can be important clues to underlying cardiac lesions.
    e. **Cardiac catheterization** can define the cardiopulmonary anatomy and quantify pulmonary and systemic shunt flows, vascular resistance, and intracardiac chamber pressures.
 2. **Premedication.** Infants younger than 6 months of age, cyanotic or dyspneic children, and patients who are critically ill should generally receive no premedication. Older or more vigorous children may be given oral midazolam (0.5 to 1.0 mg/kg) with or without oral ketamine (5 to 7 mg/kg). An alternative intramuscular regimen is ketamine (3 to 5 mg/kg) in combination with midazolam (0.5 to 1.0 mg) and glycopyrrolate (0.1 to 0.2 mg) administered in the preanesthetic holding area. With the exception of ketamine, doses of sedatives are reduced in cases where decreasing SVR would increase right-to-left shunting. Cyanotic infants are usually polycythemic and may be prone to thromboses of vital organs if they are not adequately hydrated with IV fluids preoperatively.
 3. **Monitoring and equipment.** In addition to the standard monitoring required for all patients, a precordial or esophageal stethoscope and

three temperature probes (tympanic membrane, esophageal, and rectal) should be available. Intra-arterial pressure monitoring is usually necessary. Prior surgical procedures, such as Blalock–Taussig shunt construction or coarctation repair, may influence the choice of site for radial artery cannulation. **Central venous catheters** are typically inserted. A 4-French double-lumen catheter can be used for infants weighing less than 10 kg, and a 5-French triple-lumen catheter can be used for larger children. A warming blanket, radiant heating lamps, and a heated humidifier are useful perioperatively. TEE is an important diagnostic and intraoperative management tool.

4. **Resuscitation drugs** and infusions of inotropic medications appropriate for pediatric use must be available. Commonly used inotropes include dopamine (2 to 10 µg/kg/min), epinephrine (0.01 to 0.1 µg/kg/min), and dobutamine (2 to 10 µg/kg/min). **Air bubbles** must be meticulously removed from IV tubing and syringes. **Air filters** should be used whenever possible. Even in the absence of shunts, paradoxical air emboli may traverse a probe-patent foramen ovale (PFO).

5. **Induction.** The choice between an inhalational and IV induction is based primarily on ventricular function and the degree of patient cooperation. A slow, carefully titrated induction by either technique usually provides a safe and stable anesthetic. Theoretically, patients with right-to-left shunts may have a slower rate of induction with volatile anesthetics because blood is shunted past the lungs. Similarly, arterial concentrations of IV anesthetics may increase more rapidly in patients with a significant right-to-left shunt.

E. **Cardiopulmonary bypass**
1. **Pump prime** volume ranges between 150 and 1200 mL. Packed red blood cells are frequently added to the prime to yield an initial Hct of approximately 25% when on bypass. For smaller children, the red cells may be washed to remove potassium, lactic acid, and citrate–phosphate-dextrose-adenine preservative. Cells may be leukocyte depleted to decrease patient exposure to cytomegalovirus. Typical constituents of pump prime include sodium bicarbonate (to counteract acidosis), mannitol (to promote diuresis), heparin, and calcium (to offset the effects of the citrate in blood). Albumin solutions and FFP may be added to the prime for neonates.

2. **Infants and children** generally lack vaso-occlusive disease. Consequently, blood flow during CPB is more important than arterial pressure. Flows as high as 150 mL/kg/min may be used in infants weighing less than 5 kg, while MAP as low as 30 mm Hg is well tolerated provided that SVC pressure is low (indicating that venous drainage is adequate).

3. **DHCA** is used extensively for infants weighing less than 10 kg. Up to 1 hour of circulatory arrest is tolerated without neurologic injury at a core and brain temperature of 15 °C to 20 °C. Where appropriate, low-flow CPB may offer advantages over circulatory arrest. Management points include adequate brain hypothermia (eg, packing the head with ice packs), hemodilution, acid–base balance, muscle relaxation, and blood glucose control.

F. **Procedures that do not require CPB** include PDA ligation, aortic coarctation repair, PA banding, and most procedures, which create shunts designed to increase pulmonary blood flow (eg, modified Blalock–Taussig shunt). Procedures such as pulmonary valvotomy, aortic valvotomy, and the creation of ASDs can be accomplished with percutaneous techniques.

G. **Management of specific CHD lesions** (Table 29.7)
1. **Cyanotic lesions** are secondary to **right-to-left shunting** either alone or in the presence of an obstruction to pulmonary blood flow. Typical

TABLE 29.7 Specific Congenital Cardiac Lesions

Lesion	Anatomy	Pathophysiology	Surgical Correction	Anesthetic Considerations
ASD	Three varieties: 1. Ostium secundum: defect in septum (most common) 2. Ostium primum: endocardial cushion defect 3. Sinus venosus: caval-atrial defect often with partial anomalous pulmonary venous return	Left-to-right shunt RV volume overload Potential for right-to-left shunting (eg, during Valsalva maneuver) with paradoxical embolus risk Minimal symptoms until later age, when CHF may develop	Suture or patch closure Percutaneous catheterization device closure	Inhalation or intravenous induction Potential extubation at end of procedure Avoid air bubbles
VSD	Supracristal, membranous canal, and muscular subtypes	Left-to-right shunt Increased pulmonary blood flow Pulmonary hypertension and reversal of shunt as a late effect (Eisenmenger syndrome)	Dacron patch closure of singular or multiple defects Muscular defects may be difficult to locate Selected defects may be amenable to percutaneous catheterization device closure	Hypocarbia and low FiO_2 to decrease pulmonary blood flow Avoid myocardial depressants Avoid air bubbles Potential for postoperative AV block and pacing requirement Potential need for postrepair inotropic support
Coarctation of the aorta	Narrowing usually distal to origin of left subclavian artery Maybe preductal or postductal in location Often associated with a VSD	Increased blood flow to upper extremities and head Systemic hypoperfusion Pressure overload of LV	Left thoracotomy approach Subclavian artery flap angioplasty or resection and end-to-end anastomosis	Non-CPB case Arterial line on right Suitable for regional anesthesia supplementation Potential for postrepair hypertension

(*continued*)

TABLE 29.7 Specific Congenital Cardiac Lesions (continued)

Lesion	Anatomy	Pathophysiology	Surgical Correction	Anesthetic Considerations
PDA	PDA	Right-to-left shunt when PVR is high Left-to-right shunt as PVR decreases Necessary for survival with certain lesions (eg, hypoplastic left heart syndrome)	Left thoracotomy vs. thoracoscopic approach Ligation and occasional division of PDA Potential for percutaneous catheterization coil embolization	Usually premature infants with concomitant pulmonary disease Avoid high FiO_2 (risk of retrolental fibroplasia) Risk of recurrent laryngeal nerve damage
Tetralogy of Fallot	1. VSD 2. Pulmonary outflow tract obstruction 3. RV hypertrophy Overriding aorta	Right-to-left shunting through VSD into overriding aorta Fixed (pulmonic stenosis) and dynamic (infundibular hypertrophy) RV outflow obstruction components Systemic desaturation ("Tet" spell)	Patch closure of VSD RV outflow tract reconstruction/augmentation Excision of infundibular muscle band (when appropriate)	Management of "Tet spell": augment intravascular volume, minimize PVR (increase FiO_2 and decrease $PaCO_2$), increase SVR (knee–chest position and phenylephrine), and consider negative inotropes (halothane and β-blockade) Potential need for postoperative pacing
Transposition of the great arteries	Transposition of both the aorta to the RV and the PA to the LV resulting in isolation of pulmonary and systemic circulations	ASD, VSD, and/or PDA required for pulmonary and systemic blood mixing and, hence, survival	Atrial switch procedure (Mustard and Senning): rarely performed Arterial switch procedure (Jatene) When associated with a VSD and pulmonic stenosis, a Rastelli procedure (LV to aorta baffle closure via the VSD, and RV to PA allograft conduit)	Ductus/mixing lesion-dependent CHD lesion Prostaglandin E_1 to maintain ductus patency (when appropriate)

Truncus arteriosus	Single great artery that gives rise to the aorta, PA, and coronary arteries Associated VSD	Mixing of pulmonary and systemic blood Most commonly presents with pulmonary overcirculation Valvuloplasty of truncal valve	VSD closure RV to PA valved conduit	Increase PVR or decrease pulmonary blood flow precorrection (based on the degree of pulmonary overcorrection) Normalize PVR postcorrection Potential need for inotropic support postrepair
Atrioventricular canal defect	Common AV valve. Deficiency of atrial and ventricular septae	Mixing of blood at the atrial and ventricular levels Usually presents with pulmonary overcirculation	Closure of ASD and VSD Mitral/tricuspid valvuloplasty	Manipulate PVR to balance/optimize pulmonary systemic blood flow Anticipate need for inotropic support postrepair Associated with Down syndrome (potential airway issues)
Hypoplastic left heart syndrome	Atretic/hypoplastic mitral valve, aortic valve, LV, and ascending aorta	Left-to-right shunt (obligatory) at atrial or ventricular level for mixing Ductus arteriosus dependent for right-to-left (ie, systemic) perfusion	Palliative, staged repair: 1. Norwood I: atrial septectomy, reconstruction of aortic arch, PA plasty, and creation of systemic to pulmonary shunt 2. Bidirectional Glenn: takedown of systemic to pulmonary shunt, creation of SVC to PA (cavopulmonary) shunt 3. Modified Fontan procedure: creation of an IVC to PA anastomosis via an intraatrial baffle; creates total cavopulmonary continuity Alternatively, cardiac transplantation is an option	Critically ill neonates. Preoperative (ICU) management will impact outcome. Prostaglandin E_1 to maintain ductal patency Inotropes often necessary prerepair and postrepair Avoid myocardial depressants Fentanyl >50 μg/kg prior to sternotomy. Manipulate PVR via adjustments in FiO_2 and Pco_2 to balance/optimize pulmonary vs. systemic perfusion Target goal: MAP = 40, pH = 7.40, Pao_2 = 40, $Paco_2$ = 40

ASD, atrial septal defect; AV, atrioventricular; CHD, congenital heart disease; CHF, congestive heart failure; CPB, cardiopulmonary bypass; FiO_2, fraction of inspired oxygen; ICU, intensive care unit; IVC, inferior vena cava; LV, left ventricle; MAP, mean arterial pressure; PA, pulmonary artery; Pao_2, partial pressure of oxygen; $Paco_2$, partial pressure of carbon dioxide; PDA, patent ductus arteriosus; PVR, pulmonary vascular resistance; RV, right ventricle; SVC, superior vena cava; SVR, systemic vascular resistance; VSD, ventricular septal defect.

conditions include tetralogy of Fallot, tricuspid atresia, pulmonary atresia, and pulmonary hypertension.
  a. **Management goals** are to decrease PVR, increase pulmonary blood flow, maintain SVR, and maintain central volume.
  b. **Ventilation management** include using modest hypocarbia, increasing inspired oxygen concentration, maintaining normal functional residual capacity, and avoiding acidosis.
  c. Patients with **tetralogy of Fallot** are prone to hypercyanotic spells (rapid desaturation usually in response to surgical or other stimulation). Management of these spells includes measures that reduce infundibular spasm and improve pulmonary blood flow (eg, β-blockers such as propranolol), volume loading (15 to 20 mL/kg), and use of α-agonists (eg, phenylephrine) to increase SVR. Alprostadil (prostaglandin E_1 0.05 to 0.1 µg/kg/min IV) may be used to maintain ductus arteriosus patency, decrease PVR, and increase pulmonary blood flow.
2. **Lesions with increased pulmonary blood flow** and left-to-right shunting include ASDs, VSDs, and PDA.
   a. **Management goals** are to avoid negative inotropes and excessive pulmonary blood flow.
   b. **Anesthetic maneuvers** include minimizing myocardial depressants (eg, volatile anesthetics), increasing PVR, and decreasing pulmonary blood flow in favor of systemic blood flow by maintaining normocarbia to slight hypercarbia, limiting inspired oxygen concentration, and using PEEP.
3. **Balanced shunts** have the potential for a ventricle's output to be directed to the pulmonary or systemic circulation and include hypoplastic left heart syndrome, truncus arteriosus, double-outlet RV, and complete AV canal defect. The direction of blood flow is governed by the relative resistances of the pulmonary and systemic vasculatures (PVR/SVR ratio).
   a. **Management goals** are to manipulate pulmonary blood flow to maintain adequate systemic perfusion. Often both a low–normal blood pressure (eg, MAP of 40 mm Hg) and a low PaO_2 (eg, 40 mm Hg) must be tolerated.
   b. **Anesthetic maneuvers** depend on the balance of systemic versus pulmonary blood flow, which can be affected by altering $PaCO_2$, inspired oxygen concentration, and PEEP.

VIII. OTHER CARDIAC PROCEDURES
  A. Off-bypass CABG is performed to avoid the complications associated with CPB and to minimize aortic manipulation. Proximal grafts are performed using either a partial aortic cross-clamp technique or a specifically designed proximal anastomotic device that precludes aortic clamping. Distal grafts are performed using one of several heart-stabilizing devices. Considerations for this procedure include the following:
  1. Consider tailoring anesthetic management to allow possible **early extubation** after surgery (eg, fentanyl 5 to 10 µg/kg, volatile anesthetic followed by an infusion of propofol or dexmedetomidine).
  2. **Heparin** is given to maintain ACT above 400 seconds. This allows the patient to be emergently initiated on CPB if necessary. Antifibrinolytic therapy is avoided. A small dose of protamine (50 to 100 mg) is given after the procedure.
  3. **Hemodynamic instability** is common, particularly when the surgeon is performing the distal anastomoses. Grafts to vessels with less disease

tend to be associated with more instability than those to vessels that are occluded. Increasing MAP to optimize coronary perfusion is critical for the ischemic heart during creation of the distal anastomosis. If hemodynamically intolerable ischemia results, coronary shunting may be indicated. Occasionally, repositioning of the heart is required to permit augmented right-sided filling when hemodynamic instability is due to obstruction of right heart inflow.
4. **Volume requirements** tend to be high. A full heart tends to tolerate physical manipulation better.
5. **Ventricular dysrhythmias** may be treated with an amiodarone 150-mg IV bolus and then followed with 1-mg/min infusion. Acid–base and electrolyte abnormalities should be corrected.

B. **"Redo" cardiac surgery**
1. **Mediastinal structures**, including the heart, major vessels, prior coronary bypass grafts, as well as the lungs may be adherent to the underside of the sternum. They can be lacerated during sternotomy. Usually, 2 to 4 units of blood must be in the OR before sternotomy begins. An additional 14 g IV catheter or a rapid infusion catheter should be placed to facilitate volume resuscitation. Because the patient may need to go on CPB emergently, heparin must be in a syringe ready to administer immediately. In emergency situations, venous return may be supplied from the pump suction line on the field ("sucker bypass").
2. **Insertion of a PA catheter** equipped with pacing capability is prudent as epicardial pacing may not be possible during chest opening. Transcutaneous defibrillation pads should be applied to treat malignant arrhythmias.
3. **Diffuse bleeding** from dissection of scar tissue may occur after CPB. Amicar is useful in standard doses.
4. **ECG monitoring** is imperative because manipulation of atheromatous grafts may send emboli to the coronary circulation. Because myocardial protection is more challenging in patients with previous coronary grafts, postbypass myocardial dysfunction is more likely.

C. **DHCA** may be necessary for surgery on the distal ascending aorta or aortic arch (eg, for an aneurysm or aortic dissection). Circulatory arrest provides a bloodless field for distal aortic anastomosis. Hypothermia decreases the metabolic rate and minimizes the risk of cerebral and organ ischemia during circulatory arrest. Problems associated with DHCA include increased CBP time, coagulopathy, and neurologic and end-organ dysfunction. The risk of permanent neurologic injury after aortic arch surgery using DHCA is approximately 3% to 12%. Most patients tolerate 30 minutes of DHCA without significant neurologic dysfunction. Management issues include the following:
1. **Cerebral protection during DHCA**
   a. **Hypothermia.** Systemic cooling to 18 °C produces electrical silence on the EEG in most patients. There is no outcome evidence to support topical cooling of the head in humans.
   b. **Antegrade cerebral perfusion (ACP)** via the right axillary artery or **retrograde cerebral perfusion (RCP)** via the SVC cannula can be used to extend the duration of safe circulatory arrest. ACP is thought to be superior to RCP for cerebral protection and avoid deep hypothermia.
2. **Glycemic control** is important. Glucose metabolism is impaired under DHCA. Blood glucose concentration should be maintained below 180 mg/dL to avoid worsening neurologic injury.
3. **Temperature monitoring.** It is commonly preferred to use more than one site for core body temperature monitoring. Nasopharyngeal

temperature provides the closest assessment of brain temperature for adults.

4. **Acid–base management** depends on whether α-stat or pH-stat is used (see Section IV.C.2). The pediatric literature generally recommends the use of pH-stat management during DHCA for both cerebral and myocardial protection.

D. Cardiac tamponade and constrictive pericarditis

1. Avoid decreases in myocardial contractility, peripheral vascular resistance, and heart rate. **Pericardiocentesis** prior to induction may be advisable in patients with tamponade unless the condition is secondary to aortic dissection.
2. An arterial catheter, a large-bore IV catheter should be inserted. A central venous catheter or PA catheter may be used if the patient can tolerate insertion.
3. Useful **induction agents** include etomidate and ketamine.
4. A method for **backup atrial pacing** (transesophageal or transvenous) should be available.
5. Patients should be prepped and draped for surgery prior to induction. In **severe cases**, awake intubation with maintenance of spontaneous ventilation should be considered.

E. Cardiac transplantation

1. **Anesthetic management of the donor**
   a. Basic management of donor patients and organs is discussed in Chapter 25: Anesthesia for Transplant Surgery.
   b. Donor after cardiac death organ transplantation is an emerging technique with promising initial results that serves to increase the overall number of organ donations. In donor patients, after cardiac arrest has occurred and is deemed irreversible, both heart and lungs may be harvested and transported with various preservation techniques. Outcomes in transplant recipients of these organs have been comparable with recipients of organs from donor after brain death patients.

2. **Anesthetic management of the recipient**
   a. The key to patient survival is minimizing the ischemic time of the donated heart. Consequently, expeditious preparation of the recipient and communication with the surgical team are essential.
   b. **Preoperative evaluation of** the recipient should determine whether the patient has had previous chest surgery, has an elevated PVR (>6 Wood units, transpulmonary gradient >12 mm Hg), has pulmonary hypertension responsive to vasodilators, or is coagulopathic.
   c. **Invasive monitoring** includes arterial and central lines. A PA catheter and TEE should be used. Internal cardiac defibrillator (ICD) should be turned off.
   d. **Precautions for a full stomach** may be necessary during induction. If the patient is receiving inotropic infusions, consider increasing their doses before induction. If a ventricular assist device (VAD) is present, venous return must be maintained for the pump to maintain its flow rate.
   e. **Right heart failure and coagulopathy** are common during the rewarming phase of bypass. Cellular blood products should be irradiated or leukocyte depleted to minimize foreign HLA antigen exposure. An inhaled pulmonary vasodilator, such as nitric oxide, is often empirically initiated to mitigate right heart strain.
   f. **The donor heart** may be unresponsive to drugs whose actions are mediated by the recipient's cholinergic nervous system (eg, atropine

and glycopyrrolate). Upon termination of CPB, the recipient's heart rate should be maintained between 80 and 110 beats/min. This can be accomplished with epicardial pacing or pharmacologically with dopamine (2 to 10 µg/kg/min), epinephrine (0.01 to 01 µg/kg/min), or isoproterenol infusion (0.5 to 5 µg/min).
  g. **Immunosuppressants** and steroid will be necessary and are administered in consultation with the surgeon and transplant cardiologist.
F. Lung transplantation
  1. **Indications and surgical technique:** Lung transplantation is performed for end-stage nonmalignant lung disease. Common indications are severe emphysema, α1-antitrypsin deficiency, cystic fibrosis, pulmonary fibrosis, and pulmonary hypertension. Specific operations include living-related lobar lung transplant (LRLLTx), single-lung transplant (SLTx), double-lung transplant (DLTx), sequential SLTx, and combined heart–lung transplantation. The patient's position depends on the incision required for adequate surgical exposure (lateral decub/thoracotomy for SLTx and clamshell incision/supine for DLTx or LRLLTx). Patients will have undergone preoperative counseling, exercise and cardiac testing, and a conditioning program.
  2. **Anesthetic management of the recipient**
     a. **Invasive monitoring** with arterial line, central venous line, and PA catheter. A femoral arterial line and large bore femoral venous access are contemplated for patients who have a high likelihood of requiring extracorporeal membrane oxygenation (ECMO) or CPB. TEE is useful for assessing heart function and pulmonary blood flow after implantation.
     b. **Medications** should be immediately available to treat bronchospasm, electrolyte disturbances, pulmonary hypertension, and right ventricular failure. Immunosuppressants, steroids, and antibiotics should also be administered. All blood products must be leukocyte depleted and transfused via a filter. Anticipation of a large transfusion requirement and maintenance of an ample supply of blood products are important. A total IV anesthetic is commonly administered.
     c. **Analgesia:** Intraoperative cryoablation of intercostal nerves by the surgeon is increasingly common. Alternatively, a postoperative epidural catheter may be placed for pain management, unless the patient is already on ECMO or has other contraindications.
     d. **Induction** with a technique that provides cardiovascular stability is appropriate. Most recipients are considered "full stomachs."
     e. **Lung isolation** is best achieved with a left-side DLT or less commonly large (>8 mm) single-lumen endotracheal tube with an endobronchial blocker. The DLT is exchanged for a single-lumen tube at the end of operation.
     f. **VA-ECMO** or CPB is frequently used to facilitate cardiopulmonary stability during recipient lung explantation and donor lung implantation. ECMO is typically weaned off by case end but may be continued or reconfigured to V-V to manage refractory hypoxemia. Regardless of institutional preferences, CPB or ECMO should be available to initiate should refractory hypoxemia occur. Indications for full CPB include arterial oxygen saturation of less than 90% after clamping of the PA, low cardiac index of less than 2.0 L/min/m^2 despite inotropic therapy, or a systolic blood pressure of less than 90 mm Hg.
     g. **Capnography** may be misleading because of severe mismatching of ventilation to perfusion. Frequent measurements of ABG tensions

are warranted to assess ventilation. Worsening acidemia may also signal inadequate tissue perfusion from a variety of causes (hypovolemia, air trapping, and decreased cardiac output).
h. Postoperative management
1. Pulmonary hypertension will cause increased hydrostatic pulmonary edema and worsening gas exchange and lung compliance. Serial ABGs are followed to document the function of the transplanted lung. The donor lungs should be ventilated at a low FiO_2 (21% to 30%) using a pressure control mode to achieve peak inspiratory pressures <25 cm H_2O.
2. Acute rejection may manifest as decreasing pulmonary compliance with worsening arterial oxygenation.
3. Many patients will remain intubated until the transplanted lung begins to function well, and symptoms of reperfusion edema and acute rejection are controlled. The trachea is extubated only when the patient is hemodynamically stable and breathing comfortably, which is sometimes possible in the OR.
4. Observe for signs of toxicity from the immunosuppressive regimen, including acute renal failure.
5. Repeated bronchoscopies and biopsies of the transplanted lung are necessary after surgery and are often managed under local anesthesia with IV sedation.

G. Mechanical circulatory support (MCS) may be classified as extracorporeal, percutaneously inserted, or implantable. Patients with decompensated heart failure (biventricular, LV, or RV injury) in cardiogenic shock (CS) may benefit from ECMO or temporary extracorporeal and/or percutaneously inserted VADs to support myocardial recovery before a durable implantable VAD may be appropriate.
1. Extracorporeal devices
a. **Extracorporeal centrifugal pumps** (eg, CentriMag, TandemHeart) may be implanted surgically to support univentricular function via surgical implantation to the LA or LV and aorta, or RA or RV to PA. At MGH, these devices have been supplanted by VA-ECMO and percutaneously inserted microaxial flow pumps (eg, Impella 5.5).
b. **ECMO** is an alternative form of extracorporeal life support to VADs. ECMO is indicated for the short-term management of severe but reversible CS or respiratory failure that is refractory to conventional treatment. It is an option for treatment of severe postcardiotomy ventricular dysfunction with or without hypoxemia. It consists of an external pump that pushes venous blood through a membrane allowing gas exchange before returning the blood to the circulation via a warmer.
   1. Venous drainage usually occurs from the internal jugular (IJ) vein or femoral vein. Blood is returned either to an artery (venoarterial [VA] ECMO) or a central vein (venovenous [VV] ECMO).
   2. **Venoarterial** (**VA**) ECMO bypasses the patient's heart and lungs with diversion of complete or partial flow through the ECMO circuit, providing both respiratory and hemodynamic support. It can be used for refractory postcardiotomy CS. The same cannulation setup during CPB can be used for ECMO. If considered subsequently, ECMO can be established from the femoral artery and vein. A condition called **differential hypoxemia** can occur in VA ECMO when a proportion of venous blood in a patient with some return of cardiac function is pumped into the diseased lungs, with subsequent ejection of hypoxic blood to the coronaries and

great vessels. This may be revealed by a difference in oxygenation from sampling of left-sided and right-sided arterial lines.
3. **Venovenous (VV)** ECMO provides gas exchange support in patients with good left cardiac function. Venous cannulae are usually placed in the right femoral vein for drainage and right IJ for infusion. A dual-lumen cannula (Avalon or Protek Duo) can be inserted into the IJ vein. The cannula drains blood from IVC and SVC or RA returns oxygenated blood into RA or PA.
4. Aggressive medical support is required to optimize the results of ECMO and facilitate weaning. Interventions may include the use of pulmonary vasodilators for pulmonary hypertension, lung-protective ventilation strategies; optimization of preload to provide pulmonary perfusion; and the use of renal replacement therapy. To avoid thrombus formation in the ECMO circuit, heparin is administered to maintain the ACT at 1.5 to 2.0 times normal.

2. **Percutaneously inserted devices**
    a. **Impella are percutaneously inserted microaxial VADs.** The contemporary model Impella 5.5 provides up to 6.2 L/min of flow and is an approved therapy for patients with LV failure, CS, and high-risk patients undergoing percutaneous intervention. It may be placed via retrograde approach across the aortic valve using femoral or axillary artery access.
    b. **The ProtekDuo** is a dual-lumen device inserted percutaneously via the right IJ vein to the right heart to provide RV MCS when used in conjunction with an extracorporeal centrifugal pump. Inflow ports are positioned in the RA and outflow ports in the main PA. While not actively used at MGH, the ProtekDuo is a valid alternative strategy for MCS in RV failure.
    c. The **IABP** is normally placed in the cardiac catheterization lab under sedation. It provides circulatory assistance for the failing or ischemic heart. Inflation of the intra-aortic balloon early in diastole augments aortic diastolic pressure and thus coronary perfusion. The effect is most beneficial for the LV which receives most of its blood supply during diastole. Deflation of the balloon during isovolumic contraction reduces the impedance to LV ejection, thereby reducing myocardial oxygen consumption. IABPs have fallen out of favor due to questionable mortality benefit and supplanted by Impella and VA-ECMO MCS strategies.

3. **Implantable devices** (eg, Heartmate III).
    a. These devices are used as a bridge to cardiac transplantation or destination therapy.
    b. These devices are designed for LV support only. They consist of an inflow cannula, a pump, and an outflow cannula. The inflow cannula is inserted into the LV apex while the outflow cannula is inserted into the ascending aorta. A driveline is tunneled through the skin to connect the implanted pump to the external console. CPB is always necessary for placement.
    c. The HeartMate III is an electrically driven centrifugal flow pump. A rechargeable power source fits into a holster and allows the patient to leave the hospital. The HeartMate III is the only durable VAD currently implanted at MGH.

4. **Anesthetic considerations for MCS insertion**
    a. Patients will have **marginal cardiac function.** Extreme care is required during induction to minimize decreases in contractility and preload.

b. Large-bore IV access is recommended and antifibrinolytics merit consideration depending on the type of support.
   c. If the patient is receiving the device as a bridge to transplantation, transfuse with leukocyte-depleted cellular blood products to minimize human leukocyte antigen exposure.
   d. **Transesophageal echocardiography (TEE) and/or fluoroscopy is required to assess the position and flow of the cannula** in addition to facilitating air removal. It also evaluates the position of the interventricular septum to guide the pump output and evaluate ventricular functions and volume status.
   e. Patients receiving an LVAD frequently require RV support. Inotropes, inhaled prostaglandin or nitric oxide, and occasionally an RVAD are required.
   f. The flow of the device depends largely on the volume in the ventricle. Decreased venous return or hypovolemia will be signaled by a decreased pumping rate which is typically improved with volume repletion. Vasopressors such as norepinephrine and vasopressin are typically needed to ameliorate vasodilation. Patients with an LVAD are preload dependent and afterload sensitive.
   g. Subsequent to placement of temporary MCS, continual assessment of native cardiopulmonary function is essential. If the heart and lungs do not recover within the expected timeframe (1 to 2 weeks), the decision should be made to convert to long-term support such as a durable VAD or transplant. A discussion of the goals of care is important if the disease process is believed to be nonreversible.
H. **Transcatheter aortic valve replacement (TAVR)** is conducted for patients who are not surgical candidates for aortic replacement. An expanding bioprosthetic valve is placed over the native aortic valve. The procedure may be carried out using a transfemoral arterial or open transapical approach. The procedure is typically carried out in a hybrid OR or cardiac catheterization laboratory.
   1. **Anesthetic management**
      a. **General anesthesia** is not usually required unless TEE is needed for proper positioning of the new valve. The procedure can be well tolerated under monitored anesthesia care or conscious sedation if fluoroscopy and TTE are used for valve deployment and evaluation.
      b. **Rapid ventricular pacing** is required to minimize cardiac motion during valve deployment. A temporary transvenous pacing lead is inserted into the right ventricle. A pacing rate of 140 to 200 beats/min frequently results in 1:1 ventricular capture and sufficiently lowers the pulse pressure and cardiac output. The rapid pacing periods must be minimized to avoid hemodynamic instability, especially in patients with depressed LV function and CAD.
      c. **Echocardiography** is particularly useful to assess adequate placement and function of the valve. It is crucial to ensure accurate positioning of the valve with echocardiography and fluoroscopy prior to deployment to avoid embolization of the valve or a large perivalvular leaks. Transthoracic echocardiogram or TEE can assess stability, location, and function of the valve as well as the degree of perivalvular leak.
   2. **Complications** include tamponade, cerebral vascular accident, aortic rupture or dissection, AI, conversion to emergent surgical aortic valve replacement, myocardial infarction, suboptimal valve deployment, and AV block.
I. **Transcatheter MV replacement (TMVR) and repair (TMVRep)** are effective for native primary and secondary MR in patients who are not suitable surgical

candidates. TMVR is also approved to treat MS with annular calcification or as valve-in-vale management of failed surgical bioprosthesis or ring. TMVRep may include leaflet, chordal, or annuloplasty repairs that are performed via trans-septal approach. TMVR is an evolving procedure with multiple devices available and more commonly performed via trans-septal approach than transapical approach which requires minithoracotomy.

1. **General endotracheal anesthesia** with **TEE** and fluoroscopic guidance is frequently required for the procedure. However, these procedures are increasingly done under sedation and local anesthesia.
   a. A radial arterial line is placed prior to induction and large bore access is obtained in case of complications necessitating rapid transfusion.
   b. Right heart catheterization or PA catheter placement is often performed to monitor right- and left-sided hemodynamics before and after the procedure. For TMVR, placement of a transvenous pacing wire may facilitate rapid ventricular pacing for valve deployment.
   c. Echocardiographic guidance is crucial for the trans-septal puncture and device positioning, as well as to assess severity of MR or MS pre- and postintervention.
   d. Brief periods of apnea may be required to allow precise placement of the device.
   e. Vasoactive agents and inotropes may be required to raise the blood pressure to adequately assess the severity of residual MR.
2. **Complications** include arrhythmias (especially atrial fibrillation), worsening MR, tamponade, device embolization, device entrapment in the chordal apparatus, or acute chordal rupture that may necessitate emergent open surgical repair.

IX. ANESTHESIA FOR "OFF-SITE" CARDIAC PROCEDURES

The goal of anesthesia is to provide sufficient sedation to allow the procedure to be completed without excessive movement while avoiding cardiopulmonary instability. The issues pertinent to anesthesia outside of the OR for noncardiac procedures apply to cardiac procedures as well.

A. **Aspiration thrombectomy** with the AngioVac device (Vortex Medical) combines a venous suction cannula with VV bypass to achieve filtering of aspirated thrombus and other debris. This may be utilized to remove thrombi from the pulmonary vasculature, peripheral vasculature, or right atrium without the need for concomitant thrombolytic therapy.
   1. **Anesthetic management** is driven by the indication of the procedure. Complications associated with acute PE, RV dysfunction, cardiac arrhythmias, venous embolic event, or previous failed thrombolytic therapy should be anticipated. General anesthesia with TEE and arterial line for invasive BP monitoring are indicated, with consideration given to central venous access.
   2. **VV bypass** is established for filtering of thrombotic material and other debris. Patients are heparinized to ACT of 250 to 300 seconds before initiation. Access site for VV bypass should be discussed with the proceduralist, as right IJ access may be limited if the need for more central venous access should arise.

B. **Implantable cardioverter defibrillator (ICD).** Modern ICDs consist of an endocardial lead system and a pectoral pulse generator. Older systems used epicardial lead systems and abdominal generators.
   1. ICDs are used for primary prevention of sudden cardiac death in patients with systolic heart failure (EF <35%) refractory to medical therapy or in those with high-risk conditions such as long QT

syndrome, hypertrophic cardiomyopathy, Brugada syndrome, and arrhythmogenic right ventricular dysplasia. In addition to ICD placement, patients with dilated cardiomyopathy and a widened QRS have been shown to also benefit from cardiac resynchronization therapy.

2. Devices are placed under local anesthesia in the electrophysiology laboratory. A brief period of general anesthesia is necessary for testing the device once it is implanted. A deep sedation anesthetic with propofol is suitable.

3. If intracardiac electrodes are inadequate, patients may require intraoperative epicardial electrode placement. These patients are often hemodynamically compromised. They should have an arterial catheter and catheter for vasoactive medication administration. Emergency drugs, including epinephrine, must be immediately available.

4. **Noninvasive programmed stimulation** is used to test the function of an ICD after it has been implanted. An ICD programmer is used to induce the irregular rhythm (ventricular fibrillation or tachycardia). The device is then checked for proper sensing and dysrhythmia termination.

C. **Cardioversion.** A short-acting sedative (eg, propofol or etomidate) can be administered for brief loss of consciousness. The combination of fentanyl and midazolam is an alternative but not ideal due to prolonged duration of action. Routine fasting guidelines should be followed for all elective cardioversions. Hemodynamically unstable patients often warrant immediate cardioversion, and a small dose of amnestic may be all that can be tolerated.

D. **Transcatheter ablation and electrophysiology procedures** take place in cardiac catheterization or electrophysiology labs. Common procedures include pulmonary vein isolation (PVI) for ablation of atrial fibrillation/flutter, supraventricular tachycardia (SVT), and ventricular tachycardia (VT).

1. **Anesthetic management** is determined by the type of procedure performed. PVI is performed under general anesthesia, as more durable response to therapy has been documented as compared to PVI under conscious sedation. However, SVT ablations are carried out under sedation to avoid suppression of arrhythmia by a general anesthetic.

ACKNOWLEDGMENT

We gratefully acknowledge the contributions of previous edition author, Maximilian Frank Lang, as portions of those chapters have been retained in this revision.

Suggested Readings

Alvarez CK, Zweibel S, Stangle A, Panza G, May T, Marieb M. Anesthetic considerations in the electrophysiology laboratory: a comprehensive review. *J Cardiothorac Vasc Anesth*. 2023;37(1):96-111.

Andropoulos DB, Mossad EB, Gottlieb EA, eds. *Anesthesia for Congenital Heart Disease*. 4th ed. Wiley Blackwell; 2023.

Budd AN, Wood B, Zheng W, Rong LQ. Perioperative management of direct oral anticoagulants in cardiac surgery: practice recommendations based on current evidence. *J Cardiothorac Vasc Anesth*. 2022;36(11):4141-4149.

Crowley J, Cronin B, Essandoh M, D'Alessandro D, Shelton K, Dalia AA. Transesophageal echocardiography for Impella placement and management. *J Cardiothorac Vasc Anesth*. 2019;33(10):2663-2668.

Dhruva SS, Ross JS, Mortazavi BJ, et al. Use of mechanical circulatory support devices among patients with acute myocardial infarction complicated by cardiogenic shock. *JAMA Netw Open*. 2021;4(2):e2037748.

Engelman DT, Ali WB, Williams JB, et al. Guidelines for perioperative care in cardiac surgery: enhanced recovery after surgery society recommendations. *JAMA Surg*. 2019;154(8):755-766.

Gravlee GP, Davis RF, Kurusz M, et al., eds. *Cardiopulmonary Bypass.* 2nd ed. Lippincott Williams & Wilkins; 2000.

Gravlee GP, Shaw AS, Bartels K, eds. *Hensley's Practical Approach to Cardiothoracic Anesthesia.* 6th ed. Lippincott Williams & Wilkins; 2018.

Gregory SH, Sodhi N, Zoller JK, et al. Anesthetic considerations for the transcatheter management of mitral valve disease. *J Cardiothorac Vasc Anesth.* 2019;33(3):796–807.

Hahn RT, Abraham T, Adams MS, et al. Guidelines for performing a comprehensive transesophageal echocardiographic examination: recommendations from the American Society of Echocardiography and the Society of Cardiovascular Anesthesiologists. *J Am Soc Echocardiogr.* 2013;26(9):921–964.

Kaplan JA, Augoustides JG, Gutsche JT, et al., eds. *Kaplan's Cardiac Anesthesia.* 8th ed. Elsevier; 2023.

Konstadt S, Shernan S, Oka Y. *Clinical Transesophageal Echocardiography: A Problem-Oriented Approach.* 2nd ed. Lippincott Williams & Wilkins; 2003.

Koster A, Faraoni D, Levy JH. Antifibrinolytic therapy for cardiac surgery: an update. *Anesthesiology.* 2015;123(1):214–221.

Lewis C, Parulkar SD, Bebawy J, Sherwani S, Hogue CW. Cerebral neuromonitoring during cardiac surgery: a critical appraisal with an emphasis on near-infrared spectroscopy. *J Cardiothorac Vasc Anesth.* 2018;32(5):2313–2322.

Mazzeffi MA, Rao VK, Dodd-O J, et al. Intraoperative management of adult patients on extracorporeal membrane oxygenation: an expert consensus statement from the Society of Cardiovascular Anesthesiologists-Part I, technical aspects of extracorporeal membrane oxygenation. *Anesth Analg.* 2021;133(6):1459–1477.

Pishko AM, Cuker A. Heparin-induced thrombocytopenia and cardiovascular surgery. *Hematology Am Soc Hematol Educ Program.* 2021;2021(1):536–544.

Ram H, Gerlach RM, Conte AH, Ramzy D, Jaramillo-Huff AR, Gerstein NS. The AngioVac device and its anesthetic implications. *J Cardiothorac Vasc Anesth.* 2017;31(3):1091–1102.

Ravichandran AK, Baran DA, Stelling K, Cowger JA, Salerno CT. Outcomes with the tandem protek duo dual-lumen percutaneous right ventricular assist device. *ASAIO J.* 2018;64(4):570–572.

Salter BS, Gross CR, Weiner MM, et al. Temporary mechanical circulatory support devices: practical considerations for all stakeholders. *Nat Rev Cardiol.* 2023;20(4):263–277.

Schroder JN, Patel CB, DeVore AD, et al. Transplantation outcomes with donor hearts after circulatory death. *N Engl J Med.* 2023;388(23):2121–2131.

Shore-Lesserson L, Baker RA, Ferraris VA, et al. The Society of Thoracic Surgeons, The Society of Cardiovascular Anesthesiologists, and The American Society of ExtraCorporeal Technology: clinical practice guidelines-anticoagulation during cardiopulmonary bypass. *Ann Thorac Surg.* 2018;105(2):650–662.

Thiele H, Kurz T, Feistritzer HJ, et al; SOLVE-TAVI Investigators. General versus local anesthesia with conscious sedation in transcatheter aortic valve implantation: the randomized SOLVE-TAVI trial. *Circulation.* 2020;142(15):1437–1447.

Tibi P, McClure RS, Huang J, et al. STS/SCA/AmSECT/SABM update to the clinical practice guidelines on patient blood management. *J Cardiothorac Vasc Anesth.* 2021;35(9):2569–2591.

Varshney AS, DeFilippis EM, Cowger JA, Netuka I, Pinney SP, Givertz MM. Trends and outcomes of left ventricular assist device therapy: JACC focus seminar. *J Am Coll Cardiol.* 2022;79(11):1092–1107.

Anesthesia for Head and Neck Surgery

Victoria Bass and Jeremy Goldfarb

I. ANESTHESIA FOR OPHTHALMIC SURGERY

A. General Considerations

1. **Intraocular pressure** (IOP; normal range 10 to 22 mm Hg) is principally determined by (1) aqueous volume (the rate of production of aqueous humor in relation to its rate of drainage) and (2) the blood volume within vessels of the eye. Owing to scleral inelasticity, small changes in volume result in large changes in IOP.
   a. **Factors that may increase IOP** include hypertension, hypercarbia, hypoxia, laryngoscopy and endotracheal intubation, venous congestion, vomiting, coughing, straining, bucking, external pressure on the eye, and ketamine.
   b. **Factors that may decrease IOP** include hypocarbia, hypothermia, central nervous system (CNS) depressants, ganglionic blockers, most volatile and intravenous (IV) anesthetics, nondepolarizing neuromuscular blockade (NMB), mannitol, diuretics, acetazolamide, and head elevation.

2. **Glaucoma**
   a. **Open-angle glaucoma** usually arises from chronic obstruction of the aqueous humor drainage and is characterized by a progressive, insidious course that may *be painless*.
   b. **Closed-angle glaucoma** results from acute aqueous outflow obstruction due to a narrowing of the anterior chamber. This occurs as a result of pupillary dilation or lens edema and is *painful*.

3. **Oculocardiac reflex**
   a. The oculocardiac reflex (OCR) is mediated by afferent impulses via the ophthalmic branch (cranial nerve [CN] VI) of the trigeminal nerve and efferent from the vagus nerve (CN X). Increases in IOP, manipulation of the globe, or traction on the extrinsic eye muscles may result in bradycardia, atrioventricular block, ventricular ectopy, or asystole. Administration of ocular regional anesthesia may also elicit this response.
   b. The OCR should be promptly treated by cessation of the stimulus. Atropine (0.01 to 0.02 mg/kg IV) may be administered if bradyarrhythmias persist. The reflex fatigues quickly with repeated stimulation. However, if the reflex persists, infiltration of local anesthetic near the extrinsic eye muscles or placement of a peribulbar or retrobulbar block is effective. Alternatively, pretreatment with atropine or glycopyrrolate can be helpful in preventing the reflex.

4. **Commonly used drugs**
   a. **Topical.** Most ophthalmic medications are highly concentrated solutions that are administered topically and may produce systemic effects.
      1. **Mydriatics**
         a. **Phenylephrine** eye drops may cause hypertension and reflex bradycardia, especially when administered as a 10% solution.

For this reason, a 2.5% solution is commonly used. It dilates the pupil and constricts periocular blood vessels.
- b. **Cyclopentolate, atropine, and scopolamine** are anticholinergic agents that can produce CNS toxicity (eg, confusion seizures), particularly in the elderly and young. Additional effects include flushing, thirst, dry skin, and tachycardia.
- c. **Epinephrine** 2% topical solution reduces IOP in open-angle glaucoma by decreasing aqueous secretion while improving outflow. Complications can include hypertension, tachycardia, dysrhythmias, and syncope.
2. **Miotics.** Cholinergic drugs (eg, pilocarpine 0.25% to 4% solution) may produce bradycardia, salivation, bronchorrhea, and diaphoresis.
3. **Drugs that decrease IOP**
    - a. **β-Adrenergic antagonists** (eg, timolol or betaxolol) may cause bradycardia, hypotension, congestive heart failure, and bronchospasm.
    - b. **Anticholinesterases**, such as echothiophate, depress plasma cholinesterase activity for 2 to 4 weeks and may prolong recovery from succinylcholine.
- b. **Systemic**
    1. **Acetazolamide**, a carbonic anhydrase inhibitor, is administered systemically to decrease aqueous humor secretion, thus lowering IOP. Chronic use can lead to the development of hyponatremia, hypokalemia, and metabolic acidosis.

B. Anesthetic management
1. **Preoperative evaluation.** Preoperative assessment should include evaluation of comorbid conditions and chronically administered medications (oral and ophthalmic). Tests are indicated only in patients with severe new or acutely exacerbated medical problems. Routine testing before cataract surgery has not been shown to impact outcomes.
2. **Avoidance of coughing, sudden movement, or straining is essential.** Unexpected patient or eye movements during delicate microscopic intraocular surgery can lead to increased IOP, choroidal hemorrhage, expulsion of vitreous material, or loss of vision.
3. **Regional anesthesia**
    - a. **Ophthalmic procedures** such as cataract extraction, corneal transplant, anterior chamber irrigation, oculoplastic procedures, and even vitreoretinal procedures lasting 3 to 4 hours can be performed under regional anesthesia and light sedation.
    - **b.** Patient cooperation and lack of head motion are important for the success of this technique. Patients who are unable to participate owing to extremes of age, impaired hearing, psychiatric illness, language barrier, inability to tolerate supine position or maintain a relatively motionless position may not be candidates for regional anesthesia for delicate eye surgery.
    - c. Advantages of regional anesthesia include a lower incidence of coughing, straining, and emesis on emergence, reliable postoperative analgesia, lower perioperative morbidity, and earlier discharge compared with general anesthesia (GA).
    - d. **IV sedation** may be used perioperatively. Midazolam (0.25 to 2 mg IV), fentanyl (10 to 50 μg IV), or remifentanil (0.25 to 1 μg/kg IV) can be administered just before the regional injection. Patients should have standard ASA monitors during regional block placement and receive supplemental oxygen if indicated.

e. **Technique.** Intraocular surgery requires adequate sensory and motor block of the eye and often the eyelids as well. Anesthesia of the eye is accomplished by injecting local anesthetic into the retrobulbar space, peribulbar space, or episcleral space, facilitating neural blockade of CNs II through VI.

f. **Retrobulbar block** is achieved by injecting 4 to 6 mL of a 50:50 mixture of 1% lidocaine and 0.375% bupivacaine (with 5 units hyaluronidase) within the muscle cone formed by the four recti muscles and the two oblique muscles. With the eye in a neutral position, a 23- or 25-gauge blunt Atkinson 1¼-inch needle is inserted through the lower lid or conjunctiva at the level of the inferior orbital rim in the inferotemporal quadrant. The needle is first advanced slightly inferiorly and temporally approximately 1.5 cm; once past the equator of the eye, the needle is then directed superiorly and nasally toward the apex of the orbit to a depth of approximately 3.5 cm, while feeling for a "pop" as the needle penetrates through the muscle cone (**Figure 30.1**). The retrobulbar block provides faster, more reliable anesthesia and akinesia but has a higher complication rate as compared with the peribulbar block (see section that follows.)

g. **Peribulbar block.** A shorter, 25-gauge ¾-inch Atkinson needle is advanced along the inferior orbital floor to a depth of approximately 2.5 cm. Between 5 and 7 mL of local anesthetic with hyaluronidase are administered *adjacent* to the muscle cone. Careful aspiration before injection is required for both blocks, followed by gentle massage or orbital compression to promote the spread of the anesthetic (although orbital compression should be avoided in patients with

FIGURE 30.1 Retrobulbar and peribulbar blocks.

glaucoma). If desired, the facial nerve can also be blocked by infiltrating 2 to 4 mL of additional local anesthetic along the inferior and superior orbital rim to help prevent squinting.
- h. **Episcleral block (sub-Tenon block).** This block can be administered by the surgeon after the eye has been prepped. A blunt cannula is inserted through a small incision in the conjunctiva and episcleral membrane, also known as the Tenon capsule, with subsequent deposition of local anesthetic. The episcleral block has a rapid onset, but the extent of akinesia is variable and proportional to the volume of local anesthetic injected. Serious complications are rare.
- i. **Complications of regional anesthesia** are infrequent but include direct optic nerve trauma, transient globe compression with increased IOP, retrobulbar hemorrhage, globe perforation, and stimulation of the OCR. Hyaluronidase is toxic to the eye if injected into the globe. Intravascular injection of local anesthetic may cause seizures or myocardial depression. Rarely, the local anesthetic may dissect proximally along the neural sheath of the optic nerve and a total spinal can occur; treatment is supportive.
- j. During the procedure, supplemental air may be provided to the patient. This helps to remove exhaled carbon dioxide and to offset the sense of claustrophobia some patients may experience. Oxygen may be used if indicated, but the surgeon should be notified not to use electrocautery while oxygen is flowing. Capnography is frequently used since visual inspection of respiration may be difficult while patients are draped.

4. **General anesthesia**
   - a. Goals include (1) a smooth induction and maintenance of stable IOP, (2) avoidance and treatment of OCR, (3) maintenance of a motionless field with sufficient depth of anesthesia with or without NMB since the eye is highly innervated, (4) avoidance of postoperative nausea and vomiting (PONV), and (5) a smooth emergence.
   - b. **Smooth emergence and extubation** are particularly desirable after ophthalmic surgery. This may be facilitated by thorough posterior pharyngeal suctioning while the patient is still deeply anesthetized, administration of an opioid to reduce the cough reflex, and IV lidocaine or dexmedetomidine before planned extubation. Deep extubation is also an option but does not guarantee a smooth emergence.
   - c. **Ketamine** can cause blepharospasm, nystagmus, and vomiting. For these reasons, ketamine may be a poor choice for most ophthalmic surgeries.

C. Ophthalmic procedures
1. **Open-eye injury.** Penetrating eye trauma may be a surgical emergency and needs to be addressed within 24 hours of injury to minimize the risk of infection. It requires a carefully conducted anesthetic designed to prevent aspiration and favorably affect IOP. A sudden increase in IOP can result in extrusion of ocular contents and cause permanent vision loss. Trauma to the eye and orbit often necessitates long-duration or complex surgery that is best suited for general endotracheal anesthesia.
   - a. Succinylcholine causes an increase in IOP of approximately 6 to 12 mm Hg for 10 minutes before returning to baseline. This has not been shown to be clinically significant and succinylcholine often is the drug of choice during a rapid sequence induction (RSI) in the eye surgery patient with a full stomach. Alternatively, 1.2 mg/kg of rocuronium can be used during an RSI.

b. An adequate depth of anesthesia and degree of NMB must be ensured before laryngoscopy and intubation to minimize increases in IOP (which may rise to 40 to 50 mm Hg) secondary to straining, coughing, and bucking.
   c. In children, if an IV cannot be placed, an inhalation induction along with cricoid pressure may be necessary.
2. **Strabismus repair** is a procedure to alter the lengths of the extraocular muscles.
   a. Surgical manipulation frequently elicits **the oculocardiac reflex** (see Section I.A.3).
   b. **PONV** is very common (40% to 85% incidence in untreated patients). Strategies to reduce the incidence of PONV include minimizing opioids, multimodal analgesia, combination of antiemetics with different mechanisms of action (ondansetron, dexamethasone, haloperidol, etc.), gastric decompression using orogastric tube (OGT), ensuring adequate hydration, and possible total intravenous anesthetic (TIVA).
3. **Retinal surgery for detachment and vitreous hemorrhage** often is performed on patients in extremes of age and/or with multiple comorbidities. Meticulous attention to airway management, fluid status, normothermia, and postoperative transport is crucial. Premature infants, especially those less than 60 weeks postconceptional age, are at risk for postoperative central apnea. They should demonstrate a 12-hour apnea-free interval before discharge.
   a. **Regional anesthesia** is suitable for short procedures (<3 hours) in cooperative patients, although unexpected movement during the delicate retinal repair may result in vision loss.
   b. An **intravitreal gas bubble** containing an inert, high–molecular-weight, low-diffusivity gas such as sodium hexafluoride (SF_6), perfluoropropane (C_3F_8), octofluorocyclobutane (C_4F_8), or air, may be injected at the conclusion of surgery to reduce intravitreal bleeding. Nitrous **oxide should be avoided** in surgeries where an intravitreal gas bubble is injected as it will rapidly expand the bubble and increase IOP. Because these gas bubbles remain for various periods of time, administration of nitrous oxide should be avoided for 5 days after an air injection, 3 to 4 weeks after SF_6 injection, and 6 to 8 weeks after C_3F_8 injection. *Owing to pressure changes associated with air travel, patients should be instructed to avoid air travel for up to 8 weeks after intravitreal gas injection.*

II. ANESTHESIA FOR OTORHINOLARYNGOLOGIC PROCEDURES
A. General considerations
1. **Airway.** The airway during otorhinolaryngologic (ORL) procedures is often shared with the surgeon. Pathology, scarring from previous surgery or irradiation, congenital deformities, trauma, or manipulation can produce chronic or acute airway obstruction, bleeding, and a potentially difficult airway. Preoperative discussion with the surgeon and analysis of previous anesthetic records regarding perioperative airway management, endotracheal tube (ETT) size and position, patient positioning, and use of NMB is essential. The patient may require awake examination of the airway under sedation and topical anesthesia or an awake fiberoptic intubation (FOI) before induction of GA.
2. Patients presenting for ORL surgery may have a history of heavy smoking, alcohol abuse, obstructive sleep apnea (OSA), and chronic upper

respiratory tract infections. Preoperative testing should be dictated by medical comorbidities.
3. In addition to standard monitors, intra-arterial blood pressure and urine output monitoring may be needed for major surgeries with significant anticipated blood loss.
4. **Extubation** after any upper airway surgery requires careful planning. Extubation is performed once the throat packs are removed, the pharynx is suctioned, and full protective laryngeal reflexes return.

B. Ear surgery
1. **Preoperative considerations**
   a. Ear surgery often involves dissecting and preserving the **facial nerve (CN VII)**. The need for intraoperative nerve monitoring should be discussed with the surgeon in advance. Primary anesthetic concerns include patient positioning, facial nerve preservation, use or avoidance of nitrous oxide, adequate hemostasis, smooth emergence, and prevention of PONV.
   b. The **middle ear** communicates with the oropharynx via the eustachian tube. If eustachian tube patency is compromised by trauma, edema, inflammation, or congenital deformity, normal venting of middle ear pressure cannot occur. In this situation, a high concentration of nitrous oxide can increase middle ear pressure to 300 to 400 mm Hg in 30 minutes. Conversely, acute cessation of nitrous oxide can result in rapid resorption and a net negative pressure in the middle ear. These changes may result in alteration of middle ear anatomy, rupture of tympanic membrane, disarticulation of artificial stapes, disruption of surgical grafts, and PONV.
   c. **Positioning.** During surgery, the patient's head often is elevated and turned to the side. Extremes of head position should be assessed preoperatively to determine limits of range of motion, especially in patients with arthritis or cerebrovascular disease. Furthermore, attention to adequate venous drainage is necessary with extremes of head position.
2. **Anesthetic technique.** Anesthesia is induced with a hypnotic and short-acting NMB by inhalation and can be maintained with a volatile anesthetic or TIVA. If used, nitrous oxide should be discontinued at least 30 minutes before placement of a tympanic membrane graft.
   a. Delicate microsurgery of the ear may require induced hypotension to minimize bleeding and optimize visualization of the surgical field. Volatile anesthetics, remifentanil, and α- or β-adrenergic antagonists work well to maintain mean arterial pressures of 60 to 70 mm Hg. Elevation of the head of the bed to approximately 15 degrees to decrease venous congestion and local application of epinephrine for vasoconstriction usually improve operating conditions.
   b. Myringotomy with tube placement is one of the most frequently performed outpatient pediatric surgeries. These procedures are short and can usually be performed under mask anesthesia with or without an IV placement. Deep anesthesia using volatile anesthetics alone or in combination with remifentanil can be used. If the procedure is performed without an IV line, intranasal fentanyl (1 to 2 µg/kg) and preoperative oral acetaminophen (10 to 15 mg/kg) can be used for postoperative pain management.

C. Nasal surgery
1. **Anesthetic technique.** Nasal surgery is often performed under GA, although local anesthesia can be considered for minor procedures or high-risk patients. The surgeon may apply topical cocaine to the nasal mucosa

with or without injection of lidocaine with epinephrine for vasoconstriction and hemostasis. These agents may cause tachycardia, hypertension, and arrhythmias. In a healthy adult, the cocaine dose should not exceed 1.5 mg/kg (each drop of a 4% solution contains about 3 mg of cocaine). Smaller doses should be used when administered with epinephrine or in patients with cardiovascular disease. GA may be needed to provide immobility, airway protection, or amnesia. Induced hypotension may be beneficial to facilitate endoscopic nasal surgery in particular.

2. After **nasal cosmetic surgery**, the nose is unstable, and application of a face mask is undesirable. Smooth emergence and extubation are important to decrease postoperative bleeding and to avoid laryngospasm and the need for positive-pressure ventilation by mask.

3. **Blood loss** during nasal surgery may be substantial and difficult to estimate. A throat pack may help decrease PONV by preventing passage of blood into the stomach. An OGT may be placed to evacuate the stomach of any swallowed blood.

4. Patients with **severe epistaxis** presenting for internal maxillary artery ligation or embolization often are anxious, hypertensive, tachycardic, and hypovolemic. They are assumed to have a full stomach containing blood, and induction of anesthesia and endotracheal intubation should be planned accordingly. Hypertension should be controlled to reduce blood loss. Posterior nasal packing, although helpful, can cause edema and hypoventilation. Because the extent of blood loss is difficult to assess, adequate IV access and blood for transfusion should be available. Removal of the posterior packing can be associated with substantial blood loss.

D. Upper airway surgery
1. **Tonsillectomy and adenoidectomy**
    a. **Preoperative evaluation** should seek a history of bleeding disorders, recent respiratory tract infection, and OSA. The STOPBANG questionnaire for OSA is a useful screening tool.
        1. Do you **snore** loudly at night?
        2. Do you feel **tired** during the day?
        3. Has anyone **observed** apnea?
        4. Do you have or are you being treated for high blood **pressure**?
        5. Is your **BMI** greater than 35?
        6. Is your **age** over 50?
        7. Is your **neck** circumference over 17 inches (male) or 16 inches (female)?
        8. Is your **gender** male?

        A score of 5 or greater is strongly predictive of OSA. Patients with OSA may be difficult to ventilate and intubate. Patients with diagnosed moderate-to-severe OSA (apnea–hypopnea index greater than 15 in adults and greater than 5 in children) by polysomnography or patients who screen positive with a STOPBANG score ≥5 are at increased risk for opiate-induced respiratory depression. They should be considered for prolonged observation in the postanesthesia care unit (PACU) or overnight admission to monitor for respiratory compromise.
    b. Most **children** receive an inhalation induction, followed by placement of an appropriately sized IV. Maintenance anesthetic with a volatile agent supplemented with an opioid (eg, morphine 0.05 to 0.1 mg/kg IV) is usually performed. Dexmedetomidine (0.5 to 1µg/kg) may be used to reduce opiate requirement and the risk of emergence agitation, especially in pediatric patients. NMB facilitates

intubation but is not mandatory. The ETT should be firmly secured at the midline of the mandible for surgical access.

   c. **At the end of surgery**, the throat pack is removed, an OGT is placed to empty the stomach of swallowed blood, and the pharynx is suctioned thoroughly. Administration of antiemetic agents should be considered. Extubation may be performed under deep anesthesia or when the patient is awake with intact airway reflexes. The use of an oropharyngeal airway after surgery can cause surgical wound disruption and bleeding if not carefully placed in the midline. Nasal airways are useful alternatives.

   d. Auscultate for unobstructed breathing before transport to the PACU and check for a dry pharynx before discharge.

2. Tonsillar rebleeding
   a. **Rebleeding** after a pediatric tonsillectomy occurs in approximately 5% of cases. Primary bleeds occur within 24 hours after surgery. Secondary bleeding is common 7 to 10 days postoperatively as the eschar sloughs. Hematemesis, tachycardia, frequent swallowing, pallor, and airway obstruction may be seen. The extent of blood loss is often underestimated because the blood is swallowed.
   b. **Post-tonsillectomy hemorrhage** is a surgical emergency, and induction of anesthesia in a bleeding, hypovolemic child can result in severe hypotension or cardiac arrest. Appropriate IV access is necessary, and the patient should be adequately resuscitated (with blood products if necessary) before reoperation. Hematocrit, coagulation studies, and availability of blood products should be ascertained. Doses of anesthetic agents may need to be reduced in the setting of hypovolemia.
   c. Because the stomach is full of blood, a **rapid-sequence induction** should be performed. Two working suctions and an additional styletted ETT one size smaller than anticipated should be available. The surgeon should be present. Extubation is safest with the patient awake.

3. **A tonsillar or parapharyngeal abscess** may present with trismus, dysphagia, and a distorted, compromised airway. The surgeon may be able to decompress the abscess with needle aspiration before the induction of anesthesia. If needed, an awake FOI may be performed. Anesthetic management and extubation procedures are similar to those for tonsillectomy (see Section II.D.1). In Ludwig angina, cellulitis of the submandibular and sublingual spaces may extend to the anterior compartments of the neck. Trismus, airway edema, and distorted anatomy often make visualization by direct laryngoscopy of the glottic opening difficult. Asleep intubation is contraindicated if stridor occurs at rest. *Awake FOI is the safest approach in this scenario.* If awake FOI is not possible, consider tracheostomy under local anesthesia to secure the airway.

4. **Cleft lip and palate (CLP) repair**
   a. A detailed preoperative evaluation is necessary as patients may have associated anomalies including cardiac or airway deformities.
   b. GA is required for CLP repair. An oral Ring-Adair-Elwyn (RAE) ETT is used and may become kinked or dislodged during placement of a throat pack.
   c. Prior to emergence, an OGT is used to evacuate the stomach of blood. The oropharynx is gently suctioned with soft tip catheter, while avoiding the newly repaired palate by advancing along the tongue.

d. Given concern for postoperative airway obstruction, multimodal analgesia is used to minimize opioid requirement, and the patient is extubated when fully awake. The surgeon may place a tongue stitch to allow forward tongue displacement if patient obstructs. Postoperative monitoring in the pediatric intensive care unit is required.
5. **Direct laryngoscopy** is indicated for diagnostic or therapeutic purposes and may involve potentially compromised airways. Preoperative nasal endoscopy and evaluation of imaging studies (magnetic resonance imaging or computed tomography) may help identify airway abnormalities and potential perioperative problems.
   a. **Anesthetic management** can be achieved using a TIVA or volatile gas. A TIVA is better suited for situations where the ETT may be intermittently removed. Remifentanil infusion (0.1 to 0.2 mcg/kg/min) acts to blunt the sympathetic response associated with manipulation of the larynx. NMB further prevents airway reflexes or coughing that could interfere with the surgical procedure. Placing the patient in suspension may cause an exaggerated vagal response resulting in sudden, severe bradycardia and cases of asystole have been reported. Glycopyrrolate may be given at the time of suspension to prevent this response. Oxygenation may occur through a small ETT (<6.0 mm), a jet ventilation catheter, or high-flow nasal cannula (HFNC), leaving the laryngeal structures exposed for surgical access and manipulation. The variable benefits and challenges of these approaches, as well as backup ventilation strategies, should be taken into consideration for each individual patient and procedure.
   b. **Postoperative airway edema** may develop. If anticipated, dexamethasone (4 to 10 mg IV) may be given. Additional treatment includes head elevation, humidified oxygen by mask, and nebulized racemic epinephrine. Occasionally, cessation of nebulized racemic epinephrine is associated with the return of airway edema.
6. **Laser use in ORL surgery.** Laser (light amplification by stimulated emission of radiation) produces a high-energy, high-density beam of coherent light that generates focused heat on contact with tissue. The emission media used to produce the monochromatic light determines the wavelength.
   a. **Short-wavelength (1-μm) laser** (argon gas, ruby, neodymium:yttrium aluminum garnet [Nd:YAG]) emissions in the red–green visible part of the electromagnetic spectrum are poorly absorbed by water but well absorbed by pigmented tissues such as the retina and blood vessels.
   b. **Infrared (10-μm) carbon dioxide laser** emissions are well absorbed by water and superficial surface cells and are commonly used to treat laryngeal lesions. They cannot be transmitted through fiberoptics.
   c. **Eyes must be protected** from the laser beam. Operating room personnel must wear appropriate safety goggles (green tinted for argon, amber for Nd:YAG, and clear for carbon dioxide). The patient's eyes should be taped closed and covered with safety goggles.
   d. **The most serious complication of laser airway surgery is airway fire.** The likelihood of fire depends on the gas environment of the airway, the energy level of the laser, the way the laser is used, the presence of moisture, and the type of ETT used. A safe gas mixture during laser upper airway surgery has an FiO_2 <30%. Nitrous oxide supports combustion and should be avoided.

e. **Safe laser use.** Lasers should be used intermittently, in the noncontinuous mode, and at moderate power (10 to 15 W). Surgeons should not use the laser as a cautery and should share responsibility for fire prevention by limiting the energy input, allowing time for heat dispersal, packing aside nontarget tissue and ETT cuffs with moist gauze, and maintaining moisture (as a heat sink) in the field.
f. **Airway options during laser surgery.** Specially designed, fire-resistant, impregnated, or shielded ETTs (eg, Xomed Laser-Shield II ETT) are used, and the cuff is filled with blue saline. The blue saline acts to identify laser injury to the ETT cuff and to flood the airway if ignition occurs. For some procedures, intubation is not possible because the surgeon requires free access to the surgical field. Options include the following:
   1. Jet-Venturi technique. This technique eliminates the need for an ETT, but airway fire may still occur owing to dry tissue igniting. All patients are at risk for barotrauma; pediatric patients and patients with chronic obstructive pulmonary disease are at the highest risk.
   2. HFNC may be used to provide passive oxygenation and a constant PEEP when apnea is required.
g. **If an airway fire occurs,** immediately remove the ETT, stop flow of airway gases, remove any flammable material from the airway, and pour saline into the airway. Once the fire is out, reestablish ventilation while avoiding oxidizer-enriched environment, examine the ETT for possible fragments left behind in the airway, and consider bronchoscopy. **Complications** include airway edema, inhalation injury, tracheal and laryngeal granulation tissue formation, and airway stenosis.
h. The **anesthetic goals for laser surgery** include adequate surgical exposure, fire prevention, and return of protective airway reflexes before extubation. Clear communication with the surgical team is essential. Endotracheal intubation, jet ventilation, or intermittent mask ventilation may be used. TIVA is used to maintain GA for open airway procedures. Because airway edema may occur, the patient is given humidified oxygen postoperatively and is observed closely in the PACU. Corticosteroids or aerosolized racemic epinephrine may be necessary.

III. ANESTHESIA FOR PROCEDURES OF THE NECK
A. General considerations
The primary anesthetic concerns during neck surgery are establishing and maintaining a secure airway, tissue preservation, and nerve monitoring.
1. An **armored ETT** may be necessary to prevent kinking.
2. An **elective tracheostomy** under local anesthesia may be performed before induction of GA for certain extensive procedures with anticipated difficult airway.

B. Radical neck dissection
1. **Patient condition.** These patients are often elderly, chronically debilitated, and malnourished and frequently have a history of tobacco and alcohol use. The severity of comorbidities will determine the extent of preoperative evaluation and choice of perioperative monitoring. Radical neck dissection in previously irradiated patients may be associated with large blood loss and a difficult airway.
2. **Anesthetic technique.** Airway management is of primary concern in this patient population, particularly if mass lesions exist. Awake FOI, rigid

fiberoptic scopes, video laryngoscope, or awake tracheostomy may be necessary for patients with compromised airways. Long-acting NMB is generally avoided to allow the surgeon to use a nerve stimulator. A 15- to 30-degree head-up tilt and mild hypotension (mean arterial pressure 60 to 70 mm Hg), facilitated by a volatile anesthetic, vasodilators, or remifentanil, may help reduce blood loss. However, prolonged, profound hypotension and anemia may increase the risk of end-organ damage.

3. Neck dissection often involves rotational flaps or free flaps. During dissection, traction or pressure on the carotid sinus can cause dysrhythmias such as bradycardia or asystole. Treatment is immediate cessation of the stimulus. If necessary, the surgeon can infiltrate local anesthetic near the sinus.
4. If airway compromise is anticipated postoperatively, the ETT is left in place, or an elective tracheostomy is performed.
5. Maintenance of normothermia and euvolemia and minimizing the use of vasoconstrictors are desirable during reconstructive flap transfer surgery. Intraoperative predictors of free flap compromise include significant medical comorbidity, administration of greater than 7 L of crystalloid, and prolonged operative time. Postoperatively, blood pressure should be adequate to maintain flap perfusion, but not so high that a hematoma develops.

C. Thyroid and parathyroid surgery
1. General endotracheal anesthesia is the most common technique. Approximately 40% of surgically associated recurrent laryngeal nerve (RLN) palsies are related to thyroid surgery. Use of a "nerve integrity monitor" ETT for intraoperative RLN monitoring may be considered (**Figure 30.2**). Succinylcholine is the agent of choice for intubation, and additional NMB should be avoided in the setting of RLN monitoring.
2. Injury to one RLN may cause unilateral vocal cord paralysis, leading to hoarseness, weak voice, and poor cough. Bilateral vocal cord paralysis usually leads to upper airway obstruction and stridor and requires reintubation and possible tracheostomy.
3. **Anesthetic technique.** Surgical manipulation near the trachea can be very stimulating, while postoperative pain may only be mild to moderate. Inhalational anesthetics, sometimes augmented with a remifentanil infusion, are commonly used to maintain an adequate plane of anesthesia and avoid the use of NMB.
4. **Bleeding** at the operative site after thyroid or parathyroid surgery may compress the trachea and cause acute airway obstruction. Opening the wound by placing a sterile hemostat through the incision allows egress of trapped blood. If this maneuver fails, the obstruction may be secondary to acute lymphedema and may necessitate immediate reintubation.

IV. ANESTHESIA FOR DENTISTRY AND ORAL AND MAXILLOFACIAL SURGERY
A. Anesthetic technique. Most dental and oral surgery procedures can be done under local anesthesia with or without sedation in the outpatient setting, whereas most maxillofacial surgeries require GA.
1. Patients requiring GA for dentistry may be young children, adults with severe phobias, or the developmentally or physically impaired; thus, they often require **premedication.** Oral or intranasal midazolam and intranasal dexmedetomidine can be given to cooperative patients. Intramuscular ketamine may be necessary for the agitated or uncooperative patient and can be combined with midazolam and

FIGURE 30.2 Intraoperative recurrent laryngeal nerve monitoring. **A,** Xomed NIM II endotracheal tube electrode (Medtronic Xomed). **B,** Proper intraluminal position of NIM II. NIM, nerve integrity monitor. (Redrawn from White WM, Randolph GW, Hartnick CJ, Cunningham MJ. Recurrent laryngeal nerve monitoring during thyroidectomy and related cervical procedures in the pediatric population. *Arch Otolaryngol Head Neck Surg.* 2009;135[1]:88–94.)

glycopyrrolate to combat undesirable psychological reactions and sialorrhea, respectively.

2. **Nasal intubation** is usually preferred; care must be taken not to damage the turbinates or adenoids. Prior to intubation, identification of the more patent nasal passage, topicalization of the nasal mucosa with oxymetazoline (Afrin), use of a lubricant, and warming/softening the ETT before insertion may help to reduce epistaxis. The ETT should be securely taped, pressure on the nasal septum avoided, and eyes protected and padded. *Nasal intubation is contraindicated in basilar skull fractures.*

3. A detailed airway evaluation and preoperative discussion with the surgeon are important. Patients with maxillomandibular skeletal anomalies, temporomandibular pathology, facial fractures, intermaxillary fixation, or trismus may require awake FOI and consideration for elective tracheostomy if difficult airway is anticipated.

4. If intermaxillary fixation with wires is present, the ETT is removed only when the patient is awake, edema has subsided, and bleeding is controlled. Administration of an antiemetic and decompression of the stomach with a nasogastric tube before extubation are recommended.

Wire cutters are kept at the bedside should emergent access to the mouth be necessary. The oropharynx should be suctioned before extubation and before the jaw is wired.
- B. **Hypotensive anesthesia.** Bleeding may be significant for orthognathic surgery and other major maxillofacial surgeries. Hypotensive anesthesia (mean arterial pressure 60 to 70 mm Hg) may reduce blood loss, improve operative field, and can be facilitated by volatile anesthetics, α- and β-adrenergic blockers, vasodilators, potent opioid infusion, and head elevation. Meticulous monitoring (blood pressure with possible arterial line, estimated blood loss, and urine output) is essential to ensure adequate perfusion to all vital organs. The overall medical condition of the patient, such as poorly controlled hypertension, ischemic heart disease, carotid artery stenosis, and hepatic or renal disease, may preclude the use of controlled hypotension.

Suggested Readings

Barak M, Yoav L, El-Naaj IA. Hypotensive anesthesia versus normotensive anesthesia during major maxillofacial surgery: a review of the literature. *Scientific World Journal.* 2015;2015:480728.

Choi WS, Samman N. Risks and benefits of deliberate hypotension in anaesthesia: a systematic review. *Int J Oral Maxillofac Surg.* 2008;37(8):687–703.

Chung F, Subramanyam R, Liao P, Sasaki E, Shapiro C, Sun Y. High STOP-Bang score indicates a high probability of obstructive sleep apnoea. *Br J Anaesth.* 2012;108(5):768–775.

Doyle DJ. Anesthesia for ear, nose, and throat surgery. In: Miller RD, ed. *Anesthesia.* 8th ed. Elsevier Saunders; 2015:2523–2549.

Feldman MA. Anesthesia for eye surgery. In: Miller RD, ed. *Anesthesia.* 8th ed. Elsevier Saunders; 2015:2512–2522.

Ghazal EA, Vadi MG, Coté CJ, et al. Preoperative evaluation, premedication, and induction of anesthesia. In: Coté CJ, Lerman J, Andereson BJ, et al., eds. *A Practice of Anesthesia for Infants and Children.* 6th ed. Elsevier; 2019:35–68.

Litman RS. Anesthesia for pediatric ophthalmologic surgery. In: Litman RS, ed. *Pediatric Anesthesia the Requisite in Anesthesiology.* Elsevier Mosby; 2004:267–274.

Litman RS, Samadi DS, Tobias JD. Anesthesia for pediatric ENT surgery. In: Litman RS, ed. *Pediatric Anesthesia the Requisite in Anesthesiology.* Elsevier Mosby; 2004:236–251.

McGoldrick KE, ed. *Anesthesia for Ophthalmic and Otolaryngologic Surgery.* WB Saunders; 1992.

Modest VE, Alfille PH. Anesthesia for laser surgery. In: Miller RD, ed. *Anesthesia.* 8th ed. Elsevier Saunders; 2015:2598–2611.

Pattani KM, Byrne P, Boahene K, Richmon J. What makes a good flap go bad? A critical analysis of the literature of intraoperative factors related to free flap failure. *Laryngoscope.* 2010;120(4):717–723.

Philips MB, Bendel RE, Crook JE, Diehl NN. Global health implications of preanesthesia medical examination for ophthalmic surgery. *Anesthesiology.* 2013;118(5):1038–1045.

Raafat SH, Brown KA, Verghese ST. Otorhinolaryngologic procedures. In Coté CJ, Lerman J, Anderson BJ, eds. *A Practice of Anesthesia for Infants and Children.* 6th ed. Elsevier; 2019:754–789.

Ragab SM, Hassanin MZ. Optimizing the surgical field in pediatric functional endoscopic sinus surgery: a new evidence-based approach. *Otolaryngol Head Neck Surg.* 2010;142(1):48–54.

Somerville N, Fenlon S. Anaesthesia for cleft lip and palate surgery. *Cont Educ Anaesth Crit Care Pain.* 2005;5:76–79.

Supkis DE, Dougherty TB, Nguyen DT, Cagle CK. Anesthetic management of the patient undergoing head and neck cancer surgery. *Int Anesthesiol Clin.* 1998;36(3):21–29.

Tobin JR, Weaver RG. Ophthalmology. In: Coté CJ, Lerman J, Anderson BJ, eds. *A Practice of Anesthesia for Infants and Children.* 6th ed. Elsevier; 2019:790–803.

Troll GF. Regional ophthalmic anesthesia: safe techniques and avoidance of complications. *J Clin Anesth.* 1995;7(2):163–172.

31 Anesthesia for Urologic Surgery
Lauren Peck and Daniel Ellis

I. ANESTHESIA FOR SPECIFIC UROLOGIC PROCEDURES

A. Cystoscopy and ureteroscopy are performed to diagnose and treat lesions of the lower (urethra, prostate, and bladder) and upper (ureter and kidney) urinary tracts.

1. Warmed irrigation fluids are used to improve visualization and to remove blood, tissue, and stone fragments.
   a. **Electrolyte solutions** (normal saline and lactated Ringer) are isotonic and do not cause hemolysis upon intravascular absorption. Because of ionization, normal saline and lactated Ringer cannot safely be used for procedures involving monopolar electrocautery. However, these solutions can be used with bipolar electrocautery. **Sterile water** creates optimal conditions for visibility and is nonconductive. However, intravascular absorption of sterile water may cause hemolysis and hyponatremia/hypoosmolality. **Nonelectrolyte solutions** such as glycine, sorbitol, and mannitol have good visibility and are nonconductive. Near-isotonicity also minimizes hemolysis. However, large volume absorption of glycine, sorbitol, and mannitol may cause hyponatremia (see section on transurethral resection of the prostate (TURP) syndrome that follows).

2. Anesthesia
   a. Depending on the patient and procedure, anesthesia for cystoscopy/ureteroscopy can range from topical lubrication to monitored anesthesia care (MAC), regional, and/or general anesthesia (GA). Placement of a rigid cystoscope (particularly in males) and distention of the bladder and ureters can be quite stimulating.
   b. To minimize sedation following the procedure, we recommend considering opioid-sparing pain medication regimens such as dexmedetomidine, acetaminophen, and NSAIDs (avoid in CKD).
   c. If regional anesthesia is used, a T6 level of anesthesia is required for upper tract instrumentation while a T10 level of anesthesia is adequate for lower tract surgery.
   d. GA can be effective with short-acting intravenous (IV) and inhaled anesthetics. Transient muscle relaxation may be required during general anesthesia.
   e. Lithotomy positioning is most common to facilitate surgical exposure.

B. Transurethral resection of a bladder tumor (TURBT) is performed to diagnose and treat lesions of the bladder. Anesthetic considerations are similar to TURP (see section that follows). Muscle relaxation should be considered as inadvertent stimulation of the obturator nerve, deep to the lateral bladder wall, which may result in leg adduction and risk damage to the bladder. In addition, chemotherapy instillation during TURBT for bladder cancer may impact operating room cleaning and scheduling of anesthetists.

C. Transurethral resection of the prostate (TURP) is performed to relieve urinary obstruction from benign prostatic hypertrophy (BPH). This procedure uses a modified cystoscope (resectoscope) with a wire connected to an electrocautery unit for resection of tissue and coagulation of bleeding vessels. Alternatives to TURP include medical management (α-blockers and hormonal therapies) and minimally invasive techniques such as laser ablation, microwave thermotherapy, and prostatic stents.

1. During a TURP, large prostatic venous sinuses can be opened allowing irrigant to be absorbed. The quantity of fluid absorbed depends on the following:
   a. Hydrostatic pressure related to the height of the irrigant above the patient.
   b. Surgical technique: duration of time the sinuses are exposed, rate of irrigant flow, and the size of cystoscope utilized.
   c. Number and size of venous sinuses opened during an operation (this is influenced by the prostate size).
   d. Peripheral venous pressure (lower pressure increases absorption).
2. Anesthesia
   a. If GA is used, it is essential to prevent coughing or movement as coughing and movement may increase the risk of bleeding or bladder/prostatic capsule perforation. Positive-pressure ventilation may decrease irrigant absorption by raising venous pressure.
   b. Regional anesthesia may create an atonic bladder (improved surgical visualization) and eliminate bladder spasms (more rapid postoperative hemostasis). Awake patients may also report symptoms that allow earlier detection of TURP syndrome (see below) or bladder perforation.
   c. Spinal anesthesia can be achieved with an iso- or hyperbaric solution of local anesthetic with or without opioid. A T10 sensory level of anesthesia is recommended to counteract pain from bladder distention. Lower venous pressures associated with neuraxial blockade may reduce bleeding but may increase irrigant absorption.
   d. Methods for monitoring intraoperative fluid absorption may include volumetric fluid balance, gravimetric weighing, and measurement of exhaled ethanol when a known amount of ethanol is added to the irrigating fluid.
3. **Complications**
   a. **TURP syndrome** is a collection of neurologic and cardiovascular signs and symptoms caused by excessive irrigant absorption. It may appear early (direct intravascular absorption) or after several hours (absorption from retroperitoneal and perivesicular spaces).
      1. **Central nervous system** symptoms include nausea, agitation, confusion, visual changes, seizures, and coma. These symptoms are likely multifactorial and have been attributed to hyponatremia/hypoosmolality with accompanying cerebral edema, hyperglycinemia, and hyperammonemia (glycine is hepatically metabolized to ammonia).
      2. **Cardiovascular** symptoms include hypertension or hypotension, bradycardia, dysrhythmias, pulmonary edema, and cardiac arrest likely secondary to pronounced fluid shifts and associated electrolyte disturbances. Hypervolemia initially occurs with fluid absorption followed by rapid redistribution of the irrigant to the interstitium.
      3. **Treatment involves** notifying the surgeon, completing the procedure as quickly as possible, and maintaining hemodynamic stability. There is disagreement in the literature about the most appropriate therapy. Fluid restriction and diuresis with furosemide

have been advocated to treat volume overload, and hypertonic saline is reserved for severe symptoms or severe hyponatremia (serum sodium <120 mmol/L). Others suggest that the diuretic strategy may exacerbate intravascular volume depletion and hyponatremia and recommend early use of hypertonic saline and reserving diuresis for acute pulmonary edema. Any therapy should be guided by regular measurements of serum sodium and osmolality.

b. **Bladder perforation** is a serious complication of a TURP procedure. Muscle relaxation with an adequate level of anesthesia, neuromuscular blockade, and/or spinal anesthesia minimizes this risk.

1. Extraperitoneal perforation is more common and manifests as suprapubic fullness, abdominal spasm, or pain in the suprapubic, inguinal, or periumbilical regions.
2. Intraperitoneal perforation presents as upper abdominal pain or referred pain from the diaphragm to the shoulder. This may result in hypertension, tachycardia, and abdominal distention followed by hypotension and cardiovascular collapse.

c. **Bacteremia** may occur due to absorption of bacteria through prostatic venous sinuses and is commonly associated with indwelling urinary catheters or with subclinical/partially treated prostatitis.

d. **Blood loss and coagulopathy.** Assessing blood loss is extremely difficult during a TURP because of irrigant dilution. Continuous postoperative bleeding may result from surgical bleeding, dilutional thrombocytopenia, disseminated intravascular coagulation, or the release of fibrinolytic enzymes from the prostate. Hemodynamic responses to blood loss may be masked by hypervolemia from irrigant absorption.

D. **Laser resection of the prostate** is a clinical approach to treating BPH and has less perioperative morbidity. Hemostatic properties of a laser limit tissue penetration and create a practically bloodless field. This procedure is an alternative for seriously ill patients (TURP morbidity 18%) and patients on anticoagulants. Bladder irritation (transient), delayed gross hematuria, and transient dysuria are common complications. The procedure time is relatively short in duration. GA and regional anesthesia (subarachnoid or sacral canal block) may be safely performed.

1. The **holmium** (yttrium aluminum garnet [YAG]) laser is a 60- to 80-W high-power pulse laser with a wavelength = 2140 nm. The high absorption of this laser by water limits tissue penetration. It is used to enucleate the prostate. Holmium laser preserves the histologic architecture of the prostate and facilitates prostate cancer detection.
2. The **KTP** (potassium titanyl phosphate) is a 60- to 80-W high-power laser through a crystal with a wavelength = 532 nm. It is highly absorbed by oxyhemoglobin, potentially creating a bloodless field, and is poorly absorbed by water. It is used for the enucleation of the prostate in a procedure known as "photoselective vaporization of prostate" (PVP). PVP is as effective as TURPs (2- to 4-year follow-up) for relief of BPH symptoms and has less perioperative morbidity, postoperative bladder irrigation, catheterization time, incidence of sexual dysfunction, and hospital stay. A disadvantage is that it alters prostatic histology samples. It is also important to have muscle relaxation with either an adequate level of anesthesia, neuromuscular blockade, or spinal anesthesia during PVPs. In addition, fluid absorption occurs frequently during high-power laser vaporization which may lead to volume

overload. Caution should be used in patients who present with cardiopulmonary symptoms.
E. **Radical retropubic prostatectomy (RRP)** is the operative procedure for the treatment of prostate cancer. Prostatectomy is rarely done for BPH.
 1. **Anesthesia**
    a. **Open RRP** may be performed safely using general, general/epidural, epidural, or spinal anesthesia. Several small-scale prospective randomized trials compared general with epidural techniques and found modest benefits of epidural anesthesia in reducing operative blood loss, reducing postoperative pain, and hastening recovery of bowel function. Regardless of these results, experienced surgeons routinely perform prostatectomies using GA with minimal blood loss, well-controlled intraoperative and postoperative pain, and short hospital stays. Transverse abdominis plane (TAP) blocks and rectus sheath blocks are frequently used in opioid-sparing techniques.
    b. **Laparoscopic prostatectomies (LRPs)** are promoted for their minimal invasiveness and comparable clinical outcomes. Prospective, nonrandomized trials comparing LRP to RRP show no significant differences in postoperative pain score, amount of narcotics administered, length of hospital stay, readmission rates, or complication rates. Anesthetic considerations for LRP are similar to those for other laparoscopic procedures. Retroperitoneal insufflation of carbon dioxide may be associated with increased systemic absorption compared with intraperitoneal insufflation, although reports are conflicting.
    c. **Robotic-assisted retropubic prostatectomies (RARPs)** have become increasingly more common for decreased transfusion rates, faster return of urinary continence, and decreased erectile dysfunction when compared to open and LRPs. The anesthetic plan for an RARP is similar to the anesthetic plan for an LRP. GA with standard IV induction and tracheal intubation is required. As the patient's arms will be tucked while he is in the lithotomy position, many anesthetists advocate two IV lines with a noninvasive blood pressure cuff on each of the patient's arms. These redundancies help compensate for difficulties in assessing the patient's arms and measuring blood pressure intraoperatively. Notably, trocar advancement may unexpectedly invade large vessels or enter the stomach. Therefore, a preoperative blood bank sample and decompressing the stomach with an orogastric tube are recommended. Decompressing the stomach may also decrease ocular damage caused by gastric contents draining into a patients' eyes. Neuromuscular blockade is extremely important because any movement by the patient while the robot is docked may lead to serious complications. Patients are often placed in steep Trendelenburg position to facilitate surgical exposure of deep pelvic organs. Trendelenburg positioning increases intracranial and intraocular pressures and may also result in physical objects hitting the patient's face. Therefore, clinicians must monitor patients closely to prevent harm. Fluid management is also very important during robotic prostatectomies. Too much fluid is associated with an increased risk of postoperative anastomotic leak as well as increased risk of glottic and periocular edema during Trendelenburg position. However, restrictive fluid management may cause acute tubular necrosis and compartment syndrome due to hypotension in the lower extremities.

d. **Diagnostic dyes** may be used during the procedure to demonstrate the integrity of the reconstructed urinary tract.
   1. **Methylene blue** 1% (1 mL) bolus may impact blood pressure. It may also cause transient erroneous decreases in pulse oximetry readings (SaO_2) to as low as 65%, lasting 10 to 70 seconds.
   2. **Indigo carmine** 0.8% (5 mL) is an α-agonist and may cause hypertension.
e. **Complications** are generally related to blood loss, including hypothermia, anemia, and coagulopathy. Large-bore IV access is suggested. Two IV lines and two blood pressure cuffs are recommended (see previous section on RARP). Urine output measurements are interrupted during mobilization of the prostatic urethra. Venous sinuses can be exposed during surgery, which can increase blood loss and potentially lead to air emboli.

F. **Nephrectomy** is performed for neoplasm, transplantation, chronic infection, trauma, and severe cystic or calculous disease.
   1. Patients undergoing nephrectomy for renal cell carcinoma require preoperative staging. These tumors can be quite large, and if the tumor extends into the inferior vena cava (IVC) or right atrium, then two potential complications must be considered:
      a. **The tumor may partially or fully occlude the IVC** with poor venous return and hypotension.
      b. **Tumor fragments may embolize** the pulmonary circulation. Consequently, pulmonary artery catheterization and central venous access may be risky if catheter placement dislodges tumor into the IVC or right atrium. Transesophageal echocardiogram should be considered if there is high risk of tumor embolism. Cardiopulmonary bypass may be used to minimize the risk of pulmonary emboli intraoperatively.
   2. Patients undergoing nephrectomy for transitional cell carcinoma will likely undergo an associated complete ureteral resection.
   3. **Anesthesia**
      a. The patient is positioned supine for a transabdominal approach or in the lateral decubitus position for a retroperitoneal approach. In the lateral position, the kidney rest and table flexion are often used to improve exposure. Hypotension can be produced by the kidney rest position, likely due to IVC compression, or blood pooling in dependent extremities.
      b. A thoracoabdominal incision may be required for larger or upper-pole tumors.
      c. Combined general/epidural anesthesia can maximize postoperative analgesia with an upper abdominal or thoracoabdominal incision. TAP block can also be considered for adequate pain control.
      d. Large-bore IV access with or without arterial line placement is appropriate as blood loss can be impressive due to tumor size and vascularity.

G. **Cystectomy**
   1. **Simple and partial cystectomy** is the removal of all or part of the bladder. Adjacent organs and structures, including pelvic lymph nodes, are left intact.
   2. **Radical cystectomy** is performed for invasive bladder tumors. It frequently involves removal of other pelvic organs, such as the prostate or uterus. Patients with pelvic malignancies, neurogenic bladder dysfunction, chronic lower urinary tract obstruction, or postradiation bladder dysfunction may require an ileal or colonic urinary diverting procedure.

3. **Anesthesia**
   a. Large-bore IV access may be indicated as substantial blood loss may occur.
   b. Arterial or central venous access may be indicated as large volume shifts occur while the ureters are disconnected.
   c. GA with TAP catheters is now preferred over thoracic epidurals as TAP catheters tend to be associated with less incidence of postoperative hypotension.
   d. Alvimopan (Entereg) may be used to help prevent postop ileus in cystectomy patients. Caution should be used if patient have been on opioids/opiates for longer than 7 days prior to surgery due to the risk of potential cardiovascular complications.

H. **Orchidopexy, orchiectomy, and urogenital plastic surgery procedures** are performed to treat congenital deformities, neoplasms, and impotence. Patients with testicular torsion may require emergency reduction and orchidopexy to prevent ischemia.

I. **Renal transplantation** is performed for patients with end-stage renal disease. Recipients commonly have hypertension and/or diabetes mellitus and are at increased risk for coronary artery disease and congestive heart failure. Patients may present with electrolyte and acid–base abnormalities, anemia, and platelet dysfunction. Preoperative dialysis, if possible, can improve potassium and acid–base abnormalities. The anesthesia provider must also make sure that the patient receives the proper perioperative immunosuppressants.

1. **Anesthesia**
   a. IV access may be difficult, and IV placement in extremities with fistulas or shunts should be avoided. The benefits of additional invasive monitors (arterial or central venous lines) should be weighed against the risks of catheter-related complications in immunosuppressed patients.
   b. Patients may have delayed gastric emptying from diabetes, uremia, and preoperative opioids. Rapid sequence induction should be considered for patients receiving peritoneal dialysis or patients with autonomic neuropathy.
   c. Muscle relaxation is important and should be maintained until fascial planes are closed. Coughing may dislodge a transplanted kidney from its vascular anastomosis. While cisatracurium is the preferred neuromuscular blockade agent, rocuronium has also been used to facilitate relaxation. Sugammadex, however, has not yet been approved for patients with end-stage renal disease. Of note, remifentanil has been used as an adjunct to prevent coughing at the time of extubation.
   d. Graft function depends on adequate intravascular volume before and after vascular anastomosis to maintain perfusion to the transplanted kidney. Intravascular volume expanders include crystalloid, albumin, and mannitol.
   e. Intraoperative hypotension may compromise renal perfusion and should be treated promptly by addressing mechanical factors such as IVC compression or treating hypovolemia with additional volume. If pharmacologic support is necessary, phenylephrine boluses, phenylephrine infusions, or dopamine infusions may be considered. α-agonists such as phenylephrine were previously thought to decrease renal blood flow via vasoconstriction. However, α-agonists have been used successfully in these instances. In cases of marked acidemia, sodium bicarbonate may improve hemodynamics.

f. Urine output provides an immediate gauge of renal function, which may be affected by hypovolemia, acute rejection, or patency of the anastomoses. Both mannitol and furosemide may be requested by a surgeon to promote diuresis after anastomosis.

II. LITHOTRIPSY
A. Treatment of kidney stones ranges from open surgical procedures to less invasive approaches such as cystoscopy/ureteroscopy with mechanical stone extraction and/or laser lithotripsy.
   1. Anesthetic options include regional, MAC, and GA (laryngeal mask airway vs. endotracheal tube), depending on both patient and surgical factors.
B. Extracorporeal shockwave lithotripsy, a noninvasive technique, focuses on acoustic shock waves aimed at urinary stones. At interfaces between materials of differing density, such as between soft tissues and stones, reflections of these acoustic waves set up complex patterns of internal echoes resulting in stresses that cause stones to fracture. While early-generation lithotripters required patient immersion into water baths, current models allow positioning on an operating table, have smaller cutaneous "shock entry" zones, and are more precisely focused onto the stone with less energy dissipated on surrounding structures.
C. Percutaneous nephrolithotomy (PCNL) is the preferred procedure for treating large, firm, or resistant kidney stones. The procedure is completed by making a small incision overlying the kidney followed by fluoroscopic guidance of a lithotrite into the kidney to pulverize and suction out the stone.
D. Anesthesia
   1. The patient is generally positioned supine but may be prone depending on the precise location of the stone(s). Lithotomy position may be necessary for concurrent cystoscopy or stent placement.
   2. MAC is usually adequate with newer lithotripters. Other strategies include neuraxial blockade and GA. Paravertebral blocks and/or TAP blocks with or without catheter may be used to reduce pain during and after the procedure.
   3. Adequate IV hydration may aid passage of stone fragments.
   4. Absolute contraindications are pregnancy, untreated infections, bleeding diatheses, and abdominal pacemakers. Relative contraindications are pacemakers/implantable cardioverter defibrillator, abdominal aortic or renal artery aneurysms, orthopedic prostheses, and morbid obesity.
E. Complications
   1. Ureteral colic soon after the procedure may manifest as nausea, vomiting, or bradycardia.
   2. Hematuria is common and can be treated with hydration and diuretics.
   3. Cardiac dysrhythmias such as bradycardia, premature atrial contractions, and premature ventricular contractions can occur intraoperatively secondary to mechanical (shock wave) strains on the cardiac conduction system. If premature ventricular contractions are frequent or symptomatic, they may be minimized by synchronization of the shock waves to the cardiac cycle.
   4. Hypertension can reach extreme levels in patients who have autonomic dysreflexia.
   5. Renal (subcapsular) hematoma may result from collateral damage to renal vasculature, especially in hypertensive patients.
   6. Severe pulmonary or intestinal damage is rare and occurs if the shock waves are inadvertently applied to the lung or intestines, as may occur with a patient movement during treatment.

III. PATIENTS WITH SPINAL CORD PATHOLOGY

A. Spinal cord injury frequently causes urinary retention, which promotes urinary tract infections, nephrolithiasis, and vesicoureteric reflux. Although patients with a spinal cord injury may be unable to perceive pain below the spinal cord lesion, autonomic dysreflexia is a complication that can occur during a urologic procedure if completed solely under MAC.

B. Autonomic dysreflexia is manifested by an acute onset of sympathetic hyperreactivity to certain stimuli below the level of a spinal cord lesion. Autonomic dysreflexia usually occurs when spinal cord lesions exist at or above the T6–T7 level. The syndrome may appear at any time from a few months to many years after the injury.

1. Common findings include hypertension (potentially severe), headache, diaphoresis, flushing or pallor, and bradycardia.
2. Precipitants include visceral stimulation, most commonly bladder distention, although urinary tract infection, fecal impaction, uterine contraction, bowel distention, and other intra-abdominal and cutaneous stimuli have also been reported.
3. Pathophysiology is thought to involve disorganized connections between afferent neurons and sympathetic neurons below the level of the injury that lead to vasoconstriction and hypertension. The parasympathetic nervous system is unable to counteract this vasoconstriction resulting from the spinal cord injury.
4. Treatment of autonomic dysreflexia includes removal of the inciting stimulus, increasing anesthetic depth, and pharmacologic treatment of persistent hypertension with rapidly acting agents such as IV nitroglycerin or nitroprusside.
5. In the absence of GA, neuraxial blockade may prevent autonomic dysreflexia. Neuraxial anesthesia blocks both limbs of the reflex arc and prevents dysreflexia. However, preexisting spinal cord pathology may prevent an anesthesia provider from determining the exact level of spinal or epidural anesthesia.

ACKNOWLEDGMENT

We gratefully acknowledge the contributions of previous edition author, Jenny Zhao Cheng, as portions of those chapters have been retained in this revision.

Suggested Readings

Beig Zali S, Steinhorn R, Hu V, et al. A continuous transversus abdominis plane block decreases hospital length of stay compared to thoracic epidural analgesia after open radical cystectomy surgery: a retrospective study. *Anesth Pain Med.* 2024;14(1):e143354.

Biki B, Mascha E, Moriarty DC, Fitzpatrick JM, Sessler DI, Buggy DJ. Anesthetic technique for radical prostatectomy surgery affects cancer recurrence: a retrospective analysis. *Anesthesiology.* 2008;109(2):180–187.

Carron M, Andreatta G, Pesenti E, et al. Impact on grafted kidney function of rocuronium-sugammadex vs cisatracurium-neostigmine strategy for Neuromuscular Block Management. An Italian single-center, 2014–2017 retrospective cohort case-control study. *Perioper Med (Lond).* 2022;11(1):3.

Cho JM, Moon KT, Lee JH, Choi JD, Kang JY, Yoo TK. Open simple prostatectomy and robotic simple prostatectomy for large benign prostatic hyperplasia: comparison of safety and efficacy. *Prostate Int.* 2021;9(2):101–106.

Conacher ID, Soomro NA, Rix D. Anaesthesia for laparoscopic urological surgery. *Br J Anaesth.* 2004;93(6):859–864.

Domi R, Sula H, Ohri I, et al. Anesthetic challenges of patients with cardiac comorbidities undergoing major urologic surgery. *Int Arch Med.* 2014;7:17.

Ellis DB, Albrecht M. Anesthesia for robotic surgery. In: Gropper MA, ed. *Miller's Anesthesia.* 9th ed. Elsevier; 2020:2236–2250.

Hanson RA, Zornow MH, Coulin MJ, Brambrink AM. Laser resection of the prostate: implications for anesthesia. *Anesth Analg.* 2007;105(2):475–479.

Kim KS, Kim JS, Park SW. Study on the effects and safety of propofol anesthesia during cystoscopy. *Korean J Urol.* 2006;47(11):1230.

Koo CH, Chung SH, Kim BG, et al. Comparison between the effects of deep and moderate neuromuscular blockade during transurethral resection of bladder tumor on endoscopic surgical condition and recovery profile: a prospective, randomized, and controlled trial. *World J Urol.* 2019;37(2):359–365.

Krassioukov AV, Walter M. Autonomic dysreflexia in neuro-urological practice. *Handbook of Neurourology.* 2023;663–671.

Laksita TB, Soebadi MA, Wirjopranoto S, Hidayatullah F, Kloping YP, Rizaldi F. Local anesthetics versus systemic analgesics for reducing pain during Extracorporeal Shock Wave Lithotripsy (ESWL): a systematic review and meta-analysis. *Turk J Urol.* 2021;47(4):270–278.

Łaszkiewicz J, Krajewski W, Łuczak M, et al. Pain reduction methods during transurethral cystoscopy. *Contemp Oncol (Pozn).* 2021;25(2):80–87.

Ogan F, Raphael JE. TURP syndrome and relevant considerations during anaesthesia for monopolar transurethral resection of prostate. *Am J Clin Med.* 2022;10(1):17–20.

O'Malley CMN, Frumento RJ, Hardy MA, et al. A randomized, double-blind comparison of lactated Ringer's solution and 0.9% NaCl during renal transplantation. *Anesth Analg.* 2005;100(5):1518–1524.

Pirani F, Makhani SS, Kim FY, et al. Prospective randomized trial comparing the safety and clarity of water versus Saline Irrigant in ureteroscopy. *Eur Urol Focus.* 2021;7(4):850–856.

Scavonetto F, Yeoh TY, Umbreit EC, et al. Association between neuraxial analgesia, cancer progression, and mortality after radical prostatectomy: a large, retrospective matched cohort study. *Br J Anaesth.* 2014;113(suppl 1):i95–i102.

Schmid S, Jungwirth B. Anaesthesia for renal transplant surgery: an update. *Eur J Anaesthesiol.* 2012;29(12):552–558.

Sprung J, Scavonetto F, Yeoh TY, et al. Outcomes after radical prostatectomy for cancer: a comparison between general anesthesia and epidural anesthesia with fentanyl analgesia: a matched cohort study. *Anesth Analg.* 2014;119(4):859–866.

Whalley DG, Berrigan MJ. Anesthesia for radical prostatectomy, cystectomy, nephrectomy, pheochromocytoma, and laparoscopic procedures. *Anesthesiol Clin North Am.* 2000;18(4):899–917.

Anesthesia for Obstetrics and Gynecology

A. Taylor Thomas and Emily Naoum

I. MATERNAL PHYSIOLOGY IN PREGNANCY (TABLE 32.1)
A. Respiratory system
1. **Capillary engorgement of the mucosa** may occur throughout the respiratory tract, beginning early in the first trimester and increasing throughout pregnancy. Historically, a 6.0- to 6.5-mm (inner diameter) endotracheal tube has been recommended for intubation to decrease the possibility of airway trauma in the setting of increased tissue friability. However, the use of larger tubes may be possible in most patients if required. Fluid retention may lead to an enlarged tongue, explaining the increased prevalence of Mallampati class 3 and 4 airways in term parturients compared to the general population. In addition, the airway examination may evolve during the course of labor resulting in a further increase in airway class. Hypertensive disorders of pregnancy are associated with higher Mallampati class airways. Lastly, because of mucosal engorgement, nasotracheal intubation may cause epistaxis and is best avoided in pregnant women.
2. **Minute ventilation increases by 45%** to support the high oxygen requirements of the mother and fetus and is driven by a proportional increase in tidal volume. Pulmonary resistance is decreased by 50% to accommodate these changes. As pregnancy progresses, elevation of the diaphragm from the gravid uterus leads to a 20% decrease in **functional residual capacity** (FRC). The resultant decrease in oxygen reserve mandates adequate preoxygenation prior to induction of general anesthesia.

B. Cardiovascular system
1. **Cardiac output increases** progressively by 50% from the end of the second trimester to term. This increase is primarily due to increased stroke volume, with a small contribution from heart rate. A grade II systolic ejection murmur at the left sternal border is commonly heard due to stroke volume augmentation in response to increased intravascular volume. During labor, contractions of the engorged uterus provide a 300- to 500-mL autotransfusion into the maternal circulation, further increasing cardiac output. Cardiac output is highest immediately postpartum, increasing 80% to 100% above prelabor values due to further autotransfusion from the placenta and loss of inferior vena cava (IVC) compression by the fetus. Despite this, blood pressure is not elevated at term due to decreased peripheral vascular resistance.
2. **Supine hypotension** may occur after 20 weeks of gestation when the gravid uterus compresses the IVC of the patient in the supine position. This decreases venous return, resulting in maternal hypotension and decreased uteroplacental blood flow. Left uterine displacement of at least 15 degrees may mitigate this problem.

C. Hematology
1. **Blood volume increases** markedly throughout pregnancy. Because plasma volume increases (up to 50% by 34 weeks of gestation) more than red cell mass, a relative **dilutional anemia** occurs.

Table 32.1 Physiologic Changes Associated With Pregnancy

System	Parameter Changes	Anesthetic Implications
Respiratory	*Anatomy* Upper airway edema Mucosal capillary dilation Enlarged tongue and epiglottis *Capacities/volume* ↑ Tidal volume by 45% ↑ Inspiratory reserve volume by 5% ↔ Vital capacity ↔ Closing capacity ↓ Total lung capacity by 5% ↓ Functional residual capacity by 20% ↓ Expiratory reserve volume by 20% ↓ Residual volume by 15% *Mechanics* ↑ Minute ventilation by 45% ↑ Alveolar ventilation by 45% ↔ FEV_1 ↔ FEV_1/FVC *Blood gases* ↑ Pa_{O_2} by 5–10% (100–105 mm Hg [13.3–14.0 kPa]) ↔ pH ↓ Pa_{CO_2} by 10% (28–32 mm Hg [3.7–4.2 kPa]) ↓ HCO_3 (18–22 mEq/L) *Oxygen consumption* ↑ Oxygen consumption by 20% ↑ P50 at term to 30 mm Hg	↑ risk of epistaxis ↑ risk of difficult laryngoscopy and intubation Rapid desaturation Risk of hypoxemia in the supine or Trendelenburg position ↓ time to onset of volatile anesthetics
Cardiovascular	↑ Cardiac output by 50% ↑ Stroke volume by 25% ↑ Heart rate by 20–25% ↓ Systematic vascular resistance by 20% Aortocaval compression may lead to supine hypotension syndrome	↑ risk of arrhythmia, most notably AF, pSVT, and pVT Blood loss may be more difficult to estimate Left uterine tilt after 20 wk of gestation

(*continued*)

Table 32.1 Physiologic Changes Associated With Pregnancy (*continued*)

System	Parameter Changes	Anesthetic Implications
Hematology	↑ Blood volume by 45% ↑ Plasma volume by 55% ↑ Red blood cell volume by 25% *Coagulation factors* ↑ Factors VII, VIII, IX, X, XII, fibrinogen ↔ Prothrombin ↔ or ↓ Platelet count ↓ Factors XI, XIII ↓ Total protein (albumin, globulin)	↑ risk of VTE ↓ pseudocholinesterase activity rarely causes prolongation of muscle relaxant activity ↓ protein binding ↑ volume of distribution
Central nervous system	↓ MAC Epidural venous engorgement ↑ CSF pressure	↓ Local anesthetic requirement ↑ Risk of PDPH with accidental dural puncture
Gastrointestinal	Cephalad mechanical displacement of stomach ↓ Gastric emptying during labor (to 18 h postpartum) ↓ Lower esophageal sphincter pressure	↑ risk of aspiration Rapid sequence induction in latter half of second and third trimesters
Hepatic	↑ AST, ALT, LDH, bilirubin ↑ Alkaline phosphatase ↑ Gallbladder volume and ↓ motility	↑ risk of gallbladder disease requiring nonobstetric surgery
Renal	↑ Glomerular filtration rate by 50% ↑ Renal plasma flow by 75%	Normal BUN and Cr may mask impaired renal function
Musculoskeletal	↑ joint laxity ↑ anteroposterior diameter of chest wall Exaggerated lumbar lordosis	↑ cephalad spread of local anesthetics Chest wall may hinder laryngoscopy ↑ risk of chronic back pain regardless of neuraxial analgesia/anesthesia use

AF, atrial fibrillation; ALT, alanine aminotransferase; AST, aspartate aminotransferase; CSF, cerebrospinal fluid; FEV_1, forced expiratory volume in one second; FVC, forced vital capacity; LDH, lactate dehydrogenase; MAC, minimum alveolar concentration; PDPH, postdural puncture headache; pSVT, paroxysmal supraventricular tachycardia; pVT, paroxysmal ventricular tachycardia; VTE, venous thromboembolism.

2. The pregnant patient is **hypercoagulable** throughout gestation. The concentration of most coagulation factors increases (except factors XI and XIII), as does platelet production, activation, and consumption. This hypercoagulable state helps to limit blood loss at delivery, though also increases the risk of thrombotic complications.

D. Nervous system
1. The **minimum alveolar concentration** (MAC) for inhalational anesthetics is decreased up to 40% during pregnancy. The etiology is unclear but may be related to alterations of hormone and endorphin concentrations during pregnancy, which result in an increased pain threshold. However, this increased sensitivity to volatiles may not translate to an enhanced effect on the brain nor amnesia; therefore targeting a reduced MAC is not recommended because using a reduced MAC may increase the incidence of awareness under anesthesia. The speed of induction of general anesthesia is increased in pregnancy secondary to increased cardiac output for intravenous agents, and increased minute ventilation and decreased FRC for inhalational agents.
2. The **local anesthetic** dose required for regional anesthesia is reduced in the parturient compared to the nonpregnant patient. Reasons for this include the following:
    a. **A decrease in cerebrospinal fluid (CSF) protein** results in a greater proportion of free and active drug.
    b. **Elevated CSF pH** increases the unionized fraction of the local anesthetic.
    c. **Distention of epidural veins** during pregnancy results in decreased lumbar CSF volume, enhancement of local anesthetic spread, and reduction of the segmental dose requirement for **spinal anesthesia.**
3. **Sympathetic nervous system (SNS) activity increases** from as early as 6 weeks of gestation despite decreases in diastolic pressure and total peripheral resistance. The parturient is highly dependent on the SNS for hemodynamic control, which is reflected by the significant decrease in blood pressure seen after regional anesthesia. SNS activity may return to normal by 24 to 48 hours postpartum.
4. The apex of **lumbar lordosis is shifted cephalad** with reduced thoracic kyphosis while supine. This contributes to the increased cephalad spread of spinal anesthesia.

E. Gastrointestinal system. Because of the **relaxation of the lower esophageal sphincter** and mechanical **displacement of the stomach** by the gravid uterus, gastric reflux, and heartburn are present in 30% to 50% of pregnant patients. It is not clear when during the pregnancy the risk for aspiration increases, although the difference between intragastric pressure and lower esophageal sphincter tone is decreased as early as the first trimester. Gastric emptying is not delayed during pregnancy, but it is slowed during labor, particularly following the administration of opioids. When a general anesthetic is planned, a nonparticulate antacid should be given routinely; a histamine (H_2) blocker and metoclopramide should be considered. Patients in the latter half of the second and third trimesters should have a rapid sequence induction for general anesthesia.

F. Renal system. Renal plasma flow and glomerular filtration increase by up to 50%, leading to increased creatinine clearance and decreased blood urea nitrogen and serum creatinine levels.

G. Musculoskeletal system. Increased lumbar lordosis and intra-abdominal pressure secondary to the enlarging uterus can stretch and compress the lateral femoral cutaneous nerve and produce a sensory loss over the anterolateral thigh ("meralgia paresthetica"). Carpal tunnel syndrome is also common and its etiology is likely multifactorial. Increases in the hormone relaxin result in progressive ligamentous laxity during pregnancy, peaking at 37 weeks. This allows for widening of the pubic symphysis and an increase in the anteroposterior and transverse diameters of the lower rib cage seen in parturients.

II. LABOR AND DELIVERY
   A. **Labor** is defined as the onset of regular, painful uterine contractions leading to cervical change, and may be divided into three stages:
      1. The **first stage** begins with the onset of regular contractions and ends with full cervical dilation. It is divided into a slow latent phase and a rapidly progressive active phase characterized by accelerated cervical dilation. Patients with a body mass index greater than 30 kg/m^2 and male fetuses may experience a prolonged first stage of labor, highlighting the limitations of the use of a single labor curve for all patients.
      2. The **second stage** extends from full cervical dilation until delivery of the newborn.
      3. The **third stage** begins after the delivery of the newborn, ending with the delivery of the placenta.
   B. **Pain** during the early first part of labor is primarily caused by uterine contractions and cervical dilation, and is mediated by the T10–L1 segments of the spinal cord. In the active phase of first-stage and early second-stage labor, additional pain from perineal stretching is mediated by the S2–S4 segments of the spinal cord via the pudendal nerve.
   C. **Intrapartum fetal evaluation** is most commonly accomplished with **fetal heart rate (FHR) monitoring**—either continuous or intermittent. Continuous FHR monitoring is used in up to 85% of laboring patients in the United States. The normal FHR ranges from 110 to 160 beats per minute (bpm) over 10 minutes. Fetal tachycardia may signify fetal asphyxia, maternal fever, and/or chorioamnionitis or may be the result of maternally administered drugs. Persistent fetal bradycardia is most commonly due to hypoxia, but other etiologies include fetal arrhythmias like congenital heart block, maternally administered β-blockers, or hypothermia. FHR baseline variability is defined as the fluctuation in FHR of 2 bpm or greater per minute. Minimal variability refers to less than 5 bpm fluctuation, moderate ranges from 6 to 25 bpm, and marked is greater than 25 bpm. It is modulated by fetal vagal tone and is a sign of underlying fetal health. Lack of variability may be associated with fetal hypoxia, neurogenic abnormalities, and central nervous system (CNS) depression due to side effects from opioids or other medications given throughout labor and must be interpreted in the context of FHR decelerations (decreases in FHR of 15 seconds or more from baseline to nadir). Recurrent concerning decelerations (late or deep variables), especially in the setting of minimal or absent variability, should prompt further evaluation to detect fetal compromise. Decelerations have been categorized (**Figure 32.1**) as follows:
      1. **Early decelerations** are gradual FHR decelerations (normally up to 20 bpm below baseline) that occur concomitantly with uterine contractions. They provide a mirror image of the uterine contraction, with the nadir of the deceleration occurring at the peak of the contraction. They are caused by an increase in fetal vagal tone, likely from mild hypoxia and compression of the fetal head, and do not require intervention.
      2. By definition, **variable decelerations** are variable in both duration and appearance and can occur spontaneously. Variable decelerations are

FIGURE 32.1 Patterns of periodic fetal heart rate (FHR) decelerations in relation to uterine contractions.

associated with umbilical cord compression and decreased umbilical blood flow or fetal head compression in the second stage of labor. They may indicate fetal compromise when severe and/or repetitive. Amnioinfusion (the instillation of amniotic fluid through a transcervical catheter after rupture of fetal membranes) has been demonstrated to decrease the need for emergent cesarean delivery by improving or eliminating variable decelerations.

3. **Late decelerations** are gradual decelerations that begin 10 to 30 seconds after the onset of a uterine contraction with a return of the FHR to the baseline only after the contraction has ended. Late decelerations suggest impaired maternal–fetal oxygen exchange or uteroplacental insufficiency and are observed in susceptible fetuses with intolerance of transient hypoxia. Medical interventions are tailored to improve placental oxygen delivery and include left uterine displacement, correction

of maternal hypotension, reconsideration of oxytocin dosing, and oxygen by face mask to the mother. A persistent late deceleration pattern may require prompt delivery of the fetus given the association with hypoxemia and acidemia.
 4. **Electronic FHR monitoring** has several significant limitations including a high rate of false positives and significant variability in its interpretation, and has been associated with an increase in operative deliveries. While it has not resulted in a decrease in cerebral palsy rates, it has been associated with a lower rate of neonatal seizures. To minimize intervention based on false positives, additional ancillary tests may be considered:
    a. **Fetal scalp stimulation.** An acceleration of the FHR in response to digital or instrumental stimulation of the fetal head is associated with a healthy nonacidotic fetus and a pH of at least 7.19.
    b. **Fetal pulse oximetry** can be used to continuously measure fetal oxygen saturation in the setting of nonreassuring FHR tracings. Unfortunately, it is not associated with decreased cesarean delivery rates or improved neonatal outcomes.

III. MEDICATIONS COMMONLY USED FOR LABOR AND DELIVERY

   A. **Vasopressors.** Symptoms of maternal hypotension include light-headedness, nausea, difficulty breathing, and diaphoresis. Because uterine blood flow is not autoregulated, maternal hypotension may lead to decreased placental perfusion and fetal distress. Sympathetic blockade from regional anesthesia and decreased systemic vascular resistance may cause maternal hypotension. An ideal vasopressor for obstetric anesthesia is one that increases both maternal blood pressure and placental blood flow.
   1. **Ephedrine** is an indirect agonist of α- and β-adrenergic receptors. Its inotropic and chronotropic effects increase peripheral and uterine blood flow. Historically, ephedrine was the drug of choice for the treatment of maternal hypotension, however, it has been associated with lower umbilical artery pH compared to phenylephrine.
   2. **Phenylephrine** was previously believed to decrease uteroplacental blood flow, but more recent evidence shows that phenylephrine is at least as effective in correcting maternal hypotension as ephedrine but with less risk of fetal acidemia. Phenylephrine infusions have become increasingly common to prevent and treat maternal hypotension in response to neuraxial anesthesia.
   3. Dilute **norepinephrine** may be used to counteract spinal anesthesia-induced hypotension. It increases cardiac output with a lower incidence of bradycardia compared with phenylephrine. Less commonly used than ephedrine and phenylephrine, norepinephrine use in labor and delivery continues to be an area of active investigation but findings show its short-term peripheral administration is safe.
   B. **Uterotonics** or ecbolics are agents that stimulate uterine contractions.
   1. **Indications**
      a. To induce or augment labor
      b. To control postpartum uterine atony and bleeding
      c. To induce therapeutic abortion
   2. **Uterotonic agents**
      a. **Oxytocin (Pitocin),** a synthetic posterior pituitary hormone, acts on the uterine smooth muscle to stimulate the frequency and force of contractions. Cardiovascular side effects of oxytocin include vasodilation, hypotension, tachycardia, and arrhythmias. In high doses,

oxytocin may have an antidiuretic effect and produce hyponatremia, cerebral edema, and subsequent seizures. With a half-life on the order of minutes, continuous intravenous infusion is required.
- b. **Ergot alkaloids,** like ergonovine (Ergotrate) and methylergonovine (Methergine), control postpartum bleeding following the third stage of labor by producing tetanic uterine contractions. Side effects include systemic vasoconstriction and hypertension, which may be amplified in the presence of vasopressors. IV injection has been associated with severe hypertension, seizures, stroke, myocardial infarction, and pulmonary edema. Intramuscular (IM) administration is therefore highly recommended. Ergot alkaloids should be used with caution or avoided in patients with peripheral vascular disease, preeclampsia, hypertension, heart failure, or coronary artery disease.
- c. **Prostaglandin 15-methyl $F_2\alpha$** (carboprost, Hemabate), is a treatment for uterine atony. The usual dose is 250 μg IM or by intramyometrial injection administered not more frequently than once every 15 minutes with a total maximum dose of 2 mg. Transient hypertension, severe bronchoconstriction, and increased pulmonary vascular resistance have been reported, contraindicating its use in patients with a history of asthma or pulmonary hypertension. Fever, nausea, vomiting, and diarrhea are additional side effects.
- d. **Prostaglandin E_1** (misoprostol) increases myometrial intracellular free calcium concentrations and improves uterine tone. It is available in 200-μg tablets that are placed buccally, rectally, or vaginally for the treatment of postpartum hemorrhage. The efficacy of prostaglandin E1 is lower than the other uterotonics and is most useful when other agents are unavailable or contraindicated. Side effects are less common but are similar to those of prostaglandin 15-methyl $F_2\alpha$.

C. **Tocolytics** are used to delay premature labor in patients with viable fetuses less than or equal to 34 weeks of gestation. Cervical dilation of less than 4 cm and cervical effacement of less than 80% are associated with a greater likelihood of success in terminating premature labor.
1. **Indications**
   a. To stop preterm contractions
   b. To slow or arrest labor while initiating other therapeutic measures (eg, betamethasone to accelerate fetal lung maturation)
   c. To allow transfer from a community hospital to a tertiary care center with a neonatal intensive care unit
2. **Contraindications**
   a. Chorioamnionitis
   b. Fetal distress
   c. Intrauterine fetal demise
   d. Severe hemorrhage
3. **Tocolytic Agents**
   a. **β_2-Adrenergic agonists** such as **terbutaline** produce myometrial relaxation, maternal bronchodilation, vasodilation, and tachycardia. In addition, they cause hyperglycemia, hypokalemia, hyperinsulinemia, and metabolic acidosis. Pulmonary edema and chest pain are rare with less than 24 hours of therapy. Preexisting hyperglycemia should be corrected, and a baseline electrocardiogram should be considered for patients with preexisting cardiac disease.
   b. **Cyclooxygenase inhibitors** such as **indomethacin** inhibit arachidonic acid conversion to prostaglandins. While maternal side effects

are uncommon, fetal side effects include premature closure of the ductus arteriosus and decreased urine output. They should therefore be used with caution after 32 weeks of gestation and in oligohydramnios.
  c. **Calcium channel blockers** prevent the release of calcium from smooth muscle sarcoplasmic reticulum, inhibiting uterine contractions. Calcium channel blockers are effective and well tolerated. Hypotension is an expected side effect.
  d. **Magnesium sulfate** antagonizes intracellular calcium and inhibits myometrial contraction. It is no longer recommended for tocolysis due to lack of efficacy but may be used for the prevention of eclamptic seizures and/or fetal neuroprotection to reduce the risk of cerebral palsy in preterm birth. Side effects include hyporeflexia, lethargy, and nausea; at higher serum concentrations, respiratory depression, electrocardiogram changes, and pulmonary edema are possible.

IV. PLACENTAL TRANSFER OF DRUGS
  A. **Passive diffusion** is responsible for the placental transfer of the majority of drugs, although some facilitated and active transport occurs. Factors that promote rapid diffusion include the following:
   1. Low molecular weight
   2. High lipid solubility
   3. Low degree of ionization
   4. Low protein binding
  B. Most **inhalational** and **intravenous anesthetics** readily cross the placenta due to their low molecular weight, high lipid solubility, general nonionized formation, and minimal protein binding.
  C. **Opioids** cross the placenta readily and may cause fetal neurologic and respiratory depression.
  D. **Muscle relaxants** are water-soluble, ionized molecules, with high molecular weights, and therefore do not readily cross the placenta.
  E. The transfer of **anticholinergic** drugs is variable: glycopyrrolate is poorly transferred while atropine is completely transferred. Small amounts of **acetylcholinesterase inhibitors** are transferred.
  F. **Vasoactive medications**—antihypertensives, antiarrhythmics, and vasopressors (with the exception of phenylephrine)—cross the placenta and exert some effect on the fetus.
  G. **Local anesthetics** are weak bases with low degrees of ionization and therefore may cross the placenta when absorbed into the maternal bloodstream. Fetal acidosis, exacerbated in fetal distress, favors ionization and therefore accumulation of basic drugs in the fetal circulation through a process known as "ion trapping." However, under normal circumstances, these concentrations rarely result in clinical toxicity.

V. ANALGESIA FOR LABOR AND VAGINAL DELIVERY
  A. **Natural childbirth.** Some women favor a delivery plan with minimal medical intervention. Nonetheless, it is important to evaluate each patient's medical history and physical findings so as to facilitate informed and expedient care in an emergency.
  B. **Systemic analgesia**
   1. **Mixed opioid agonist–antagonists.** Nalbuphine or butorphanol are often the initial choice for systemic analgesia due to their efficacy as well as their ceiling effect on maternal ventilatory depression.

2. **Opioids.** Meperidine, morphine, remifentanil, and fentanyl are commonly used opioids. Maternal side effects, including dose-dependent respiratory depression, sedation, and rapid placental diffusion, limit their overall use. These drugs may also contribute to neonatal respiratory depression, decreased FHR variability, a need for active neonatal resuscitation, and possible neurobehavioral effects in the neonate. Of note, remifentanil and fentanyl have the advantage of self-administration via PCA. Remifentanil is rapidly metabolized by the fetus and parturient. Fentanyl is preferred to meperidine due to lower rates of respiratory depression and nausea.
3. **Inhalational analgesia.** Nitrous oxide has limited analgesic efficacy and is used most commonly in a 50% mixture with oxygen. Environmental pollution and possible hypoxemia when given with systemic opioids are concerns. Neonatal depression is rare.

C. **Epidural** anesthesia provides the most effective labor analgesia and allows for a transition to effective neuraxial anesthesia if a cesarean delivery becomes necessary. Existing evidence does not show an increased rate of cesarean delivery when compared to systemic analgesia. The duration of the second stage of labor is about 15 minutes longer, and historically, the instrumental delivery rate was increased with epidural analgesia. Modern management with high volume, dilute local anesthetic solutions reduces the risk of motor block and associated instrumental delivery rate.

1. **Technique**
   a. Initial IV access should be established. Prehydration with 500 mL of fluid may be routine among some anesthetists, but data from small studies have provided conflicting results regarding the effect on FHR.
   b. Vital signs and FHR should be monitored according to institutional protocol.
   c. Specific physiologic and anatomic features of term pregnancy—for example, epidural venous distention, increased abdominal size, and intermittent uterine contractions—must be taken into account for positioning. A patient may be seated or in the lateral decubitus position.

2. **Advantages**
   a. Epidurals offer continuous analgesia for the duration of labor and cesarean section if necessary.
   b. Drug dose and delivery mode (eg, continuous epidural infusion [CEI], programmed intermittent epidural bolus [PIEB] with or without patient-controlled epidural analgesia [PCEA]) may be individualized.
   c. The hyper-/hypoventilation cycle during a contraction and associated decrease in PaO_2 or O_2 saturation are favorably modified by epidural analgesia.
   d. Effective epidural analgesia is associated with decreased peripheral catecholamines.
   e. Memory, alertness, and emotional perception are preserved.

3. **Disadvantages**
   a. Patient cooperation is necessary.
   b. Providers skilled in neuraxial technique in pregnant women are required.
   c. Vital signs must be regularly monitored and systemic hypotension corrected.
   d. Accidental dural puncture complicates approximately 1.5% of placements.

4. **Contraindications**
   a. Patient refusal or inability to cooperate during placement.
   b. Coagulation disorder or significant thrombocytopenia—either acquired or inherited.
   c. Infection at the site of catheter placement.
   d. Severe hypovolemia.
   e. Space-occupying lesion with increased intracranial pressure predisposing the patient to herniation after accidental dural puncture and CSF loss.
5. **Anesthetics**
   a. **A test dose** of 3 mL of 1.5% lidocaine (45 mg) with 1:200,000 epinephrine (15 µg) aids in the detection of intrathecal or intravascular placement. Signs of intrathecal placement include motor weakness, inability to flex at the hip, and/or immediate relief of contraction pain. Signs of intravascular placement include hypertension (SBP >20 mm Hg from baseline) and tachycardia (HR >20 bpm from baseline), however, the utility of the intravascular test dose in obstetrics remains a point of debate given low sensitivity and specificity.
   b. The ideal analgesia in labor provides adequate pain relief and minimizes motor blockade. The combination of a local anesthetic and opioid helps to achieve this goal. Our current practice is to administer an epidural mix of 0.0625% (0.625 mg/mL) bupivacaine with 2 µg/mL of fentanyl. Epidural administration is now preferred through PIEB instead of CEI with PCEA. There is a greater spread of anesthetic with intermittent bolus compared to the continuous infusion which results in a local anesthetic–sparing effect, less dense motor block, and greater patient satisfaction. Additional clinical boluses typically range from 5 to 10 mL. Over the course of labor, it is not uncommon to administer supplemental boluses of concentrated local anesthetics—for example, 0.125% to 0.2% bupivacaine or 0.8% to 1.5% lidocaine—to meet analgesic requirements. Malfunction and malposition of the epidural catheter must be considered when the observed analgesic effect is lower than expected and should be adjusted or replaced promptly if suspected.
   c. Blood pressure monitoring must be more frequent at the onset of epidural analgesia and after local anesthetic boluses since hypotension may cause impaired placental perfusion. Hypotension treatment includes crystalloid volume expansion, phenylephrine 80 µg IV, and/or ephedrine 5 to 10 mg repeated as necessary.
   d. **Continuous epidural infusion** for labor is also possible but not common practice in our hospital as it is associated with increased risk of motor blockade and need for rescue boluses.
6. **Complications**
   a. Epidural failure—Epidural catheter replacement rates due to inadequate analgesia range between 5% and 13%.
   b. **Dural puncture** complicates 1.5% of labor epidural placements. The frequency of accidental dural puncture is increased with increasing depth to epidural space and number of attempts whereas the frequency is decreased with increased practitioner skill and experience and use of loss of resistance to saline. Accidental intrathecal catheters may be kept and dosed accordingly in patients with particularly difficult epidural placements, but careful attention must be paid to label the catheter accordingly and educate the patient, nursing team, and anesthesia colleagues regarding dosing to reduce the risk of high spinal.

c. **Postdural puncture headache (PDPH)**. Approximately 52% of inadvertent dural punctures with an epidural needle will cause frontal or occipital headaches of variable intensity with possible radiation to the neck within 5 days postpuncture. The headache is often orthostatic with symptoms that appear within seconds of being upright and resolve quickly after becoming horizontal. Risk factors for PDPH include young age (<40 years), female gender, low BMI, history of PDPH, use of a needle with a cutting bevel, and vaginal delivery. In mild PDPH, hydration, bed rest, analgesics, caffeine, and avoidance of heavy lifting may be helpful in treating, though not preventing, symptoms. Severe PDPH may warrant an **epidural blood patch (EBP)**. Immediate symptomatic relief occurs in up to 75% of cases. A second EBP might be considered in refractory cases. There is mounting literature supporting the use of sphenopalatine ganglion block (SPG) for PDPH, however, it should not take the place of EBP and large-scale prospective studies are lacking. Rare complications of PDPH include meningitis, subdural hematoma, diplopia, hearing loss, and cerebral venous thrombosis. These serious complications should be considered if the headache does not respond to conservative measures or EBP. There is increasing evidence that untreated PDPH may result in chronic headaches, chronic back pain, and long-term adverse outcomes and therefore should be actively managed if it does occur.
d. **Intravascular injection.** The total dose and rate of intravascular injection are correlated with signs and symptoms of local anesthetic toxicity. When intravascular injection is suspected, the infusion should be discontinued and appropriate therapy immediately instituted, including the administration of Intralipid. Cardiovascular collapse must be treated with cardiopulmonary resuscitation (CPR), left uterine displacement, and, potentially, perimortem cesarean delivery (PMCD).
e. **Intrathecal injection.** Aspiration before each epidural dose helps to detect intrathecal catheters. Large epidural doses inadvertently injected into the intrathecal space may produce high or total spinal anesthesia. Nausea, hypotension, and loss of consciousness may precede cardiopulmonary arrest. Critical interventions include IV crystalloid, vasopressors, inotropes, left uterine displacement, and 100% oxygen administration. Cardiac and respiratory arrest associated with a total spinal must be emergently treated in accordance with the advanced cardiac life support (ACLS) principles, and PMCD may be necessary.
D. **Spinal anesthesia.** A small single intrathecal dose of 0.25% bupivacaine (1 to 2.5 mg) ± 10 to 25 mcg fentanyl provides prompt analgesia lasting up to 90 minutes. Single-shot spinals are not preferred for laboring women due to the prolonged duration of labor and fixed duration of the spinal. They may be used if delivery is imminent due to their rapid onset. In a subset of patients for whom labor pain inhibits active participation in the epidural placement process, initiation of spinal analgesia may improve the success of a subsequent epidural placement and reduce the risk of unintended dural puncture. However, it may prevent paresthesia identification during placement and immediate verification of epidural function.
E. **Combined spinal-epidural analgesia (CSE)** offers both a rapid onset (2 to 5 minutes) of sacral analgesia for advanced labor and the benefit of leaving an epidural catheter in place. The use of CSE analgesia is associated

with decreased epidural failure rate, despite the historical concern for the "untested catheter." Addition of a lipophilic opioid may decrease the dose of local anesthetic required, thereby limiting the motor blockade and hypotension associated with local anesthetics. This may be particularly helpful in patients who are preload dependent. Despite the dura being punctured, there has not been an increase in PDPH noted when a small-gauge pencil point needle is used. However, dural puncture may theoretically increase the risk of a neuraxial infection. Intrathecal opioid administration is associated with a higher incidence of pruritus and transient FHR abnormalities compared to epidural administration.

F. **Dural puncture epidural (DPE)** is a technique in which the dura is punctured with a spinal needle, but unlike a CSE, no medication is injected into the intrathecal space. Studies have shown a shorter time for pain relief and more frequent blockade of the sacral dermatomes compared to a straight epidural due to migration of local anesthetic into the intrathecal space. Data are conflicting, but some studies suggest DPE produces improved analgesia compared with straight epidural and fewer side effects compared with CSE.

VI. ANESTHESIA FOR CESAREAN DELIVERY

The anesthetic technique for cesarean delivery must be planned according to the urgency of the delivery. Indications may be either maternal (eg, prior cesarean delivery, arrest of labor, failed induction, placental or uterine pathology) or fetal (eg, malpresentation, concern for fetal well-being).

A. Positioning should include a **15- to 30-degree left table tilt** to relieve aortocaval compression and prevent maternal hypotension and uteroplacental insufficiency.

B. **Aspiration prophylaxis** should be carried out with a nonparticulate antacid, H_2 receptor antagonist, and/or metoclopramide. In the case of elective cesarean delivery, clear liquids may be consumed until 2 hours prior to surgery. While parturients may be allowed moderate amounts of clear liquids throughout labor, those patients at additional risk for aspiration (eg, morbid obesity) or operative delivery (eg, nonreassuring fetal heart tracing) should be subject to additional restrictions on oral intake.

C. **Anesthetic technique**

1. **Regional anesthesia** is more commonly employed and offers maternal and fetal benefits, including avoidance of airway manipulation, minimal fetal drug exposure, improved postoperative pain control, and decreased blood loss.

    a. **Spinal anesthesia** provides rapid onset of surgical anesthesia, but its duration is time limited. A T4 sensory level is required for adequate coverage of abdominal viscera. The use of hyperbaric bupivacaine (0.75% in dextrose 8.25%) allows positional control over the cephalad spread of the local anesthetic. The ED_{95} for spinal bupivacaine in cesarean delivery is 11.2 mg. Common adjuvants include a lipophilic opioid (eg, fentanyl or sufentanil) for intraoperative pain control and a hydrophilic opioid (eg, morphine or hydromorphone) for postoperative analgesia. Concomitant fluid load and prophylactic phenylephrine or norepinephrine may reduce sympathectomy-associated hypotension. Postoperatively, patients should be monitored for delayed respiratory depression, nausea, vomiting, and pruritus.

    b. **Epidural anesthesia** is most commonly used during cesarean delivery when a preexisting labor epidural is already in use. In comparison with spinal anesthesia, epidural anesthesia is slower in onset,

requires higher local anesthetic doses, and may be redosed as necessary. Epidural anesthesia is associated with increased breakthrough pain and need for intraoperative supplementation compared to spinal or CSE anesthesia. Commonly used local anesthetics include 2% lidocaine with epinephrine and 3% 2-chloroprocaine; the utility of bupivacaine is limited by the slow onset time. The addition of sodium bicarbonate to lidocaine or 2-chloroprocaine may speed their onset. Epidural fentanyl 100 mcg may enhance the quality of the surgical block. After delivery, 2 to 3 mg of epidurally administered preservative-free morphine may improve postoperative analgesia. Monitoring for postoperative respiratory depression and pruritus is indicated.
    c. **CSE** combines the advantage of rapid anesthetic onset with the option to prolong its duration. Although the function of the epidural catheter is not tested at the start, literature has shown that positioning of the epidural catheter is usually correct and more likely to be successful than straight epidural placement.
2. **General anesthesia**
    a. Indications
        1. Failure of neuraxial technique
        2. Insufficient time to implement neuraxial anesthesia
        3. Maternal preference
        4. Medical contraindication to regional anesthesia
    b. The potential for a difficult airway and increased risk of aspiration mandate careful preparation of alternative airway plans and immediate availability of advanced airway equipment. The rate of difficult intubation in a parturient ranges from 1 in 50 to 1 in 250, which is 8 to 10 times higher than the general population. Preoxygenation followed by rapid sequence intravenous induction with succinylcholine 1 to 1.5 mg/kg followed by endotracheal intubation is the technique of choice.
    c. To minimize fetal exposure to anesthetics, cesarean delivery should begin immediately upon securing the airway. Halogenated agents antagonize uterine contracture, therefore, to avoid atony, it is customaray to either decrease the concentration to 0.5 to 0.75 MAC and increase the N2O fraction after delivery or transition to a propofol infusion. To reduce risk of awareness, which is elevated in emergency cesarean delivery, consider processed EEG monitoring or midazolam administration after delivery.
    d. Additional neuromuscular blockade following induction is not usually necessary.
    e. Emergence and extubation are high-risk, especially if the patient had a difficult intubation or large fluid shifts occurred intraoperatively. Gastric decompression with an orogastric tube is recommended prior to emergence. Strict extubation criteria should be applied and delayed extubation may be considered.
    f. In the absence of long-acting neuraxial opioid, adequate postoperative pain control may require a regional block (eg, transversus abdominis plane or quadratus lumborum block, assuming no contraindication), multimodal analgesia, and/or initiation of intravenous opioid patient-controlled analgesia.

VII. PREECLAMPSIA

Preeclampsia occurs in approximately 5% of pregnancies, particularly in nulliparous, diabetic, and hypertensive patients or those with chronic disease.

Although the etiology is incompletely understood, possible mechanisms include exaggerated maternal immune and inflammatory responses and chronic uteroplacental ischemia leading to upregulation of angiogenic factors.

A. Diagnosis

1. Persistent hypertension after 20 weeks of gestational age should prompt a diagnostic workup for preeclampsia.
2. The American College of Obstetricians and Gynecologists defines a diagnosis of preeclampsia as a single blood pressure measurement of >160/110 mm Hg or two measurements more than 4 hours apart of >140/90 mm Hg combined with *either* proteinuria or evidence of end-organ damage (thrombocytopenia, pulmonary edema, renal insufficiency, or impaired liver function).
3. Preeclampsia with severe features is defined as a blood pressure of >160/110 mm Hg on two occasions at least 4 hours apart in addition to visual disturbances, new-onset headache, or the end-organ sequelae listed in the previous section.
4. **Eclampsia** and **HELLP syndrome,** are also part of this disease spectrum.
    a. **Eclampsia** describes the new onset of seizures in a parturient with preeclampsia and is observed in approximately 50% of preeclampsia-related deaths.
    b. **HELLP syndrome** (**h**emolysis, **e**levated **l**iver enzymes, and **l**ow **p**latelets) involves a constellation of laboratory abnormalities and is generally regarded as a subset of severe preeclampsia. The diagnosis of HELLP syndrome is also associated with an increased risk of adverse outcomes including placental abruption, renal failure, hepatic subcapsular hematoma formation and liver rupture, and fetal and maternal morbidity and mortality.

B. Management

1. **Obstetric management**
    a. **Expectant management** and monitoring until 37 weeks of gestation is preferred for women with a preterm fetus and preeclampsia without severe features.
    b. **Delivery** is recommended for preeclampsia with severe features at 34 weeks of gestation or beyond. Delivery of the placenta is the accepted treatment.
2. **Pharmacologic therapy**
    a. **Seizure prophylaxis** may be carried out with **magnesium sulfate.** Magnesium is administered during labor and delivery and 24 to 48 hours postpartum via an IV loading dose of 4 g over 30 minutes, followed by an infusion of 1 to 2 g/h. Because of its smooth muscle relaxation, magnesium may decrease maternal blood pressure and predispose them to postpartum uterine atony and hemorrhage.
    b. **Antihypertensives** such as **labetalol, hydralazine,** and **calcium channel blockers** are frequently administered for blood pressure control. The goal is not to normalize blood pressure but to prevent progression to hypertensive crisis, encephalopathy, or stroke. Because the placenta has minimal ability to autoregulate flow, a sudden drop in blood pressure may decrease placental perfusion and result in fetal compromise.
    c. **Fluid management.** Volume assessment is challenging. Intravascular depletion should be corrected with judicious administration of crystalloid, as preeclamptic patients are at increased risk for the development of pulmonary edema, particularly with concomitant administration of magnesium.

d. **Coagulation abnormalities.** A platelet count of less than 100,000/μL is the most common coagulation abnormality. Per the 2021 SOAP Consensus Statement on Thrombocytopenia, the risk of epidural hematoma is likely very low in obstetric patients with platelet counts greater than 70,000/μL in the setting of known gestational thrombocytopenia, immune thrombocytopenia, or hypertensive disorders of pregnancy without additional risk factors (Class IIa, Level C-LD evidence). There is limited data available for platelet counts between 50,000/μL and 70,000/μL, but it may be reasonable to proceed with neuraxial anesthesia depending on competing clinical risks (Class IIb, Level C-LD evidence). Vigilance for epidural hematoma and availability of neurosurgical consultation are essential. Viscoelastic and repeated coagulation testing may be advisable. The coexistence of other hemostatic abnormalities (eg, prolonged prothrombin time or partial thromboplastin time, low fibrinogen) should be taken into account.

C. Anesthesia

1. **Neuraxial** anesthesia.
    a. Neuraxial anesthesia is the preferred type of anesthesia for labor, vaginal delivery, or cesarean delivery.
    b. A platelet count of <150,000 × 10^9/L is present in about 20% of preeclamptic patients overall and up to 50% of patients with severe disease. Investigation of platelet count is advisable prior to any instrumentation of the neuraxis (including epidural catheter removal).
    c. **Epidural anesthesia.** Early epidural placement offers possible improved uteroplacental perfusion, reduction in circulating maternal catecholamines, and assessment of epidural catheter function prior to the development of fetal intolerance to labor and urgent cesarean section.
    d. **Spinal anesthesia.** Growing evidence shows spinal anesthesia is not associated with more severe hypotension in preeclamptic patients, supporting its safe use.
2. **General anesthesia** is usually reserved for emergent cesarean sections or for patients with coagulopathy or other contraindications to regional techniques. Disadvantages of general anesthesia include autonomic stimulation and possible hypertension with intubation and extubation, increasing the risk of intracranial bleeding. The sympathetic response to laryngoscopy can be blunted with remifentanil or esmolol. Diffuse, severe interstitial edema of the airway may also increase the likelihood of a difficult intubation. The interaction of magnesium with nondepolarizing muscle relaxants might prolong their duration of action in preeclamptic patients.

VIII. PERIPARTUM HEMORRHAGE

Peripartum hemorrhage is the leading cause of maternal mortality worldwide, accounting for approximately 15% of deaths.

A. Antepartum hemorrhage threatens oxygen transfer to the fetus since it is most commonly due to hemorrhage originating along the uteroplacental interface.

1. **Placenta previa** occurs when the placenta implants in advance of the fetal presenting part. A placenta that covers the cervical os is considered a true placenta previa. If it is near the cervical os, it is classified as a low-lying placenta. The hallmark presentation is painless vaginal

bleeding in the second or third trimester. The first hemorrhage is usually self-limiting and does not compromise the fetus. Patients with a previous cesarean section and placenta previa have a higher incidence of **placenta accreta** with a subsequent need for a gravid hysterectomy. A minimum distance of 1 cm from placental edge to the internal os is recommended to proceed with vaginal delivery. The amount and rate of blood loss and severity of associated signs and symptoms are the primary considerations in the anesthetic choice.

2. **Placental abruption** is the premature separation of part or all of a normally implanted placenta. Classically, an abruption is painful and associated with either vaginal bleeding or hemorrhage concealed behind the placenta. Hypertension, preeclampsia, advanced maternal age, and abdominal trauma are associated with an increased risk for abruption. Patients may deliver vaginally or via cesarean section depending on the degree of compromise. Anesthetic management is similar to that of placenta previa. One-third of coagulopathies in pregnancy are a result of abruption, which increases the risk for disseminated intravascular coagulation (DIC).

3. **Vasa previa** is a condition in which the fetal vessels are in front of the presenting part of the fetus and are not protected by the umbilical cord. Trauma during vaginal examination, artificial rupture of membranes, or descent of the presenting part might tear the vessels causing fetal hemorrhage. Immediate cesarean delivery is warranted.

4. **Vaginal birth after cesarean (VBAC) section.** Patients with a singleton fetus in vertex presentation and a history of a single low transverse uterine incision might be candidates for a trial of labor and VBAC. Although induction with prostaglandins is contraindicated, oxytocin augmentation may be administered. Uterine scar dehiscence occurs in 0.7% of VBAC and does not compromise the fetus nor cause excessive hemorrhage. Uterine rupture (0.65% of VBAC), however, may result in fetal compromise, maternal hemorrhage, or both, necessitating cesarean section or postpartum exploratory laparotomy. If uterine rupture occurs, the presence of a functioning epidural may provide a means for establishing a quick, safe anesthetic for cesarean section. If uterine rupture causes massive hemorrhage, anesthetic management is the same as for any actively bleeding patient.

B. **Postpartum hemorrhage:** Redefined in 2017 by the American College of Obstetricians and Gynecologists (ACOG) as >1000 mL blood loss following a vaginal or cesarean delivery.

1. **Uterine atony**, the inadequate contractile response of the uterus after delivery, is the most common cause of postpartum hemorrhage. Risk factors include induced labor, prolonged labor, cesarean delivery, hypertension, diabetes, and advanced maternal age. Uterotonics should be initiated, and oxytocin is typically the first-line agent. Patients should receive adequate resuscitation with crystalloid, colloid, and blood products as clinically indicated. If conservative measures fail, intrauterine balloon tamponade, surgical management, and/or arterial embolization may be necessary.

2. **Retained placenta** occurs in up to ~3% of all vaginal deliveries and often requires manual exploration of the uterine cavity facilitated by epidural or spinal block. Nitroglycerin in 50 to 100 µg IV boluses can be used for additional uterine relaxation. For analgesia, small doses of opioids and/or ketamine may be administered. Volatile anesthetic via facemask should be avoided due aspiration risks. If there has been significant

bleeding and the patient is hypovolemic, general endotracheal anesthesia with a volatile agent to help relax the uterus may be necessary. When the placenta has been removed, the volatile anesthetic must be discontinued to reverse uterine relaxation. Many patients require additional uterotonics to improve uterine tone.
3. **Retained products of conception** may cause significant postpartum bleeding. Uterine relaxation is usually not necessary for uterine curettage to remove remaining placental fragments. Anesthetic options are augmentation of an existing labor epidural, spinal, or general anesthesia.
4. **Laceration of the vagina, cervix, or perineum** is a common cause of postpartum hemorrhage. Bleeding may be insidious and difficult to estimate. Patients require adequate analgesia to facilitate repair that may involve augmentation or placement of regional blocks, infiltration of local anesthetics, or a general anesthetic.
5. **Uterine inversion** is a rare cause of postpartum hemorrhage (~1 in 3400) that represents a true obstetric emergency. Nitroglycerin in small IV boluses may produce adequate uterine relaxation and avoid the need for general anesthesia. Atony often follows the replacement of the uterus, and uterotonic medications are indicated.
6. **Placenta accreta spectrum** refers to an abnormally adherent placenta with increasing incidence in patients with prior cesarean sections or placenta previa. The rising prevalence is directly related to the increase in cesarean delivery rate. The condition may be divided into three types: accreta vera (abnormal placental attachment to the myometrium), increta (invasion into the myometrium), and percreta (invasion through the myometrium into the serosa and adjacent organs). Placenta accreta generally necessitates peripartum hysterectomy with antenatal diagnosis improving the chance of favorable outcomes. Anesthetic management should include close interdisciplinary communication and planning as well as preparation for massive hemorrhage.

IX. AMNIOTIC FLUID EMBOLISM
A. **Amniotic fluid embolism (AFE)** is a rare and catastrophic condition unique to pregnancy that should be considered during any sudden cardiorespiratory collapse or seizure during the peripartum period. It commonly presents with hypotension, hypoxia, and coagulopathy. While AFE is a diagnosis of exclusion, there must be evidence of coagulopathy. US estimates range from 1.7 to 5.4 per 100,000 live births with mortality rates as high as 80%, usually occurring within the first hours of onset. Permanent neurologic dysfunction affects up to 85% of survivors. Other diagnoses to consider include myocardial infarction, pulmonary embolism, anaphylaxis, eclampsia, and sepsis.
B. **Pathophysiology.** The pathophysiology of AFE is poorly understood but seems to involve a breach in the barrier between the maternal and fetal compartments. This results in an abnormal maternal systemic response to fetal tissue, the activation of proinflammatory mediators, and a consequent syndrome similar to systemic inflammatory response syndrome with right heart dysfunction.
C. **Clinical presentation.** Risk factors include advanced maternal age, placental abruption, eclampsia, and induction of labor. The diagnosis is made based on clinical features of acute peripartum hypoxia and hypotension, with rapid deterioration leading to cardiovascular collapse, coagulopathy, and death. AFE remains a clinical diagnosis, and laboratory tests are not recommended to either confirm or rule out the diagnosis.

D. **Manifestations.** AFE affects multiple organ systems, and the presentation may vary.
   1. **Cardiovascular.** Hypotension is a key feature, present in 100% of patients with severe disease. A biphasic model of shock has been proposed with initial transient pulmonary hypertension—likely from the release of vasoactive substances—resulting in hypoxia and right-sided heart failure. The patients who survive the initial insult develop left heart failure and pulmonary edema due to left ventricular ischemic injury or direct myocardial depression.
   2. **Respiratory.** Hypoxia is an early manifestation of AFE, thought to arise from acute pulmonary hypertension, decreased cardiac output, and ventilation–perfusion mismatch. Later, pulmonary edema develops in association with left ventricular failure. Many patients will also manifest noncardiogenic pulmonary edema when the left ventricular function improves.
   3. **Coagulation.** Disruption of the normal clotting cascade occurs in most patients, resulting in DIC and hemorrhage after the initial cardiopulmonary instability.
E. **Management** of AFE involves aggressive resuscitation. Right heart failure from pulmonary artery hypertension can be treated with inotropes such as epinephrine, dobutamine, and/or milrinone. Patients may respond to sildenafil, inhaled or IV prostacyclin, or inhaled nitric oxide to decrease pulmonary vascular resistance. To address abnormalities in coagulation, maintaining a platelet count >50,000, fibrinogen >200 mg/dL, and a normal international normalized ratio is recommended. Uterine atony should be treated with oxytocin, ergot derivatives, and prostaglandins when indicated. Serious AFE will result in total cardiovascular collapse requiring intubation and CPR. Extracorporeal membrane oxygenation may be the most immediately available rescue method. Intra-aortic balloon counterpulsation and cardiopulmonary bypass have also been used. The decision for immediate delivery of the fetus should be made by the obstetrician to maximize chances of fetal survival and aid maternal resuscitation, but is recommended after only 23 weeks.

X. ANESTHESIA FOR NONOBSTETRIC SURGERY DURING PREGNANCY
A. Approximately 1% to 2% of women undergo nonobstetric surgery during pregnancy. Purely elective surgical procedures are relatively contraindicated in pregnancy and should be postponed until 6 weeks postpartum. If a procedure must be performed, the second trimester is the preferred time. Anesthetic management objectives include the following:
   1. **Maternal safety.** Induction and emergence from general anesthesia are more rapid in pregnant patients due to the increase in minute ventilation and decrease in FRC. Uterine displacement to minimize aortocaval compression should be considered as early as the second trimester and after 20 weeks of gestation. During any anesthetic, oxygen transport to the placenta must be maintained.
   2. **Teratogenicity.** In 2016, the U.S. Food and Drug Administration released a Drug Safety Communication warning that "repeated or lengthy use of general anesthetic or sedation drugs during surgeries or procedures in children younger than 3 years or in pregnant women during their third trimester may affect the development of children's brains." However, no data from pregnant women were included among the clinical studies cited, and subsequent studies showed no evidence of neurodevelopmental effects in young children exposed to anesthesia. Nitrous oxide

may interfere with DNA synthesis and is often avoided by practitioners in the first and second trimesters.
3. **Fetal well-being.** Women who undergo surgery while pregnant have a higher rate of preterm labor. Laparoscopy is not associated with a higher rate of adverse pregnancy outcomes.
4. **Reversal of residual neuromuscular blockade.** The use of the combination of neostigmine and glycopyrrolate has been postulated to expose the fetus to unopposed neostigmine and cause fetal bradycardia, as the placenta is more permeable to neostigmine than glycopyrrolate. However, there is little data to support the use of alternative antimuscarinic agents such as atropine given the wealth of clinical experience and demonstrated safety utilizing traditional reversal with neostigmine and glycopyrrolate. Because of a computer-generated model demonstrating Sugammadex binding and encapsulating progestogen, in 2019 the Society for Obstetric Anesthesia and Perinatology released a warning that Sugammadex is best avoided during early pregnancy and used with caution in late pregnancy. Animal studies have not demonstrated increased risk of preterm labor and there is no human data to suggest this either. Since this statement, many obstetric anesthesiologists have advocated reconsidering this warning as the risk of postoperative pulmonary complications is increased in pregnancy and Sugammadex is superior to traditional reversal.

B. **Procedures directly related to pregnancy**
1. **Ruptured ectopic pregnancy** is the leading cause of maternal death in the first trimester and is a surgical emergency. Intra-abdominal hemorrhage is common, and it is prudent to have blood available in the operating room even without hemodynamic instability.
2. **Abortion or miscarriage.** Spontaneous abortion refers to the loss of pregnancy before 20 weeks or at a fetal weight of less than 500 g (**Table 32.2**). A dilation and evacuation is often indicated for incomplete and missed abortions. Monitored anesthesia care, spinal, epidural, or general anesthesia can be used after careful assessment of the patient's NPO status, volume status, and presence of DIC or sepsis. Consideration to airway protection should be given in the second half of the second trimester and beyond.

TABLE 32.2 Spontaneous Abortion Classification

Type	Vaginal Bleeding	Cervix	Products of Conception	Management
Threatened	Y	Closed	In utero	Observation
Inevitable	Y	Dilated	In utero	Await spontaneous passage or induce labor
Missed	N	Closed	In utero	Await spontaneous passage, induce labor, or D&C
Incomplete	Y	Dilated	Partial expulsion	Emergent D&C
Complete	Y	Dilated	Complete expulsion	Observation

D&C, dilation and curettage.

3. **Cerclage placement.** An incompetent cervix might lead to early pregnancy loss and is treated with cerclage placement. A prophylactic cerclage is placed early in the second trimester to prevent preterm birth. A spinal anesthetic is recommended for this ~30-minute procedure, and a sensory block to T10 is required to cover the cervix, vagina, and perineum. In the case of rescue cerclage placement, which may be complicated by prolapse of membranes and cervical dilation, regional blockade may be utilized or an inhalational anesthetic may be preferred due to associated myometrial relaxation.
4. **Anesthesia for postpartum sterilization.** Elective postpartum tubal ligation is performed through an infraumbilical incision typically within 48 hours after delivery. The labor epidural may be dosed to achieve a T4 sensory level, although adequate epidural function decreases, the longer the interval after delivery. Spinal anesthesia is also common. Our practice is to use an intrathecal dose of 15 mg of 0.75% hyperbaric bupivacaine with 10 to 15 µg fentanyl. Increased neuraxial local anesthetic requirements are noted as soon as 12 hours postpartum secondary to the changes in intra-abdominal pressure following delivery. General anesthesia is reserved for rescue of intraoperative neuraxial failure. All patients should receive aspiration prophylaxis.

C. Procedures incidental to pregnancy
1. When a nonemergent procedure must be performed, the second trimester is preferred since organogenesis is complete and the risk of preterm labor is minimized.
2. The most common urgent/emergent procedures in pregnancy include appendicitis, cholecystitis, and bowel obstruction.
3. **Consultation with an obstetrician** preoperatively improves the assessment of risks and benefits to the patients and guides the choice of perioperative monitoring. Most commonly, FHR is measured before and after surgery. In select cases, continuous intraoperative FHR monitoring and uterine tocometry might be indicated.
4. **Use regional techniques when possible.**

XI. CPR DURING PREGNANCY
A. Cardiac arrest during pregnancy occurs in 1 per 9,000–12,000 admissions for delivery. CPR is more difficult in individuals who are pregnant, but survival to hospital discharge is as high as 58.9%. The American Heart Association recommends the following changes in the ACLS algorithm for cardiac arrest in pregnancy:
1. Standard **basic life support** and activation of the maternal cardiac arrest team (if present in the institution) should be initiated immediately upon discovery of a pregnant patient in cardiac arrest.
2. The patient should be placed **supine** for chest compressions. If the uterus is palpated at or above the umbilicus, or if the uterus cannot be assessed, **manual left uterine displacement** should be employed to relieve aortocaval compression. Left lateral tilt is no longer recommended due to the hindrance of effective chest compressions.
3. **No change in the hand position** for chest compressions is recommended. There is no evidence supporting prior guidelines to perform compressions higher on the sternum.
4. When indicated, **defibrillation should not be delayed to allow for removal of invasive fetal monitors.** Defibrillation energy does not change in pregnancy. Anterolateral pad placement is recommended, with attention to placement of the lateral pad underneath the breast tissue.

5. **Rapid development of hypoxemia** should be anticipated in the pregnant patient due to lower oxygen reserve and higher metabolic demand. Difficult airway management should also be expected.
6. Intravenous or intraosseous **access** should be obtained **above the diaphragm** due to possibly impeded lower extremity venous return due to aortocaval compression.
7. Resuscitation drugs should be administered per ACLS guidelines without alteration.
8. Evaluation of fetal well-being during maternal cardiac arrest should not be carried out due to the risk of interference with maternal resuscitation or monitoring.
9. **Perimortem cesarean delivery** (PMCD) should be completed **within 5 minutes** of maternal arrest with unsuccessful resuscitation in a woman with fundal height at or above the umbilicus. PMCD may facilitate maternal resuscitation while also limiting fetal anoxia. Delivery should be performed at the site of arrest.
10. Causes of maternal cardiac arrest may be remembered with mnemonics like **BEAUCHOPS** (**b**leeding/DIC, **e**mbolism, **a**nesthetic complications, **u**terine atony, **c**ardiac disease, **h**ypertension, **o**ther [common etiologies as in standard ACLS guidelines], **p**lacenta previa or placental abruption, **s**epsis).

XII. ANESTHESIA FOR GYNECOLOGIC SURGERY

A. **Abdominal procedures** are performed under general anesthesia, whereas **pelvic surgery** can be performed using either regional or general anesthesia. For pelvic procedures, duration of the procedure, intraoperative blood loss, fluid shifts, laparoscopic approach, and Trendelenburg positioning might require control of the airway and general anesthesia. Rescue IV and radial artery access may be limited by draping and positioning.

B. **Vaginal and intrauterine surgeries** may be performed using regional or general anesthesia. A T10 level is sufficient for these procedures, while a T4–T6 level is necessary for vaginal hysterectomy.

XIII. ANESTHESIA FOR OOCYTE RETRIEVAL

A. Oocytes are retrieved with a transvaginal needle under ultrasound guidance. Immobility during the procedure minimizes risks and improves the quality of retrieval.

1. **Monitored anesthesia care** with moderate-to-deep sedation is the most common anesthetic choice. Midazolam, fentanyl, remifentanil, and meperidine do not appear to affect fertility.
2. **General anesthesia.** There is no conclusive evidence that the commonly used inhalational anesthetics adversely affect pregnancy or live birth rates for in vitro fertilization procedures. However, nitrous oxide might be avoided due to its interference with DNA synthesis. Volatile halogenated anesthetics may interfere with DNA synthesis and mitosis. While propofol is found in follicular fluid, no DNA damage has been observed and fertility outcomes are comparable to regional anesthetic techniques.
3. **Spinal anesthesia** can provide excellent surgical conditions and provides the advantage of minimizing oocyte exposure to anesthetic agents. Postoperative recovery is often longer than with general anesthesia.

Suggested Readings

Bauer ME, Arendt K, Beilin Y, et al. The Society for Obstetric Anesthesia and Perinatology Interdisciplinary Consensus statement on neuraxial procedures in obstetric patients with thrombocytopenia. *Anesth Analg.* 2021;132(6):1531–1544.

Bollag L, Lim G, Sultan P, et al. Society for Obstetric Anesthesia and Perinatology: consensus statement and recommendations for enhanced recovery after cesarean. *Anesth Analg.* 2021;132(5):1362–1377.

Chestnut D, Wong C, Tsen L, et al., eds. *Chestnut's Obstetric Anesthesia: Principles and Practice.* 6th ed. Elsevier; 2020.

Committee on Practice Bulletins – Obstetrics. ACOG Practice Bulletin No. 202: gestational hypertension and preeclampsia. *Obstet Gynecol.* 2019;133(1):1.

Devroe S, Bleeser T, Van de Velde M, et al. Anesthesia for non-obstetric surgery during pregnancy in a tertiary referral center: a 16-year retrospective, matched case-control, cohort study. *Int J Obstet Anesth.* 2019;39:74–81.

Jeejeebhoy FM, Zelop CM, Lipman S, et al; American Heart Association Emergency Cardiovascular Care Committee, Council on Cardiopulmonary, Critical Care, Perioperative and Resuscitation, Council on Cardiovascular Diseases in the Young, and Council on Clinical Cardiology. Cardiac arrest in pregnancy: a scientific statement from the American Heart Association. *Circulation.* 2015;132(18):1747–1773.

Lim G, Facco FL, Nathan N, Waters JH, Wong CA, Eltzschig HK. A review of the impact of obstetric anesthesia on maternal and neonatal outcomes. *Anesthesiology.* 2018;129(1):192–215.

Lipman S, Cohen S, Einav S, et al; Society for Obstetric Anesthesia and Perinatology. The Society for Obstetric Anesthesia and Perinatology consensus statement on the management of cardiac arrest in pregnancy. *Anesth Analg.* 2014;118:1003–1016.

Meng ML, Arendt KW. Obstetric anesthesia and heart disease: practical clinical considerations. *Anesthesiology.* 2021;135(1):164–183.

Mhyre JM, Sultan P. General anesthesia for cesarean delivery: occasionally essential but best avoided. *Anesthesiology.* 2019;130(6):864–866.

Mushambi MC, Kinsella SM, Popat M, et al; Obstetric Anaesthetists' Association; Difficult Airway Society. Obstetric Anaesthetists' Association and Difficult Airway Society guidelines for the management of difficult and failed tracheal intubation in obstetrics. *Anaesthesia.* 2015;70(11):1286–1306.

Practice guidelines for obstetric anesthesia: an updated report by the American Society of Anesthesiologists Task Force on Obstetric Anesthesia and the Society for Obstetric Anesthesia and Perinatology. *Anesthesiology.* 2016;124:270.

Sultan P. A narrative review of the literature relevant to obstetric anesthesiologists: the 2023 Gerard W. Ostheimer lecture. *Int J Obstet Anesth.* 2024;58:103973.

Tamirisa K, Elkayam U, Briller J, et al. Arrhythmias in pregnancy. *J Am Coll Cardiol EP.* 2022;8(1):120–135.

U.S. Food and Drug Administration. *FDA Drug Safety Communication: FDA Review Results in New Warnings about Using General Anesthetics and Sedation Drugs in Young Children and Pregnant Women.* FDA; 2016.

33 Anesthesia for Pediatric Surgery and Care of the Neonate

Christopher Bean and Chang A. Liu

I. FETAL DEVELOPMENT
   A. Organogenesis is virtually complete after the 12th gestational week.
   B. Respiratory development
   1. **Anatomic**
      a. **The lungs** begin as a bud on the embryonic gut in the 4th week of gestation. Failure of separation of the lung bud from the gut later results in the formation of a **tracheoesophageal fistula (TEF)**.
      b. **The diaphragm** forms during the 4th through 10th week of gestation, dividing the abdominal and thoracic cavities.
         1. If the diaphragm is not completely formed when the midgut reenters the abdomen from the umbilical pouch, the abdominal contents can enter the thorax.
         2. The presence of abdominal contents within the thorax is associated with arrested lung growth.
         3. The lungs from patients with **congenital diaphragmatic hernia (CDH)** have a decreased number of arterioles and alveoli in the hypoplastic lung. In addition, the pulmonary arteries of both lungs are abnormally thick and reactive, resulting in increased pulmonary vascular resistance.
   2. **Physiologic**
      a. **Lung development** is generally insufficient for survival at less than the 23rd week of gestation, prior to the saccular stage of lung development. This is when thinning of the pulmonary interstitium due to decreased collagen fiber deposition, increased cellular differentiation, and capillary development begins the capacity for gas exchange.
      b. Secretion of **surfactant,** which reduces alveolar wall surface tension and promotes alveolar aeration, is often inadequate until the last month of gestation.
         1. Birth before 32 weeks of gestation is associated with **respiratory distress syndrome (RDS)**.
         2. Because glucose metabolism affects lung surfactant maturation, infants of diabetic mothers are at increased risk of RDS when prematurely born at later stages of gestation.
         3. Antenatal treatment with steroids is associated with a decrease in the incidence of RDS in prematurely born infants.
      c. After birth, the onset of breathing is stimulated by hypoxemia, hypercarbia, tactile stimulation, and a decrease in plasma prostaglandin E_2. After aeration and distension of the lung, the pulmonary vascular resistance decreases, and pulmonary blood flow increases nearly 10-fold. Failure of the reduction of pulmonary vascular resistance after birth is associated with extrapulmonary shunting of blood and severe hypoxemia and is called **persistent pulmonary hypertension of the newborn (PPHN)**.

C. Cardiovascular development
1. Anatomic
  a. **The cardiovascular system is the first organ system to function in utero. Its formation consists of three developmental stages including tube formation, looping, and septation. Heart formation is complete by approximately 8 weeks of gestation.**
  b. The primitive **cardiac tube** consists of the sinoatrium, the ventricle, the bulbus cordis (primitive right ventricle), and the truncus (primitive main pulmonary artery). During the 2nd month of gestation, a heart with two parallel pumping systems develops out of this initially tubular system. During this process, various structures divide and migrate. Failure of structural maturation at this stage of development causes numerous cardiac malformations. For example:
     1. Failure of division of the sinoatrium into the two atria results in a single atrium. Improper closure results in an **atrial septal defect.**
     2. Failure of migration of the ventricular septum and atrioventricular valve between the primitive ventricle and the bulbus cordis results in a **double-outlet left ventricle** (single ventricle). Minor migrational defects result in **ventriculoseptal defects.**
     3. Failure of division of the truncus into the pulmonary artery and the aorta results in **truncus arteriosus.**
  c. The aortic arch system initially consists of six pairs of arches.
     1. The sixth arches produce the pulmonary arteries. The **ductus arteriosus** develops from the distal portion of the right sixth arch. Although the left proximal sixth arch usually degenerates, it can persist and form an aberrant left ductus arteriosus.
     2. Failure of regression of various portions of the aorta and arch system also can result in aberrant vessels and vascular rings. For example, failure of regression causes a **double aortic arch.** Regression of the left-sided but not the right-sided arches can result in a right-sided aortic arch.

2. Physiologic
  a. **Fetal circulation.** After the 12th week, the circulatory system is in its final form. Oxygenated blood from the placenta passes through the umbilical vein and the ductus venosus and returns to the heart. Subsequently, 85% to 95% of fetal cardiac output bypasses the pulmonary circulation by flowing right to left through the foramen ovale and the ductus arteriosus into the aorta.
  b. **At birth,** umbilical placental circulation ceases with the clamping of the umbilical cord, and blood flow through the ductus venosus ceases. However, the ductus venosus often remains patent for up to a week. Also, the interruption of umbilical blood flow at birth reduces right atrial pressure and causes functional closure of the foramen ovale. Moreover, pulmonary resistance decreases as the lungs are distended and ventilated at birth, while systemic resistance increases with removal of the high-capacitance placental circulation. Constriction of the ductus arteriosus occurs with increasing PaO_2. Cessation of ductus arteriosus blood flow often occurs within several hours to days in term infants but may be delayed in premature or sick infants.

D. Body composition
  1. **Extracellular fluid** (ECF) and total body water decrease as the fetus grows, while intracellular fluid increases with gestational age. ECF is 90% of total body weight at 28 weeks, 80% at 36 weeks, and 75% at term.

2. After birth, a physiologic diuresis occurs, with the term infant losing 5% to 10% of ECF in the first few days of life. Premature infants may lose up to 15% of ECF.
3. Before 32 weeks of gestation, the **neonatal kidney is immature** and has a relatively low glomerular filtration rate and altered tubular function. This leads to difficulties in excreting water loads and diminished capacity to reabsorb sodium and water and thereby concentrate urine. In part, this is due to incomplete glomerular development, tubule insensitivity to vasopressin, loops of Henle that have not yet penetrated into the medulla, low osmolality in the medullary interstitium, and low serum urea levels. Renal tubular function increases with postnatal age, and the concentrating ability of the kidney reaches adult levels at 6 to 12 months postnatal age.

II. ANATOMY AND PHYSIOLOGY
A. Upper airway
1. **Neonates are obligate nose breathers** due to weak oropharyngeal muscles and increased compliance of the pharynx, larynx, and bronchial tree. Their nares are relatively narrow, and a significant fraction of the work of breathing is needed to overcome nasal resistance. Occlusion of the nares by bilateral choanal atresia or tenacious secretions can cause complete airway obstruction; however, some infants will convert to mouth breathing. Placement of an oral airway, a laryngeal mask airway, or an endotracheal tube may be necessary to reestablish airway patency during sedation or anesthesia.
2. **Infants have relatively large tongues**, which can make mask ventilation and laryngoscopy challenging. Studies have called tongue size into question and found the tongue to be proportional in children aged 1 to 12. Clinically, the tongue can easily obstruct the airway if excessive submandibular pressure is applied during mask ventilation.
3. **Infants and children have a more cephalad glottis** (C3 vertebral level in premature infants, C4 in infants, and C5 in adults) and **a narrow, long, angulated epiglottis,** which can make laryngoscopy difficult.
4. In infants and young children, functionally **the narrowest part of the airway is at the cricoid cartilage** (recent studies have questioned this; see suggested readings), rather than at the glottis (as in adults). An endotracheal tube that passes through the cords may still be too large distally.
5. **Deciduous teeth** erupt within the first year and are shed between ages 6 and 13 years. To avoid dislodging a loose tooth, it is safest to open the mandible directly, without introducing a finger or appliance into the oral cavity. Loose teeth should be documented on the preoperative evaluation. In some instances, unstable teeth should be removed before laryngoscopy. Parents and patients should be informed of this possibility in advance.
6. **Airway resistance** in infants and children can be increased dramatically by subtle changes in an already small-caliber system. Even a small amount of edema can significantly increase airway resistance and cause airway compromise.

B. Pulmonary system (Table 33.1)
1. Neonates have **higher metabolic rates,** resulting in an elevated oxygen consumption (6 mL/kg/min) when compared with adults (3 mL/kg/min).
2. **Neonatal lungs have high closing volumes,** which fall within the lower range of their normal tidal volume. Below closing volume, alveolar collapse and shunting occur.

TABLE 33.1 Age Dependence of Typical Respiratory Parameters

Variable	Newborn	1 Y	3 Y	5 Y	Adult
Respirations (breaths/min)	40–60	20–30	Gradual decrease to 18–25	18–25	12–20
Tidal volume (mL)	15	80	110	250	500
Functional residual capacity (mL/kg)	25		35		40
Minute ventilation (L/min)	1	1.8	2.5	5.5	6.5
Hemoglobin(g/dL)	14–20	10–11	—	—	13–17
Hematocrit (%)	47–60	33–42			38–50
Arterial pH	7.30–7.40	7.35–7.45	—	—	—
$Paco_2$ (mm Hg)	30–35	30–40	—	—	—
Pao_2 (mm Hg)	60–90	80–100	—	—	—

3. To meet the higher oxygen demand, infants have a **higher respiratory rate and minute ventilation.** An infant's functional residual capacity (FRC) is nearly equivalent to that of an adult, on a per weight basis. Their higher minute ventilation to FRC ratio results in rapid inhalational induction. The tidal volume for infants and adults is equivalent (6 to 7 mL/kg).
4. **Anatomic shunts** including patent ductus arteriosus (PDA) and patent foramen ovale may develop significant right-to-left flow with increases in pulmonary artery pressure (eg, hypoxia, acidosis, or high positive airway pressure). This may predispose to air emboli if care is not taken to remove it from the IV tubing.
5. The characteristics of the infant's pulmonary system contribute to **rapid desaturation during apnea.** Profound desaturation can occur when an infant coughs or strains and alveoli collapse. Treatment may require deepening anesthesia, using neuromuscular relaxants, as well as alveolar recruitment.
6. The **diaphragm** is the infant's major muscle of ventilation. Compared with the adult diaphragm, the newborn has only half the number of type I, slow-twitch, high-oxidative muscle fibers essential for sustained increased respiratory effort. Thus, the infant's diaphragm fatigues earlier than the adult's. By 2 years of age, the child's diaphragm would have attained mature levels of type I fibers.
7. The **pliable rib cage** (compliant chest wall) of an infant cannot maintain negative intrathoracic pressure easily. This diminishes the efficacy of the infant's attempts to increase ventilation.
8. An infant's **dead space** is 2 to 2.5 mL/kg, equivalent to an adult's.
9. Infants' high baseline minute ventilation limits their ability to increase their ventilatory effort further. End-tidal CO_2 concentrations should be followed if spontaneous ventilation is permitted under anesthesia; assisted or controlled ventilation may be necessary.
10. **Alveolar maturation** occurs by 8 to 10 years of age when alveoli number and size reach adult ranges.

Table 33.2 Cardiovascular Variables

Age	Heart Rate (beats/min)	Blood Pressure (mm Hg)	
		Systolic	Diastolic
Preterm neonate	120–180	45–60	30
Term neonate	100–180	55–70	40
1 y	100–140	70–100	60
3 y	84–115	75–110	70
5 y	84–100	80–120	70

11. **Retinopathy of prematurity (ROP)** (discussed later in the chapter).
12. **Apnea and bradycardia** after general anesthesia occur with increased frequency in infants who are premature and in infants who have anemia, sepsis, hypothermia, central nervous system disease, hypoglycemia, or other metabolic derangements. These patients should have cardiorespiratory monitoring for a minimum of 24 hours postoperatively. Such infants are not candidates for ambulatory day surgery. The guidelines for discharge vary among institutions. Most hospitals agree that infants who are <45 to 60 weeks of postconceptual age are monitored postoperatively. Any full-term infant who displays apnea after general anesthesia should also be monitored.

C. Cardiovascular system
1. **Heart rate** and **blood pressure** vary with age and should be maintained at age-appropriate levels perioperatively (**Tables 33.2**).
2. **Cardiac output** is 180 to 240 mL/kg/min in newborns, which is two to three times that of adults. This higher cardiac output is necessary to meet the higher metabolic oxygen consumption demands.
3. The **ventricles** are less compliant and have a relatively smaller contractile muscle mass in newborns and infants. The ability to increase contractility is limited; increases in cardiac output occur by increasing heart rate rather than stroke volume. Bradycardia is the most deleterious dysrhythmia in infants, and hypoxemia is a frequent cause of bradycardia in infants and children.
4. Neonates have immature calcium signaling and handling in the sarcoplasmic reticulum and myocardium and are more dependent on ionized calcium concentrations for myocardial function.

D. Fluid and electrolyte balance
1. The **glomerular filtration rate** at birth is 15% to 30% of the normal adult value. Adult value is reached by 1 year of age. Renal clearance of drugs and their metabolites is diminished during the first year of life.
2. Neonates have an intact renin–angiotensin–aldosterone pathway, but the distal tubules resorb less sodium in response to aldosterone. Thus, newborns are "obligate sodium losers," and IV fluids should contain sodium.
3. The **total body water** in the preterm infant is 90% of body weight. In term infants, it is 80%; at 6 to 12 months, it is 60%. This increased percentage of total body water affects drug volumes of distribution. The dosages of some drugs (eg, propofol, succinylcholine, pancuronium, and rocuronium) are >20% to 30% are equally effective dose for adults.

E. Hematologic system
1. Normal values for hemoglobin and hematocrit are listed in **Table 33.1**. The nadir of physiologic anemia is at 3 months of age, and the hemoglobin may reach 10 to 11 g/dL in an otherwise healthy infant. Premature infants may demonstrate a decrease in hemoglobin concentration as early as 4 to 6 weeks of age.
2. At birth, **fetal hemoglobin** (HbF) predominates, but β-chain synthesis shifts to the adult type (HbA) by 3 to 4 months of age. HbF has a higher affinity for oxygen; that is, the oxyhemoglobin dissociation curve is shifted to the left, but debate exists regarding the clinical relevance.
3. See Section X.B for calculations of blood volume and red cell mass.

F. Hepatobiliary system
1. **Liver enzyme systems,** particularly those involved in phase-II (conjugation) reactions, are immature in the infant. Drugs metabolized by the P-450 system may have prolonged elimination times.
2. **Jaundice** is common in neonates and can be physiologic or have pathologic causes.
3. **Hyperbilirubinemia** and displacement of bilirubin from albumin by drugs can result in kernicterus. Premature infants develop kernicterus at lower levels of bilirubin than do term infants.
4. **Plasma levels of albumin** are lower at birth and as a result, drugs that are protein bound may have a higher free fraction and higher effective concentration.

G. Endocrine system
1. **Newborns,** particularly premature babies and those small for gestational age, have decreased glycogen stores and are more susceptible to **hypoglycemia**. Infants of diabetic mothers have high insulin levels because of prolonged exposure to elevated maternal serum glucose levels and are prone to hypoglycemia. Infants who fall into these groups may have dextrose requirements as high as 5 to 15 mg/kg/min. Normal glucose concentrations in the full-term infant are ≥45 mg/dL (2.5 mmol/L).
2. **Hypocalcemia** is common in infants who are premature, are small for gestational age, have a history of asphyxia, are offspring of diabetic mothers, or have received transfusions with citrated blood or fresh-frozen plasma. Serum calcium concentration should be monitored in these patients and calcium administered if the ionized calcium is <4.0 mg/dL (1.0 mmol/L).

H. Temperature regulation
1. Compared with adults, infants and children have a greater surface area to body weight ratio, which increases loss of body heat.
2. Infants have significantly less muscle mass and cannot compensate for cold by shivering or adjusting their behavior to avoid the cold.
3. Infants respond to cold stress by increasing norepinephrine production, which enhances metabolism in brown fat. Norepinephrine also produces pulmonary and peripheral vasoconstriction, which can lead to right-to-left shunting, hypoxemia, and metabolic acidosis. Sick and preterm infants have limited stores of brown fat and therefore are more susceptible to cold. Strategies to prevent cold stress are discussed later in the chapter.

III. THE PREANESTHETIC VISIT
General principles of the preanesthetic visit are discussed in Chapter 1. The preoperative visit is an excellent opportunity to address the concerns of the child and parents.

A. **History** should include the following:
   1. Maternal health during gestation, including alcohol or drug use, smoking, diabetes, hypertension, and viral infections
   2. Prenatal concerns (Poly- or oligohydramnios, abnormal α-fetoprotein, maternal infections, and premature labor are often associated with neonatal problems)
   3. Gestational age and weight
   4. Events during labor and delivery, including Apgar scores and length of hospital stay
   5. Hospitalizations/emergency room visits
   6. Congenital, chromosomal, metabolic anomalies or syndromes
   7. Recent upper respiratory infections, tracheobronchitis, "croup," reactive airway disease (asthma), exposure to communicable diseases, cyanotic episodes, or history of snoring
   8. Sleeping position (prone, side, or supine)
   9. Respiratory quality and pattern (ie, noisy breathing that increases with sleep; periods of apnea with sleep)
   10. Growth history
   11. Vomiting and gastroesophageal reflux
   12. Siblings' health
   13. Parents who smoke
   14. Past surgical and anesthetic history
   15. Allergies (environmental, drugs, food, and latex)
   16. Bleeding tendencies
B. **Physical examination** of the pediatric patient should include:
   1. General appearance, alertness, color, tone, congenital anomalies, head size and shape, activity level, and social interaction
   2. Vital signs, height, and weight
   3. Loose teeth, craniofacial anomalies, or large tonsils that could complicate airway management
   4. Respiratory pattern and quality. Signs of upper respiratory infection and/or reactive airways disease (excessive secretions may predispose patients to laryngospasm and bronchospasm during induction and emergence of anesthesia)
   5. Cardiac exam including age-appropriate heart rate, rhythm, and heart murmurs (which may indicate flow through anatomic shunts)
   6. Potential vascular access sites
   7. Strength, developmental milestones, activity level, and motor and verbal skills
   8. Additional exam(s) pertinent to specific anesthetic/surgical condition
C. **Preoperative evaluation and physical examination of the neonate** should include the following:
   1. A complete, systematic evaluation is needed. No assumptions should be made about the development, location, or function of organ systems. An abnormality in one system may be associated with abnormalities in another.
   2. **Vital signs** provide a useful physiologic screen of organ function. If a cardiac abnormality is suspected, a chest x-ray (CXR), electrocardiogram (ECG), and four extremity blood pressure measurements are required. Postductal oxygen saturation should be >94%. In addition, an echocardiogram and pediatric cardiology consultation should be considered. Normal vital signs are summarized in **Table 33.2**.
   3. **Gestational age** influences care, management, and survival potential of the neonate. An infant is considered preterm if the gestational age is

<37 weeks, term if it is 37 to 41 weeks, late term if it is 41 to 42 weeks, and post term if the gestational age is more than 42 weeks. Although the date of conception and ultrasound examination can be used to predict gestational age, a physical examination to determine gestational age should be performed. **The Dubowitz–Ballard scoring system** involves evaluation of physical characteristics of the skin, external genitalia, ears, breasts, and neuromuscular behavior to assess gestational age.

4. **Weight determination.** Similar to gestational age, birth weight is an important prognostic factor for premature infants. By convention, low–birth-weight (LBW) infants weigh <2500 g, very low–birth-weight infants (VLBW) <1500 g, and extremely low–birth-weight (ELBW) infants <1000 g. Intrauterine growth restriction (IUGR) is defined as a rate of growth less than a fetus' predetermined genetic potential. **Small-for-gestational age (SGA) infants at birth are <10th percentile of the standard population–based weight.** This may be the result of chromosomal defects, maternal hypertension, chronic placental insufficiency, maternal cigarette or drug use, or congenital infection. These infants have a high incidence of hypoglycemia, hypocalcemia, and polycythemia. Infants who are **large for gestational age** (LGA) are >90th percentile of standard population–based weight and may have mothers with diabetes. In the immediate postnatal period, LGA newborns should be evaluated for hypoglycemia and polycythemia. Infants of diabetic mothers and LGA infants are at risk of complications from fetal macrosomia, including shoulder dystocia and brachial plexus injuries.

5. **Respiratory.** Signs of respiratory distress include tachypnea, grunting, nasal flaring, intercostal and subcostal retractions, rales, rhonchi, asymmetry of breath sounds, and apnea. **Pulse oximetry** is used to screen the levels of systemic oxygenation in neonates. Blood gas tensions should be measured in patients with suspected cardiopulmonary abnormalities.

6. **Cardiovascular.** Central cyanosis and capillary refill should be assessed. Distal pulses should be palpated, noting whether they are bounding. A delay between brachial and femoral pulses is suggestive of **coarctation of the aorta.** Note the character and location of murmurs and splitting of the second heart sound. During the first 48 hours after birth, murmurs may appear as intracardiac pressure gradients change and disappear as the ductus arteriosus closes.

7. **Abdominal exam.** A scaphoid abdomen suggests **diaphragmatic hernia.** A normal umbilical cord has two arteries and one vein. In nearly 40% of cases, the existence of a single umbilical artery is associated with renal abnormalities. The size of the liver, spleen, and kidneys and the presence of hernias or abdominal masses should be determined by inspection and palpation. The location and patency of the anus should be assessed.

8. **Neurologic.** A thorough examination includes evaluation of motor activity, muscle strength and tone, and newborn reflexes (Moro, tonic neck, grasp, suck, and stepping reflexes). Full-term newborns should have an up-going Babinski reflex and brisk deep tendon reflexes.

9. **Genitourinary.** The gonads may be differentiated or ambiguous, and in males, the testes should be palpable. The location of the urethra should be determined, remembering that hypospadias precludes a circumcision. A male infant with hypospadias and bilateral cryptorchidism must be evaluated for congenital adrenal hyperplasia.

10. **Musculoskeletal.** Any deformities, unusual posturing, or asymmetric limb movement should be noted, and the hips should be examined

for possible dislocation with congenital hip dysplasia, particularly in breech infants. A clavicle or humerus may be fractured during a difficult delivery.
11. **Craniofacial.** One should determine head circumference, the location and size of the fontanelles, the presence of a cephalohematoma or caput, and ensure the palate is intact. Observing nasal gas flow despite occluding each naris or passage of a nasogastric tube will rule out choanal atresia.

D. **Laboratory studies.** Routine initial laboratory studies may include hematocrit and serum glucose. Additional studies should be guided by the individual problem. For example, blood type and Coombs determination may be indicated in infants at risk for hyperbilirubinemia such as those whose mothers who are blood type O. In addition, a complete blood count (CBC) and blood culture should be checked and wide spectrum antibiotic therapy initiated if there is suspicion of neonatal sepsis or maternal chorioamnionitis. For older children, laboratory studies appropriate for the child's illness and proposed surgery should be obtained. Most centers agree that a "routine hemoglobin" is unnecessary for healthy children. If indicated, laboratory tests can often be obtained after induction of general anesthesia (eg, blood bank sample).

E. **Fluids**
   1. **The total fluid requirement** varies with birth weight.
      a. <1.0 kg, use 100 mL/kg/d.
      b. 1.0 to 1.5 kg, use 80 to 90 mL/kg/d.
      c. 1.5 to 2.5 kg, use 80 mL/kg/d.
      d. >2.5 kg, use 60 mL/kg/d.
   2. **Isosmolar solutions** should be used.
      a. **Electrolyte supplementation** is not required within the first day of life for maintenance fluids in full-term infants. For premature infants, check the electrolytes at 8 to 12 hours of life and consider adjusting the fluid infusion rate and/or adding electrolytes as indicated.
      b. **10% Dextrose** in water is typically used as the initial IV fluid in preterm and term infants. Blood glucose concentrations should be monitored closely in high-risk infants and the dextrose concentration of IV fluids should be adjusted as required to maintain serum glucose levels described below.
   3. Additional fluids may be required **for insensible water loss.**
      a. Fluid requirements increase with lower birth weight and gestational age, as well as with many neonatal interventions including phototherapy, radiant warmer use, and support of infant with respiratory distress.
      b. Insensible losses from pathologic causes (eg, omphalocele, gastroschisis, neural tube defect, bladder exstrophy) must similarly be taken into account and replaced. The electrolyte composition of the replacement fluid should match that of what is lost.
      c. Infants who are mechanically ventilated absorb free water through their respiratory system.
   4. Several signs will determine the adequacy of fluid infusions.
      a. Urine output at least 1 mL/kg/h.
      b. Only a 1% loss in body weight per day for the first 10 days of life.
      c. Stable hemodynamics and good perfusion.

F. **Electrolytes**
   1. The usual electrolyte requirements after the first 12 to 24 hours of life are as follows:

a. Na^+, 2 to 4 mEq/kg/d.
b. K^+, 1 to 2 mEq/kg/d.
c. Ca^{+2}, 150 to 220 mEq/kg/d.
2. The frequency of laboratory tests for serum electrolyte levels will be determined by the rate of insensible loss.

G. Glucose. Supplemental glucose should be given after birth to keep blood glucose levels between 50 and 125 mg/dL.
1. In most infants, 10% D/W at maintenance fluid rates will provide adequate glucose. This infusion rate provides the 5 to 8 mg/kg/min of glucose that is required for basal metabolism.
2. Infants with hyperinsulinism, intrauterine growth restriction, or metabolic defects can require glucose infusion rates as high as 12 to 15 mg/kg/min.
3. In peripheral intravenous lines, up to 12.5% D/W may be infused. In central lines, 15% to 20% D/W may be infused.
4. **Hypoglycemia** (glucose <50 mg/dL) is treated with a bolus of glucose at 200 mg/kg IV over 1 min and increased glucose infusion rate. Serial blood tests are necessary to determine the effectiveness of the increased glucose.

H. Nutrition. The gastrointestinal tract is functional after 28 weeks of gestation but is of limited capacity. Requirements vary with each neonate.
1. **Calories.** Requirements are 100 to 130 kcal/kg/d.
2. **Protein.** Requirements are 2 to 4 g/kg/d.
3. **Fat.** Initiate at 1 g/kg/d and increase gradually as tolerated up to 3 to 4 g/kg/d so that the fat provides 40% of the daily calories.
4. **Vitamins** A, B, C, D, E, and K should be provided.
5. **Iron.** Requirements are 2 to 4 mg/kg/d of elemental iron. The adequacy of iron supplementation can be assessed by measuring the hemoglobin or hematocrit and the reticulocyte count.
6. **Minerals.** Calcium, phosphate, magnesium, zinc, copper, manganese, selenium, and iron need to be replaced. Premature infants, in particular, have increased calcium and phosphate requirements in order to prevent metabolic bone disease of prematurity.
7. **Enteral feedings.** Feedings are usually initiated with breast milk or a formula that contains the whey-to-casein ratio that is contained in breast milk. For infants that exhibit lactose intolerance, non- or low-lactose containing formulas are available. Infants <32 weeks of gestation often have poor suck and swallow reflexes and require gavage feedings. For premature infants or ill full-term neonates, small volume enteral feedings are generally initiated once the baby is stable. Subsequently, the volumes of the feedings are gradually increased every 12 to 24 hours as they are tolerated. Once the desired goal volume of enteral feedings is reached, the breast milk or formula is supplemented with additional calories, as needed, to attain the desired weight gain.
8. **Parenteral feeding.** If enteral feeding is impossible, parenteral nutrition should be started as soon as possible to promote positive nitrogen balance and growth. The metabolic status of the infant should be assessed frequently so that the parenteral formulation can be adjusted to meet the infant's needs and to identify signs of toxicity from hyperalimentation. Usual studies include serum glucose, electrolytes, osmolality, liver function tests, blood urea nitrogen, creatinine, lipid levels, and platelet count.

I. Thermoregulation. It is critical to measure the newborn's body temperature and use active measures to maintain it in a euthermic range. Babies exhibit thermal instability because of decreased epidermal and dermal thickness, minimal subcutaneous fat, immature nervous system, and increased surface area to body weight ratio with a relatively large head size. Moreover, premature newborns are particularly susceptible to hypothermia because they lack thermogenic brown fat cells. Measures to maintain the newborn's body heat include using a warm incubator during transport to and from the nursery; keeping the ambient operating room temperature at 85 °F (30 °C); using warming blankets, radiant warmers, and a head cover; and prewarming intravenous fluids. Neonates with significant cold stress are particularly prone to hypoglycemia.

IV. PERIPROCEDURAL CONSIDERATIONS AND FASTING GUIDELINES
A. Periprocedural considerations
1. Children face multiple stressors in the perioperative period. They may not understand the specific disease; the concept of anesthesia, or the procedure itself. Honesty about the procedure(s), associated pain, and the sequence of events is essential in maintaining the trust of children regardless of their level of development.
   a. Approaches to optimize the periprocedural experience include the use of nonpharmacologic techniques. Examples of these strategies include distraction, humor, sharing control (eg, would you like to sit up or lie down for induction?), and medical reinterpretation of equipment. The use of a child life specialist, tablet, and/or a teaching module may decrease the need for preprocedure pharmacologic therapy and improve a child's experience.
2. Infants <8 months old generally tolerate short periods of separation from parents and usually do not require premedication.
3. Children 8 months to 5 years of age likely have developed separation anxiety and may require sedation before the induction of anesthesia (see Section VI.B).
4. Older children generally respond well to information and reassurance. Parental and patient anxiety may be reduced by having parents accompany their children to the operating room. An especially anxious child may benefit from premedication.
5. Premedication with intramuscular (IM) **anticholinergics** generally is not recommended. If vagolytic drugs are indicated, they are usually administered intravenously (IV) at the time of induction of anesthesia.
6. In the presence of **gastroesophageal reflux, ranitidine** (2 to 4 mg/kg PO, 2 mg/kg IV) along with **metoclopramide** (0.1 mg/kg) can be administered 2 hours before surgery to increase gastric pH and reduce gastric volume. Children receiving medications for medical problems such as reactive airway disease, seizures, or hypertension should continue to take these medications preoperatively.

B. Fasting guidelines
1. Milk, breast milk, formula, and solid foods should be restricted as outlined in **Table 33.3**.
2. The **last feeding** should consist of clear fluids or sugar water. Studies document that there is no increased risk of aspiration if clear fluids are offered up to 2 hours preoperatively. This policy minimizes preoperative dehydration and hypoglycemia and contributes to a smooth induction and stable operative course. We recommend that patients receive clear fluids until 2 hours before surgery is scheduled. Oral intake is then restricted (see **Table 33.3**).
3. If schedule delays occur, clear fluids may be given. Some patients may require IV placement for hydration and/or glucose administration.

TABLE 33.3 Fasting Guidelines

Type of Food	Fasting Guidelines (Hours)
Clear fluids	2
Breast milk	4
Nonhuman milk	6
Solid food	8

V. PREPARATION OF THE OPERATING ROOM
  A. Perioperative/procedure huddle is a useful meeting to confirm procedure details, anesthetic requirements, special concerns, patient-specific factors, and nonroutine steps.
   1. Conditions that require emergent surgery in neonates are often accompanied with medical problems. As a result, the care for these critically ill newborns requires careful coordination of medical, surgical, and nursing management. In some cases, surgical procedures might occur at the bedside in the neonatal intensive care unit (NICU). In these instances, before the surgical procedure is initiated, it is important to identify and integrate the key resources and care measures provided by the NICU team into the anesthetic management of the surgical procedure.
  B. **Anesthetic circuit**
   1. The **semiclosed circuit** normally used in adults has some disadvantages if used in infants or small children:
      a. The inspiratory and expiratory valves increase resistance during spontaneous ventilation: This can be overcome by closing the adjustable pressure-limiting (APL) valve to 3 to 5 cm of water and providing adequate gas flow rates to maintain pressure, or the use of pressure support).
      b. The large volume of the absorber system acts as a reservoir for anesthetic agents.
      c. The breathing circuit tubing has a large compression volume; however, neonatal and pediatric tubing are available that help compensate for this, as well as decrease the circuit dead space volume.
         1. The **nonrebreathing, open circuit (Mapleson D)** solves these problems (see Chapter 10: The Anesthesia Machine). **Rebreathing** is prevented by using fresh gas flows 2.0 to 2.5 times the minute ventilation to wash out carbon dioxide. Capnography is essential in recognizing rebreathing (inspired CO_2 >0) and avoiding excessive hyperventilation. This circuit is useful for very small infants who are allowed to breathe spontaneously and during transport. The specialized ventilators used in the NICU (eg, high-frequency oscillator ventilator) and continuous infusions of anesthetics and analgesics are often used for the patient during bedside surgery.
         2. A passive heat and moisture exchanger may be used with either circuit.
         3. The **reservoir bag volume** should be at least as large as the child's vital capacity but small enough so that a comfortable squeeze does not overinflate the chest. General guidelines for bag volumes are as follows: infants, 500-mL bag; 1 to 3 years, 1000-mL bag; and more than 3 years, 2000-mL bag.

4. For **most infants and children,** the semiclosed circuit-absorber system can be used with a smaller reservoir bag and a pediatric breathing circuit with small-caliber tubing (ie, circle system).

C. Airway equipment

1. A **mask** with minimal dead space should be chosen. A clear plastic type is preferred because the lips (for color) and mouth (for secretions and vomitus) can be visualized.
2. The appropriate size of **oral airway** can be estimated by holding the airway in position next to the child's face. The tip of the oral airway should reach to the angle of the mandible with the base at the lips.
3. **Laryngoscopy**
   a. A **narrow handle** is often preferred because it has a more natural feel when using a smaller blade.
   b. **Straight blade** (Miller or Wis-Hipple) is recommended for children <2 years old. The smaller flange and long tapered tip of the straight blade provide better visualization of the larynx and manipulation of the epiglottis in the confined spaces of a small oral cavity (see Section VII.A)
   c. **Curved blades** are generally used for patients more than 5 years old.
   d. **Guidelines for laryngoscope blade sizes (Table 33.4)**
   e. **Special consideration should be given to the use of video laryngoscopy in infants and neonates, as a recent Cochrane review suggests that video laryngoscopy may decrease the number of intubation attempts and increase the success of intubation on the first attempt.**
4. **Endotracheal tubes**. Traditionally, uncuffed tubes were used for children under 6 to 7 years of age (5.5-mm inner diameter endotracheal tube or smaller). However, the risk of tracheal stenosis is minimal with modern low-pressure cuffs, and cuffed tubes are more commonly used currently and provide additional benefit against aspiration in airway and abdominal surgeries. The size of the endotracheal tube is a significant factor for postoperative recovery in the pediatric patients. In our institution, we primarily use cuffed tubes. The size of cuffed endotracheal

TABLE 33.4 Guidelines for Choice of Laryngoscope Blades

Age	Blade
Premature and neonate	Miller 0
Infant up to 6–8 mo	Miller 0–1
9 mo to 2 y	Miller 1
	Wis-Hipple 1.5
2–5 y	Macintosh 1
	Miller 1–1.5
	Wis-Hipple 1.5
Child over 5 y	Macintosh 2
	Miller 2
Adolescent to adult	Macintosh 3
	Miller 2

Table 33.5 Guidelines for Uncuffed Endotracheal Tube Sizes

Age	Size (mm Internal Diameter)
Premature newborn	2.5–3.0
Full-term newborn	3.0
6–12 mo	3.5
12–20 mo	4.0
2 y	4.5
Over 2 y	4+ (age [years]/4)
6 y	5.5
10 y	6.5

Tube length at mouth (cm) = (10 + age [years])/2.

tube can be estimated with the equation: ET tube size (mm internal diameter) = (age/4) + 3.5.

5. Care must be taken not to overinflate the cuff and to realize that N_2O can diffuse into the cuff which can increase cuff pressure. At the time of intubation, endotracheal tubes that are one size larger and smaller than the estimated size should be available. Special techniques of endotracheal intubation are discussed in Section VII. **Table 33.5** provides guidelines for endotracheal tube sizes.

D. Temperature control
1. The **operating room should be warmed** to 80 °F to 90 °F before the child's arrival and an underbody warmer placed on the operating room table. Infants should be kept covered with a blanket and a hat.
2. **A servocontrolled radiant warmer** will keep infants warm during the induction of anesthesia and positioning. Skin temperature should be measured and should not exceed 39 °C.
3. **Passive heat and moisture exchangers** can be used for most routine cases. Some practitioners prefer to actively heat and humidify inspired gases during prolonged surgery.
4. Fluids, blood products, and irrigation solutions should be warmed.

E. Monitoring
1. In addition to standard monitoring (Chapter 15: Monitoring), a **precordial or esophageal stethoscope** provides information about heart and respiratory function.
2. **Blood pressure**
   a. A blood pressure cuff should cover at least two-thirds of the upper arm but not encroach on the axilla or antecubital space.
   b. The cuff can be placed on the leg if the arms are inaccessible (eg, cast present).
   c. Several manufacturers of oscillometric blood pressure cuffs have different preset initial pressure settings and cycle durations, for neonate, pediatric, and adult sized cuffs. Care should be taken to choose the appropriate size/setting to avoid inadvertent injury.
3. **Pulse oximetry** is one of the best indicators for the early detection of desaturation. It can also provide plethysmographic data on perfusion and respiratory variation.

Chapter 33 Anesthesia for Pediatric Surgery and Care of the Neonate

4. Observed **end-tidal carbon dioxide measurements** usually will be lower than expected when a nonrebreathing circuit is used, because exhaled gas will be diluted with high flows of fresh gases.
5. **Temperature** should routinely be monitored. In small infants esophageal, rectal, or axillary probes are acceptable. Once the drapes are placed, the warming blanket and room temperature should be adjusted so that children (especially small infants) do not become hyperthermic.
6. **Urine output** can provide a good reflection of volume status in children. In newborns, 0.5 mL/kg/h is adequate; for infants over 1 month of age, 1.0 mL/kg/h usually indicates adequate renal perfusion.
7. **Noninvasive cardiac output monitoring** is a developing technology that may provide earlier identification of hemodynamic changes in the pediatric patient when compared to the current monitoring methods. When this monitor was compared with transthoracic echocardiography, it was shown to have variability with absolute cardiac output; however, it has been shown to accurately predict volume responsiveness.
8. **EEG** utilization and density spectral array data (see Chapter 16: Monitoring Anesthetic Brain States) to determine depth of anesthesia can be a useful tool(s) to monitor the cortical biorhythm in the pediatric patient and prevent anesthetic overdose. Caution is advised in children under 2 years of age due to developmental changes in the EEG signal.

F. IV setup and supplies
1. For children <10 kg, a control chamber (burette) should be used to prevent inadvertent fluid administration and to quantify the fluid volume given.
2. Extension tubing (low volume) used as a drug push-line connected proximally to the patient facilitates drug administered as close to the IV insertion site as possible and prevents excessive flush fluid administration.
3. For older children, a pediatric infusion set is used where 60 drops equal 1 mL.
4. Extra care should be taken to purge IV tubing of air because right to left shunting of blood (and possibly air) can occur in infants with a patent foramen ovale. An air filter should be used in infants and children with known or suspected intracardiac shunts (some drugs are not compatible with these filters; ie, propofol).

VI. INDUCTION TECHNIQUES
A. Infants <8 months old can often be transported to the operating room without premedication; anesthesia can then be induced by an inhalation technique (see Section VI.C). The vessel-rich organs are proportionately larger, and the muscle and fat groups are smaller in neonates than in adults, affecting uptake and distribution of inhalation agents (see Chapter 11: Administration of General Anesthesia).

B. Preoperative sedation options for children 8 months to 5 years old (without established IV access) include the following:
1. Often children who are older than 5 to 6 years old are able to proceed to the procedure without sedation (see Section IV.A); however, these techniques are useful in special circumstances where sedation in an older child are required (ie, developmental delay, extreme anxiety, etc.)
2. **Oral midazolam,** 0.5 to 0.75 mg/kg, dissolved in sweet syrup, usually produces sedation within 20 minutes, although the time to onset of action can be quite variable. Patients often remain awake but sedated, and, generally, they will have no recall of leaving their parents or of induction of anesthesia.

3. **Oral ketamine,** 5 mg/kg given orally, produces sedation within 10 to 15 minutes and is synergistic with oral midazolam. Emergence time may be prolonged.
4. **Intranasal dexmedetomidine** (0.5 to 2 μg/kg) is an effective sedative given 30 to 75 minutes prior to induction with relatively preserved respiratory function. It has also been used to reduce emergence delirium, as an adjunct to postoperative pain management, and for opioid withdrawal. Side effects can include decreased sympathetic activity, including bradycardia and hypotension. Delayed emergence time should also be anticipated.
5. **Pulse oximetry** is used routinely once a patient is sedated.

C. Inhalation induction

1. This is the most common approach for pediatric patients, except when a rapid sequence IV induction is indicated.
2. An **excitement stage or "stage two"** of anesthesia with disconjugate gaze, injected conjunctiva, increased airway obstruction, altered breathing pattern, increased risk for laryngospasm and bronchospasm, muscular jerkiness, as well as sympathetic discharge as reflected by elevated heart rate and blood pressure is often encountered during inhalation induction. This is the critical period during induction of anesthesia; therefore, noise and activity in the operating room should be minimized during this stage. This stage should be explained to parents if they will be present during induction.
3. **Techniques**
    a. **Children 8 months to 5 years old** may be anesthetized after premedication. The inhalational induction can begin with nitrous oxide initially (eg, 4 L/min O_2 and 6 L/min nitrous oxide). Once the effect of the nitrous oxide is apparent, characterized by loss of attention and lack of patient response, the concentration of sevoflurane can be gradually increased in 0.5% to 1% increments.
    b. A **slow inhalation induction** may be used in cooperative toddlers and older children who have not received premedication. Children are shown how to breathe through a clear anesthetic mask. O_2 and N_2O are delivered via facemask, and sevoflurane is gradually added to the mixture. An engaging story incorporating breathing instructions can be very useful.
    c. A **"single-breath induction"** may be accomplished with a mixture of a volatile anesthetic with nitrous oxide.
        1. Loss of consciousness can be achieved with a single vital capacity breath of 8% sevoflurane and 70% N_2O in O_2. Desflurane and isoflurane are pungent volatile anesthetics that are not recommended for inhalation induction.
        2. The circuit is primed with 70% N_2O–O_2 and 7% to 8% sevoflurane. The end of the circuit should be occluded with a plug or another reservoir bag. Care should be taken to avoid environmental exposure of anesthetic gas to personnel in the room.
        3. Painting the mask with flavor extracts or flavored lip balm may increase acceptance by children.
        4. The child is instructed to take a deep breath approaching vital capacity of room air, blow it all out as a forced expiration, and then hold their breath. At this point, the anesthetist gently places the mask on the patient's face. The child then takes a deep inspiration of the anesthetic mixture and again holds their breath. This sequence is repeated for four or five breaths.

5. Most children will be anesthetized with an adequate vital capacity single breath sevoflurane inhalational induction within 60 seconds; a few children will need longer.
    d. Children can become frightened, uncooperative, and even combative during an inhalation induction. Should this occur, it is imperative to have a backup plan, such as an IM injection of a sedative or hypnotic medication.
D. **IM induction.** For the extremely uncooperative or developmentally delayed child, anesthesia may be induced with ketamine (4 to 8 mg/kg IM), which takes effect in 3 to 5 minutes. Atropine (0.02 mg/kg IM) or glycopyrrolate (0.01 mg/kg IM) should be mixed with the ketamine to prevent excessive salivation. Midazolam, 0.2 to 0.5 mg/kg IM, may also be given to reduce the chance of emergence delirium.
E. **IV induction**
    1. **For children more than 8 years old.** Often, older children may prefer an IV technique rather than a mask. Anesthesia can be induced with propofol (3 to 4 mg/kg). Ketamine (1 to 2 mg/kg) is a useful inductive agent in patients requiring hemodynamic stability upon induction. Etomidate (0.2 to 0.3 mg/kg) can be used in children with major trauma associated with hemodynamic instability or children with cardiomyopathy.
    2. IV induction at this age is often preferable to a mask induction because many older children do not like the smell of volatile anesthetics. Local anesthesia before IV placement can be achieved with subcutaneous injection of lidocaine 1%. Alternatively **EMLA cream** (a eutectic mixture of 2.5% lidocaine and 2.5% prilocaine), **LMX cream** (lidocaine 4%), or Synera (a heated topical patch with a eutectic mixture of lidocaine and tetracaine) can be applied to the skin approximately 45 minutes before IV placement. EMLA cream is also useful to reduce the pain of accessing a Portacath. The use of the jet injection lidocaine applicator is another method for achieving analgesia for IV placement.
F. **Children with "full stomachs"**
    1. For **rapid sequence induction,** in general, the same principles apply to infants and children as for adults.
        a. **Atropine** (0.02 mg/kg) may be given IV to prevent bradycardia, especially if succinylcholine will be given.
        b. Children often require larger doses propofol (3 to 4 mg/kg) and succinylcholine (1 to 2.0 mg/kg) because of a larger volume of distribution for these drugs.
        c. Infants with gastric distention (eg, pyloric stenosis) should have their stomachs decompressed with an orogastric tube before induction of anesthesia. This gastric tube should be suctioned again before the trachea is extubated.
        d. **Ranitidine** (2 to 4 mg/kg) can be given to decrease gastric volume and increase gastric pH. **Ondansetron** (0.1 mg/kg) can be given for postoperative nausea and vomiting prophylaxis.
        e. **Metoclopramide** should not be given if gastric outlet or bowel obstruction is suspected.
    2. **An awake laryngoscopy and intubation** is an option for the moribund infant or an infant with a grossly abnormal airway (eg, severe craniofacial anomaly) and a "full stomach."
    3. **A cuffed endotracheal tube** should be considered for a child with a full stomach. This option minimizes the need for replacing an uncuffed tube that proves too small. The cuff volume can be adjusted to ensure an appropriate air leak.

VII. ENDOTRACHEAL INTUBATION
A. Oral approach
1. Older children are placed in the "sniffing" position using a blanket or shoulder roll. Infants and small children have large occiputs, and a small rolled towel placed under the scapulae can be helpful.
2. During laryngoscopy, the tip of the blade is used to elevate the epiglottis. If this technique does not provide a good view of the glottis, the laryngoscope blade can be placed in the vallecula even with a straight blade.
3. In a previous study done by Hochman and Zeitels et al., it was demonstrated that complete exposure of vocal cord can be achieved by positioning the patient in an alternative flexion–flexion position during intubation. This technique has been practiced in our institution under certain circumstances when clear view of vocal cord cannot be achieved with sniffing position.
4. The distance from the glottis to the carina is about 4 cm in a term neonate. Pediatric endotracheal tubes have a single black line located 2 cm from the tip and a double black line at 3 cm; these markings should be observed while the tube is passed beyond the vocal cords.
5. If resistance is met during intubation, a half-size smaller tube should be tried.
6. After intubation, the chest should be examined for bilateral equal expansion, end tidal CO_2, and the lungs auscultated for equal breath sounds. There should be a leak around an uncuffed tube when 15 to 20 cm H_2O positive pressure is applied. If the leak is present at <10 cm H_2O pressure, the endotracheal tube should be exchanged for the next larger size.
7. The chest should be auscultated after every change in head or body position to verify equal bilateral breath sounds. Extension of the head can result in extubation, while flexion can result in tube advancement into either mainstem bronchus.
8. Endotracheal tubes should be securely taped and the numerical marking on the tube closest to the gingiva noted; migration of the endotracheal tube will be apparent from any change in this relation.

B. Nasal approach
1. This method is generally similar to that for adults (see Chapter 13: Airway Evaluation and Management).
2. The cephalad position of the infant larynx makes unaided intubation difficult; Magill forceps or a fiberoptic scope are frequently needed to guide the tip of the tube through the vocal cords.
3. Nasal intubation should be performed only when specifically indicated (eg, oral surgery) because of the risk of epistaxis from enlarged adenoids.

C. Muscle relaxants
1. **Muscle relaxants** often are used to facilitate endotracheal intubation. Muscle relaxants may be contraindicated in infants and children with abnormal airway anatomy.
2. **Succinylcholine** can cause bradycardia and may be exaggerated with repeated doses. Atropine (0.02 mg/kg) may be given before administration of succinylcholine in infants or children with immature respiratory and autonomic nervous systems. The use of succinylcholine in children with occult myopathies may result in life-threatening hyperkalemia, manifesting as wide complex bradycardia, ventricular tachycardia, ventricular fibrillation, or asystole. A history of mild muscle

weakness or failure to attain age-appropriate physical milestones may be absent, as the Duchenne and Becker types of muscular dystrophy may not be apparent until the child is 4 years of age. Any suspicion of muscle weakness, particularly in male infants, should warrant a preoperative creatine kinase level. The FDA "black box" warns that "succinylcholine in children should be reserved for emergency intubation or instances where immediate securing of the airway is necessary, for example, laryngospasm, difficult airway, full stomach." Succinylcholine should be avoided in children with a close family history of malignant hyperthermia (see Chapter 14: Neuromuscular Blockade).

3. **Rocuronium** (0.6 to 1.2 mg/kg) has a quick onset of action (40 to 90 seconds), and in most cases, this drug has replaced succinylcholine when a rapid sequence induction is mandated. Reduced dosing (0.25 to 0.5 mg/kg) is recommended in infants due to pharmacokinetic/dynamic properties.
4. Routine neuromuscular relaxation can be achieved with **cisatracurium** (0.1 to 0.2 mg/kg).
5. For very long cases (eg, craniotomy and cardiac surgery), **pancuronium** (0.1 mg/kg) is an option which has the wanted side-effect of supporting the heart rate in pediatric patients.
6. Reversal of neuromuscular blockade with **neostigmine** (0.05 to 0.06 mg/kg) and an anticholinergic drug (eg, atropine or glycopyrrolate) should occur if the twitch monitor (train of four ratio is <0.9) or clinical examination suggests weakness. The use of **sugammadex** (2 to 4 mg/kg depending on number of twitches returned) is an accepted practice at many institutions for pediatric patients, infants, and neonates, although this is an off-label use as sugammadex is only FDA approved for use in ages 2 and older.

D. The **laryngeal mask airway** (see Chapter 13: Airway Evaluation and Management) has revolutionized pediatric anesthesia. It has replaced the mask airway for simple cases (eg, herniorrhaphy) and the endotracheal tube for many procedures (eg, magnetic resonance imaging or computed tomography scan).

VIII. ANALGESIA
Perioperative/periprocedural pediatric pain evaluation, treatment, and monitoring are essential to mitigate biologic and psychological stresses and improve long-term outcomes. Multiple methods are used for treatment of pediatric pain and include nonpharmacologic and pharmacologic techniques. These include neuraxial, regional, nonopioid, and opioid pharmacotherapy.

IX. PHARMACOTHERAPY
A. **Nonopioid pharmacotherapeutic agents** can be used as sole or adjuvant therapy for the treatment of pain. Common medications include the following:
   1. **Acetaminophen** 10 to 15 mg/kg PO (IV administration is also 10 to 15 mg/kg) and 30 to 45 mg PR. Daily dosing should not exceed 75 mg/kg for children, 60 mg/kg for neonates, and 45 mg/kg for preterm infants.
   2. **Ketorolac** given 0.5 mg/kg IV or 1 mg/kg IM (given q6h). Caution is used in patients <2 years old.
   3. Additional agents include ketamine, gabapentin, dexmedetomidine, clonidine, and magnesium.
B. **Opioid therapy** is summarized in **Table 33.6**. There are multiple PO and IV agents to achieve analgesia. Codeine received a black box warning by the

Table 33.6 Guidelines for Opioid Administration in Pediatric Patients

Drug	Starting IV Dose and Interval	Parenteral: Oral Dose Ratio	Starting Oral Dose and Interval
Codeine	—	—	0.5–1 mg/kg q 3–4 h
Morphine	0.05–0.1 mg/kg q2–4h	1:3	0.3 mg/kg q 3–4 h
Oxycodone	—	—	0.1–0.2 mg/kg every 3–4 h
Methadone	0.1 mg/kg every 4–8 h	1:2	0.1 mg/kg every 4–8 h
Fentanyl	0.5–1.0 µg/kg every 1–2 h Infusion: 0.5–2.0 µg/kg/h	—	—
Hydromorphone	0.02 mg/kg every 2–4 h	1:4	0.04–0.08 mg/kg every 3–4 h
Meperidine	0.8–1.0 mg/kg every 2–3 h	1:4	2–3 mg/kg every 3–4 h
Remifentanil	0.1–0.25 µg/kg 1–4 µg/kg for intubation Infusion 0.05–0.15 µg/kg/min	—	—

FDA in 2013 and warning in 2012 for tonsillectomy and adenoidectomy and caution in postsurgical pediatric for rare but adverse events (rapid metabolism to morphine), respectively. Controversy exists surrounding the use of remifentanil and the induction of rapid tolerance and hyperalgesia. It should also be noted that clearance is higher in neonatal patients. As previously discussed, remifentanil can be used to facilitate endotracheal intubation; caution should be taken due to the side effects of hypotension and bradycardia, especially with elevated dosing.

C. Regional and neuraxial anesthesia for pediatric patients has gained acceptance because of a better understanding of the pharmacokinetics and pharmacodynamics of local anesthetics in infants and children and the availability of specifically designed equipment. In addition, regional anesthesia has been demonstrated to be safe when performed during general anesthesia, and complication rates are comparable under general anesthesia versus sedated or awake children.

D. Pharmacology of local anesthetics

1. **Protein binding** of local anesthetics is decreased in neonates because of decreased levels of serum albumin. Free drug concentration may be increased, especially for bupivacaine.
2. **Plasma cholinesterase activity** may be decreased in infants <6 months old, which theoretically diminishes clearance of amino esters.
3. **Hepatic microsomal enzyme systems** are immature in the neonate, and this will decrease the clearance of amino amides.
4. **The increased volume of distribution** in the infant and child acts to decrease free local anesthetic concentrations in the blood.
5. **Systemic toxicity** is the most frequent complication of regional anesthetics, and doses should be carefully calculated on a weight basis. The

risk of accumulation of free drug after repeated doses of local anesthetics is increased in infants and children.

E. Brachial plexus block and additional regional blocks

Brachial plexus blocks (for upper extremity surgery), **penile blocks** (for circumcision), and **ilioinguinal blocks** (for inguinal herniorrhaphy) are particularly useful and common regional techniques in the pediatric population. In addition, regional techniques as performed in pediatric patients as in the adult population have yielded great postoperative analgesia and are discussed in Chapter 21: Regional Anesthesia.

F. Spinal anesthesia

1. **Indications**
   a. Premature infants <60 weeks postmenstrual age and infants with a history of apnea and bradycardia, bronchopulmonary dysplasia (BPD), or need for long-term ventilatory support are at increased risk for apnea and cardiovascular instability after general anesthesia. Spinal anesthesia may decrease the likelihood of these postoperative anesthetic complications. The benefit of spinal anesthesia is beyond postoperative pain management. These techniques in infants can avoid airway instrumentation, decrease the risk of early postoperative apnea and maintain hemodynamic stability. In the Cochrane review done by Jones LJ et al., it was demonstrated that moderate-quality evidence supports that spinal anesthesia is preferred compared to general anesthesia with the risk of postoperative apnea reduced up to 47% in preterm infants. The number needed to treat (NNT) is estimated at four. In the recently published study done by Liu et al., it is demonstrated that infants that received spinal anesthesia for hernia repair have significantly lower r-FLACC score (the revised Face, Legs, Activity, Cry, and Consolability score) and less requirement for acetaminophen postoperatively in infants younger than 60 weeks postmenstrual age compared to general anesthesia. These infants still require a minimum of 24 hours of cardiorespiratory monitoring postoperatively, regardless of the anesthetic technique. Intravenous or inhalational medications during spinal anesthesia may negate the potential benefits of protection against early postoperative apnea.
   b. Children at risk for malignant hyperthermia.
   c. Children with chronic airways disease such as reactive airway disease or cystic fibrosis.
   d. Cooperative older children and adolescents with full stomachs undergoing peripheral emergency surgery (eg, fractured ankle).

2. **Anatomy.** The spinal cord in an infant terminates at approximately L3 and does not assume the adult L1–L2 termination until approximately 12 months.

3. **Technique**
   a. The procedure may be performed with the patient in the lateral decubitus or sitting position in the OR using a team approach. All infants undergoing spinal anesthesia had EMLA cream applied to the L4–L5 interspace and covered with a Tegaderm for 30 minutes before coming into operation room. An assistant is present for positioning the infant (refer to **Figure 33.1** below). Premature infants and neonates are positioned in the sitting position to limit rostral spread of drug. The head is supported upright to prevent upper airway obstruction. A 22-gauge 1.5-inch spinal needle is used for infants, because cerebrospinal fluid (CSF) flow can be very slow especially

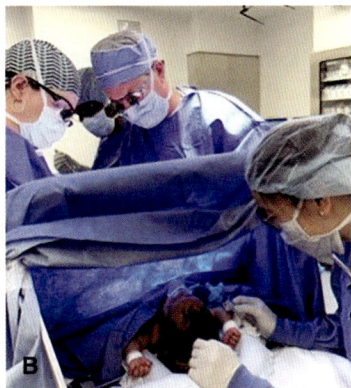

FIGURE 33.1 Awake infant spinal anesthetic. A, Placement of awake spinal anesthesia. **B,** Awake infraumbilical surgery under spinal anesthesia in an infant.

with a smaller needle. In children older than 2 years, a 25-gauge needle is acceptable. A timer is started as soon as the spinal is placed. We place IV catheter in one of the extremities following the placement of spinal anesthesia. Absence of infant response to attempted IV placement in the lower extremity or detection of lower extremity motor paralysis was used as an indication for successful onset of spinal anesthesia. If an IV was unable to be placed in the lower extremities, it was then attempted in the upper extremities. The surgeons are informed of the time since spinal placement at 30 minutes, 45 minutes, and 60 minutes to help track progression of the surgery.

b. Patient should be monitored throughout the procedure. Maintaining normothermia is essential, especially for premature infants and neonates. The infant should remain supine after placement of the spinal anesthetic; the Trendelenburg position and leg raising should be avoided because of possible cephalad migration in the subarachnoid space. Special attention should be paid to the tone of crying in the infants under spinal anesthesia. Muffled or weakened crying is a sign of high spinal in this population. Rarely, transient Horner syndrome has been reported in this population without long term effect.

4. **Drugs and dosage**
   a. Hyperbaric solutions of bupivacaine or tetracaine are used most frequently.
   b. The dosage requirements are increased, and the duration of action is decreased in infants.
   c. **Recommended dosages** for infants, for a T6 level of anesthesia:
      1. **Bupivacaine** 0.5% (isobaric solution): 0.5 to 1 mg/kg
      2. **Bupivacaine** 0.75% in 8.25% dextrose: 0.5 to 1 mg/kg
      3. **Tetracaine,** 1% in 5% dextrose: 0.8 to 1.0 mg/kg in an infant and 0.25 to 0.5 mg/kg in a child. This dose is large compared with adult dosage, but it is necessary in infants.
   d. **Duration of surgical anesthesia** averages 90 minutes with both tetracaine and bupivacaine. Multiple agents have been added to the local anesthetic in attempts to prolong the block. **Epinephrine** 2 to 5 µg/kg

and **clonidine** 1 µg/kg have been shown to prolong duration of spinal block.
5. **Complications and contraindications**
   a. **The anesthetic level** recedes more quickly in children than in adults. If the block subsides, supplemental sedation must be used cautiously, especially in premature infants and neonates. If subarachnoid anesthesia is inadequate, it is best to initiate general anesthesia before positioning.
   b. **Hypotension** is rare in children <7 to 10 years old, perhaps because resting sympathetic vascular tone is lower than in adults. A high spinal anesthetic may be heralded only by mottled skin or apnea and bradycardia.
   c. **Contraindications** are similar to those in adults, with particular attention to congenital anatomic defects of the central nervous system and a history of intraventricular hemorrhage.

G. **Caudal and epidural anesthesia**
  1. **Indications.** These techniques are useful in combination with general anesthesia for minor and major procedures of the thorax, abdomen, pelvis, bladder, and lower extremities, particularly when significant postoperative pain is anticipated (eg, orthopedic surgery).
  2. **Anatomy** is outlined in Chapter 20: Spinal, Epidural, and Caudal Anesthesia. Note that the dural sac ends at the level of the S3 vertebra in the neonate; care is required to avoid dural puncture during placement of the caudal needle.
  3. **Technique** is outlined in Chapter 20: Spinal, Epidural, and Caudal Anesthesia. Most caudal and lumbar epidural anesthetics are placed after induction of general anesthesia.
     a. **Caudal anesthesia** may be administered as a single injection of local anesthetic through a 1.5-inch, short-bevel styletted needle placed into the caudal epidural space. This technique is ideally suited for short procedures with mild-to-moderate postoperative pain such as inguinal herniorrhaphy, orchiopexy, and circumcision. For longer procedures or prolonged postoperative analgesia, a catheter may be advanced from the sacral epidural space. Intermittent boluses or a continuous infusion of local anesthetic with or without an opioid may be used. In infants, 22-gauge caudal catheters are placed through 20-gauge, 40- to 50-mm Tuohy needles; older children require 20-gauge catheters placed through 17- or 18-gauge, 90- to 100-mm Tuohy needles.
     b. **Caudal catheters** can be advanced to lumbar or thoracic levels in young children because the epidural space is not yet extensively vascularized. The recommended levels are T6–T9 vertebral level for thoracic surgery (eg, pectus excavatum repair), T10–T12 vertebral level for abdominal surgery (eg, Nissen fundoplication or bowel resections), and L3–L4 vertebral level for pelvic procedures. Usually, these catheters advance easily; resistance may indicate malpositioning. If necessary, confirmation of catheter placement can be done with contrast dye, stimulation, ECG, and fluoroscopy techniques. While easy to place when compared with a lumbar catheter, the caudal catheter has a greater potential to become contaminated from stool. Also, the catheter may become dislodged postoperatively.
     c. **Epidural catheters** may be placed via lumbar or thoracic approaches. The distance from the skin to the epidural space is short (1 to 2 cm) in children, and, again, care must be taken to avoid dural

puncture. Loss of resistance is usually accomplished with saline. In older children, 18-gauge Tuohy needles and 20-gauge catheters are used. Thoracic catheters are useful for pectus excavatum repair or thoracotomy.

4. **Drugs and doses**
   a. In **single-dose caudal anesthesia,** a long duration of sensory blockade with minimal motor blockade is desirable. Bupivacaine, 0.125% to 0.25% with epinephrine, is administered according to the formula of 0.06 mL of local anesthetic per kg per segment, where the number of segments is counted from the S5 spinal level to the desired level of analgesia. A simple alternative dosing scheme is to administer 0.125% bupivacaine with epinephrine at a dose of 1 to 1.25 mL/kg. Increasing the concentration of bupivacaine above 0.25% does not appear to improve analgesia. Dosages of bupivacaine 2.5 mg/kg without epinephrine and 3 mg/kg with epinephrine result in plasma levels in infants and children below the toxic range determined for adults. Ropivacaine 0.2% has been successfully used in caudal anesthesia at doses of 1 mL/kg for minor elective surgery. The addition of **clonidine** 0.5 to 2 µg/kg to bupivacaine prolongs the duration of analgesia by 2 to 3 hours. It may cause increased sedation postoperatively and should be avoided in babies at risk of apnea (neonates and ex-preterm infants).
   b. **Continuous infusion.** Bupivacaine 0.05% to 0.1% or ropivacaine 0.2% can be infused epidurally at a dose of 0.2 to 0.3 mg/kg/h in infants and 0.2 to 0.4 mg/kg/h in children. Opioids may be added in µg to the local anesthetic solution: fentanyl (1 to 3 µg/mL), infused at 0.3 to 1 µg/kg/h; morphine 5 to 10 µg/mL, infused at 1 to 5 µg/kg/h; or hydromorphone 3 to 7 µg/mL, infused at 1 to 2.5 µg/kg/h. Infants younger than 6 to 12 months generally do not receive opioids in the epidural infusion, unless they are in a closely monitored setting.
   c. **Postoperative analgesia** may be provided by infusion through the caudal or epidural catheter. Generally, an infusion of 0.1% bupivacaine with fentanyl, 1 to 3 µg/mL at 0.3 to 1 µg/kg/h, will provide good analgesia without motor blockade. However, some patients benefit from omission of local anesthetic from the infusion, and fentanyl, 0.5 to 1 µg/kg/h, can be used in these patients. Because of concern about postoperative respiratory depression, infants younger than 6 to 12 months generally do not receive epidural opioids unless they are in a closely monitored setting. These infants receive an infusion of 0.1% bupivacaine, 0.2 to 0.4 mL/kg/h.
   d. **Contraindications** are the same as for spinal anesthesia (see Section IX.F.5.c.). Chlorhexidine use in infants <2 months old or with skin breakdown is controversial due to systemic absorption and risk of burn injury.
   e. **Complications** of epidural and caudal anesthesia are discussed in Chapter 20: Spinal, Epidural, and Caudal Anesthesia.

H. Combined spinal caudal catheter anesthesia
   1. A well-known caveat for spinal anesthesia in infants is its short duration limiting its utility for longer-duration surgeries (>90 minutes). Studies have shown that an awake combined spinal and caudal anesthetic in infants and older children is a safe option for providing surgical anesthesia for longer-duration surgeries.
   2. **Description of anesthetic.** After the infant spinal is completed utilizing the above described technique and the IV is placed, a caudal catheter

is inserted through a 20 g angiocatheter under ultrasound guidance in the lateral decubitus position. Up to 1 mL of saline is used to expand the caudal space to confirm placement of the catheter up to the L5–S1 level and expansion of the epidural/caudal space under ultrasound. Commonly, infants fall asleep following spinal placement and IV sedation is avoided for preference for soothing methods. When clinical signs of receding spinal anesthetic are noted (waking of the previously sleeping infant, an increasingly louder cry, return of palpable abdominal tone, etc.), the caudal catheter is activated with 1 mL/kg of 2% chloroprocaine with 1:200,000 epinephrine slowly over 15 minutes, followed by an infusion of 1 mL/kg/h of the same. The infusion is continued throughout the procedure until <15 minutes remain. At the end of the procedure, a calculated remaining dose of 0.2% ropivacaine with 1:200,000 epinephrine, as allowable by total maximum safe local anesthetic dose(<2.5 mg/kg), is given through the caudal catheter prior to removal.
   3. This technique allows for avoidance of additional IV sedatives or inhalational anesthetics, instrumentation of the airway, and use of opioid pain medications for longer duration infraumbilical surgeries.
   4. Important caveats to this technique include parental, surgical, nursing, and anesthesia buy-in and support. Contraindications and complications of the technique are listed above.

X. FLUID MANAGEMENT
The following calculations may be used to estimate fluid requirements for infants and children. Other reflections of volume status, including clinical exam, blood pressure, heart rate, urine output, central venous pressure, pulse pressure variation, straight leg raise, noninvasive cardiac output monitoring, point-of-care ultrasound (POCUS), fluid challenge, and osmolarity may guide further adjustments.
A. Maintenance fluid requirements
   1. Historically, the 4/2/1 rule has been the basis for calculating maintenance fluids in pediatric patients. The rule is as follows: administer 4 mL/kg/h for the first 10 kg of body weight (100 mL/kg/d), 2 mL/kg/h for the second 10 kg (50 mL/kg/d), and then add 1 mL/kg/h for more than 20 kg (25 mL/kg/d). For example, maintenance fluids for a 25-kg child would be ([4 mL/kg × 10 kg] + [2 mL/kg × 10 kg] + [1 mL/kg × 5 kg]) = 65 mL/h.
   2. The usual solution for replacement of fluid deficits and ongoing losses in the healthy child is **lactated Ringer solution**. A second solution of 5% dextrose is frequently used in the perioperative period for premature infants, septic neonates, infants of diabetic mothers, and those receiving total parenteral nutrition. These patients should have their blood glucose levels measured periodically.
B. Estimated blood volume (EBV) and blood losses
   1. **EBV** is 95 mL/kg in premature neonates, 80 to 90 mL/kg in full-term neonates, 75 to 80 mL/kg in infants up to 1 year old, and 70 mL/kg thereafter.
   2. **Acceptable blood loss (ABL).** ABL can be estimated with a simple formula. This should be used with caution if fluid redistribution/equilibration has not occurred.

   $$ABL = EBV \times (Hct_{initial} - Hct_{acceptable})/Hct_{initial}$$

   General guidelines are as follows:
   a. If the amount of the blood loss is less than one-third of the ABL, it can be replaced with lactated Ringer solution.

b. If the amount of blood loss is greater than ABL, replace with packed red blood cells (leukoreduced, CMV negative, and irradiated). Fresh frozen plasma and platelet transfusions should be guided by the results of coagulation tests, estimates of the present and anticipated blood losses, and adequacy of clot formation in the wound.
c. For infants and young children, blood loss should be measured using small suction containers and by weighing sponges. Because it is sometimes difficult to measure small-volume blood losses precisely in young children, monitoring of hemoglobin and hematocrit will help avoid unnecessary transfusions and also alert the anesthetist to the need for blood transfusion.
d. The **"acceptable hemoglobin and hematocrit"** is no longer considered to be 10 g/dL and 30%. Each patient is evaluated with regard to the need for red blood cell transfusion. A healthy child with normal cardiac function can compensate for acute anemia by increasing cardiac output. A premature infant, a debilitated child, a child with sepsis, a child receiving chemotherapy, or one facing massive surgery may require a higher hemoglobin.

C. Estimated fluid deficit = (maintenance fluid per hour) × hours since the last oral intake. The entire estimated fluid deficit replaced during all major cases; the first half is administered during the first hour, and the remaining deficit is infused over the next 1 to 2 hours.

D. Third-space losses may require up to an additional 10 mL/kg/h of lactated Ringer solution or normal saline if there is extensive exposure of the intestine or a significant ileus.

XI. EMERGENCE AND POSTANESTHESIA CARE

A. Extubation
1. **Laryngospasm** may occur during emergence, especially during the critical period of the excitement stage before consciousness returns.
2. In most cases, the trachea is extubated after emergence from anesthesia. Coughing is not a sign that the child is ready for extubation. Instead, children should demonstrate purposeful activity (eg, reaching for the endotracheal tube) or eye opening before extubation. In the infant, hip flexion, strong grimaces, and purposeful movements are useful indications of awakening.
3. Alternatively, the trachea may be extubated while the patient is in a deep plane of anesthesia with spontaneous ventilation. This can be done in operations such as inguinal herniorrhaphy where coughing on emergence is undesirable or in patients with reactive airways disease. Extubation under deep anesthesia is not appropriate for the child with a full stomach, a child whose trachea was difficult to intubate, or the child who had oral or laryngeal surgery. Clinical judgment is essential.
4. **Emergence delirium** is a relatively common postanesthetic event and can be difficult to differentiate from pain. Common risk factors include age (1 to 5 years old), surgery type (ENT/ophthalmic procedures), preoperative anxiety, preoperative medication, rapid emergence, and pain. Treatment options after treating pain include early reunion with parents, fentanyl (1 μg/kg), propofol (1 mg/kg), and dexmedetomidine (0.5 μg/kg).

B. During transport to the postanesthesia care unit (PACU), the child's color and ventilatory pattern should be continuously monitored. Supplemental oxygen may be administered if indicated (eg, the child with anemia or pulmonary disease).

C. In the PACU, early reunion of the child and parents is desirable. Discharge criteria often follow the Aldrete Scoring System (motor function, breathing, blood pressure, consciousness, and oxygenation) as well as pain control. In addition, extended postoperative/procedural monitoring of infants and children should be considered on a case-by-case basis (obstructive sleep apnea, prematurity, children <3 years who underwent airway surgery including tonsillectomy, etc.).

XII. SPECIFIC PEDIATRIC ANESTHESIA PROBLEMS
A. The compromised airway
1. **Etiologies**
   a. Congenital abnormalities (eg, choanal atresia, Pierre Robin syndrome, tracheal stenosis, or laryngeal web).
   b. Inflammation (eg, tracheobronchitis or "croup," epiglottitis, and pharyngeal abscess).
   c. Foreign bodies (FBs) in the trachea or esophagus.
   d. Neoplasms (eg, congenital hemangioma, cystic hygroma, or thoracic lymphadenopathy).
   e. Trauma.
2. **Initial management**
   a. Administer 100% oxygen by face mask (continually assess oxygenation and ventilation).
   b. Keep the child as calm as possible. Evaluation should be efficient, because it may increase agitation and cause further airway compromise. Parents are invaluable in their ability to pacify their children and should remain with them as long as feasible.
   c. An anesthetist must be present during transport to the operating room. Oxygen, a resuscitation bag and mask, laryngoscope, atropine, succinylcholine, drugs suitable for sedation and hypnosis, appropriate endotracheal tubes and laryngeal mask airways, oral airways, and pulse oximetry must be available.
3. **Induction of anesthesia with a compromised airway**
   a. **Minimize manipulation of the patient.** A precordial stethoscope and pulse oximeter are adequate monitors during the initial induction of anesthesia.
   b. The child may remain in a **semisitting position,** with the parents present, if indicated. A **gradual inhalation induction** with sevoflurane is the next step (see Section VI.C.3). Airway obstruction and poor air exchange will prolong induction.
   c. Parents are asked to leave when the child becomes unconscious, and an IV is started. If indicated, atropine may be given at this time. Alternatively, a preinduction IV may be started if there is concern for acute decompensation and proceed with IV or inhalational induction.
   d. **Patients with croup** may benefit from gentle application of continuous positive airway pressure (CPAP), but any positive pressure can cause acute airway obstruction in patients with epiglottitis or an FB.
   e. The **oral endotracheal tube** should have a stylet and be at least one size smaller than the predicted size. If postoperative ventilation is anticipated (eg, epiglottitis), a cuffed endotracheal tube may be indicated.
   f. At this point, patients usually are hypercarbic ($ETCO_2$ between 50 and 60 mm Hg), but generally, this is well tolerated. Bradycardia is an indication of hypoxemia and requires immediate establishment of a patent airway.

616 Part II Administration of Anesthesia

g. Perform laryngoscopy only when the child is deeply anesthetized. The decision to give a muscle relaxant depends on the situation. A muscle relaxant facilitates intubation and obviates the need for deep anesthesia in certain circumstances. In other cases, muscle relaxation may further compromise the airway. In general, orotracheal intubation should be accomplished before any further airway procedures are attempted. **Bronchoscopy** is indicated before intubation in cases of large upper airway FBs or friable subglottic tumors (eg, hemangioma).

h. **A nasal tube** may be more appropriate for illnesses that require several days of intubation (eg, epiglottitis). An orotracheal tube may be changed to a nasotracheal tube at the end of the procedure, provided the oral intubation was easily accomplished. Never jeopardize a secure oral endotracheal tube for the sake of changing it to a nasal endotracheal tube.

i. Children should be sedated during transport to the intensive care unit. A combination of a narcotic and a benzodiazepine, propofol infusion, or dexmedetomidine infusion or bolus can be effective. Breathing may be spontaneous or assisted during the immediate postoperative period. Propofol is not approved by the FDA for sedation of pediatric intensive care patients due to the risk of propofol infusion syndrome and its associated metabolic derangements.

4. Management of the inhaled FB

a. FB aspiration usually occurs between 7 months and 4 years of age. About 75% of FBs lodge in the proximal airway (larynx, trachea, mainstem bronchus). Most deaths occur at the time of aspiration, and the mortality in most series is zero if the child reaches the hospital alive.

b. Choking and wheezing following a witnessed aspiration event is the most common **presentation**. The triad of coughing, wheezing, and reduced breath sounds is present in only 50% of cases. CXR may show radiopaque objects, postobstructive emphysema, or a localized pneumonia but has a false-negative rate of 40%.

c. **Management** is prompt rigid bronchoscopy regardless of CXR findings. It is vital to communicate with the bronchoscopist before and during the procedure. An emergency tracheotomy and thoracotomy kit should be prepared. There are two approaches to the anesthetic: spontaneous ventilation and controlled ventilation.

d. **Spontaneous ventilation.** After preoxygenation and IV atropine or glycopyrrolate, a sevoflurane/100% oxygen induction is performed. Sevoflurane is preferred for inhalational induction, and spontaneous ventilation is maintained. Once an adequate depth is achieved, the vocal cords and subglottic space are sprayed with topical lidocaine (2% for school age children and 1% for small infants). The trachea is then intubated with a ventilating bronchoscope. A sufficient depth of anesthesia is required to prevent moving and coughing. Consider a small dose of muscle relaxant just before removal of the FB through the vocal cords. The stomach is then suctioned, and the patient is allowed to emerge breathing through either a mask or an endotracheal tube placed after FB removal. Advantages of this technique are better air flow distribution and ventilation–perfusion matching, uninterrupted ventilation, and the ability to immediately assess ventilatory mechanics after FB removal. Disadvantages are the risks of patient movement, coughing, laryngospasm, and prolonged emergence.

e. **Controlled ventilation.** Anesthesia is commenced with a rapid sequence induction using propofol and a muscle relaxant. Maintenance anesthesia can be provided with propofol and remifentanil infusions and muscle relaxant. The trachea is intubated with a ventilating bronchoscope, and ventilation is performed in concert with the bronchoscopist's interventions. When the bronchoscope is in place, ventilation is achieved with high inspiratory pressures, and long expiratory times are necessary to prevent barotrauma. Emergence is achieved in a manner similar to the spontaneous ventilation technique. The advantages of controlled ventilation are rapid control of the airway, no patient movement, and lower anesthetic requirements. However, ventilation is intermittently interrupted, and there are risks of displacing the FB distally and causing barotrauma with ball-valve hyperinflation.
f. A large retrospective study showed that **ventilatory technique** did not affect the success of FB removal or influence adverse outcomes (hypoxia, hypercarbia, bradycardia, and hypotension).
g. Subglottic edema resulting in postextubation croup can be treated with humidified oxygen. If symptoms are severe, then racemic epinephrine (0.5 mL of a 2% solution in 2 to 4 mL of volume) can be given. In addition, dexamethasone (0.25 to 0.5 mg/kg up to 8 mg) should be considered.

B. Respiratory disorders
1. **Differential diagnosis.** The following diseases present similarly as pulmonary parenchymal disease and should be considered when evaluating an infant with respiratory distress.
    a. **Airway obstruction.** Choanal atresia, vocal cord palsy, laryngomalacia, tracheal malacia or stenosis, and compression of the trachea by external masses (eg, cystic hygroma, hemangioma, vascular ring).
    b. **Developmental anomalies.** TEF, CDH, congenital lobar emphysema, pulmonary sequestration, bronchogenic cysts and congenital pulmonary airway malformations (CPAMs)/congenital cystic adenomatoid malformations (CCAMs).
    c. **Nonpulmonary.** Cyanotic heart disease, PPHN, congestive heart failure, and metabolic disturbances.
2. **Apnea**
    a. **Etiology and treatments**
        1. **Central apnea** is due to immaturity or depression of the respiratory center (eg, narcotics). It is related to the degree of prematurity and is exacerbated by metabolic disturbances (eg, hypoglycemia, hypocalcemia, hypothermia, hyperthermia, or sepsis). Before 34 weeks of gestational age, central apnea is often treated with **methylxanthines** such as caffeine citrate.
        2. **Obstructive apnea** is caused by inconsistent maintenance of a patent airway. It can result from incomplete maturation and poor coordination of upper airway musculature. This form of apnea may respond to changes in head position, insertion of an oral or nasal airway, or placement of the infant in a prone position. Occasionally, administration of **CPAP** or a high-flow oxygen nasal cannula may be beneficial. These therapies especially may be effective in infants with a large tongue, such as with trisomy 21 or Beckwith–Wiedemann syndrome.
        3. **Mixed apnea** represents a combination of both central and obstructive apnea.

b. Postoperative apnea in the neonate

1. Apnea is associated with anesthesia in infants that are born prematurely. The etiology of postoperative apnea is multifactorial. Risk factors have been identified including postconceptual age <60 weeks at time of surgery, anemia, LGA infants, hypothermia and altered ventilatory response to hypoxemia and hypercarbia induced by general anesthesia.
2. If it is not possible to delay surgery until the patient is more mature, it is prudent to use **postoperative apnea monitoring** for 24 hours in neonates who undergo anesthesia at <60 weeks postconceptual age. In the previous meta-analysis done by Cote CJ et al., it was demonstrated that the incidence of apnea following hernia repair remains above 5% until postconceptual age of 48 weeks and the incidence is reduced to <1% beyond postconceptual age of 56 weeks. Infants with a history of apnea are at increased risk for postoperative apnea, and should be actively monitored.

3. Respiratory distress syndrome (RDS)

a. **Pathophysiology.** RDS results from physiologic surfactant deficiency. This causes decreased lung compliance, alveolar instability, progressive atelectasis, and hypoxemia resulting from intrapulmonary shunting of deoxygenated blood.

b. Prematurely born infants have an increased incidence of RDS. Newborns at risk for RDS can be identified prenatally by amniocentesis and evaluation of the amniotic fluid phospholipid profile. Lung surfactant maturity in the fetus is associated with a lecithin-to-sphingomyelin ratio >2, saturated phosphatidylcholine level >500 µg/dL, or presence of phosphatidylglycerol in the specimen.

c. **Glucocorticoid (betamethasone) treatment** of the mother at least 48 hours prior to delivery decreases the incidence and severity of RDS. Only one full course of a glucocorticoid treatment regimen during a pregnancy is necessary. This is accomplished by giving one dose of glucocorticoid to the pregnant woman per day for 2 days.

d. **Clinical features** of RDS include tachypnea, nasal flaring, grunting, and retractions. Cyanosis appears shortly after birth. Because of the intrapulmonary shunt across atelectatic lung units, infants with RDS remain hypoxemic despite breathing at high FiO_2.

e. The **CXR** will show low lung volumes. A "ground-glass" pattern of the lung fields and air bronchograms may also be evident.

f. **Initial treatment** includes warmed, humidified oxygen administered by hood or nasal cannula. The FiO_2 should be adjusted to maintain the PaO_2 between 50 and 80 mm Hg (SaO_2 between 88% and 92%). If an FiO_2 >60% is required to keep the patient oxygenated, **nasal CPAP** should be administered. With more severe disease, or if the nasal CPAP is poorly tolerated, intubation and ventilation with positive end-expiratory pressure may be required. In intubated newborns with RDS, endotracheally administered exogenous **surfactant** decreases the morbidity and mortality of the disease. In babies with severe RDS, **high-frequency oscillatory ventilation** (HFOV) decreases the incidence of air leaks and chronic lung disease (CLD).

g. **Broad-spectrum antibiotics** are often begun after appropriate cultures are obtained because the clinical signs and CXR of patients with RDS are indistinguishable from pneumonia.

h. In more mature newborns, RDS may be self-limited. Clinical improvement often occurs after 2 to 3 days and is associated with a

spontaneous diuresis. In extremely premature newborns, RDS may progress to CLD.
   i. The **morbidity and mortality** of patients with RDS are directly related to the degree of prematurity, perinatal resuscitation, and the coexistence of other complications of prematurity (eg, PDA, infection, intraventricular hemorrhage). **Pneumothoraces, pulmonary interstitial emphysema, and pulmonary hemorrhage** may complicate the recovery and can be associated with the evolution to CLD.
4. **Bronchopulmonary dysplasia (BPD)**
   a. **Etiology.** BPD is defined as the continued need for oxygen therapy or mechanical ventilation beyond 36 weeks postconceptual age. BPD is also referred to as CLD of prematurity and is associated with oxygen toxicity, chronic inflammation, and mechanical injury in the lung. BPD can be worsened by the presence of a PDA or infection. However, in some premature infants, BPD occurs in the absence of significant lung injury. Recent studies suggest that BPD is associated with excessive transforming growth factor-beta (TGF-β) signaling in the injured developing lung. Preventive strategies include vitamin A or caffeine administration and early initiation of CPAP.
   b. **Clinical features** include retractions, rales, and areas of lung hyper- and hypoinflation. Because of nonhomogeneous ventilation, an intrapulmonary shunt may produce hypoxemia and hypercarbia in patients with BPD. Hypoxia and hypercarbia may also be associated with bronchospasm in many patients with severe BPD. Many patients with severe BPD have growth failure and require high-caloric feeds.
   c. **Treatment** consists of supportive respiratory care, aggressive nutrition, and diuretic therapy. Because patients with BPD may have lung segments with long time constants, a ventilatory pattern with low respiratory rates and increased inspiratory and expiratory time may decrease gas trapping and improve gas exchange. Permissive hypercapnia is typically utilized to minimize further lung injury. In addition, **bronchodilator therapy** may be lifesaving in patients with BPD and bronchospasm. Systemic steroids sometimes are used to treat patients with CLD. However, because of adverse long-term neurodevelopmental outcomes observed in infants treated with systemic steroids, this therapy is typically reserved for the most severe cases. In some patients with severe BPD, pulmonary hypertension might be observed. In these cases, pulmonary vasodilators including inhaled nitric oxide (INO) and type 5 phosphodiesterase inhibitors have been used.
   d. **Prognosis** of BPD varies with the severity of the disease. Of severely affected infants, 20% die within the first year. Most infants are generally asymptomatic by 2 years of age but additional morbidities include recurrent respiratory infections, increased pulmonary reactivity and asthma, repeated hospitalizations, pulmonary hypertension, and neurodevelopmental abnormalities.
5. **Pneumothorax**
   a. **Etiology.** Pneumothorax can occur in infants requiring positive pressure or mechanical ventilation. In addition, spontaneous pneumothorax can occur in 1% to 2% of otherwise healthy full-term infants who often remain asymptomatic or mildly symptomatic and require no intervention. The incidence increases up to 5% to 10% of full-term infants with meconium staining or prematurely born infants with RDS.

b. **Clinical features.** The diagnosis should be considered in any neonate with an acute deterioration in clinical condition (eg, sudden cyanosis and hypotension). Occasionally, asymmetric chest movement with ventilation and asymmetric breath sounds may be appreciated; however, endobronchial intubation should be ruled out.
c. **Laboratory studies.** Transillumination of the chest with a strong light usually will show a hyperlucent hemithorax. Absence of lung sliding may be seen on lung ultrasound. If the patient is stable, a CXR may be obtained to confirm the diagnosis.
d. **Treatment**
   1. In otherwise stable and well-oxygenated term infants with minimal respiratory distress, a nitrogen washout by breathing a high concentration of oxygen has historically been used to assist with resolution of the pneumothorax. However, the data supporting this mode of therapy are minimal and should be weighed against newer ones suggesting that hyperoxia is associated with end-organ injury.
   2. In the **unstable infant,** immediate aspiration of the pleural space with an IV catheter should be performed. Reaccumulation of clinically significant air after aspiration warrants placement of a chest tube.

6. **Meconium aspiration syndrome**
   a. **Meconium staining of amniotic fluid** occurs in 12% of all births and may be associated with fetal distress and perinatal depression.
   b. To **decrease the effects of aspiration,** it is prudent to intubate and suction the airways of infants with meconium-stained fluid who are born with depressed respirations and poor tone.
   c. **Meconium aspiration** may produce lung airspace disease by mechanical obstruction of the airways with fecal matter and chemical inflammation and surfactant inactivation causing pneumonitis. Complete obstruction of the airways by meconium results in distal atelectasis. Partial obstruction of the airways may produce overinflation of distal air spaces by a ball-valve effect, leading to pneumothorax. The bile in meconium may cause chemical pneumonitis and airway edema.
   d. **Meconium aspiration syndrome** is also associated with PPHN (see Section XII.D.5.).
   e. Chest radiographic findings can include diffuse, patchy intraparenchymal densities with areas of hyper- and hypoinflation.
   f. **Respiratory support** for meconium aspiration is dependent on the etiology of the poor gas exchange. Obstruction of airways with meconium may require mechanical ventilation with long expiratory times to decrease gas trapping. Pneumothorax is treated by placement of a chest tube. Sometimes high-frequency oscillatory ventilation can recruit closed lung segments and improve gas exchange. Alkalosis and **INO** have been useful to decrease pulmonary vasoconstriction. Exogenous **surfactant** has also been observed to be beneficial as meconium inhibits endogenous surfactant activity

7. **Recent upper respiratory infection.** Infants and children can have 6 to 10 upper respiratory infections each year. It is important to balance the severity of symptoms with the urgency of surgery. Wheezing, fever, and cough are signs of lower respiratory inflammation and are associated with an increased risk of perioperative airway complications. Conversely, myringotomy and ear tube placement may relieve the rhinorrhea associated with chronic otitis media.

C. Gastrointestinal disorders. Intra-abdominal malformations include pyloric stenosis, gastroschisis, omphalocele, necrotizing enterocolitis (NEC), duodenal atresia, and volvulus.
  1. **Duodenal atresia**
     a. **Clinical features.** Duodenal atresia usually presents with bile-stained emesis, abdominal distention, and increased volume of gastric aspirates. It is associated with trisomy 21 and may coexist with other intestinal malformations.
     b. Prenatal ultrasound or a postnatal **abdominal x-ray** often reveals a **"double bubble,"** representing air in the stomach and proximal duodenum.
     c. **Treatment** consists of avoiding oral feeds, use of nasogastric suction, ensuring adequate hydration, and managing electrolytes. Anesthesia consists of an awake or rapid sequence intubation, avoidance of nitrous oxide, and often the use of muscle relaxants.
  2. **Pyloric stenosis**
     a. **Clinical features.** Pyloric stenosis usually presents in the 3rd to 5th week of life and is characterized by hypertrophy of the pylorus, which causes gastric outlet obstruction. The patient may present with persistent nonbilious emesis. Although the infant may exhibit hypochloremic, hypokalemic metabolic alkalosis from loss of hydrochloric acid, protracted vomiting may result in metabolic acidosis, intravascular volume depletion, and shock. An abdominal mass consisting of the hypertrophic pylorus or "olive" may be palpable.
     b. An **abdominal x-ray** usually shows gastric dilatation. The diagnosis is confirmed by abdominal ultrasound. In the past, x-ray examinations with contrast were performed to confirm this disease.
     c. **Treatment** consists of rehydration, correction of metabolic alkalosis, and nasogastric or orogastric drainage before surgical repair via pyloromyotomy.
     d. **Anesthetic considerations.** It is critical to empty the stomach before anesthetic induction. Since the patient's nasogastric tube is often blocked with gastric secretions, it is best replaced just before induction and the patient suctioned while they are positioned supine, lateral, and prone. A rapid-sequence or awake intubation may then be performed. Inhalation anesthetics or muscle relaxants can be used as needed. Opioids often are not necessary, and the patient may be prone to respiratory depression from opioids due to CSF alkalosis. Rectal acetaminophen and local anesthetic infiltration of the surgical incision may be sufficient for analgesia. The neonate should be fully awake and breathing adequately before removing the endotracheal tube.
  3. **Omphalocele and gastroschisis**
     a. **Clinical features.** An **omphalocele** is caused by failure of the migration of the intestine into the abdomen and subsequent closure of the abdominal wall at 6 to 8 weeks of gestation. The viscera remain outside the abdominal cavity and are covered with intact peritoneum. Associated defects are present in 45% to 80% of patients with an omphalocele and can include genetic abnormalities (50%), cardiac defects (28%), exstrophy of the bladder and other genitourinary abnormalities (20%), craniofacial defects (20%), and CDH (12%). **Gastroschisis** occurs later in fetal life (12 to 18 weeks of gestation) from interruption of the omphalomesenteric artery. The resulting paraumbilical defect allows exposure of the bowel to the

intrauterine environment without peritoneal coverage. Bowel loops are often edematous and covered with an inflammatory exudate. In contrast to omphalocele, gastroschisis is associated with other congenital abnormalities in only 10% to 20% of cases but may be complicated by intestinal atresia/stenosis or midgut volvulus in up to 16% of cases.

b. **Medical stabilization** includes nasogastric drainage, IV hydration, and protection of the viscera before surgical repair. If the peritoneal sac is intact, the omphalocele should be covered with sterile, warm, saline-soaked gauze to decrease heat and water loss and the risk of infection. If the sac has ruptured or if the infant has gastroschisis, warm saline-soaked gauze should be used to wrap the exposed viscera or the infant can be placed in a sterile plastic bag with careful ongoing monitoring of intestinal perfusion. The infant should then be wrapped in warm sterile towels before surgical repair.

c. **Anesthetic considerations.** In the operating room, special measures are directed at compensating for the increased insensible water and heat loss associated with the abdominal surgery. After carefully emptying the stomach, a rapid-sequence induction is performed to minimize gaseous distension of the gastrointestinal tract. Muscle relaxation aids the surgeons in placing the organs into the abdominal wall or silo placement. Special attention is required to maintain ventilation and systemic blood flow after the organs are placed in the abdomen, which can be facilitated by measuring ventilatory pressures, urine output, and lower body blood pressure and oxygen saturation. These data aid in the decision of whether the lesion should be corrected in a single or staged procedure. It is essential to assess ventilation and oxygenation of the patient prior to extubation. The increased intra-abdominal pressures associated with the procedure can compromise the pulmonary function of the patient and perfusion of the abdominal contents.

4. **Necrotizing enterocolitis (NEC)**
    a. **NEC** is an acquired intestinal necrosis that appears in the absence of functional or anatomic lesions. It occurs predominantly in premature infants with an increased incidence at lower gestational ages. It usually develops during the first few weeks of life and almost always after the institution of enteral feedings. Mortality may be as high as 40%.
    b. **Pathogenesis** is unclear but involves critical stress of an immature gut by ischemic, infectious, or immunologic insults. Enteral feedings seem to potentiate mucosal injury, though feeding with breast milk may be protective.
    c. **Clinical features** include abdominal distention, feeding intolerance with gastric aspirates or emesis, ileus, abdominal wall erythema, and bloody stool. The infant may demonstrate temperature instability, lethargy, respiratory and circulatory instability, apnea, oliguria, and disseminated intravascular coagulation (DIC).
    d. **Laboratory studies** should include an abdominal x-ray (which may show **pneumatosis intestinalis,** fixed loops of bowel, portal venous air, or free intraperitoneal air), CBC (revealing leukocytosis, leukopenia, thrombocytopenia), arterial blood gases (demonstrating acidosis), electrolytes (showing hyponatremia or acidosis), stool guaiac (often showing occult blood), and stool Clinitest (showing evidence of carbohydrate malabsorption). Because the differential diagnosis

includes sepsis, cultures of blood and urine should also be obtained. If the patient is stable and disseminated intravascular coagulation is not evident, CSF should be obtained by lumbar puncture for Gram stain and culture.
- e. **Treatment.** When NEC is suspected, enteral feedings are discontinued, and the stomach is decompressed with a nasogastric tube. Oral feeds are withheld for at least 10 to 14 days, and the patient is supported with parenteral nutrition. Broad-spectrum antibiotics (ampicillin, an aminoglycoside and, if perforation is suspected, metronidazole or clindamycin) are administered empirically.
- f. **Surgical consultation** is indicated, although laparotomy or abdominal drain placement is usually reserved for intestinal perforation, a fixed loop on serial abdominal x-rays, or persistent metabolic acidosis.
- g. **Anesthetic concerns** include hemodynamic instability due to abdominal sepsis, increasing abdominal girth leading to ventilation challenges and profound metabolic acidosis which is associated with severe NEC. It is also important to prevent aspiration of gastric contents and maintaining organ perfusion in the presence of significant third-space fluid losses.

5. **Volvulus**
   - a. **Volvulus** may occur as a primary lesion or, more commonly, as the result of intestinal malrotation, which can rapidly compromise blood flow to the intestine causing ischemia. If present in utero, intestinal necrosis may be present at birth, and immediate resection is indicated.
   - b. **Clinical features** may include abdominal distention, bilious emesis, and signs of dehydration, acidosis, sepsis, or shock.
   - c. **The diagnosis** of malrotation is made by upper gastrointestinal and small bowel follow-through examination, which demonstrates an abnormally positioned ligament of Treitz.
   - d. **Treatment** involves volume resuscitation, placement of a nasogastric tube, cessation of feeding, antibiotic administration, and surgical repair.
   - e. **Anesthetic considerations.** After evacuation of the stomach, a rapid sequence induction should be performed and anesthesia maintained with inhalation or IV anesthetics as tolerated. Nitrous oxide should be avoided to prevent further distention of the bowel.

D. Thoracic disorders
1. **Esophageal atresia (EA) and TEF.** EA is usually associated with TEF. The location of the fistula in patients with TEF is variable, with the most common configuration consisting of a proximal esophageal pouch and a distal TEF. EA/TEF is often accompanied by other congenital abnormalities, particularly cardiac defects.
   - a. **Pathophysiology.** The proximal esophageal pouch has a small capacity, resulting in overflow aspiration. Aspiration leads to the classic clinical triad of coughing, choking, and cyanosis in patients with EA. Occasionally, copious secretions with drooling requiring frequent suctioning may be the only early symptom.
   - b. The **diagnosis** is confirmed by the inability to pass a nasogastric tube into the stomach. A CXR that includes the neck with air or water-soluble contrast agent will confirm the existence of EA.
   - c. **Medical treatment** is directed at reducing aspiration. Neonates should be kept NPO. A nasogastric tube is placed on continuous low suction and the head of the bed is elevated. Aspiration pneumonia should

be treated with antibiotics and oxygen as required. Endotracheal intubation and ventilation may be required for severe pneumonia. However, ventilation may be difficult when a TEF exists.
   d. **Surgical treatment** depends on the stability of the infant. In newborns with severe aspiration pneumonia, surgery may be delayed until the lungs improve. If gastric distension because of air transiting the TEF into the GI track compromises pulmonary function, a gastrostomy tube may be placed under local anesthesia. After initial stabilization, definitive repair of the esophagus and fistula may occur.
   e. **Anesthetic considerations.** It is critical, and sometimes difficult, to establish an airway in patients with a TEF. Surgeons should be readily available during the induction should emergent decompression of the stomach be required. The patient should be fully monitored; a precordial stethoscope should be placed over the left thorax to aid in the assessment of ventilation. If the patient has a gastrostomy tube, it should be placed to water seal. Spontaneous ventilation should be maintained throughout induction and intubation until the time of surgical ligation of the fistula. To facilitate placement of the endotracheal tube so that its tip resides between the fistula and the carina, the tube may be placed first into the right mainstem bronchus. The tube then may be withdrawn slowly until breath sounds are heard over the left thorax. Decreased breath sounds and insufflation of the stomach or gas exiting from the gastrostomy tube suggest that the end of the endotracheal tube is above the fistula and that it should be advanced. Once the tube is in a good location, it must be carefully secured and monitored for dislodgement during the surgical procedure.
2. **Congenital diaphragmatic hernia (CDH)**
   a. **CDH** is a defect of the diaphragm allowing abdominal contents to herniate into the chest. CDH occurs in 1 in 5000 live births and has a high mortality, with 40% not surviving infancy.
   b. **Clinical features.** CDH is usually detected during a prenatal ultrasound. Eighty-five percent of defects occur in the left posterior lateral region of the diaphragm through the foramen of Bochdalek. The neonate often has a scaphoid abdomen with absent breath sounds on the involved side. Rarely, bowel sounds are heard in the affected hemithorax. The clinical spectrum of CDH may vary and is probably related to the degree of lung hypoplasia and associated pulmonary hypertension and cardiac dysfunction.
   c. The **diagnosis** is confirmed by CXR. The intestines and stomach are typically observed in the thorax. The liver, spleen, and/or kidneys may also be involved. Approximately 40% of infants with CDH have associated anomalies including cardiac, gastrointestinal, genitourinary, or renal anomalies that significantly increase the risk of mortality.
   d. **Treatment is geared toward decreasing pulmonary vascular resistance and facilitating CO_2 elimination prior to surgical correction.** Insufflation of the stomach and intestines is minimized by intubating the patients while they are spontaneously breathing and may often take place in the delivery room. However, if necessary, ventilation with bag and mask should be accomplished with minimal airway pressures. Continuous gastric suction also decreases air insufflation. Conventional ventilation or HFOV is used. Ventilation with INO has been observed to decrease pulmonary vasoconstriction

and cyanosis in some patients with CDH. The main causes of mortality are respiratory insufficiency and pulmonary hypertension. Pneumothorax in the unaffected lung can occur and is often the cause of death during resuscitation. Hypotension and shock are frequently seen secondary to prolonged systemic hypoxemia, cardiac impairment caused by shifting of the mediastinal contents by the hernia, and gastrointestinal fluid losses.

  e. **Surgical repair** involves replacing the abdominal contents and repairing the diaphragm. Current evidence supports first stabilizing the patients with medical therapy and gentle ventilation, using **extracorporeal membrane oxygenation** (ECMO) as a last resort. During the stabilization period, pulmonary artery pressures fall, and the patient is subsequently taken to the OR for repair.

  f. **Anesthetic considerations.** Decompression of the gut with continuous nasogastric suction is helpful. An arterial catheter is indicated for the frequent assessment of acid–base balance, oxygenation, and ventilation. Sodium bicarbonate and hyperventilation are used to treat metabolic and respiratory acidosis, respectively. In addition, alkalosis and INO may decrease pulmonary vasoconstriction. Although spontaneous ventilation may prevent gastric inflation and lung compression, ventilator support is often needed. Using the lowest effective inflating pressures reduces the risk of pneumothorax and ventilator-induced lung injury (VILI). Nitrous oxide is avoided because it may distend the gut and compromise lung function. Muscle relaxation, narcotics, and oxygen therapy are often used during anesthesia.

  g. Postoperative morbidities include feeding difficulty, gastroesophageal reflux, hearing loss, neurodevelopmental disability, and potential recurrence of the diaphragmatic hernia, particularly in those infants with a large defect requiring a patch repair.

E. Cardiovascular disorders

1. **Congenital heart disease** should be suspected in the setting of persistent cyanosis, hypotension, respiratory distress, murmur, hypoxemia, poor perfusion, or shock. Congenital heart disease occurs with an overall incidence of 8 per 1000 live births with 2 per 1000 presenting in the first year of life. The most common congenital heart disease lesions include ventricular septal defects, pulmonary stenosis with intact ventricular septum, tetralogy of Fallot, atrial septal defects, and transposition of the great arteries.

2. **Cyanosis**

   a. **Etiology.** There are many causes of cyanosis, including diffusion abnormalities in the lung, intracardiac and extracardiac shunts, and polycythemia. The pulmonary causes of cyanosis are described above.

   b. **Cardiac lesions** may cause systemic hypoxemia by decreasing pulmonary blood flow or by causing admixture of systemic and pulmonary venous blood via shunts.

   c. Several factors allow the majority of fetuses to tolerate congenital heart lesions in utero. Fetal oxygenation occurs via the placenta, rather than being dependent on pulmonary blood flow. Both the left and right ventricles contribute to systemic blood flow, and mixing occurs at atrial and ductal levels. Furthermore, the fetus has greater oxygen carrying capacity because of HbF and an elevated hemoglobin concentration.

d. In the newborn, the **ductus arteriosus may initially permit pulmonary blood flow** in patients with transposition of the great arteries, pulmonic stenosis or atresia, tetralogy of Fallot, or ventricular hypoplasia. Most of these infants become symptomatic as the ductus arteriosus closes at 2 to 3 days of life. If a ductal-dependent cardiac lesion exists, prevention of ductal closure is critical to maintain pulmonary blood flow. This may be accomplished with a **prostaglandin E_1** infusion. Side effects of prostaglandin treatment include apnea, hypotension, and seizure activity.

e. Many patients with **septal defects** are asymptomatic during the fetal and neonatal period. However, with increased pulmonary vascular resistance, right-to-left shunting of deoxygenated blood may produce systemic hypoxemia. Later in life, the normal decrease in pulmonary vascular resistance increases blood flow to the lung and potentially causes pulmonary vascular overcirculation and pulmonary hypertension.

f. **Laboratory studies.** In the infant with signs and symptoms of cardiovascular disease, relevant studies include an arterial blood gas, pre- and postductal oxygen saturations, four extremity blood pressures, an ECG, CXR, hemoglobin or hematocrit, and determination of arterial blood gas tension during inhalation of pure oxygen ("**hyperoxia test**"). A PaO_2 that remains below 150 mm Hg while the infant breathes 100% oxygen is suggestive of an intracardiac shunt. Cardiology consultation is indicated, and echocardiography is frequently performed to detect potential structural heart lesions.

3. **Patent ductus arteriosus (PDA)**
   a. **Clinical features.** PDA is commonly encountered in the premature infant and is characterized by a murmur at the left sternal border radiating to the back, bounding pulses, widened pulse pressure, evidence of increased pulmonary blood flow by CXR, respiratory distress, and excessive weight gain. The PDA often can be confirmed by cardiac ultrasound. In some cases, cardiac dysfunction associated with a PDA may decrease systemic blood pressure, peripheral perfusion, and urine output and may be associated with metabolic acidosis.
   b. Although **early treatment** of a PDA consists of fluid restriction and supportive care, it is important to maintain systemic perfusion. If the degree of shunt through the ductus arteriosus is significant, and renal and platelet function are adequate, pharmacologic closure of the ductus with **indomethacin** or **ibuprofen** may be attempted.
   c. **Surgical closure** of a PDA is indicated in symptomatic infants for whom medical therapy has either failed, is contraindicated, such as those with decreased renal or platelet function, or thought not to be effective.
   d. **Anesthetic considerations.** Often these infants are critically ill, requiring high levels of oxygen support, ventilator support and vasopressor therapy. They may have renal dysfunction, because of decreased cardiac output caused by the PDA and fluid restriction, and platelet dysfunction because of medical therapies. Many PDA closures may take place in the NICU to avoid the risk of transporting the infant to the OR. In addition to a preductal pulse oximeter that is used to assess cerebral oxygen delivery, a postductal oximeter can be helpful during the surgical procedure for detecting inadvertent occlusion of the aorta during assessment of the anatomy of the central circulation.

An opiate-based anesthetic (eg, fentanyl) with muscle relaxation is a common technique used for infants undergoing PDA ligation. Infants should be monitored closely in the postoperative period for complications including pneumothorax, hypotension, and oliguria.

4. **Dysrhythmias**
   a. **Supraventricular tachycardia** (SVT) is the most frequent dysrhythmia seen in fetuses and neonates. The associated heart rate >250 beats/min is often self-limited and well tolerated. However, if the SVT is associated with hypotension or oxygen desaturation, prompt treatment is required.
   b. **SVT treatment** consists of vagal maneuvers such as nasopharyngeal stimulation or placement of a cold pack glove or ice-filled glove on the infant's face. Massage of the eye should be avoided, as this may lead to disruption of the lens in neonates. **Adenosine** and **esophageal pacing** are also useful for acute management of symptomatic SVT.
   c. Synchronized cardioversion is indicated if the patient is hemodynamically unstable.

5. **Persistent pulmonary hypertension of the newborn (PPHN)**
   a. **Pathophysiology.** PPHN, previously referred to as persistent fetal circulation, is manifested by an increase in lung vascular resistance with resulting pulmonary arterial hypertension, right-to-left shunting across the foramen ovale and the ductus arteriosus, and systemic hypoxemia.
   b. **Etiology.** It is suspected that many newborns with PPHN have abnormal muscularization of the distal lung vascular bed and reactivity of the pulmonary arteries. Although PPHN is associated with perinatal depression, meconium aspiration, bacterial pneumonia, or sepsis, the exact role of these in the etiology of PPHN is unknown.
   c. **Clinical features.** Typically, term or near-term newborns with PPHN have severe systemic hypoxemia unrelieved by breathing at high FiO_2. They may have shunt evidenced by higher oxygen saturations in the upper versus lower extremities. ECG may reveal right ventricular hypertrophy, and CXR may show decreased pulmonary vascular markings. Echocardiography may demonstrate shunting of blood at the level of the PDA and/or PFO.
   d. **Treatment** of PPHN
      1. Specific treatments include intubation and mechanical ventilation with high FiO_2, induced respiratory or metabolic alkalosis, and INO administration. In nearly 50% of cases, carefully administered INO gas rapidly vasodilates the pulmonary vasculature, decreases shunt, and increases systemic oxygenation. In babies breathing NO gas, the levels of methemoglobin and INO oxides need to be measured.
      2. Nonspecific and supportive treatments include aggressive blood pressure support, sedation with narcotics (eg, fentanyl), and occasionally muscle relaxants.
      3. **ECMO** may be lifesaving for some patients with PPHN refractory to ventilatory and medical therapy.

F. **Head and neck procedures**
   1. Strabismus repair. See Chapter 30: Anesthesia for Head and Neck Surgery.
   2. Tonsillectomy, adenoidectomy, and emergency surgery in the child with bleeding tonsils. See Chapter 30: Anesthesia for Head and Neck Surgery.

G. Neurologic disorders
1. Intracranial hemorrhage
  a. **Intraventricular hemorrhage** occurs in more than 30% of infants with birth weights below 1000 g typically within the first 7 days of life. Subdural and subarachnoid hemorrhages are much less common.
  b. **Clinical features.** Intraventricular hemorrhage is often asymptomatic, although it may present with unexplained lethargy, apnea, or seizures. On examination, the head circumference can be increased, and the fontanelle may be bulging.
  c. **Laboratory studies.** Laboratory examination may show anemia and acidosis. Screening head ultrasounds are generally performed in infants under 32 weeks of gestational age.
  d. **Grading of intraventricular hemorrhage**
     1. **Grade I.** Subependymal or choroid plexus bleeding only.
     2. **Grade II.** Intraventricular bleeding without dilatation of ventricles.
     3. **Grade III.** Intraventricular bleeding with dilatation of ventricles.
     4. **Grade IV.** Intraparenchymal bleeding.
  e. The **major complication** of intraventricular hemorrhage is CSF obstruction resulting in **hydrocephalus.** This is followed by measuring daily head circumferences and by serial cranial ultrasounds. Serial lumbar punctures or intraventricular shunting is often required.
  f. Hypertonic agents (eg, 25% dextrose in water) that had previously been advocated in the treatment of hypoglycemia have been implicated in the etiology of intraventricular hemorrhage and should be avoided.

2. Myelodysplasia
  a. Abnormal neurulation of the embryo can result in failed closure of the posterior neural tube by the 4th week of gestation. A **meningocele** is caused when the meninges herniate through a bony abnormality in the spine (spina bifida) and form a sac filled with CSF. The spinal cord and nerve roots are generally not involved. A **myelomeningocele** is the result of spinal cord and meninges herniating through a defect in the spinal canal. Eighty percent of myelomeningoceles involve the lumbar spinal region. Hydrocephalus may affect as many as 90% of newborns with myelomeningocele because the cord lesion can displace the cerebellum and interfere with CSF flow.
  b. Myelomeningoceles occur with an incidence of 4 to 10 per 10,000 live births. The incidence has significantly decreased with maternal folic acid supplementation. Women with diabetes or taking certain medications (eg, antiepileptics) are at increased risk of having a child with myelodysplasia.
  c. **Postnatal management** includes covering the defect with a warm, normal saline-soaked sterile dressing to prevent adhesion of the dressing to the defect. The infant should be kept prone, and latex exposure should be avoided. Preoperatively, the infant should undergo assessment for additional abnormalities (eg, scoliosis, hydrocephalus, Arnold–Chiari malformation), and neuroimaging is recommended. Early surgical repair significantly decreases the risk of infection. Postoperatively, infants must be monitored closely for seizures and hydrocephalus that may require shunt placement. Prognosis ultimately depends on the level of the lesion and the presence of other congenital anomalies.
  d. **Anesthetic considerations.** During intubation of the patient in a supine position, special care must be taken to pad the exposed

neural tissue to prevent injury. In some cases, intubation of the patient in the left lateral decubitus position may be preferred to protect the lesion. Many patients with myelomeningocele may have a short trachea, creating an increased risk for endobronchial intubation. Blood loss tends to be minimal unless extensive subcutaneous tissue dissection is required to mobilize the skin so that it can cover a large lesion. If hydrocephalus is present, the neonate may have a diminished response to hypoxia, causing an increased risk of apneic episodes in the postoperative period.

3. **Retinopathy of prematurity (ROP)**
   a. **Etiologies**
      1. **The risk of ROP** is increased in premature neonates requiring oxygen therapy. ROP is seen in infants with birth weights <1500 g and gestational age <30 weeks. There is an 80% incidence in infants weighing <1000 g. To decrease the incidence of ROP, **hyperoxia should be avoided.**
      2. Factors other than hyperoxic exposure and prematurity may produce ROP, as it has been demonstrated in full-term infants, infants with cyanotic heart disease, stillborn infants, and infants without hyperoxic exposure. Factors that may increase risk include anemia, infection, intracranial hemorrhage, acidosis, and PDA.
   b. **Pathophysiology.** ROP begins in the temporal peripheral retina, which is the last part of the retina to vascularize. An elevated ridge demarcating vascularized and nonvascularized retina is initially seen. **Fibrovascular proliferation** from this border extends posteriorly, and in 90% of patients, gradual resolution occurs from this stage. These patients may develop strabismus, amblyopia, myopia, or peripheral retinal detachment in later life.
   c. In 10% of patients, fibrovascularization extends into the vitreous, resulting in vitreous hemorrhage, peripheral retinal scarring, temporal dragging of the disk and macula, and partial retinal detachment. In severe disease, extensive fibrovascular proliferation can result in a retrolental white mass (leukocoria), complete retinal detachment, and loss of vision.
   d. **Infants ≤32 weeks of gestational age, birth weight ≤1500 g, or with additional risk factors should undergo** indirect ophthalmoscopy at 34 weeks of corrected gestational age. If ROP is identified, the infant is reexamined at 1- to 2-week intervals until spontaneous resolution occurs. New cases of ROP do not occur after 3 months of age.
   e. **Treatment** for severe manifestations of ROP has included photocoagulation, diathermy, cryotherapy, vitrectomy, and bevacizumab injection.

H. **Potential for neurotoxicity of general anesthetics**
   1. In vivo and in vitro animal models of neuronal cell death have been demonstrated with almost all commonly used anesthetic agents (ie, propofol, ketamine, desflurane, halothane, isoflurane, sevoflurane, xenon, diazepam, midazolam, chloral hydrate, pentobarbital). However, the long-term outcomes regarding neurodevelopmental effects and tests of memory and cognitive processing in animal studies are mixed and call into question the effects of anesthetic drugs. Furthermore, significant limitations in animal studies (ie, developmental equivalence, dosing/duration of exposure controlled for life span, study design, etc.) preclude extrapolation to our pediatric patient.
   2. Due to the in vitro and animal evidence, there has been growing concern regarding the long-term developmental effects of general

anesthesia on our pediatric patients. The data regarding the long-term outcomes of pediatric patients exposed to general anesthesia early in development are mixed and have several limitations (ie, study design, anesthetic used, surgical exposure, comorbidities, etc.). The first prospective randomized control trial (GAS; NCT00756600) investigating the effects of general versus regional anesthesia on neurodevelopmental outcomes in infants undergoing inguinal hernia repair has concluded in two publications, Davidson et al. and McCann et al. The "GAS study" showed that in healthy children receiving a single sevoflurane exposure of slightly <1 hour in duration, there is no change in intelligence scores at 2 years and 5 years of age. The long-term developmental effects of longer exposure duration, multiple exposures, and in children who have comorbidities remains unclear.

3. In advising a parent or caregiver concerned about the neurodevelopmental effects of general anesthesia, it may be helpful to discuss several points below:
    a. Alternatives, if possible, to general anesthesia (eg, spinal anesthesia)
    b. Necessity of surgical/procedural intervention
    c. Necessity of anesthesia if surgery is indicated
    d. Not exceeding the required amount of anesthesia for the indicated procedure to accomplish procedural and patient comfort goals
    e. Uncertainty regarding the human and animal data

Suggested Readings

Anand KJS, Hickey PR. Pain and its effects in the human neonate and fetus. *N Engl J Med.* 1987;317:1321–1329.

Arant BS Jr. Developmental patterns of renal functional maturation compared in the human neonate. *J Pediatr.* 1978;92:705–712.

Bahrami KR, Van Meurs KP. ECMO for neonatal respiratory failure. *Semin Perinatol* 2005;29:15–23.

Bean C, Low S, Novak A, Chen A, Elder J, Liu CA. Awake combined spinal caudal anesthesia for longer-duration urologic surgery in infants: a case series. *A & A Pract.* 2024;18(6):e01792.

Bell EF, Warburton D, Stonestreet BS, Oh W. Effect of fluid administration on the development of symptomatic patent ductus arteriosus and congestive heart failure in premature infants. *N Engl J Med.* 1980;302:598–604.

Berde CB, Sethna NF. Analgesics for the treatment of pain in children. *N Engl J Med.* 2002;347(14):1094–1103.

Chen AL, Elder JS, Liu CA. Awake neuraxial anesthesia for infants undergoing infraumbilical surgery. *Pediatric Anesthesia.* 2022;32(7):e14606.

Cloherty JP, Eichenwald EC, Hansen AR, Stark AR. *Manual of Neonatal Care.* 7th ed. Lippincott Williams & Wilkins; 2011.

Constant I, Sabourdin N. The EEG signal: a window on the cortical brain activity. *Paediatr Anaesth.* 2012;22(6):539–552.

Coté CJ, Zaslavsky A, Downes JJ, et al. Postoperative apnea in former preterm infants after inguinal herniorrhaphy. A combined analysis. *Anesthesiology.* 1995;82(4):809–822.

Coté CJ, Lerman J, Anderson BJ. *A Practice of Anesthesia for Infants and Children.* 5th ed. Saunders Elsevier; 2013.

Coté CJ, Sui J, Anderson TA, et al. Continuous noninvasive cardiac output in children: is this the next generation of operating room monitors? Initial experience in 402 pediatric patients. *Paediatr Anaesth.* 2015;25(2):150–159.

Dalal PG, Murray D, Messner AH, Feng A, McAllister J. Pediatric laryngeal dimensions: an age-based analysis. *Anesth Analg.* 2009;108(5):1475–1479.

Dalens B, Khandwala R. *Regional Anesthesia in Infants, Children, and Adolescents.* Williams & Wilkins; 1995.

Dorsch JA, Dorsch SE. *Understanding Anesthesia Equipment.* 5th ed. Wolters Kluwer Health, Lippincott Williams & Wilkins; 2008.

Fanaroff AA, Wald M, Gruber HS, Klaus MH. Insensible water loss in low birth weight infants. *Pediatrics.* 1972;50:236–245.

Fluge G. Clinical aspects of neonatal hypoglycaemia. *Acta Paediatr Scand.* 1974;63:826–832.

Gallagher TM, Crean PM. Spinal anaesthesia for infants born prematurely. *Anaesthesia.* 1989;44:434–436.

Gersony WM, Peckham GJ, Ellison RC, Miettinen OS, Nadas AS. Effects of indomethacin in premature infants with patent ductus arteriosus: results of a national collaborative study. *J Pediatr.* 1983;102:895–906.

Greeley WJ. *Pediatric Anesthesia.* Churchill Livingstone; 1999.

Gregory GA. *Pediatric Anesthesia.* 4th ed. Churchill Livingstone; 2001.

Johns Hopkins Hospital, Custer JW, Rau RE, Lee CK. *The Harriett Lane Handbook.* 18th ed. Elsevier Health Sciences; 2008.

Hall BD. Choanal atresia and associated multiple anomalies. *J Pediatr.* 1979;95:395–398.

Keith CG, Doyle LW. Retinopathy of prematurity in extremely low birth weight infants. *Pediatrics.* 1995;95:42–45.

Kliegman RM, Behrman RE, Jenson HB, et al. *Nelson Textbook of Pediatrics.* 18th ed. WB Saunders Elsevier; 2007.

Koehntop DE, Rodman JH, Brundage DM, Hegland MG, Buckley JJ. Pharmacokinetics of fentanyl in neonates. *Anesth Analg.* 1986;65:227–232.

Krane EJ, Haberkern CM, Jacobson LE. Postoperative apnea, bradycardia, and oxygen desaturation in formerly premature infants: prospective comparison of spinal and general anesthesia. *Anesth Analg.* 1995;80:7–13.

Kurth CD, Spitzer AR, Broennle AM, Downes JJ. Postoperative apnea in preterm infants. *Anesthesiology.* 1987;66:483–488.

Marks KH, Devenyi AG, Bello ME, Nardis EE, Seaton JF, Ultman JS. Thermal head wrap for infants. *J Pediatr.* 1985;107:956–959.

Lin EP, Soriano SG, Loepke AW. Anesthetic neurotoxicity. *Anesthesiol Clin* 2014;32(1): 133–155.

Lingappan K, Neveln N, Arnold JL, Fernandes CJ, Pammi M. Videolaryngoscopy versus direct laryngoscopy for tracheal intubation in neonates. *Cochrane Database Syst Rev.* 2023.

Miller RD, ed. *Anesthesia.* 8th ed. Elsevier-Churchill Livingstone; 2009.

Motoyama EK, Davis PJ. *Smith's Anesthesia for Infants and Children.* 8th ed. St. Elsevier Mosby–Saunders; 2007.

Moya FR, Lally KP. Evidence-based management of infants with congenital diaphragmatic hernia. *Semin Perinatol.* 2005;29:112–117.

O'Neill JA, Rowe MI, Grosfeld J, et al. *Pediatric Surgery.* 5th ed. Mosby-Year Book; 1998.

Philippart AI, Canty TG, Filler RM. Acute fluid volume requirements in infants with anterior abdominal wall defects. *J Pediatr Surg.* 1972;7:553–558.

Roberts JD Jr, Fineman JR, Morin FC III, et al. Inhaled nitric oxide and persistent pulmonary hypertension of the newborn. The Inhaled Nitric Oxide Study Group. *N Engl J Med.* 1997;336:605–610.

Roberts JD Jr, Polaner DM, Lang P, Zapol WM. Inhaled nitric oxide (NO): a selective pulmonary vasodilator for the treatment of persistent pulmonary hypertension of the newborn (PPHN). *Circulation.* 1991;84:A1279.

Roberts JD, Polaner DM, Lang P, Zapol WM. Inhaled nitric oxide in persistent pulmonary hypertension of the newborn. *Lancet.* 1992;340:818–821.

Sola A. Oxygen in neonatal anesthesia: friend or foe? *Curr Opin Anaesthesiol.* 2008;21: 332–339.

Srinivasan G, Jain R, Pildes RS, Kannan CR. Glucose homeostasis during anesthesia and surgery in infants. *J Pediatr Surg.* 1986;21:718–721.

Touloukian RJ, Higgins E. The spectrum of serum electrolytes in hypertrophic pyloric stenosis. *J Pediatr Surg.* 1983;18:394–397.

Tyszczuk L, Meek J, Elwell C, Wyatt JS. Cerebral blood flow is independent of mean arterial blood pressure in preterm infants undergoing intensive care. *Pediatrics.* 1998; 102:337–341.

Vergnaud E, Vidal C, Montmayeur Verchere J, et al. Noninvasive cardiac output measurement using bioreactance in postoperative pediatric patients. *Paediatr Anaesth.* 2015;25(2): 160–166.

Wessel DL, Keane JF, Parness I, Lock JE. Outpatient closure of the patent ductus arteriosus. *Circulation.* 1988;77:1068–1071.

Wright TE, Orr RJ, Haberkern CM, Walbergh EJ. Complications during spinal anesthesia in infants: high spinal blockade. *Anesthesiology.* 1990;73:1290–1292.

Yaster M, Buck JR, Dudgeon DL, et al. Hemodynamic effects of primary closure of omphalocele/gastroschisis in human newborns. *Anesthesiology.* 1988;69:84–88.

34 Non-Operating Room Anesthesia
Anastasia P. Piersa and Rafael Vazquez

I. GENERAL CONSIDERATIONS
The number of non-operating room anesthesia (NORA) procedures continues to increase rapidly. Technologic advancements and innovations in percutaneous image-guided procedures have continued to rapidly evolve and, in conjunction with an aging patient population, have resulted in an increased technical complexity of NORA interventions. This has been paired with innovations in anesthetic care for complex cases such as advanced ventilation techniques. NORA locations typically include the following suites: interventional radiology (IR), diagnostic radiology (magnetic resonance imaging [MRI] and computerized tomography [CT]), electrophysiology (EP), cardiac catheterization, endoscopy, nuclear medicine, and others. Although the same principles and considerations apply to patients who are having monitored anesthesia care (MAC) or general Anesthesia (GA) outside of the main operating room, three distinctive features characterize NORA: location, operator, and distinctive workflows. Ergonomics, lack of anesthesia resources and personnel, and lack of familiarity with the environment are perhaps the biggest and most underestimated considerations when working in NORA locations. Team communication and robust crisis resource management (CRM) awareness are paramount to promote patient safety and procedural success in NORA.

A. Required equipment in remote locations
1. Each location should be equipped with medical gas systems. Depending on where the anesthesia machine will be stationed, more than one gas outlet may be installed. The common gas outlets should include oxygen, vacuum, waste anesthetic gas disposal (WAGD), vacuum, and medical air. A full reserve tank of O_2 should be available as a backup. An air tank may be necessary but is not mandatory.
2. Functioning suction is necessary.
3. Adequate monitoring equipment that adheres to the American Society of Anesthesiologists (ASA) standards is required.
4. Adequate electrical outlets and lighting that are connected and a power source are mandatory.
5. Functioning anesthesia machine appropriate for the anesthetic must be made available. Extra-long gas supply hoses may be necessary; anesthesia breathing circuit tubing may require extensions to reach the patient. If inhalational anesthetic is administered, an adequate and reliable scavenging system is required via WAGD.
6. Resuscitation equipment must be immediately available. This includes a defibrillator, Ambu Bag, as well as emergency medications (this may include sugammadex if using nondepolarizing neuromuscular blockers, lipid emulsion if performing regional anesthesia, and dantrolene if using malignant hyperthermia-triggering agents).
7. Dedicated NORA supply cart or Omnicell that can dispense controlled substances are necessary to ensure that adequate supplies and medications are available to provide anesthetic care.

Chapter 34 Non-Operating Room Anesthesia

8. Dedicated advanced emergency airway equipment (eg, video laryngoscope and/or an airway cart with a fiberoptic scope) can be helpful given the high-risk nature of emergent airway management outside of the OR.
9. A NORA-specific cognitive aid such as an emergency manual which includes most common emergent situations specific to the NORA location may be valuable to serve as a resource during a crisis.

B. Ergonomics and patient access
1. Ensure adequate space to deliver a safe anesthetic with a plan to access the patient if the layout and equipment positioning (eg, moving C-arm, CT gantry, etc.) is less than ideal.
2. Ensure a means to remotely monitor patient and vital signs (eg, visible anesthesia display in control room) during intraprocedural points where additional irradiation or other workflow considerations warrant anesthesia team exiting the room.
3. Plan in advance for positioning on hard surfaces when anesthetizing in the CT scanner and MRI suite. To avoid positioning injuries during prolonged procedures, consider additional blankets, pillows, prone face foam, etc. Ensure easy access to the airway by positioning the head of patient away from gantry, if possible, for CT-guided cases.
4. Imaging, especially for MRI-guided studies/procedures, often requires the patient moving great lengths frequently in and out of the gantry. Prepare to have additional length on circuit/O_2 tubing, end-tidal CO_2 ($EtCO_2$) tubing, intravenous (IV) tubing, and monitoring cables. A "test scan" of full excursion is helpful prior to starting the procedure to ensure the equipment has sufficient slack.

C. Radiation safety
1. "As low as reasonably achievable" (ALARA) is the main principle of radiation safety. The goal is to minimize radiation exposure to patients, practitioners, and the environment. Three measures can help achieve ALARA:
   a. Time (minimize amount of time exposed to radiation)
   b. Distance (maximize distance to the radiation source)
   c. Shielding (shield yourself from radiation source with appropriate barriers)
2. Radiation exposure is inversely proportional to the square of the distance from the source. Given radiation dose is cumulative, standing as far away as possible from source is recommended to limit exposure. Extension IV tubing can decrease the radiation exposure to anesthesia clinicians during medication administration, especially when biplane is used for fluoroscopic procedures.
3. The use of mobile lead shields and wraparound lead with a properly fitting thyroid shield is strongly recommended. A personalized radiation badge should also be used. Lead goggles can be used to decrease radiation to the cornea, an organ highly vulnerable to radiation.

II. ANESTHESIA TECHNIQUES
A. Procedural sedation.
Sedation and analgesia comprise a continuum of states ranging from minimal sedation (anxiolysis) through GA. Specially trained nurses provide procedural sedation for the majority of procedures outside of the operating room for patients deemed ASA physical status (PS) I and ASA PS II. Procedural sedation encompasses moderate sedation (or conscious sedation) and deep sedation. The ASA defines moderate sedation as a state of depressed consciousness where a patient responds

purposefully to verbal commands or light touch. Common medications used to achieve moderate sedation include midazolam and fentanyl. Deep sedation occurs when a deeper level of consciousness depression is reached, and patients can only be aroused with repeated painful stimuli. Deep sedation requires special privileges and providers skilled in airway management, as airway manipulation may be needed and unintended GA may occur. The ASA, Joint Commission on Accreditation of Health care Organizations, and state agencies (licensing boards) have a set of guidelines on provision and supervision of moderate and deep sedation by nonanesthesiologist physicians and other health care professionals.

B. **MAC** is an anesthesia service performed by a qualified anesthesia clinician for a diagnostic or therapeutic procedure. It does not describe the continuum of depth of sedation. MAC allows provision of levels of analgesia and sedation that are appropriate for a given patient and procedure. As part of the MAC service, patients must have a formal preoperative/preprocedural evaluation. This enables for proper evaluation of the various elements that factor into the decision on depth of sedation necessary, including procedure, patient comorbidities, and clinical experience. Depending on the depth of sedation, ventilation may be affected, rescue airway maneuvers may need to be performed, and appropriate equipment should be available if inadvertent conversion to GA occurs. MAC may be associated with less hemodynamic perturbations and may be a better choice for a subset of patients with severely compromised cardiovascular function. For patients and/or procedures with a high aspiration risk, MAC can be performed after careful consideration, and anxiolytic and analgesic techniques should focus on preserving airway reflexes.

C. **GA** is used when a secured airway is necessary, when there is a need for a patient to be still (eg, long complex procedures), and when the procedures involve painful portions that would be difficult to manage under MAC. The cardiopulmonary risk/benefit ratio of GA in high-risk patients undergoing minimally invasive procedures has to be carefully considered on a case-by-case basis.

D. **Ultrasound-guided peripheral nerve blocks (PNBs)** may be used as the primary anesthetic or as an adjunct for procedural and/or postprocedural analgesia.
   1. **Brachial plexus nerve blocks (BPBs)** are options for specific dysfunctional arteriovenous access procedures of the distal upper extremity in end-stage renal disease (ESRD) patients.
   2. **Paravertebral nerve block (PVBs)** may be beneficial for procedures on the liver and kidney (eg, transhepatic biliary drains, liver ablations and embolizations, and renal ablations). Bilateral T7 to T10 PVB can be beneficial for liver lesions (as the liver is innervated bilaterally) while a unilateral PVB suffices for renal procedures.

E. **High-frequency jet ventilation (HFJV)** may be utilized to achieve a semiquiescent field superior to GA with conventional ventilation for intrathoracic or peridiaphragmatic percutaneous procedures such as pulmonary vein isolation (PVI), basilar pulmonary ablations and embolizations, or ablations of liver dome lesions.

F. **Selective lung isolation** utilizing a double-lumen tube or bronchial blockers has been used to achieve a static lung. In addition, these techniques are useful for lung protection of the nonaffected lung from hemorrhage for procedures such as bronchial artery embolizations of patients with hemoptysis and ablations of large lung tumors. A fiberoptic bronchoscope should be available to verify positioning.

G. Enhanced recovery after procedure (ERAP) is an extension of enhanced recovery after surgery (ERAS) and has been applied to select procedures in NORA. Application of evidence-based opioid sparing techniques can decrease post procedural pain and opioid requirements. Preprocedure analgesics such as acetaminophen and celecoxib can be beneficial. Administration of high-dose dexamethasone and antiemetics may be useful to prevent postembolization and ablation syndrome in the interventional oncology patient population undergoing procedures such as transarterial chemoembolization and microwave ablations (MWA).

III. CONTRAST MEDIA
A. Types of contrast media. Ionic and nonionic iodine-based contrast media are administered intravenously and intra-arterially to supplement x-ray–based imaging. Nonionic media are better tolerated than ionic media. High-osmolality contrast media are no longer used intravascularly due to higher rates of adverse events. Nonionic low-osmolality contrast media are most commonly used. Gadolinium-based contrast media are primarily used for MRI imaging.
   1. **Contrast-induced nephropathy (CIN)** is defined as a deterioration in kidney function following intravascular contrast administration. Of note, recent studies on the topic have called into question the prevalence of CIN and the true risk of CIN may be lower than previously thought.
      a. Main risk factor for development of CIN is preexisting severe renal insufficiency with estimated glomerular filtration rate (eGFR) <30, while patients with eGFR between 30 and 45 are at intermediate risk. Diabetes mellitus may provide additive risk, particularly in the intermediate-risk population by eGFR. Coronary angiography and percutaneous coronary procedures may be associated with a higher incidence of CIN.
      b. Baseline eGFR should be obtained in patients considered at risk.
      c. Precontrast IV volume expansion with isotonic normal saline is the mainstay of prophylaxis for CIN, and is indicated for patients with baseline eGFR <30 not on hemodialysis and with no contraindications to IV fluid administration. The ideal infusion rate and volume is unknown. Benefits of oral hydration have not been well studied. Sodium bicarbonate administration to prevent CIN is less studied and often impractical. Administration of N-acetylcysteine (NAC) is not effective and is not recommended.
   2. **Nephrogenic systemic fibrosis** is a sclerosing skin condition with systemic manifestations and poor prognosis that occurs after gadolinium exposure in patients with advanced or end-stage renal disease, with or without dialysis. This typically occurs days to months following exposure.
B. Contrast media reactions. Acute contrast media reactions to modern contrast agents are rare (rates of hypersensitivity reactions range from 0.6% for iodinated and 0.01% to 0.22% for gadolinium-based agents). Most acute contrast media reactions are not considered to be hypersensitivity reactions, and hypersensitivity reactions to contrast may involve direct release of histamine and other mediators or more typical IgE-mediated pathways. Prior exposure to contrast is not required for a reaction to occur. Intravascular contrast administration is more likely to elicit a reaction compared to other routes of administration.
   1. **Risk factors** for allergiclike hypersensitivity reactions include personal and family history of a previous adverse reaction, other allergies, asthma, and hyperthyroidism.

2. **Symptoms** are most commonly mild with a feeling of warmth/flushing, nausea, vomiting, pruritus, or mild urticaria. More severe reactions may present with severe urticaria, vomiting, and bronchospasm, and may progress to angioedema, hypotension, loss of consciousness, and cardiovascular collapse. Almost all severe reactions typically present within 20 minutes of exposure to the contrast media.
3. **Treatment** is supportive and should aim at presenting symptoms. In addition to targeted pharmacologic treatment, consider positioning the patient supine and administering supplemental O_2. In severe cases, intubation for airway protection, inhaled beta agonists, epinephrine, and vasopressors may be necessary.

C. **Contrast premedication strategies** are aimed at reducing the likelihood of a contrast reaction. Although definitive data in high-risk patients is lacking, the risks of premedication are small, and premedication may therefore be considered. Oral premedication is preferable to IV premedication as most studies on this topic used oral medications. Oral premedication regimens recommended by the American College of Radiologist (ACR) Manual on Contrast Media span 12 to 13 hours and involve oral methylprednisolone or prednisone with diphenhydramine as an adjunct. This should be initiated by the scheduling clinicians ahead of time. Accelerated protocols are less than ideal, however, under urgent and emergent circumstances they may be considered. The ACR Manual on Contrast Media recommends the following accelerated IV premedication regimens (in decreasing order of desirability):
1. Methylprednisolone 40 mg IV or hydrocortisone 200 mg IV immediately followed by every 4 hours until contrast medium administration, plus diphenhydramine 50 mg IV 1 hour before contrast administration.
2. Dexamethasone 7.5 mg IV immediately followed by every 4 hours until contrast administration, plus diphenhydramine 50 mg IV 1 hour before contrast administration.
3. Methylprednisolone 40 mg IV or hydrocortisone 200 mg IV, plus diphenhydramine 50 mg IV, each 1 hour before contrast administration.

Of note, the efficacy of premedication regimens <4 to 5 hours in duration has not been shown, and these regimens should be considered in emergency situations only.

IV. ANESTHESIA FOR DIAGNOSTIC RADIOLOGY

CT and MRI scans are usually performed without GA. Children and uncooperative adults (eg, patients with severe head injuries, claustrophobia, or severe chronic back pain) may require sedation or GA to minimize motion artifacts.

A. **CT**
1. **Adults.** Small IV doses of benzodiazepines, narcotics, or short-acting hypnotics (eg, propofol or dexmedetomidine) are useful for sedation; continuous infusions should be titrated to effect.
2. **Infants and children** <3 months of age may not need sedation; most children, however, will require some level of sedation or GA. Children provide specific challenges to the anesthetist as outlined in Chapter 31: Anesthesia for Urologic Surgery.
   a. **Sedation.** Small IV doses of benzodiazepines, narcotics, or short-acting hypnotics (eg, propofol, dexmedetomidine) may be used for sedation as either bolus or continuous infusions titrated to effect.
   b. **GA** maintained with either IV or inhalational agents may be required. The airway may be maintained naturally, using a laryngeal mask airway (LMA) or by endotracheal intubation as necessary. Considerations include type of study and motion artifact generated by ventilation

technique (ie, large motion artifact from irregular ventilation for certain brain MRI sequences).

B. MRI
1. The **physical environment** of the MRI suite presents several challenges for anesthetizing patients.
   a. The long, narrow bore of the magnet where the patient reclines does not allow ready access to the patient during imaging. Scanners are located in shielded rooms that contain the magnetic field and shield against radiofrequency noise that would produce image artifacts.
   b. The static magnetic field is always present and exerts a force on all ferromagnetic materials (eg, steel gas tanks, batteries, and standard stethoscopes). Ferromagnetic objects brought near the magnetic field can be forcibly pulled toward the magnet, potentially injuring people and equipment in their path. Standard anesthesia equipment such as noninvasive blood pressure monitors, ventilators, and infusion pumps are often non-MRI compatible; specialized compatible equipment is necessary. Only plastic stethoscopes and commercially available magnet-compatible laryngoscopes should be used in the magnet area. Credit cards, watches, and pagers must be left outside the scanning room.
   c. Non-MRI compatible metallic implants (eg, joint prostheses, aneurysm clips, and cochlear implants) or implanted devices (eg, pacemakers, implantable cardioverter defibrillators [ICDs], insulin infusion pumps, intrathecal pumps, or spinal cord stimulators) may potentially be dislodged, dysfunction, or suffer permanent damage by the magnetic field. In addition, equipment heating may occur from radiofrequency signals generated during scanning. Some specific pacemakers, ICDs, or pulmonary artery catheters are considered "MRI safe," and scanning can proceed. Imaging of patients with these devices should not be considered routine, and individual cases should be carefully reviewed for medical necessity. Imaging may require that the pacemaker be turned off while the patient is in the magnetic field; the device is interrogated and turned on after scanning. Cerebral aneurysm clips are not considered an absolute contraindication to MRI; it is important, however, to identify the type of clip present to determine MRI compatibility. Each MRI site carries a list of medical devices designated MRI compatible by the U.S. Food and Drug Administration (FDA). Because medical devices may be upgraded or altered by a manufacturer without notifying the FDA, MRI centers should, in addition, contact the manufacturer about specific devices when questions arise.
2. **Monitors and equipment** must be safe for the patient, function within the magnetic field, and have a minimal effect on imaging. Specialized compatible monitoring equipment is available so that equipment can remain in the magnetic field and communicate to an additional monitor outside the shielded magnet area.
   a. Radiofrequency signals and shifting magnetic fields generated during scanning may create significant artifacts on the standard ECG monitor, and special MRI-compatible monitoring devices are needed.
   b. Similarly, scanning interferes with standard pulse oximeters. Specialized "MRI-compatible" monitoring systems utilizing fiberoptic cables are available.
   c. A large amount of noise can be generated during imaging.
   d. Temperature probes are not used because of the potential for thermal burns.
   e. Visualization of patients during scanning is imperative and may occur via a shielded window or closed-circuit video.

f. Electrical currents induced in coiled cables during scanning can burn patients; cables should be kept as straight as possible to minimize this risk.

3. General issues. The duration of an MRI scan varies. Immobility is required only during the actual scanning, 3 to 12 minutes at a time. GA is necessary for most infants and children, usually utilizing an LMA or endotracheal tube. GA can be induced in the magnet area. Alternatively, induction can be performed in an area outside of the static magnetic field and the anesthetized patient moved into the scanner. Maintenance of anesthesia is provided with specially modified anesthesia machines that contain only nonferrous metals. The patient must be removed from the magnetic field if cardiopulmonary resuscitation is required. Challenges may also arise in developmentally delayed adults. A special pathway that may include oral sedative premedication prior to arrival to the scanner and a special induction area can be beneficial for these patients. Coordination with the patient's primary care physician is important. Intramuscular medications may be needed in patients unable to tolerate oral sedative.

V. ANESTHESIA FOR CT-GUIDED THERMAL ABLATIONS

Microwave, radiofrequency, and cryoablation are procedural modalities that utilize extreme thermal energy to induce cell death, primarily via coagulative necrosis. Applicators/probes are guided using CT to the tumor tissue and emit the energy to achieve locoregional tumor treatment of lesions of a certain size (<3.0 cm for liver). The heat modalities include radiofrequency ablation (RFA) and MWA. RFA involves application of radiofrequency electrical current that passes through tissue with resulting thermal energy deposition and local temperature increase via resistive heating, which causes tissue damage. Its cost effectiveness makes it very popular worldwide, however, it is limited by electrical and thermal tissue conductivity and is therefore better suited for smaller targets. MWA involves dielectric heating. During cryoablation, room temperature gas (typically argon) is applied to the probe at high pressure, and rapid expansion of argon cools the gas and achieves temperatures low enough to freeze the tumor cells. Each procedure consists of 1 to 3 cycles of freezing and thawing per lesion, and produces tissue damage via cell damage from ice crystals, osmotic fluid shifts with thawing, and apoptosis. Unlike with other techniques, the ablation zone can be visualized real time with CT during treatment. In addition, cryoablation tends to be less painful than other ablation methods. However, the risk of bleeding may be increased due to lack of coagulation effect to adjacent vessels. If the targeted lesions are adjacent to delicate tissue structures such as bowel or the diaphragm, physical separation can be achieved by fluid hydrodissection or pneumoperitoneum with CO_2 to prevent collateral damage.

A. CT-guided thermal ablations of liver, renal, bone, and soft tissue

1. The anesthetic can be performed with GA or MAC ± regional anesthesia.
   a. HFJV can be utilized for hepatic dome lesions to minimize diaphragm movement.
   b. ERAP can be beneficial as postprocedural pain can result from large ablations.
   c. Ultrasound-guided bilateral PVB can be beneficial for hepatic and unilateral renal ablations. Short-acting PNB can be used for musculoskeletal procedures.

2. Discuss positioning with the proceduralist. Pad bony prominences and support the arms in pillow or blankets to be in an extended position without exaggerated abduction. The typical positioning for specific

procedures is outlined below; however, it is important to communicate and confirm with the interventional radiology (IR) team.
- a. Liver ablations: supine with arms above head on towel rolls. Take care to not overextend the arms and prevent exaggerated abduction.
- b. Renal ablations: usually lateral decubitus with targeted lesion typically dependent side down. This positioning decreases kidney mobility secondary to respiratory motion. For deep lesions the patients are positioned prone.
- c. Bone and soft tissue ablations: These procedures involve heterogeneous lesions in the body including abdomen, retroperitoneum, chest wall, bones of upper extremities, vertebrae, and lower extremity. Patient positioning and anesthetic is variable as is anesthetic technique. Some centers use neuromonitoring when ablations are in delicate areas prone to nerve damage.

3. Postablation syndrome (PAS) may occur in up to 30% of patients undergoing liver MWA or RFA, and has been described after renal ablations and cryoablations as well. Symptoms are usually self-limited and may include nausea, fever, malaise, and delayed postprocedure pain.

B. CT-guided lung biopsies and ablations

1. Percutaneous procedures of the lung are becoming more common. Biopsies and ablations are suitable for small tumor lesions in patients who are poor candidates for surgical intervention due to underlying comorbidities or anatomical reasons (eg, previous chest surgery or location of small tumor). These present special considerations for the anesthesiologist as some procedures can benefit from a static lung field to facilitate ablation, while others can benefit from lung isolation to induce pneumothorax to separate pleural lesions from the chest wall. Treatment modalities include both heat ablations and cryoablations. Irrespective of modality, hemoptysis is a real concern, particularly for large ablations.
   - a. When anesthesia support is provided, the cases can be done with either MAC or GA. Lung biopsy is a relatively painless procedure amenable to procedural sedation or MAC. However, the pleura is well innervated, and penetration with a needle may be painful.
   - b. MAC techniques should focus on keeping the patient immobile during needle placement and breathing in a normal pattern. Rapid and shallow or deep and slow breathing can make procedures challenging.
   - c. Ablation procedures require the use of large bore probes and are more painful, especially during the actual ablation portion of the case. GA can be performed, but positive pressure can lead to higher risk of pneumothorax progressing to tension pneumothorax. GA is often required for cases involving complex lesions for advanced airway support.

2. Positioning is dependent on the location of tumor and planned trajectory. Supine, prone, or lateral positioning may be requested depending on the laterality and lesion location. Prone positioning in the CT scanner is challenging under GA. Pillows and abdominal rolls can be used to elevate the body, to keep the abdomen free, and allow the head and face to be supported with the neck midline and neutral.

3. HFJV or a double-lumen tube can be utilized as previously described.
   - a. Possible starting HFJV settings include driving pressure (DP) 10 to 15 psi, inspiratory time (IT) 30%, frequency 100 to 120 bpm.
   - b. For these procedures, if positive pressure is utilized, it is prudent to set pressures as low as possible and consider chest tube placement

by interventionalist either prophylactically or if there is evidence of pneumothorax on CT.

4. Post procedure, the probe is removed and the wound immediately covered to prevent a sucking chest wound and pneumothorax. This necessitates turning the patient prone or supine, depending upon the insertion site, immediately after removal of the probe. Extubation considerations include hemoptysis (particularly important for large ablations), tension pneumothorax, or hemothorax (if not chest tube in place). It is prudent to have two suctions and a brochoscope readily available. Ensure the patient has fully recovered airway protection reflexes prior to extubation. Reintubation for airway protection may be necessary.

VI. ANESTHESIA FOR NEUROINTERVENTIONS

Anesthetic management may be necessary for both diagnostic (eg, angiography, balloon test occlusion) and therapeutic (eg, aneurysm embolization) procedures. Access to the patient after start of the procedure may be limited to the left arm and leg.

- **A. Endovascular embolization** is performed to treat ruptured as well as unruptured cerebral aneurysms, to interrupt blood supply to intracranial and extracranial arteriovenous fistulas (AVFs) and malformations, vascular tumors, and bleeding vessels in the nose or pharynx.
  1. Embolization requires access to the vascular tree, commonly via the femoral artery, and advancement of a small catheter into the aneurysm or blood vessels supplying the area of pathology. Once position is confirmed by angiography, the vascular occlusive material (detachable metal coils, glue, or small particles) is deployed via the catheter.
     a. Anesthetic goals include provision of a still field during placement of the microcatheter and deployment of the occlusive material, stable hemodynamics, and rapid recovery after the procedure to test neurologic function. This often necessitates GA to provide amnesia in addition to paralysis. Anesthesia can be accomplished with IV medications (propofol, muscle relaxant, and narcotics) and/or volatile anesthetics. Nitrous oxide is avoided to minimize consequences of inadvertent arterial air emboli. These procedures are relatively painless with little stimulation from the procedure.
        1. If hypertonic contrast agents are used, bladder catheterization and fluid replacement may be necessary as these agents may produce diuresis.
        2. Invasive arterial blood pressure monitoring via a radial artery is often necessary for control of hemodynamics; alternatively, blood pressure may be transduced from the femoral artery sheath placed during the procedure.
        3. Judicious blood pressure control is important during embolization procedures. Hypotension should be avoided to ensure adequate cerebral perfusion, however vasoactive drugs such as phenylephrine should be used with great caution in patients with unprotected cerebral aneurysms. Hypertension should also be avoided because it may increase the risk of hemorrhage or aneurysm rupture.
        4. Procedures may be lengthy and place the patient at risk for thromboembolic events. Patients often require anticoagulation (typically with unfractionated heparin) during the procedure to minimize propagation of thrombus from the embolization coils or microcatheters; anticoagulation is monitored by activated clotting time (ACT). For some procedures, patients may receive

aspirin and/or clopidogrel before the procedure. Aspirin can be given by suppository during procedures if necessary. In addition, intra-arterial administration of eptifibatide may reduce the rate of thromboembolic events and can be considered.
5. Intraprocedural complications include rupture of the aneurysm, AVF or malformation, dissection or rupture of a blood vessel, and inadvertent occlusion of a blood vessel. If intracranial hemorrhage is suspected, immediate placement of a ventriculostomy may be necessary to drain cerebrospinal fluid (CSF) emergently to reduce intracranial pressure (ICP). Unlike intraoperative aneurysm rupture in open procedures, (Chapter 23: Anesthesia for Neurosurgery), there is no significant blood loss because the cranium is closed. Elevation of ICP may require immediate interventions such as hyperventilation or osmotic agents, up to barbiturate coma. An immediate CT scan may be necessary to determine the extent of hemorrhage and need for emergency surgery.

B. **Embolization for control of epistaxis and extracranial vascular lesions** presents potential problems of hemorrhage, hemodynamic instability, large amounts of blood in the airway, and aspiration. Typed and cross-matched blood should be available; large-bore IV access may be necessary if acute hemorrhage is a potential threat. Endotracheal intubation is optimal especially for urgent cases, though it could be difficult if the pathology involves the airway and/or face. The nose and nasopharynx may be packed as temporizing treatments.

C. **Balloon test occlusion** of the internal carotid artery is performed to determine whether permanent obstruction of the vessel will lead to neurologic deficit. Occlusion is performed endovascularly by temporarily obstructing blood flow with inflation of a balloon in the vessel; if no deficit is apparent on neurologic examination, hypotension is induced and maintained for 20 to 30 minutes to elicit signs of ischemia. Often, cerebral blood flow is evaluated during the hypotensive period by IV injection of a positron emission tomography (PET) isotope; PET scan is obtained after the procedure, when the vessel is open and blood pressure is back to normal. If there is any deterioration in neurologic function, the balloon is immediately deflated, and blood pressure is returned to normal. While sedation is appropriate during initial angiography and placement of the balloon, a completely awake, nonsedated patient is necessary for neurologic testing during occlusion; short-acting agents are preferred. Hypotension is induced with rapidly reversible agents (eg, nitroprusside or nitroglycerine). These agents may cause tachycardia. Emergency airway management including endotracheal intubation may be required if complications (eg, seizures, loss of the airway) occur during test occlusion.

D. **Intracarotid sodium amobarbital procedure (ISAP)** or the Wada test is performed for planned epilepsy surgery or, less commonly, for tumor resection. Sodium amobarbital, a short-acting barbiturate, is carefully injected into the internal carotid artery to limit spread beyond the brain hemisphere of interest. This test is considered to be gold standard for lateralizing speech and assessing memory function prior to planned surgery. Patient must be completely awake during this procedure in order to participate in the battery of neurocognitive tests. Emergency airway management including endotracheal intubation may be required if seizures, drastic disinhibition, or loss of the airway occur during the injection.

E. **Cerebral angiography and spinal angiography** are generally painless diagnostic procedures. Only children or uncooperative adults usually require GA for angiography, though GA for comfort may be a consideration because of the potentially long duration of these procedures. Adult patients requiring GA for intracranial angiography may have depressed mental status because of elevated ICP, encephalopathy, recent stroke, or intracerebral hemorrhage. Meticulous attention to hemodynamics may be necessary, which may require invasive blood pressure monitoring. Spinal angiography requires several hours for each vessel supplying the spinal cord to be identified and the angiogram to be performed. The duration of the procedure may need to be limited because the upper limit of contrast agent dosing may be reached. Patients are often anesthetized for their comfort; invasive hemodynamic monitoring is not necessary unless dictated by comorbidities.

F. **Carotid artery stenting (CAS)** with an embolic protection device can be considered as an alternative to carotid endarterectomy in high-risk symptomatic patients with high-degree stenosis. Transcarotid artery revascularization (TCAR) is an updated approach to CAS which requires surgical exposure of the common carotid artery and dynamic flow reversal for cerebral protection. These procedures can be performed under sedation with MAC or GA, however there is emerging evidence that MAC may be associated with better outcomes compared to GA for patients undergoing CAS. Tight hemodynamic control is important; stroke is a risk. Bradycardia may occur during the procedure and can be preemptively treated with an anticholinergic.

G. **Vertebroplasty and kyphoplasty** are percutaneous procedures performed to treat painful acute and subacute vertebral compression fractures or sacral fractures refractory to medical therapy via injection of acrylic bone cement. Vertebroplasty involves introducing a hollow needle via a transpedicular or parapedicular approach into the desired posterior vertebral body under fluoroscopic visualization. The cement is then deposited at a controlled rate. Multiple levels can be performed at one sitting. Kyphoplasty involves a similar approach, with the addition of a balloon inflation to create a cavity for cement deposition and restore vertebral height. These procedures are performed in the prone position. As high-quality studies on MAC versus GA for these procedures are lacking, either approach can be used based on patient preferences and comorbidities. Patients presenting for vertebroplasty/kyphoplasty are often frail, elderly, have cardiopulmonary comorbidities, and chronic pain, all of which should be considered when forming an anesthetic plan. GA may significantly impact cardiovascular stability in this patient population. Positioning can present challenges as patients may have limited neck and shoulder mobility. Sedation often involves titration of judicious doses of anxiolytic(s) and providing analgesia for stimulating portions of the procedure (eg, introduction of vertebroplasty needle). Sedatives and analgesics should have minimal residual effects as postprocedural pain is minimal. Post procedure, patients typically remain supine for several hours to permit the cement to harden.

H. **Endovascular therapy for acute ischemic stroke** may be indicated in appropriate patients, but should not delay or interfere with IV alteplase administration. Mechanical thrombectomy may be indicated within up to 24 hours of last known normal for patients with a large vessel occlusion in the anterior circulation, if they fall within appropriate National Institutes of Health (NIH) stroke scale and Alberta Stroke Programme Early CT Score (ASPECTS) parameters. Angioplasty of atherosclerotic plaque or placement of an intra-arterial stent may be used to supplement thrombolytic therapy to maintain patency of the occluded vessel. Hemorrhagic conversion is a feared complication of thrombolytic and endovascular therapies, and longer time lapse between stroke onset and treatment is one of the risk factors.

1. Anesthetic management is guided by the individual assessment of the patient. There is insufficient evidence to recommend GA versus MAC for these procedures, as the quality of evidence on functional outcomes based on anesthetic technique remains low. However, the quality of evidence for target artery recanalization appears to be higher with GA. Either GA or MAC would therefore be reasonable, as long as anesthetic management does not delay endovascular therapy. MAC can be performed with a wide array of anxiolytics and analgesics including midazolam and fentanyl. Dexmedetomidine may be beneficial for these cases, however, the impact on hemodynamics has to be taken into account.
2. Blood pressure must be maintained to ensure adequate cerebral perfusion. Hypotension after acute ischemic stroke is associated with poor neurologic outcomes, and it is recommended to maintain systolic blood pressure ≤180 mm Hg in patients who received endovascular therapy.
3. Hypovolemia should be corrected.
4. Hyperthermia (>38 °C) and hypoglycemia (<60 mg/dL) should be promptly treated.
5. Patients presenting for endovascular therapy for acute stroke may have received alteplase previously. Complications arising from alteplase include:
    a. Intracranial bleeding. Management is largely supportive, and general principles of management of acute intracranial hemorrhage apply. Cryoprecipitate and potentially antifibrinolytic therapy (eg, tranexamic acid) should be considered.
    b. Angioedema. This may present with mild facial swelling but can progress to severe airway obstruction. Patients on angiotensin-converting enzyme (ACE) inhibitors are at an increased risk of this complication. Management includes stopping alteplase and supportive care with methylprednisolone, antihistamines, and nebulized epinephrine. Preparation for awake fiberoptic intubation should be made if the airway is severely obstructed. Icatibant, a selective bradykinin receptor antagonist, and C1 esterase inhibitor have been suggested for severe cases of alteplase-induced angioedema in case reports.

I. **Cerebral vasospasm** is a common and potentially devastating late complication of subarachnoid hemorrhage. Patients may require angiography and local intra-arterial infusion of vasodilating drugs (eg, papaverine, nicardipine, or verapamil) or even angioplasty to increase the diameter of segments of cerebral blood vessels that are critically constricted. Medical management has traditionally focused on hypervolemia, hemodilution, and hypertension to increase blood flow through stenotic segments of feeding vessels, however, the focus has shifted on maintenance of euvolemia and hypertensive therapy. ICP may be elevated from brain edema secondary to initial injury or evolving ischemic injury.

1. ICP monitoring may be helpful in the perioperative setting because intracranial hypertension is common, and ICP may increase with therapy. Intraventricular catheter is preferable because it permits drainage of CSF to treat increased ICP; "Camino" bolt is adequate for monitoring, but CSF cannot be withdrawn.
2. Anesthetic goals are to optimize cerebral perfusion by maintaining systemic hypertension and intracranial normotension and to provide a rapidly reversible general anesthetic so that neurologic examination can be performed immediately after intervention.

3. ICP may rise, and systemic blood pressure may fall dramatically with intra-arterial infusions of papaverine, nicardipine, or verapamil. High doses of vasopressors such as phenylephrine or norepinephrine may be necessary.
4. Because hyperglycemia may worsen consequences of cerebral ischemia, patients may be receiving an insulin infusion in conjunction with 5% dextrose in normal saline to maintain tight control of glucose.
5. Patients are often febrile. Normothermia can be maintained with surface cooling; hyperthermia may worsen consequences of cerebral ischemia.

VII. ANESTHESIA FOR GASTROINTESTINAL, GENITOURINARY, AND VASCULAR RADIOLOGY PROCEDURES

A. Embolization for gastrointestinal bleeding and hemoptysis. Arterial embolization can be used to treat acute nonvariceal gastrointestinal (GI) hemorrhage of the upper or lower GI tracts that is not amenable to endoscopic treatment. Bronchial artery embolization is an effective treatment for massive hemoptysis. Both procedures are performed under angiographic guidance, through arterial access that allows delivery of embolic agents such as gelatin sponges, beads, microcoils, or glue, to selected arteries through microcatheters. These procedures are typically performed under GA with the patient intubated for airway control with lung isolation for patients with hemoptysis. Breath holds and muscle relaxation are helpful to minimize motion artifacts during digital subtraction angiography.

B. Transjugular intrahepatic portosystemic shunt (TIPS) decompresses the portal system in patients with decompensated portal hypertension (hepatic venous pressure gradient ≥10 mm Hg). Often, patients may have advanced liver disease with its stigmata, which may include actively bleeding esophageal varices, massive recurrent ascites, and hypoxemia. Oliguria from hepatorenal syndrome is common. Liver failure patients are often hyperdynamic with low systemic vascular resistance, which may result in a vasodilatory shock state. Preprocedural hypoxemia may be multifactorial from ventilation/perfusion (V/Q) mismatch or hepatopulmonary syndrome with associated intrapulmonary vascular dilations. The patient with actively bleeding varices may be on an octreotide infusion to decrease mesenteric blood flow.

1. The liver is commonly accessed via cannulation of the right internal jugular vein. Access to the portal circulation is achieved by sequentially placing a guidewire, needle, and sheath through the hepatic vein and through the liver parenchyma. A conduit is thus created to allow for egress of portal blood flow into the systemic circulation. Portal pressures are transduced to assess portosystemic gradient with a target portosystemic gradient of <12 mm Hg.
2. Sedation under MAC can be performed for patients without complex anatomy. GA, however, may be preferred due to the duration and discomfort.
   a. If a concomitant large volume paracentesis is performed, it is recommended that albumin be replenished 6 to 8 g per each liter of ascites fluid removed exceeding 5 L drain. This reduces the risk of paracentesis-induced circulatory dysfunction that may result from decreased circulating blood volume. At our institution, the goal is to avoid concomitant large volume paracentesis and TIPS due to large fluid shifts.
   b. Patients with bleeding or massive ascites are considered to have full stomachs and receive a rapid sequence induction. It is preferable to perform paracentesis to drain ascites before induction of GA, if possible, to reduce intra-abdominal pressure.

3. Post-TIPS complications can include acute hepatic encephalopathy, acute hepatic failure, stent migration or occlusion, biliary injury, and stent infection.
C. **Balloon-occluded retrograde transvenous obliteration (BRTO)** is a less invasive alternative to TIPS that allows to control of gastric variceal bleeding. In a 2020 meta-analysis, BRTO appeared equally as effective as TIPS in treatment of gastric varices but was associated with lower rates of certain postoperative complications including 1-year mortality. In BRTO, balloon occlusion venography followed by injection of sclerosant into gastric varices is achieved through either a transjugular or transfemoral venous approach. While it is an effective treatment for gastric varices, BRTO may increase the risk of esophageal varices and ascites. This procedure can be lengthy and GA is preferred due to the high risk of variceal bleeding.
D. **Selective internal radiation therapy (SIRT) and transarterial chemoembolization (TACE)** are procedures performed in patients presenting with large hepatic tumors not amenable for surgical excision or percutaneous ablation. Treatment relies on taking advantage of the arterial hepatic blood flow to the tumor tissues to selectively deliver tumoricidal medications. SIRT involves guiding a microcatheter to the terminal arterial branches supplying the tumor with placement of radioactive microspheres or beads. TACE procedure combines the local delivery of chemotherapy with embolization of the tumor to disrupt the blood supply to the tumor. Access can be via the left radial or femoral artery.
   1. These procedures are amenable to MAC as they are relatively painless. However, they can be long and may require prone positioning, which some patients may not tolerate under sedation.
   2. TACE procedures can result in postprocedural pain secondary to ischemia of the hepatic tissues. These patients can benefit from ERAP.
E. **Transhepatic percutaneous biliary and nephrostomy drains.** These procedures are performed when there is the need for diversion of biliary or urinary flow due to the presence of obstruction from either anomalous anatomy, stones, malignancy, or infections of the biliary tree or renal collecting system. The procedures involve ultrasound guidance and fluoroscopy for access of the tract. Once access is obtained, small flexible drain catheters are placed.
   1. These patients can present under a wide variety of conditions ranging from nonurgent to emergent in the case of cholangitis.
   2. Positioning for biliary drain placement is supine. Optimal positioning for nephrostomy drain placement is prone, however, lateral positioning is possible.
   3. Sedation under MAC or GA may be appropriate for anesthetic care of these patients, and the optimal anesthetic plan largely depends on the clinical context and patient condition. For complex anatomy and an unstable patient, it may be prudent to secure the airway and consider invasive blood pressure monitoring.
   4. Elective primary placement of large biliary drains can be stimulating and painful postprocedure. ERAP can be beneficial.
   5. Catheter exchange or upsizing are quick procedures and can be amenable to MAC, however, large dilations and upsizes can be stimulating and deep sedation may be required.
F. **Percutaneous gastrostomy (G) or gastrojejunostomy (GJ) tubes** placement is indicated in patients with dysphagia unable to meet nutritional requirements. A GJ-tube is preferred in cases where there is reflux of gastric tube feeds due to an incompetent lower esophageal sphincter or inability to tolerate gastric tube feeds, however GJ-tube placement is associated with a higher complication rate compared to G-tube placement. The patient

population requiring these interventions includes patients with depressed mental status secondary to a neurologic insult, most commonly stroke, head and neck cancer patients undergoing radiation therapy, or amyotrophic lateral sclerosis (ALS) patients. Patients with gastric outlet obstruction from abdominal malignancy may require a G-tube as a vent for stomach contents and/or a jejunostomy tube for nutritional support; such patients must be treated with full stomach precautions. These procedures may be done endoscopically with fluoroscopy or a gastroscope. Alternatively, in cases with altered anatomy, a G-tube may be placed under CT guidance.

1. Airway exam is particularly important in this patient population as tumors, prior surgeries, and radiation can make mask ventilation and intubation potentially difficult.
2. G-tube placements can be performed under MAC or GA depending on the patient comorbidities, GI anatomy, and institutional preference.
3. Fluoroscopic and CT-guided procedures require gastric insufflation to expand stomach below inferior costal margin. This is achieved by placement of a 5-French nasogastric tube. Prior to insufflation, glucagon is administered to prevent the gastric air from escaping the stomach through the pyloric opening. Small amounts of contrast are injected to verify stomach access.
4. After fluoroscopic identification of the stomach, the feeding tube is placed with care to avoid the liver edge and/or transverse colon. In certain circumstances, a contrast enema may be placed to identify the transverse colon.
5. For patients with severe neurodegenerative diseases such as ALS, anesthetic care presents a challenge. These patients may present with significant procedural anxiety. MAC with minimal sedation is ideal to avoid airway obstruction and hypercarbia. The nasopharynx may be anesthetized with 2% lidocaine for nasogastric tube placement, and sedation may be supplemented with judicious use of midazolam and fentanyl. Succinylcholine is contraindicated due to potential lethal hyperkalemia.

G. Fistulograms/graftrograms, thrombectomies, and tunneled dialysis catheter (TDC) placements. Most of the patients who present for these procedures have ESRD and accompanying comorbidities. These patients require maintenance of their dialysis access, which may include AVF, AV graft (AVG), and TDCs. Vascular access dysfunction may occur due to failure of maturation of an AVF or stenosis at various sites along the AVF/AVG and may necessitate a reintervention to reestablish dialysis access.

1. It may be prudent to assess patients' electrolytes, particularly potassium, before proceeding with the anesthetic. Hyperkalemia, especially with ECG changes, calls for immediate temporizing medical management and emergent hemodialysis via placement of a nontunneled dialysis catheter.
2. MAC is sufficient for most procedures, however, some patients may be better candidates for GA due to the inability to stay still or cooperate for a variety of reasons including respiratory insufficiency or back pain.
3. Angioplasty can vary in discomfort from minimal with angioplasty of central veins to very painful for angioplasty of stenotic regions located in the distal arm. Pain is proportional to the size and duration of the angioplasty procedure, and no residual pain is usually expected. Well-timed small propofol boluses can be administered to mitigate painful stimulation, however, close attention to hemodynamics is required.
    a. Regional anesthesia (RA) techniques can be used for procedures involving significant angioplasty in the mid-distal arm, specifically

for radiocephalic fistulas in patients with limited cardiopulmonary reserve. Short-acting local anesthetics should be used as procedures can last 1 to 3 hours. Extreme care must be taken to weigh risks and benefits and to select the most appropriate regional anesthetic technique to avoid compromising pulmonary reserve.
4. Thrombectomies are performed for clotted dialysis access. This procedure involves a combination of pharmacologic and mechanical thrombolysis. Fibrinolysis is achieved with alteplase and mechanical thrombectomy techniques may include embolectomy and/or aspiration devices. Although prompt intervention to restore dialysis access is indicated, these patients need to be optimized and carefully assessed. A feared complication is pulmonary embolism with cardiogenic shock due to thrombus microemboli. Vulnerable populations include patients with large clot burden, compromised right ventricle or significant pulmonary hypertension with previous AV thrombectomies in a relatively short span. Caution should also be advised in patients with a right-to-left shunt, increasing the risk of systemic embolization. Anesthetic choice can be MAC or GA with invasive monitoring depending on patient comorbidities. Alternatively, if the patient is deemed high risk, they may be referred for open surgical thrombectomy to decrease the clot burden.
5. TDCs are indicated in situations where prolonged hemodialysis access is needed, but AVF/AVG cannot be placed or is awaiting maturation. The catheter is commonly placed into the right internal jugular vein and tunneled under the skin overlying the chest wall. Anesthetic approach may include MAC sedation or GA, and should be selected based on patient comorbidities.

VIII. ANESTHESIA FOR PROTON BEAM THERAPY AND RADIATION THERAPY
A. Proton beam radiation therapy is used to treat arteriovenous malformations, central nervous system tumors, and a large number of pediatric tumors. Irradiation is painless, but planning sessions and creation of molds may take many hours, while each individual therapy session is much shorter. During irradiation, the target area must remain in a fixed position using a stereotactic frame locked to a positioning device.
1. In adults, placement of small pins or screws in the skull can be performed under local anesthesia with 2% lidocaine with epinephrine. If "ear bars" are used, a satisfactory ear block can be performed by subcutaneous injection of 3 mL of 2% lidocaine with epinephrine in the outer ear canal. Sedation is usually not recommended because patient cooperation is required.
2. In children, a general anesthetic is usually administered to ensure the child remains still during the session. The detailed anesthetic considerations for these procedures are discussed in Chapter 33: Anesthesia for Pediatric Surgery and Care of the Neonate.
B. Radiation therapy can be used to treat a variety of tumors in adults and children. Children receiving radiation therapy often require GA, and detailed anesthetic considerations for these procedures are discussed in Chapter 33: Anesthesia for Pediatric Surgery and Care of the Neonate.
1. External beam radiation treatments in adults do not typically require anesthesia care, unless patient comorbidities make it challenging to remain still for the duration of the procedure. If anesthesia care is required, sedation with propofol is typically sufficient. Typical treatment course is three or four times a week for 4 weeks. It is desirable to

choose an anesthetic that allows rapid recovery with minimal risk of nausea and vomiting.
2. The first radiation procedure may be time consuming (one to several hours) because measurements must be performed and molds fitting the patient are made. Subsequent treatments are typically <30 minutes.
3. Intraoperative radiation therapy (IORT) is typically delivered in the OR with a mobile electron accelerator and is discussed in detail in other chapters.
4. Brachytherapy is commonly performed in NORA settings. When interstitial brachytherapy for prostate or gynecologic cancer treatment is required, neuraxial techniques can be effective to provide analgesia for the procedure and may be associated with improved pain control and decreased need for rescue analgesics compared to GA. Depending on the procedure duration and the number of required brachytherapy treatments, combined spinal epidural (CSE), epidural, or, more rarely, spinal anesthesia may be utilized. Appropriate neuraxial monitoring and management guidelines should be available to guide neuraxial placement and postprocedure recovery considerations.

IX. ANESTHESIA FOR ELECTROCONVULSIVE THERAPY

Electroconvulsive therapy (ECT) is used to treat severe depression, catatonia, treatment-resistant mania, and schizophrenia, and may be considered in patients who have not responded to medications, are debilitated by serious side effects, or are acutely suicidal. ECT involves unilateral or bilateral electrode placement followed by a brief electrical stimulus applied through the electrodes with a goal of eliciting a controlled seizure. Usually, a series of 6 to 12 treatments over 2 to 4 weeks is required for a clinical response, and maintenance ECT may be considered for patients with severe psychiatric disease.

A. Physiologic effects of ECT
1. The electrical stimulus applied transcutaneously produces a generalized tonic–clonic seizure which will be detected on electroencephalogram (EEG) monitoring. Optimal duration of seizure is unknown, but a duration of longer than 20 seconds is typically desired, and seizures lasting longer than 120 seconds may need to be terminated pharmacologically.
2. An initial vagal discharge may result in severe bradycardia and mild hypotension. Subsequent sympathetic nervous system activation produces hypertension and tachycardia, which can persist for 5 to 10 minutes. ECG changes are common and may include atrial or ventricular arrhythmias and ST segment and T wave changes. A second postictal parasympathetic surge may also occur and may lead to severe bradycardia and asystole, most commonly in young otherwise healthy men.
3. Increased cerebral blood flow and metabolic rate lead to increased ICP. Increased intraocular and intragastric pressure may occur.

B. Anesthetic goals
include amnesia for the duration of the seizure with a rapid return to consciousness, prevention of damage from tonic–clonic contractures (eg, long bone fractures and other musculoskeletal injuries), control of hemodynamic response to induced seizure, and avoidance of interference with initiation and duration of induced seizure.

C. Contraindications.
The only absolute contraindication to ECT is known history of pheochromocytoma, however multiple relative contraindications should be considered. Among the most important relative contraindications to ECT are intracranial hypertension (particularly with

a space-occupying lesion and mass effect), recent cerebrovascular accident or myocardial infarction, unprotected cerebral aneurysm, myocardial ischemia, major unstable fractures, uncontrolled glaucoma, retinal detachment, and untreated active venous thromboembolism. Patients on maintenance treatment with benzodiazepines or lithium may need to discontinue these medications before ECT; benzodiazepines are anticonvulsants that may abolish or attenuate the seizure; lithium is associated with worsened post-ECT cognitive dysfunction and delirium.

D. Anesthetic management

1. Sedative premedication is not indicated and may prolong emergence. Anticholinergic drugs may be used to reduce secretions and to minimize bradycardia. Ondansetron may be useful in patients with a history of nausea and vomiting.
2. A small-gauge IV cannula is placed for drug administration, and standard monitors are applied.
3. The patient is preoxygenated with 100% oxygen; anesthesia may be induced with methohexital, etomidate, or propofol and succinylcholine. Patients are ventilated with 100% oxygen via mask and Ambu bag. Small doses of short-acting nondepolarizing muscle relaxant can be used in patients with contraindications to succinylcholine. Pretreatment with labetalol or esmolol blunts the hypertensive response and may be useful in patients with hypertension or coronary artery disease.
4. Ketorolac may decrease muscle pains after ECT.
5. Rolled gauze pads placed bilaterally as bite blocks protect gums and lips from biting from electrical stimulus and subsequent seizure.
6. Nature and duration of induced seizures can be monitored by EEG or by "isolated arm" technique. With the latter, inflation of a blood pressure cuff interrupts blood supply to one arm before injecting muscle relaxant; seizure activity is apparent in the isolated arm.
7. Patients are ventilated with oxygen by facemask until spontaneous ventilation resumes. They are then placed in a lateral decubitus position and monitored in a recovery area until awake and alert. Agitated delirium may occur after ECT and can be treated with small doses of propofol or benzodiazepine.
8. Patients with underlying medical conditions may require special attention:
   a. Patients with gastroesophageal reflux may require aspiration prophylaxis and rapid sequence intubation.
   b. Patients with severe cardiac dysfunction may require invasive monitoring.
   c. Patients with intracranial mass lesions may require invasive blood pressure monitoring for tight hemodynamic control; hyperventilation before inducing a seizure may reduce the ICP response.
   d. Pregnant patients may require endotracheal intubation, fetal monitoring, and left uterine displacement.
9. Rarely, an induced seizure will not spontaneously terminate. Ventilation with 100% oxygen is continued, and seizure is terminated within 3 minutes with propofol or benzodiazepines.

E. Psychiatric drug interactions.
Patients requiring ECT may be treated with psychotropic drugs that have potent side effects and interactions with anesthetic drugs.

1. Tricyclic antidepressants (eg, amitriptyline, nortriptyline, desipramine, imipramine, and doxepin) potentiate effects of norepinephrine and serotonin by preventing reuptake. Untoward effects include postural hypotension, sedation, dry mouth, urinary retention, and tachycardia.

2. Monoamine oxidase inhibitors (MAOIs) (eg, phenelzine and isocarboxazid) increase availability of norepinephrine at postsynaptic receptors; orthostatic hypotension and severe hypertension may occur. Tyramine, present in certain foods, may produce a hypertensive crisis in patients taking MAOIs. Although it has been recommended previously that MAOI therapy be discontinued at least 10 days before elective surgery, the risk of severe depression outweighs the risks of discontinuing the drug. Important interactions between MAOIs and anesthetics include severe hypertension with indirectly acting vasopressors (ephedrine). Administration of meperidine (and meperidine derivatives) to patients receiving MAOIs has been associated with serotonin syndrome (SS) characterized by severe hemodynamic instability, respiratory depression, and malignant hyperpyrexia.
3. Selective serotonin reuptake inhibitors (eg, fluoxetine, sertraline, fluvoxamine, and paroxetine) are associated with mild adverse effects with no known significant interactions with anesthetic drugs.

X. ANESTHESIA FOR GASTROENTEROLOGY PROCEDURES

Gastroenterology procedures are the most common and fastest growing NORA procedures performed in the United States. Unique to these procedures is the ability to be performed bedside in the ICU or in the OR for unstable or medically complex patients. Anesthetic approach is dictated by patient comorbidities, including body habitus, nature of procedure, and clinical context.

A. Esophagogastroduodenoscopy (EGD) permits assessment and treatment of esophageal, gastric, and duodenal structures. Indications include evaluation of dysphagia, abdominal pain, gastroesophageal reflux disease (GERD), persistent nausea/vomiting, and upper GI bleeding. It is also used to clear foreign bodies including food impaction. Endoscopy is not painful, and stimulation is limited to insertion of the endoscope. It requires sharing the airway with the endoscopist.

1. Esophageal banding uses elastic bands to ligate large bleeding esophageal varices, stigmata of portal hypertension often secondary to hepatic cirrhosis. Risks of the procedure include bleeding and esophageal perforation. The procedure can be very stimulating with high aspiration risk, and the airway should be secured. If the patient is on octreotide, the infusion should be continued throughout the procedure.

B. Endoscopic ultrasound (EUS) is a diagnostic and therapeutic procedure for malignancies of the GI tract and pancreaticobiliary disease. EUS uses high-frequency ultrasound to produce detailed images of the GI tract walls and adjacent organs. Combination of EUS with fine needle aspiration (FNA) allows to take samples from tissue or fluid-filled cystic neoplasms. Therapeutic EUS can be utilized to drain symptomatic pancreatic pseudocysts or provide imaging guidance for celiac plexus blocks.

1. A deep MAC or GA may be employed with the goal to ensure the patient does not move during FNA, if planned. Aspiration risk should be considered when deciding on the appropriate anesthetic plan for patients undergoing EUS. For example, if the GI tract is to be irrigated with fluid to improve imaging, a secured airway is prudent to prevent aspiration.

C. Endoscopic retrograde cholangiopancreatography (ERCP) is a procedure allowing to evaluate the biliary tree, gallbladder, and pancreatic duct for diagnosis and treatment of malignancy and/or obstruction. These

structures are accessed via the catheterization of the sphincter of Oddi through a side channel of the endoscope. A combination of contrast media and fluoroscopy is used to achieve calculi retrieval, stent placement(s), and/or sphincterotomy to facilitate drainage.
1. The vast majority of these procedures are performed with the patient in the prone position.
2. Sedation with MAC may be considered if a relatively straightforward procedure is anticipated and the patient is a low–aspiration risk with a favorable airway exam.
3. GA is performed if there is concern for aspiration and/or anticipated complex procedure.

D. **Endoscopic sleeve gastroplasty (ESG)** is an endoscopic procedure performed to achieve weight loss by reducing the size of the stomach. The target population are patients with a BMI of >30.
1. GA is required for these procedures. They are typically performed with the patient prone or in lateral decubitus position. Given the patient population, considerations include preparing for possible difficult airway with appropriate equipment.
2. Nausea and vomiting occur at high frequency with these procedures. As such, anesthetics should be tailored to reduce the risk. Aprepitant can be included in the medication strategy to decrease the rates of postprocedure nausea and vomiting.
3. Complications include gastric perforation.

E. **Colonoscopy** evaluates and treats pathologies of the large intestine and rectum such as polyps, cancer, inflammatory bowel disease, and may be required as a part of a diagnostic workup evaluating abdominal pain or rectal bleeding. Successful procedure is predicated on an adequate bowel prep for visualization. It is performed in the lateral decubitus position.
1. MAC with a natural airway is a sufficient anesthetic choice in situations where there is not a concern for aspiration. However, in situations where bowel obstruction is considered, precautions should be taken to secure the airway.
2. Colonoscopic perforation is one of the most serious complications following colonoscopies and is associated with a high rate of morbidity and mortality. The incidence is estimated around 0.2% following diagnostic colonoscopies and could be up to 5% following some colonoscopic interventions. Patients present with persistent abdominal pain due to peritonitis. Prompt surgical evaluation and intervention is necessary.
3. Flexible sigmoidoscopy is a limited examination of the rectum and lower sigmoid colon. It may be performed to rule out lower GI bleeding in situations where an adequate bowel prep is not possible. It can be done bedside or in the ICU. Anesthetic choice is dictated by the patient's hemodynamic status and clinical situation.

XI. ANESTHESIA FOR BRONCHOSCOPY PROCEDURES
The anesthetic considerations for bronchoscopy procedures are discussed in detail in Chapter 27: Anesthesia for Thoracic Surgery.

XII. ANESTHESIA FOR NORA CARDIAC PROCEDURES
The anesthetic considerations for cardiac procedures in the NORA setting (eg, EP and catheterization lab procedures) are discussed in Chapter 29: Anesthesia for Cardiac Surgery.

XIII. SAFETY IN NORA

With the increasing volume of NORA cases, the safety of NORA care has become an important issue. Patients who present for NORA procedures tend to be older and sicker with higher ASA PS scores, while the environment of NORA presents unique safety challenges. Large national database studies suggest that NORA sites had a higher proportion of reported deaths and respiratory events compared to main OR locations, highlighting the importance of addressing NORA anesthetic care specifically. The ASA has recently updated its guidelines on ensuring safety in NORA locations, however additional studies and guidelines are needed to ensure that care provided in NORA locations is safe, high quality, and takes into account the unique nature of procedures and the physical environment of NORA.

ACKNOWLEDGMENT

We gratefully acknowledge the contributions of previous edition author, Stephanie L. Counihan, as portions of those chapters have been retained in this revision.

Suggested Readings

Abu Dayyeh BK, Bazerbachi F, Vargas EJ, et al. Endoscopic sleeve gastroplasty for treatment of class 1 and 2 obesity (MERIT): a prospective, multicentre, randomised trial. *Lancet.* 2022;400(10350):441–451.

American College of Radiology. ACR Manual on Contrast Media 2023 version 2023 ACR Committee on Drugs and Contrast Medial. *American College of Radiolgy.* 2023. Accessed June 9, 2023. https://www.acr.org/-/media/ACR/Files/Clinical-Resources/Contrast_Media.pdf?1695112539584

American Society of Anesthesiology. Advisory on granting privileges for deep sedation to non-anesthesiologist physicians committee of origin: quality management and departmental administration (Approved by the ASA House of Delegates on October 20, 2010 and last amended on October 25, 2017).

American Society of Anesthesiology. Practice Guidelines for Moderate Procedural Sedation and Analgesia 2018. *Anesthesiology.* 2018;128(3):437–479.

American Society of Anesthesiology. Statement on nonoperating room anesthetizing locations. Reaffirmed October 18, 2023. https://www.asahq.org/standards-and-guidelines/statement-on-nonoperating-room-anesthetizing-locations

Amin A, Lane J, Cutter T. An anesthesiologist's view of tumor ablation in the radiology suite. *Anesthesiology Clinics.* 2017;35(4):611–615.

Anastasian ZH, Strozyk D, Meyers PM, Wang S, Berman MF. Radiation exposure of the anesthesiologist in the neurointerventional suite. *Anesthesiology.* 2011;114(3):512–520.

Bhagavatula SK, Lane J, Shyn P. A radiologist's view of tumor ablation in the radiology suite. *Anesthesiology Clinics.* 2017;35(4):617–626.

Bhavani SS, Abdelmalak B. Nonoperating room anesthesia: anesthesia in the gastrointestinal suite. *Anesthesiology Clinics.* 2019;37(2):301–316.

Brott TG, Halperin JL, Abbara S, et al. ASA/ACCF/AHA/AANN/AANS/ACR/ASNR/CNS/SAIP/SCAI/SIR/SNIS/SVM/SVS guideline on the management of patients with extracranial carotid and vertebral artery disease: executive summary: a report of the American College of Cardiology Foundation/American Heart Association Task Force on Practice Guidelines, and the American Stroke Association, American Association of Neuroscience Nurses, American Association of Neurological Surgeons, American College of Radiology, American Society of Neuroradiology, Congress of Neurological Surgeons, Society of Atherosclerosis Imaging and Prevention, Society for Cardiovascular Angiography and Interventions, Society of Interventional Radiology, Society of NeuroInterventional Surgery, Society for Vascular Medicine, and Society for Vascular Surgery. *J Am Coll Cardiol.* 2011;57(8):1002–1044.

Chun JY, Morgan R, Belli AM. Radiological management of hemoptysis: a comprehensive review of diagnostic imaging and bronchial arterial embolization. *Cardiovasc Intervent Radiol.* 2010;33(2):240–250.

Chung M, Vazquez R. Non-operating room anesthesia. In: M Gropper et al. *Miller's Anesthesia.* 10th ed. Elsevier, 2024;2284–2312.

Continuum of Depth of Sedation: Definition of General Anesthesia and Levels of Sedation/Analgesia Committee of Origin: Quality Management and Departmental Administration (Approved by the ASA House of Delegates on October 13, 1999, and last amended on October 23, 2019).

Coté CJ. Anesthesia outside the operating room. In: Coté CJ, Lerman J, Anderson BJ. *A Practice of Anesthesia for Infants and Children*. 6th ed. Elsevier; 2018:1077–1094.

Dougherty TB, Nguyen DT. Anesthetic management of the patient scheduled for head and neck cancer surgery. *J Clin Anesth*. 1994;6(1):74–82.

Finlay JE, Leslie K. Sedation/analgesia techniques for nonoperating room anesthesia: new drugs and devices. *Current Opinion in Anesthesiology*. 2021;34(6):678–682.

Friedberg SR, Lachter J. Endoscopic ultrasound: current roles and future directions. *World J Gastrointest Endosc*. 2017;9(10):499–505.

Herman AD, Jaruzel CB, Lawton S, et al. Morbidity, mortality, and systems safety in non-operating room anaesthesia: a narrative review. *British Journal of Anaesthesia*. 2021;127(5):729–744.

Joung KD, Yang HK, Shin WJ, et al. Anesthetic consideration for neurointerventional procedures. *Neurointervention*. 2014;9(2):72–77.

Lin OS, Weigel W. Nonoperating room anesthesia for gastrointestinal endoscopic procedures. *Current Opinion in Anesthesiology*. 2018;31(4):486–491.

Mason KP, Roback MG, Chrisp D, et al. Results from the adverse event sedation reporting tool: a global anthology of 7952 records derived from >160,000 procedural sedation encounters. *Journal of Clinical Medicine*. 2019;8(12):2087.

Nay MA, Fromont L, Eugene A, et al. High-flow nasal oxygenation or standard oxygenation for gastrointestinal endoscopy with sedation in patients at risk of hypoxaemia: a multicentre randomised controlled trial (ODEPHI trial). *British Journal of Anaesthesia*. 2021;127(1):133–142.

Practice advisory on anesthetic care for magnetic resonance imaging: an updated report by the American Society of Anesthesiologists Task Force on Anesthetic Care for Magnetic Resonance Imaging. *Anesthesiology* 2015;122(3):495–520

Petitt MS, Ackerman RS, Hanna MM, et al. Anesthetic and analgesic methods for gynecologic brachytherapy: a meta-analysis and systematic review. *Brachytherapy*. 2020;19(3):328–336.

Powers WJ, Rabinstein AA, Ackerson T, et al. Guidelines for the early management of patients with acute ischemic stroke: 2019 update to the 2018 guidelines for the early management of acute ischemic stroke: a guideline for healthcare professionals from the American Heart Association/American Stroke Association. *Stroke*. 2019;50(12):e344–e418

Prabhakar A, Owen CP, Kaye AD. Anesthetic management of the patient with amyotrophic lateral sclerosis. *J Anesth*. 2013;27(6):909–918.

Raiten J, Elkassabany N, Gao W, Mandel JE. Medical intelligence article: novel uses of high frequency ventilation outside the operating room. *Anesth Analg*. 2011;112(5):1110–1113.

Routman J, Boggs SD. Patient monitoring in the nonoperating room anesthesia (NORA) setting: current advances in technology. *Current Opinion in Anesthesiology*. 2021;34(4):430–436.

Runyon BA, AASLD. Introduction to the revised American Association for the Study of Liver Diseases Practice Guideline management of adult patients with ascites due to cirrhosis 2012. *Hepatology*. 2013;57(4):1651–1653.

Tobin CD, Bridges KH. Systems safety in nonoperating room anesthesia locations. *Current Opinion in Anesthesiology*. 2022;35(4):502–507.

Uppal V, Doursish J, Macfarlance AJR. Anaesthesia for electroconvulsive therapy. *Continuing Education in Anaesthesia Critical Care & Pain*. 2010;10(6):192–196.

Vazquez R. Peripheral nerve blocks. In: McCarthy CJ, Walker TG, Vazquez R. *Specialty Imaging: Acute and Chronic Pain Intervention*. 1st ed. Elsevier; 2020:36–45

Vazquez R, Beermann SL, Fintelmann FJ, Mullen EM, Chitilian H. High-frequency jet ventilation in the prone position to facilitate cryoablation of a peridiaphragmatic pulmonary neoplasm. A case report. *A & A Practice*. 2019;13(5):169–172.

Walker TG, Salazar GM, Waltman AC. Angiographic evaluation and management of acute gastrointestinal hemorrhage. *World J Gastroenterol*. 2012;18(11):1191–1201.

Wong T, Georgiadis PL, Urman RD, Tsai MH. Non-operating room anesthesia: patient selection and special considerations. *Local and regional anesthesia*. 2020;13:1–9.

Anesthesia for Trauma and Burns

Carl Jn Pierre and Jamie L. Sparling

I. INITIAL EVALUATION OF THE TRAUMA PATIENT

Rapid assessment of injuries and institution of resuscitative measures are particularly important in trauma patients. Life-threatening injuries should be identified immediately based on **A**irway, **B**reathing, **C**irculation, **D**isability (neurologic evaluation), and **E**xposure (hypothermia, smoke inhalation, chemical substances). Treatment measures should be initiated simultaneously. Assume that all patients have a cervical spine injury, a full stomach, and hypovolemia until proven otherwise.

A. Airway

1. Airway assessment should include inspection for foreign bodies, facial and laryngeal fractures (palpable fracture and subcutaneous emphysema), and expanding cervical hematomas. Dyspnea, hemoptysis, dysphonia, stridor, and air leaking through the neck wound may also be signs of airway injury. Remove all secretions, blood, vomitus, and any existing foreign bodies (eg, dentures or teeth).

2. **Minimize movement of the cervical spine during airway manipulation.** If immobilizing devices must be removed temporarily, an assistant should keep the head in a neutral position with manual in-line stabilization.

3. **Establish** a definitive airway if there is any doubt about the patient's ability to maintain airway integrity. With blunt or penetrating injuries to the neck, endotracheal intubation may worsen a laryngeal or bronchial injury. Functional suction equipment should always be immediately available to prevent aspiration if the trauma patient with a full stomach vomits.

   a. **The awake patient.** Depending on the patient's injuries, the ability to cooperate, and cardiopulmonary stability, several options are available. Choice of technique for securing the airway should be individualized based on operator preference and level of experience, as well as patient circumstances.

      1. Intubation **after a rapid sequence induction** is the most common approach to the airway. Video laryngoscopy may be helpful in patients with suspected cervical spine injury.
      2. **Awake nasal or orotracheal intubation** with the use of a laryngoscope or fiberoptic bronchoscope is an alternative.
      3. **Blind nasal intubation** may be performed on the spontaneously breathing patient.
      4. **Awake cricothyroidotomy** or **tracheostomy** may be necessary for patients with severe facial trauma that might be contraindications to other methods of intubation.

   b. **The combative patient.** A rapid sequence orotracheal intubation is often the most expedient approach. Preoxygenation may be difficult, and any delay in securing the airway will cause progressive hypoxemia.

   c. **The unconscious patient.** Orotracheal intubation is usually the safest and most expeditious approach.

d. The patient with a prehospital supraglottic airway. If the patient arrives with a supraglottic airway, prioritize establishing a definitive airway with endotracheal intubation. Ventilating via a supraglottic airway may force air into the stomach, leading to gastric inflation and subsequent emesis. Common prehospital supraglottic airways include laryngeal mask airways, King laryngeal tubes, and Combitubes.

e. The intubated patient. Verify the position of an endotracheal tube by auscultating for breath sounds bilaterally and by detecting end-tidal CO_2. Secure the endotracheal tube and ensure adequate ventilation and oxygenation. If there are any problems with oxygenation, consider bronchoscopy to assess endotracheal tube placement and patency.

B. Breathing. Adequate function of the lungs, diaphragm, and chest wall should be evaluated rapidly. Supplemental oxygen should be provided to all trauma patients, either by mask or by endotracheal tube.

1. Assess the chest wall excursion. Auscultate the lungs to ensure adequate gas exchange. Visual inspection and palpation may rapidly detect injuries such as a pneumothorax.
2. Tension pneumothorax, massive hemothorax, and pulmonary contusion are three common conditions that may acutely impair ventilation and should always be identified.
   a. Treatment of tension pneumothorax. Perform needle decompression on the affected side with a large-bore 14-gauge, 3.25-inch/8-cm catheter in the fourth or fifth intercostal space, anterior axillary line. The second intercostal space midclavicular line is no longer recommended in adults as use of the fourth or fifth intercostal space has shown significantly better success in accessing the thoracic cavity. The second intercostal space at the midclavicular line is still the primary recommended site in children. Effective treatment will result in a normalization of physiologic parameters but rarely cause the classically taught "whoosh" of air. Needle thoracocentesis is, however, only a temporizing measure and insertion of a chest tube remains the definitive treatment.
3. Positive-pressure ventilation may worsen a tension pneumothorax and/or cardiac tamponade, which can rapidly lead to cardiovascular collapse.
4. **Lung protective ventilation.** Use tidal volumes of 6 to 8 mL/kg. In patients with metabolic acidosis or suspected traumatic brain injury, increase the respiratory rate to achieve a $PaCO_2$ of 35 to 40 mm Hg. In patients with hemorrhagic shock, be wary that high levels of positive end-expiratory pressure (PEEP) and auto-PEEP will increase intrathoracic pressure and subsequently decrease venous return, cardiac output, and systemic blood pressure.
5. The trauma patient's breathing and gas exchange should continue to be periodically reevaluated after intubation or initiation of positive-pressure ventilation.

C. Circulation

1. In the severely injured trauma patient, rapid initiation of resuscitation measures is important to prevent and control the lethal triad: hypothermia, acidosis, and coagulopathy.
2. **Hemodynamics** are initially assessed by palpating pulses and measuring the blood pressure. Consider placing an intra-arterial catheter for continuous blood pressure measurement in unstable patients.
3. **Intravenous (IV) access.** Check IV lines already in place to ensure proper function. At least two large-bore catheters should be placed, preferably

16 gauge or larger. These lines should be placed above the level of the diaphragm in patients with injuries of the abdomen, where there is a potential for major venous disruption. IV access below the level of the diaphragm is helpful when obstruction or disruption of the superior vena cava, innominate, or subclavian vein is suspected.

4. **Peripheral venous cannulation failure.** In this event, percutaneous subclavian or femoral vein cannulation should be carried out. Although the internal and external jugular veins remain options, access to these structures is frequently hindered by immobilization of the head and neck for a suspected cervical spine injury. If these approaches prove unsuccessful, **surgical cutdowns** can be performed. The saphenous vein at the ankle and the antecubital venous system are acceptable options. When emergent access for vasoactive medications or fluid resuscitation is needed, intraosseous (IO) access to the vasculature is also an option for personnel trained in this technique.
   a. IO access locations: proximal tibia (most common), distal tibia, proximal humerus, iliac crest, and sternum.
   b. IO flowrates vary by site but are roughly 165 mL/min and can be optimized by initially flushing the line and then using a pressure bag. In awake patients, flushing the line under pressure is usually much more painful than initial placement.
   c. IO access can be used for blood and fluid resuscitation, as well as vasoactive medications.

5. **Volume resuscitation should be individualized.** The concept of "damage control" emphasizes multiple approaches to control and prevent tissue hypoperfusion, acidosis, coagulopathy, and hypothermia.
   a. **Damage control resuscitation (DCR)** refers to the strategy of limiting crystalloid use, early resuscitation with packed red blood cells and clotting factors, and maintenance of a systolic blood pressure at approximately 90 mm Hg or mean arterial pressure at 50 to 65 mm Hg. The disadvantages to crystalloid infusion include dilution of coagulation factors, hemodilution, and clot disruption. The infusion of >1.5 L of crystalloid has been shown to be associated with increased mortality. Early administration of blood and clotting factors serves to treat trauma-induced coagulopathy that can occur early after injury. In a patient in whom hemorrhage has not been definitively controlled, elevation in blood pressure and cardiac output can cause dislodgement of a clot and further bleeding. DCR blood pressure parameters should not be used in certain subsets of patients, such as patients with head trauma. Avoiding hypotension is a priority in patients with moderate and severe traumatic brain injury. In this patient population, maintain a systolic blood pressure ≥100 mm Hg for patients 50 to 69 years old and ≥110 mm Hg for patients 15 to 49 or >70 years old.
   b. **Massive blood transfusion** is defined as the transfusion of more than 10 units of blood in 24 hours, or more than 4 units in 1 hour in response to massive and uncontrolled hemorrhage. In an emergency, type-specific uncross-matched blood or type O–negative blood may be given before cross-matched blood becomes available. A ratio of 1:1:1 or 2:1:1 (RBCs:plasma:platelets) is targeted for blood product administration. Although this ratio mirrors the content of whole blood, superior clot formation is achieved with transfusion of whole blood compared with 1:1:1 component transfusion. Therefore, fresh whole blood has been used for combat injuries in the military.

R	Period of latency from when blood is placed into the TEG analyzer until the initial fibrin formation. Represents the enzymatic portion of coagulation.
K	Measures the speed to reach a certain level of clot strength (20 mm above baseline). This represents clot kinetics.
α	Measures the rapidity of fibrin built up and cross-linking (clot strengthening). This represents fibrinogen level.
MA	Maximum amplitude, is a direct function of the maximum dynamic properties of the fibrin and platelet binding via GPIIb/IIIa and represents the ultimate strength of the fibrin clot. This represents platelet function/aggregation.
LY30	Measures the rate of amplitude reduction 30 min after MA. This represents clot lysis.

FIGURE 35.1 Overview of thromboelastogram parameters. (Reprinted with permission from Handa RR, Turnbull IR, Ismail O. Hemostasis, anticoagulation, and transfusions. In: Klingensmith ME, Wise PE, Courtney CM, et al., eds. *The Washington Manual of Surgery.* 8th ed. Wolters Kluwer; 2019. Figure 6.2.)

Some civilian institutions have now adopted its use in trauma. An intraoperative blood salvage system (cell saver) can also be used to help in the reduction of allogenic red blood cell administration. Aggressive resuscitation with blood products can lead to hypothermia, hyperkalemia, and hypocalcemia. Empiric treatment is often indicated as the laboratory results may lag behind the clinical scenario when massive transfusion resuscitation is undertaken.

c. **Management of coagulopathy** is guided by point-of-care (POC) and standard laboratory testing. POC tests, such as the thromboelastogram (**Figure 35.1**), provide rapid, near–real-time information regarding clot initiation, kinetics of clot formation, clot strength, and fibrinolysis. Standard tests of hemoglobin levels, platelet counts, fibrinogen levels, prothrombin time, partial thromboplastin time, and international normalized ratio are useful but may lag behind rapidly evolving clinical situations. Utilizing dynamic parameters, such as transesophageal echocardiography (TEE) and the intra-arterial pressure waveform, can also assist in judicious blood and fluid administration.

d. Severely injured trauma patients do not tolerate prolonged surgical procedures. **Damage control surgery** refers to the concept of employing initial short surgical procedures immediately after injury with the goals of controlling hemorrhage and preventing contamination (eg, due to GI tract injury) through temporary measures. Patients then undergo definitive corrective surgery at a later date after they have been stabilized.

6. **Vasopressor infusions** should not substitute for adequate volume replacement during initial resuscitation. Vasopressors may be necessary as a temporizing measure if perfusion pressure is clearly inadequate during ongoing volume resuscitation.
7. **Antifibrinolytics**, such as tranexamic acid (TXA), can reduce mortality in a bleeding trauma patient when started as soon as possible within 3 hours of injury. The safety of antifibrinolytics after 3 hours has yet to be fully elucidated. Immediate antifibrinolytic therapy is also associated with a decrease in mortality in patients presenting with traumatic brain injury. Administer a loading dose of 1 g of TXA over 10 minutes, followed by an IV infusion of 1 g over 8 hours.

D. **Disability/neurologic evaluation.** A brief neurologic examination yields useful information in assessing cerebral perfusion or oxygenation and can provide a simple and quick means of predicting a patient's outcome.
1. The level of consciousness can be described by the AVPU method (A, **a**lert; V, responds to **v**erbal stimuli; P, responds only to **p**ainful stimuli; and U, **u**nresponsive to all stimuli). A more detailed and quantitative assessment of neurologic function is with the Glasgow Coma Scale (**Table 35.1**) that is the sum of the best eye opening, verbal, and motor responses.
2. An altered level of consciousness dictates immediate reevaluation of the patient's oxygenation and circulation, even though it can be of central nervous system origin (trauma or intoxication).

TABLE 35.1 Glasgow Coma Scale

Eye Opening	Score
Spontaneous	4
To speech	3
To pain	2
No response	1
Best Verbal Response	
Oriented	5
Confused conversation	4
Inappropriate words	3
Incomprehensible sounds	2
None	1
Best Motor Response	
Obeys commands	6
Localizes pain	5
Normal flexion (withdrawal)	4
Abnormal flexion (decorticate)	3
Extension (decerebrate)	2
None (flaccid)	1

3. Neurologic deterioration can rapidly occur in trauma patients and necessitates frequent neurologic reevaluation.
E. **Exposure.** Trauma patients are often hypothermic upon arrival at the hospital and require aggressive efforts to maintain normothermia (temperature ≥35.5 °C). Hypothermia can exacerbate coagulopathy.
  1. External warming devices should be applied, IV fluids and blood products warmed before infusion, and a warm environment maintained.
  2. If there is any suspicion of exposure to chemical agents, decontamination of the patient must be carried out before entrance into the hospital. This terminates exposure, protects the health care provider, and allows the hospital to function effectively.
F. **Diagnostic studies**
  1. **Laboratory studies** include blood type and cross-match, complete blood count, platelet count, prothrombin time, activated partial thromboplastin time, electrolytes, glucose, blood urea nitrogen, creatinine, urinalysis, and, if indicated, toxicologic screening.
  2. **Radiographic studies** should include a lateral cervical spine film, a chest radiograph (CXR), and an anteroposterior view of the pelvis on all patients with blunt trauma. At a minimum, a CXR is obtained in all patients with penetrating injuries of the trunk. Additional studies include thoracic, lumbar, and sacral spine films, and chest and abdominal computed tomography (CT) studies.
      a. **Lateral radiographs of the cervical spine** must include the C7–T1 interface and must be of sufficient quality to delineate the structures of interest (ie, soft tissues and bones).
      b. If the patient's clinical condition allows time for additional studies, **open-mouth odontoid and anteroposterior views of the neck** (standard trauma cervical spine series) may be obtained.
      c. If the clinical evaluation demonstrates a patient with significant neck pain and tenderness but no evidence of fracture or dislocation on the plain radiographs, CT and magnetic resonance imaging may help delineate an occult injury.
  3. A **12-lead electrocardiogram (ECG)** should be performed on all major trauma patients to help evaluate the presence of myocardial injury (eg, contusion, tamponade, ischemia, and arrhythmia).
  4. **F**ocused **A**ssessment with **S**onography in **T**rauma (**FAST, Figure 35.2**) is a rapid ultrasound examination evaluating for bleeding or free fluid around the heart or abdominal organs. The four areas that are examined are the perihepatic space (including Morison pouch or hepatorenal recess), perisplenic space, pelvis, and pericardium. A negative FAST examination, however, cannot completely rule out significant intraperitoneal bleeding in patients with blunt abdominal trauma.
  5. The extended FAST (eFAST) examination includes the ultrasound examination of a patient's bilateral lungs. It can be used to detect a pneumothorax with the absence of normal lung sliding.
G. **Monitoring** is dictated by the severity of the patient's injuries and preexisting medical problems.
  1. **An arterial line** is useful in patients with hemodynamic instability or respiratory failure.
  2. **A central venous catheter (CVC)** may be required to assess volume status via central venous pressure (CVP) measurements. Vasoactive medications can also be administered through a CVC.
  3. A **pulmonary artery catheter** may be helpful in patients with ventricular dysfunction, severe coronary artery disease, valvular heart disease,

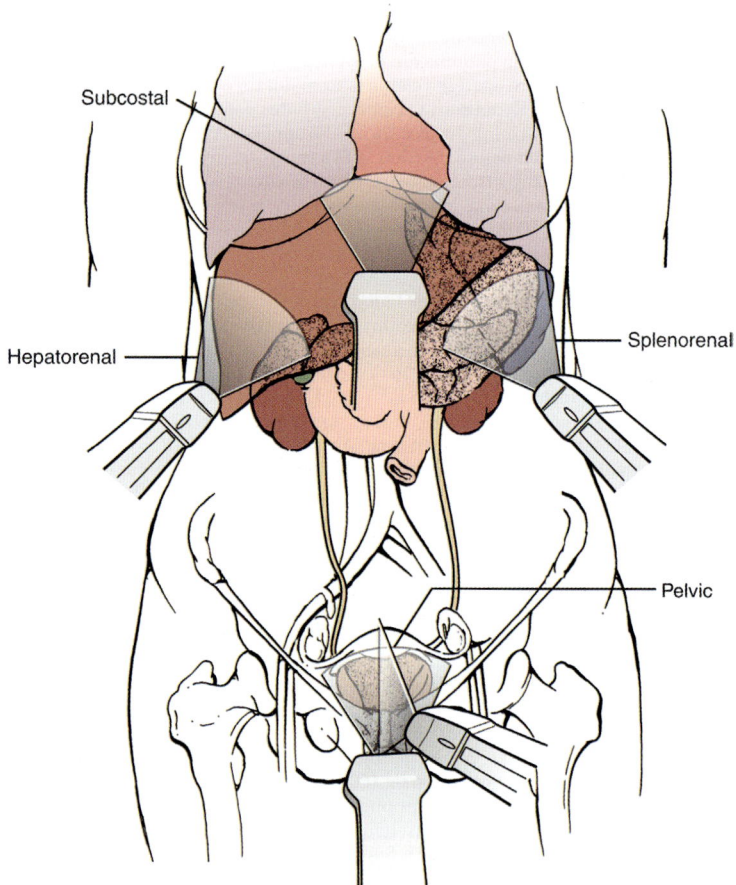

FIGURE 35.2 FAST examination ultrasound locations. (Reprinted with permission from Berg SM, Bittner EA, Zhao KH. *Anesthesia Review: Blasting the Boards.* Wolters Kluwer; 2016. Figure 19.1.)

multiple organ system involvement, or hemodynamics that seem disproportionate to their trauma burden. Placement is planned according to the time available and the clinical status of the patient.

II. SPECIFIC INJURIES

A. Intracranial and spinal cord trauma (see Chapter 23: Anesthesia for Neurosurgery)

B. Facial trauma. Considerable force is required to produce facial fractures. Accordingly, these injuries often are associated with other injuries such as intracranial and spinal cord trauma, thoracic injury, myocardial contusion, and intra-abdominal bleeding. Brisk oral or nasal bleeding, limited mouth opening, broken teeth, vomitus, or tongue or pharyngeal injury may occlude the airway, obscure visualization, and complicate airway

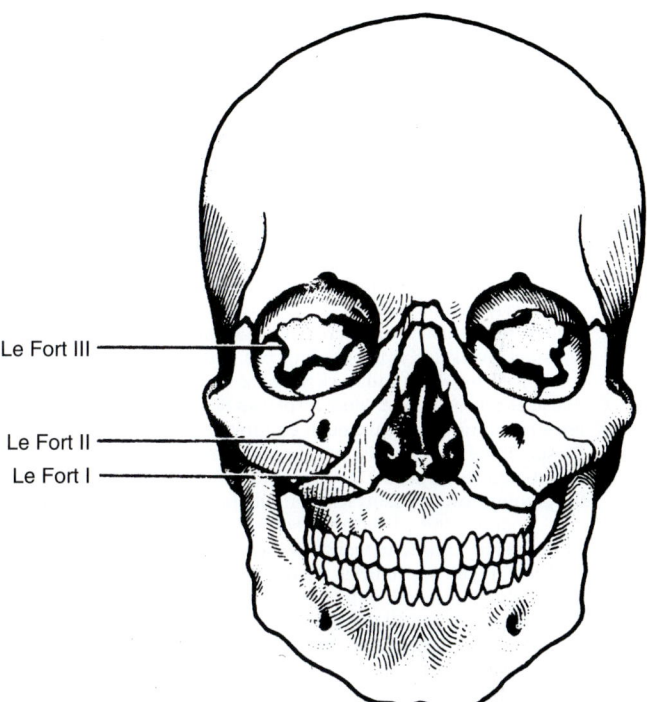

FIGURE 35.3 The Le Fort classification. (Reprinted from Rosen P, Baker FJ, Barkin RM, et al., eds. *Emergency Medicine: Concepts and Clinical Practice.* 2nd ed. Mosby; 1988. Copyright © 1988 Elsevier. With permission.)

management. Trismus may be associated with these injuries and should be assessed before the induction of anesthesia. Emergency cricothyroidotomy or tracheostomy done under local anesthesia may be lifesaving.
1. **Maxillary fractures** are grouped by the **LeFort classification** (**Figure 35.3**).
   a. **Type I (transverse or horizontal).** The body of the maxilla is separated from the base of the skull above the level of the palate and below the level of the zygomatic process.
   b. **Type II (pyramidal).** Vertical fractures through the facial aspects of the maxilla extend upward through the nasal and ethmoid bones.
   c. **Type III (craniofacial separation).** Fractures extend through the frontozygomatic suture lines bilaterally, across the orbits, and through the base of the nose and the ethmoid region.
   d. **Le Fort and related fractures** are frequently associated with skull fractures and **cerebrospinal fluid (CSF) rhinorrhea.** Evaluation of radiographic images may help determine anatomic distortion and airway integrity. Nasotracheal intubation and placement of nasogastric tubes are relatively contraindicated under these circumstances. Elective nasal intubation (or tracheostomy) may be necessary, however, before operative repair. A fiberoptic bronchoscope may be used in these cases to guide an endotracheal tube into the trachea.

e. In the presence of a CSF leak (rhinorrhea), positive-pressure mask ventilation can potentially cause pneumocephalus.

2. **Mandibular fractures**
   a. Malocclusion, limitation of mandibular movement, loose or missing teeth, sublingual hematoma, and swelling at the fracture site complicate airway management.
   b. **Posterior displacement of the tongue** producing airway obstruction is associated with bilateral condylar or parasymphyseal fractures of the mandible. Simple forward traction on the tongue often provides relief.
   c. Reestablishment of normal occlusion may necessitate intermaxillary fixation, which can also be combined with rigid fixation. Awake nasotracheal intubation is recommended if the nose has not been severely traumatized.

3. **Ocular trauma** usually requires general anesthesia for repair. Special considerations for open-eye injuries are discussed in Chapter 30: Anesthesia for Head and Neck Surgery.

4. **Anesthetic management.** Most displaced facial fractures require general anesthesia for repair. Although children usually require general anesthesia, many soft tissue injuries can be treated with local anesthesia. Maintenance of a patent airway is the principal concern, and induction may require awake nasotracheal intubation, fiberoptic laryngoscopy, or tracheostomy under local anesthesia.

C. **Neck trauma** may cause cervical spine injury, esophageal tears, major vascular injuries, and airway injuries. Airway injuries may present with obstruction, subcutaneous emphysema, hemoptysis, dysphonia, or hypoxemia.

1. The neck is divided into three anatomic zones when describing penetrating neck trauma (**Figure 35.4**). These zones guide surgical or conservative management:
   a. Zone 1: clavicles and sternal notch to cricoid cartilage. Greatest potential for injuries to intrathoracic great vessels. Important structures

FIGURE 35.4 Zones of the neck. (Reprinted with permission from Fiser SM. *The ABSITE Review.* 3rd ed. Wolters Kluwer Health/Lippincott Williams & Wilkins; 2010. Figure 16.6.)

include the aortic arch, proximal common carotid arteries, vertebral arteries, subclavian vessels, innominate vessels, lung apices, esophagus, trachea, brachial plexus, and thoracic duct.
- **b.** Zone 2 (80% of injuries): cricoid cartilage to angle of mandible. Important structures include the common, internal and external carotid arteries, internal and external jugular veins, larynx, hypopharynx, and proximal esophagus.
- **c.** Zone 3: angle of mandible to base of skull. Important structures include internal carotid artery, vertebral artery, external carotid artery, jugular veins, prevertebral venous plexus, and facial nerve trunk.

2. "**Clothesline**" injuries occur from direct trauma to the upper airway and can result in separation of the larynx from the trachea or separation between the cricoid cartilage and the first tracheal ring. These injuries do not always present with an open neck wound. Additional injuries include laryngotracheal transection, laryngeal fractures, and vascular injury.

3. Blunt injury over the carotid arteries may result in intimal disruption and dissection, even in the absence of initial symptoms. Angiography or ultrasonography may be required to exclude these injuries.

4. Initial management of **penetrating trauma** includes direct compression of involved vessels to control hemorrhage and prevent air embolism.

5. Associated **thoracic injuries**, such as pneumothorax and hemorrhage from injury to the great vessels, may occur with lower neck injuries.

6. Anesthetic management
- **a. Securing the airway** is the central issue in these patients. A coordinated approach among members of the trauma team is necessary. A surgical airway or direct intubation of an open airway defect can be lifesaving. Anesthesia induction via spontaneous ventilation of a potent inhalational agent can be useful in the presence of airway disruption with the caveat that the patient likely has a full stomach and is a high risk for aspiration. Preparations should be made for fiberoptic intubation, rigid bronchoscopy, and a surgical airway below the level of injury.
- **b. Great vessel injuries** in the neck may necessitate lower extremity IV access.

D. Chest trauma can involve injuries to the trachea or larynx, heart, great vessels, thoracic duct, esophagus, lung, or diaphragm.

1. Rib fractures are a common feature of major thoracic trauma and mandate assessment for pneumothorax by CXR. First-rib fractures should alert the clinician to the potential for associated internal injuries due to severe forces needed to fracture the first rib. Multiple rib fractures most commonly involve ribs 7 to 10 and often accompany lacerations of the spleen or liver.

2. The hypoxemia and respiratory failure that accompany **flail chest** and other major chest injuries are indicative of underlying pulmonary contusion. IV fluids should be administered judiciously because the injured lung is sensitive to fluid overload.

3. The presence of **subcutaneous emphysema** may indicate the presence of a pneumothorax or laryngeal, tracheobronchial, or esophageal trauma. Pneumothorax and hemothorax may lead to respiratory and cardiovascular collapse. If these conditions are present or highly suspected, chest tubes should be placed before the induction of general anesthesia. Avoid central line insertion (particularly by the subclavian route)

on the side opposite an injury because of the potential consequence of bilateral pneumothorax. Avoid the ipsilateral side if a concomitant major venous injury is suspected.
4. **Traumatic diaphragmatic injury** can present as an elevated diaphragm, gastric dilatation, loculated pneumothorax, or subpulmonic hematoma. An upper gastrointestinal contrast study should be considered if the diagnosis is not clear.
5. **Anesthetic management**
   a. Patients with significant chest injuries almost always require general anesthesia.
   b. The necessity for mechanical ventilation may extend into the postoperative period.
   c. Avoid nitrous oxide when a pneumothorax is suspected and a chest tube has not yet been placed. Airway pressures must be closely monitored during positive-pressure ventilation.
   d. Pulmonary hemorrhage into the main conducting airways calls for isolation of the uninjured side before it is flooded with blood. Double-lumen endotracheal tube placement, mainstem intubation, or endobronchial blockade may be needed to prevent blood from spilling into the noninjured side (see Chapter 27: Anesthesia for Thoracic Surgery).
   e. Regional anesthesia (ie, intercostal nerve blockade, thoracic epidural anesthesia, or paravertebral blocks) may provide analgesia for multiple painful rib fractures. Adequate pain relief can reduce chest wall splinting, regional hypoventilation, and progressive hypoxemia.

E. Cardiac and major vascular trauma
1. **Blunt cardiac injury** can result in myocardial muscle contusion, chamber rupture, valvular disruption, tamponade, or dysrhythmias.
2. **Cardiac trauma** may be associated with a fractured sternum, hemothorax, pericardial tamponade, myocardial dysfunction, valvular dysfunction, and ECG changes (persistent sinus tachycardia, multiple premature ventricular contractions and other dysrhythmias, bundle branch block, nonspecific ST-segment and T-wave changes, and overt ischemia).
   a. **Beck triad** of distended neck veins, muffled heart sounds, and hypotension is present in only 30% of patients with pericardial tamponade, and pulsus paradoxus is even less reliable. The diagnostic test of choice is cardiac ultrasound.
   b. **Pericardiocentesis** may be used to stabilize the patient until surgical repair can be performed. A subxiphoid pericardial window is ideally performed in the operating room.
3. A widened mediastinal profile, lack of clarity of the aortic knob, rightward tracheal shift, or widening of the left paraspinal line without associated fracture on the CXR mandate further workup to rule out traumatic aortic injury. CT is the diagnostic test of choice and is more sensitive than angiography. Potentially salvageable patients with aortic rupture often have an incomplete laceration near the ligamentum arteriosum. An intact adventitial layer or contained hematoma prevents immediate death. An arterial line should be placed in the right arm since the compromised aorta may not transmit a normal pulse distal to the left subclavian and the flow through the left subclavian may be occluded during the course of surgical repair.
4. **The subclavian artery** is subject to injury with hyperextension of the neck and shoulder.

5. **Anesthetic management**
   a. These patients are often **severely hypovolemic** and may have compromised cardiac function. Cardiopulmonary bypass may be required for certain repairs.
   b. **Resuscitative endovascular balloon occlusion of the aorta (REBOA)** is an option for patients presenting with noncompressible torso hemorrhage. REBOA does not provide definitive hemorrhage control. This temporary measure supports vital organ perfusion, decreases the amount of bleeding distal to the occluded site, and provides a window of opportunity for resuscitation and hemorrhage control.
   c. Monitors should include **intra-arterial catheter** placed in an upper extremity since lower-extremity arterial perfusion is lost during balloon inflation and occlusion of the aorta, CVC, and **TEE** to assess ventricular function, volume status, and position of the endovascular balloon.
   d. Clear communication with the surgical team is essential in preparation for the physiologic changes of reperfusion following balloon deflation: hypoxemia, hypercarbia, acidosis, hyperkalemia, anemia, and disorders of hemostasis.
   e. Etomidate and ketamine both provide hemodynamic stability for induction. However, ketamine use is cautioned in patients with concomitant head injury and those with cocaine abuse.
   f. Cross-matched type-specific blood or O-negative blood should be available before induction. Inotropic and vasopressor agents should be immediately available to treat severe hypotension.
   g. For refractory cardiogenic shock or acute respiratory distress syndrome, either venoarterial or venovenous extracorporeal membrane oxygenation, respectively, may be considered.

F. **Peripheral vascular trauma**
   1. Check **peripheral pulses** in all extremities during the evaluation of trauma patients. Arteriography can be used to further define injuries.
   2. **Anesthetic management** should focus on the recognition of hypovolemia secondary to uncontrolled hemorrhage. Regional anesthetic techniques may be considered in stable patients.

G. **Abdominal trauma**
   1. In stable patients without peritonitis, **penetrating abdominal wounds** (with the exception of gunshot wounds) are initially evaluated by local wound exploration. If the exploration is equivocal, diagnostic peritoneal lavage, abdominal ultrasound, or an abdominal CT scan may be performed.
   2. All patients with **gunshot wounds of the abdomen** are surgically explored.
   3. With **impalement injuries** (eg, stab wounds or falls onto sharp objects), the penetrating object, if still present in the wound, will usually be removed in the operating room after anesthesia has been induced and the patient stabilized. Removal may result in exsanguination.
   4. **Blunt trauma** may result in intra-abdominal or retroperitoneal bleeding.
      a. The **spleen** is the most frequently injured abdominal organ in blunt trauma. Signs and symptoms include abdominal or referred shoulder pain, abdominal rigidity, a falling hematocrit, or hypotension. Minor splenic hematomas are often managed nonoperatively, but grade IV (active bleeding) and V (shattered/avulsed spleen) injuries require splenectomy.
      b. The **liver** frequently fractures with blunt abdominal trauma. Minor injuries are managed nonoperatively unless other injuries mandate

laparotomy. Thus, liver injuries that require operation are often complex with large blood loss and high mortality. Manual compression can temporarily control bleeding and allow time for volume resuscitation. Perihepatic packing **("damage control surgery")** with planned reexploration is sometimes considered for patients with severe injuries.

5. **Abdominal compartment syndrome** (ACS) can occur in the setting of direct injury as well as after massive fluid resuscitation.
    a. ACS often presents with a clinical triad of:
        1. tense, distended abdomen
        2. respiratory distress or high peak pressure if the patient is intubated
        3. oliguria
    b. Intra-abdominal pressure >12 mm Hg is indicative of abdominal hypertension. ACS is defined as a sustained intra-abdominal pressure >20 mm Hg that is associated with new organ dysfunction. ACS often warrants immediate decompression. Systemic hypotension is common because of a decrease in preload by compression of the inferior vena cava.
    c. Retroperitoneal hematomas and aortic rupture may present with ACS. Bowel perforation can occur from ischemia, and peritonitis can lead to further tissue edema. Electrolyte disorders, myoglobinuria, and renal failure can occur.
    d. Surgical decompression may be necessary. These patients are often **intravascularly depleted** and may **become severely hypotensive** after decompression owing to the newly uncompressed abdominal vasculature. Cross-matched type-specific blood or O-negative blood should be available before induction. Inotropic and vasopressor agents should be immediately available to treat severe hypotension.

H. Genitourinary trauma

1. All multiple trauma patients should have a **Foley catheter** placed. If pelvic or perineal injury has occurred, as evidenced by blood at the urethral meatus, or a perineal hematoma, retrograde urethrography should be performed before urethral catheterization. Digital rectal exam for evaluation for the presence of a high-riding prostate is no longer recommended.
2. All patients with penetrating abdominal or back injuries and those with significant hematuria after blunt trauma should have a radiographic evaluation for damage to the kidneys, ureter, and bladder.
3. Eighty-five percent of renal injuries can be managed nonoperatively, but patients with refractory hypotension should go directly to the operating room for exploration.
    a. **Ureteral laceration** is managed by surgical intervention after locating the disruption by retrograde urography.
    b. **Bladder** contusions may be treated nonoperatively, but rupture usually requires exploration.
    c. The inability of the patient to void or clinical signs of injury indicate **injury to the urethra** (see Section II.H.1). Diagnostic urethrography should precede treatment with suprapubic cystostomy for urinary diversion and control of hemorrhage. Most disruptions can undergo delayed repair.

I. Orthopedic trauma

1. All **fractures or dislocations** that compromise nerve or vascular function may constitute surgical emergencies (eg, radial nerve injury with humeral shaft fractures and aseptic necrosis of the femoral head with

hip dislocation) and must be reduced immediately. It is important to document the neurovascular examination immediately before anesthesia and upon awakening. Regional anesthesia may delay diagnosis of compartment syndrome and is relatively contraindicated if compartment syndrome is anticipated.

2. **Upper extremity**
   a. Severe **depression or hyperabduction of the shoulder girdle** can stretch or tear the brachial plexus. A damaged cervical sympathetic chain may present as Horner syndrome.
   b. When the shoulder is struck hard from the side, the medial end of the clavicle may be dislocated upward or retrosternally. Pressure on the trachea in a retrosternal dislocation may cause life-threatening airway compromise.
   c. Dislocation of the glenohumeral joint can cause axillary nerve injury.
   d. **Fractures of the humeral shaft,** especially the middle or distal part, are frequently associated with radial nerve injury.
   e. Neurovascular compromise of the forearm can occur with **fracture or dislocation of the elbow.** Peripheral ischemia is often complicated by edema of the anterior compartment with risk for nerve and muscle necrosis. Fasciotomy may be indicated.
   f. Median nerve compression is possible with **fractures at the wrist** or with carpal dislocation and may require division of the transverse carpal ligament.

3. **Pelvis**
   a. Patients who have sustained pelvic injuries can be divided into three major categories:
      1. **Exsanguinating hemorrhage** from external bleeding in open fractures or from retroperitoneal hematoma in closed fractures (0.5% to 1.0%). These patients almost always present with severe hypotension or cardiac arrest and rarely respond to resuscitative measures.
      2. **Hemodynamically stable** with a relatively uncomplicated course (75%). Urgent or elective surgery for repair of bony and ligamentous pelvic disruptions may be required.
      3. An **intermediate group** in critical condition with various degrees of overall injury, hemorrhage, and hemodynamic instability (25%).
   b. **Initial management** for these injuries may include the application of a compressive pelvic binder for "open-book" fractures, pelvic angiography (with or without therapeutic embolization to control hemorrhage), and external pelvic fixation.
   c. Pelvic fractures without major disruption, such as type I anterior–posterior compression (APC) injury or type I lateral compression injury, can be treated with bed rest and delayed open reduction and internal fixation (ORIF). More complex injuries such as APC II (widened sacroiliac joint with hemorrhagic and vascular consequences) require acute external fixation with delayed conversion to internal fixation, acute ORIF, or arterial embolization.
   d. **Fat embolism** can occur with pelvic and major long-bone fractures (see Chapters 17: Intra-anesthetic Problems and Chapter 22: Anesthesia for Orthopedic Surgery).
   e. **Crush injuries** may be associated with **myoglobinuria.** Aggressive and early hydration may help prevent acute renal failure.

4. **Lower extremity**
   a. Fractures of the **tibia and fibula,** the most common major skeletal injuries, can be associated with neurovascular trauma and attendant compartment syndrome.
   b. With a fracture of the **femur,** blood loss can be much greater than is evident from superficial inspection.
   c. **Hip fractures** are common in the elderly, whose clinical picture is often dominated by other complicating medical illnesses. Traction is used initially for pain relief, but most fractures require ORIF to ensure adequate healing and function and to avoid the complications of prolonged immobilization.
   d. Regional, general anesthesia, and combined techniques can be considered for patients with isolated lower-extremity injuries without concern for compartment syndrome.
5. **Extremity reimplantation**
   a. **Indications.** In general, these procedures are performed on the upper extremities and only in patients who are otherwise stable. An amputated arm, hand, or digit will not be reimplanted if it has sustained a severe crush injury or has been raggedly torn from major nerves and blood vessels. Reimplantations may be extremely lengthy procedures, occasionally in excess of 24 hours.
   b. **Anesthetic management**
      1. General anesthesia is usually chosen because of the long duration of these procedures. A combined technique will reduce anesthetic requirements and provide for postoperative analgesia (especially with catheter placements, rather than single-dose brachial plexus blocks). Regional anesthesia may improve blood flow via the induced sympathectomy.
      2. During general anesthesia, the head and pressure points must be evaluated every 1 to 2 hours to avoid pressure-induced injury (eg, scalp ulceration and hair loss). Low-pressure mattresses and padded sponge blocks should be used to minimize pressure on susceptible peripheral nerves (eg, ulnar, sciatic, peroneal, or sural). The endotracheal tube cuff pressure should be periodically assessed because nitrous oxide will diffuse into the cuff and increase the pressure on the tracheal mucosa.
      3. Patients should be kept warm and adequately hydrated. Avoid hyperventilation or the use of vasoconstrictors.
      4. Consider invasive hemodynamic monitoring for optimization of the perfusion pressure and for prolonged cases. If a noninvasive blood pressure cuff is used, it should be rotated among multiple sites. The need for anticoagulation is determined intraoperatively.
      5. Blood loss can be vastly underestimated. Blood samples should be sent periodically to assess hemoglobin levels.

III. THE PEDIATRIC TRAUMA PATIENT
A. General considerations
1. A clear understanding of the salient anatomic and physiologic differences among adults, children, and infants and a working knowledge of the specific anesthetic considerations for this patient population are required (see Chapter 33: Anesthesia for Pediatric Surgery and Care of the Neonate).
2. **Blunt trauma,** usually from falls or motor vehicle accidents, predominates in children. Multiple injuries are the rule rather than the

exception, but diagnosis is often more difficult because of the child's inability to provide an accurate history.

B. Specific considerations
1. Although the pediatric trauma patient frequently presents with significant blood loss, initially, the **vital signs** may be minimally altered. **Reliance on vital signs alone may seriously underestimate the severity of the injury.**
2. Orotracheal intubation with protection of the cervical spine is the preferred method of obtaining airway control. Nasotracheal intubation is **not** recommended in children under the age of 12 years. **Surgical cricothyroidotomy** is rarely performed in an infant or a small child because of technical difficulties. If airway control and ventilation cannot be accomplished, needle cricothyroidotomy is an appropriate temporary approach for oxygenation.
3. **IO** is an acceptable procedure for critically injured pediatric patients in whom venous access cannot be established.
4. The small child who is **hypothermic** may be refractory to therapy for shock. During initial evaluation and management, overhead heaters or thermal blankets will be needed to maintain body temperature.
5. Avoidance of hypoxemia is pertinent in the pediatric population. Owing to high metabolic rate and oxygen consumption, desaturation can occur rapidly, followed by severe bradycardia. **Atropine IV 10 to 20 μg/kg or IM 20 to 30 μg/kg** should be prepared to treat bradycardia.

IV. THE PREGNANT TRAUMA PATIENT
A. General considerations
1. Pregnancy must always be suspected in any female trauma patient of childbearing age until proven otherwise by a definitive pregnancy test or ultrasound scan (see Chapter 32: Anesthesia for Obstetrics and Gynecology for management of the pregnant patient). All pregnant women >24 weeks of gestation should have cardiotocographic monitoring for a minimum of 4 to 6 hours.
2. **Airway, breathing, and ventilation**
   a. Pregnant patients are at increased risks of developing hypoxemia. Oxygen supplementation should be provided liberally with the goal of maintaining oxygen saturation above 95%.
   b. If unable to achieve adequate maternal oxygenation, consider early intubation. A rapid sequence induction is recommended with a smaller-sized endotracheal tube and use of cricoid pressure. Advanced airway equipment (video laryngoscope, fiberoptic bronchoscope) should be readily available in anticipation of a difficult airway. Placement of a nasal or orogastric tube prior to induction of anesthesia should be considered to decompress the patient's stomach and reduce the risk of aspiration.
   c. If thoracostomy tube insertion is needed, it should be inserted 1 to 2 intercostal spaces above the usual recommendation (fifth intercostal space) as the diaphragm is elevated in pregnancy.
3. **Circulation**
   a. Because the fetus depends on its mother for oxygen, an **uninterrupted supply of oxygenated blood** must be provided to the fetus at all times. The resuscitation of the fetus thus depends on the optimum resuscitation of the mother. The uterus remains an intrapelvic organ until the 12th week of gestation and reaches the umbilicus by 20 weeks. **Compression of the vena cava by the gravid uterus** after 20 weeks of gestation reduces venous return to the heart, thereby decreasing

cardiac output and exacerbating shock. The pregnant patient should be transported and evaluated with **left uterine displacement**.
- **b.** Any pregnant patient suspected of having serious injuries should have two large bore IVs (14 g or 16 g) for intravascular volume replenishment. Transfusion guidelines for pregnancy are similar to nonpregnant patients with the exception of added attention to fibrinogen levels. Fibrinogen levels should be measured in addition to routine blood test as hypofibrinogenemia (<2 g/L) may indicate disseminated intravascular coagulation (DIC) which may be a complication of uterine rupture or placental abruption or raise concern for severe hemorrhage.
- **c. Kleihauer–Betke analysis helps in determining the amount of fetomaternal hemorrhage and should be performed.** O-negative blood should be transfused in a Rh-negative pregnant patient until crossmatched blood becomes available. Fetomaternal hemorrhage in a Rh-negative patient warrants Rh immunoglobulin therapy.
- **d.** Vasopressor use should be reserved only for cases of hypotension refractory to fluid resuscitation as their use may decrease placental perfusion.
  4. Although diagnostic irradiation poses a risk to the fetus, necessary radiographic studies should always be obtained. Consultation with a radiologist may be obtained for estimation of the total radiation dose to the fetus if multiple diagnostic imaging studies with ionizing radiation have been obtained.
  5. If the amniotic fluid gains access to the intravascular space, it can be a source of amniotic fluid embolism and resultant disseminated intravascular coagulation.

B. Treatment
  1. If the mother's condition is stable, the status of the fetus and the extent of uterine injury will determine further management. Obstetrical consultation is advisable.
  2. A potentially viable fetus at ≥24 weeks' gestation that shows no signs of distress should be monitored by external ultrasound. Premature labor is always a possibility in these patients, and tocolytic therapy should be initiated in consultation with the obstetrics team if premature labor develops.
  3. When a viable fetus shows signs of distress despite successful resuscitative measures, a cesarean delivery must be performed expeditiously. A nonviable fetus may be managed conservatively in utero to optimize maternal oxygenation and circulation.
  4. Primary repair of all maternal wounds should be attempted in a critically injured mother carrying a viable gestation, even at the expense of the fetus.
  5. Perimortem cesarean section/resuscitative hysterotomy is recommended for pregnant woman with fundus height at or above the umbilicus (20 weeks' gestation) or who are perimortem or after 4 minutes of advanced cardiac life support. If maternal viability is not possible (from fatal injury or pulselessness), it should be performed immediately.

V. MAJOR BURN INJURIES
A. Physical implications of burn injury
  1. Thermal injury destroys skin, the body's barrier to the external environment. Skin plays a vital role in thermal regulation, fluid and electrolyte homeostasis, and protection against bacterial infection. Significant heat and protein loss, massive fluid shifts, and infections all commonly

occur in patients with severe thermal injuries. Microvascular injury results from local damage by heat and from the release of vasoactive substances from the burned tissue.

B. Physiologic implications of burn injury

1. In major burns, circulating mediators trigger systemic inflammation, hypermetabolism, and immune suppression. There is also diffuse alteration in the permeability of cell membranes to sodium, resulting in generalized cellular swelling. Therefore, edema occurs in both burned and unburned tissues.

   ### a. Cardiovascular effects
   1. Alterations in microvascular permeability result in a transcapillary fluid flux and significant tissue edema 12 to 24 hours after a thermal injury. Large amounts of water, electrolytes, and proteins are lost into the extravascular space leading to intravascular fluid depletion and hypovolemic shock (burn shock).
   2. Immediately after a burn injury, the cardiac output is frequently reduced owing to decreased preload and myocardial depression, possibly due to circulating humoral factors. Blood pressure may be normal owing to increased systemic vascular resistance (SVR). The magnitude of these pathophysiologic changes depends on the size and the depth of the burn injury.
   3. The cardiovascular response 24 to 48 hours after successful resuscitation of a major burn is characterized by an *increase* in cardiac output and *reduced* SVR, consistent with the pathophysiology of the systemic inflammatory response syndrome.

   ### b. Metabolic effects
   1. "Ebb phase": During the first 2 days after severe, acute burns, a **hypo**metabolic state may be seen, accompanied by decreased oxygen consumption, cardiac output, and metabolic rate. This is also known as the "resuscitative phase" of the burn injury, where effective fluid resuscitation is guided by formulas targeted to achieve a urine output of 0.5 to 1 mL/kg/h.
   2. "Flow phase": Starting days 2 to 5, there ensues a catecholamine, inflammatory, and hormonally mediated **hyper**metabolic–hyperdynamic state, which can persist for more than a year. It is frequently accompanied by high cardiac output, decreased SVR, increased oxygen consumption and carbon dioxide production, and protein wasting and catabolism. Treatment during the flow phase should be multifactorial and directed at the various physical and physiologic changes:
      a. Early skin grafting to aid thermal regulation, electrolyte homeostasis, and protect against bacterial infection.
      b. Strict temperature regulation with ambient temperature kept within the thermoneutral range to avoid shivering and a further increase in metabolic rate.
      c. Early nutrition with enteral feeding decreases muscle catabolism, promotes wound healing and may reduce bacterial translocation through the intestinal mucosa.
      d. Pharmacologic interventions, such as adrenergic blockade with propranolol, reduce resting energy expenditure, insulin resistance, and muscle–protein catabolism. Other pharmacologic interventions are areas of ongoing interest and research.

   ### c. Capillary leakage results in **hemoconcentration** immediately after injury. Despite apparent adequate fluid resuscitation, the hematocrit

level often remains increased during the first 48 hours after injury. Bleeding from wounds and a shortened erythrocyte half-life, however, can result in anemia.

  d. Microaggregation of the platelets in the skin and smoke-damaged lung and aggressive volume resuscitation result in early **thrombocytopenia** after major burns. Thrombotic and fibrinolytic mechanisms are activated, and disseminated intravascular coagulation may complicate the course of a massive burn injury. A decrease in antithrombin III, protein C, and protein S levels can increase the thrombogenicity of these patients later in their clinical course and theoretically can cause venous thrombosis and pulmonary embolism.

  e. **Acute renal failure** is not uncommon in patients with major burn injury and is associated with high mortality. Decreased renal blood flow secondary to hypovolemia and decreased cardiac output, as well as increased levels of catecholamines, aldosterone, and vasopressin, can contribute to renal failure. Other mechanisms include nephrotoxic effects of drugs, rhabdomyolysis, hemolysis, and sepsis (see Chapter 5: Specific Considerations With Renal Disease).

  f. **Gastrointestinal function** is diminished immediately after burn injury, secondary to the development of gastric and intestinal ileus. The stomach should be adequately vented with a nasogastric tube.

      1. **Curling ulcers (mucosal erosion)** will occur at variable times after major burns and may lead to gastric hemorrhage or perforation. These ulcers seem to be more common in children than in adults. Therapy consists of antacids, histamine (H_2) receptor antagonists, and proton pump inhibitors.

      2. **Other gastrointestinal complications of burns** include esophagitis, tracheoesophageal fistula (from prolonged intubation and the presence of a nasogastric tube), hepatic dysfunction, pancreatitis, acalculous cholecystitis, and mesenteric artery thrombosis.

  g. **Infection** of burned areas delays healing and prevents successful skin grafting. Bacterial invasion of underlying tissue may result in septicemia. Common organisms involved are staphylococci, β-hemolytic streptococci, and gram-negative rods such as *Pseudomonas* and *Klebsiella* species. Local treatment with topical antimicrobials and early skin grafting are important measures to reduce risk of infection.

2. In **electrical burns,** current creates thermal energy that destroys tissue, particularly tissues with high resistance such as skin and bone. Exposure to high voltage can result in compartment syndromes, fractures of long bones and the axial spine, myocardial injury, and rhabdomyolysis with subsequent renal injury.

3. In **chemical burns,** the degree of injury depends on the chemical, its concentration, duration of contact, and the penetrability and resistance of the tissues involved. Some substances producing chemical burns, such as phosphorus, are absorbed systemically, producing significant and often life-threatening injury. Hydrofluoric acid exposure will cause severe hypocalcemia and requires close monitoring of serum calcium levels. Subeschar injection of calcium gluconate and emergent wound excision may be indicated. Many chemical agents can be safely and copiously irrigated with water. Chemicals that should *not* be irrigated include dry lime, elemental metals, and phenol. If the name of the offending chemical agent can be determined, websites, including OSHA, as well as Poison Control provide Safety Data Sheets (formerly

known as Material Safety Data Sheets) that provide relevant chemical information and first aid care.
C. Classification of burn injury
1. Burns are classified according to the total body surface area (TBSA) burned, depth of burn, and the presence or absence of inhalational injury. Superficial burns (first degree) should not be included in the TBSA assessment.
2. **The extent of a burn** (TBSA) is calculated by using a Lund–Browder or other burn diagram.
   a. The **rule of nines** guides estimation (**Figure 35.5**).
      1. **Adults:** The head and each upper extremity each represent 9% TBSA. The anterior trunk, posterior trunk, and each lower extremity each represent 18% TBSA.
      2. **Infants and children:** Because of the different proportions of body surface area relative to patient age, reference must be made to the proper burn chart when calculating percent TBSA to avoid significant errors (**Figure 35.5**).
   b. Another practical method to estimate percent TBSA is that the area of the patient's palm will cover about 1% TBSA.
3. The **depth of the burn** determines therapy (ie, conservative management vs. excision and grafting). Burn depth is difficult to determine visually; however, there are some useful guidelines:
   a. The area under a **partial-thickness burn** should have normal or increased sensitivity to pain and temperature, and should blanch with pressure.
   b. A **full-thickness burn** will be anesthetic and will not blanch with pressure. Commonly, the wound bed has varying depth of burn, so the presence of pain can still be common around areas of full-thickness burn where partial-thickness burns with surviving nerve tissue are also present.

D. Initial evaluation of the burn patient
1. **Airway and breathing**
   a. Brief exposure of the epiglottis or larynx to either dry air at 300 °C or steam at 100 °C leads to massive edema and rapid airway obstruction. Chemical products of combustion such as ammonia, sulfur oxide, and chlorine dissolve in the tracheobronchial tree, forming acids and irritating the mucous membrane of the respiratory tract.
   b. When airway burns are suspected, early endotracheal intubation should be performed before airway edema occurs. Continued swelling and distortion of the soft tissues may progress at a rapid rate, rendering intubation difficult if not impossible. Upper airway edema usually resolves within the first week and can be reduced by avoiding excessive fluid administration and elevating the head of the bed.
   c. **Circumferential full-thickness burns** of the thorax will decrease chest wall compliance, which can lead to hypoxemia and respiratory failure. Emergency escharotomies may be required.
   d. **Ventilation strategies** involve avoidance of further respiratory compromise from barotrauma caused by increased alveolar distention and shearing forces. Low-tidal volume ventilation is recommended. Bronchospasm is frequently present, and bronchodilator therapy with β_2-agonists is warranted. Intraoperatively, minimize retained secretions and cellular debris by attention to body positioning and frequent suctioning.

FIGURE 35.5 Rule of nines (Lund and Browder chart). (Modified from Ryan JF, Todres ID, Cote CJ, et al., eds. *A Practice of Anesthesia for Infants and Children*. WB Saunders; 1986:230. Copyright © 1986 Elsevier. With permission.)

e. **Smoke inhalation injury** may occur during a fire within a closed space or when heated noxious vapors are inhaled.
   1. An inhalation injury should be suspected in the presence of burns of the head or neck; singed nasal hairs; swelling of the mucosa of the nose, mouth, lips, or throat; a brassy cough; or carbonaceous sputum. Both the upper airway and pulmonary parenchyma may be affected.
   2. **Chemical products** of combustion combine with water in the respiratory tract to form strong acids and alkali, causing bronchospasm, edema, and mucous membrane ulceration. Inhalation of gases such as phosgene and sulfuric acid can damage the alveolar membrane and cause partial or complete airway obstruction. Aldehydes such as acrolein impair ciliary function and damage mucosal surfaces.
   3. Combustion of polyurethane-containing products (eg, insulation and wall paneling) releases **hydrogen cyanide,** which causes tissue asphyxia by inhibiting cytochrome oxidase activity. Patients may present with an anion gap metabolic acidosis and an elevated mixed venous PO_2. Plasma lactate levels correlate with the cyanide levels. Antidotal treatment of cyanide poisoning involves three strategies: binding of cyanide, induction of methemoglobinemia, and use of sulfur donors.
      a. Binding cyanide: Hydoxocobalamin/Cyanokit (dose 70 mg/kg IV, maximum dose 5 g) binds CN and forms cyanocobalamin, a less toxic substance.
      b. Induction of methemoglobinemia provides an alternative binding site for cyanide, rather than the cytochrome electron transport chain complex. Sodium nitrite is the drug of choice (300 mg IV over 5 minutes in 100 mL of 5% dextrose). Amyl nitrate (0.3 mL ampule, crushed and inhaled over 15 to 30 seconds, repeated every minute) is more technically challenging to administer and induces a much weaker methemoglobinemia, thus should be considered a second-line, temporizing agent. Treatment with amyl nitrite or sodium nitrite is **contraindicated** in cases of concurrent carbon monoxide toxicity.
      c. Sulfur donors aid the rhodanese enzyme in detoxifying cyanide and resulting in thiocyanate, which can be renally excreted. Usual dosing is sodium thiosulfate 12.5 g in a 50-mL solution.
   4. **Carbon monoxide** binds hemoglobin, displacing oxygen and shifting the oxyhemoglobin curve to the left. Tissue hypoxia ensues.
      a. All burn-injured patients, especially those burned within a closed space, may have sustained some degree of CO exposure with their thermal injury. Oxygen administration should begin at the scene.
      b. Because oxyhemoglobin and carboxyhemoglobin absorb light at the same wavelength, conventional pulse oximetry cannot be used as an indicator of CO poisoning. Diagnosis is made on clinical suspicion and the level of arterial or venous carboxyhemoglobin, measured spectrophotometrically with a CO-oximeter.
      c. The half-life of CO is inversely related to the inspired oxygen concentration (FIO_2); it is 5 to 6 hours when breathing room air but 30 to 60 minutes when breathing 100% oxygen.
      d. Treatment is supportive and consists of supplemental oxygen until the carbon monoxide is eliminated. Hyperbaric oxygen

should be considered in comatose patients and in those with severe carbon monoxide poisoning.
   e. **Indirect respiratory injury** and pulmonary edema may occur in burn patients without an inhalational injury. Mechanisms involved include the effect of burn wound mediators on the lung, decreased plasma oncotic pressure, and complications of burn therapy.
2. **Cardiovascular resuscitation**
   a. **Fluid replacement** consists of crystalloid, usually lactated Ringers, with or without the addition of colloid. Standard protocols for fluid replacement exist using body weight (in kilograms) and percent TBSA burned, but modern practices have moved away from formula-based strategies (such as the Parkland formula, Brooke formula, and Rule of Tens) toward individualized fluid management based on trending markers of end organ perfusion and assessment of volume responsiveness.
   b. Adult patients with deep-partial and full-thickness burns involving more than 20% TBSA should receive initial fluid resuscitation of 2 mL/kg/% TBSA. In children with burns, 3 mL/kg/% TBSA should be used and 4 mL/kg/% TBSA should be used in electrical burns.

   The first half of the fluids should be given over the course of 8 hours, and the remaining half over the span of 16 hours. Fluid boluses should be reserved for use in unstable patients only.
   c. The end points of fluid therapy are hemodynamic stability, which should be assessed by trending markers of end-organ perfusion, and maintenance of an adequate urine output. A urine output of 0.5 mL/kg/h should be targeted in adults and 1 mL/kg/h in children. In extensive burns, fluid management is adjusted according to appropriate invasive monitors and laboratory studies.

E. **Management of the burn wound**
   1. **Early excision and grafting of burned areas** is a widely accepted procedure and appear to decrease mortality and hospital length of stay. It consists of the removal of all devitalized, lacerated and/or contaminated tissue (eschar) that is not compatible with healing, followed by wound coverage. Patients may be brought to the operating room in the acute phase of injury, with hemodynamic instability and respiratory dysfunction. Special emphasis should be placed on correcting acid-base and electrolyte disturbances, temperature normalization, and treatment of anemia and coagulopathy. Blood loss during wound excision and grafting can be massive. Adequate colloid and blood products should be ordered in advance. IV access should be adequate for resuscitation.
   2. **Wound coverage**
      a. **Skin grafting** involves transplanting healthy avascular skin tissue to the burn site. It can be divided into split-thickness versus full-thickness autografting depending on layers of the skin involved. Other options include:
         1. Allograft: skin graft from deceased donor
         2. Xenograft: skin grafts harvested from animals for use as temporary grafts in humans
         3. Biosynthetic products as temporary coverage.
      b. **Flap reconstruction** surgery consists of transplantation of tissue with blood supply from donor site to the burn site. For this type of surgery, the transplanted tissue does not rely on the recipient bed for blood supply, for healing.

c. Other procedures such as Z-plasty, tissue expansion, and laser therapy may be used for management of burn scars, surgical scars, or contractures.
3. Topical agents are used to minimize the colonization of healing wounds. Burns should be kept moist, and many centers use petroleum-based agents with or without antibiotics (such as Bacitracin) and nonadherent, petroleum-impregnated dressings (such as Xeroform gauze). Other topical agents and their side effects include:
   a. **Silver nitrate** may cause hyponatremia or, rarely, methemoglobinemia.
   b. **Silver sulfadiazine** may cause leukopenia, which is reversible upon discontinuing the drug.
4. The incidence of **sepsis** may be reduced by using temporary biologic dressings, either allografts (cadaver skin or amnion) or xenografts (porcine). Artificial skin (eg, Integra) bioengineered from collagen and cultured epidermis can be used when a conventional autograft is not available.
5. The use of **systemic antibiotics** is limited to treatment of documented systemic infection (as opposed to colonization), and they are also used as prophylaxis before surgical procedures.

F. Anesthetic considerations
1. **Burn-injured patients may also suffer from nonthermal traumatic injuries** and should initially be assessed as a trauma patient (see Sections I.A to I.E). The patient's age, preexisting disease, and the extent of burn injury provide an index of the patient's likely physiologic condition. Altered pharmacokinetics, drug tolerance, difficult IV access, and anatomic derangements of the airway (neck scar or mouth contracture) are primary considerations.
2. **Airway.** Obtaining an adequate mask fit may be difficult because of edema in the early phases of burn injury or because of scars and contractures later on. The same processes can render endotracheal intubation extremely difficult in burn patients.
3. **Monitoring and IV access** (**Table 35.2** and **Figure 35.6**)
   a. Often IV access will still be in place from the initial resuscitation. Large-bore IVs are mandatory to allow for massive fluid replacement.

| | Intraoperative Monitoring Challenges in Patients With Major Burn Injury | |

Monitor	Possible Challenges of Burn Injury	Possible Solutions
Electrocardiogram (ECG)	ECG electrodes may not adhere	Consider needle electrodes or stapling of electrodes
Noninvasive blood pressure monitor	Edema or extensive burns in the extremities may limit use of cuff	Consider alternative location, use dressing or gauze under cuff Consider invasive monitoring
Invasive blood pressure monitor	Hypothermia, hypovolemia, initial decreased cardiac output, vasoconstriction	Consider alternative location, trend values, confirm with noninvasive blood pressure
Pulse oximetry	Extensive burn injury may limit placement Carboxyhemoglobin will falsely elevate oxygen saturation reading	Consider alternative location, trend values, assess partial pressure of oxygen by arterial blood gas (ABG)

Acute Burns Intra-operative Protocol
Apply "Burn" macro in Epic to trigger communication reminders

Monitor cables untangled and draped ABOVE the blankets	**Temperature management:** • Warm OR to 100°F prior to transport • 2 Bair Huggers • Fluid warmer primed • Goal patient temp 37-37.5°C	Infusion tubing untangled and draped to the side of CVC

Neuro
- Patients will come from ICU with sedative and analgesic infusions
- *Confirm volume/dose accounted for at pre/post-op handoffs*
- Consider multimodal analgesia: regional, ketamine, dexmedetomidine, magnesium, acetaminophen, lidocaine, others

CV
- Review hemodynamics/pressors with ICU team prior to transport
- Transport with appropriate push pressors prn
- Conventional hemodynamic targets, MAP >65 (unless specific patient factor)
- Assure adequate venous access prior to start

Pulm
- Transport on travel vent; in-line suction prior to transport
- Consider clamping ETT during transition to avoid derecruitment
- Ensure FULL O₂ tank, Ambu Bag w/PEEP valve, mask, airway bag
- In trached patients, travel with spare trach of appropriate size
- Maintain minute ventilation from ICU (often high 2/2 hypermetabolism)
- Monitor for kinking of tube due to warming measures

GI
- Follow DACCPM Pre-Procedural Fasting Guidelines for Tube Feeds (see back)
- Minimize fasting times or continue enteral feeding intra-operatively if no high-risk features (patient, operative site, positioning)
- TPN should always be continued intra-operatively

GU
- Non-HD patients: target 0.5-1.0 mL/kg/hr UOP
- Consider diuretics with blood product/colloid administration
- CVVH patients: continue intra-op (with SICU RN) vs. minimize downtime

Heme
- Discuss estimated EBL in huddle
- Scan ID bracelet and send for blood upon arrival
- Begin transfusion EARLY and follow 1:1:1 or 2:1:1
- Recognize EBL in drapes and check-in frequently

ID
- Review scheduled antimicrobials and continue as scheduled
- ICU will send antimicrobials that require ID approval

Endo
- Obtain baseline blood glucose + at least q2h if on gtt
- Ensure sufficient insulin gtt for case

Communication is CRITICAL

Check-in hourly (and prn) to review critical labs, I&O, hemodynamics, & temp
Use the white-board next to anesthesia station to record check-in
Send full set of labs as dressings being applied prior to transport

Version 1.0

FIGURE 35.6 Cognitive aid detailing intraoperative burn anesthesia considerations. (Used with permission by Dr. Jamie Sparling and Dr. Jonathan Friedstat.)

    b. In massive burns, ECG electrodes may be placed directly on debrided tissue. Alternatively, needle electrodes can be used.

    c. **Arterial lines** are indispensable for continuous blood pressure monitoring and frequent blood sampling. The cannulation site will depend on the availability of unburned areas. If all appropriate sites are burned, the line may have to be placed through the burn wound after the area has been prepared in a sterile fashion.

    d. **CVP lines** are useful both for monitoring central pressures and for central access for drug infusions.

    e. A **pulmonary artery catheter** may be required for management of patients with myocardial dysfunction or undifferentiated shock.

4. **Muscle relaxants. Extrajunctional nicotinic receptors** proliferate in muscle at the burn site and at sites distant from the burn injury. Succinylcholine is only safe in the immediate 24 hours after thermal injury. An increase in acetylcholine receptors is usually associated with resistance to nondepolarizing neuromuscular-blocking agents, increased sensitivity to depolarizing muscle relaxants, and life-threatening hyperkalemia when succinylcholine is used.
5. **Anesthetics**
   a. There is no single preferred agent or combination of agents; however, ketamine and etomidate may have advantages in patients with a tenuous hemodynamic status.
   b. These patients may have **greatly increased opioid requirements** owing to tolerance, hypermetabolic physiology, and an increase in the apparent volume of distribution for drugs. It is important to provide adequate analgesia, which may necessitate massive doses of opiates.
6. **Temperature regulation.** The most comfortable body temperature for a burn patient is about 100 °F (38 °C). In the burn intensive care unit, patients are cared for in warmed, humidified rooms. Every effort should be made to maintain normothermia during transport and surgery. The operating room, IV fluids, and blood products should be warmed and inspired gases heated and humidified. Pediatric patients should be placed under a radiant heat source and on a warming blanket whenever possible.
7. **Immunosuppression.** The immune system is suppressed for weeks to months after burn injury, and the wound itself serves as an excellent medium for bacterial growth. Every attempt should be made to practice aseptic technique when handling patients, suctioning airways, and inserting intravascular lines.
8. **Postanesthetic care.** It is important to maintain normothermia while transporting patients back to the intensive care unit because shivering results in vasoconstriction and could contribute to graft loss. Supplemental oxygen should be given until patients are fully recovered from anesthesia. Severe pain is common, and patient responses vary, necessitating individual titration of analgesics and frequent reassessment of the effect.

ACKNOWLEDGMENTS

We gratefully acknowledge the contributions of previous edition authors, Evan Hodell, Stephanie Lankford, and Ilan Mizrahi, as portions of those chapters have been retained in this revision.

Suggested Readings

American College of Surgeons. *Advanced Trauma Life Support (ATLS) Student Manual.* 10th ed. American College of Surgeons; 2019.

Bickell WH, Wall MJ Jr, Pepe PE, et al. Immediate versus delayed fluid resuscitation for hypotensive patients with penetrating torso injuries. *N Engl J Med.* 1994;331(17):1105–1109.

Bittner EA, Martyn JA, Sjöberg F. Chapter 87. Acute and anesthetic care of the burn-injured patient. In: Gropper MA, Miller RD, eds. *Miller's Anesthesia*. Elsevier/Churchill Livingstone; 2020.

Bittner EA, Shank E, Woodson L, Martyn JAJ. Acute and perioperative care of the burn-injured patient. *Anesthesiology.* 2015;122(2):448–464.

Bowen DK, Antevil JL, Gurney JM, et al. *Wartime Thoracic Injury. Joint Trauma System Clinical Practice Guidelines.* 2018. Accessed April 2, 2020. https://jts.amedd.army.mil/index.cfm/PI_CPGs/cpgs

Charbit B, Mandelbrot L, Samain E, et al. The decrease of fibrinogen is an early predictor of the severity of postpartum hemorrhage. *J Thromb Haemost.* 2007;5(2):266–273.

Chung KK, Salinas J, Renz EM, et al. Simple derivation of the initial fluid rate for the resuscitation of severely burned adult combat casualties: in silico validation of the rule of 10. *J Trauma.* 2010;69(1):S49–S54.

Driscoll IR, Mann-Salinas EA, Boyer NL, et al. *Burn Care. Joint Trauma System Clinical Practice Guidelines.* 2016. Accessed February 12, 2021. http://jts.amedd.army.mil/index.cfm/PI_CPGs/cpgs

Duchesne JC, Barbeau JM, Islam TM, et al. Damage control resuscitation: from emergency department to the operating room. *Am Surg.* 2011;77(2):201–206.

Jain V, Chari R, Maslovitz S, et al. Guidelines for the management of a pregnant trauma patient. *J Obstet Gynaecol Can.* 2015;37(6):553–574.

Kaiser HE, Kim CM, Sharar SR, et al. Advances in perioperative and critical care of the burn patient. *Adv Anesth.* 2013;31(1):137–161.

Martyn JA, Richtsfeld M. Succinylcholine-induced hyperkalemia in acquired pathologic states: etiologic factors and molecular mechanisms. *Anesthesiology.* 2006;104(1):158–169.

Neschis DG, Scalea TM, Flinn WR, Griffith BP. Blunt aortic injury. *N Engl J Med.* 2008;359(16):1708–1716.

Orgill DP, Ogawa R. Current methods of burn reconstruction. *Plastic and Reconstructive Surgery.* 2013;131(5):827e–836e.

Roberts I, Shakur H, Ker K, et al. CRASH-2 Trial collaborators. Antifibrinolytic drugs for acute traumatic injury. *Cochrane Database Syst Rev.* 2012;12:CD004896.

Theusinger OM, Madjdpour C, Spahn DR. Resuscitation and transfusion management in trauma patients: emerging concepts. *Curr Opin Crit Care.* 2012;18(6):661–670.

Wang C, Zhang F, Lineaweaver WC. Clinical applications of allograft skin in burn care. *Annals of Plastic Surgery.* 2020;84(3S):S158–S160.

Transfusion Therapy
Andrew D. Siemens and Marvin G. Chang

I. THE DECISION TO TRANSFUSE

The decision to initiate transfusion is complex. There are many risks to transfusion (see Section VIII), and transfusion is ultimately indicated when the potential benefits outweigh these risks. In most civilian settings, transfusion therapy utilizes blood components rather than whole blood. The benefits of blood component transfusion stem from the correction of conditions that result in decreased production; increased utilization, destruction, or loss; or dysfunction of a specific blood component (usually red blood cells, platelets, or coagulation factors). Although many attempts at creating universal transfusion protocols have been introduced, few have successfully demonstrated definitive thresholds or clear superiority. The aim of this chapter is to provide the background to help clinicians make these decisions on an individual basis. A condensed summary of approaches to perioperative transfusion therapy and decision making may be found in **Table 36.1**.

A. Assessing red cell mass and oxygen-carrying ability

1. **The decision to transfuse red blood cells** (also called erythrocytes, red cells, or RBCs). Most evidence suggests that higher red cell transfusion thresholds (eg, 10 to 12 g/dL) do not confer a mortality benefit and may even be harmful. Nonetheless, maintaining adequate red cell mass is essential for adequate oxygen-carrying capacity to the tissues. Further, it has been shown that perioperative anemia may increase the risk of acute kidney injury, acute coronary or cerebrovascular events, and prolonged postoperative hospital stays. The decision to transfuse, therefore, must be weighed carefully based on a variety of patient and situational factors rather than rigid guidelines.

2. **Patient factors.** The main reason for transfusing red cells is to maintain the oxygen-carrying capacity of the tissues, a primary determinant of which is the hemoglobin (Hb) level.

    a. **Healthy individuals** or **individuals with chronic anemia** can usually tolerate lower Hb levels of 6.5 to 8 g/dL, assuming normal intravascular volume. The use of a "restrictive" transfusion practice, aiming for Hb of 7 to 9 g/dL, is generally safe and has been shown to reduce the risk of death compared with transfusing toward a "liberal" Hb goal of 10 to 12 g/dL. The precise reasons for reduced mortality in the restrictively transfused group have not been clearly delineated, but the effects of allogeneic transfusion on diminished immune function have been substantiated in animal and human studies (see Section VIII.D).

    b. For **patients with coronary artery disease (CAD)**, the risk of myocardial ischemia due to anemia has resulted in many practitioners transfusing to a higher (9 to 10 g/dL) Hb target. As the incidence of CAD rises substantially with age, many practitioners also opt to use a higher transfusion threshold in the elderly. Studies to support this practice, however, are lacking, and those that exist have produced contradictory results. For example, a study of medical patients with acute

TABLE 36.1 Summary of Perioperative Transfusion Considerations

Preoperative Decision Making
1. Evaluate indications for and contraindications to blood product transfusion, including patient history and comorbidities, surgical considerations, and allowable blood loss.
    a. Address preoperative anemia by administering iron, EPO, and blood products or adjuvants as appropriate.
    b. Hold nonessential anticoagulants and address preoperative coagulopathies.
    c. Consider preoperative autologous blood donation or acute normovolemic hemodilution strategies.
2. Perform a preoperative examination and review relevant laboratory tests to determine perioperative indications for blood products or adjuvants.
    a. Consider the need for a preoperative type and screen or crossmatch.
3. Discuss the risks and benefits of transfusion with the patient and obtain informed consent.
4. Prepare the operating room or anesthetizing location for blood product transfusion.
    a. Set up and prime an infusion circuit incorporating a fluid warmer and blood filter using calcium-free crystalloid, colloid, or blood components.
    b. Prepare rapid or pressure infusion devices as appropriate.
    c. Coordinate use of blood salvage and other devices with operating room staff.
5. Initiate discussion with the surgical team during a standardized huddle or time-out regarding how much blood loss is anticipated.

Intraoperative Decision Making
1. Consider available blood-sparing measures, but do not withhold blood products when they may significantly improve patient outcomes.
    a. Administer adjuvant agents, particularly antifibrinolytics, to select patients when major blood loss is possible.
    b. Implement a controlled hypotension strategy if indicated.
    c. Replace simple fluid losses with nonblood product volume expanders (eg, crystalloid or colloid) prior to initiating transfusion.
    d. Consider recommending the use of hemostatic agents in the surgical field.
    e. Reinfuse perioperatively salvaged blood as appropriate.
2. Assess for clinical signs of adequate oxygen delivery and surgical blood loss using visual inspection and standard monitors.
    a. Consider additional hemodynamic monitoring techniques such as transesophageal echocardiography if substantial blood loss is present or expected.
3. Obtain point-of-care assessments of blood counts and coagulation (eg, TEG) to guide blood product and adjuvant administration.
4. Adhere to institutional and society-recommended transfusion thresholds and blood ordering protocols.
    a. Consider administration of leukoreduced red cells to patients at risk for CMV transmission and nonhemolytic transfusion reactions.
5. Monitor for and treat any early complications of transfusion therapy.

Postoperative Decision Making
1. Maintain ongoing clinical and laboratory assessments of blood loss in the Post-Anesthesia Care Unit (PACU) or postoperative destination.
    a. Implement periodic evaluations of the operative site and drain outputs.
    b. Keep PACU phase I monitors applied until bleeding slows and vitals remain stable.
    c. Follow hemoglobin or hematocrit values serially if anemia is suspected.
2. Continue evaluation for and treatment of delayed complications of transfusion therapy.
3. Consider escalation of care or disposition to an intensive care setting if bleeding continues to be excessive, if the patient's status remains unstable, or if ongoing significant transfusion may be required.

coronary syndromes also found a higher mortality rate attributable to red cell transfusion in otherwise stable patients with a hematocrit (Hct) greater than 25%. Meanwhile, a recent 2023 meta-analysis of patients with acute coronary syndrome suggested that liberal transfusion thresholds may decrease the risk of long-term major adverse cardiac events and myocardial infarction.

The most recent 2021 STS/SCA/AmSECT/SABM Clinical Practice Guidelines recommend a restrictive over liberal transfusion strategy, while not providing a specific transfusion threshold. This is consistent with the 2019 Society of Cardiovascular Anesthesiologists Clinical Practice Advisory Statement that stated that a Hb transfusion threshold of 7.5 g/dL as reasonable for most cardiac surgery patients. The most recent 2023 Association for the Advancement of Blood and Biotherapies (AABB) International Guidelines recommend a restrictive over liberal transfusion strategy, and that transfusions for a Hb greater than 10 g/dL is not recommended and unlikely to improve oxygen transport.

3. **Situational factors**
   a. **Intraoperative red cell transfusion** depends on red cell loss. This can be roughly estimated by measuring blood in suction canisters, weighing sponges, and checking blood loss in the drapes. In the perioperative period, suspected or confirmed hemorrhage remains the most common indication for transfusion. During periods of ongoing blood loss, transfusion may be indicated even with a Hb >10 g/dL if bleeding is brisk enough that the clinician expects a substantial drop in Hb without treatment.
   b. If a patient is anemic preoperatively, the etiology should be clarified and then used to guide perioperative therapy. It may be secondary to decreased production (marrow suppression or nutritional deficiencies), increased loss (hemorrhage), or destruction (hemolysis).

4. **Estimating blood volumes (BVs)**
   a. **Estimated allowable blood loss** (EABL) can be calculated as follows, using either Hcts (as shown) or Hbs:

   $$\text{EABL} = [(\text{Hct}_{starting} - \text{Hct}_{allowable}) \times \text{BV}] / [(\text{Hct}_{starting} + \text{Hct}_{allowable})/2]$$

   BV in an adult is approximately 7% of lean body mass. This may be calculated as approximately 70 mL/kg of body weight in an average adult man and approximately 65 mL/kg of body weight in an average adult woman (see Chapter 33: Anesthesia for Pediatric Surgery and Care of the Neonate for Pediatric Considerations). Obese patients have a lower relative lean body mass and a lower relative BV; thus, the greater the degree of obesity, the lower the BV estimate relative to total body weight (TBW). For example, a patient with a body mass index (BMI) of 40 may have an estimated BV of 53 mL/kg TBW, whereas patients with a BMI of 70 may have an estimated BV of 40 mL/kg TBW.
   b. **The volume of blood to transfuse** can be calculated as follows:

   $$\text{Volume to transfuse} = [(\text{Hct}_{desired} - \text{Hct}_{present}) \times \text{BV}] / \text{Hct}_{transfused\ blood}$$

   c. One unit of packed red blood cells (PRBCs) has a Hct of 70% to 85% when stored with the standard Adsol preservative.

B. **Thrombocytopenia** is due to either decreased bone marrow production (eg, chemotherapy, tumor infiltration, or alcoholism) or increased utilization or destruction (eg, trauma or surgery creating a large wound, hypersplenism, idiopathic thrombocytopenia purpura [ITP], disseminated intravascular coagulation [DIC], or drug effects). It also results from dilution and loss associated with massive transfusion (see Section IX.A.1). Spontaneous bleeding is unusual with platelet counts above 20,000/mm^3. Platelet counts above 50,000/mm^3 are preferable for surgical hemostasis. However, as in the case of red cell administration, the decision to transfuse must be made based on clinical factors rather than platelet count alone. For example, patients with ITP have a high rate of platelet turnover and will often exhibit normal coagulation despite a low platelet count. In addition, as this form of thrombocytopenia is primarily due to platelet destruction, patients with ITP will not respond adequately to platelet transfusion. Instead, treatments should be aimed at halting the underlying destructive process.

C. **Coagulopathy.** Bleeding associated with documented factor deficiencies or prolonged clotting studies (prothrombin time [PT] and partial thromboplastin time [PTT]) mandates replacement therapy to maintain normal coagulation function. See Sections II and IX for a discussion of coagulopathy.

II. COAGULATION STUDIES

The most important clues to a clinically significant bleeding disorder in an otherwise healthy patient may be obtained from a thorough history. In particular, a personal or family history of anemia requiring iron replacement or blood products may suggest a bleeding diathesis. Prior excessive surgical bleeding, gingival bleeding, easy bruising, epistaxis, or menorrhagia should raise concern. Many laboratory tests are available to assess the coagulation system. However, the clinician must remember that coagulation depends on a complex interplay of platelets and coagulation factors that may not be fully captured by any single test.

A. **Activated partial thromboplastin time (aPTT or PTT)** is measured by adding particulate matter such as silica or kaolin to a blood sample to activate the coagulation system. Normal values for the PTT are 22 to 34 seconds but vary according to the reagent and instruments used by the specific laboratory. The PTT assesses factors in the intrinsic (VIII, IX, XI, XII, and contact factors) and the common (II, V, X, and fibrinogen) coagulation pathways. The test is sensitive to decreased amounts of coagulation factors, and the value is elevated in patients on heparin therapy. The PTT will also be abnormally elevated in patients with hemophilia or a circulating anticoagulant (eg, lupus anticoagulant or antibodies to factor VIII). The clinician should remember that an abnormal PTT does not necessarily correlate with clinical bleeding severity. Therefore, aggressive correction of an abnormal PTT in surgical patients is not universally indicated unless the patient is actively bleeding.

B. **PT** is measured by adding tissue factor (thromboplastin) to a blood sample to activate coagulation. It serves as a measure of factors of the extrinsic (VII and tissue factor) and common (see above) coagulation pathways. Although both PT and PTT are affected by levels of factors V and X, prothrombin, and fibrinogen, the PT is specifically sensitive to deficiencies of factor VII. The PT is also normal in deficiencies of intrinsic pathway factors VIII, IX, XI, XII, prekallikrein, and high–molecular-weight kininogen. Normal values fall between 10 and 15 seconds, although the international normalized ratio (INR) (see below) is more commonly reported given the variability of PT results between laboratories.

C. The **INR** represents a means of standardizing PT values to allow reliable comparison among different laboratories. It is defined as the ratio of the patient's PT to the control PT value that would be obtained if international reference reagents had been used to perform the test. Oral warfarin anticoagulation therapy may therefore be guided by a target INR value that is independent of the laboratory variability of the PT. For example, an INR of 2.0 to 3.0 is recommended for prophylaxis against thromboembolism in atrial fibrillation. Higher INR values may be targeted in specific populations at increased risk for thromboembolic phenomena (eg, 2.5 to 3.5 in patients with mechanical mitral valves).

D. **Activated clotting time (ACT)** is a modified whole blood clotting time in which diatomaceous earth (celite) or clay (kaolin) is added to a blood sample to activate the intrinsic pathway. The ACT is the time until clot formation. A normal ACT is 90 to 130 seconds depending on the instrument used. Compared with the PTT, the ACT is a relatively easy and expedient test to perform and is useful in monitoring heparin therapy rapidly in the operating room (see Chapter 24: Anesthesia for Spine Surgery). However, because the ACT is relatively insensitive to lower levels of heparin anticoagulation, it is typically reserved for settings that require higher doses of heparin, particularly cardiopulmonary bypass (CPB) and extracorporeal membrane oxygenation.

E. **Platelet counts** can be measured to determine the risk of excessive bleeding due to platelet depletion. Commonly accepted normal values range between 150,000 and 450,000/mm^3, and a clinical threshold for perioperative platelet transfusion is often less than 50,000/mm^3. However, platelet counts do not provide a qualitative metric of platelet function and thus may not reliably reflect the risk of bleeding in certain populations.

F. **Platelet function tests** range from simple assessments of bleeding time to sophisticated optical aggregometry techniques. In circumstances involving elements of platelet dysfunction, including uremia and the use of antiplatelet agents, point-of-care tests of platelet activation and aggregation—such as that generated by the platelet function analyzer 100 (PFA-100) device—may provide insight into bleeding risk. However, these tests remain largely unvalidated for routine perioperative use. Thromboelastography (TEG) (see below) may also allow for rapid assessment of platelet function.

G. **Fibrinogen** is the precursor protein that is activated to form fibrin and then cross-linked to strengthen clots. Assaying fibrinogen levels can be helpful when coagulopathy is present or suspected. Although the diagnostic specificity of the fibrinogen level is low, it can be helpful to guide further transfusion support (ie, the administration of fresh frozen plasma [FFP] or cryoprecipitate).

H. **Thromboelastography (TEG)** is available in some centers for clinical use, often as a point-of-care test. TEG is performed by placing a small aliquot of blood into a heated oscillating cup, into which a pin on a torsion wire is suspended. Clot formation in the oscillating cup generates torque on the pin, and the torque is measured and converted to an electrical signal. The signal is then recorded by a computer, creating a characteristic trace (**Figure 36.1**) that may be analyzed for abnormalities of clot formation. By measuring clot formation and viscoelastic clot strength, TEG provides information about the adequacy of clotting factors, fibrin levels, and platelets. In general, R time represents the activity of coagulation factors, the alpha angle and K time represent acceleration of fibrin formation, maximum amplitude represents platelet function, and percent lysis in 30 minutes (LY30) represents the rate of fibrinolysis. Thromboelastometry

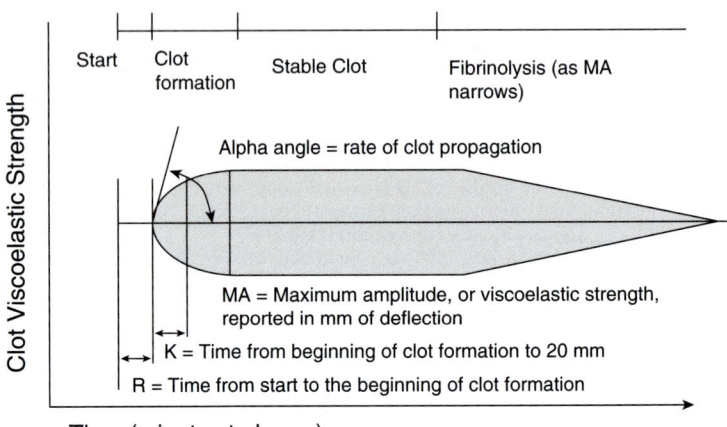

FIGURE 36.1 Thromboelastography.

(TEM, previously ROTEM) uses similar technology with similarly measured parameters.

III. BLOOD TYPING AND CROSS-MATCHING

A. **Donor blood and recipient blood** are typed using the red cell surface **ABO and Rh systems** and screened for antibodies to other cell antigens. "Direct" cross-matching involves directly mixing the patient's plasma with the donor's red cells to establish that hemolysis does not occur from any undetected antibodies. An individual's red cells display A antigen, B antigen, both antigens (AB), or no surface antigens (O). If the patient's red cells do not display either surface antigen A or surface antigen B, then antibodies will be produced upon exposure to the absent antigen(s). Thus, a person who is type B may develop anti-A antibodies in the serum, and a type O individual may develop circulating anti-A and anti-B antibodies. A type AB individual will not produce antibodies to either A or B antigens and therefore can receive red cells from any donor blood type. People with type O blood display neither A nor B surface antigens and can donate blood cells to any other type (universal red cell donor; **Table 36.2**). The universal FFP

TABLE 36.2 Transfusion Compatibility

Recipient Blood Type	RBC Donor	FFP Donor
AB	AB, A, B, or O	AB
A	A or O	A or AB
B	B or O	B or AB
O	O	A, B, AB, or O
Rh+	Rh+ or Rh+	Rh+ or Rh−
Rh−	Rh−	Rh+ or Rh−

donor, conversely, has type AB blood, which will contain neither anti-A nor anti-B antibodies to antigens on recipient RBCs. Whole blood donors and recipients must be exact ABO matches because whole blood contains both RBCs and serum. For example, a unit of type O whole blood will contain serum with anti-A and anti-B antibodies and therefore cannot be used to transfuse patients who are A, B, or AB blood types.

B. Rh surface antigens are either present (Rh positive) or absent (Rh negative). Individuals who are Rh negative will develop antibodies to the Rh factor when exposed to Rh-positive blood. Although this does not usually have clinical consequences at the time of the initial exposure, subsequent exposures to Rh-positive RBCs may cause circulating antibodies to produce hemolysis. This can pose a particular problem during pregnancy. Maternal anti-Rh antibodies belong to the IgG class and freely cross the placenta. Rh-negative mothers who have developed Rh antibodies will therefore transmit these antibodies to the fetus. If the fetus is Rh positive, massive hemolysis may occur (a phenomenon referred to as hemolytic disease of the newborn or erythroblastosis fetalis). **Rh immune globulin** (*RhoGAM*), an Rh-blocking antibody, prevents the Rh-negative patient from developing anti-Rh antibodies. It should be administered to Rh-negative individuals who receive Rh-positive blood and to Rh-negative mothers delivering Rh-positive babies (as some fetomaternal blood mixing often occurs at delivery). The recommended dose is 300 μg intramuscularly for every 15 mL of Rh-positive blood transfused, although administration of Rh-negative blood to Rh-negative mothers is preferred when available.

C. Recipient antibodies against other donor RBC antigens (such as those from the Kell, Kid, Duffy, or Lewis groups) can also cause hemolytic transfusion reactions. When a patient's blood sample is screened and found to contain antibodies against antigens found on donor RBCs, it complicates cross-matching and can delay the availability of blood products. When a patient's antibody screen is positive, it is advisable to discuss anticipated transfusion needs with the blood bank.

D. If an emergency blood transfusion is needed, type-specific (ABO) red cells can often be obtained within minutes at large centers if the patient's blood type is known. If type-specific blood is unavailable, type O Rh-negative red cells should be transfused (although type O–positive blood can be used emergently in males and postmenopausal women). Type-specific blood should be substituted as soon as possible to minimize the amount of type O plasma (containing anti-A and anti-B antibodies) transfused.

IV. BLOOD COMPONENT THERAPY
A. General considerations
   1. One unit of **PRBCs**, which has a Hct of about 70% and a volume of about 250 mL, will usually increase the Hct by 2% to 3% or the Hb by 1 g/dL in the euvolemic adult once equilibration has taken place. In euvolemic children, PRBC volumes of 4 mL/kg will also increase the Hb by approximately 1 g/dL. PRBCs must be ABO compatible with the recipient.
   2. One unit of **platelets** increases the platelet count by 5000 to 10,000/mm^3. A usual platelet transfusion is 1 unit per 10 kg of body weight. If thrombocytopenia is caused by a destructive or consumptive process or if platelets are dysfunctional, platelet transfusions will be less efficacious (see Section I.B). Transfusion of ABO-compatible platelets is not obligatory, although they may provide a better posttransfusion platelet count. Single-donor or human leukocyte antigen (HLA)-matched platelets may be required for patient's refractory to platelet transfusion. A unit

of single-donor platelets provides the equivalent of approximately six random donor units of platelets. Owing to inactivation at low temperatures, **platelets should be stored at room temperature** and never placed in a cooler or refrigerator.

3. **FFP,** which is stored in volumes of about 250 to 300 mL/U and administered at doses of 10 to 15 mL/kg, should increase plasma coagulation factors to 30% of normal, the minimum necessary for hemostasis (except for fibrinogen, of which 50% of the normal 200 to 400 mg/dL concentration is required). Fibrinogen levels increase by 1 mg/dL per mL of plasma transfused. Acute reversal of warfarin is often achieved with only 5 to 8 mL/kg of FFP, although the PT may remain modestly prolonged. FFP transfusions must be ABO compatible, but Rh compatibility and cross-matching are not required (**Table 36.1**).

4. **Cryoprecipitate** is prepared via centrifugation of the plasma and contains concentrated factor VIII, factor XIII, fibrinogen, von Willebrand factor (vWF), and fibronectin. Indications for cryoprecipitate include hypofibrinogenemia, von Willebrand disease, hemophilia A (when recombinant factor VIII is unavailable), and preparation of fibrin glue. The usual dosage of 1 unit per 7 to 10 kg should raise the plasma fibrinogen by about 50 mg/dL in a patient without massive bleeding. ABO compatibility is not mandatory for cryoprecipitate transfusion.

B. Technical considerations

1. **Compatible infusions.** Normal saline (0.9%) solution, albumin (5%), and FFP are compatible with RBCs and may be preferred in diluting blood products or priming blood delivery systems. Coadministration of blood products with Plasmalyte solutions is probably safe. Coadministration with calcium-containing lactated Ringer's solution was historically discouraged given concerns for calcium precipitating with citrate, however, recent studies have suggested against this risk; nevertheless, concern persists. Blood products should not be infused with hypotonic (eg, 5% dextrose) solutions, as these may cause hemolysis.

2. **Blood filters.** Standard blood filters (170 to 200 μm) remove debris and should be used for all blood components. However, manufacturer recommendations for specific bedside blood filters should be followed with respect to the component to be filtered and the number of units administered per filter.

   a. **Leukocyte reduction (leukoreduction)** is achieved by filtration, either in the blood bank or at the bedside. Microaggregate filters (20 to 50 μm), which should not be used for platelets, remove 70% to 90% of leukocytes. Third-generation or adhesion filters remove more than 99.9% of leukocytes via a combination of filtration and adhesion of white blood cells. These filters are recommended for use in patients with a history of febrile nonhemolytic transfusion reactions (FNHTRs), for prevention of alloimmunization to foreign leukocyte antigens (eg, in the oncologic patient expected to require multiple platelet transfusions), or to prevent cytomegalovirus (CMV) transmission in organ transplant recipients. Other potential but unproven benefits of leukocyte reduction include a diminished immunomodulatory effect of allogeneic transfusion; reduced transmission of bacterial, viral, or prion diseases; prevention of transfusion-related acute lung injury (TRALI); and decreased incidence of graft-versus-host disease (GVHD). Several countries have implemented universal leukoreduction protocols for transfused cellular blood products. The proposed benefits and cost efficiency of universal leukoreduction have

generated significant controversy within transfusion medicine and are not mandatory in the United States at this time.
- b. **Hypotensive reactions** associated with the use of bedside leukocyte reduction filters have been reported. The pathophysiology may involve activation of bradykinin by the leukocyte filter, and the hypotensive effect may be exaggerated in patients taking angiotensin converting enzyme (ACE) inhibitors. When this reaction occurs, the transfusion should be stopped and the blood pressure supported. These interventions usually result in rapid resolution of hypotension. Products that are leukoreduced in the blood bank may carry a lower risk of this hypotensive reaction, as bradykinin is rapidly metabolized in stored blood.

C. Massive transfusion is traditionally defined as transfusion of 10 or more units of PRBCs, or one BV, within a 24-hour period. When anticipating or initiating a large-volume transfusion, coordination with the blood bank is crucial; therefore, many institutions have developed massive transfusion protocols to ensure availability and rapid mobilization of blood products when activated. The decision to activate a massive transfusion protocol may be complex but can be guided by validated clinical scoring systems such as the ABC score. Initial management should be aimed at correcting drivers of hemorrhage (eg, giving several units of FFP to correct a greatly elevated INR) prior to administering blood components according to any standard ratio. Some evidence suggests that transfusion of platelets, FFP, and PRBCs in a 1:1:1 ratio may be superior to a 1:1:2 ratio in promoting hemostasis and reducing mortality related to hemorrhage in the setting of trauma (see Chapter 35: Anesthesia for Trauma and Burns for further discussion). Platelet counts may also be expected to fall by approximately 50% for each BV that is hemorrhaged; therefore, the early transfusion of platelets and consideration of antifibrinolytics may be beneficial.

D. Blood substitutes. Despite years of research intent on finding a blood substitute capable of oxygen transport, none provides significant clinical usefulness at this time. Hb-based oxygen carriers trialed to date have been shown to scavenge nitric oxide (NO), provoke inflammation, and produce other harms that outweigh their potential benefits. These products continue to be an area of research.

V. PLASMA SUBSTITUTES

Although various colloid products are available commercially, their use remains limited by cost, potential allergic reactions, adverse effects on coagulation, and a lack of clear benefits relative to crystalloids.

A. Albumin is available as either an isotonic 5% or a hypertonic 20% or 25% solution. Albumin has an intravascular half-life of 10 to 15 hours. Although albumin is frequently used to avoid high volumes of crystalloid infusion and fluid creep, evidence of superiority with routine use over crystalloids is lacking, and its cost is substantially higher than that of crystalloids. For these reasons, many authors argue against the routine use of albumin except in particular circumstances, which may include volume expansion for patients with substantial fluid third spacing (eg, severe hepatic dysfunction) or replacement of rapid albumin losses (eg, after large-volume paracentesis).

B. Hydroxyethyl starches (hetastarch, Voluven [R]) are manufactured from amylopectin. Hetastarch effects on coagulation include decreased fibrinogen, vWf, and factor VIII levels as well as impaired platelet function. It has also been shown to increase rates of renal failure and mortality in patients with severe sepsis and is now rarely used.

VI. PHARMACOLOGIC THERAPY

   A. **Erythropoietin (EPO)** increases RBC mass by stimulating the proliferation and development of erythroid precursor cells. Recombinant EPO can be administered before elective surgery, ideally 3 to 4 weeks prior, to increase RBC production. However, its role in the perioperative period is unclear, and its use may be associated with an increased incidence of hypertension and adverse thrombotic events.

   B. **Desmopressin (DDAVP)** is a V2 receptor-selective analog of antidiuretic hormone (or vasopressin) that may be beneficial in patients with mild hemophilia A, von Willebrand disease (type 1), and uremic platelet dysfunction. DDAVP increases endothelial cell release (but not production) of vWF, factor VIII, and tissue plasminogen activator to promote coagulation. The standard dosage is 0.3 µg/kg diluted in normal saline and administered over 30 minutes. Tachyphylaxis is possible if doses are more frequent than every 48 hours. The intravenous (IV) dose should be administered slowly to avoid hypotension or hypertension. Hyponatremia may occur with excessive DDAVP use.

   C. **Lysine analogues** such as epsilon-aminocaproic acid (EACA) and tranexamic acid (TXA) inhibit fibrinolysis, the endogenous process by which fibrin clots are broken down. They act by displacing plasminogen from fibrin, inhibiting plasminogen conversion to plasmin, and preventing plasmin from binding to fibrinogen or fibrin monomers. Trials have shown that TXA may be useful in the early treatment of trauma victims to reduce bleeding and mortality as well as in modestly reducing bleeding-related mortality in women with postpartum hemorrhage (see Chapter 32: Anesthesia for Obstetrics and Gynecology and Chapter 35: Anesthesia for Trauma and Burns). However, TXA has been associated with the development of perioperative tonic–clonic seizures, likely as a result of off-target gamma-aminobutyric acid (GABA) receptor inhibition, at therapeutic doses. Uses of EACA may include prophylaxis for dental surgery in hemophiliacs, reduction of bleeding in prostatic surgery, and reduction of hemorrhage in cases of excessive fibrinolysis. Because CPB has been shown to initiate fibrinolysis, EACA has been used during cardiac surgery to decrease postoperative chest tube drainage. However, the drug's efficacy in reducing blood transfusion requirements has been demonstrated only when the transfusion threshold is restrictive (Hb approximately 7 g/dL). Theoretical risks of thrombosis with EACA have not been demonstrated clinically; nevertheless, caution should be taken when administering these agents to treat DIC. The dosage of EACA in adults is a 5 to 10 g IV load over 1 hour followed by 1 to 2 g/h IV infusion, whereas the standard dosage of TXA is 1 g (or 10 to 30 mg/kg depending on the surgery) over 10 to 30 minutes. Dose reduction is commonly required in patients prone to drug accumulation, particularly those with renal insufficiency or failure.

   D. **Serpins** (serine protease inhibitors) such as aprotinin function to directly inhibit the activity of plasmin and other proteases involved in fibrinolysis. Although these agents were previously used to reduce massive hemorrhage in cardiac surgery, they have been associated with increased mortality rates and have largely disappeared from use in the United States.

   E. **Topical hemostatic agents** such as fibrin glue, thrombin gel, and oxidized regenerated cellulose (*Surgicel*) have been shown in trials to reduce perioperative transfusion requirements and time to hemostasis. Their use is now recommended for patients with potential or active excessive bleeding.

VII. CONSERVATION AND SALVAGE TECHNIQUES

A. Autologous donation usually begins 6 weeks before surgery and can greatly reduce the amount of homologous blood transfused. The length of the predonation period is limited by the length of time that blood can be stored, currently 42 days, unless the blood is frozen. Current blood bank guidelines require a predonation Hb of at least 11 g/dL, donations no more frequently than every 3 days, and no donations in the 72 hours before surgery. Most patients tolerate autologous donation without complication. Patients with severe aortic stenosis or unstable angina are not candidates for autologous donation. Patients donating autologous blood should receive supplemental iron because depleted iron stores frequently limit RBC recovery. Recombinant EPO treatment (see Section VI.A) also may be considered. Because a risk of transfusion reactions due to clerical error still exists, autologous blood should not be transfused unless transfusion is clinically indicated.

B. Acute normovolemic hemodilution (ANH) entails removing one or more units of fresh whole blood from a patient while replacing the lost volume with either colloid or crystalloid. By implementing an ANH strategy in anticipation of intraoperative blood loss, fresh autologous blood is available for later reinfusion as surgical blood loss is complete. Any bloodshed after hemodilution will also contain a smaller proportion of red cells relative to plasma, thus reducing the loss of Hb and oxygen-carrying capacity. Hemodilution may be helpful in situations in which platelets are lost or altered intraoperatively (eg, CPB), as autologous blood retains normal platelet and clotting factor concentrations when reinfused. It should also be remembered that the autologous blood retains a Hct value similar to the patient's preoperative Hct (ie, approximately 40% to 50% if normal); this is in contrast to a standard unit of PRBCs, which has a Hct of approximately 70%. Although ANH alone may not eliminate the need for allogeneic transfusion, it may decrease the need for allogeneic units when used in combination with preoperative autologous donation. In most cases, however, ANH will only modestly diminish the need for allogeneic transfusion unless the preoperative Hct is high, the patient can tolerate a low-target Hct, and the expected blood loss is large.

C. Intraoperative autotransfusion (cell salvage) utilizes blood collected from the surgical field by a double-lumen suction device. As the shed blood is suctioned from the surgical field into one lumen, it is mixed with an anticoagulant (citrate–phosphate–dextrose or heparin) solution from the other lumen to prevent clotting of the blood in the filtered collecting reservoir. The blood then undergoes a series of steps including filtration, centrifugation, and washing; this process is designed to remove debris, plasma, free Hb, and anticoagulant factors. The final product is a collection bag of RBCs with a Hct of 50% to 70% that is ready for reinfusion after about 3 minutes of processing time. Although this technique remains highly useful, the clinician must note that blood collected via intraoperative salvage is deficient in plasma, clotting factors, and platelets. The technique is also generally restricted to procedures with clean surgical fields and nononcologic procedures because of the theoretical risks of reinfusing bacteria or tumor cells into the bloodstream.

D. Controlled hypotension (or induced hypotension) involves deliberate maintenance of a patient's blood pressure in a lower range than usual, often allowing a mean arterial pressure of 55 to 65 mm Hg or 30% less than the patient's baseline. This technique is most appropriate when performed in carefully selected patients for brief periods during specific procedures (eg, clipping of cerebral aneurysms). Short-acting, easily titratable vasodilator infusions are ideal for the maintenance of the hypotensive state. Although this technique may limit bleeding and potentially avoid the need for additional blood products, it has significant potential drawbacks including end-organ ischemia and thrombosis due to decreased forward blood flow. As these risks are amplified in states of preexisting cardiovascular disease and sensitivity to diminished perfusion, controlled hypotension is contraindicated in patients with severe atherosclerotic burdens in the coronary and cerebral circulations as well as those with increased intracranial pressure.

VIII. COMPLICATIONS OF BLOOD TRANSFUSION THERAPY
A. Transfusion reactions
1. **Acute hemolytic transfusion reactions** most commonly occur when ABO-incompatible blood is transfused, resulting in recipient anti-A and/or anti-B antibodies attaching to donor RBC antigens and forming antigen–antibody complexes. These antigen–antibody complexes activate complement, precipitating intravascular hemolysis with the release of RBC stroma and free Hb. Immune system activation also results in endothelial and mast cell activation, stimulating the release of serotonin, histamine, and bradykinin; these mediators set off a cascade of widespread vasodilation, diffuse inflammation, and acute hypotension. The net results may include shock, kidney injury due to Hb precipitation in renal tubules, and DIC (see Section IX.B). Many signs and symptoms of an acute hemolytic transfusion reaction appear immediately and include fever, chest pain, anxiety, back pain, and dyspnea. While many signs are masked by general anesthesia, intraoperative clues to the diagnosis include fever, hypotension, hemoglobinuria, unexplained bleeding, or failure of the Hct to increase after transfusion. **Table 36.3** outlines steps to take if a transfusion reaction is suspected. The incidence of fatal hemolytic transfusion reactions in the United States is approximately 1 in every 250,000 to 1,000,000 units transfused. Most reactions occur

Approach to Suspected Acute Hemolytic Transfusion Reaction

1. Stop the transfusion.
2. Quickly check for error in patient identity or donor unit.
3. Send the donor unit and a newly obtained blood sample to blood bank for repeat cross-match.
4. Treat hypotension with fluids and vasopressors as necessary.
5. If ongoing transfusion is required, administer type O-negative PRBC and type AB FFP as necessary.
6. Insert a Foley catheter and support renal function with fluids to correct hypovolemia and, if needed, alkaline diuresis (sodium bicarbonate + furosemide ± mannitol) to maintain brisk urine output.
7. Monitor for signs of DIC clinically and with appropriate laboratory studies; treat supportively (see Section IX.B).
8. Send patient blood sample for direct antiglobulin (Coombs) test, free Hb, and haptoglobin; send urine for Hb.

DIC, disseminated intravascular coagulation; FFP, fresh frozen plasma; PRBC, packed red blood cells.

because of administrative errors, with the majority caused by improper identification of the blood unit or patient. The importance of adhering to strict policies of checking blood and matching to the correct patient in the operating room cannot be overemphasized.

2. **Delayed hemolytic transfusion reactions** occur because of antibodies targeting minor RBC antigens (eg, Kidd) and are characterized by extravascular hemolysis. Delayed hemolytic transfusions reactions are most common in patients with a history of multiple prior transfusions, especially those with chronic anemias or hemoglobinopathies. These reactions often present days to weeks after transfusion. Patients may experience minimal symptoms but may display signs of anemia and jaundice. Laboratory studies reveal a positive direct antiglobulin test, hyperbilirubinemia, decreased haptoglobin levels, and hemosiderin in the urine. Treatment is aimed at correcting the anemia.

3. **Febrile nonhemolytic transfusion reactions** (**FNHTRs**) are the most common transfusion reactions, occurring in approximately 1% of RBC transfusions and up to 30% of platelet transfusions. These may occur in response to cytokines in the stored product or may occur when antileukocyte or anti-HLA antibodies in the recipient react with donor white blood cells or platelets in the transfused blood product, thus producing pyrogen and proinflammatory cytokine release. Signs and symptoms include fever, chills, rigors, tachycardia, malaise, nausea, and vomiting. Approach to treatment involves first stopping the transfusion and excluding an acute hemolytic transfusion reaction or bacterial contamination of the donor unit. Acetaminophen and meperidine may diminish fever and rigors, respectively. Once the diagnosis of FNHTR has been made, future reactions may be avoided or diminished by administering leukoreduced blood products (see Section IV.B.2), premedicating at-risk patients with acetaminophen and hydrocortisone (50 to 100 mg IV), and administering the transfusion slowly.

4. **Allergic transfusion reactions** are common, occurring in 1% to 3% of transfusions. They arise from recipient IgE-mediated antibody responses to donor plasma proteins. Urticaria with pruritus and erythema is the most common manifestation, but bronchospasm or anaphylaxis may occur in rare instances. Many patients also develop fevers. Patients with IgA deficiency may be at an increased risk of allergic transfusion reactions and anaphylaxis because of the presence of anti-IgA antibodies that react with transfused IgA; this is best prevented by administering plasma-free blood products (eg, washed PRBCs) to patients with known IgA deficiency. Treatment involves stopping the transfusion, excluding more severe reactions (see above), and administering antihistamines (eg, diphenhydramine 50 mg IV and ranitidine 50 mg IV). A significant reaction may warrant administration of a corticosteroid (methylprednisolone 80 mg IV). Bronchospasm and anaphylaxis should be treated as described in Chapter 17: Intra-Anesthetic Problems.

5. **TRALI** is a condition involving rapid-onset respiratory insufficiency following blood, FFP, cryoprecipitate, or platelet transfusion. Signs and symptoms include fevers, dyspnea, hypoxemia, hypotension, and low-pressure pulmonary edema developing within 4 hours of transfusion. TRALI is thought to occur when anti-HLA and antileukocyte antibodies present in donor plasma target recipient neutrophils, which damage the lung parenchyma. This mechanism also accounts for the transient leukopenia that may be observed in recipients who develop TRALI. TRALI may rapidly progress to hypoxemic respiratory failure

and acute respiratory distress syndrome (ARDS) and is currently the leading cause of transfusion-related mortality in the United States. Most cases are traced to plasma-containing blood products from multiparous female donors who have developed anti-HLA antibodies; therefore, measures to prevent plasma donation by women who have been pregnant may reduce the incidence of TRALI-related episodes.

6. **Transfusion-associated circulatory overload (TACO)** is a condition of circulatory congestion secondary to the fluid volumes administered during massive transfusion. Symptoms often mimic those of decompensated congestive heart failure and include dyspnea, high-pressure pulmonary edema, tachycardia, and jugular venous distention. While TRALI usually produces pulmonary edema in the absence of overt hypervolemia, signs of hypervolemia and increased left ventricular filling pressures may be observed in TACO. TACO often affects patients at risk for congestive heart failure and occurs in less than 1% of transfusions. If a patient is at risk for fluid overload with high-volume transfusion, diuretics or volume-reduced blood products may be administered prophylactically. However, as TACO is often traced to overly aggressive transfusion in patients with preexisting myocardial dysfunction, the clinician should also be judicious with respect to the volume transfused.

7. **GVHD** is a rare and serious complication of blood transfusion resulting from an attack of immunocompetent donor lymphocytes on the host's tissues. In a great majority of transfusions, donor lymphocytes are destroyed by the recipient's immune system, thus preventing GVHD. However, if the host is immunodeficient or if a specific type of partial donor–recipient HLA matching occurs, the risk of GVHD is increased. The condition often develops 4 to 30 days after transfusion, with patients typically presenting with fever and an erythematous rash that may become generalized. Other symptoms include anorexia, vomiting, abdominal pain, and cough. The diagnosis is made by skin biopsy and confirmed by demonstrating the presence of circulating lymphocytes with a different HLA phenotype, verifying their origin from the donor. GVHD is poorly responsive to most available treatments. Therefore, prevention is of utmost importance and is achieved by exposing lymphocyte-containing components to gamma radiation, thereby inactivating donor lymphocytes. In addition to immunocompromised recipients, patients receiving blood products from family donors or HLA-matched platelets are viable candidates for transfusion of irradiated blood components owing to an associated risk of partial HLA matching.

B. Metabolic complications of blood transfusions
1. **Hyperkalemia** is common with rapid blood transfusion but most often becomes clinically significant in cases involving massive transfusion or renal failure. During storage, red cells leak potassium into the extracellular environment, elevating potassium levels to greater than 20 mEq/U PRBCs after approximately 2 weeks. However, this state is rapidly corrected with transfusion and repletion of cellular energy stores.
2. **Hypocalcemia.** Citrate, which chelates calcium, is used as an anticoagulant in stored blood products. Consequently, rapid transfusion decreases ionized calcium levels in the recipient, potentially producing neuromuscular or cardiovascular complications. Although hypocalcemia is usually insignificant owing to efficient hepatic metabolism of the infused citrate, it may become problematic in small children, in patients with impaired liver function, in hypothermic or alkalemic patients, in patients with decreased hepatic blood flow, and during the

anhepatic phase of liver transplantation. It is also more common with the transfusion of FFP, which contains higher concentrations of citrate. Ionized calcium levels should be followed to gauge timing for repletion, as total serum calcium includes inactive citrate-bound calcium and thus may not accurately reflect free serum calcium.
3. **Acid–base abnormalities.** Banked PRBCs become acidic because of accumulated red cell metabolites, with pH decreasing linearly to approximately 6.6 after 2 weeks in storage. However, the actual acid load delivered to the patient is minimal. Metabolic acidosis in the face of severe blood loss is more likely due to hypoperfusion and will typically improve with volume resuscitation. The development of a metabolic alkalosis is also common following massive blood transfusion because citrate is rapidly metabolized in the liver to bicarbonate.
4. **Hypothermia.** With the exception of platelets, blood products are typically refrigerated to a standard temperature of 4 °C. Rapid administration of a large volume of PRBCs and other cooled blood products may precipitate hypothermia, which may have adverse effects on immune function, wound healing, coagulation, myocardial function, and maintenance of electrolyte balance. Therefore, blood products, particularly when administered rapidly, other than platelets are best transfused through a primed warming device.
5. **Iron overload.** Repeated or high-volume transfusion of red cells has the potential to produce or worsen a state of hemochromatosis (systemic iron overload with consequent organ impairment). Although this is typically of little immediate concern in the setting of acute surgical or traumatic hemorrhage, patients with preexisting hereditary or transfusion-related hemochromatosis may exhibit progressive hepatic dysfunction, cardiomyopathy, and insulin resistance in addition to other endocrine abnormalities. As the body lacks a finely tuned mechanism for the elimination of excess iron, serial phlebotomy and iron chelation may be required as therapeutic measures. To minimize the buildup of excess iron in high-risk patients, perioperative blood-conserving approaches such as cell salvage and ANH may be appropriate (see Section VII).
6. **Derangements from blood storage.** It is known that stored red blood cells undergo progressive structural and functional alterations that decrease their functionality and viability following transfusion. For example, prolonged storage may diminish microvascular flow as red cells lose their deformability. A decrease in oxygen delivery also occurs secondary to depletion of 2,3-diphosphoglycerate, which results in a leftward shift of the oxyhemoglobin dissociation curve as well as increased adhesion and aggregation of red cells. In addition, there is an accumulation of proinflammatory substances and priming of the nicotinamide adenine dinucleotide phosphate ($NADP^+$) system with reduction in concentrations of NO and adenosine triphosphate (ATP). Some studies have suggested increased rates of complications and mortality following cardiac surgery in patients who received blood that was stored for more than 2 weeks, highlighting the potential clinical consequences of prolonged blood storage.

C. **Infectious complications of blood transfusions** have decreased with improved laboratory testing for transmissible diseases. Exposure to pooled products (eg, cryoprecipitate) increases the risk in proportion to the number of donors. See Chapter 8: Infectious Diseases and Infection Control in Anesthesia for all infectious diseases transmitted by blood transfusion.

1. **Hepatitis B virus.** The risk of hepatitis B infection from a blood transfusion has decreased since testing donated blood for hepatitis B antigen became routine in 1971. The current risk is estimated to be 1:60,000 to 1:120,000 units transfused.
2. **Hepatitis C virus (HCV).** The institution of routine testing for antibodies to HCV in 1990 (and recently nucleic acid testing) has reduced the risk of transfusion-related HCV to approximately 1:800,000 to 1:1.6 million units transfused.
3. **Human immunodeficiency virus (HIV).** Because of improved screening and testing of patients and blood products, the risk of transfusion-associated HIV has been estimated to be about 1:1.4 to 1:2.4 million units transfused in the United States.
4. **CMV.** The prevalence of antibodies to CMV in the general adult population is approximately 70%. The incidence of transfusion-associated CMV infection in previously noninfected patients is quite high, and CMV remains the most common infectious agent transmitted via blood product administration. Infection is typically asymptomatic; however, because immunosuppressed patients and neonates may develop severe disease, CMV-negative or leukoreduced blood products may be recommended.
5. **West Nile virus (WNV).** Following the 2002 epidemic of WNV in the United States, it was found that transfusion of red cells, platelets, and FFP can transmit WNV. With universal screening, the risk of WNV from transfusion has decreased to less than 1:1 million.
6. **Bacterial sepsis** caused by transfused blood products remains rare. Donors with evidence of infectious disease are excluded from transfusion, and the storage of PRBCs at 4 °C minimizes the risk of infection. Nonetheless, PRBCs may become contaminated, most frequently with *Yersinia enterocolitica*. Platelets, which are stored at room temperature, are more problematic, with an estimated infection rate of 1:1,000 to 1:2,000 units. The most common organisms associated with platelet contamination are *Staphylococcus* species (especially *S. aureus* and *S. epidermidis*) and diphtheroids. The risk of infection is directly related to the storage time of the product, with 15% to 25% of infected units causing severe sepsis in the recipient. Signs of infection usually become apparent during transfusion and should trigger immediate discontinuation of the transfusion and testing of the unit for contamination. Individual outcomes from transfusion-related sepsis depend on the size of the bacterial inoculum and the immunocompetence of the recipient, but overall mortality remains high at approximately 60%.

D. **Transfusion-related immunomodulation.** Transfusion of allogeneic blood is known to suppress the immune system. Although the exact mechanism is unknown, theories suggest that transfusion of donor leukocytes may induce an "immune-tolerant" state in the recipient. Thus, allogeneic blood transfusion has been used preoperatively and intraoperatively in renal transplant recipients to improve graft viability, although studies supporting this practice were largely performed prior to the advent of modern immunosuppressants such as cyclosporine. More controversial are the potential detrimental effects of intraoperative allogeneic blood transfusion on cancer recurrence rates, postoperative infections, activation of latent viral infections, and postoperative mortality. Some experts contend that many of the adverse immunomodulatory effects of allogeneic blood transfusion may be diminished by universal blood product leukoreduction, and promising research suggests that the use of leukoreduced blood products may improve survival in cardiac surgery. Universal leukoreduction protocols have therefore been increasingly adopted in various institutions.

IX. PERIOPERATIVE COAGULOPATHY
A. Coagulopathy of massive transfusion is unusual with transfusions less than 1 to 1.5 BVs, assuming the patient has a normal coagulation profile, platelet count, and platelet function initially.
   1. **Thrombocytopenia.** Diffuse oozing and failure to form clots after massive transfusion may be precipitated in part by thrombocytopenia, which is typically due to the transfusion of platelet-poor blood products. However, clinically significant bleeding is unlikely with platelet counts above 50,000 cells/mm^3. If the loss of one BV or more is expected, platelets should be transfused to maintain a count of 50,000 cells/mm^3 or greater.
   2. **Coagulation factor deficiencies.** The normal human body has tremendous reserves of clotting factors. In addition, the patient receives small amounts of the most stable clotting factors in the plasma of each unit of red cells. Bleeding from factor deficiency in the face of massive transfusion is therefore typically due to decreased levels of fibrinogen and labile factors with shorter storage half-lives (especially factors V, VIII, or IX). Bleeding from hypofibrinogenemia is unusual unless the fibrinogen level is below 75 mg/dL. In some patients, factor VIII levels increase with massive transfusion due to increased release from endothelial cells. Additional labile clotting factors are best repleted in the form of FFP. Six units of platelets contain coagulation factor levels equivalent to one unit of FFP. Cryoprecipitate may also provide a source of concentrated fibrinogen for the patient who cannot tolerate FFP owing to volume overload.
B. DIC refers to the abnormal, diffuse systemic activation of the clotting system. The pathophysiology involves excessive generation of thrombin (factor IIa), resulting in unrestrained fibrin cross-linking throughout the circulation accompanied by platelet activation, fibrinolysis, and coagulation factor consumption. The profound consumptive coagulopathy produced by DIC often results in hemorrhage.
   1. **Causes** of DIC include infection, shock, trauma, burns, pancreatitis, and fat or cholesterol embolism. DIC is also common in extensive head injury and complications of pregnancy (eg, amniotic fluid embolism, placental abruption, or septic abortion) because of the high concentrations of tissue factor (thromboplastin) in brain and placental tissues, respectively. A chronic form of DIC may accompany cirrhotic liver disease, nephrotic syndromes, aortic dissection, and malignancy.
   2. **Clinical features** include petechiae, ecchymoses, bleeding from venipuncture sites, and frank hemorrhage from operative incisions. Although the hemorrhagic manifestations of DIC are clinically most obvious, complications related to diffuse microvascular and macrovascular thromboses are more common, more difficult to treat, and more potentially life threatening because of the resulting ischemia of vital organs. Systemic bradykinin release in DIC may also cause acute hypotension. Estimates for the mortality for DIC are approximately 50%.
   3. **Laboratory features** of DIC universally include an elevated D-dimer level and increased fibrin degradation products, although these abnormalities are nonspecific. The PT and PTT are typically prolonged, and serial measurements reveal decreased fibrinogen levels and platelet counts.

After an initial PTT value is obtained, the waveform used to generate the PTT result can be reviewed for an early negative slope that is suggestive of DIC. Various TEG parameters, usually first indicating a hypercoagulable state followed by severe coagulation factor deficiencies, can also be followed as point-of-care assessments of a patient's coagulation profile.

4. **Treatment of DIC** involves addressing the precipitating cause and transfusing appropriate blood products (eg, FFP, platelets, and cryoprecipitate) to correct bleeding. It is now generally recommended that blood products not be withheld out of concern for "feeding the fire" of the consumptive coagulopathy, particularly if significant hemorrhage is present. However, inhibitors of fibrinolysis (eg, TXA) are contraindicated in DIC owing to the risk of exacerbating or precipitating further thrombotic complications.

C. **Chronic liver disease.** With the notable exceptions of factor VIII and vWF, which are produced by the endothelium, the liver synthesizes all coagulation factors. Assessment of serum factor VIII levels may thus be useful in distinguishing hepatic synthetic dysfunction from other coagulopathies. Patients with hepatic dysfunction may simultaneously exhibit decreased production of inactive coagulation factors and decreased clearance of activated factors. If circulating levels of activated clotting factors are increased, patients may develop an ongoing consumptive coagulopathy similar to that seen in DIC. Because the liver is also instrumental in removing the byproducts of fibrinolysis, levels of fibrin degradation products may be elevated. Note that, although the INR provides a reliable indicator of hepatic synthetic dysfunction, it does not correlate well with surgical bleeding risk in patients with significant liver disease.

D. **Vitamin K deficiency.** The fat-soluble vitamin K (phylloquinone) is required by the liver as a cofactor for the gamma-carboxylation of factors II, VII, IX, and X as well as anticoagulant proteins C and S. Because vitamin K cannot be synthesized endogenously, decreased vitamin K intake or malabsorption may cause a coagulopathy with a prolonged PT (see Chapter 6: Specific Considerations With Liver Disease). In addition, because humans rely on gastrointestinal (GI) flora for some production of vitamin K, vitamin K deficiency is also commonly found in patients receiving broad-spectrum antibiotics, neonates who lack a mature GI microbiome, and patients with short bowel syndrome. Patients on warfarin therapy also exhibit a functional vitamin K deficiency (see Section IX.E.3). Patients with poor absorption or limited GI flora can be treated with subcutaneous vitamin K (eg, 10 mg daily for 3 days), whereas malnourished patients or those on warfarin may be given vitamin K orally. IV administration of vitamin K (2.5 to 10 mg) may result in a faster correction of the PT but is accompanied by a greater risk of anaphylaxis. If used, IV vitamin K should be administered slowly. If faster correction of PT than can be achieved with vitamin K is required (as in active intracranial hemorrhage), FFP (5 to 8 mL/kg) or other blood products such as prothrombin complex concentrate (PCC or *Kcentra*) should be coadministered.

E. **Coagulopathy associated with CPB** has long been recognized as a consequence of abnormal activation of the coagulation cascade and platelet dysfunction, which are likely precipitated by contact of blood with CPB circuit components. This increases the likelihood of bleeding in patients after cardiac surgery despite a lack of clear correlation with coagulation studies such as platelet counts. More recently, there has been an increased interest in the use of point-of-care platelet function assays as a metric of the risk of hemorrhagic complications associated with CPB.

F. Pharmacologic interventions

1. **Heparin** acts by accelerating the effects of antithrombin III, thus inhibiting both factors IIa (thrombin) and Xa. It prolongs the PTT and has a short half-life; therefore, its anticoagulant effect is usually reversed approximately 4 to 6 hours after discontinuation of the infusion. If faster reversal is required, protamine sulfate, a natural antagonist, may be administered. Special attention must be given when administering protamine as severe reactions (hypotension, pulmonary vasoconstriction, anaphylaxis, etc.) can occur.
2. **Low–molecular-weight heparins (LMWHs)** such as enoxaparin (*Lovenox*) are commercially prepared by fractionating heparin into molecules of 2000 to 10,000 Da. They exert their anticoagulant effect primarily by inhibiting factor Xa and usually do not require monitoring of the PTT. These drugs have longer half-lives than heparin and are incompletely reversed by protamine, yet protamine reversal may be indicated in the setting of a major bleeding episode. Faster reversal may require FFP transfusion.
3. **Warfarin (*Coumadin*)** is an oral vitamin K antagonist that inhibits vitamin K epoxide reductase. This produces a deficiency of activated vitamin K, preventing the hepatic gamma-carboxylation of factors II, VII, IX, and X and proteins C and S to their active forms. The PT and the INR are prolonged in patients taking warfarin. The onset and offset of warfarin's effects are slow due to the drug's half-life and the half-lives of vitamin K–dependent factors. Initiation of warfarin is associated with a period of paradoxical hypercoagulability due to the short half-life of protein C. If quick reversal of warfarin is required, vitamin K–dependent factors can be repleted in the form of FFP (5 to 15 mL/kg) or PCC. Vitamin K (2.5 to 10 mg by mouth, intravenously, or subcutaneously) can also be given to accelerate warfarin reversal.
4. **Platelet inhibitors** (or antiplatelet agents) target multiple pathways of platelet adhesion, activation, and aggregation. Irreversible inhibitors such as aspirin and clopidogrel generally impair the function of the platelets throughout their 7- to 10-day lifespan. Thus, immediate reversal of certain platelet inhibitors may require platelet transfusion and may not be effective if the inhibitor is still present in the plasma.
5. **Aspirin** and **nonsteroidal anti-inflammatory drugs (NSAIDs)** inhibit platelet aggregation by interfering with cyclooxygenase function. Nonaspirin NSAIDs reversibly inhibit the cyclooxygenase pathway, and their effects typically dissipate within 3 days of discontinuation.
6. **Ticlopidine, clopidogrel, prasugrel, ticagrelor,** and **cangrelor** are agents that inhibit ADP-mediated platelet aggregation by antagonizing the $P2Y_{12}$ receptor. Clopidogrel remains the most commonly coprescribed antiplatelet agent with aspirin in patients requiring dual antiplatelet therapy; although ticagrelor, a more potent reversible inhibitor, may have greater clinical efficacy in certain contexts. Ticlopidine is now rarely prescribed owing to the associated risk of neutropenia.
7. **Eptifibatide, abciximab,** and **tirofiban** are inhibitors of the platelet glycoprotein IIb/IIIa receptor. Abciximab, notably, is an IV monoclonal Fab antibody fragment directed against the receptor and thus also has the potential to produce thrombocytopenia. Although the drug's plasma half-life is short, impairment of platelet function may last for days, and reversal of its effects may require multiple platelet transfusions owing to ongoing adsorption of the antibody to donor platelets.
8. **Dipyridamole** and **cilostazol** are selective phosphodiesterase 3 inhibitors that increase platelet and endothelial cyclic adenosine monophosphate

(cAMP) levels, thereby inhibiting platelet aggregation and producing a degree of vasodilation. Cilostazol is commonly used in the management of symptomatic peripheral arterial disease.
9. **Thrombolytic agents** act by dissolving thrombi via direct conversion of plasminogen to plasmin, which lyses fibrin clots. They are intended to rapidly antagonize thrombosis and thus recanalize blood vessels occluded as a result of thrombotic phenomena (eg, thromboembolic stroke). Two thrombolytic agents, recombinant **tissue plasminogen activator** and **streptokinase,** are most commonly used in clinical practice. Each of these drugs results in a hypofibrinogenemic state and carries a substantial risk of bleeding. Therefore, they are generally contraindicated perioperatively, and the benefits of their administration should be carefully weighed against their considerable risks. If emergent surgery is required after thrombolytic therapy, the effect may be antagonized by administration of aminocaproic acid or TXA. Fibrinogen levels may also be restored by transfusion of cryoprecipitate or FFP.
10. **Direct thrombin inhibitors (DTIs)** such as **dabigatran, argatroban,** and **bivalirudin** inhibit thrombin (factor IIa). Dabigatran is an oral DTI often used for stroke prevention in atrial fibrillation and, unlike warfarin, does not require frequent INR monitoring. It also carries the advantage of the availability of a novel reversal agent called idarucizumab, a monoclonal antibody that targets and inactivates drug. Argatroban (often preferred in renal insufficiency) and bivalirudin are IV medications used for anticoagulation as alternatives to heparin in patients with heparin-induced thrombocytopenia. At this time, argatroban and bivalirudin lack specific reversal agents and can thus cause life-threatening bleeding if administered without due caution.
11. **Direct factor Xa inhibitors** such as **apixaban, edoxaban,** and **rivaroxaban** inhibit factor Xa. This mechanism lies in contrast to that of LMWHs and synthetic agents such as fondaparinux, which inhibit factor Xa indirectly via interaction with antithrombin III. Like dabigatran, these oral agents are also typically used for the prevention and treatment of thromboembolic events, and they have been demonstrated to be efficacious, safe, and convenient alternatives to warfarin therapy in patients with adequate renal function. Although direct factor Xa inhibitors were traditionally irreversible, a novel reversal agent called andexanet alfa (*Andexxa*), a recombinant derivative of factor Xa that acts as a decoy receptor for the anticoagulant drug, has gained U.S. Food and Drug Administration (FDA) approval. Additional antidotes such as ciraparantag, a "universal" reversal agent potentially capable of counteracting a wide variety of anticoagulants, remain under investigation.

G. **Reversal of perioperative coagulopathy** can often be achieved with blood component therapies such as cryoprecipitate, platelets, and FFP, although the choice of therapy depends on the underlying cause of the coagulopathy. In addition, specific clotting factors are available for patients who require rapid reversal of coagulopathy and may not tolerate the large volumes or other risks associated with transfusion of conventional blood products.
1. **Recombinant factor VIIa (rFVIIa)** is FDA approved for the treatment of hemophiliacs with antibody inhibitors that prevent factor VIII or IX from normalizing their coagulation. Rather than replenishing factor VII levels directly, it produces direct and rapid platelet activation and can trigger the coagulation cascade with a "thrombin burst." The apparent efficacy of rFVIIa in massive surgical or traumatic bleeding, primarily shown in case studies, has generated interest in wider applications for

the drug. A major trial of rFVIIa administration demonstrated reduced expansion of intracerebral hematoma in cases of nontraumatic hemorrhagic stroke, although a follow-up study showed no improvement in mortality or functional outcome. rFVIIa is expensive and has been associated with adverse thrombotic events.

2. **PCCs** are preparations of vitamin K–dependent factors II, VII, IX, X, and proteins C and S that are derived from FFP. They are useful for the urgent reversal of warfarin or other serious coagulopathies resulting from specific factor deficiencies. PCCs are expensive, and their use is currently restricted to particular clinical circumstances requiring immediate reversal of anticoagulation. Standard inactive PCC (*Kcentra*) is currently approved for the rapid reversal of warfarin anticoagulation in patients with severe acute bleeding or those requiring major surgery, whereas an activated form (factor eight inhibitor bypass activity or FEIBA) is primarily administered for uncontrolled hemorrhage in patients with hemophilia A. Key adverse effects include thrombotic sequelae, especially with the use of activated PCC.

X. SPECIAL CONSIDERATIONS

A. **Hemophilias** are rare, mainly X-linked diseases affecting males almost exclusively. **Hemophilia A** is due to an abnormality or deficiency of factor VIII, whereas **hemophilia B (Christmas disease)** is due to an abnormality or deficiency of factor IX. The incidences in the United States are 1:10,000 males for hemophilia A and 1:100,000 males for hemophilia B. An even rarer autosomal recessive variant, hemophilia C (Rosenthal syndrome), is caused by a deficiency or dysfunction of factor XI.

1. **Clinical features.** Patients usually present early in childhood with deep bleeding manifestations such as hemarthroses and soft tissue (eg, skeletal muscle) hematomas after minor trauma. Such events may be painful and recurrent, potentially resulting in significant complications such as hemophilic arthropathy. Laboratory tests demonstrate a markedly prolonged PTT with a normal PT and platelet count.

2. **Treatment** with the appropriate factor (in the form of a recombinant or lyophilized concentrate) should be coordinated perioperatively with the patient's hematologist. Hemophilia A is treated with recombinant factor VIII to achieve preoperative activity levels of 25% to 100%, depending on the extent of the procedure. Some patients with mild hemophilia A may also respond to DDAVP therapy, which promotes release of factor VIII (with vWF) from the endothelium. If factor VIII is unavailable in an emergent situation, cryoprecipitate transfusion can provide the deficient factor, and antifibrinolytics such as TXA can reduce bleeding. Hemophilia B is treated with factor IX to achieve at least 30% to 50% activity before surgery.

B. **Von Willebrand disease** is caused by a deficiency or abnormality of vWF, a protein involved in anchoring platelets to injured endothelium and stabilizing factor VIII. It is the most common inherited bleeding disorder, affecting 1% to 2% of the population. It is inherited in an autosomal dominant pattern and affects both sexes equally. The disease is classified into three main phenotypes: type 1, characterized by mild to moderate quantitative deficiencies of vWF and factor VIII; type 2, characterized by a qualitative abnormality of vWF; and type 3, characterized by very low or undetectable levels of vWF in plasma with low but detectable levels of factor VIII.

1. **Clinical presentation.** The phenotypic expression is variable, and clinical manifestations may range from very mild to life-threatening hemorrhage.

Usually, patients have a history of easy bruising and superficial bleeding from mucosal surfaces (eg, epistaxis or menorrhagia), but some patients are not diagnosed with a bleeding disorder until they suffer major trauma or undergo surgery complicated by abnormal bleeding. Laboratory tests may reveal a prolonged bleeding time with normal PT, PTT, and platelet counts.

2. **Treatment** of vWD depends on the subtype. Many patients respond to DDAVP treatment (type 1), but others (types 2 and 3) may require cryoprecipitate or a purified, lyophilized complex of vWF and factor VIII derived from pooled human plasma (*Humate-P*). There is evidence that administration of DDAVP in certain patients with various subtypes (particularly type 2B) of vWD type 2 may precipitate paradoxical thrombosis or thrombocytopenia; therefore, empiric administration of DDAVP in patients with uncharacterized vWD is not recommended. Antifibrinolytics such as TXA also have been used in some patients to reduce surgical bleeding. Preoperative consultation with the patient's hematologist is recommended.

C. **Sickle cell disease** (or sickle cell anemia) is an inherited hemoglobinopathy that is particularly prevalent in patients of African descent, affecting 1:600 African Americans. The disease is caused by the substitution of valine for glutamic acid at the sixth position (E6V) on the β-chain of Hb. Homozygotes for this substitution (as well as double heterozygotes for sickle-type hemoglobin variant [HbS] and hemoglobin C [HbC], or β-thalassemias) produce significant quantities of an abnormal HbS and thus have clinical sickle cell disease. Patients who are heterozygous for the E6V substitution are said to have sickle cell trait, which is largely asymptomatic but may produce hyposthenuria or hematuria due to intermittent sickling in the relatively hypoxic and hypertonic renal medulla.

1. **Clinical features.** In sickle cell disease, abnormal HbS molecules polymerize and cause a sickling deformity of the red cell under certain conditions, notably hypoxia, hypothermia, acidosis, and dehydration. Sickled cells are poorly deformable and may become lodged in small vessels, producing microvascular occlusion with tissue ischemia and infarction. A sickle cell crisis typically presents with excruciating bone or abdominal pain, fever, tachycardia, leukocytosis, and hematuria. Particularly concerning is the development of acute chest syndrome, which manifests with dyspnea, hypoxia, chest pain, fevers, and new pulmonary infiltrates on chest radiography. Many traditional signs and symptoms of a sickle cell crisis may be masked by anesthesia. Sickled RBCs exhibit a shortened survival time of 12 days, leading to chronic anemia and extramedullary hematopoiesis.

2. **Anesthetic management** of patients with sickle cell disease includes avoiding conditions that promote sickling (especially hypoxia, hypovolemia, acidemia, and hypothermia). Conservative transfusion management to a preoperative Hct of approximately 30% prevents postoperative complications as effectively as the traditional "exchange transfusions" that sought to reduce the amount of HbS to 30% of total Hb. If acute chest syndrome is suspected perioperatively, the patient may require broad-spectrum antibiotics, ongoing respiratory support, and PRBC transfusions or exchange transfusion to rapidly reduce the proportion of sickled red cells.

D. **Jehovah's Witness (JW)** patients generally refuse to receive allogeneic as well as certain autologous blood products because of their religious beliefs, even if such refusal results in death. Special considerations apply if the patient is a minor, does not have the capacity to make health care related decisions, or has responsibilities for dependents as well as in certain emergency circumstances (see also Chapter 1: Evaluating the Patient Before Anesthesia). However, under elective conditions, a physician is not required to agree to treat a patient who refuses a transfusion if doing so is contrary to the physician's ethical beliefs. Blood conservation measures are crucial in these patients (see Section VII). Jehovah Witnesses may allow transfusion of intraoperatively phlebotomized blood (see Section VII.B) as long as the blood remains in continuity with the body (ie, the blood tubing must always remain connected to the patient). EPO is sometimes used to increase red cell mass perioperatively. A more conservative transfusion threshold (eg, transfusing only at a Hb of 6 g/dL) may sometimes be used intraoperatively to reduce the need for blood administration. The use of colloid instead of crystalloid has not been shown to help reduce the need for transfusions despite its theoretical benefit in expanding intravascular volume. In all major surgical procedures planned for a JW patient, it is crucial that the anesthesiologist fully discuss the patient's beliefs and decisions concerning transfusion and document these decisions clearly in the medical record as well as on operative consent forms.

ACKNOWLEDGMENT

We gratefully acknowledge the contributions of previous edition author, Lukas H. Matern, as portions of those chapters have been retained in this revision.

Suggested Readings

- American Society of Anesthesiologists Task Force on Perioperative Blood Management. Practice guidelines for perioperative blood management: an updated report by the American Society of Anesthesiologists Task Force on Perioperative Blood Management. *Anesthesiology*. 2015;122(2):241–275.
- Carson JL, Stanworth SJ, Guyatt G, et al. Red Blood Cell Transfusion: 2023 AABB International Guidelines. *JAMA*. 2023;330(19):1892–1902.
- Carson JL, Stanworth SJ, Roubinian N, et al. Transfusion thresholds and other strategies for guiding allogeneic red blood cell transfusion. *Cochrane Database Syst Rev*. 2016;10(10): CD002042.
- Cotton BA, Dossett LA, Haut ER, et al. Multicenter validation of a simplified score to predict massive transfusion in trauma. *J Trauma*. 2010;69(1):S33–S39.
- Crash-2 Trial Collaborators. Effects of tranexamic acid on death, vascular occlusive events, and blood transfusion in trauma patients with significant haemorrhage (CRASH-2): a randomised, placebo-controlled trial. *Lancet*. 2010;376(9734):23–32.
- Fergusson DA, Hebert PC, Mazer CD, et al. A comparison of aprotinin and lysine analogues in high-risk cardiac surgery. *N Engl J Med*. 2008;358(22):2319–2331.
- Goodnough LT. Risks of blood transfusion. *Crit Care Med*. 2003;31(12):S678–S686.
- Goodnough LT, Brecher ME, Kanter MH, AuBuchon JP. Transfusion medicine. I. Blood transfusion. *N Engl J Med*. 1999;340(6):438–447.
- Goodnough LT, Brecher ME, Kanter MH, AuBuchon JP. Transfusion medicine: II. Blood conservation. *N Engl J Med*. 1999;340(7):525–533.
- Hebert PC, Wells G, Blajchman MA, et al. A multicenter, randomized controlled clinical trial of transfusion requirements in critical care. *N Engl J Med*. 1999;340(6):409–417.
- Holcomb JB, Tilley BC, Baraniuk S, et al. Transfusion of plasma, platelets, and red blood cells in a 1:1:1 vs a 1:1:2 ratio and mortality in patients with severe trauma: the PROPPR randomized clinical trial. *J Am Med Assoc*. 2015;313(5):471–482.
- Kopko PM, Holland PV. Transfusion-related acute lung injury. *Br J Haematol*. 1999;105(2): 322–329.
- Lake CL, Moore RA, eds. *Blood: Hemostasis, Transfusion, and Alternatives in the Perioperative Period*. Raven Press; 1995.

Mistry N, Hare GMT, Shehata N, et al. Transfusion thresholds for acute coronary syndromes-insights from the TRICS-III randomized controlled trial, systematic review, and meta-analysis. *J Am Heart Assoc.* 2023;12(1):e028497.

O'Connell NM, Perry DJ, Hodgson AJ, et al. Recombinant FVIIa in the management of uncontrolled hemorrhage. *Transfusion.* 2003;43(12):1711–1716.

Rao SV, Jollis JG, Harrington RA, et al. Relationship of blood transfusion and clinical outcomes in patients with acute coronary syndromes. *J Am Med Assoc.* 2004;292(13): 1555–1562.

Raphael J, Mazer CD, Subramani S, et al. Society of cardiovascular anesthesiologists clinical practice improvement advisory for management of perioperative bleeding and hemostasis in cardiac surgery patients. *Anesth Analg.* 2019;129(5):1209–1221.

Shaw AD, Stafford-Smith M, White WD, et al. The effect of aprotinin on outcome after coronary-artery bypass grafting. *N Engl J Med.* 2008;358(8):784–793.

Tanaka KA, Bader SO, Görlinger K. Novel approaches in management of perioperative coagulopathy. *Curr Opin Anaesthesiol.* 2014;27(1):72–80.

Tibi P, McClure RS, Huang J, et al. STS/SCA/AmSECT/SABM update to the clinical practice guidelines on patient blood management. *Ann Thorac Surg.* 2021;112(3):981–1004.

WOMAN Trial Collaborators. Effect of early tranexamic acid administration on mortality, hysterectomy, and other morbidities in women with post-partum haemorrhage (WOMAN): an international, randomised, double-blind, placebo-controlled trial. *Lancet.* 2017;389(10084):2105–2116.

PART III: PERIOPERATIVE ISSUES

The Postanesthesia Care Unit
Alfredo Valdivia and Ryan J. Horvath

I. GENERAL CONSIDERATIONS
For most patients, recovery from anesthesia is uneventful. Nevertheless, when postoperative complications occur, they may be sudden and life-threatening. The **postanesthesia care unit (PACU)** is designed to provide close monitoring and care to patients recovering from general anesthesia (GA) and sedation. This care covers the transition period from one-on-one monitoring in the operating room (OR) to a hospital floor or the patient's home. Medical oversight may range from oversight by anesthesia providers also covering operating areas, but near the PACU, to a team consisting of intensivists, residents, and other clinicians (NPs and PAs) with critical care experience dedicated to the PACU. The PACU should ideally be located in immediate proximity to the OR, with access to radiology, laboratory services, medications, and equipment for routine care and advanced support.

II. ADMISSION TO THE PACU
A. Transport from the OR should only be considered once a patent and stable airway is confirmed. The patient should be transported under direct supervision of the anesthetist, preferably with the head of the bed elevated or with the patient in the lateral decubitus position to maximize airway patency. Oxygen delivered via face mask is indicated in most patients to prevent hypoxemia. Unstable patients, such as those receiving vasoactive medications, may require monitoring of oxygenation and hemodynamics during transport. The anesthetist may elect to bring rescue medications and airway management tools as the clinical situation dictates.

B. A complete **report** should be provided to the PACU team upon arrival. The anesthetist remains in charge of the care of the patient until the PACU team is prepared to assume responsibility.

C. As clinically indicated, the anesthetist may speak directly to the anesthesiologist in charge of the PACU, the surgeon, or a consultant about issues of particular importance for the patient. The report from the anesthetist to the PACU team is often the only formal account of the intraoperative events between the OR team and the personnel who will manage the immediate postoperative care. The report should include the following:

1. Clinical history. Patient identification, age, surgical procedure, diagnosis, medical history (including hearing and visual impairments, psychiatric conditions, and precautions for infection control), medications, allergies, preoperative vital signs, and language preference.

2. **Intravascular access.** Location and size of catheters.
3. **Intraoperative pharmacology.** Premedication, antibiotics, anesthesia induction and maintenance agents, opioids, muscle relaxants, reversal agents, vasoactive drugs, bronchodilators, and other clinically relevant agents administered.
4. **Surgical procedure.** Exact nature of the surgery and relevant surgical issues (eg, adequacy of hemostasis, care of drains, restrictions on positioning); the surgeon may present these details to the PACU team.
5. **Anesthetic course.** Emphasis on problems that may affect the immediate postoperative period including laboratory values, difficult intravenous (IV) access, airway management issues, intraoperative hemodynamic instability, and electrocardiographic (ECG) changes.
6. **Fluid balance.** Amount, type, and reason for fluid replacement, urine output, and estimated fluid and blood losses.

III. MONITORING

Close observation of the patient's level of consciousness, breathing pattern, oxygen saturation, and hemodynamics is of utmost importance. The nurse-to-patient ratio for routine cases and postoperative care is one nurse to two or three patients and increases to single coverage for high-acuity patients, such as those with significant comorbidities, intraoperative complications, or particularly complex procedures. Vital signs are monitored and recorded at regular intervals according to clinical necessity. Standard monitoring includes **respiratory rate** measurement, continuous **electrocardiogram**, noninvasive **blood pressure**, and **pulse oximetry. Temperature** should be monitored and recorded.

A. Invasive monitoring, such as arterial catheters, central venous catheters, and pulmonary artery catheters, can be instituted, if necessary. Arterial catheters provide continuous measurement of the systemic blood pressure and provide access for blood sampling. Central venous and pulmonary artery catheters should be considered when the etiology of hemodynamic instability is unclear (see Chapter 15) or when there is a requirement for vasopressors that can be administered only in the central venous system. Bedside transthoracic echocardiography may provide a less invasive alternative to assessing cardiac function and intravascular volume status. If monitoring and care requirements are escalating, and a prolonged or complicated recovery is expected, plans should be made to transfer the patient to an intensive care unit (ICU).

IV. GENERAL COMPLICATIONS

The incidence of overall PACU complications has been found to be as high as 24%, although this number varies with specific patient populations and is likely dependent upon a patient's medical history as well as the anesthesia and procedure performed. The most frequent issues encountered in the PACU setting include the following:
A. Respiratory and airway complications
B. Hemodynamic perturbations
C. Postoperative nausea and vomiting (PONV)
D. Renal complications
E. Neurologic compromise

V. EFFECTS OF ANESTHETICS AND SEDATIVES

GA affects the respiratory system by altering respiratory drive and mechanics via the following mechanisms, all of which are relevant in the immediate postoperative period:

A. **Reduction in respiratory drive.** Volatile anesthetics, sedatives, and opioids are respiratory depressants. They exert their effects by blunting central and peripheral chemoreceptor responsiveness to hypoxemia and hypercapnia, suppressing normal reflexive responses to negative upper airway pressure, and decreasing wakefulness.
   1. **Opioids,** the most commonly prescribed analgesics for postoperative pain control, are potent inhibitors of the hypercapnic ventilatory drive. Respiratory failure secondary to postoperative opioid use peaks during the first 24 hours. Patients treated with opioids have a decreased respiratory rate and may become apneic if not stimulated. **Benzodiazepines** also inhibit ventilatory drive, but to a lesser extent than opioids. The effects of these drugs are dose dependent and influenced by age and comorbidities such as intracranial pathology, obstructive sleep apnea (OSA), or chronic obstructive pulmonary disease (COPD).
B. **Residual neuromuscular blockade** often persists despite reversal of muscle relaxants. The upper airway dilator muscles are particularly sensitive to the effects of muscle relaxants, increasing the risk of upper airway obstruction, aspiration, and reintubation when not fully reversed. Neuromuscular blocking agents should be avoided or administered judiciously in patients with neuromuscular disorders such as Guillain–Barré syndrome, myasthenia gravis, and muscular dystrophies.
C. **Modified respiratory mechanics.** GA alters lung and chest wall mechanics, causing reductions in lung volume and compliance, and chest wall compliance. Immediately after induction of GA, functional residual capacity (FRC) decreases by as much as 20%, resulting in atelectasis of dependent regions of the lung. Atelectasis is further exacerbated by supine positioning of patients, intra-abdominal insufflation, as well as absorption of alveolar gas (absorption atelectasis) caused by high concentrations of oxygen. Reduced FRC and atelectasis cause ventilation perfusion mismatch, shunting, and hypoxemia.
D. **Intraoperative mechanical ventilation.** Ventilator-induced lung injury results from repetitive overdistention and collapse of dependent lung tissue. Lung protective ventilation with low tidal volumes, low plateau pressures, and the administration of positive end-expiratory pressure (PEEP) is the cornerstone of mechanical ventilation in intensive care unit (ICU) patients with acute respiratory distress syndrome (ARDS). Patients at risk for acute lung injury or with evidence of lung pathology undergoing surgery under GA may also benefit from low tidal volumes, low plateau pressures, higher levels of PEEP, and intraoperative recruitment maneuvers.

VI. RESPIRATORY AND AIRWAY COMPLICATIONS

Respiratory complications occur in 2% to 19% of postoperative patients, with atelectasis and alveolar hypoventilation being the most commons causes of these events. Additional causes of arterial hypoxemia include upper airway obstruction, laryngospasm, bronchospasm, and aspiration.
A. **Hypoxemia.** GA is associated with inhibition of hypoxic and hypercapnic ventilatory drive and a reduction in the lung's FRC. These changes may persist for a variable period of time postoperatively and predispose the patient to hypoventilation and hypoxemia. Supplemental oxygen can delay the detection of hypoventilation by pulse oximetry; however, it also reduces the incidence of hypoxia in the postoperative period. The decision to administer supplemental oxygen should be clinically determined for each patient but should generally be applied when transporting the patient from the OR to the PACU. Signs of hypoxemia include dyspnea,

cyanosis, altered mental status, agitation, obtundation, tachycardia, hypertension, and arrhythmias. Hypoxemia should be ruled out before undertaking specific treatment for these symptoms.

B. Causes of hypoxemia
   1. **Upper airway obstruction** is most often caused by inadequate recovery of the pharyngeal tone and is seen commonly in patients recovering form sedating medications and anesthesia and especially with obesity, preexisting OSA, or residual neuromuscular blockade.
   2. **Atelectasis** is a predictable effect of the reduction in the FRC during GA and can lead to increased intrapulmonary shunting. Obese patients and those undergoing thoracic or upper abdominal procedures are more susceptible to atelectasis. Epidural anesthesia without GA is associated with little or no atelectasis formation. Deep breathing, intermittent positive-pressure breathing, and incentive spirometry are effective in rapidly reexpanding small areas of alveolar collapse, although their ability to reduce respiratory complications is uncertain. Noninvasive ventilation (NIV) has been shown to decrease atelectasis and improve oxygenation in postoperative patients. Occasionally, hypoxemia may persist, and a chest radiograph (CXR) may reveal a segmental or lobar collapse. Chest physiotherapy or fiberoptic bronchoscopy may help with reinflating the collapsed segment.
   3. **Hypoventilation** causes hypoxemia through decreased minute ventilation and mismatch between oxygen delivery and consumption.
   4. **Diffusion hypoxia** may occur during washout of nitrous oxide upon emergence from GA. High-inspired O_2 fraction (FiO_2) by face mask can prevent hypoxemia.
   5. **Bronchospasm** may cause hypoventilation, CO_2 retention, and hypoxemia.
   6. **Aspiration of gastric contents** can lead to aspiration pneumonitis and pneumonia.
   7. **Pulmonary edema** may occur from cardiac failure, increased pulmonary capillary permeability, exposure to significant negative pressure, or iatrogenic volume overload. Cardiogenic edema occurs mostly in individuals with preexisting cardiac disease and is characterized by hypoxemia, dyspnea, orthopnea, jugular venous distention, wheezing, and an S_3 gallop. It may be precipitated by fluid overload, dysrhythmias, and myocardial ischemia. A CXR, arterial blood gas, 12-lead ECG, and troponin level should be obtained. Evaluation by a cardiologist may be indicated, particularly when aggressive management of conditions such as unstable angina or acute valvular disease is being considered. Inotropic agents, diuretics, and vasodilators are the mainstay of treatment. The use of NIV can obviate the need for intubation in patients with severe hypoxia, pending the response to the medical treatment. Noncardiogenic pulmonary edema secondary to sepsis, head injury, aspiration, transfusion reaction, anaphylaxis, negative-pressure pulmonary edema (NPPE), or upper airway obstruction is characterized by hypoxemia without the signs of left ventricular overload. NPPE can transpire secondary to persistent upper airway collapse such as laryngospasm, biting or kinking of the endotracheal tube, or hypopharyngeal collapse, with continued diaphragmatic activity. Young, healthy, athletic patients with good muscle strength are at an increased risk for NPPE, which commonly develops immediately after airway obstruction is relieved. It is characterized by hypoxemia, pink frothy sputum, and bilateral infiltrates on CXR that usually resolve within 24 to 48 hours. Treatment for pulmonary edema generally includes positive pressure

ventilation (via BiPAP or reintubation) and often needs to be continued in an ICU setting.
8. **Pneumothorax** may cause hypoventilation, hypoxemia, and hemodynamic instability.
9. **Pulmonary embolism** can occur in the immediate postoperative period and must be considered in patients with deep venous thrombosis, cancer, multiple trauma, or extended periods of immobility. Additional, non-thrombotic causes of pulmonary embolism include amniotic fluid embolism and bone cement implantation syndrome can also present in the immediate postoperative period.

C. **Hypoventilation** is characterized by inadequate minute ventilation resulting in hypercapnia and acute respiratory acidosis. When severe, hypoventilation can result in hypoxemia, mental status changes, and, ultimately, apnea. Supplemental oxygen may mask early detection of hypoventilation through pulse oximetry. Therefore, monitoring the ventilatory status of postoperative patients should not rely entirely on pulse oximetry. Etiologies of postoperative hypoventilation may be divided into two groups:
  1. **Decreased ventilatory drive**
     a. All inhaled **halogenated agents** depress ventilatory drive (see Chapter 12: Intravenous and Inhalation Anesthetics) and may produce hypoventilation in the postoperative period. **Opioids** are also potent respiratory depressants. All μ-receptor agonists increase the apneic threshold. Narcotized patients typically appear pain-free, take slow, deep breaths, have constricted pupils, and tend to become apneic if left unstimulated. Large doses of **benzodiazepines** also inhibit ventilatory drive. The safest treatment of anesthetic-related hypoventilation is to continue mechanical ventilation until breathing is adequate. Alternatively, pharmacologic reversal may be used.
        1. Opioid-induced hypoventilation can be reversed by **naloxone**, an opioid antagonist with the greatest affinity for the μ-receptor. Doses of 40 to 80 μg IV are titrated to effect. Reversal occurs within 1 to 2 minutes and lasts for 30 to 60 minutes. Naloxone treatment may induce significant side effects such as pain, tachycardia, hypertension, and pulmonary edema. It can also precipitate acute withdrawal in patients with history of chronic opioid use. The respiratory depressant effects of the opioids may outlast a single dose of naloxone. Thus, the patient should be monitored for recurrence of opioid-induced hypoventilation. A naloxone infusion may be helpful in large overdoses, or in the setting of long-acting opioids, like methadone.
        2. Hypoventilation secondary to benzodiazepines can be reversed by **flumazenil** (increments of 0.2 to 1 mg IV over 5 minutes, up to a maximum of 5 mg). The onset of reversal occurs within 1 to 2 minutes, with peak effect at 6 to 10 minutes. Patients should be monitored closely after administration of flumazenil because resedation may occur owing to its short 7- to 15-minute half-life. Flumazenil should be used cautiously in patients with chronic benzodiazepine use because it may precipitate seizures.
     b. Less common, but potentially life-threatening, causes of decreased ventilatory drive include complications of **intracranial** and **carotid artery** surgery, **head injuries**, high spinal, and intraoperative **stroke**.

2. **Pulmonary and respiratory muscle insufficiency**
   a. **Preexisting respiratory disease** is the most important risk factor for postoperative respiratory complications. COPD alters the match of ventilation and perfusion, resulting in hypoxemia and hypercapnia. Impaired gas exchange and expiratory flow limitation cause a high ventilatory workload under normal circumstances. **Restrictive disease** (eg, pulmonary fibrosis, pleural effusions, obesity, scoliosis, massive ascites, and pregnancy) is associated with fewer complications than COPD, particularly when respiratory muscle strength is preserved, and the restrictive defect is extrapulmonary. NIV can be beneficial in COPD and in restrictive pulmonary disease by decreasing the work of breathing, augmenting the ventilatory parameters, and avoiding intubation.
   b. **Residual neuromuscular blockade (NMB)** is defined as a train-of-four ratio less than 0.9 and suggested by the clinical observations of spasmodic twitching, generalized weakness, upper airway obstruction, or by more subtle signs such as hypoxemia or shallow breathing. The incidence of residual NMB in the PACU using the above definition has been found to be as high as 64%. Adequacy of muscle strength can only be definitively assessed with the aid of a **quantitative neuromuscular transmission monitor** (see Chapter 14: Neuromuscular Blockade). If muscle weakness persists after adequate pharmacologic reversal (eg, **sugammadex** 2 to 4 mg/kg for aminosteroids **or neostigmine** 20 to 60 µg/kg up to 5 mg, and **glycopyrrolate** 0.2 mg per 1 mg of neostigmine administered), consider redosing the reversal agent, institute or continue mechanical ventilation, administer adequate sedation, and wait for the muscle strength to recover. Redosing of sugammadex (at half the initial reversal dose) is relatively benign. However, resdosing neostigmine (at hald the initial dose up to a maximum of 60 µg/kg) and glycopyrolate carries more risk given the potential for inducing weakness. If recovery of muscle strength remains elusive, special situations such as myasthenia gravis and myasthenic syndromes, pseudocholinesterase deficiency, succinylcholine-induced phase II block, hypothermia, acid–base and electrolyte imbalance, and anticholinesterase inhibitor–induced weakness should be considered. The use of quantitative train-of-four significantly reduces the incidence of complications related to residual neuromuscular blockade.
   c. **Inadequate analgesia** after thoracic or upper abdominal surgery may cause splinting and decreased minute ventilation, resulting in alveolar collapse, hypercapnia, and hypoxemia. This is preventable with early analgesia and encouragement of deep breathing and coughing. Compared with systemic opioids, epidural analgesia may reduce the incidence of respiratory complications (atelectasis, pulmonary infections, or hypoxia).
   d. **Bronchospasm** is common in the pediatric population as well as patients with COPD, asthma, or a recent respiratory tract infection. It is often precipitated by manipulation of the airway, particularly tracheal intubation. Wheezing may also be heard upon chest examination of patients with pulmonary edema, endobronchial intubation, aspiration pneumonitis, and pneumothorax.
   e. **Pneumothorax** may complicate certain procedures such as thoracotomy, mediastinoscopy, bronchoscopy, high retroperitoneal dissection for nephrectomy or adrenalectomy, laparoscopic surgery, and spinal fusion. Insertion of central venous lines and nerve blocks of the upper extremities are other possible iatrogenic etiologies.

Diagnosis is made with a CXR in the upright position. In the presence of hemodynamic instability (tension pneumothorax), a needle decompression or tube thoracostomy must be performed emergently even without CXR diagnosis.
D. **Upper airway obstruction** may occur during recovery from anesthesia. Principal signs are the lack of adequate air movement, intercostal and suprasternal retractions, and paradoxical abdominal and chest wall motion during inspiration. Complete upper airway obstruction is silent. Partial obstruction is accompanied by either snoring (if the obstruction is above the larynx) or stridor (if perilaryngeal). Obstruction is more commonly seen in patients with OSA, obesity, tonsillar or adenoidal hypertrophy, or craniofacial abnormalities. Often times, airway obstruction may be relieved with a chin lift or jaw thrust. Patients with OSA may benefit from the use of continuous positive airway pressure. Common etiologies for upper airway obstruction include the following:
   1. **Incomplete recovery** from GA and/or neuromuscular blockade. Decreased strength and coordination of the intrinsic and extrinsic airway musculature causes the tongue to fall backward and occlude the airway. Patency is reestablished by inserting a nasal or oral airway, by manually assisting ventilation, or by intubating the trachea.
   2. **Laryngospasm is actually** a "protective reflex," which involves involuntary contraction of the vocal cords (VCs) after stimulation of the superior laryngeal nerve by noxious stimuli such as blood and airway secretions, particularly while under light anesthesia. It is characterized by stridor or the absence of breath sounds and air movement. Children, smokers, and obese patients are at increased risk for laryngospasm.
   3. **Airway edema** may be caused by laryngoscopy, bronchoscopy, nasogastric tube insertion, esophagoscopy, allergic reactions, or surgery on the head and neck. It may also follow a traumatic intubation, allergic reaction, the administration of large amounts of IV fluids, or prolonged prone position. Children are particularly susceptible to airway obstruction from edema because of the small diameter of their upper airway. The cuff leak test is neither sensitive nor specific and should not be used as the sole determinant for extubation of a patient with suspected airway edema. Video and flexible laryngoscopy have been used to assess the airway, although there are no universal guidelines for this practice. Treatment of upper airway edema includes the following:
      a. Administration of warmed, humidified **100% O$_2$** by face mask.
      b. **Head elevation, fluid restriction**, and possible **diuresis**.
      c. Nebulization of racemic **epinephrine** 2.25% solution, 0.5 to 1.0 mL in normal saline, or L-epinephrine, 2 mL of a 1:1000 solution, which may be repeated in 20 minutes if needed.
      d. **Dexamethasone**, 4 to 8 mg IV every 6 hours for 24 hours.
      e. Administration of **Heliox** (helium:oxygen, 80:20) can dramatically improve gas exchange and the work of breathing by establishing laminar airflow and improving gas exchange at distal alveoli.
      f. **Reintubation** of the trachea must be considered early in the course of suspected airway obstruction as distortion of airway anatomy may occur rapidly, particularly in the setting of allergic reactions.
   4. **Wound hematoma** caused by bleeding at the surgical site may complicate thyroid and parathyroid surgery, neck dissections, and carotid endarterectomy. The pressure caused by an expanding hematoma within the neck tissue planes causes obstruction of venous and lymphatic drainage and massive edema. Patients complain of local pain and pressure,

dysphagia, and variable degrees of respiratory distress and may have drainage from the surgical site. Signs of a neck wound hematoma may be subtle, so it is important to involve the surgery team at the earliest sign of concern. They must be treated immediately by emergency reexploration and evacuation in the OR. The anesthesiologist must support the airway by mask ventilation with 100% O_2, followed by endotracheal intubation. If tracheal intubation cannot be rapidly accomplished, opening the wound at the bedside can relieve soft tissue compression of the airway and improve airway patency and visualization.

5. **VC paralysis** may occur after thyroid, parathyroid, thoracic, tracheal, and neck surgery or a traumatic endotracheal intubation. VC paralysis may be transient, resulting from manipulation of the recurrent laryngeal nerve, or permanent, from severing the nerve. Unilateral transient VC paralysis is relatively common, and the primary concern is potential aspiration of gastric contents. Permanent unilateral VC paralysis can occur without clinical symptoms as compensatory action of the contralateral VC minimizes the occurrence of aspiration. Bilateral VC paralysis can occur after radical surgery for thyroid or tracheal cancer when neoplastic infiltration makes identification of the recurrent laryngeal nerves difficult. Bilateral VC injury is a rare and serious complication that can lead to complete upper airway obstruction after extubation in the immediate postoperative period. It requires emergency endotracheal intubation (which may be more difficult owing to disrupted airway anatomy) and possibly a tracheostomy.

E. **The intubated patient** presents special considerations. The ability to take intubated patients in the PACU depends on institution-specific capacity, comfort, and protocols. The anesthesiologist in the PACU should establish a plan regarding weaning and extubation or, alternatively, transfer the patient to an ICU. Conditions that could delay the extubation at the end of the surgery include the following:

1. **Delayed emergence** from GA due to volatile or IV agents. Reversal may be facilitated pharmacologically for some agents, but it is generally prudent to support ventilation and allow the respiratory depression to resolve spontaneously. The presence of a full stomach mandates additional vigilance in ensuring the recovery of consciousness and pharyngeal reflexes before extubation.

2. **Deep intraoperative neuromuscular blockade** is not appropriate to pharmacologically reverse with **neostigmine and glycopyrrolate**. The steroidal neuromuscular blockers vecuronium and rocuronium can be reversed with appropriately dosed **sugammadex**. Absent the availability of sugammadex, the patient should remain intubated until the patient can be safely, and permanently, reversed. In addition, if muscle weakness persists after adequate pharmacologic reversal, the patient needs mechanical ventilation until full recovery is achieved.

3. **Inadequate O_2 and CO_2 exchange** often resolve as the effects of anesthesia, surgery, and positioning fade. While supporting ventilation, possible etiologies, discussed in Sections VI.A and VI.B, must be considered.

4. **Potential for airway obstruction** exists after any extubation but especially when the patient has had a head and neck procedure, drainage of pharyngeal abscesses, mandibular wiring, large fluid resuscitation, or a prolonged surgery in the prone position. These patients should not be extubated until fully awake.

5. **Hemodynamic instability**, when severe, may be associated with a variable degree of impaired gas exchange and/or consciousness that mandate

continuation of mechanical ventilation. Transfer to an ICU should be arranged for patients who fail to improve.
   6. **Hypothermia** has numerous adverse effects that may make extubation undesirable immediately after surgery.
F. **Guidelines for extubation.** There is no single value or ventilatory parameter that will predict a successful extubation with certainty. Unlike extubation in the OR, extubation of patients in the PACU should follow similar guidelines to the ICU. These include ensuring adequate oxygenation on minimal ventilatory support, breathing frequency and tidal volumes, level of consciousness, and muscle strength.

VII. HEMODYNAMIC AND CARDIOVASCULAR COMPLICATIONS

Hemodynamic and cardiovascular complications are frequent occurrences in the PACU, with hypotension, arrhythmias, myocardial ischemia, and pulmonary edema being the most common complications recorded.

A. **Hypotension** should prompt a review of the patient's history and the intraoperative management to generate a differential diagnosis. The anesthetist who performed the case can be contacted to help interpret postoperative events. Hemorrhage must remain a primary consideration in the evaluation of hypotension in the postoperative patient.
   1. **Hypovolemia** is the most common cause of hypotension in the PACU, and administration of a fluid bolus during the initial assessment is generally appropriate. Ongoing hemorrhage, inadequate fluid replacement, osmotic polyuria, and fluid sequestration (eg, intestinal obstruction and ascites) are among the causes of hypovolemia in the PACU. Nonspecific signs include tachycardia, dry mucous membranes, oliguria, and thirst. A meaningful volume challenge (250 to 1000 mL of crystalloid or an equivalent volume of synthetic colloid, blood products, or both) should be considered for specific indications. Persistent hypotension after a seemingly adequate volume replacement mandates further assessment, starting with placement of a urinary catheter and consideration of ongoing surgical bleeding. Additional diagnostics may include transthoracic echocardiogram, a pulmonary artery catheter, or noninvasive cardiac output monitoring.
   2. **Impaired venous return** occurs when mechanical forces decrease the venous return to the heart in the absence of a reduction of circulating blood volume. Common causes include **positive-pressure ventilation**, dynamic hyperinflation of the lungs resulting in **auto-positive end-expiratory pressure (auto-PEEP)**, tension **pneumo/hemothorax**, high abdominal pressures from bleeding and/or abdominal compartment syndrome, and **pericardial tamponade.** Signs of obstruction to venous return are similar to those of true hypovolemia except for the presence of jugular vein distention, an elevated central venous pressure, and possibly decreased breath sounds and heart tones. Volume administration is the mainstay of symptomatic therapy, but treatment of the underlying cause is the definitive intervention.
   3. **Vasodilation** leading to hypotension can be caused by neuraxial anesthesia, residual inhalation agents, rewarming after hypothermia, transfusion reactions, adrenal insufficiency, anaphylaxis, systemic inflammation, sepsis, recent use of pharmacologic renin-angiotensin-aldosterone pathway modifiers, and the administration of vasodilating drugs. Hypovolemia accentuates the hypotension due to vasodilatation, but volume replacement alone cannot fully restore the blood pressure. Pharmacologic treatment includes α–adrenergic receptor agonists

such as **phenylephrine, norepinephrine**, and **epinephrine**. Diagnosis and treatment of the specific etiology should be concurrent with symptomatic treatment.

4. **Decreased cardiac output** can be caused by myocardial ischemia and infarction, dysrhythmias, congestive heart failure, administration of negative inotropic drugs (anesthetics, β-adrenergic blockers, calcium channel blockers, and antiarrhythmics), sepsis, and hypothyroidism (see Chapters 3, 7, and 17). Symptoms include dyspnea, diaphoresis, cyanosis, jugular vein distention, oliguria, rhythm disturbances, wheezing, dependent crackles, and an S_3 gallop on auscultation. A CXR, 12-lead ECG, and basic laboratory tests may help with diagnosis. Invasive monitoring may be necessary to guide pharmacologic therapies, including: ionotropic support, afterload reduction, diuresis, antiarrhythmics, or electrical cardioversion (see Chapter 3: Specific Considerations for Cardiac Disease).

B. **Hypertension** is most commonly observed in patients with preexisting hypertensive disease, particularly if antihypertensive medications were held preoperatively. Certain types of surgery such as carotid, vascular, endocrine, and intrathoracic procedures are more likely to be followed by hypertensive events. Specific postoperative etiologies for hypertension may include pain, bladder distention, fluid overload, hypoxemia, hypercarbia, hypothermia, increased intracranial pressure (ICP), and administration of vasoconstrictive agents. Hypertension is usually asymptomatic, but patients with malignant hypertension may have headache, visual disturbances, dyspnea, restlessness, and even chest pain. In the initial assessment, one should verify the accuracy of blood pressure measurement by checking cuff size and placement, review the patient's history and operative course, and rule out correctable etiologies. The management of hypertension is aimed at restoring blood pressure close to the patient's baseline. Strict blood pressure control is extremely important after surgery for intracranial aneurysm, creation of vascularized muscular flaps, microvascular surgery, and in patients with severe vascular disease. If possible, resumption of chronic antihypertensive oral therapy is ideal. If needed, this can be supplemented or substituted with a fast-onset, short-acting IV medication including β-adrenergic blockers, calcium channel blockers, smooth muscle relaxants, and nitrates.

C. **Dysrhythmias** in the perioperative period can be caused by increased sympathetic outflow, hypoxemia, electrolyte and acid–base imbalance, myocardial ischemia, increased ICP, drug toxicity, thyrotoxicosis, and malignant hyperthermia. Premature atrial contractions and unifocal premature ventricular contractions (PVCs) generally do not require treatment. In the presence of more worrisome rhythm disturbances, supplemental O_2 and supportive management should be administered while the etiology is investigated.

1. **Common supraventricular dysrhythmias** encountered in the PACU include:
    a. **Sinus tachycardia** may be secondary to pain, agitation, hypovolemia, fever, hyperthermia, hypoxemia, hypercarbia, congestive heart failure, and pulmonary embolism. Symptomatic treatment with β-blockers should be instituted only after its etiology is addressed, unless the patient is at risk of myocardial ischemia.
    b. **Sinus bradycardia** may result from a high neuraxial anesthetic block, opioid administration vagal stimulation, β-adrenergic blockade, and increased ICP. Symptomatic treatment with anticholinergic muscarinic agents, **glycopyrrolate**, 0.2 mg IV, or **atropine**, 0.5 to 1 mg IV, is indicated for hemodynamically significant bradycardia (see Chapter 39: Adult, Pediatric, and Newborn Resuscitation).

c. **Paroxysmal supraventricular tachydysrhythmias** occur with a higher incidence in patients over 70 years of age; after abdominal, thoracic, or major vascular procedures; and in patients with preoperative premature atrial contractions. These rhythms may cause significant hypotension. Treatment options include synchronized cardioversion (if unstable), adenosine, nondihydropyridine calcium channel blockers like verapamil or diltiazem, amiodarone, and β-blockers. See Chapter 39: Adult, Pediatric, and Newborn Resuscitation for more information on using these interventions.
2. **Stable ventricular dysrhythmias** such as PVCs and stable nonsustained ventricular tachycardia generally do not require treatment; however, a search for reversible causes (hypoxemia, myocardial ischemia, acidosis, hypokalemia, hypomagnesemia, and irritation due to a central venous catheter) should be conducted. Stable sustained ventricular tachycardia can be treated with synchronized cardioversion or pharmacologic modalities. PVCs that are multifocal and occur in runs, or are close to the preceding T wave, should be treated, especially in patients with structural heart disease, owing to the risk of developing an unstable ventricular rhythm. Treatment usually consists of β-blockers and amiodarone.
    a. Management for **unstable ventricular tachycardia** and **ventricular fibrillation** are described in the Advanced Cardiac Life Support (ACLS) protocol (see Chapter 39: Adult, Pediatric, and Newborn Resuscitation).
D. **Myocardial ischemia and infarction**
  1. **T-wave changes** (inversion, flattening, and pseudonormalization) may be associated with myocardial ischemia and infarction, electrolyte changes, hypothermia, surgical manipulation of the mediastinum, or incorrect lead placement. Isolated T-wave changes must be considered within the clinical context because they are common postoperatively and do not always indicate myocardial ischemia.
  2. **ST segment changes** including depressions and elevations are generally indicative of myocardial ischemia and infarction, respectively. Unlike myocardial infarctions in the nonsurgical setting, in the postoperative period, most myocardial infarctions are associated with ST depression and have a non–Q-wave pattern. As supplemental O_2 is administered and a 12-lead ECG and cardiac enzymes are obtained, possible precipitating factors for the ST segment changes must be reviewed and corrected. Common etiologies include hypoxemia, anemia, tachycardia, hypotension, and hypertension. If ischemia is present, and the patient is hemodynamically stable, patients should be rate controlled with a **β-blocker.** Aspirin and statins may decrease the mortality of patients with acute coronary syndrome in the perioperative period. IV nitroglycerin is a good option for cases with ST segment elevations. Cardiology consultation and transfer to an ICU should be considered.
E. **The patient with a permanent pacemaker (PPM) or an intracardiac defibrillator (ICD)** requires special care. Information about the patient's pacemaker dependency state and the features of the device must be obtained from the OR team. Continuous ECG monitoring with special attention to the patient's rhythm, rate, and hemodynamic status is indicated. Electrocautery used during the surgery can potentially trigger arrhythmia responses in PPM and ICD. Modern devices are less likely to be affected by intraoperative electromagnetic interference. Placing a magnet over the PPM or ICD should not be standard practice without precise knowledge of its effects. Communication with the electrophysiology service before and after surgery is highly recommended for interrogation of the device.

Interrogation and reprogramming of the device to the original parameters may be required in the PACU after the operation. Temporary pacing devices can be supported in the PACU as long as the institutions supports this practice, the PACU caregivers have training on these devices, and there is a destination plan for the patient after recovery from anesthesia.

VIII. RENAL COMPLICATIONS

Acute renal failure in the postoperative period significantly increases the morbidity and mortality of the surgical patient. The physiology, diagnosis, and treatment of renal abnormalities are described in Chapter 5: Specific Considerations with Renal Disease. Three common conditions encountered in the PACU that can indicate renal malfunction include oliguria, polyuria, and electrolyte disturbances. For more information on the management of these conditions, see Chapter 5.

- **A. Oliguria** is defined as a urine output of less than 0.5 mL/kg/h over 6 or more hours; however, reduced urine output in the PACU often precedes the official diagnosis. **Hypovolemia** is the most frequent cause of postoperative oliguria. Administration of a fluid bolus (250 to 500 mL of crystalloid or colloid), even when other etiologies are not yet excluded, is acceptable, as well as placement of a urinary catheter. Further diagnostic tests (eg, plasma and urine electrolytes) and invasive monitoring should be considered when oliguria persists. **Diuretics** (see Chapter 5: Specific Considerations with Renal Disease) should be used only when deemed necessary, such as in congestive heart failure and chronic renal insufficiency. Modern enhanced recovery after surgery (ERAS) protocols emphasize conservative intraoperative fluid management, and thus hypovolemia should be considered in the oliguric ERAS patient in the PACU.
- **B. Polyuria**, defined as a urine output disproportionately high for a given fluid intake, occurs less frequently. Symptomatic treatment is based on volume replacement to maintain hemodynamic stability and adequate fluid balance. Electrolyte and acid-base equilibrium may be perturbed secondary to the etiology or to large volume loss. The differential diagnosis includes excessive volume, pharmacologic diuresis, osmotic diuresis, postobstructive diuresis, acute tubular necrosis, and diabetes insipidus.
- **C. Electrolyte disturbances** such as **hyperkalemia** and acidemia can develop within hours and must be corrected emergently to avoid ventricular dysrhythmias and death (see Chapter 5). Polyuria may cause profound dehydration, with massive potassium losses and resulting alkalemia. **Hypokalemia**, often associated with **hypomagnesemia**, may also trigger atrial and ventricular dysrhythmias, although not as severe as those associated with hyperkalemia. Potassium should be replaced cautiously to avoid overdose. Magnesium replacement may effectively treat atrial and ventricular dysrhythmias, especially if the latter are in the form of torsade de pointes.

IX. NEUROLOGIC COMPLICATIONS
A. Delayed awakening
1. The most frequent cause of delayed awakening is **persistent effects of anesthetics**. Less common but possibly life-threatening causes include the organic cerebral events described in the section that follows.
2. **Decreased cerebral perfusion** of sufficient duration, during or after surgery, may cause diffuse or localized cerebral damage responsible for obtundation and delayed awakening. In patients with cerebrovascular disease, short periods of hypotension may cause a critical reduction of cerebral perfusion resulting in brain damage. If such an event

is suspected, a neurologic consultation should be obtained as soon as possible, and specific tests (eg, computed tomography [CT], magnetic resonance imaging [MRI], or angiography) should be considered. If cerebral edema is suspected, treatment should be started immediately (see Chapter 23: Anesthesia for Neurosurgery).
3. **Metabolic causes** of delayed awakening include hypothermia, sepsis, preexisting encephalopathies, hypoglycemia, and electrolyte or acid–base derangements.

B. **Neurologic damage** may be the result of a **stroke** or may be due to peripheral nerve injury. Strokes in the perioperative period have an incidence of 0.1% to 2.2% and may be ischemic or hemorrhagic. Early diagnosis of a stroke may be difficult because symptoms such as slurred speech, visual changes, dizziness, agitation, confusion, psychosis, numbness, muscular weakness, and paralysis may overlap with the manifestations of residual anesthetics. **Ischemic strokes** are more common in patients with cerebrovascular disease, hypercoagulable states, and atrial fibrillation, and they may be associated with intraoperative hypotension. Fat emboli secondary to long-bone fractures can also lead to strokes. **Hemorrhagic strokes** are more common in patients with coagulopathies, uncontrolled hypertension, cerebral aneurysms, arteriovenous malformations, and head trauma. Strokes are more frequent after intracranial surgery, carotid endarterectomy, cardiac surgery, and trauma. Neurologic consultation followed by brain CT or MRI is mandatory to guide immediate, and possibly brain-saving, treatment options.

C. **Emergence delirium** occurs in 5% to 20% of patients and is characterized by excitement alternating with lethargy, disorientation, and inappropriate behavior. Delirium may occur in any patient, but specific risk factors include age (<5 and >64 years old), preexisting anxiety or psychiatric diagnosis, type of surgery (breast, abdominal, ENT, and ophthalmic procedures), severe postoperative pain, and benzodiazepine premedication. Many drugs used perioperatively may precipitate delirium: ketamine, opioids, benzodiazepines, large doses of metoclopramide, and anticholinergics (atropine or scopolamine). Delirium may be a symptom of ongoing pathology such as hypoxemia, acidemia, hyponatremia, hypoglycemia, intracranial injury, sepsis, severe pain, and alcohol withdrawal. Along with addressing the underlying causes, treatment is symptomatic: supplemental O_2, fluid and electrolyte replacement, and adequate analgesia. **Dexmedetomidine** (0.5 to 1 mcg/kg over 10 minutes), an alpha-2 agonist, may be effective in preventing or treating delirium in the perioperative period. Antipsychotic medications such as **haloperidol** (2.5 to 5 mg IV increments every 20 to 30 minutes) may be indicated. Benzodiazepines (**diazepam**, 2.5 to 5 mg IV, and **lorazepam**, 1 to 2 mg IV) may be added if agitation is severe; however, benzodiazepines carry an inherent independent risk of worsening delirium. **Physostigmine** (0.5 to 2.0 mg IV) may reverse delirium due to anticholinergic agents.

D. **Local anesthetic systemic toxicity (LAST)** may present with neurologic symptoms including tinnitus, perioral numbness, metallic taste, agitation, seizures, respiratory depression, and unresponsiveness. Cardiovascular effects include hypertension, hypotension, and arrythmias. Prompt initiation of intralipid is the cornerstone of treatment. Dosing of intralipid 20% is 1.5 mL/kg (max 100 mL) given over 1 to 3 minutes, followed immediately by an infusion of 0.25 mL/kg/minute (max 200 to 250 mL given over 15 to 20 minutes).

E. **Peripheral neurologic lesions** may follow improper intraoperative positioning or direct surgical damage or may be a complication of regional anesthetic techniques. They are often discovered in the PACU, so it is essential to understand the common injuries and their presentations. Early identification, documentation, and neurologic consultation is crucial for a full recovery. In the American Society of Anesthesiologists (ASA) closed-claim analysis, ulnar nerve injury accounted for about one-third of the cases of nerve injury, followed by damage of the brachial plexus and the common fibular nerve. The risk factors for nerve injury after surgery include thin body habitus, previous history of neuropathy, smoking, and diabetes. Other sites of possible nerve damage are the wrist (median and ulnar nerve), internal aspect of the arm (radial nerve), and the points of emergence of the main branches of the VII cranial nerve, which can be compressed during mask-airway cases. Lithotomy position, especially when prolonged, may result in sciatic, femoral, common peroneal, and saphenous nerve injury. Improper positioning leads to compression or stretching of the nerve with demyelination. Remyelination often occurs in 6 to 8 weeks and results in complete recovery. Nevertheless, recovery may be more prolonged and, in some instances, the deficits are permanent.

F. Intraoperative awareness and recall are rare complications of GA (0.13% in a large multicenter trial) that can be first detected in the PACU. These are often the consequences of "light" anesthetic techniques and occur especially after trauma, cardiac, and obstetric surgery. Risk factors include genetic or acquired (history of substance abuse or prescribed medications) resistance, ASA physical status III to V, and the use of muscular relaxants. The long-term effects of awareness under GA range from mild anxiety to overt posttraumatic stress disorder. A short interview (such as the modified Brice protocol) can be conducted in the PACU to identify patients with recall. Patients with recall should receive reassurance and close inpatient and outpatient follow-up. Referral for psychological counseling should be offered.

X. POSTOPERATIVE NAUSEA AND VOMITING

PONV is a common complication of GA and less often of regional anesthesia. Patients should be stratified preoperatively with regard to their risk of PONV. The incidence of PONV is higher in women, nonsmokers, and patients with a history of PONV or motion sickness and when nitrous oxide and volatile anesthetics are used under GA. Certain types of surgery (cholecystectomy, laparoscopy, and gynecologic) may also increase the risk for PONV.

A. PONV prophylaxis is recommended in individuals with one or more risk factors (female sex, younger age, nonsmoker, receipt of opioid analgesia, higher risk surgery, and history of PONV or motion sickness). Some antiemetics can be dosed after induction, and others are more appropriate at the end of surgery. If appropriate, patients with higher risk for PONV should be offered a regional anesthetic technique. A combination of two or three antiemetic drugs from different classes is recommended along with measures aimed to diminish the baseline risk factors for PONV: preoperative anxiolysis, use of propofol for induction and maintenance of anesthesia, total IV anesthesia, adequate hydration, and minimization of perioperative opioids. If PONV occurs in a patient who has not received prophylaxis, therapy should be initiated with a serotonin antagonist and supplemented, if necessary, with medications from other classes. In patients who have received prophylaxis, rescue therapy should consist of drugs from classes other than the ones already administered. Administration of drugs from the same class within the first 6 hours after surgery has not been found to be effective in treating PONV. Nonmedication treatments for PONV include smelling alcohol swabs and benzoin, and these may buy some time until

the patient receives rescue medication. Common antiemetic classes and agents include the following:
- B. **Serotonin antagonists** (**ondansetron** 4 mg IV bolus) are well studied as prophylactic antiemetics when administered at the end of surgery, and rescue antiemetics when nausea and emesis have occurred postoperatively. However, if a serotonin antagonist has already been given prophylactically, there is no observed benefit of readministration as a rescue agent within 6 hours of the prophylactic dose.
- C. **Corticosteroids** are commonly used for the prevention of PONV. **Dexamethasone** (4 to 8 mg IV bolus) is the best studied. It is most effective for prophylaxis if administered at induction of anesthesia. Methylprednisolone (40 mg IV bolus) can also be used for PONV prevention.
- D. **Butyrophenones** include haloperidol and droperidol. **Haloperidol** (0.5 to 2 mg IV bolus) is likely as effective as ondansetron (4 mg IV bolus) in preventing PONV. **Droperidol** is no longer used as a first-line agent owing to a 2001 U.S. Food and Drug Administration boxed warning associating it with QT segment prolongation and torsade de pointes. Several studies have however suggested that antiemetic doses of droperidol are safe, are associated with only a transient prolongation in QTc comparable to that of ondansetron, and are not associated with changes in transmural dispersion of repolarization. The QT prolongation induced by the combination of ondansetron and droperidol is not different from that induced by each drug alone. A large retrospective study involving 20,122 patients who received droperidol 0.625 mg for PONV prophylaxis also found no increase in the risk of polymorphic ventricular tachycardia. Droperidol is still recommended as an alternative treatment for established PONV.
- E. **Transdermal scopolamine** (1.5 mg) is effective in prophylaxis if applied 2 hours before the start of the surgery. It may, however, cause visual changes and sedation in the PACU postoperatively. The patient should also be counselled to avoid touching the patch and then their eyes as it could precipitate mydriasis, which in the perioperative setting could be misconstrued for a cerebrovascular accident (CVA).
- F. **Phenothiazines** include **promethazine** (6.25 mg IV bolus) and **perphenazine** (5 mg IV bolus), which have been used for the prevention and treatment of PONV. Promethazine should be injected carefully as extravasation, or subcutaneous injection could result in tissue necrosis.
- G. **Antihistamines** including **dimenhydrinate** (1 mg/kg IV bolus), and **diphenhydramine** (50 mg IV) can be used for PONV prophylaxis. The major side effect is sedation.
- H. **Propofol** (20 mg IV bolus or 10 mg bolus followed by an infusion at 17 mcg/kg/min) can be used as a rescue agent in the PACU. This may have implications regarding airway management and nursing supervision requirements **that could necessitate ICU admission**.
- I. **NK-1 receptor antagonists** are a newer class of antiemetic agents. **Aprepitant** (40 to 80 mg PO), should be taken within 3 hours prior to induction for maximal effect, with some studies showing utility for rescue.

XI. PRINCIPLES OF PAIN MANAGEMENT
Principles of pain management are described in Chapter 38: Pain Management. Adequate analgesia begins preoperatively and continues in the OR and in the PACU.
- A. **Opioids** (IV or epidural) are the most common form of postoperative analgesia.

1. **Fentanyl**, a potent synthetic opioid with a rapid onset of action, small IV doses (25- to 50-μg IV bolus) can be titrated postoperatively to establish rapid analgesia.
2. **Hydromorphone** (0.2 to 0.5 mg IV bolus) may also be repeated every 10 to 20 minutes until adequate analgesia is achieved. It is a synthetic opioid approximately eight times more potent than morphine and associated with significantly less histamine release.
3. **Morphine** (2 to 4 mg IV bolus) may be repeated every 10 to 20 minutes until adequate analgesia is achieved. In children above 1 year of age, 15 to 20 μg/kg can be safely administered IV or intramuscularly at 30- to 60-minute intervals.
4. **Meperidine** (25 to 50 mg IV bolus) is similarly effective. It lacks the vagotonic effect of other opiates and is frequently used to reduce postanesthetic shivering. **Meperidine must be avoided in patients taking monoamine oxidase inhibitors** (serotonin syndrome) and must be administered cautiously in patients with renal insufficiency (toxic metabolite normeperidine is associated with seizures).
B. **Nonsteroidal anti-inflammatory drugs** (NSAIDs) and **acetaminophen** are effective complements to opioids. **Ketorolac** (15 mg IV bolus followed by 15 mg IV bolus every 6 to 8 hours in the perioperative period) provides potent postoperative analgesia. Other nonselective NSAIDs (**ibuprofen, naproxen**, and **indomethacin**) are also effective. Potential toxicities of all NSAIDs include decreased platelet aggregation resulting in increased bleeding risk, although newer studies suggest this may not be the case. NSAIDS may also increase nephrotoxicity.
C. **Adjuvant analgesics** include spasmolytics **(cyclobenzaprine)** and small doses of benzodiazepines.
D. **Regional sensory blocks** can be very effective postoperatively (see Chapter 21: Regional Anesthesia).
E. **IV patient-controlled analgesia** has been shown to be superior in patient satisfaction compared with intermittent analgesia administered by the medical staff.
F. **Continuous epidural analgesia** should be continued postoperatively or promptly initiated in the PACU if not used in the OR.

XII. BODY TEMPERATURE CHANGES
A. Postoperative **hypothermia** causes vasoconstriction with secondary elevation of blood pressure, increased myocardial contractility, and tissue hypoperfusion; it impairs platelet function and clot formation and may increase the risk of bleeding. Changes in cardiac repolarization such as prolongation of the QT interval may induce dysrhythmias. In addition, the metabolism of various drugs is slowed and may result in prolonged recovery from the neuromuscular blockade. During rewarming, shivering significantly increases O_2 consumption and CO_2 production, which may be undesirable in patients with limited cardiopulmonary reserve. Hypothermia in the perioperative period can increase the length of stay in PACU, wound infection rates, and cardiac morbidity. Heated blankets, forced warm air blankets, and warm IV solutions should be used to correct hypothermia (see Chapter 17: Intra-anesthetic Problems).
B. Etiologies of **hyperthermia** include infection, transfusion reaction, hyperthyroidism, **malignant hyperthermia**, serotonin syndrome, and neuroleptic malignant syndrome. Symptomatic treatment should be limited to situations in which hyperthermia is potentially dangerous, such as in young children or patients with compromised respiratory or cardiac reserve. **Acetaminophen** (suppositories 650 to 1300 mg or 10 mg/kg in children) and cooling blankets are commonly used.

XIII. RECOVERY FROM REGIONAL AND NEURAXIAL ANESTHESIA

A. Uncomplicated regional blocks may not require recovery in the PACU. Postoperative monitoring is indicated when heavy sedation was administered, when a complication from the block occurred (eg, intravascular injection of a local anesthetic and pneumothorax), or when required by the nature of the surgery (eg, carotid endarterectomy).

B. Recovery from spinal and epidural anesthesia occurs gradually. Patients should show signs of regression of both sensory and motor blockade before discharge. If recovery seems delayed, a neurologic examination should be performed to investigate the possibility of epidural hematoma or nerve injury.

XIV. CRITERIA FOR DISCHARGE

At the Massachusetts General Hospital, all patients who undergo GA are observed until ready for discharge, with no mandatory minimum recovery time. At least 30 minutes of observation after the last dose of opioids (or other respiratory depressant medication) is required to ensure the adequacy of ventilation and oxygenation. The criteria for recovery room discharge within a health care facility may differ depending on the procedural location (main OR, cath lab, endoscopy, interventional radiology, etc.), the resources available, and the comfort of the staff. This can be a potential source of confusion and errors, so the protocols at each site must be clear and understood by all members of the team.

A. To be discharged from the PACU, patients must meet several criteria. They should be easily arousable and oriented, or at their baseline. Vital signs should be stable and within normal limits. Pain and nausea should be under control. The requirement for urination or ability to tolerate clear liquids before discharge may be required in select patients. There should be no obvious surgical complications (eg, active bleeding) present. Effective communication with both the surgical team and the ward to which the patient is to be transferred can expedite the discharge of patients from the PACU. Outpatients should be discharged to a responsible adult with written instructions regarding postoperative diet, medications, etc., and with a phone number to call in case of emergency.

B. Fast-track recovery may be utilized for patients who meet certain criteria upon leaving the OR and are deemed ready to bypass the traditional PACU at the discretion of the anesthesia provider. These patients may be transferred directly to a second-stage recovery unit if they are ambulatory patients or to the floor if they are to be admitted as inpatients. Fast-track recovery criteria include the following:
  1. The patient should be awake, alert, and oriented (or at the baseline state).
  2. Vital signs should be stable (unlikely to require pharmacologic intervention).
  3. Oxygen saturation should be 94% or higher on room air (3 minutes or longer) or at baseline.
  4. If a muscular relaxant has been used, the patient should show no clinical signs of muscle weakness and/or the quantitative train-of-four monitoring should be greater than 0.9.
  5. Nausea and pain should be minimal (unlikely to require parenteral medications).
  6. There should be no active bleeding.

C. The intraoperative use of short-acting pharmacologic agents (midazolam, propofol, dexmedetomidine, remifentanil, succinylcholine, desflurane, and sevoflurane) and certain surgeries (orthopedic or simple gynecologic procedures) may make the fast-track recovery more likely.

XV. ENHANCED RECOVERY AFTER SURGERY

ERAS Society promotes a series of evidence-based interventions and treatments encompassing the entire perioperative period. When these recommendations are applied, they lead to better clinical outcomes, including reduced mortality and shorter hospital lengths of stay. The foundational efforts were performed in patients who had elective colonic surgery, but additional guidelines have been presented for pancreaticoduodenectomies, rectal and pelvic surgeries, and radical cystectomies. In the PACU, specific attention can be given toward minimizing PONV, applying multimodal analgesia strategies, reducing opioid administration while maintaining adequate pain control, and judicious application of balanced crystalloids for resuscitation.

XVI. CONSIDERATIONS FOR PEDIATRIC RECOVERY

A. PONV is more common in the pediatric surgery population than in adults; however, children under the age of 2 years are exceptions and have a reduced incidence relative to adults. Certain operations (adenotonsillectomy, strabismus repair, hernia repair, orchidopexy, and penile surgery) are associated with increased incidence for PONV. Risk factors, as well as the general principles for prevention and treatment, are similar to those described in adults. There is reasonable evidence to suggest **ondansetron** (100-μg/kg IV bolus for <6 months old; 150-μg/kg IV bolus >6 months old up to 4 mg) and **dexamethasone** (62.5 to 500 μg/kg up to 8 mg) are superior to other drugs in the prevention of PONV in children.

B. Airway obstruction results from similar etiologies and responds to similar treatments in children as in adults. Active or recent upper respiratory infections increase the risk of postoperative laryngospasm, especially in children with a history of prematurity or reactive airway disease. Subglottic edema after extubation (postextubation croup) is associated with concurrent upper respiratory infections; traumatic, repeated, or prolonged intubations; tight-fitting endotracheal tubes; and surgeries of the head and neck. Placement of the children in the lateral decubitus position after emergence from anesthesia improves the patency of the upper airway and efficacy of chin lift and jaw thrust maneuvers, and it also minimizes the risk of aspiration of gastric contents should vomiting occur.

C. Agitation in children may be a normal response upon emergence from anesthesia in a strange, unfamiliar environment and in the absence of their parents. Intraoperative use of volatile anesthetics, ketamine, and atropine as well as inadequately treated pain may increase the incidence of agitation and anxiety. Other causes such as hypoxemia, hypercarbia, hypothermia, hypotension, metabolic disorders, and central nervous system pathology should be considered, investigated, and treated appropriately. Adequate pain control, reassurance, cuddling, and the presence of the parents at the bedside may mitigate the symptoms in most children.

XVII. CRITICAL CARE IN THE POSTANESTHESIA RECOVERY UNIT

Increasingly, patients are admitted to the postanesthesia recovery unit for short-term delivery of ICU level of care. Patients undergoing uncomplicated thoracic (eg, thoracotomies, lobectomies, and wedge resections) and vascular procedures (eg, infrarenal abdominal aortic aneurysm repairs, carotid endarterectomies), as well as other procedures involving large volume shifts, require a closer level of postoperative care. Care issues range from aggressive blood pressure management with IV medications to continued mechanical ventilation and hemodynamic resuscitation. It is important for the PACU care providers to establish a plan for continued monitoring and care. If longer-than-expected critical care needs arise, or respiratory and/or hemodynamic perturbations continue, transfer to the ICU should occur.

XVIII. PACU ROLE IN HOSPITAL CAPACITY CHALLENGES
A. Flex procedural space
The PACU is unique in that the combination of equipment, layout, and staff skillset allow it to be used for more than just recovery from OR procedures. In fact, the PACU can be set up to allow for certain procedures to be performed in the PACU itself. This can improve hospital efficiency by using beds that would otherwise be empty and saving on costly OR time. For example, electroconvulsive therapy (ECT), cardioversion, and other simple elective outpatient or inpatient nonelective procedures can be performed safely in a PACU setting with the appropriate resources and personnel training. Perioperative procedures including postop chest tubes, wound vac changes, and vascular access can be performed in the PACU, potentially avoiding a return trip to the OR.

B. Flex postop recovery space
The broad capability inherent to the PACU can be leveraged to serve as capacity buffer that offsets capacity limitations in other hospital floors during times of increased demand. The PACU can often accommodate patients who would otherwise be in the ICU, step down units, or the cardiology floor. For instance, patients requiring airway monitoring, or recovering from electrophysiology procedures, may be monitored in the PACU. When hospital floors are stretched for capacity, especially overnight, the PACU can serve as flex poor space, accommodating patients who would not otherwise have a bed due to bed capacity remaining at 100%. This flexibility allows hospital capacity administrators to focus on areas of highest demand.

XIX. PACU AS SURGE ICU CAPACITY IN PANDEMICS
Many lessons were learned from necessities that arose during the COVID-19 pandemic. One of the most notable ones was how to use the PACU to add surge capacity during acute increases in demand. In many institutions, PACU space is the easiest to convert to ICU space, as they had advanced monitors (with central alarming), O_2, suction, and an architectural layout with designed for increased visibility that is conducive to intensive monitoring. Other advantages of the PACU that make it readily convertible to ICU surge capacity include its advanced supplies, its colocalization with ORs, and the relative ease of obtaining and using OR supplies. The use of anesthesia machines during periods of ventilator shortages is one such example.

Suggested Readings

Apfelbaum JL, Silverstein JH, Chung FF, et al; American Society of Anesthesiologists Task Force on Postanesthetic Care. Practice guidelines for postanesthetic care: an updated report by the American Society of Anesthesiologists Task Force on postanesthetic care. *Anesthesiology*. 2013;118(2):291–307.

Apfelbaum JL, Walawander CA, Grasela TH, et al. Eliminating intensive postoperative care in same-day surgery patients using short-acting anesthetics. *Anesthesiology*. 2002; 97(1):66–74.

Bartels K, Karhausen J, Clambey ET, Grenz A, Eltzschig HK. Perioperative organ injury. *Anesthesiology*. 2013;119(6):1474–1489.

Chenitz KB, Lane-Fall MB. Decreased urine output and acute kidney injury in the postanesthesia care unit. *Anesthesiol Clin*. 2012;30(3):513–526.

Daley MD, Norman PH, Colmenares ME, Sandler AN. Hypoxaemia in adults in the postanesthesia care unit. *Can J Anaesth*. 1991;38(6):740–746.

Fu ES, Downs JB, Schweiger JW, Miguel RV, Smith RA. Supplemental oxygen impairs detection of hypoventilation by pulse oximetry. *Chest.* 2004;126(5):1552–1558.

Gan TJ, Belani KG, Bergese S, et al. Fourth consensus guidelines for the management of postoperative nausea and vomiting. *Anesth Analg.* 2020;131(2):411–448.

Gustafsson UO, Scott MJ, Hubner M, et al. Guidelines for perioperative care in elective colorectal surgery: Enhanced Recovery After Surgery (ERAS®) Society Recommendations: 2018. *World J Surg.* 2019;43(3):659–695

Hines R, Barash PG, Watrous G, O'Connor T. Complications occurring in the postanesthesia care unit: a survey. *Anesth Analg.* 1992;74(4):503–509.

Kluger MT, Bullock MFM. Recovery room incidence: a review of 419 reports from the Anaesthetic Incident Monitoring Study (AIMS). *Anaesthesia.* 2002;57(11):1060–1066.

Mashour GA, Orser BA, Avidan MS. Intraoperative awareness: from neurobiology to clinical practice. *Anesthesiology.* 2011;114(5):1218–1233.

Munk L, Andersen LP, Gögenur I. Emergence delirium. *J Perioper Pract.* 2013;23(11):251–254.

POISE Study Group; Devereaux PJ, Yang H, Yusuf S, et al. Effects of extended-release metoprolol succinate in patients undergoing non-cardiac surgery (POISE trial): a randomised controlled trial. *Lancet.* 2008;371(9627):1839–1847.

Priebe HJ. Perioperative myocardial infarction–aetiology and prevention. *Br J Anaesth.* 2005;95(1):3–19.

Rose DK, Cohen MM, DeBoer DP. Cardiovascular events in the postanesthesia care unity: contribution of risk factors. *Anesthesiology.* 1996;84(4):772–781.

Sebel PS, Bowdle TA, Ghoneim MM, et al. The incidence of awareness during anesthesia: a multicenter United States study. *Anesth Analg.* 2004;99(3):833–839.

Thilen SR, Weigel WA, Todd MM, et al. 2023 American Society of Anesthesiologists Practice Guidelines for monitoring and antagonism of neuromuscular blockade: a report by the American Society of Anesthesiologists Task Force on Neuromuscular Blockade. *Anesthesiology.* 2023;138(1):13–41

Thompson A, Balser JR. Perioperative cardiac arrhythmias. *Br J Anaesth.* 2004;93(1):86–94.

Wang K, Asinger RW, Marriott HJL. ST-segment elevations in conditions other than acute myocardial infarction. *N Engl J Med.* 2003;349(22):2128–2135.

Pain Management

Rachel Padilla Judge and Peter Stefanovich

I. DEFINITION AND TERMINOLOGY

Pain is an unpleasant sensory and emotional experience associated with actual or potential tissue damage or described in terms of such damage. Different categories of pain can be defined according to the duration, etiology, or perception of the painful experience.

A. **Acute pain** is caused by damage, ongoing inflammation, or physiologic malfunction after a physical injury to body tissues and usually resolves as the wound heals. The intensity and duration of acute postoperative pain is a major risk factor in the development of chronic postsurgical pain. Improved control of acute pain following surgery has become a focus for practice improvement measures leading to a more timely and diversified approach to pain. Studies demonstrate that techniques that effectively reduce acute pain, including "prehabilitation," multimodal preventative analgesia, and the use of regional anesthetics are also associated with a lower incidence of subsequent chronic postsurgical pain and is a target as a primary prevention measure.

B. **Chronic pain** is pain that persists beyond the time of healing, often defined as pain persisting beyond 3 to 6 months. Common chronic pain conditions include chronic postsurgical pain, chronic low back pain, complex regional pain syndrome, postherpetic neuralgia, temporomandibular disorders, cancer pain, and myofascial pain. Current research suggests that mechanisms in the development of chronic pain involve signaling at both the site of tissue trauma and central sensitization at the level of the spinal cord and above.

C. **Neuropathic pain** results from pathologic function of the somatosensory system, either in peripheral elements (receptors or peripheral nerves) or in the central nervous system. The abnormal somatosensory function of neuropathic pain is a direct result of injury to the nervous system, and this type of pain persists even after tissue healing appears to be complete. It is most frequently described as burning, radiating, lancinating, or shooting in nature and can be accompanied by *allodynia*, or the perception of pain from a normally innocuous stimulus.

D. **Nociceptive pain** results from an injury that activates peripheral nociceptors, which can be somatic or visceral in origin, and is the pain associated with most acute injuries. **Somatic pain** typically reflects injury to the superficial structures of the musculoskeletal system and skin. Somatic pain is typically well localized in contrast to that of **visceral pain**, which arises from distention or injury to the viscera, owing to the less dense sensory innervation of the organs as compared with other tissues.

E. **Inflammatory pain** is categorized as nociceptive pain in the presence of acute inflammation, but chronic inflammatory states can play mechanistic roles in neuropathic pain states. Inflammation resulting from tissue damage can lead to *hyperalgesia*, which is the exaggerated painful perception of a known noxious stimulus.

II. TREATMENT OF ACUTE PAIN IN THE PERIOPERATIVE SETTING
A. Pharmacologic treatment of pain
1. **Nonsteroidal anti-inflammatory drugs (NSAIDs, Table 38.1)** can effectively treat mild to moderate pain, particularly pain associated with inflammatory conditions. Drugs classified as NSAIDs have diverse chemical structures, but all share the ability to inhibit the enzyme cyclooxygenase (COX) and thereby inhibit the formation of prostaglandins from arachidonic acid. Combination therapy with the addition of NSAIDs to opioid during the perioperative period can often provide synergistic analgesia and reduce opioid-related side effects. Although it is important to avoid NSAIDs in patient populations at significant risk for toxicity, many patients having surgery can benefit from their addition.
    a. **Mechanism of action.** The apparent mechanism for analgesia produced by the NSAIDs is the prevention of neuronal sensitization by diminishing prostaglandin production. Type I cyclooxygenase (COX-1) is a constitutively expressed enzyme that is present in varying amounts in most cells at a constant level. COX-1 serves a key role in cellular homeostasis and is the primary form of the enzyme present in platelets, the kidney, stomach, and vascular smooth muscle. COX-2-selective inhibitors, developed with the goal to reduce side effects such as gastrointestinal (GI) bleeding associated with NSAIDs, have also been associated with an increase in the risk of adverse cardiovascular effects (eg, myocardial infarction and stroke). COX-2 inhibitors should be used with caution when cardiovascular risk factors are present and are contraindicated during coronary artery bypass graft surgery. Celecoxib is now the only available COX-2 inhibitor in the United States. For an overview of the NSAIDs according to their inhibition of COX and their selectivity for the COX-2 isoenzyme, see **Table 38.1**.
    b. **Toxicity** from NSAIDs impacts primarily the GI, renal, hematologic, and hepatic systems.
        1. **GI system.** Dyspepsia is the most common side effect, and nonselective NSAIDs lead to asymptomatic ulcers in 20% to 25% of users within 1 week of administration. Complicated ulcers, including perforated ulcers, upper GI bleeding, and obstruction occur in a significant number of long-term NSAID users. Factors that increase the risk of NSAID-induced GI toxicity are shown in **Table 38.2**.
        2. **Renal impairment** occurs in some patients taking NSAIDs and results from reduction in renal perfusion due to inhibition of prostaglandin synthesis. In patients with contraction of their intravascular volume (eg, congestive heart failure, acute blood loss,

Classification of Common NSAIDs Based on COX Inhibition and Selectivity

Aspirin	Irreversible inhibition of both COX-1 and COX-2
Ibuprofen, naproxen	Reversible, competitive inhibition of both COX-1 and COX-2
Ketorolac	Nonselective COX-1 and COX-2 inhibition
Indomethacin	Slower, time dependent, but reversible inhibition of both COX-1 and COX-2
Celecoxib	Slow, time dependent, and highly selective COX-2 inhibition

Table 38.2 Risk Factors That Increase the Risk of NSAID-Induced GI Toxicity

Age over 60 y

Prior history of peptic ulcer disease

Steroid use

Alcohol use

Use of multiple NSAIDs

The first 3 mo of use

---

and hepatic cirrhosis), renal perfusion is maintained through the vasodilatory effects of prostaglandins. Renal toxicity may manifest as acute interstitial nephritis or nephrotic syndrome. Acute renal failure occurs in as many as 5% of patients using NSAIDs; renal impairment typically resolves with the discontinuation of NSAID therapy but, rarely, progresses to end-stage renal disease. Factors that increase the risk of NSAID-induced renal toxicity are shown in **Table 38.3**.

3. **Hematologic toxicity** associated with NSAIDs takes the form of inhibition of normal platelet function. Platelet activation is blocked by the inhibitory effects of NSAIDs on COX and the secondary decrease of prostaglandin conversion to thromboxane A_2 (platelet activator). Aspirin irreversibly acetylates COX, and thus, the platelet inhibition resulting from aspirin use persists for the 7 to 10 days required for new platelet formation. Nonaspirin NSAIDs induce reversible platelet inhibition that resolves when most of the drug has been eliminated. A recent meta-analysis suggests that the effect of ketorolac on platelet function does not necessarily result in clinically appreciable postoperative bleeding.

4. **Hepatic toxicity** may also result from NSAID use. Minor elevations in hepatic enzyme levels appear in 1% to 3% of patients. The mechanism appears to be immunologic or metabolic-mediated direct hepatocellular injury, with dose-related toxicity occurring with both acetaminophen and aspirin. Periodic assessment of liver function is recommended in those on long-term NSAID therapy.

Table 38.3 Factors That Increase the Risk of NSAID-Induced Renal Toxicity

Preexisting renal insufficiency

Hypovolemia
- Acute blood loss
- Chronic diuretic use

Low cardiac output (congestive heart failure)

Hepatic cirrhosis

5. **Inhibition of normal bone formation** has been reported in both clinical and animal models by inhibiting osteogenesis. There is some evidence that NSAIDs have a negative effect regarding bone healing, but this is associated with longer duration and higher doses.
   c. **Clinical uses.** NSAIDs are used most widely to treat the pain and inflammation associated with rheumatic and degenerative arthritis. They also serve as a useful adjunct to opioids for providing control of acute pain, often reducing opioid requirements and opioid-related side effects in the postoperative period. Numerous agents are available for oral administration, and several are available without prescription. Thus, they are among the most common first-line analgesics.
   d. **Available formulations.** Ketorolac and diclofenac are parenteral NSAIDs approved for clinical use in the United States. Both are potent analgesics and antipyretics, and several studies have demonstrated their usefulness in treating moderate postoperative pain. Ketorolac and diclofenac are nonselective NSAIDs, and despite a parenteral form, intravenous (IV) administration is still associated with GI toxicity like other orally administered NSAIDs. Familiarity with the dosing and administration of several oral NSAIDs as well as the parenteral formulations is an important tool for those treating acute pain. For a summary of comparative efficacy and dosages of commonly used nonopioid analgesics, see **Table 38.4.**
2. **Acetaminophen** is a para-aminophenol derivative with analgesic and antipyretic properties similar to NSAIDs. The exact mechanism by which acetaminophen exerts its effects has yet to be fully understood, but it is known to act peripherally (COX inhibition) and centrally (multiple pathways). Acetaminophen does not produce any significant peripheral inhibition of prostaglandin production. Acetaminophen causes no significant GI toxicity or platelet dysfunction, and there are few side effects within the normal dose range. Acetaminophen is entirely metabolized by the liver, and minor metabolites are responsible for the hepatotoxicity associated with overdose. The most common oral analgesics used to treat moderate to severe pain incorporate acetaminophen in combination with one of the opioids. Standing per os, per rectum, or IV dosing of 1 g of acetaminophen every 6 hours (<4 g/d) can be a very useful adjunct in the postoperative setting and can significantly improve pain and reduce opioid requirements.
3. **Ketamine** is an atypical dissociative anesthetic and potent analgesic that is an N-methyl-D-aspartate receptor (NMDA) receptor antagonist, which may play a role in decreasing central sensitization in the development of chronic pain. In contrast to opioids, spontaneous respiration and airway reflexes are relatively well maintained. Hypersalivation is a common side effect that can be eased by coadministration of an antisialagogue such as glycopyrrolate. Ketamine causes indirect stimulation of the sympathetic nervous system by inducing a catecholamine release. In high doses, ketamine causes a "dissociative" state and is associated with unpleasant side effects such as nightmares, which may be attenuated by concomitant administration of benzodiazepines. Use of ketamine as an adjuvant anesthetic has been shown to result in decreased opioid requirements in the immediate postoperative period in a majority of studies without a significant increase in adverse outcomes and is especially useful in the management of perioperative pain in patients on chronic opioid therapy. Ketamine infusions (2.5 to 10 µg/kg/min)

TABLE 38.4 Selected Nonopioid Analgesics and Comparative Efficiency

Special Nonopioid Analgesic Dosage and Comparative Efficiency to Standards

Drug	Common Brand Names	Average Analgesic Dose (mg)	Dose Interval (h)	Maximum Daily Dose (mg)	Analgesic Efficacy Compared With Standards	Plasma Half-Life (h)	Comments
Acetaminophen	Tylenol numerous	500–1000 PO, PR, or IV	4–6	4000	Comparable to aspirin 650 mg	2–3	Use with caution in presence of alcoholism or liver disease. Rectal suppository available
Aspirin (*Salicylate*)	Numerous	500–1000 PO	4–6	4000		0.25	Because of risk of Reye syndrome, do not use in children under 12 y with possible viral illness. Rectal suppository available
Ibuprofen (*Propionic acid*)	Advil numerous	200–400 PO	4–6	2400	Superior at 200 mg to aspirin 650 mg	2–2.5	
Naproxen	Naprosyn	500 PO initial 250 PO	6–8	1250		12–15	

(*continued*)

TABLE 38-4 Selected Nonopioid Analgesics and Comparative Efficiency (continued)

Special Nonopioid Analgesic Dosage and Comparative Efficiency to Standards

Drug	Common Brand Names	Average Analgesic Dose (mg)	Dose Interval (h)	Maximum Daily Dose (mg)	Analgesic Efficacy Compared With Standards	Plasma Half-Life (h)	Comments
Indomethacin	Indocin	25 PO	8–12	100	Comparable to aspirin 650 mg	2	Not routinely used because of high incidence of side effects
Ketorolac (*Pyrrole acetic acid*)	Toradol	15–30 IV or IM	6	150 first day, 120 thereafter	Comparable to 6–12-mg morphine	6	Do not take >5 d
Diclofenac (*Phenyl acetic acid*)	Dyloject	75–150 IV or IM	24	150 daily		1–2 h	Do not take >2 d
Celecoxib (*COX-2 inhibitor*)	Celebrex	100–200 PO	12	400			Not to be taken if allergic to sulfa

can be used as an intraoperative anesthetic adjunct for pain and has been shown to reduce opiate consumption in complex spine surgery up to 48 hours postoperatively. A Cochrane review of perioperative ketamine demonstrated both reduced pain and opioid consumption, increased time to first analgesic, and decreased postoperative nausea and vomiting, at the consequence of increased dysphoric side effects (hallucinations, unpleasant dreams, nystagmus). Ketamine bolus (10 to 30 mg) can also be used in the immediate postoperative period as a rescue analgesic, especially after opioid rescue has failed. Patients should be premedicated with a benzodiazepine to mitigate dysphoria and be monitored on telemetry. Ketamine infusions can be useful in patients with significant acute pain refractory to multimodal analgesia, and are especially helpful in opioid-tolerant patients.

4. **Opiates and opioids. Opiates** are among the most universally effective agents available for treating acute pain. Morphine, the prototypical opiate, is derived from the milk of the scored seed pod of the Oriental poppy, *Papaver somniferum*. Several other compounds can be derived directly through the chemical modification of morphine. Those drugs derived directly from morphine are termed the opiates. Other synthetic compounds have been produced that act via opiate receptors—all compounds that act via opiate receptors are termed **opioids**. Although opioids form the cornerstone of effective acute pain management, they have significant side effects, and their long-term effectiveness is limited by tolerance, physical dependence, and the possibility of addiction. Opioids are extremely useful for treating acute pain; although they are in widespread clinical use, their long-term effectiveness for treating chronic, noncancer pain is less clear. Common prescribing practices in the United States have led to an epidemic of prescription opioid misuse and abuse. Overdoses involving opioids killed nearly 47,000 people in 2018, and 32% of those deaths involved prescription opioids. Significant reform in physician's prescribing patterns represents the first step in addressing this public health issue.

   a. **Metabolism.** Following injection, morphine rapidly undergoes hepatic conjugation with glucuronic acid; morphine remains largely in the ionized form at physiologic pH and is highly protein bound. The plasma concentration attained after an identical dose of morphine increases progressively with increasing age of patients. The plasma concentration of morphine correlates poorly with its pharmacologic effect. Analgesia and respiratory depression correlate more closely with the cerebrospinal fluid (CSF) concentration. Of the metabolites morphine-3-glucuronide (M-3-G) and morphine-6-glucuronide (M-6-G), M-6-G, although produced in smaller amounts (a ratio of 1:9 in M-6-G:M-3-G), is pharmacologically active producing both analgesia and respiratory depression via interaction with μ-opioid receptors. As a result, prolonged respiratory depression can occur in patients with renal failure as M-6-G elimination is significantly impaired. Unlike fentanyl, histamine release follows IV morphine administration resulting in a decrease in systemic vascular resistance and blood pressure.

   b. **Side effects** associated with opioid analgesics:
      1. **Respiratory depression.** Opioids cause a dose-dependent reduction in the responsiveness of the brain stem respiratory centers to increases in arterial carbon dioxide tension ($PaCO_2$) that manifests as a reduction in breathing rate and at high doses, apnea.

2. **Sedation.** Mediated through the limbic system.
3. **Pupillary constriction.** Excitatory action on the autonomic segment of the Edinger–Westphal nucleus of the oculomotor nerve.
4. **Nausea and vomiting.** Direct stimulation of the chemoreceptor trigger zone within the area postrema in the medulla.
5. **Constipation.** Reduction in the propulsive peristaltic contractions of the small and large intestines.
6. **Bradycardia.** Central stimulation of the vagal nucleus within the medulla.
  c. **Tolerance.** With continued use of substantial amounts of opioids, larger doses of the drug are required over time to produce the same physiologic effects. This phenomenon is called tolerance and is characteristic of the entire class of opioids.
  d. **Physical dependence.** The precipitation of a distinct withdrawal (abstinence) syndrome when the opioid is discontinued. Manifestations of opioid withdrawal include diaphoresis, hypertension, tachycardia, abdominal cramping, and nausea and vomiting. Physical dependence occurs in any individual given sufficient doses of opioid for extended periods of time and is *not* synonymous with the complex disease that is addiction, although it can contribute to the neurobiologic mechanisms driving compulsive opioid-seeking behaviors.
  e. **Opioid-induced hyperalgesia (OIH).** There can be a paradoxical increase in painful stimuli with opioid administration thought to be secondary to the upregulation of compensatory pain pathways, of which the central glutaminergic system plays a central role. Discerning between OIH and tolerance is challenging, and as such, one must rule out an exacerbation of the patient's pain syndrome before considering OIH as a contributor. Strategies to address OIH once it occurs include opioid rotation and gradual dose reduction.
f. **Forms of opioids**
  1. **Oral opioids** are common agents used for the control of mild to moderate pain in those who are able to continue oral intake. Many agents are available as combination preparations containing an opioid along with acetaminophen. The duration of analgesic action for the orally administered opioids is similar and in the range of 3 to 4 hours. Commonly used oral opioids are listed in **Table 38.5**. In those with opioid tolerance or greater than average opioid requirements, oral opioid alone (without acetaminophen) should be used to avoid hepatic toxicity.
  2. **IV opioids.** Control of moderate to severe pain or treatment of those who are unable to tolerate oral intake often requires the use of IV opioids. The pharmacokinetic profiles of opioid analgesics administered intramuscularly are similar but somewhat more erratic owing to variations in the muscle blood flow compared with that seen with IV administration; however, there is significant discomfort with intramuscular (IM) administration. There is no maximum dose for any of the pure opioid agonists (either orally or parenterally), and the dose can be increased until acceptable analgesia is produced, or intolerable side effects ensue. Patients who require large doses of opioids should be closely monitored during initial dose titration, as marked respiratory depression and apnea may occur. Commonly used IV opioids include fentanyl, hydromorphone, morphine, methadone. Fentanyl is typically used for severe acute breakthrough pain. Hydromorphone

TABLE 38.5 Common Oral Opioid and Opioid/Acetaminophen Combinations Used to Treat Mild to Moderate Pain

Drug	Equianalgesic Oral Dose (mg)	How Supplied
Codeine	60	15-, 30-, 60-mg tabs; 15-mg/5-mL elixir
Acetaminophen with codeine	—	300–15-, 300–30-, 300–60-mg tabs; 120–12/5-mL elixir
Hydrocodone	60	(Available only in combination with acetaminophen)
Acetaminophen with hydrocodone	—	500–2.5-, 500–5-, 500–7.5-, 660–10-mg tabs; 500–7.5/15-mL elixir
Oxycodone	10	5-mg tabs; 5-mg/5-mL elixir
Acetaminophen with oxycodone	—	325–5-, 500–5-mg tabs; 325–5/5-mL elixir
Morphine	10	15-, 30-mg tabs; 10-, 20-mg/5-mL elixir
Hydromorphone	2	2-, 4-, 8-mg tabs; 5-mg/5-mL elixir

is the most common IV opioid with an onset time of 20 minutes and duration of 2 to 4 hours. IV methadone, a long-acting opioid, can be used in patient-controlled analgesia (PCA) for opioid-tolerant patients, or perioperatively. Perioperatively IV methadone is beneficial for long surgeries, or surgeries that create high pain requirements, specifically it decreases postoperative pain scores in posterior spinal fusion surgeries compared to IV hydromorphone.

3. **Intrathecal opioids (see section that follows).**
4. **Epidural opioids (see section that follows).**
5. **Muscle relaxants.** Medications used in the treatment of pain associated with musculoskeletal systems and spasms have varying mechanisms of action and unique safety and side-effect profiles. These include but are not limited to GABA-B agonists such as baclofen, α_2-agonists such as tizanidine, 5-HT2 antagonists such as cyclobenzaprine, and benzodiazepines such as diazepam. The mechanisms of action, side effects, and suggested dosing can be found in **Table 38.6**.

B. **Adjuncts used with opioids**
   1. **Gabapentinoids.** Meta-analyses of preoperative use of gabapentin (250 to 500 mg) has shown decreased opioid use for 24 hours (by 35%), decreased pain at rest and with movement, decreased pruritus, nausea, and vomiting, but at the cost of increased dizziness, sedation and prolonged PACU time. Gabapentin and pregabalin are helpful for neuropathic and some chronic pain syndromes.
   2. **α_2-Agonists.** α_2-Agonists such as dexmedetomidine have been shown to decrease the risk of nausea and morphine consumption in the first 24 hours postoperatively without increased recovery times in abdominal surgery. It has also shown benefits in reducing pain scores and morphine consumption in the first 24 hours after cardiothoracic, breast, and bariatric surgery.

TABLE 38.6 Muscle Relaxants Used in the Management of Pain Related to Muscular Spasm

Name	Mechanism	Suggested Dose	Caution
Baclofen	GABA-B receptor agonist	Starting dose: 5 mg PO up to 3 times daily Increase by 5 mg every 3 d, to max dose of 80 mg daily No hepatic or renal dose adjustments	Transient dizziness, withdrawal syndromes, interactions with CNS depressants
Tizanidine	Central α-2 receptor agonist	2–4 mg PO 3 times daily Increase as tolerated up to maximum dose of 36 mg daily Caution in renal or hepatic impairment; dose adjustments necessary	Hypotension, mild LFT elevation, and transient withdrawal syndrome with abrupt discontinuation
Diazepam	GABA-A receptor agonist	2 mg PO 2–3 times daily Contraindicated in hepatic impairment	Sedation, potential for dependence, withdrawal syndromes with abrupt discontinuation, interaction with CNS depressants
Cyclobenzaprine	Centrally acting 5HT2 receptor antagonist	5 mg PO 3 times daily Can be increased to 7.5 or 10 mg PO 3 times daily for up to 3 wk Use avoided in hepatic impairment, elderly patients. Long-term use not recommended	Anticholinergic effects including dizziness, dry mouth, visual disturbances, ocular hypertension, constipation, urinary retention, cardiac conduction disturbances

3. **Lidocaine (IV).** Meta-analyses of IV lidocaine infusion demonstrate decreased morphine consumption in both open and laparoscopic abdominal surgery. In addition, this review found moderate decreases in pain at both rest and with movement, time to first flatus and bowel movement (7 and 12 hours, respectively), as well as hospital stay. Proposed mechanisms suggest that lidocaine exerts its effects not only through sodium channel blockade but also through interactions with inflammatory signaling cascades and inhibition of excitatory responses in wide dynamic range neurons. Additional studies have shown benefits in reducing opioid consumption in the ambulatory surgery setting and in thoracic surgery patients who are not candidates for neuraxial anesthesia. Of note, although lidocaine did not show remarkable differences in opioid consumption in the perioperative setting in breast surgery, patients had a lower rate of chronic pain at 3 and 6 months, respectively. Similar studies in spine surgery show a decrease in postoperative pain 1 and 3 months after complex spine

surgery. Lidocaine infusions can also be continued postoperatively for inpatient management of pain in conjunction with interdisciplinary support between pain service anesthesiologists, surgeons, and nursing staff, to ensure appropriate monitoring for signs of lidocaine toxicity. Intralipid emulsion should be readily available if lidocaine infusions are used. At our institution, the acute pain service is routinely consulted on these patients, and nurses are given specific instructions for monitoring patients and on how to reach the service at any time.

C. Specific pain treatment modalities used in the postoperative setting

1. **PCA** utilizes patient self-administration of opioid analgesia via a patient-activated infusion device. This method for delivering analgesics has evolved with the introduction of computer-controlled, programmable infusion pumps. The PCA paradigm holds that the timely administration of small intermittent doses of analgesics will allow maintenance of optimal plasma drug concentration while minimizing side effects and periods of poor analgesia associated with intermittent IV or IM administration. Typical PCA devices can be programmed to deliver a specified dose of opioid and then "lockout" further administration for a specified interval. Guidelines for PCA administration of common opioid analgesics are shown in **Table 38.7**. PCA provides superior analgesia in many settings where hospitalized patients experience acute pain. Patients are very accepting of this technology and are typically quite satisfied with the close degree of control of pain that PCA allows. The addition of a basal infusion to the PCA dosing regimen for opioid-tolerant patients is generally not recommended. Routinely including a basal infusion does not improve analgesia but increases the total opioid dose used and the frequency of opioid-related side effects.

    a. **Advantages** of PCA. PCA allows each patient to control their own pain relief, provides for rapid administration of analgesic immediately on patient request, has a high degree of patient acceptance and satisfaction, and reduces total opioid dose and related side effects.

    b. **Disadvantages** of PCA. PCA requires the patient's ability to understand and follow directions, requires enough mobility to utilize the PCA option, requires availability of specific infusion pumps, and is subject to programming errors that can cause overdosing or underdosing.

2. **Neuraxial analgesia.** In this section, we will focus on the practical aspects of using neuraxial techniques to provide postoperative analgesia. The combined use of thoracic epidural analgesia with general anesthesia

TABLE 38.7 Guidelines for Opioid Administration via IV PCA

Drug (Concentration)	Typical Demand Dose (Range)	Typical Lockout Interval (Range)
Morphine (10 mg/mL)	1 mg (0.5–3 mg)	10 min (5–12 min)
Meperidine[a] (10 mg/mL)	10 mg (5–30 mg)	10 min (5–12 min)
Fentanyl (50 µg/mL)	10 µg (10–20 µg)	10 min (5–10 min)
Hydromorphone (1 mg/mL)	0.2 mg (0.1–0.5 mg)	10 min (5–10 min)

[a]Use of meperidine has diminished, as this agent has an active metabolite, normeperidine, which can accumulate and lead to central nervous system excitation and seizures at very high doses.

(when compared with **general anesthesia** with IV opioids) has demonstrated many advantages for abdominal and thoracic surgery including decreased length of hospitalization, improved postoperative pain control with less sedation, improved respiratory function, accelerated recovery of bowel function, improved lower-extremity blood flow, and reduced stress response. In addition, the use of thoracic epidurals has shown to decrease mortality in elderly thoracic trauma patients as compared with parenteral medications in the setting of two or more rib fractures. If neuraxial analgesia is contraindicated, erector spinae plane, serratus anterior, or paravertebral blocks can provide regional analgesia in patients at risk for respiratory failure from rib fractures.

a. **Intrathecal opioids** can provide prolonged analgesia after a single injection. When a surgical procedure is to be carried out using spinal anesthesia, the addition of an opioid to the local anesthetic serves as a practical and effective means for improving postoperative analgesia. The technique is limited by the frequency of side effects at higher doses and the inability to provide complete analgesia for more extensive and painful procedures. There are two general classes of opioids used for spinal analgesia: those that are hydrophilic (eg, morphine) and those that are lipophilic (eg, fentanyl and sufentanil).

  1. Hydrophilic opioids are slower in onset (peak analgesic effect occurs between 20 and 60 minutes) but persist at significant levels within the CSF for prolonged periods of time. The prototypic hydrophilic agent is morphine. Although it produces prolonged analgesia, it has also been associated with a small incidence of delayed respiratory depression occurring as late as 18 to 20 hours after administration. This is believed to be due to the persistence of significant levels of the drug within the CSF for up to 24 hours and the rostral spread of the drug within the CSF. Morphine 0.1 to 0.3 mg can provide analgesia for up to 8 to 24 hours; however, patients should remain hospitalized and observed periodically to detect and promptly treat delayed respiratory depression with this agent. The depression of ventilation can be difficult to detect because patients may demonstrate a relatively normal respiratory rate; however, hypoxemia detected by pulse oximetry, $PaCO_2$ (with bimodal peak of approximately 6 and 18 hours) detected by blood gas, and clinically depressed level of consciousness can point to undesired respiratory effects.

  2. Lipophilic opioids have a rapid onset (peak analgesic effect within 5 to 10 minutes), greater systemic absorption, and a short duration of analgesic action (2 to 4 hours). Delayed respiratory depression has not been observed with the lipophilic opioids. Fentanyl 10 to 25 µg or, less commonly, sufentanil 2.5 to 10 µg is often combined with small doses of local anesthetic to provide surgical anesthesia and postoperative analgesia for outpatient surgery.

b. **Epidural opioids.** Opioid analgesics also provide effective analgesia when administered into the epidural space. They can be administered as single-bolus injections, but it is far more common to place a catheter and administer combinations of opioid and low-dose local anesthetic to provide for continuous analgesia following surgery. It is imperative to understand the dermatomal extent of analgesia that can be expected from each agent and to place the injection at or near the midpoint of the dermatomal location of the surgical incision.

1. Hydrophilic agents such as morphine or hydromorphone can be placed in the lumbar region and still provide analgesia for incisions that extend to the thoracic region, whereas fentanyl will not spread to the same extent.
2. Local anesthetics provide analgesia only within the dermatomes adjacent to the site of injection. When administering combined opioid and local anesthetic infusions via an epidural catheter, we suggest an initial bolus to establish analgesia, prior to starting an infusion.

c. **Continuous epidural infusion and patient-controlled epidural analgesia** (PCEA). Continuous epidural infusions of opioids or opioid–local anesthetic combinations result in fewer fluctuations in the concentration of the analgesic drug and allows for patient-controlled supplementation via PCEA using programmable infusion pumps identical to those used for IV PCA. In contrast to the IV PCA, when using PCEA, the continuous infusion provides most of the analgesia, and small intermittent patient-administered doses are used to supplement its effect. There is evidence that patients can safely receive epidural opioids while on the regular hospital ward, provided that an anesthesiology-based acute pain service is responsible for all adjustments of analgesic and sedative medications.

d. **Adverse effects** associated with neuraxial opioid administration including sedation, pruritus, nausea, and vomiting, and urinary retention are common in patients receiving epidural or intrathecal opioids. Standing orders should be in place for addressing these common, minor side effects. Suggested standing orders for management of common side effects associated with neuraxial opioid administration are shown in **Table 38.8**.

e. Treatment of **inadequate analgesia** in patients receiving continuous epidural infusions requires a systematic approach. A member of the acute pain service should be immediately available to assess the patient and determine the cause for inadequate analgesia. A common algorithm for responding to inadequate analgesia in patients receiving epidural analgesia is shown in **Table 38.9**. Daily

Pharmacologic Management of Common Side Effects Associated With Neuraxial Opioid Administration

Adverse Effect	Standing Orders for Treatment
Nausea	• Ondansetron 1–4 mg IV or dolasetron 12.5 mg IV • Nalbuphine 1–3 mg IV or butorphanol 0.25–0.5 mg IV every 4 h as needed
Pruritus	• Diphenhydramine 25–50 mg IV every 4 h as needed • Nalbuphine 1–3 mg IV or butorphanol 0.25–0.5 mg IV every 4 h as needed
Urinary retention	• Keep indwelling urinary catheter in place until discontinuation of the epidural analgesia
Sedation or respiratory depression	• Notify acute pain service immediately, for respiratory rate less than 6/min • Place supplemental oxygen 4 L/min via nasal cannula • Administer naloxone 0.4 mg IV

Table 38.9 Suggested Management of Inadequate Analgesia in Patients Receiving Continuous Epidural Analgesia

1. Assess the patient directly at the bedside to determine the cause for inadequate analgesia. If the patient is unable to respond in a timely fashion, consider alternate means for providing analgesia (eg, order a one-time IV dose of opioid by telephone; consider discontinuing epidural infusion and beginning IV PCA).
2. Examine the patient for signs of a unilateral block or a dislodged or disconnected epidural catheter.
3. Administer a bolus dose of the opioid or opioid–local anesthetic combination in use for continuous infusion. Choose the dose based on the severity of pain and use between ½ and 1 h worth of the medication (eg, 4- to 8-mL bolus of fentanyl 4 μg/mL/bupivacaine 0.0625% in a patient receiving 8 mL/h).
4. If there is no improvement in pain relief within 20–30 min, consider test dosing the epidural catheter with 10 mL of 2% lidocaine. *Do not* administer a test dose unless the patient can be attended continuously and monitored with blood pressure checks at least every 5 min for 20 min after the bolus is given. Means for treating hypotension must be readily available (IV access and ready availability of a vasopressor such as ephedrine or phenylephrine).
5. If no sensory or motor block appears within 20 min, replace or discontinue epidural catheter and begin an alternate means for providing analgesia (eg, IV PCA).
6. If a bilateral sensory or motor block develops, readminister an epidural bolus of the medication in use for continuous infusion and increase the epidural infusion rate. Be alert for causes of inadequate analgesia (eg, a lumbar epidural catheter in use for pain following thoracotomy). Consider changing the opioid in use if the catheter location is suboptimal or there is an extensive incision.

management of the patient receiving epidural analgesia requires a systematic approach aimed at assuring safe and effective pain treatment. A suggested daily checklist that will guide patient management is shown in **Table 38.10**.

  f. **Complications** associated with epidural analgesia. Although the goal of epidural analgesia is to provide pain relief and minimize side effects, there are several serious complications associated with its use.

Table 38.10 Suggested Daily Checklist for Daily Management of Patients Receiving Epidural Analgesia

1. Examine the nursing record for adjustments and supplemental analgesics as well as medications for side effects. Check vital signs for evidence of persistent fever or hypotension.
2. Assess for adequate analgesia and side effects by directly questioning the patient. Be alert for sedation, pruritus, nausea and vomiting, and urinary retention.
3. Examine the patient to detect signs of unilateral block or excessive sensory or motor block.
4. Examine the epidural catheter site for signs of infection and the presence of an intact occlusive dressing.
5. Interrogate the infusion pump to assess the patient's use of supplemental doses, assure that it is properly programmed. Examine the infusion bag directly to be certain the medication ordered is what the patient is receiving.
6. Document your interaction in detail in the patient's chart and order any changes needed. Include when you anticipate changing or discontinuing therapy.

1. Catheter migration into the intrathecal space can lead to increasing levels of sensory block and total spinal anesthesia.
2. Indwelling epidural catheters can become infected directly at the skin entry site or through hematogenous seeding of the catheter tip within the epidural space. Superficial site infection is common and rarely needs treatment beyond the removal of the catheter. Extension of a superficial infection or direct seeding of the catheter tip to produce an epidural abscess is rare.
3. Epidural hematoma formation is uncommon but the risk is higher in patients receiving systemic anticoagulants. Both epidural abscess and hematoma present with worsening back pain and neurologic deficit (urinary retention and sensory and motor loss in the lower extremities).

3. **Continuous peripheral nerve blocks** using catheters are commonly used in inpatient and ambulatory settings. The focus in this chapter is to outline a strategy for the management of continuous nerve catheters in the postoperative period. The availability of lightweight and sophisticated infusion pumps has greatly facilitated the use of continuous perineural infusions of local anesthetics. Advances in technology, integration of ultrasound use, and the emergence of the literature supporting continuous perineural infusions for improved postoperative analgesia and recovery have led to the widespread use of continuous perineural infusions of local anesthetics.

   a. **Specific indications** for continuous peripheral nerve blocks vary in terms of surgical site. For example, femoral and **popliteal** fossa nerve catheters **are commonly used** following below-the-knee amputations. **Similarly**, brachial plexus blocks using continuous infusion have also proven effective for surgery on the shoulder and upper extremity.

   b. **Choice of drug**, concentration, and infusion rate will depend on the target nerve or plexus, the surgical procedure, as well as the individual patient's response. Infusion rates can be fixed or variable, including the possibility of a bolus (patient-controlled regional anesthesia). Continuous peripheral nerve blocks are carried out by infusing local anesthetic alone (for example, 0.1% bupivacaine or 0.2% ropivacaine) at a rate of 5 to 10 mL/h.

   c. **Management of continuous peripheral nerve catheters.** Since the extremity will have decreased sensitivity for the duration of the block, care should be taken to prevent injury to exposed nerves. A properly fitted sling, brace, and thorough patient education are paramount to provide adequate protection. Given the high cumulative dose of local anesthetic, caution should be used in patients with renal failure and the drug should be avoided in those with hepatic failure. Daily follow-up of hospitalized patients with a perineural catheter should include close attention to specific aspects shown in **Table 38.11**.

   d. **Use of perineural catheters in ambulatory patients.** Perineural catheters have been successfully employed in the ambulatory care setting. This requires careful patient selection, comprehensive patient education, and the implementation of a protocol for patient follow-up. Patient education should involve the patient and the patient's caregiver and include instructions on how to operate the pump, signs of catheter-related complications (such as infection, migration, and leak), and signs of local anesthetic toxicity. Patients should be aware of the expected time for resolution of the block and should understand the necessity to abstain from driving or operating machinery. A plan for breakthrough pain management should be in place. Daily

Table 38.11 Checklist for Daily Follow-Up of Patients With Perineural Catheters

1. Inspect the catheter insertion site to assess for signs of infection, leaks, and catheter dislocation.
2. Assure that ongoing analgesia is adequate.
3. Assess the patient for signs of excessive motor and/or sensory block.
4. Assess the patient for signs or symptoms of local anesthetic toxicity (local anesthetic toxicity is rare in the context of continuous perineural infusion, but the daily dose and any associated side effects should be assessed daily).

follow-up should be arranged, and provisions for immediate contact with an anesthesiologist should be available.

D. Acute pain management in patients with opioid tolerance or dependence

1. Patients with opioid tolerance or dependence represent a unique challenge to the anesthesiologist in the perioperative period. In contrast to the term addiction, dependence is defined by the World Health Organization as a cluster of physiologic, behavioral, and cognitive phenomena in which the overwhelming desire and use of a substance, such as an opioid, takes on higher priority than other behaviors that once had value. Tolerance may or may not be present.
2. **Perioperative management of patients with opioid tolerance or a history of opioid dependence.** Concepts to consider when managing patients who have been taking large doses of opioids for chronic pain and those with current or previous history of opioid use disorder are shown in **Table 38.12**. Communication with the patient's prescribing physician is recommended.

Table 38.12 Managing Patients With Opioid Tolerance or With Current or Previous Dependence

Consider use of regional anesthesia (spinal opioids and epidural infusions) to improve analgesia and minimize systemic opioid effects.

Use adjunctive analgesics whenever possible to reduce total opioid requirements (eg, NSAIDs, ketamine).

Administer opioids liberally to control pain in the immediate postoperative period. *Do not* attempt to limit opioid dose or wean opioid analgesics in the immediate postoperative period. Those with significant tolerance will probably require higher-than-average doses to control acute pain.

Use preoperative opioid doses as a baseline requirement and administer additional doses beyond this to control acute pain. This baseline requirement can be administered by continuing the preoperative long-acting opioid in addition to the use of a PCA.

Consider consultation with a substance abuse specialist during hospitalization for those with ongoing opioid abuse or a history of addiction.

Closely coordinate (communicate) the pain management with the patient's primary care provider or prescribing provider before hospital discharge. Although acute escalation in the opioid requirement is often necessary in the perioperative period, a plan for weaning the opioids to their previous levels should be established *before* the patient is discharged from the hospital.

a. **Managing acute pain in patients on buprenorphine maintenance therapy.** Buprenorphine, a semisynthetic, potent, and long-acting opioid, has been introduced for ambulatory treatment of patients with opioid dependence. It is a high-affinity partial agonist at the μ-opioid receptor and antagonist at the μ-opioid receptor that exhibits a plateau effect for euphoria and respiratory depression at higher doses. When prescribed in the outpatient setting, buprenorphine is often mixed with naloxone (Suboxone) to be taken sublingually. Naloxone has poor bioavailability after oral and sublingual administration; however, if the drug combination is administered intravenously in an attempt to abuse, naloxone is present in high-enough concentrations to precipitate acute withdrawal symptoms in opioid-dependent patients. The addition of naloxone aims at limiting both abuse and diversion of the drug. Buprenorphine alone (Subutex) is used for initial testing prior to initiating a buprenorphine therapy–based maintenance regimen in the opioid-addicted patient. Subutex has also gained some popularity for use in the treatment of chronic pain, owing to its limited abuse potential and significant efficacy as an analgesic agent. In addition to the general principles for managing patients with opioid tolerance or addiction discussed above, specific considerations for the patient receiving buprenorphine are shown in **Table 38.13**.
b. **Managing acute pain in patients on methadone maintenance therapy.** Methadone, a synthetic mixed μ-opioid and δ-receptor agonist, with

Table 38.13 Perioperative Considerations for the Patient Receiving Long-Term Buprenorphine Treatment

For patients undergoing elective surgery, data from clinical studies suggest a possible synergistic and additive effect between buprenorphine at low to moderate analgesic doses (8–12 mg SL or less) and full μ-opioid receptor agonists. Our institutional policy is as follows: If a patient is on 8 mg or less per day, the regimen should be continued. For surgeries in which minimal to mild postoperative pain is expected, home dose buprenorphine is recommended to be continued. For those in which moderate to severe pain is expected, the management depends on the buprenorphine dose. For those managed on 16-mg buprenorphine or less, it is recommended to continue the home dose until the day before surgery, and to continue patients on a regimen of 8 mg daily plus additional full opioid agonists and adjunctive pain medications as needed to manage pain postoperatively. Once postoperative pain subsides, patients can resume their home dose. For those managed on greater than 16 mg of buprenorphine, it is recommended that patients titrate down their therapy over time with the goal of 16 mg on the day before surgery with the assistance of the physician responsible for prescribing their opioid agonist therapy. Patients are then maintained on 8 mg daily plus full opioid agonists as needed until the period of acute pain resolves and the home regimen can be reinstated after full agonists are tapered off. Discontinuation of buprenorphine is not recommended as it increases risk of illicit opioid use in persons with opioid use disorder and can complicate perioperative pain management and restarting home buprenorphine dose.

For patient requiring urgent or emergent surgery or when prior conversion to a full agonist is not feasible, a short-acting full agonist such as fentanyl can be titrated to effect. As is the case for patients maintained with other opioid agonists, higher-than-usual doses to achieve adequate analgesia are likely to be required. The appropriate dose of fentanyl in a patient taking buprenorphine might also be higher because of the strong affinity of buprenorphine for the μ receptor.

NMDA receptor antagonist and serotonin norepinephrine reuptake inhibitor activity, has been used in the treatment of opioid-dependent patients for over 60 years and has found increasing applications in the treatment of cancer-related pain, neuropathic pain, and other chronic pain states. Its long half-life with a biphasic elimination profile exerts an effect both on pain control (8 to 12 hours) and on withdrawal (30 to 60 hours). However, variable oral bioavailability (40% to 99%), variable hepatic elimination, and the phenomena of incomplete cross tolerance, or lack of tolerance to the effects of opioids of other classes, make conversion from oral to IV formulations and calculating equianalgesic doses very challenging. Considering these attributes and its long half-life, titration to reach steady-state levels over days to weeks should only be done with assistance of a pain specialist owing to the risk of delayed respiratory depression. Furthermore, pretreatment EKG should be checked in any patient initiated or titrated on methadone, as QT_C prolongation remains a significant concern. Patients who present for surgery should continue their baseline dose methadone on the morning of surgery, and pain should be managed proactively and aggressively in the perioperative period. The general principles for managing patients with opioid tolerance or addiction discussed above apply to these patients as well.

c. **Managing acute pain in patients on naltrexone.** Naltrexone, a semisynthetic opioid antagonist is a competitive antagonist at the μ-opioid receptor and partial agonist at the κ-opioid receptor which is used to treat alcohol use disorder and opioid use disorder. It comes in two forms, daily oral tablets, or monthly IM formulations. For elective surgery, it is recommended to hold the oral form for 72 hours prior to surgery, and the IM form for 4 weeks prior to surgery. Patients should not take opioids 7 to 10 days prior to restarting naltrexone after surgery.

III. MULTIMODAL ANALGESIA

Multimodal analgesia is the incorporation of multiple therapies with different targets for a patient. The goal is to achieve adequate analgesia, reduce opioid requirements and minimize side effects. Different classes of medications and regional or neuraxial analgesia are essential to achieve multimodal analgesia, as long as the patient does not have any contraindications. Complementary and alternative medicine (CAM) can also be incorporated to reduce pain perioperatively, especially if the patient incorporates these methods into their lifestyle preoperatively. Multimodal analgesia is especially helpful in patients who take methadone, buprenorphine, and naltrexone as these patients are more tolerant to opioid medications, more susceptible to opioid side effects, and may have increased pain requirements.

IV. COMPLEMENTARY AND ALTERNATIVE MEDICINE IN PAIN MANAGEMENT

CAM encompasses a broad range of therapeutic modalities that are often integrated into western medicine in the management of chronic conditions, including, but not limited to, pain.

A. Definitions of CAM
1. Practices that are not accepted as correct or in conformity with the beliefs of the dominant group of medical practitioners in a society.
2. Complementary practices are those that are used in conjunction with other medical practices, while alternative medicine is used in place of conventional medical practices.

B. **Categories of CAM practices.** The National Center for Complementary and Integrative Health, a subdivision of the National Institutes of Health, has grouped CAM practices into several major subdivisions:
   1. **Mind–body interventions** use techniques to facilitate the mind's ability to affect bodily functions. Examples include hypnosis, mindfulness meditation, art therapy, and music medicine and therapy.
   2. **Natural products** refer to products such as herbs, botanicals, probiotics, and special diets designed to promote wellness and manage symptoms.
   3. **Alternative medicine** includes homeopathic medicine, Ayurvedic medicine, traditional Chinese medicine (acupuncture, massage, herbs), and other systems of belief typically used in place of conventional medicine.
   4. **Manipulative therapies** include chiropractic manipulation, osteopathic manipulation, and massage.
   5. **Energy- and biofield-based therapies** include qi gong and reiki, among other therapies that purport to direct healing by manipulating a body's perceived energy.

C. **Perioperative acupuncture**
   1. **Definition. Acupuncture** involves the insertion of fine needles into specific points on the body to produce therapeutic results. The analgesic effects of acupuncture have been attributed to the presynaptic release of enkephalins and dynorphin along the afferent fibers of the spinothalamic tract, the stimulation of norepinephrine and serotonin release in midbrain structures and in the periaqueductal gray matter to dampen nociceptive signaling, and the stimulation of the hypothalamus pituitary axis to effect systemic ACTH and endorphin release.
   2. **Preoperative use.** Numerous studies using preoperative acupuncture, including ear points, show significant relaxation. In two double-blinded studies, preoperative auricular acupuncture reduced anxiety up to 48 hours compared with sham acupuncture. This reduction in anxiety correlates with less pain and analgesic consumption postoperatively. Acupuncture may complement the use of preoperative anxiolytics and has also been shown in a few studies to reduce the incidence of postoperative nausea and vomiting.
   3. **Intraoperative use.** Intraoperative acupuncture does not provide muscle relaxation, suppress autonomic reflexes, or provide unconsciousness. Available data show that acupuncture has little or no effect on anesthetic requirements—in some studies, it slightly increased anesthetic requirements.
   4. **Postoperative use.** Studies regarding the effect of acupuncture on postoperative pain requirements remain conflicting and controversial, partially in part due to variances in study design, patient population, practitioner experience level, and acupuncture methods. However, several studies do reveal a substantial reduction in postoperative opioid consumption. In one study, acupuncture performed 20 minutes prior to induction reduced 24-hour morphine consumption by PCA after total abdominal hysterectomy. Other studies show similar opioid-reducing effects in abdominal surgery, in addition to significant decreases in serum plasma cortisol levels in the first 24 hours postoperatively.

D. **Hypnosis**
   1. **Definition.** Hypnosis involves the induction of a state of mind that allows for a heightened receptivity to suggestion. It is generally a state of relaxation in which critical thought is bypassed. The mechanism by which hypnosis can contribute to analgesia is thought to be mediated by a perceptual dissociation of the sensory and affective components of the pain experience.

2. **Mechanism.** Hypnosis influences the affective (cognitive/evaluative) component of pain. Functional magnetic resonance imaging and positron emission tomography scans during hypnosis suggest that this affective processing of pain occurs in part in areas of the anterior cingulate gyrus, modulating pain unpleasantness without significant changes in perceived intensity encoded by activity in the primary and secondary somatosensory cortices.
3. **Possible applications.** Many studies focus on the use of hypnosis to alleviate perioperative pain, anxiety, and nausea. Although findings vary, the use of preoperative hypnotic suggestion has often been found to reduce emesis and narcotic requirements postoperatively. Children are often receptive to hypnosis-guided imagery. Hypno-analgesia has emerged as a combination of hypnotic techniques with pharmacologic analgesics and sedation. In one study of 241 patients undergoing hypnosis as compared with standard IV conscious sedation and focused attention during percutaneous vascular and renal procedures, hypnosis showed the greatest reduction in intraoperative anxiety and the least pain over procedure time, as well as a lessened need for IV anxiolytics and opioid medications. It has been used effectively for dressing changes in burn patients, with the concurrent suggestions of improved appetite and nutrition. Positive suggestions to anesthetized patients may also promote fewer postoperative complications.

E. Mindfulness meditation
1. **Definition.** A "nonelaborative, nonjudgmental awareness of the present moment experience," the recognition of such experiences as fleeting, and a resultant lack of emotional or cognitive reactions to such.
2. **Mechanism.** Although studies of the interplay between meditative practices and pain produced mixed results, they suggest that cognitive modulation reduces the influence of expectation and catastrophizing in the processing of painful stimuli in a manner that develops over time and experience. In one study, functional and structural MRI in experienced Zen meditation practitioners have exhibited increased activation in areas associated with sensory processing of pain, but reduced activity in the amygdala, caudate, and hippocampus suggesting decreased emotional reactivity to and appraisal of painful stimuli despite increased attention to such stimuli. Meditation's mechanism appears to not involve endogenous opioids in the perceived reduction of pain. In a randomized, double-blind study conducted in 2016 where 78 participants separated into mindfulness meditation and control groups were subjected to a noxious stimulus and given naloxone, mindfulness meditation produced significantly greater reductions in pain intensity and unpleasantness than the control groups in a manner that could not be reversed with naloxone, providing further support for the use of meditation as an adjunct to manage chronic pain.
3. **Preoperative use.** Studies are currently being conducted regarding the role of meditation in postoperative neurocognitive outcomes and pain as part of a "prehabilitation" program prior to cardiac surgery.
4. **Postoperative use.** Although a recent study examining postoperative pain scores in 52 patients receiving mindfulness meditation therapy via virtual reality (VR) headsets was underpowered to show any significance in narcotic utilization as compared with control, it highlights the potential for meditation to be utilized in postoperative period.

F. Music medicine and music therapy
1. **Definitions. Music medicine** is the practice of passive listening to prerecorded music; it is generally administered by physicians and nurses.

Music therapy is the application of an individualized music intervention and therapeutic process based on music preferences administered by a trained music therapist.
  2. **Preoperative use.** Music interventions offer a safe and inexpensive nonpharmacologic intervention for reduction of preoperative stress and anxiety that may complement the effect of other anxiolytics.
  3. **Intraoperative use.** Several small studies show music interventions in patients undergoing neuraxial anesthesia for childbirth and for total knee replacement significantly decreased the need for intraoperative sedatives.
  4. **Postoperative use.** Patients report increased satisfaction regarding their care and the postanesthesia care unit recovery period.
G. **Virtual reality (VR)**
  1. **Definitions.** VR is a fully immersive, engaging experience that incorporates a head-mounted display with an audio source and another device to allow for manipulation of a computer-generated environment, with applications in the attenuation and modulation of acute pain as well as procedural anxiety. The effectiveness of VR in reducing the intensity of perceived pain may stem from the engaging attention away from the painful stimulus using multisensory distraction, reflecting both gate control and multiple resources theories of pain perception.
  2. **Perioperative use.** It has been studied as a nonpharmacologic, noninvasive adjunct to pain medications in the management of acute burn patients, particularly in pediatric patients. Small studies have shown reductions in pain and anxiety scores during physiotherapy and wound dressing changes by various pain scales when used in conjunction with opioid pain medication as compared with medications alone. Other applications have included use of VR for unpleasant routine medical procedures such as phlebotomy, IV insertion, port access, and lumbar puncture as well as an adjunct to regional anesthesia and light sedation in orthopedic procedures.

ACKNOWLEDGMENT

We gratefully acknowledge the contributions of previous edition author, Gloria Nadayil Berchmans, as portions of those chapters have been retained in this revision.

Suggested Readings

Alford DP, Compton P, Samet JH. Acute pain management for patients receiving maintenance methadone or buprenorphine therapy. *Ann Intern Med*. 2006;144(2):127–134.

Angst MS, Clark JD. Opioid-induced hyperalgesia: A qualitative systematic review. *Anesthesiology*. 2006;104(3):570–587.

Astin JA. Why patients use alternative medicine: Results of a national study. *J Am Med Assoc*. 1998;279(19):1548–1553.

Blaudszun G, Lysakowski C, Elia N, Tramèr MR. Effect of perioperative systemic α2 agonists on postoperative morphine consumption and pain intensity: Systematic review and meta-analysis of randomized controlled trials. *Anesthesiology*. 2012;116(6):1312–1322.

Boezaart AP. Perineural infusion of local anesthetics. *Anesthesiology*. 2006;104(4):872–880.

Chernyak GV, Sessler DI. Perioperative acupuncture and related techniques. *Anesthesiology*. 2005;102(5):1031–1049.

Gobble RM, Hoang HLT, Kachniarz B, Orgill DP. Ketorolac does not increase perioperative bleeding: a meta-analysis of randomized controlled trials. *Plast Reconstr Surg*. 2014;133(3):741–755.

Grant JA, Rainville P. Pain sensitivity and analgesic effects of mindful states in Zen meditators: a cross sectional study. *Psychosom Med*. 2009;71(1):106–114.

Haisley KR, Straw OJ, Müller DT, et al. Feasibility of implementing a virtual reality program as an adjuvant tool for peri-operative pain control; results of a randomized controlled trial in minimally invasive foregut surgery. *Compl Ther Med*. 2020;49:102356.

Harrison TK, Howard K, Aggarwal AK, Lembke A. Perioperative considerations for the patient with opioid use disorder on buprenorphine, methadone, or naltrexone maintenance therapy. *Anesthesiology Clinics*. 2018;36(3):345–359

Ilfeld BM, Enneking FK. Continuous peripheral nerve blocks at home: a review. *Anesth Analg*. 2005;100(6):1822–1833.

Joshi GP, Gertler R, Fricker R. Cardiovascular thromboembolic adverse effects associated with cyclooxygenase-2 selective inhibitors and nonselective antiinflammatory drugs. *Anesth Analg*. 2007;105(6):1793–1804.

Lang EV, Benotsch EG, Fick LJ, et al. Adjunctive non-pharmocological analgesia for invasive medical procedures: a randomized trial. *Lancet*. 2000;355(9214):1486–1490.

Manion SC, Brennan TJ. Thoracic epidural analgesia and acute pain management. *Anesthesiology*. 2011;115(1):181–188.

Mitra S, Sinatra RS. Perioperative management of acute pain in the opioid-dependent patient. *Anesthesiology*. 2004;101(1):212–227.

Quaye AN, Zhang Y. Perioperative management of buprenorphine: solving the conundrum. *Pain Med*. 2019;20(7):1395–1408.

Rainville P, Duncan GH, Price DD, Carrier B, Bushnell MC. Pain affect encoded in human anterior cingulate but not somatosensory cortex. *Science*. 1997;277(5328):968–971.

Rathmell JP, Lair TR, Nauman B. The role of intrathecal drugs in the treatment of acute pain. *Anesth Analg*. 2005;101(5 suppl):S30–S43.

Rathmell JP, Neal JM, Viscomi CM. *Regional Anesthesia. The Requisites in Anesthesiology*. Elsevier Mosby; 2004.

Stewart JH. Hypnosis in contemporary medicine (review). *Mayo Clin Proc*. 2005;80(4):511–524.

Straube S, Derry S, Moore RA, Wiffen PJ, McQuay HJ, et al. Single dose oral gabapentin for established acute postoperative pain in adults. *Cochrane Database Syst Rev*. 2010;2010(5):CD008183.

Sun Y, Li T, Wang N, Yun Y, Gan TJ. Perioperative systemic lidocaine for postoperative analgesia and recovery after abdominal surgery: a meta-analysis of randomized controlled trials. *Dis Colon Rectum*. 2012;55(11):1183–1194.

Wobst AH. Hypnosis and surgery: past, present, and future. *Anesth Analg*. 2007;104(5):1199–1208.

Zhang Y, Peck K, Spalding M, Jones BG, Cook RL. Discrepancy between patients' use of and health providers' familiarity with CAM. *Patient Educ Couns*. 2012;89(3):399–404.

39 Adult, Pediatric, and Newborn Resuscitation

John H. Nichols and Christopher Di Capua

I. OVERVIEW

Circulatory collapse and the need for cardiopulmonary resuscitation (CPR) is one of the more stressful crises that can occur in the operating room (OR). In such an emergency, it is the responsibility of the anesthesiologist to swiftly recognize and intervene to ensure recovery of spontaneous circulation (ROSC) without further injury. Success requires the necessary reflexive clinical skills, awareness of surrounding equipment, understanding of reversible etiologies, appropriate task delegation, and a composed demeanor. Fortunately, intraoperative cardiac arrest in noncardiac surgery is rare (1 to 7 cases per 10,000, ~40% 30-day survival) and an OR serves as an almost ideal location for such an event given its advanced monitoring, immediate medication availability, proximity to invasive line equipment, airway management tools, and pacemaking/defibrillation equipment. In addition, timely access to advanced imaging and treatment modalities such as transthoracic and transesophageal echocardiography, extracorporeal membrane oxygenation (ECMO), and cardiac catheterization (eg, emergent coronary stent, thrombectomy, intra-aortic balloon pump) enhances the likelihood of a successful outcome.

In addition to the availability of physical resources, cognitive aids can help ensure successful resuscitation. The recent development of easily consulted emergency manuals within reach of the anesthesiologist has greatly facilitated accurate recall of critical resuscitation management steps during highly stressful situations. MGH includes an emergency manual adopted from the Stanford Cognitive Aid Working Group in all of its anesthetizing locations. In addition, simulation of intraoperative code events has become more integrated into the training curriculums of MGH and other institutions, which provides a structured, supportive environment to rehearse decision making, enhance communication, and establish reflexive mental models. Together, simulation and easy access to emergency manuals promote a calm, quick adherence to optimal protocols during otherwise difficult circumstances.

Essential to the swift return of spontaneous circulation after sudden cardiac arrest (SCA) are defibrillation for ventricular fibrillation (VF) or pulseless ventricular tachycardia (VT); prompt delivery of effective, minimally interrupted chest compressions to maintain cerebral and cardiac perfusion; and maintenance of effective oxygenation/ventilation. Effective compressions deliver oxygen and energy substrates to the myocardium and increase the likelihood that a perfusing rhythm will return after defibrillation. Appropriate oxygenation and ventilation are critical as hypoxemia inhibits oxygen delivery while sustained hyperoxia following ROSC has been associated with increased mortality and poor neurologic outcomes. The most recent American Heart Association (AHA) guidelines recommend against hyperoxia in the postcardiac arrest period. Likewise, hypo/hypercarbia during CPR can create decreased cerebral perfusion and unwanted sympathetic surges, respectively. Excessive tidal volumes can also reduce venous return, which

TABLE 39.1 Classification System for Recommendation and Levels of Evidence

Class of Recommendation			Level of Evidence
I	Strongly recommended	A	High quality, >1 RCT or meta-analyses of high-quality RCTs
IIa	Moderate	B-R	Moderate quality from 1+ RCT or meta-analysis of moderate-quality RCTs
IIb	Weak	B-NR	Moderate quality without RCT
III (NB)	No benefit (Moderate)	C-LD	Limited data such as observational/registry studies
III (H)	Causes harm (Strong)	C-EO	Expert opinion

Note that the recommendation class and quality of evidence are separate, independently determined factors. For instance, a class I recommendation may not have an A quality.

RCT, randomized controlled trial.

inhibits cardiac output during CPR. CPR is more successful the earlier it is started; thus, prompt and clear communication with all team members about the emergency is essential. In the OR, the patient is often poorly positioned for CPR (prone/lateral/elevated) and may have open surgical sites requiring rapid packing. Quick recognition and communication will facilitate optimal positioning and preparation for effective CPR.

There is a tendency after delivering defibrillating shocks to watch the monitors or check pulses for return in cardiac output, but CPR should be resumed immediately after defibrillation as the myocardium has been depleted of oxygen and metabolic substrates and is stunned. When possible, early consideration for patients with presumably reversible causes of cardiac arrest should include alerting the hospital ECMO and emergency echocardiography teams in accordance with institutional capabilities and policy.

The management and algorithms that follow are derived from evidence-based guidelines established through systematic reviews by the AHA in collaboration with the International Liaison Committee on Resuscitation, which has switched to a continuous review process since the last edition of this book. This section is current with respect to the 2020 *AHA Guidelines for Cardiopulmonary Resuscitation and Emergency Cardiovascular Care* and its yearly supplements up to 2023 for adult and pediatric management, which incorporates basic life support (BLS), advanced cardiac life support (ACLS), and pediatric advanced life support (PALS), which includes neonatal resuscitation.

Table 39.1 lists the AHA classifications used for the strength of recommendation and the quality of evidence used to support most of the protocol interventions presented in this chapter. Note that the recommendation class and quality of evidence are independently established. When helpful, the AHA recommendation class and quality will be provided next to suggestions in the form of *Class/Evidence*.

II. CARDIAC ARREST
A. Diagnosis. The absence of a palpable pulse in a major peripheral artery (carotid, radial, or femoral) for >10 seconds in an unconscious, unmonitored patient, is diagnostic. Within the OR, monitoring equipment might

show a precipitous drop in end-tidal CO_2 (ETCO$_2$), loss of pulse oximetry waveform, a low or nondetectable noninvasive blood pressure, or a flattening and drop in the arterial pressure waveform. Nonperfusing cardiac rhythms on EKG include tachyarrhythmias such as VF and VT as well as nontachyarrhythmias such as asystole, pulseless electrical activity (PEA), or severe bradycardia.
- **B. Etiologies.** Commonly recognized causes of cardiac arrest, the five Hs and Ts, are:
  1. **H**ypovolemia.
  2. **H**ypoxemia.
  3. **H**ydrogen ion/acid-base disturbances.
  4. **H**yper/hypokalemia/electrolyte derangements (K, Ca, Mg).
  5. **H**ypothermia.
  6. **T**oxins (drug toxicity).
  7. **T**amponade (cardiac).
  8. **T**ension pneumothorax.
  9. **T**hrombosis (pulmonary embolus).
  10. **T**hrombosis (cardiac/myocardial infarction).
  11. Hypoglycemia (not in the "5 Hs and Ts," but a critical assessment).

  Within the OR, additional etiologies to consider are:

  1. Local anesthetic systemic toxicity.
  2. Neuraxial anesthesia causing severe sympathectomy.
  3. Anaphylaxis (eg, paralytics, antibiotics).
  4. Malignant hyperthermia.
  5. Excessive vagal tone during surgical manipulation or laparoscopy.
  6. Embolism of air, fat, amniotic fluid, or procedural cement.
  7. Excessive anesthetic.
  8. Coronary stent thrombosis (in setting of holding antiplatelet medication).
  9. Postreperfusion syndrome in liver transplantation.
- **C. Pathophysiology.** If CPR is not immediately started after cardiac arrest, the cessation of blood flow causes tissue hypoxia, anaerobic metabolism, accumulation of cellular wastes, depletion of ATP, and ion-gradient breakdown (eg, uncontrolled calcium flow into cells that is excitotoxic and may trigger apoptosis). Widespread anaerobic metabolism leads to a sudden, severe acidemia with effects including systemic vasodilation, pulmonary vasoconstriction, and decreased response to catecholamines. Neurologic injury can become irreversible in as little as 4 to 6 minutes of absent circulation. After restoration of cardiac output, patients can have ischemia reperfusion injury with the generation of reactive oxygen species, mitochondrial dysfunction, and an immune/inflammatory cascade for which targeted temperature management (formerly therapeutic hypothermia) may be beneficial. The cumulative effects of absent flow and reperfusion injury result in variable multiorgan damage and neurologic disability.
- **D. Epidemiology.** There are roughly 350,000 yearly out-of-hospital arrests in the United States, of which half are witnessed and only 1 in 10 survive to hospital discharge. Even fewer (~8.4%) survive with good functional status. Shockable rhythms (pulseless VT/VF) represent around 20% of the initial observed rhythms.

III. ADULT RESUSCITATION
- **A. BLS** refers to the skill set of CPR, activation of the emergency response system, and expedient use of an automated external defibrillator (AED). BLS certification is offered to the public and is required for health care

providers with variations in management suggestions based on level of training and comfort.

Any person found unresponsive or with absent or gasping/agonal breath sounds should be suspected to be in cardiac arrest (*I/C-LD*). Pulse checks by a health care provider in this setting should last at most 10 seconds (*I/C-LD*). If the person cannot be aroused, the AHA guidelines for CPR and emergency cardiac care stress immediate activation of the emergency response system for out-of-hospital arrests and initiation of chest compressions to provide **C**irculation prior to **A**irway management and **B**reathing, or **C-A-B**. This was changed from **A-B-C** in 2010 to emphasize the initial focus on restoring circulation based on survival studies.

The C-A-B sequence emphasizes circulation first to minimize delays in chest compressions associated with establishing a patent airway. Beginning with chest compressions may also increase likelihood that bystanders will perform CPR on persons who have suffered from SCA as lay persons may find airway management challenging and hesitate to initiate CPR. In fact, the guidelines changed in 2017 to emphasize that untrained lay rescuers may provide compression only CPR (*I/B-NR*), and dispatchers should offer compression-only CPR instructions (*I/C-LD*). Lay persons trained in CPR should still add rescue breaths when trained or able.

For lone rescuers, the public is taught the "phone first/phone fast" rule. For adults, children aged 8 years and older, and all children known to be at high risk for arrhythmias, the emergency medical system (911; EMS) should be activated (phone first) before attempts at resuscitation by a lone rescuer (*I/C-LD*). An initial resuscitation attempt followed by the activation of EMS ("phone fast") is indicated for children less than 8 years old and for all ages in cases of submersion or near drowning, arrest secondary to trauma, and drug overdose. Owing to the increased rate of opioid overdoses nationwide, the BLS Task Force suggests that CPR be started without delay in any unresponsive person who is not breathing normally, and that naloxone be administered by rescuers if there is suspicion that respiratory or circulatory arrest is opioid-related (*I/C-EO*).

1. **Circulation (chest compressions).** It is estimated that chest compressions can provide up to one-third of the normal cardiac output. To ensure sufficient circulation, especially coronary and cerebral flow, compressions should occupy a minimum 60% of the arrest event time (*IIb/C-LD*) with a target of 80% and minimal pauses between shocks (*I/C-LD*). The patient should be on a firm surface, preferably a backboard when possible, and flat with their head at the level of the thorax. This is especially true in an OR where the soft surgical table padding/gel absorbs energy from compressions, which can decrease their effectiveness. For a prone, intubated patient in the OR who cannot be quickly turned supine for CPR, one member can place a clenched fist between the subxiphoid area and the OR table with compressions over the corresponding region of the back (*IIb/C-LD*).

   Proper positioning involves placing the heel of the hand in the center of the patient's chest at the intermammary line with the heel of the other hand on top of the first so that the hands are overlapped and parallel (*IIa/B*). Shoulders can be positioned directly over the patient and elbows locked. The chest should depress a minimum of 2 inches in adults (*I/B-NR*) and at least one-third of the anterior–posterior chest diameter for pediatric patients (roughly 2 inches in children, 1.5 inches in infants) (*IIa/C-LD*). For children, single responders can use the heel of one or both hands (*IIb/C-LD*). In infants, single responders should use a two-finger technique, whereas the two-thumb encircling hands technique is used with multiple responders (*I/C-LD*).

The chest compression rate should be 100 to 120/min and allow for complete chest recoil by targeting equal compression and relaxation times (*IIb/C*). While rate and depth tend to err on the lower side, compressions quality can also suffer from being too deep or too fast, thus upper bounds of 2.4 inches for depth and 120 for rate were introduced. Given this notably small range of 2 to 2.4 inches (5 to 6 cm), compression feedback devices that optimize performance should be used when available (*IIb/B-R*).

The target compression–ventilation ratio is 30:2 for single responders with two breaths being delivered over less than 10 seconds (*IIa/B-R*). With two or more people, the 30:2 ratio is preserved, and providers should switch every 2 minutes (five cycles) in less than 5 seconds (*IIa/B*). In children, the compression–ventilation ratio is 15:2 when there are two rescuers to reflect the more respiratory driven arrest incidence. If an advanced airway such as an endotracheal tube (ETT) or laryngeal mask airway (LMA) is in place during two-rescuer CPR, ventilations should be given at a rate of 10 breaths/min simultaneously with compressions without pauses (IIb/C-LD).

There is growing evidence that $ETCO_2$ monitoring can be used to guide the delivery of effective chest compressions. While cutoff values have varied by study, it is generally accepted that an $ETCO_2$ <10 mm Hg during CPR is associated with poor outcome and >20 mm Hg has a stronger association with ROSC. As such, the AHA recommends $ETCO_2$ monitoring when feasible (IIb/C-LD).

Another described maneuver is the precordial "thump" whereby the rescuer slams the underside of their fist to the mid-sternum to depolarize the heart. This maneuver can be considered for monitored patients with unstable or pulseless VT if a defibrillator is not immediately available (*IIb/C*). This method of triggering depolarization with swift mechanical impulses should not be used to "pace" the heart.

2. **Airway and breathing.** Although recent guideline changes have focused on circulation, including compression-only CPR, maintaining a patent airway with adequate ventilation and oxygenation remains critical (*I/C*). It becomes more vital as arrest time increases owing to exhaustion of alveolar oxygen reserve and accumulation of carbon dioxide. Spontaneous ventilation is evaluated by observation and auscultation and aided by repositioning, most commonly through a head tilt–chin lift technique (*IIa/B*). If a cervical spine injury is suspected based on the scene or nature of injury, a jaw thrust without head extension should be attempted (*IIb/C*), although if unsuccessful at establishing airway patency, a head tilt should still be used (*I/C*). If ventilation remains impossible after these maneuvers and an advanced airway is not available, efforts to clear the airway of a suspected foreign body should be attempted. In primary foreign body obstruction, abdominal thrusts (Heimlich maneuver) should be attempted (*IIb/B*) and chest thrusts considered when unsuccessful (*IIb/B*). This differs for infants for whom back blows are delivered in succession with chest compressions for foreign body obstruction.

When an adult has spontaneous circulation by palpable pulses but ineffective breathing alone, rescue breaths should be provided at a rate of about 1 breath every 6 seconds, or about 10 times per minute

(*IIb/C-LD*). Breaths should be delivered over 1 second with enough volume for visible chest rise, roughly 500 to 600 mL in adults (*IIa/C-LD*). Rescue breaths during cardiac arrest should be similarly provided over 1 second with visible chest rise. In the absence of an advanced airway, compressions are briefly paused for breaths at the 30:2 ratio whether there are one or more providers. With an advanced airway in place, breaths should be given every 6 seconds (10/min) concurrent with compressions as mentioned in the previous section.

Hyperventilation (*III/C-LD*) from excess respiratory rate or tidal volume should be avoided as it can cause gastric insufflation provoking aspiration and, more importantly, it can increase intrathoracic pressure, impair venous return, and lower cardiac output, which ultimately worsens outcomes.

3. **Defibrillation** in BLS refers to the use of AEDs, which should be retrieved as part of the initial activation of the emergency response system. Timely defibrillation and CPR are major determinants of a successful resuscitation. Defibrillation is the definitive management for pulseless VT and VF (*I/A*). When an arrest is witnessed and an AED is within reach, the defibrillator should be used as soon as possible (*IIa/C-LD*). For unwitnessed arrests, CPR should be initiated while the AED is being retrieved (*IIa/B-R*).

   Public access defibrillation programs have enabled public safety professionals (eg, fire personnel, police, security guards, and airline attendants) to employ readily accessible AEDs. The devices themselves are small and lightweight and use adhesive electrode pads for both sensing and delivering shocks. Visual and voice prompts are provided to assist the operators with the goal of making it usable by an untrained bystander. After analysis of the frequency, amplitude, and slope of the ECG signal, the AED *advises* either "shock indicated" or "no shock indicated." The AED is manually triggered and does not automatically defibrillate the patient as an automatic shock could injure someone touching the patient. AEDs are now also equipped with pediatric pad-cable systems that attenuate the adult dose to a smaller dose appropriate for children. The dose attenuators should be used in children less than 8 years of age and less than 25 kg in weight. For infants, manual defibrillation is recommended, but if unavailable, an AED with or without an attenuator can be used. There are efforts to make AED analysis more sophisticated such as incorporating artifact filtering so that compressions can be continued during rhythm analysis. At this point, these technologies are not reliable enough to promote (*IIb/C-EO*).

4. **Reassessment.** Although it is tempting to see if the defibrillation worked by checking for a pulse immediately after a shock, the heart still needs time to establish sufficient forward flow and compressions should be resumed immediately after shock delivery (*IIb/C-LD*) with a rhythm check after five cycles of CPR (2 minutes). For health care providers, if there is evidence of a perfusing rhythm, the pulse can be checked to determine if there is ROSC. If a nonshockable rhythm or no pulse is detected, CPR should be resumed with rhythm checks after every five cycles as before.

B. **ACLS** describes the definitive, medically exhaustive treatment for cardiac arrest taught exclusively to health care professionals. It builds upon BLS skills and can be provided in the field by paramedics or in a hospital setting. As OR and intensive care unit (ICU) providers, anesthesiologists should keep themselves up to date with their certification and with changes to management protocols, which are amended yearly. Interventions described in ACLS include advanced airway management, manual defibrillation, synchronized cardioversion, pharmacologic management, and decisions toward more invasive mechanical circulatory support or withdrawal of care.

1. **Advanced airway.** Swift control of the airway optimizes oxygenation and the removal of carbon dioxide during resuscitation. Options are bag–mask ventilation or an advanced airway such as an ETT or LMA (*IIb/B-R*). The goal is to secure the airway via endotracheal intubation, which should be performed by the most experienced provider, often a trained anesthesiologist. Insertion of an oropharyngeal or nasopharyngeal airway can improve ventilation in an obstructed airway before intubation (*IIa/C*). Although cricoid pressure is sometimes used during bag–mask ventilation to decrease gastric insufflation, routine use is discouraged (*III/B*) as it tends to be performed incorrectly or in a manner that impairs ventilation.

   Endotracheal intubation during an in-hospital arrest can be difficult given confined space, poor patient positioning, suboptimal visualization, and interference from chest compressions. Waveform capnography, which is often a component of modern defibrillators, is the most reliable method to confirm correct placement (*I/C-LD*), although a color-changing in-line CO_2 detector is frequently the most readily available. The ETT may be used to deliver certain lipophilic drugs like naloxone, atropine, vasopressin, epinephrine, or lidocaine (NAVEL, now known as LEAN with removal of vasopressin) if intravenous (IV) access has not been established. Higher doses of these drugs are needed (2 to 3 times as much) owing to lower peak blood concentrations and should be diluted in 10 mL of sterile saline.

2. **Defibrillation.** Pulseless VT and VF are shockable dysrhythmias associated with cardiac arrest (see **Figure 39.1**). As the duration of SCA increases, cardiac ischemia worsens, and it becomes more difficult to achieve ROSC. Rapid defibrillation is critical in this situation before the rhythm degenerates into PEA or asystole. It is the responsibility of the person operating the defibrillator to ensure that members of the resuscitation team are not in contact with the patient during defibrillation. Defibrillators deliver energy in a biphasic pulse that alternates current flow. The optimal dose to terminate VF is 150 to 200 J and is indicated on the front of the defibrillator. In children, an initial dose of 2 to 4 J/kg is advised (*IIa/C-LD*). The pediatric dose can be increased with successive shocks but should not exceed 10 J/kg or the maximum adult dose (*IIb/C-LD*). The large adult pads/paddles (8 to 13 cm) are recommended in children above 1 year of age and at least 10 kg in weight. Infant pads/paddles (4.5 cm) are used in children less than 10 kg in weight.

   Double sequential external defibrillation (DSED) is a technique that involves the provision of rapid sequential shocks via two defibrillators with defibrillation pads placed in both planes (anterior–lateral and anterior–posterior). It has been explored for patients with shock refractory VT. However, on the basis of current evidence, the AHA does not support its use. Pads are preferred to paddles, as they can aid in rhythm detection and pacing. The defibrillator should be charged while compressions continue, and once ready to discharge, the provider calls "clear" to alert everyone to remove their hands from the patient and the shock is delivered, and compressions are resumed.

FIGURE 39.1 Algorithm for pulseless arrest. VF, ventricular fibrillation; VT, ventricular tachycardia. [a]When rhythm is unclear and could be VF, treat as shockable rhythm. [b]Biphasic. One cycle of CPR should follow any successful defibrillation. [c]Amiodarone bolus should be administered in 20 to 30 mL saline or D5W. This is followed by an infusion of 1 mg/min for 6 hours and then 0.5 mg/min thereafter. An additional dose of 150 mg IV can be readministered for recurrence of VF or VT. [d]Lidocaine can be bolused again at a dose of 0.5 to 0.75 mg/kg. [e]Magnesium sulfate 1 to 2 g can be considered for torsades (long-QT-associated polymorphic VT) but trials have not demonstrated an advantage. Vasopressin is no longer used in the ACLS protocol as its use had no added benefit relative to or in combination with epinephrine.

    a. Cardioversion using synchronized biphasic shocks are used for unstable tachyarrhythmias with pulses (rates generally >150 bpm) such as paroxysmal supraventricular tachycardia (PSVT), atrial fibrillation, reentrant arrhythmias, or unstable VT. The recommended initial energy dose for synchronized cardioversion of atrial fibrillation is 120 to 200 J (*IIa/A*). Dosing can be increased in a stepwise fashion if the initial shock is ineffective. Hemodynamically stable VT can be treated by synchronized cardioversion using 100 J as the starting point (*IIb/C*). The initial dose for cardioversion in children is 0.5 to 1 J/kg followed by subsequent doses of 2 J/kg. See **Figure 39.3** for management of tachyarrhythmias in adults.

  3. Pacing. High-grade heart block with profound bradycardia is one etiology of cardiac arrest. Temporary pacing should be used when the bradyarrhythmia does not improve with medication (primarily atropine) and there are signs of instability (eg, altered mental status, severe hypotension) (*IIa/B*). Transcutaneous pacing is the easiest method to increase the ventricular rate but may require high currents for consistent capture, which can be very uncomfortable for awake patients. Transesophageal atrial pacing is efficacious for sinus bradycardia with maintained atrioventricular (AV) conduction and is useful intraoperatively for bradycardia-related hypotension in otherwise stable

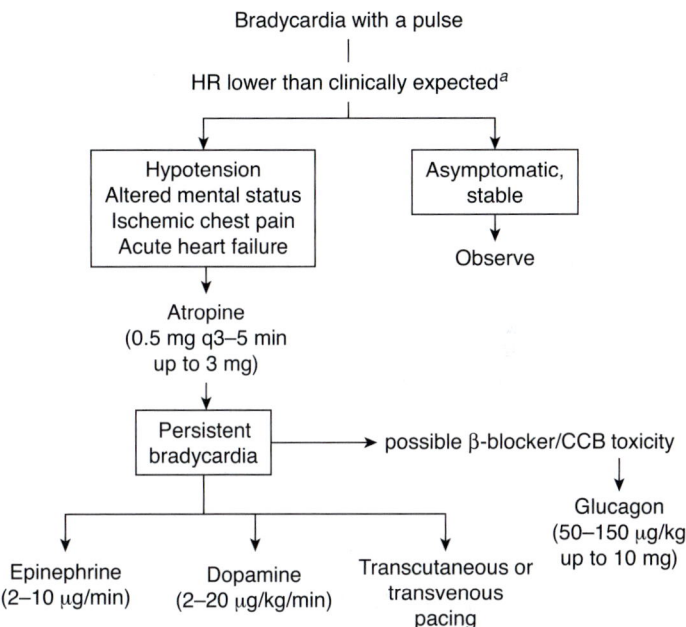

FIGURE 39.2 Algorithm for bradycardia. HR, heart rate; bpm, beats per minute; CCB, calcium channel blocker. ^aNormal heart rate goal may be <60 bpm for patients receiving therapeutic nodal agents (eg, β-blocker). When IV access or medications are not immediately available, can jump to transcutaneous pacing.

patients. Transvenous pacing via a temporary wire into the right heart is a third option to increase heart rate while CPR continues. Special pacing pulmonary artery catheters are capable of AV pacing. See **Figure 39.2** for management of symptomatic bradycardia.

4. **Vascular access** is imperative for successful resuscitation, but establishment of venous access should not delay chest compressions or defibrillation when appropriate. The most desirable route is into the central circulation, which should be prioritized when possible (*IIb/C*). The insertion site (internal jugular, external jugular, subclavian, or femoral vein) is predicated on the anatomy of the patient, experience of the physician, and what is least disruptive to resuscitation. Peripheral IV catheters in antecubital veins are adequate when an appropriate volume is used to flush medications toward the central circulation (~20-mL bolus). While peripheral vascular access should be prioritized, intraosseous (IO) cannulation should be attempted if venous cannulation attempts are unsuccessful (*IIa/B-NR*). IO access can be done in less than a minute in children. All drugs and fluids can be given through an IO route until good IV access is found.

Another form of vascular access to strongly consider is an arterial line, which is beneficial for sending arterial blood gases to aid in management and for evaluating compression quality (via pulsatile waveform visualization) and return of spontaneous circulation.

5. **Drugs.** The drugs described in the section that follows are used in ACLS protocols for the treatment of hemodynamic instability, myocardial ischemia/infarction, and arrhythmias. The doses of drugs used for PALS are in parentheses following the adult doses. Drugs should be provided centrally whenever possible given the slow circulation times during CPR but can be given peripherally (IV or IO) or via ETT (LEAN medications as described previously).

   a. **Adenosine** is an endogenous purine nucleoside with a half-life of 5 seconds. Adenosine slows or blocks anterograde AV node conduction and interrupts AV node reentry pathways to convert a stable PSVT to sinus rhythm. It can also slow the heart rate enough to identify an underlying rhythm that may be difficult to differentiate at elevated heart rates such as atrial fibrillation or atrial flutter. Adenosine can also be considered in the treatment of stable, regular, wide complex monomorphic VT. The initial dose is always a 6-mg rapid IV bolus immediately followed by a 20-mL saline flush (*I/B*). A brief asystole ensues, followed by P waves, flutter waves, or fibrillation waves that are initially without ventricular responses. The PSVT is sometimes converted to sinus rhythm by the initial dose, but a second injection of 12 mg may be required to terminate the PSVT if there is no effect of the first dose after 1 to 2 minutes. These doses are based on peripheral IV administration.

   Recurrent PSVT, AF, and atrial flutter will require longer-acting nodal agents for definitive treatment. The required dose of adenosine may need to be increased in the presence of methylxanthines like theophylline owing to competitive inhibition and decreased if dipyridamole has been administered owing to potentiation via blockage of nucleoside transport (although such adjustments are usually made for infusions during stress tests to induce vasodilation and not in ACLS protocols) (PALS: 0.1 mg/kg; repeat dose 0.2 mg/kg; maximum dose 12 mg). Adenosine should not be used for preexcitation syndromes like Wolff–Parkinson–White (WPW) as exclusive accessory tract conduction can precipitate VF (*III/C*). Atrial fibrillation with preexcitation can present as an irregular wide-complex tachycardia. For this reason, adenosine use in wide-QRS tachycardias should be limited to those which are regular.

   b. **Amiodarone** is the most versatile drug in ACLS algorithms. It has the properties of all four classes of antiarrhythmics: lengthening of the action potential, sodium channel blockade at high frequencies of stimulation, noncompetitive antisynaptic actions, and negative chronotropism. Because of its high efficacy and low incidence of proarrhythmic effects, it is the preferred antiarrhythmic for patients with severely impaired cardiac function. For shock-refractory pulseless VT/VF, 300 mg diluted in 20 to 30 mL of saline or 5% dextrose in water (D5W) is administered as a bolus. To treat stable dysrhythmias (eg, hemodynamically stable AF, VT), 150 mg is administered over 10 minutes, followed by an infusion of 1 mg/min for 6 hours, and then 0.5 mg/min. The maximum daily dose is 2 g. Immediate side effects can be bradycardia and hypotension (PALS: loading dose 5 mg/kg; maximum dose 15 mg/kg/d). Amiodarone is indicated in the following situations:
   1. Unstable VT (*IIb/C*).
   2. VF or pulseless VT after failed electrical defibrillation and epinephrine treatment (*IIb/B-R*).

3. Attempted rate control during stable monomorphic VT, polymorphic VT (*IIb/B*), or AF.
4. Need for an adjunct to electrical cardioversion of refractory PSVT (*IIa*) or atrial tachycardia (*IIb*).

c. **Atropine** is an anticholinergic used as the first-line agent for hemodynamically significant bradycardia (*IIa/B*) or AV block occurring at the nodal level. It increases the rate of sinus node discharge and enhances AV node conduction by its vagolytic activity. It is not effective for Mobitz type II heart block, for complete heart block, or in transplanted hearts missing vagal innervation. It is also not indicated for asystole or PEA (*IIb/B*) but should be considered for treatment of profound bradycardia that may appear as asystole but with a preserved pulse. The dose of atropine for bradycardia or AV block is 1 mg repeated every 3 to 5 minutes to a total dose of 3 mg (PALS: 0.02 mg/kg; minimum dose, 0.1 mg; maximum single dose, 0.5 mg in child, maximum total dose for adolescent 3 mg).

d. **β-Adrenergic antagonists** (eg, atenolol, metoprolol, esmolol, propranolol) have established utility for patients with unstable angina or myocardial infarction. Their competitive inhibition of adrenergic receptors reduces heart rate, AV node conduction, blood pressure, and the effects of catecholamines. This action serves to reduce the rate of recurrent ischemia, nonfatal reinfarction, and postinfarction VF. In contrast to calcium channel blockers, β-blockers are not direct negative inotropes.

β-Blockers are useful for the acute treatment of stable PSVT, AF, atrial flutter (*I*), and ectopic atrial tachycardia (*IIb*). Initial and subsequent IV doses, if tolerated, are atenolol, 5 mg over 5 minutes, repeated once at 10 minutes; metoprolol, three doses of 5 mg every 5 minutes; propranolol, 0.1 mg/kg divided into three doses given every 2 to 3 minutes; esmolol, 0.5 mg/kg over 1 minute followed by an infusion starting at 50 µg/min and titrated as needed up to 200 µg/min. Contraindications include second- or third-degree heart block, hypotension, and severe congestive heart failure. When a β-blocker might trigger bronchospasm in a patient with chronic lung disease, metoprolol with selective β1-blockade at therapeutic doses may be preferred.

e. **Calcium** is indicated during cardiac arrest only when hyperkalemia, hypermagnesemia, hypocalcemia, or toxicity from calcium channel blockers is suspected. Calcium chloride can be given as a dose of 8 to 16 mg/kg IV (usually 0.5 to 1 g) and repeated as necessary (PALS: calcium chloride 10%: 20 mg/kg = 0.2 mL/kg). Although calcium plays a role in myocardial contraction, studies have not shown any benefit with routine use in cardiac arrest (*III/B-R*).

f. **Calcium channel blockers (nondihydropyridine)** such as verapamil and diltiazem depress AV nodal conduction and increase refractory time. These are used to treat hemodynamically stable, narrow complex PSVT unresponsive to vagal maneuvers or adenosine (*IIa/B*). The initial verapamil dose is 2.5 to 5.0 mg IV, with subsequent doses of 5 to 10 mg IV administered every 15 to 30 minutes. Diltiazem is given as an initial bolus of 15 to 20 mg over 2 minutes. An additional dose of 20 to 25 mg and an infusion of 5 to 15 mg/h can be administered if needed. Their vasodilator and negative inotrope properties can cause hypotension, exacerbation of congestive heart failure, bradycardia, and enhancement of accessory conduction in patients with WPW syndrome. The hypotension can often be reversed with calcium chloride, 0.5 to 1.0 g IV. They are contraindicated for wide complex tachyarrhythmias (*III/B*).

g. **Dopamine** has dopaminergic (1 to 5 μg/kg/min), β-adrenergic (5 to 10 μg/kg/min), and α-adrenergic (>10 μg/kg/min) activity. Although those listed are "traditional" ranges for dose-dependent receptor agonism, the pharmacodynamics are not reliable (eg, tachycardia may occur with the lowest doses). Dopamine should be started at a low dose and titrated to the desired effect such as increased urine output, increased heart rate/inotropy, increased blood pressure or when undesired side effects limit further increases. It is the second-line agent to atropine for symptomatic bradyarrhythmias (*IIa/B*), alongside epinephrine and transcutaneous pacing. Infusions can range from 5 to 20 μg/kg/min.

h. **Epinephrine** continues to be the mainstay of pharmacologic therapy for all forms of cardiac arrest (*I/B-R*) given its demonstrated survival benefits. Its α-adrenergic vasoconstriction of noncerebral and noncoronary vascular beds produces compensatory shunting of blood toward the brain and heart. Its β1- and β2-agonism stimulates the heart and relaxes the bronchial tree. In normal circulation, its half-life is a few minutes. The recommended dose in SCA is 1 mg IV repeated every 3 to 5 minutes (*IIa/C-LD*). Epinephrine is second line to atropine for symptomatic bradycardia with a target dose range of 2 to 10 μg/min (*IIb/B*). It is the first-line agent, however, for bradycardia associated with neuraxial anesthesia (PALS: bradycardia with a pulse but poor perfusion, 0.01 mg/kg; pulseless arrest, 0.01 mg/kg).

The optimal dose timing around defibrillation is not clear, but it is reasonable to give after the initial defibrillating shock fails (*IIb/C-LD*). In shock-refractory rhythms, epinephrine is combined with antiarrhythmics, including amiodarone or lidocaine. It is also commonly used in the OR in smaller, escalating doses for managing anaphylaxis and hypotension.

Studies have trialed high-dose epinephrine as high as 0.2 mg/kg but have not shown any advantage, and such doses are discouraged (*III/B-R*). High doses can contribute to myocardial dysfunction or even precipitate a stress cardiomyopathy.

i. **Isoproterenol** is a $β_1$ and $β_2$-adrenergic agent. It is another second-line drug used to treat hemodynamically significant bradycardia unresponsive to atropine and dobutamine in the event that a temporarily pacemaker is not available. It is not stocked in code carts. Its $β_2$ activity can cause hypotension. Isoproterenol is administered by IV infusion at 2 to 10 μg/min, titrated to achieve the desired heart rate.

j. **Lidocaine** acts on voltage-gated sodium channels and functions as both a local anesthetic and a class Ib antiarrhythmic. In the 2018 ACLS guidelines, lidocaine was added alongside amiodarone for VF/pulseless VT unresponsive to defibrillation, especially for witnessed arrests (*IIb/B-R*). It may be useful for the control (not prophylaxis) of ventricular ectopy during an acute myocardial infarction. The initial dose is 1 to 1.5 mg/kg IV and may be repeated as a 0.5 to 0.75 mg/kg bolus every 3 to 5 minutes to a total dose of 3 mg/kg followed by a continuous infusion of 2 to 4 mg/min. The lidocaine dose should be decreased for patients with reduced cardiac output, hepatic dysfunction, or advanced age (PALS: 1 mg/kg; infusion, 20 to 50 μg/kg/min).

k. **Magnesium** is a divalent cation with a myriad of regulatory roles such as being a cofactor in enzyme reactions including that of the Na^+, K^+-ATPase, decreasing nerve and muscle conduction, relaxing bronchial smooth muscle, acting as a vasodilator, and even effecting N-methyl-D-aspartate antagonism through competition at calcium-binding sites. That said, magnesium is not recommended for general use in cardiac arrest (*III/C-LD*) except in specific circumstances such as for preventing recurrent long QT associated polymorphic VT (Torsades de Pointes) (*IIb/C-LD*). The dose for emergent administration is 1 to 2 g in 10 mL D5W over 1 to 2 minutes. Hypotension and bradycardia are side effects of rapid administration (PALS: 25 to 50 mg/kg; maximum dose, 2 g).

l. **Oxygen** (100%) should be administered during CPR by bag-valve-mask or advanced airway and to hemodynamically stable, breathing patients by unpressurized face mask. For neonates and infants not in cardiac arrest, high FiO_2 can be deleterious and is carefully titrated to preductal SpO_2. In the care of adult patients following ROSC, FiO_2 should be titrated to a SpO_2 of 92% to 98% with avoidance of unnecessary hyperoxia.

m. **Procainamide** is a class Ia antiarrhythmic that can be used to convert atrial fibrillation/atrial flutter to sinus rhythm and control the ventricular response to supraventricular tachycardia secondary to accessory pathways and is useful during cardioversion of wide complex tachycardias of unknown origin. It has essentially been replaced by amiodarone. The loading dose is a continuous infusion of 20 to 30 mg/min that is terminated when the arrhythmia is suppressed, hypotension occurs, the QRS complex is widened by 50% of its original size, or a total dose of 17 mg/kg is reached. When the arrhythmia is suppressed, a maintenance infusion of 1 to 4 mg/min should be initiated, with a reduced dose considered in the presence of renal dysfunction. An ECG should be examined for QRS widening at least daily (PALS: 15 mg/kg over 30 to 60 minutes).

n. **Sodium bicarbonate** administration is detrimental in most cardiac arrests (*III/B*) because it creates a paradoxical intracellular acidosis. It can be considered when the standard ACLS protocol has failed in the presence of severe preexisting metabolic acidosis and for the treatment of hyperkalemia or tricyclic antidepressant overdose. The initial dose of bicarbonate is 1 mEq/kg IV, with subsequent doses of 0.5 mEq/kg given every 10 minutes (as guided by arterial blood pH and partial pressure of carbon dioxide [$PaCO_2$]) (PALS: 1 mEq/kg).

o. **Sotalol**, a type III antiarrhythmic and nonselective β-blocker can be considered alongside amiodarone and procainamide and is primarily used for atrial fibrillation/flutter and stable monomorphic VT (*IIb/B*). A dose of 1.5 mg/kg is given over 5 minutes for hemodynamically stable arrhythmias. Like procainamide, it should be avoided in patients with prolonged QT as it can precipitate Torsades de Pointes (*III/B*). Other side effects include bradycardia and hypotension.

p. **Vasopressin**, a hormone from the neurohypophysis, has pressor (V_1) and antidiuretic (V_2) activities. Endogenous levels of vasopressin are increased in patients undergoing CPR who eventually have ROSC. It is more effective than epinephrine in maintaining the coronary perfusion pressure, has a longer half-life of 10 to 20 minutes, and was previously considered as a substitute for either the first or second dose of epinephrine in the treatment of pulseless arrest at doses of 40 units IV. Although vasopressin may still be considered as a substitute or in combination with epinephrine (*IIb/C-LD*), it has not been shown to offer any clear advantage and is no longer part of the ACLS protocol (PALS: 0.4 to 1 U/kg bolus with a maximum dose of 40 units for cardiac arrest and 0.0002 to 0.002 U/kg/min for catecholamine-resistant hypotension).

6. **Specific ACLS protocols** are shown in **Figures 39.1** to **39.3**.
   a. Pulseless arrest (**Figure 39.1**).
   b. Bradycardia with pulse (**Figure 39.2**).
   c. Tachycardia with pulse (**Figure 39.3**).
7. **Open-chest direct cardiac compression** is an intervention used at institutions with appropriate resources to manage penetrating chest trauma, abdominal trauma with cardiac arrest, pericardial tamponade, hypothermia, or pulmonary embolism. Direct cardiac compressions also are indicated for individuals with anatomic deformities of the chest that prevent adequate closed-chest compression (*IIb/C*).
8. **ECMO** is a portable form of advanced mechanical cardiopulmonary support through invasive cannulation of large vessels. Recently, it has

FIGURE 39.3 Algorithm for tachycardia with pulse. If there are signs of instability with hemodynamic compromise, the treatment of choice is immediate cardioversion. A useful estimate for peak heart rate is 220–Age. When stable, EKG analysis and appropriate pharmacologic interventions should be attempted. [a]Adenosine should not be prioritized over cardioversion with unstable patients. It is given as a 6 mg IV push with a potential second dose of 12 mg (avoid with history or evidence of WPW). [b]Consider vagal stimulation before adenosine for stable, regular, narrow tachyarrhythmias. [c]Generally metoprolol, esmolol infusion, or diltiazem push. [d]Amiodarone given as 150 mg IV over 10 minutes followed by an infusion of 1 mg/min. [e]Alternatives to amiodarone for regular, wide complex include procainamide or sotalol.

been referred to as extracorporeal cardiopulmonary resuscitation (eCPR). There are two forms of eCPR, venovenous (VV) and venoarterial (VA). Both provide respiratory support through external gas exchange, whereas VA provides additional circulatory (hemodynamic) support. eCPR is indicated when traditional CPR has failed, but it has many contraindications including, but not limited to, unwitnessed arrest, >30 minutes of traditional CPR without ROSC, severe bleeding, and the inability to tolerate systemic anticoagulation.

Although eCPR can achieve normal cardiac output in situations where ROSC is not attainable through traditional CPR, it is not recommended as a routine intervention and should be reserved for patients who would likely recover (*I/C-EO*). Institutions that offer ECMO services should have a separate emergency consult team that screens, selects, and cannulates patients.

9. **Termination of CPR.** There are no absolute guidelines based on outcome studies to determine when to stop an unsuccessful resuscitation, but there is a very low probability of survival after 30 minutes. One objective measure is the failure to attain an $ETCO_2$ of 10 mm Hg after 20 minutes of CPR (*IIb/C-LD*). It is at the discretion of the physician in charge to determine when the failure of the cardiovascular system to respond to adequately applied BLS and ACLS indicates that the patient has died. There should be meticulous documentation of the resuscitation, including the reasons for terminating the effort.

10. **Advanced directives,** such as "Do Not Resuscitate" **(DNR)**, places the anesthesiologist in a key position with respect to intraoperative and postoperative care. It is often incorrectly *assumed* that a DNR order is suspended in the perioperative period. Each institution's written guidelines should be reviewed. In advance of a procedure, physicians and the patient with the DNR status or the patient's health care proxy should clarify any resuscitative measures that would be compatible with the patient's wishes. For example, the use of a pressor to control hypotension following induction of general anesthesia might be permitted while defibrillation and CPR for spontaneous VF might be prohibited. When asked to perform an emergent intubation outside of the OR, the anesthesiologist should ask about the patient's code status and is ethically and legally bound to documented and known decisions to limit treatment.

IV. PEDIATRIC RESUSCITATION

A. BLS. The need for CPR in the pediatric age group is rare after the neonatal period. Pediatric cardiac arrests usually result from hypoxemia linked to respiratory failure or airway obstruction. Initial efforts should be directed toward the establishment of a secure airway and adequate ventilation. The pediatric guidelines apply to infants between the ages of about 1 month and 1 year and to children more than 1 year of age. For newborns, see the Neonatal Resuscitation section of this chapter. The definition of "children" for health care providers is patients between the ages of 1 year and the start of puberty; for the lay public, a child is defined as aged 1 to 8 years.

In contrast to the guideline of "phone first" for adult CPR, one should "phone fast" for infants and children. That is, the lone rescuer should perform five cycles (about 2 minutes) of CPR before phoning 911. The "phone fast" rule also applies to pediatric resuscitation from drowning, traumatic arrest, or drug overdose. Exceptions include witnessed and sudden arrests (eg, an athlete who collapses on the playing field) or situations in which a

Table 39.2 Adult and Pediatric Cardiopulmonary Resuscitation

Age	Ventilations/Min	Compressions/Min	Ventilation:Compression Ratio	Depth of Compressions
Neonate	30	90	3:1[a,b]	1/3 depth of chest
Infant (<1 y)	12–20	100–120	30:2[a]/15:2[b]	1/3–1/2 depth of chest
Child (1–8 y)	12–20	100–120	30:2[a]/15:2[b]	1/3–1/2 depth of chest
Adult and child >8 y	10–12	100–120	30:2[a,b]	1.5–2 inches

[a]One-person rescue.
[b]Two-person rescue.

child is known to be at high risk for a sudden arrhythmia. Modifications to the rate and magnitude of compressions and ventilations, as well as to the hand positions for compressions are necessary because of anatomic and physiologic differences (**Table 39.2**). Differences between pediatric and adult resuscitation techniques are detailed below.

Airway and breathing. Maneuvers to establish an airway are the same as in the adult, with a few caveats. For children less than 1 year of age, abdominal thrusts are not used in the setting of airway foreign body obstruction since the gastrointestinal tract can be damaged easily. Hyperextension of an infant's neck for the head tilt–chin lift may lead to airway obstruction because of the small diameter and ease of compression of the immature airway. Submental compression while performing the chin lift can also lead to airway obstruction by pushing the tongue into the pharynx. Ventilations should be given slowly and with low airway pressures to avoid gastric distention and should be of sufficient volume to cause visible chest rise and fall. While previous guidelines recommended rescue breaths be administered at about 12 to 20/min (1 breath every 3 to 5 seconds), the most recent recommendations support a ventilatory rate of 1 breath every 2 to 3 seconds (20 to 30 breaths/min).

B. Circulation. The brachial or femoral artery is used for pulse assessment in infants (<1 year old) because the carotid artery is difficult to palpate. Upon determination that a pulse is absent, chest compressions should be initiated. Chest compressions in infants are delivered using two fingertips applied to the sternum or by encircling the chest with both hands and using the thumbs to depress the sternum one fingerbreadth below the intermammary line (*Ib/C-LD*). If the rescuer is unable to achieve the recommended chest-compression depth using the two-finger or thumb-encircling hand technique, it may be reasonable to use the heel of one hand for infant CPR (2b/C-EO). In older children, the correct hand position is determined as for adults, but with one or two hands depressing the sternum (2b/C-LD). The chest should be compressed at least one-third of the anterior–posterior depth, roughly 1.5 in (4 cm) in infants and 2 in (5 cm) in children (*IIa/C-LD*). The compression–ventilation ratio is 30:2 for one-rescuer CPR of infants and children and 15:2 when two rescuers are available. If an advanced airway is in place during two-person CPR, there is no need to synchronize breaths between compressions. Ventilations should be given at a rate of approximately 1 breath every 2 to 3 seconds (20 to 30 breaths/min) (*IIb/C-LD*), and chest compressions should be given at a rate of 100 to 120/min without pauses for ventilation (*IIa/C-LD*).

1. **PALS.** Most pediatric cardiac arrests present as asystole and bradycardia, rather than ventricular arrhythmias, as they primarily occur secondary to respiratory failure or shock. In infants less than 1 year old, respiratory and idiopathic (sudden infant death syndrome) etiologies predominate. Anatomic and physiologic differences from the adult require weight-based defibrillator settings and drug dosing.

    a. **Intubation.** Low-pressure high-volume cuffed ETT have mostly replaced uncuffed ones as the ETT of choice in children owing to improved capnography accuracy and more reliable tidal volume delivery. Achieving an appropriate airway seal with an uncuffed ETT often requires multiple intubation attempts, which may predispose a child to iatrogenic airway edema. For these reasons, the most recent AHA guidelines favor use of cuffed versus uncuffed ETTs when intubating infants and children (*IIa/C-LD*). However, whether using an uncuffed or cuffed ETT, a correctly sized tube should have an air leak at a driving pressure between 15 and 30 cm of water. For a cuffed ETT, this leak should be tested with the cuff deflated. Once the appropriately sized cuffed ETT has been selected, the cuff can be inflated and maintained at a pressure (as measured with a manometer) between 20 and 30 cm of water.

    The internal diameter (ID) of an ETT required for children less than 1 year of age is 3.5 mm uncuffed or 3 mm cuffed and for children 1 to 2 years of age, the size is 4 mm uncuffed or 3.5 mm cuffed. The formula for the size of ETT (ID in millimeters) in children above 2 years of age is as follows: age in years/4 + 4 for uncuffed tubes and age in years/4 + 3.5 for cuffed tubes. Appropriate oral ETT depth (centimeters at teeth) for infants and neonates can be calculated by the formula: inner diameter (millimeters) × 3. For children >1 year, appropriate oral ETT depth (centimeters at teeth) can be calculated using the formula: age (in years)/2 + 12. Correct ETT positioning should be confirmed with capnography, auscultation, and radiographic confirmation when available. If an intubated patient's condition deteriorates, the provider must rule out displacement or obstruction of the ETT, pneumothorax, or equipment failure (mnemonic DOPE).

    Cricoid pressure had previously been recommended during intubation to minimize risk of pulmonary aspiration. However, recent data showing lower intubation success rates when cricoid pressure was applied have resulted in updated guidelines against its use in pediatric patients (*III/C-LD*).

    b. **Defibrillation.** Defibrillator pads/paddles used for infants are 4.5 cm in diameter, and those used for older children (>8 years, >25 kg) are 8 cm in diameter (adult size). In an emergency, and if no pediatric sizes are available, adult pads on the chest and back will suffice. The energy level is 2 J/kg for the initial biphasic shock and 4 J/kg, or the lowest level that was previously successful for any subsequent shocks (*IIa/C-LD*). Hypoxemia, acidosis, or hypothermia should be considered as treatable causes of an arrest if the defibrillation attempts are unsuccessful. For synchronized cardioversion, the starting energy is 0.5 to 1 J/kg, which can be increased up to 2 J/kg

(*IIb/C*). The configuration for pediatric pads/paddles varies among defibrillators.

c. **IV access.** During resuscitation, peripheral IV access is preferred over central venous access as central IV-line placement may require an interruption in chest compressions. If central IV access is in place, it is the preferred route for the delivery of drugs and fluids. All drugs by peripheral route should be flushed with saline to ensure delivery to the central circulation. Intraosseous (IO) access can be used in all age groups if needed.

d. **Medications.** Many of the drugs described in the adult ACLS section apply to PALS, with doses adjusted to the child's weight. Weight estimations can be obtained using a body length tape with precalculated weights (Broselow tape) or formulas like the European pediatric life support formula ([age in years + 4] × 2 kg).

e. **eCPR, targeted temperature management, and electroencephalography (EEG) monitoring.** eCPR and postarrest targeted temperature management can both be utilized in pediatric patients. eCPR may be considered for in-hospital cardiac arrest, but its utility is questioned in out-of-hospital cardiac arrest. For pediatric patients who remain comatose after cardiac arrest, either targeted temperature management of 32 °C to 34 °C followed by targeted temperature

FIGURE 39.4 Algorithm for pediatric cardiac arrest. CPR, cardiopulmonary resuscitation; VF, ventricular fibrillation; VT, ventricular tachycardia. [a]Provide oxygen, establish intravenous or intraosseous access. [b]First shock, 2 J/kg; second shock, 4 J/kg; subsequent shocks ≥4 up to 10 J/kg or adult dose (200 J). [c]May repeat up to two times for VF or refractory VT. [d]Lidocaine can be used alternatively to amiodarone and following the bolus a maintenance of 20 to 50 µg/kg/min infusion may be used.

management of 36 °C to 37.5 °C or simply targeted temperature management 36 °C to 37.5 °C are acceptable. Updated recommendations do not specify a length of treatment. For patients with persistent postarrest encephalopathy, continuous EEG should be considered to detect possible nonconvulsive status epilepticus.
  f. Specific PALS algorithms are shown in **Figures 39.4** to **39.6**.
     1. Pediatric cardiac arrest (**Figure 39.4**).
     2. Pediatric bradycardia with pulse (**Figure 39.5**).
     3. Pediatric tachycardia with pulse (**Figure 39.6**).
  g. **Family presence.** Family presence during pediatric resuscitation is common in most institutions. Studies have shown that this is beneficial to family members, and parents should be offered the opportunity to observe the resuscitative efforts (*I/B*). One person should be assigned to stay with the family to explain the ongoing efforts, answer questions, and provide comfort and support. Parents can be requested to leave if they are disruptive (*IIa/C*). The resuscitation team should be aware of the presence of a family member.

FIGURE 39.5 Algorithm for pediatric bradycardia. HR, heart rate; AV, atrioventricular. [a]May repeat every 3 to 5 minutes. If vascular access is not available, may give 0.1 mg/kg via endotracheal tube. [b]May repeat once. Minimum atropine dose is 0.1 mg; maximum 0.5 mg. If vascular access is not available, may give 0.04 to 0.06 mg/kg atropine via ETT. [c]Transcutaneous pacing is effective for bradycardia secondary to complete heart block or sinus dysfunction associated with a congenital heart disease, but is not useful for asystole or hypoxic bradycardia. If pulse is lost, proceed to pulseless arrest PALS algorithm (Figure 39.4).

FIGURE 39.6 Algorithm for pediatric tachycardia with pulse and poor perfusion. HR, heart rate; SVT, supraventricular tachycardia; VT, ventricular tachycardia. [a]If not effective, increase to 2 J/kg. [b]Alternative to amiodarone is procainamide, 15 mg/kg over 30 to 60 minutes, but should not be given together and given with caution as can precipitate torsades. [c]Vagal stimulation should be attempted unless hemodynamically unstable or if it would delay medical or electrical cardioversion. Can be performed with ice applied to the face of infants/young children or carotid massage/Valsalva in older children.

V. NEONATAL RESUSCITATION

The neonatal period refers to the time from when a child is born and adjusting from the intrauterine environment/physiology through the first month of life. About 10% of newborns require brief resuscitation at birth such as assistance with respiration, whereas 1% require more extensive interventions. At least one person who is skilled in the resuscitation of newborns should be present at every delivery. Rapid assessment of term gestation, respiration/crying, and good muscle tone ("yes" to all three predicts good outcome) helps identify babies who may require ongoing resuscitation from those who can stay with the mother. Resuscitation is often needed during an emergent cesarean section for fetal distress. In the event that the anesthesiologist is the only provider available to treat the newborn, the neonatal warmer should be brought to the head of the OR table to facilitate the treatment and monitoring of both the mother and child until a second provider (pediatrician) arrives (**Figure 39.7**).

A. Assessment. Immediate neonatal resuscitation is crucial, since profound hypoxemia can occur rapidly and may lead to persistence of the fetal circulation and resulting right-to-left shunting, which will exacerbate hypoxemia. A neonate who requires resuscitation will likely have a significant right-to-left shunt.

The **Apgar score** is an objective assessment of the physiologic well-being of the child as it relates to heart rate, respiration, tone, reflexes, and color and is taken between 1 and 5 minutes after birth.

B. An Apgar score of 0 to 2 mandates immediate CPR. Neonates with scores of 3 to 4 will need bag–mask ventilation and may require more extensive

FIGURE 39.7 Algorithm for newborn resuscitation. HR, heart rate; PPV, positive pressure ventilation. [a]Target SpO$_2$ refers to preductal saturation (eg, right arm) as opposed to postductal (eg, feet). For access can place IV/IO but can consider umbilical venous catheter (UVC) placement as well.

resuscitation. Supplemental oxygen and stimulation are normally sufficient for newborns with Apgar scores of 5 to 7. Respiratory activity should be evaluated by watching chest excursions and by auscultation. The heart rate is assessed by auscultation or by palpation of the umbilical pulse.

C. If rapid assessment at birth is "yes" regarding term gestation, crying/breathing, and good muscle tone, then in most cases drying the baby and providing warmth (mother/wrapping) is sufficient. If the answer is "no" to any of those categories, the following four interventions should be followed in sequence.
1. Initial steps in stabilization (dry, provide warmth, position, clear airway, stimulate to breathe).
2. Ventilation.
3. Chest Compressions.
4. Medications/volume expansion.

D. Resuscitation. The first 60 seconds is referred to as the "Golden Minute" and is the time allotted for the initial steps and evaluation to decide if the baby requires ventilation. The decision to progress depends on the simultaneous assessment of two vital characteristics: appropriate respiration and heart rate. Once ventilation is required owing to inappropriate respiration or heart rate, ongoing assessment is based on three vital characteristics: heart rate, respiration, and oxygenation (pulse oximetry is used to avoid hyperoxia, and hence color is not recommended). An increase in heart rate with each intervention is the most valuable and sensitive indicator of a successful response.

1. **Initial steps.** The cold-intolerant neonate should be dried thoroughly after birth and warmth provided by placing the baby under a radiant heat source. Temperature on admission to a neonatal ICU is a strong mortality predictor (*I/B-NR*) and should be maintained between 36.5 °C and 37.5 °C (*I/C-LD*). Risks of hypothermia include intraventricular hemorrhage, hypoglycemia, or delayed recognition of sepsis. Hyperthermia should also be avoided (*III/C-EO*). In the OR, a thermal mattress or warmed gases can be used in addition to the radiant warmer (*IIb/B-R*). It is unclear if there are risks with rapid rewarming (>0.5 °C/h) for newborns (*IIb, C-LD*).

   Placement in the lateral Trendelenburg position with the head in a "sniffing" position helps to open the airway and allow secretions to drain. Routine suctioning of the oro/nasopharyngeal area is not recommended (meconium-stained *or* clear amniotic fluid) and should be reserved for babies with clear airway obstruction or who need positive-pressure ventilation (*IIB/C*). Suctioning the nasopharynx can induce bradycardia, reduce cerebral blow flow, and worsen pulmonary compliance. When necessary, clear the airway with a bulb syringe or suction catheter and use supplementary oxygen or bag–mask ventilation as needed. Drying and suctioning, however, usually provide adequate respiratory stimulation. Infants with meconium-stained amniotic fluid (vigorous or nonvigorous) are no longer routinely intubated for tracheal suctioning unless there are other reasons for intubation such as severe airway obstruction, slow heart rate or compromised breathing (*IIb/C-LD*).

   Pulse oximetry is recommended during resuscitation to avoid hyperoxia, which has proved to be detrimental. Pulse oximetry (SpO_2) and heart rate are reliably measured 90 seconds after birth with a neonatal probe. Preductal values (right upper limb) are higher than postductal. Oximetry should be used in conjunction with and not replace clinical assessment of heart rate.

2. **Ventilation.** Positive-pressure ventilation is initiated if the baby is apneic/gasping within 60 seconds after birth and/or if the heart rate is less than 100 beats/min. The initial peak inspiratory pressure required for chest movement and increase in heart rate is variable. If airway pressure is monitored, an initial peak pressure of 20 to 25 cm of water may be required (*IIa/C-LD*). Occasionally, higher peak inflation pressures are required. However, excessive peak pressures could create lung injury so should be avoided (*III/C-LD*). Similarly, sustained inflations to initiate resuscitation are potentially harmful and should be avoided (*III/B-R*). Assisted ventilation should be delivered at 40 to 60 breaths/min for a goal heart rate of above 100 (*IIa/C-EO*).

   PEEP at 5 cm H_2O has been shown to be beneficial and should be used if proper equipment is available for its delivery (*IIb/B-R*). Continuous positive airway pressure is recommended for preterm babies breathing spontaneously with difficulty, thus avoiding intubation (*IIa/A*).

Endotracheal intubation is indicated in prolonged or ineffective bag–mask ventilation, during chest compression, and in special circumstances like a diaphragmatic hernia. Exhaled CO_2 monitoring should be used for confirmation of correct ETT placement including in very–low-birth weight neonates (*IIa/B*). An LMA can be considered as an alternative to an ETT (*IIb/B-R*) and is suggested for infants greater than 34 weeks gestation when ETT placement is unsuccessful (*I/C-EO*), although their efficacy during chest compressions is unclear.

Based on studies comparing air (21% O_2) and 100% oxygen for newborn resuscitation, air has been shown to have a higher survival rate and similar neurocognitive outcomes. Therefore, in term and late-preterm newborns air is most reasonable (*IIa/B-R*) and 100% O_2 should be avoided (*III/B-R*). In preterm newborns (<35 weeks gestational age), it is reasonable to start with an FiO_2 between 21% to 30% and titrate to achieve the targeted range of preductal oxygen saturation (*IIb/C-LD*; target SpO_2 table in **Figure 39.7**). If blended oxygen is unavailable, resuscitation should be started with air and if there is no improvement in 90 seconds, 100% oxygen should be used.

3. **Chest compressions** are indicated if the heart rate is **less than 60 beats/min** despite adequate ventilation with oxygen for 30 seconds (*IIa/C-EO*). Compressions should be delivered on the lower third of the sternum, and the chest should be compressed approximately one-third of its anterior–posterior depth (*IIb/C-LD*). Compressions and ventilations should be alternated and delivered at a 3:1 ratio, with a total of 90 compressions and 30 breaths per minute (*IIa/C-LD*). This 3:1 ratio reflects the predominant cardiopulmonary collapse secondary to poor gas exchange in infants, although if the arrest has a clear cardiac origin, a higher ratio such as 15:2 can be used (*IIb/C-EO*). There are two techniques, two thumb encircling hands and the two-finger with second hand on the back. The two thumb encircling hands are recommended as it generates higher pressures and is less exhausting to the provider (*IIb/C-LD*).

   Frequent interruption of compressions should be avoided. Periodic assessment of ventilation, heart rate, and oxygenation should be done, and compressions are stopped when the spontaneous heart rate is greater than 60 beats/min. The optimal FiO_2 during neonatal CPR is uncertain. However, current recommendations based upon expert opinions support a higher initial FiO_2, which should then be reduced as soon as possible (*IIb/C-EO*).

4. **Delivery of resuscitation drugs and fluids.** Resuscitation drugs should be administered when the heart rate remains below 60 beats/min despite adequate ventilation with 100% oxygen and chest compressions. The umbilical vein, the largest and thinnest of the three umbilical vessels, provides the best vascular access for resuscitation of the newborn. It is cannulated with a 3.5- to 5.0-French umbilical catheter after the umbilical cord stump has been prepped with an antiseptic and trimmed. Sterile umbilical tape placed at the base of the cord will prevent bleeding. The catheter should be placed below the skin level with blood aspirated freely, and care must be taken not to permit air into the system. If vascular access is unavailable, the ETT or IO access can be used to administer drugs.

5. **Medications and volume expansion**
   a. **Epinephrine.** The β-adrenergic effect of epinephrine increases the intrinsic heart rate during neonatal resuscitation. Epinephrine should be used for asystole and for heart rates less than 60 despite adequate oxygenation and chest compressions. The dose of 0.01 to

0.03 mg/kg per dose of a 1:10,000 solution is recommended intravenously (*IIb/C*). Higher IV doses are not recommended. If the drug is given via the endotracheal route, a dose of 0.05 to 0.1 mg/kg of 1:10,000 (0.1 mg/mL) should be considered.
- b. **Naloxone** is a specific opiate antagonist used for neonatal respiratory depression secondary to narcotics administered to the mother. The initial dose is 0.1 mg/kg. Naloxone is not recommended as part of the initial resuscitative efforts in newborns. Depressed respiration due to narcotics should be treated with assisted ventilation. Studies have shown misuse of naloxone in newborns and association of seizures following administration.
- c. **Sodium bicarbonate** is not recommended for newborn resuscitation unless specifically considered during prolonged arrests in an attempt to relieve depression of myocardial function and reduced action of catecholamines induced by marked acidemia. Intraventricular hemorrhage in premature infants has been associated with the osmotic load occurring with bicarbonate administration. A neonatal preparation of sodium bicarbonate (4.2% or 0.5 mEq/mL) should be used to prevent this from occurring. The initial dose is 1 mEq/kg IV given over 2 minutes. Subsequent doses of 0.5 mEq/kg may be given every 10 minutes and should be guided by arterial blood pH and $PaCO_2$.
- d. **Atropine, calcium, and glucose** are not recommended for use in neonatal resuscitation unless specifically indicated.
- e. **Fluids.** Hypovolemia should be considered in the setting of peripartum hemorrhage, hypotension, weak pulses, and persistent pallor, despite adequate oxygenation and chest compressions. The fluid of choice for volume expansion in the delivery room is an isotonic crystalloid or blood (*IIb/C*). The volume infused should be 10 mL/kg and repeated as necessary. The administration of volume expanders too rapidly to premature infants has been associated with intraventricular hemorrhage (*IIa/C*).
6. **Postresuscitation care.** After resuscitation, the baby should be in an environment where continuous monitoring and anticipatory care are provided. Maintenance of normothermia and normoglycemia is important in preventing any further injury to the brain. Therapeutic hypothermia should be offered to near-term babies with evolving moderate to severe hypoxic–ischemic encephalopathy (*I/A*). It should be conducted and initiated under clearly defined protocols in centers with facilities and capabilities of a multidisciplinary team.
7. **Guidelines for withholding and discontinuing resuscitation**
    - a. It is considered reasonable to withhold resuscitative efforts when the conditions are known to be associated with high mortality and poor outcome especially with parental consent.
    - b. The following guidelines should be interpreted according to current regional outcomes.
        1. Gestation (<23 weeks), birth weight (<400 g), and congenital anomalies (anencephaly, trisomy 13) are associated with high mortality (*IIb/C*). Resuscitation is not generally indicated.
        2. High rate of survival and acceptable morbidity. Resuscitation is usually indicated. Includes gestational age >25 weeks and most congenital malformations (*IIb/C*).
        3. In conditions with an uncertain prognosis, borderline survival, high morbidity, and anticipated large burden to the child, parental desires concerning initiation of resuscitation should be supported (*IIb/C*).

E. Discontinuation of resuscitation is appropriate if no heart beat is detectable after 20 minutes of efficient resuscitation (*I/C-LD*). The decision to continue after 20 minutes is influenced by presumed etiology of arrest, gestational age, potential reversibility of the situation, and parents' request.

ACKNOWLEDGMENT

We gratefully acknowledge the contributions of previous edition author, Paul D. Guillod, as portions of those chapters have been retained in this revision.

Suggested Readings

Aziz K, Lee HC, Escobedo MB, et al. Part 5: neonatal resuscitation: 2020 American Heart Association Guidelines for Cardiopulmonary Resuscitation and Emergency Cardiovascular Care. *Circulation*. 2020;142(suppl 2):S524–S550.

Merchant RM, Topjian AA, Panchal AR, et al; on behalf of the Adult Basic and Advanced Life Support, Pediatric Basic and Advanced Life Support, Neonatal Life Support, Resuscitation Education Science, and Systems of Care Writing Groups. Part 1: executive summary: 2020 American Heart Association Guidelines for Cardiopulmonary Resuscitation and Emergency Cardiovascular Care. *Circulation*. 2020;142(suppl 2): S337–S357.

Panchal AR, Bartos JA, Cabañas JG, et al; on behalf of the Adult Basic and Advanced Life Support Writing Group. Part 3: Adult basic and advanced life support: 2020 American Heart Association Guidelines for Cardiopulmonary Resuscitation and Emergency Cardiovascular Care. *Circulation*. 2020;142(suppl 2):S366–S468.

Perman SM, Elmer J, Maciel CB, et al; on behalf of the American Heart Association. 2023 American Heart Association focused update on adult advanced cardiovascular life support: An update to the American Heart Association Guidelines for Cardiopulmonary Resuscitation and Emergency Cardiovascular Care. *Circulation*. 2024;149(5):e254–e273.

Topjian AA, Raymond TT, Atkins D, et al; on behalf of the Pediatric Basic and Advanced Life Support Collaborators. Part 4: Pediatric basic and advanced life support: 2020 American Heart Association Guidelines for Cardiopulmonary Resuscitation and Emergency Cardiovascular Care. *Circulation*. 2020;142(suppl 2):S469–S523.

Wyckoff MH, Greif R, Morley PT, et al. 2022 International Consensus on Cardiopulmonary Resuscitation and Emergency Cardiovascular Care Science With Treatment Recommendations: Summary From the Basic Life Support; Advanced Life Support; Pediatric Life Support; Neonatal Life Support; Education, Implementation, and Teams; and First Aid Task Forces. *Circulation*. 2022;146(25):e483–e557. Epub 2022 Nov 3.

Yamada NK, Szyld E, Strand ML, et al. American Heart Association and American Academy of Pediatrics; 2023 American Heart Association and American Academy of Pediatrics Focused Update on Neonatal Resuscitation: an update to the American Heart Association Guidelines for Cardiopulmonary Resuscitation and Emergency Cardiovascular Care. *Pediatrics*. 2024;153(2):e2023065030.

Vascular Access

James S. Cho and Omar Hyder

I. OVERVIEW
Vascular access is essential and must be tailored to the patient, procedure, and clinical setting. This chapter focuses on ultrasound-guided peripheral intravenous (IV) and arterial access in adults using the short-axis approach. Procedures for central venous and peripheral arterial access are discussed in Chapter 15: Monitoring.

II. APPLIED VASCULAR ANATOMY
A. Peripheral venous system
1. Preferred sites for ultrasound-guided IV placement are in order of preference, the cephalic vein in the mid-to-distal forearm, the antecubital veins, and the basilic vein in the upper arm. The cephalic vein follows a consistent, linear, and superficial path along the anterolateral aspect of the forearm, making it the easiest to cannulate (**Figure 40.1**).
2. The antecubital veins are less ideal due to venous confluences, branching, changes in depth, and the risk of accidental brachial artery injury.
3. The basilic vein in the upper arm is a large and consistent target. However, its proximity to the brachial artery and nerve increases the risk of complications, and extravasation in the deep tissues of the arm can occur undetected.

B. Peripheral arterial system
The distal portion of the radial artery is the first choice for arterial line placement due to its superficial location and compressibility. Alternatively, femoral, brachial, or axillary arterial cannulation can be performed.

III. VASCULAR ACCESS DEVICES
A. Structure
Vascular access devices in anesthesia and critical care are typically a combination of needles, catheters, wires, and dilators.

B. IV catheters
1. The flow rate through an IV catheter depends on its diameter (Gauge; G) and length. For use in adults, sizes range from 24G to 14G, each available in multiple lengths.
2. Sheath introducers and rapid infusion catheters (RICs) are large-bore IV access catheters placed percutaneously. They can be used for high-flow fluid resuscitation. Hemodialysis catheters (Quinton) allow high flow rates and can be used for resuscitation in an emergency.
3. **Table 40.1** shows the flow rates of commonly used sizes and lengths of IV catheters and access devices. Users are advised to review the device's packaging for flow rates.

IV. PRINCIPLES OF ULTRASOUND-GUIDED VASCULAR ACCESS
A. Ultrasound basics relevant to vascular access
1. **Linear array probe.** High-frequency probes are ideal for imaging superficial structures such as veins and arteries in extremities. Use presets for

FIGURE 40.1 Venous anatomy of the upper extremity. Area highlighted in green is preferred site for ultrasound-guided IV placement. (Courtesy of Osman Hyder, MFA and redrawn from Lewis WH. *Anatomy of the Human Body*. 20th ed. Lea and Fabiger; 1918.)

vascular access on silicon-chip–based whole-body ultrasound systems (Butterfly IQ, Butterfly Network, Inc, Guilford, CT).
2. **Depth setting.** Adjust depth setting to place the vessel of interest in the middle of the screen.
3. **Gain.** Use higher gain to distinguish between the dark lumen (blood is hypoechoic) and the lighter walls of the vein and surrounding structures.

TABLE 40.1 Maximal Flow Rates of Common Venous Access Catheters

Size	Length (mm)	Flow Rate (mL/min)
24G[a]	19	22
22G[a]	25	35
20G[a]	32	60
18G[a]	45	100
16G[a]	50	210
14G[a]	50	345
7-Fr triple lumen distal 16G port[b]	160	56
MAC proximal 12G (no catheter)[b]	100	216
Dual-lumen dialysis line (12 Fr)[c]	200	400
9-Fr PSI/MAC distal lumen (no catheter)[b]	100	550
8.5-Fr RIC[d]	64	N/A

MAC, multilumen access catheter; PSI, percutaneous sheath introducer; RIC, rapid infusion catheter.
[a]B. Braun Medical Inc, Allentown, PA.
[b]Teleflex, Morrisville, NC.
[c]Covidien LLC, Mansfield, MA.
[d]Manufacturer of RIC (Teleflex) does not list flow rate with standard measure. 8.5-Fr RIC can flow @ 1000 mL/min of saline with pressure head of 300 mm Hg.

Listed by Manufacturer, Based on ISO 10555-1:2014 Annex E:100 cm Head Height Gravity Saline Flow.
Reprinted from Greer C, Delaney W, Hamm J, Chavez R, John S. The need for speed—rapid infusion catheters versus central venous catheters for large volume infusions: a preliminary study and literature review. *Ann Emerg Med.* 2021:S17–S18, with permission from Elsevier.

4. **Using the bevel as a specular reflector.** Flat, solid structures that are held perpendicular to the ultrasound beam act as specular reflectors, reflecting acoustic waves directly back to the probe and appearing bright (hyperechoic) compared to surrounding structures. The bevel of the needle is the only relatively flat structure in cross-section, making it the ideal target for guiding vascular access.

B. **Description of procedure**

The following description highlights the use of real-time ultrasound guidance for peripheral IV placement, emphasizing the importance of the needle bevel. Similar principles apply to using ultrasound for arterial and central line placements.

1. **Scanning technique.** Apply a tourniquet to the upper arm. Apply sterile gel to the probe and cover it with a sterile probe cover. First map the venous anatomy of the ventral forearm, starting from the antecubital fossa and scanning down toward the wrist. Keep the vessel in the center of the screen. Veins are easily compressible and without pulsation.
2. **Evaluation of vessel structure and choice of puncture site.** Larger, thin-walled, superficial vessels with a straighter course are easier to cannulate than smaller, thick-walled vessels with turns and branches. Identify a linear segment that is at least 5 cm long. The preferred location for ultrasound-guided IV placement is the cephalic vein in the middle half of the forearm (**Figure 40.1**). IVs placed close to wrists and elbows are more likely to be positional.
3. **Setup.** Materials needed are clean gloves, skin disinfectant, syringe of local anesthetic with a 27G or 30G needle, IV in the plastic sheath, gauze, securement materials. Clean off previously used ultrasound gel; vigorously disinfect skin at and around the planned needle entry site.
4. **Skin infiltration with local anesthetic.** Vessels accessed with ultrasound guidance may be deep; therefore, infiltrating 0.5 to 1 mL of 1 to 2% lidocaine is highly recommended. Place the clean probe over the planned vein entry site. Enter the skin in line with the center marker, 5 to 10 mm away from the probe. If there is no center marker, use the approximate middle of the probe. Infiltrate the anesthetic down to the vein.
5. **Insertion steps** (Video 40.1). Like most surgical procedures, ultrasound-guided IV placement is best learned with hands-on practice. The following description highlights key steps of the procedure.
    a. **Skin entry and sonographic identification of the needle tip.** The most challenging part of this procedure is sonographically locating the IV tip in soft tissue immediately after skin entry. This can be optimized by using a shallow needle entry angle, approximately 30 degrees relative to the skin surface. Once the entire bevel is under the dermis, ensure that the bevel is facing the ultrasound probe and then tilt the ultrasound probe away from the IV. This adjustment aligns the ultrasound beam nearly perpendicular to the bevel's plane. Subsequently, a slow, controlled, sliding movement of the probe toward the IV helps accurately locate the bevel beneath the skin surface (**Figure 40.2**, left panel).
    b. **Advancement to the top of the vein.** After identifying the needle tip, the next crucial step is to determine the needle's trajectory toward the vein. Gently moving the needle's hub from side to side causes corresponding movements of the tip, which can be observed using ultrasound to confirm the intended direction. At this stage, the angle between the needle and the skin should be made steeper. Once the path is confirmed, advance the needle in 1- to 2-mm increments, verifying the needle tip position with each step.

FIGURE 40.2 Technical considerations in positioning the probe and needle and representative ultrasound images. **Left panel:** Tilting the ultrasound probe to visualize the bevel (*solid red arrow*) above the cephalic vein (*yellow arrow*). **Right panel:** Sliding the ultrasound probe to visualize the bevel (*solid red arrow*) and tip of the needle (*interrupted red arrow*).

   c. **Vein entry and advancement inside vessel lumen.** Once the needle tip is positioned directly above the middle of the vein, introduce it into the vessel lumen with a short, controlled motion. Hold the ultrasound probe perpendicular to the skin to ensure a clear cross-sectional view of the vessel lumen. The body of the needle bevel will appear as a bright white object within the lumen. Position the needle tip in the center of the vessel and advance the IV apparatus until the bevel is fully visible within the lumen. Slide the ultrasound probe away from the needle till only a small cross section of the tip is visible. Advance the needle in 1- to 2-mm increments, until the bright middle of the bevel appears on the screen. Continue advancing by repeating this process until at least half to three-fourths of the catheter is inside the vein (**Figure 40.2**, right panel).
   d. **Deployment of the catheter in the vein.** For catheter deployment, visualize and center the needle tip in the vessel lumen using ultrasound. Retract the needle hub slightly (approximately 2 to 3 mm) to pull the bevel inside the catheter. Fully advance the catheter into the vein. Withdraw the needle completely, leaving the catheter in place.

V. COMMON ISSUES AND TROUBLESHOOTING
A. Inadequate visualization or insufficient catheter length
1. Use ≥18G catheters that are at least 1.5 inches long. Large bevels are easier to visualize.
2. Longer length provides a margin of safety against an inadequate length of catheter in the vein.

B. No reasonable venous targets in the forearm
1. **Scan contralateral forearm.** Use veins in antecubital fossa or basilic vein as a backup site.
2. An experienced operator is recommended for upper arm basilic vein cannulation to reduce the risk of neurovascular injury.

C. Cannulating thick-walled veins
Veins that resemble arteries—characterized by a small diameter, round shape, and thick walls—are prone to spasm, extravasation, and becoming obscured (isoechoic). These veins are challenging for ultrasound-guided IV placement. Meticulous visualization of the needle tip typically improves first-pass success rates.

D. Use of wires for venous cannulation
Wires can tunnel subintimally and create a false passage in small peripheral veins, posing a significant risk of unrecognized infiltration. This technique should be used with caution.

E. Verifying intravascular placement
Injecting agitated saline through the IV and observing it on ultrasound as it passes through the basilic vein system is an effective method for verifying vascular placement of a catheter.

F. Venous leakage
1. **Venous leakage can result from posterior vessel wall puncture, catheter dislodgement, or leakage around the access site.** Infiltration refers to leakage of nonvesicant solutions, for example crystalloid IV fluids, while extravasation involves vesicants. Tissue injury may arise from the infusate's pharmacologic properties, volume effects, or inflammatory responses. Signs of leakage include poor fluid flow, perivascular swelling or bruising, lack of expected medication response, and patient discomfort. Leakage detection may be delayed with ultrasound-guided deep IV catheter placement.
2. **Upon suspicion of infiltration or extravasation, immediately stop the infusion and initiate treatment specific to the agent involved.** Attempt to aspirate the infusate. Administer antidotes through the catheter, via needle, or topically. For example, use phentolamine for α-adrenergic agonist extravasation and hyaluronidase for vancomycin extravasation. Apply cold compresses to cause vasoconstriction, warm compresses to cause vasodilation, and elevate the affected site to reduce swelling and discomfort.

Suggested Readings

Blanco P. Ultrasound-guided peripheral venous cannulation in critically ill patients: a practical guideline. *Ultrasound J.* 2019;11(1):27.

Gottlieb M, Sundaram T, Holladay D, Nakitende D. Ultrasound-guided peripheral intravenous line placement: a narrative review of evidence-based best practices. *West J Emerg Med.* 2017;18(6):1047–1054.

Le A, Patel S. Extravasation of noncytotoxic drugs: a review of the literature. *Ann Pharmacother.* 2014;48(7):870–886.

APPENDIX

Drugs With Narrow Therapeutic Ranges and Potential for Harm

Hiu Ling (Karen) Wong

Anesthetists frequently administer intravenous (IV) medications with narrow therapeutic windows and the potential for critical events. The drugs described in this section are not routinely administered by anesthetists but may be requested by others. It does not include agents that fall within the scope of the training and practice of anesthetists, for example, neuromuscular blockers.

A. **Alprostadil** (prostaglandin E1 [PGE_1]): Vasodilator; decreases peripheral and pulmonary arterial resistance, which causes reflexive increase in cardiac output and heart rate.
   1. **Indications**
      a. Primary nonfunctional liver transplant characterized by rising transaminases, minimal bile production, and coagulopathy from 4 to 34 hours after transplantation.
      b. Pulmonary hypertension.
      c. Distal ischemia (limb or digit) refractory to conventional revascularization or drug therapy.
      d. Vasospastic disorders (Raynaud disease), vasculitis, Buerger disease, and atheroembolic diseases.
      e. Protection against tacrolimus nephrotoxicity.
   2. **Administration guidelines**
      a. Standard concentration: 500 μg of alprostadil in 1000 mL NS (0.5 μg/mL = 500 ng/mL)
      b. Infusion rates should be titrated to patient response.
         1. Remove rings/tight-fitting jewelry during the infusion since most experience extremity swelling. Patients often experience a "flushing" feeling during the initiation that is not necessarily an indication to stop the infusion, unless there is a drop in blood pressure (BP).
         2. Start the infusion at 1 ng/kg/min. If the patient becomes hypotensive, wean back to the previous dose. A starting dose of 0.4 ng/kg/min is recommended for patients with borderline low BP and/or poor left ventricular (LV) function.
         3. The infusion rate (dose) may be doubled every 30 minutes as tolerated to a peak dose of 16 ng/kg/min.

B. **Alteplase** (Activase): Tissue plasminogen activator (tPA)
   1. **Indications**
      a. Acute myocardial infarction (MI).
      b. Pulmonary embolism.
      c. Peripheral arterial or venous thrombosis.
      d. Catheter occlusion.
   2. **Administration guidelines**
      a. **Acute MI**
         1. Concentration (1 mg/mL): 100 mg/100 mL and 50 mg/50 mL.

2. Patient weight less than 67 kg: 15 mg bolus; then 0.75 mg/kg (maximum 50 mg) over 30 minutes. Initiate heparin therapy with a bolus; then alteplase 0.5 mg/kg (maximum 35 mg) over the next hour.
3. Patient weight greater than 67 kg: 15 mg bolus; then 50 mg over the next 30 minutes. Institute heparin therapy with a bolus. Infuse remaining 35 mg of tPA over the next hour (total maximum dose of tPA = 100 mg).

b. Pulmonary embolus
1. Standard concentration: 100 mg/100 mL.
2. Maintenance infusion: 100 mg continuous infusion over 2 hours.

c. Peripheral venous thrombosis (systemic thrombolysis approach)
1. Concentration (0.1 mg/mL): 50 mg/500 mL, 25 mg/250 mL.
2. Loading dose: none.
3. Maintenance infusion: 0.5 to 4 mg/h for 24 hours (recommended maximum 50 mg/24 h). Heparin (no loading dose) should be started after alteplase infusion is completed to maintain activated partial thromboplastin time (aPTT) in a therapeutic range.

d. Peripheral arterial thrombosis and peripheral venous thrombosis catheter-directed thrombolysis
1. Concentration (0.1 mg/mL): 50 mg/500 mL, 25 mg/250 mL.
2. Loading dose: 4 to 10 mg.
3. Maintenance infusion: 0.5 to 4 mg/h for 4 to 24 hours intracatheter. Recommended cumulative maximum of 50 mg (load plus infusion). Heparin should be used at a low non–weight-adjusted dose (eg, 250 units/h) keeping aPTT less than 1.5 times baseline during alteplase infusion.

C. Argatroban: Direct thrombin inhibitor
  1. Indications
  a. Anticoagulation in patients with suspected or confirmed heparin-induced thrombocytopenia (HIT type II).
  b. Anticoagulation during and immediately following percutaneous coronary interventions (PCIs).

  2. Administration guidelines
  a. Standard concentration (1 mg/mL): 50 mg/50 mL premixed vial and 250 mg/250 mL in NaCl for large volume infusion pump.
  b. Low concentration (0.05 mg/mL): 2.5 mg/50 mL bag.
  c. Bolus: None.
  d. Maintenance
  1. Start 0.5 to 2 µg/kg/min as a continuous infusion.
  2. Reduce initial dose to 0.25 µg/kg/min for moderate hepatic dysfunction, and critically ill.
  3. Check the aPTT 2 hours after the start of the infusion and after any rate change until stable (ie, two consecutive values within the goal range). Goal: aPTT 1.5 to 3× baseline, not to exceed a PTT of 100 seconds.

D. Bivalirudin (Angiomax): Direct thrombin inhibitor
  1. Indication: Anticoagulation in patients with strongly suspected or confirmed HIT (type II).
  2. Administration guidelines
  a. Standard concentration (5 mg/mL): 250 mg/50 mL bag.
  b. Low concentration (1 mg/mL): 100 mg/100 mL bag.
  c. Bolus: None.
  d. Maintenance
  1. Starting dose: 0.15 mg/kg/h (CrCl ≥60 mL/min).
  2. If CrCl 30 to 59 mL/min: 0.05 mg/kg/h.

Appendix I Drugs With Narrow Therapeutic Ranges and Potential for Harm **779**

3. If CrCl less than 30 mL/min or renal replacement therapy: 0.025 mg/kg/h.
4. Goal aPTT: 1.5 to 2.5 times baseline. Check the aPTT 2 hours after the start of the infusion and after any rate change until two consecutive aPTT values are within the goal range.

E. **Cangrelor**: Antiplatelet agent. It is a direct $P2Y_{12}$ platelet-receptor inhibitor that blocks adenosine diphosphate (ADP)–induced platelet activation and aggregation.
  1. **Indication:** Use in PCI to reduce risk of MI, repeat coronary revascularization, and stent thrombosis for patients not previously treated with $P2Y_{12}$ inhibitor or glycoprotein IIb/IIIa inhibitor.
  2. **Administration guidelines**
     a. Standard concentration: 50 mg/250 mL.
     b. **Bolus:** 30 µg/kg. Administer over 1 minute (<100 kg); 2 minutes (100 to 200 kg); or 3 minutes (>200 kg).
     c. Starting rate: 4 µg/kg/min.

F. **Epoprostenol (Veletri):** Potent vasodilator that also inhibits platelet aggregation.
  1. **Indication:** Pulmonary hypertension.
  2. **Administration guidelines**
     a. Do not give with other parenteral medications or carriers.
     b. A dedicated central venous catheter is required for administration with a 0.22 micron air-eliminating filter.
     c. **Do not flush catheter with epoprostenol in-line.**
     d. **Bolus: None.**
     e. Maintenance infusion
        1. Initial dose: 1 to 2 ng/kg/min IV.
        2. Titrate in 1 to 2 ng/kg/min increments every 15 to 30 minutes.
     f. If the catheter needs to be flushed, measure the catheter volume by withdrawing blood until it gets into the syringe and discard. This is the dead space volume, which is the maximum amount of prime to be given. The line can then be flushed with saline and thereafter primed with reconstituted epoprostenol from the medication bag.
     g. Avoid abrupt withdrawal that may cause rebound pulmonary artery hypertension.
     h. Bag is stable for 24 hours at room temperature.

G. **Eptifibatide (Integrilin)**
  1. **Indication:** Prevention of thrombus formation after PCI.
  2. **Dosage:** Bolus of 180 µg/kg (maximum dose: 22.6 mg); then 2 µg/kg/min continuous infusion.
  3. **Effect:** Inhibits glycoprotein IIb/IIIa; prevents platelet adhesion and aggregation.
  4. **Comments:** Bleeding complications and thrombocytopenia are common side effects.

H. **Insulin, regular (human):** Humulin R, Novolin R
  1. **Indications:** Hyperglycemia, hyperkalemia, diabetic ketoacidosis.
  2. **Administration guidelines**
     a. Regular insulin is the only insulin that can be administered intravenously.
     b. Insert infusion below any inline filters.
     c. Standard concentration: 100 units/100 mL normal saline.
     d. Loading dose: 0 to 10 units intravenous push (IVP) or bolus (usually given prior to starting maintenance).
     e. Maintenance infusion: 0.5 to 25 units/h IV titrated according to blood glucose level.

f. Once under control, blood glucose should be monitored at a minimum of every 2 hours and more often as needed.
I. **Potassium chloride (KCl)**
 1. **Indication:** Correction of hypokalemia.
    a. **Caution: Hypokalemia is not usually treated in the operating room (OR).**
    b. The decision to administer KCl requires **anesthesia attending approval** in advance of administration.
 2. **Administration guidelines**
    a. **Bolus dose: None. May cause cardiac arrest.**
    b. Peripheral concentration: 10 mEq/100 mL.
    c. Central concentration: 20 mEq/50 mL.
    d. Rate: Not to exceed 20 mEq/h.
J. **Tenecteplase** (TNKase): tPA
 1. **Indications:** Acute ST-elevation MI, pulmonary embolism with cardiac arrest, and acute ischemic stroke.
 2. **Administration guidelines**
    a. Standard concentration: 5 mg/mL.
    b. Reconstitute the 50 mg IV kit of TNKase using the provided 10 mL syringe along with the TwinPak Dual Cannula Device and 10 mL of sterile water for injection. Gently swirl the mixture; avoid shaking. Some foaming may occur.
    c. Dosing for ST-elevation MI and pulmonary embolism with cardiac arrest
       1. Less than 60 kg: 30 mg.
       2. 60 kg to less than 70 kg: 35 mg.
       3. 70 kg to less than 80 kg: 40 mg.
       4. 80 kg to less than 90 kg: 45 mg.
       5. 90 kg or more: 50 mg.
    d. Give as IV push over 5 seconds and flush line with normal saline following TNKase.
    e. Acute ischemic stroke dosing
       1. 0.25 mg/kg IV push over 5 seconds (with a maximum total dose of 25 mg).

ACKNOWLEDGMENT

We gratefully acknowledge the contributions of previous edition author, Richard M. Pino, as portions of those chapters have been retained in this revision.

APPENDIX III

Commonly Used Drugs
Audrey Kennedy

The drugs listed in this section are those that are commonly used or encountered by anesthetists during perioperative patient care. Anesthetics and muscle relaxants are not included and are covered in respective chapters.

I. ACETAMINOPHEN
   A. **Indications:** Antipyretic, analgesic, adjunct to opioid therapy.
   B. **Dosage:** Adult >50 kg: 1000 mg IV/PO q6h, <50 kg: 500 mg IV/PO q6h. Pediatric <40 kg: 7.5 to 15 mg/kg IV/PO q6h.
   C. **Effect:** Nonopioid analgesic and nonsalicylate antipyretic.
   D. **Comments**
      1. Adult daily dosage limit: <4 g.
      2. Pediatric daily dosage limit: <2 years, 60 mg/kg/d, ≥2 years, 75 mg/kg/d <50 kg: not to exceed 3750 mg/d, ≥50 kg: not to exceed 4000 mg/d.

II. ADENOSINE
   A. **Indications:** Paroxysmal supraventricular tachycardia.
   B. **Dosage:** Adult: 6 to 12 mg peripheral intravenous (IV) bolus followed by rapid 10 mL saline IV flush. Central line: initial dose, 3 mg. Pediatric: 50 µg/kg IV. Maximum initial dose 6 mg.
   C. **Effect:** Slows or temporarily blocks atrioventricular (AV) node conduction and conduction through reentrant pathways (especially those involving the AV node).
   D. **Comments**
      1. Contraindicated in patients with second- or third-degree heart block or sick sinus syndrome.
      2. Not effective in terminating atrial flutter or fibrillation, but may aid in diagnosis by slowing ventricular response.
      3. Asystole for 3 to 6 seconds after administration is common and resolves spontaneously.
      4. May cause bronchospasm or hypotension.
      5. Use with caution in patients with preexcitation syndromes (eg, Wolff–Parkinson–White).

III. ALBUTEROL
   A. **Indications:** Bronchospasm, hyperkalemia.
   B. **Dosage**
      1. Bronchospasm, aerosolized via nebulizer: 2.5 mg in 3 mL saline; or via metered dose inhaler (MDI): 2 puffs (180 µg).
      2. Hyperkalemia, aerosolized via nebulizer: 10 to 20 mg over 10 minutes.
   C. **Effect:** β_2-Receptor agonist, causing bronchial smooth muscle relaxation, translocation of potassium into cells.

D. Comments: Possible β-adrenergic overload, tachydysrhythmias. Increased dose required when using MDI for intubated patients (four to six puffs).

IV. ALPROSTADIL (SEE APPENDIX I)

V. ALTEPLASE (SEE APPENDIX I)

VI. AMINOCAPROIC ACID (AMICAR)
A. Indications: Prevention of bleeding due to fibrinolysis.
B. Dosage: 5 g/100 to 250 mL of normal saline (NS) IV to load, followed by 1 g/h infusion.
C. Effect: Stabilizes the formed clot by inhibiting plasminogen activators and plasmin.
D. Comments: Contraindicated in disseminated intravascular coagulation.

VII. AMIODARONE
A. Indications: Refractory or recurrent atrial and ventricular tachydysrhythmias.
B. Dosage: Advanced Cardiac Life Support (ACLS): For stable ventricular tachycardia (VT) or atrial fibrillation (AF), 150 mg over 10 mins. For unstable VT, or ventricular fibrillation (VF), 300 mg intravenous push (IVP), then 1 mg/min for 6 hours (360 mg), then 0.5 mg/min for 18 hours (540 mg).
C. Effect: Depresses the sinoatrial node and prolongs the PR, QRS, and QT intervals; produces α- and β-adrenergic blockade.
D. Comments
1. May cause severe sinus bradycardia, ventricular arrhythmias, AV block, liver and thyroid function test abnormalities, hepatitis, cirrhosis, and may cause hypotension.
2. Pulmonary fibrosis can result from long-term use.
3. Increases serum levels of digoxin, oral anticoagulants, diltiazem, quinidine, procainamide, and phenytoin.

VIII. APREPITANT
A. Indications: Prevention of postoperative nausea and vomiting (PONV).
B. Dosage: Aponvie IV: 32 mg prior to induction of anesthesia. Aprepitant PO: 40 mg within 3 hours prior to anesthesia induction.
C. Effect: Substance P/neurokinin 1 (NK 1) receptor antagonist.
D. Comments
1. Clinically significant CYP3A4 drug interactions. Contraindicated in patients taking pimozide due to possible QT prolongation.
2. Concomitant use with warfarin may result in clinically significant decrease in International Normalized Ratio (INR) of prothrombin time. After a single 40 mg dose, monitor INR in 2-week period following administration.
3. Risk of reduced efficacy of hormonal contraceptives during administration and for 28 days following last dose.

IX. ARGATROBAN (SEE APPENDIX I)

X. ATENOLOL
A. Indications: Hypertension, angina, and postmyocardial infarction (post-MI).
B. Dosage: Oral (PO) 50 to 100 mg/d.
C. Effect: $β_1$-Selective adrenergic receptor blockade.

D. Comments
1. Relatively contraindicated in acute congestive heart failure and heart block.
2. Caution in patients on calcium channel blockers and other agents prolonging AV conduction.

XI. ATROPINE
A. Indications: Antisialagogue; bradycardia; cardiac arrest (ACLS protocol).
B. Dosage
1. Antisialagogue, adult, 0.2 to 0.4 mg IV; pediatric, 0.01 mg/kg/dose IV/intramuscular (IM) (<0.4 mg).
2. Bradycardia, adult, 0.2 to 0.4 mg IV; pediatric, 0.02 mg/kg/dose IV (<0.4 mg).
3. Cardiac arrest, adult, 1 mg IV; pediatric, 0.01 to 0.02 mg/kg/dose IV.

C. Effect: Competitive blockade of acetylcholine at muscarinic receptors.
D. Comments
1. Low doses may cause paradoxical bradycardia.
2. May cause tachydysrhythmias, AV dissociation, premature ventricular contractions, dry mouth, or urinary retention.
3. Central nervous system (CNS) effects occur at high doses.

XII. BICARBONATE, SODIUM ($NaHCO_3$)
A. Indications: Metabolic acidosis; urinary alkalinization.
B. Dosage: IV dose in mEq $NaHCO_3$ = (base deficit × weight [kg] × 0.3) (subsequent doses titrated against patient's pH).
C. Effect: H^+ neutralization.
D. Comments
1. Not compatible with many IV medications.
2. May cause metabolic alkalosis, hypercarbia, and hyperosmolality.
3. In neonates, can cause intraventricular hemorrhage.
4. Crosses placenta.
5. An 8.4% solution is approximately 1.0 mEq/mL; a 4.2% solution is approximately 0.5 mEq/mL.

XIII. BIVALIRUDIN (SEE APPENDIX I)

XIV. CALCIUM CHLORIDE; CALCIUM GLUCONATE
A. Indications: hypocalcemia, hyperkalemia, and hypermagnesemia.
B. Dosage:
1. Calcium chloride: 5 to 10 mg/kg IV prn (10% $CaCl_2$ = 1.36 mEq Ca^{2+}/mL).
2. Calcium gluconate: 15 to 30 mg/kg IV prn (10% calcium gluconate = 0.45 mEq Ca^{2+}/mL).

C. Effect: Maintains cell membrane integrity, muscular excitation–contraction coupling, glandular stimulation–secretion coupling, and enzyme function. Increases blood pressure.
D. Comments
1. May cause bradycardia or arrhythmia (especially with digitalis).
2. Irritating to veins. Ca^{2+} less available with calcium gluconate than with calcium chloride owing to the binding of gluconate.
3. Rapid infusion may cause coronary vasoconstriction.

XV. CARBOPROST (PROSTAGLANDIN $F_{2\alpha}$; HEMABATE)
A. Indications: Refractory postpartum hemorrhage.

B. **Dosage:** 250 µg IM; may repeat every 15 to 90 minutes, maximum total dose 2 mg.
C. **Effect:** Causes uterine muscle contraction.
D. **Comments**
  1. May cause hypertension.
  2. May cause significant bronchospasm, especially in patients with reactive airways.

XVI. CELECOXIB
A. **Indications:** Management of acute pain in adults.
B. **Dosage:** 100 to 400 mg PO.
C. **Effect:** Nonsteroidal anti-inflammatory; exhibits anti-inflammatory, analgesic, and antipyretic actions.
D. **Comments**
  1. Contraindicated for treatment of perioperative pain in setting of coronary bypass graft (CABG) surgery.
  2. Avoid in patients with significant renal impairment.
  3. Consider using 100 mg dose in patients >65 years old or <50 kg.

XVII. CLEVIDIPINE (CLEVIPREX)
A. **Indications:** Treatment of acute hypertension when oral therapy is undesirable/unavailable.
B. **Dosage:** IV infusion: 1 to 2 mg/h; double the dose q90 seconds until approaching goal, then adjust q5–10 minutes. Maximum dose 32 mg/h.
C. **Effect**
  1. Dihydropyridine calcium channel blocker; causes blood pressure reduction ± reflex tachycardia via decreased systemic vascular resistance.
  2. May have negative inotropic effects. Does not affect preload.
  3. No dose adjustments for hepatic/renal dysfunction.
  4. Lasts 5 to 15 minutes after discontinuation.
D. **Comments**
  1. Rapidly titratable. In lipid emulsion.
  2. Discard unused portion after 4 hours.
  3. Contraindicated in soy/egg allergic patients, defective lipid metabolism, or severe aortic stenosis.
  4. Risk of rebound hypertension with prolonged infusion; risk of atrial fibrillation.

XVIII. CLOPIDOGREL (PLAVIX)
A. **Indications:** Antiplatelet agent.
  1. Acute coronary syndrome.
  2. Percutaneous coronary intervention (PCI).
  3. Recent MI, recent thromboembolic stroke, or established arterial disease.
  4. Coronary stent stenosis prophylaxis.
B. **Dosage:** Load, 300 to 600 mg PO; maintenance, 75 mg every day (qd).
C. **Effect:** Irreversible platelet adenosine diphosphate (ADP) receptor blockade.
D. **Comments**
  1. Major side effect is bleeding.
  2. Proton pump inhibitors may reduce clopidogrel efficacy.
  3. Recommend discontinuing 5 to 7 days prior to neuraxial anesthesia.

XIX. DANTROLENE
  A. Indications: Malignant hyperthermia (MH); neuroleptic malignant syndrome.
  B. Dosage: At first signs of MH, 2.5 mg/kg IV bolus; repeat dose, up to 10 mg/kg. Prophylactic IV treatment is not recommended.
  C. Effect: Reduces Ca^{2+} release from sarcoplasmic reticulum; relaxes skeletal muscles.
  D. Comments
  1. Revonto or Dantrium, mix each 20 mg vial with 60 mL of sterile water. Dissolves slowly into solution.
  2. Ryanodex, mix each 250 mg vial with 5 mL sterile water.
  3. Avoid extravasation as it is a tissue irritant.

XX. DESMOPRESSIN ACETATE (DDAVP)
  A. Indications
  1. Treatment of coagulopathy in von Willebrand disease, hemophilia A (but contraindicated if factor VIII >5% activity), renal failure.
  2. Central diabetes insipidus (DI).
  B. Dosage
  1. Coagulopathy; 0.3 μg/kg IV (diluted 50 mL NS), infused over 15 to 30 minutes.
  2. Central DI; 5 to 20 μg intranasally qd/bid.
  C. Effect: Increases plasma levels of factor VIII activity by causing release of von Willebrand factor from endothelial cells; increases renal water reabsorption (antidiuretic hormone [ADH] effect).
  D. Comments: Chlorpropamide, carbamazepine, and clofibrate potentiate the antidiuretic effect. Repeat doses q12–24h will have diminished effect compared with initial dose. Can cause hyponatremia. Can cause hypo- or hypertension if delivered too rapidly.

XXI. DEXAMETHASONE (DECADRON)
  A. Indications: Cerebral edema; airway edema; prophylaxis to reduce PONV; reduced narcotic requirement, pain adjunct.
  B. Dosage
  1. Edema: 10 to 16 mg IV, 4 to 6 mg IV q6h (tapered over 6 days).
  2. Nausea and vomiting (N/V): 4 mg IV.
  3. Pain adjunct: 0.12 mg/kg.
  C. Effect: See Hydrocortisone. Has 20 to 25 times the glucocorticoid potency of hydrocortisone. Minimal mineralocorticoid effect.
  D. Comments: See Hydrocortisone. Can cause perineal burning or itching if injected rapidly IV.

XXII. DILTIAZEM (CARDIZEM)
  A. Indications: Angina pectoris, variant angina from coronary artery spasm, atrial fibrillation/flutter, paroxysmal supraventricular tachycardia, hypertension.
  B. Dosage: 20 mg IV bolus then 10 mg/h infusion; PO 30 to 60 mg q6h.
  C. Effect: Calcium channel antagonist that slows conduction through sinoatrial and AV nodes, dilates coronary and peripheral arterioles, and reduces myocardial contractility.
  D. Comments
  1. May cause bradycardia and heart block.
  2. Possible impairment of contractility by interaction with β-blockers and digoxin.
  3. Causes transiently elevated liver function tests.

4. Avoid use in patients with accessory conduction tracts, AV block, IV β-blockers, or ventricular tachycardia (VT).

XXIII. DOBUTAMINE
A. **Indications:** Inotropy for heart failure.
B. **Dosage:** Begin infusion at 2 µg/kg/min and titrate to effect, up to 40 µg/kg/min.
C. **Effect:** α_1-, β_1-, β_2-Adrenergic agonist.
D. **Comments:** May cause hypotension, arrhythmias, or myocardial ischemia. Can increase ventricular rate in atrial fibrillation.

XXIV. DOPAMINE
A. **Indications:** Hypotension, heart failure, bradycardia.
B. **Dosage:** 5 to 20 µg/kg/min IV; titrate to effect.
C. **Effect:** dopaminergic; α- and β-adrenergic agonist.
D. **Comments**
  1. May cause hypertension, dysrhythmias, or myocardial ischemia.
  2. Primarily dopaminergic effects (increased renal blood flow) at 1 to 5 µg/kg/min.
  3. Primarily α- and β-adrenergic effects at greater than or equal to 10 µg/kg/min.

XXV. ENOXAPARIN (LOVENOX)
A. **Indications**
  1. Prophylaxis of DVT.
  2. Treatment of DVT.
  3. Acute coronary syndromes.
B. **Dosage**
  1. DVT prophylaxis, 30 mg SC bid or 40 mg SC qd.
  2. DVT treatment, 1 mg/kg SC q12h or 1.5 mg/kg SC qd.
  3. ACS, 1 mg/kg SC bid for a minimum of 2 days, in conjunction with aspirin therapy.
C. **Effect:** Anticoagulant; inhibits both factor Xa and factor IIa. See Heparin.
D. **Comments**
  1. Equally effective as unfractionated heparin with more predictable dose-response characteristics.
  2. Spinal and epidural hematomas have been associated with spinal and lumbar punctures, or epidural catheter placement or removal.
  3. Only partially reversed by protamine.
  4. For CrCl <30 reduce dose or consider using heparin.

XXVI. EPHEDRINE
A. **Indication:** Treatment of hypotension, especially with concomitant bradycardia.
B. **Dosage:** 5 to 10 mg IV.
C. **Effect:** α- and β-adrenergic stimulation; norepinephrine release at sympathetic nerve endings.
D. **Comments**
  1. May cause hypertension, dysrhythmias, myocardial ischemia, CNS stimulation, decrease in uterine activity, and mild bronchodilation.
  2. Minimal effect on uterine blood flow. Crosses the placenta.
  3. Avoid in patients taking monoamine oxidase inhibitors (MAOI).
  4. Tachyphylaxis with repeated dosing.

XXVII. EPINEPHRINE
A. Indications
1. Heart failure.
2. Cardiac arrest (ACLS).
3. Bronchospasm, anaphylaxis.
4. Airway edema.

B. Dosage
1. Heart failure, 1 to 12 µg/min titrated to effect.
2. ACLS, 0.1 to 1 mg IV or 1 mg intratracheal q5min prn. Pediatric, 0.01 mg/kg IV up to 0.5 mg. 0.01 mg/kg SC q15min × 2 doses up to 1 mg/dose.
3. Bronchospasm, anaphylaxis, 0.1 to 0.5 mg SC, 0.1 to 0.25 mg IV, or 0.25 to 1.5 µg/min IV infusion.
4. Airway edema, nebulized: 0.5 mL of 2.25% solution in 2.5 to 3.5 mL of NS q1–4h prn.

C. Effect: α- and β-Adrenergic agonist.

D. Comments
1. May cause hypertension, arrhythmias, or myocardial ischemia. Topical or local injection (1:80,000 to 1:500,000) causes vasoconstriction. Crosses the placenta.
2. Reduce dose when treating local anesthetic systemic toxicity (LAST), 1 µg/kg.

XXVIII. EPOPROSTENOL (FLOLAN) (SEE APPENDIX I)

XXIX. EPTIFIBATIDE (INTEGRILIN) (SEE APPENDIX I)

XXX. ESMOLOL (BREVIBLOC)
A. Indications: Supraventricular tachydysrhythmias and myocardial ischemia.
B. Dosage: Start with 5 mg to 10 mg IV bolus and increase q3min prn to total 100 to 300 mg; infusion 1 to 15 mg/min.
C. Effect: Selective β_1-adrenergic blockade.
D. Comments: May cause bradycardia, AV conduction delay, hypotension, congestive heart failure; β_2 activity at high doses.

XXXI. FLUMAZENIL (MAZICON)
A. Indications: Reversal of benzodiazepine overdose.
B. Dosage: 3 to 5 mg IV at 0.2 mg/min. Maximum rate of 3 mg/hour.
C. Effect: Competitive antagonism of CNS benzodiazepine receptor.
D. Comments
1. Duration of action shorter than midazolam and other agonists.
2. May induce CNS excitation including seizures, acute withdrawal, nausea, dizziness, and agitation.
3. Only partial reversal of midazolam-induced ventilatory depression.

XXXII. FOSPHENYTOIN
A. Indication: Seizure prophylaxis, treatment of seizures (see Phenytoin).
B. Dosage
1. It is a prodrug; active metabolite is phenytoin.
2. 1.5 mg fosphenytoin is equivalent to 1 mg phenytoin and is referred to as 1 mg phenytoin equivalent (PE).
3. Dilute fosphenytoin in 5% dextrose or 0.9% saline solution for injection to a concentration ranging from 1.5 to 25 mg PE/mL.

4. The loading dose of fosphenytoin is 10 to 20 mg PE/kg given IV.
5. Maximum rate, 150 mg PE/min.
C. **Effect:** Anticonvulsant.
D. **Comments**
   1. IV bolus may cause bradycardia, hypotension, respiratory arrest, cardiac arrest, or CNS depression.
   2. Determination of unbound phenytoin levels may be helpful in patients with renal failure or hypoalbuminemia 2 hours after infusion has been completed.
   3. Multiple drug interactions that may change the effective concentration of phenytoin.

XXXIII. FUROSEMIDE (LASIX)
A. **Indications:** Edema, intracranial hypertension, renal failure, and hypercalcemia.
B. **Dosage:** 2 to 40 mg IV (initial dose, dosage individualized).
C. **Effect:** Increases excretion of Na^+, Cl^-, K^+, PO_4^{3-}, Ca^{2+}, and H_2O by inhibiting reabsorption in loop of Henle.
D. **Comments:** May cause electrolyte imbalance, dehydration, transient hypotension, deafness, hyperglycemia, or hyperuricemia. Sulfa-allergic patients may exhibit hypersensitivity to furosemide.

XXXIV. GLUCAGON
A. **Indications**
   1. Duodenal or choledochal relaxation.
   2. Refractory β-adrenergic blocker toxicity.
B. **Dosage**
   1. GI effects, 0.25 to 1 mg IV q20 min prn.
   2. β-Blocker toxicity, 5 mg IV bolus, with 1 to 10 mg/h titrated to patient response.
C. **Effect:** Catecholamine release. Positive inotrope and chronotrope.
D. **Comments**
   1. May cause anaphylaxis, nausea, vomiting, hyperglycemia, or positive inotropic chronotropic effects.
   2. High doses potentiate oral anticoagulants.
   3. Use with caution in the presence of insulinoma or pheochromocytoma.

XXXV. GLYCOPYRROLATE
A. **Indications:** Decrease GI motility, antisialagogue, bradycardia.
B. **Dosage:** 0.1 to 0.2 mg IV/IM/SC.
C. **Effect:** Competitive blockade of acetylcholine at muscarinic receptors.
D. **Comments:** Longer duration, possibly less chronotropic effect than atropine. Does not cross the blood-brain barrier or placenta.

XXXVI. HALOPERIDOL (HALDOL)
A. **Indications:** Psychosis, delirium, agitation, and PONV.
B. **Dosage:** 0.5 to 10 mg IM/IV prn (dosage individualized); antiemetic, 1 mg IV.
C. **Effect:** Antipsychotic effects due to dopamine (D_2) receptor antagonism. CNS depression.
D. **Comments**
   1. May cause mild α-adrenergic antagonism.
   2. Can prolong QT interval and produce ventricular arrhythmias, notably torsade de pointes, and lower seizure threshold.
   3. May precipitate neuroleptic malignant syndrome.
   4. Contraindicated in Parkinson's disease.

XXXVII. HEPARIN—UNFRACTIONATED
A. Indications: Anticoagulation for:
1. Thrombosis, thromboembolism.
2. Cardiopulmonary bypass (CPB).
3. Disseminated intravascular coagulation.
4. Thromboembolism prophylaxis.

B. Dosage
1. Thrombosis, load: 50 to 150 units/kg IV; maintenance: 15 to 25 units/kg/h IV; titrate dosage with activated partial thromboplastin time.
2. CPB, load: 300 units/kg IV; maintenance: 100 units/kg/h IV; titrate with activated clotting time (ACT).
3. Disseminated intravascular coagulopathy (DIC), load: 50 to 100 units/kg IV; maintenance: 15 to 25 units/kg/h IV; titrate with coagulation tests.
4. DVT prophylaxis, 5000 units q8–12h SC.

C. Effect: Potentiates action of antithrombin III; blocks conversion of prothrombin and activation of other coagulation factors.

D. Comments
1. May cause thrombocytopenia, allergic reactions.
2. Half-life increased in renal failure and decreased in thromboembolism and liver disease.
3. Does not cross the placenta.
4. Reversed by protamine.
5. Spinal and epidural hematomas have been associated with neuraxial anesthesia (single-shot, or catheter placement or removal) and lumbar punctures in patients on heparin infusions.

XXXVIII. HYDRALAZINE
A. Indication: Hypertension.
B. Dosage: 2.5 to 5 mg IV. Repeat as needed up to total dose of 20 mg.
C. Effect: Reduces arterial smooth muscle tone; diastolic pressure more affected than systolic pressure.
D. Comments: May cause reflex tachycardia, systemic lupus erythematosus syndrome. Increases coronary, splanchnic, cerebral, and renal blood flows.

XXXIX. HYDROCORTISONE (SOLU-CORTEF)
A. Indications
1. Adrenal insufficiency.
2. Inflammation and allergic reaction.
3. Cerebral edema from CNS tumors.
4. Asthma.

B. Dosage: 10 to 100 mg IV q8h. Physiologic replacement: IV: 0.25 to 0.35 mg/kg/d; PO: 0.5 to 0.75 mg/kg/d.

C. Effect
1. Anti-inflammatory.
2. Mineralocorticoid effect.
3. Stimulates gluconeogenesis.
4. Inhibits peripheral protein synthesis.

D. Comments
1. May cause adrenocortical insufficiency (Addisonian crisis) with abrupt withdrawal.
2. Delayed wound healing.
3. CNS disturbances, osteoporosis, or electrolyte disturbances.
4. Can cause perineal pruritus after rapid IV administration.

XL. IPRATROPRIUM BROMIDE
A. Indications: Anticholinergic agent, bronchodilator.
B. Dosage: 0.5 mg via nebulization q4–8h.
C. Effect: Blocks the action of acetylcholine at parasympathetic sites in bronchial smooth muscle causing bronchodilation.
D. Comments: Typically used in combination with inhaled short-acting beta agonist (albuterol).

XLI. ISOPROTERENOL
A. Indications: Heart failure; bradycardia.
B. Dosage: 2 μg/min titrated up to 20 μg/min.
C. Effect: β-Adrenergic agonist; positive chronotrope and inotrope.
D. Comments: May cause dysrhythmias, myocardial ischemia, hypertension, hypotension, or CNS excitation.

XLII. KETOROLAC (TORADOL)
A. Indications: Nonsteroidal anti-inflammatory drug (NSAID) for moderate pain. Useful adjunct for severe pain when used with parenteral or epidural opioids.
B. Dosage: 15 to 30 mg q6h.
C. Effect: Limits prostaglandin synthesis by cyclooxygenase inhibition.
D. Comments
  1. Adverse effects are similar to those with other NSAIDs: peptic ulceration, bleeding, decreased renal blood flow.
  2. Duration of treatment not to exceed 5 days.
  3. Caution when used in the elderly or in patients with preexisting renal dysfunction or significant hypovolemia.
  4. Use half recommended dose in patients that are <50 kg, and/or >65 years old and/or moderately renally impaired CrCl 30 to 50 mL/min.

XLIII. LABETALOL
A. Indications: Hypertension, controlled hypotension.
B. Dosage: 5 to 10 mg IV increments at 5-minute intervals, to 40 to 80 mg/dose. Infusion: titrate to desired response, 10 to 180 mg/h.
C. Effect: Selective α_1-adrenergic blockade with nonselective β-adrenergic blockade. Ratio of α/β-blockade = 1:7.
D. Comments: May cause bradycardia, AV conduction delays, and postural hypotension. Crosses the placenta.

XLIV. LEVETIRACETAM (KEPPRA)
A. Indication: Seizure prophylaxis; treatment of seizures.
B. Dosage: 500 to 1000 mg IV push over 2–5 minutes.
C. Effect: Suppression of seizure activity.
D. Comments: Adjustment for renal insufficiency.

XLV. LIDOCAINE (XYLOCAINE)
A. Indications
  1. Ventricular dysrhythmias.
  2. Cough suppression.
  3. Local anesthesia.
B. Dosage
  1. Dysrhythmias, 1 mg/kg IV × 2 (second dose 20 to 30 minutes after first dose) followed by 15 to 50 μg/kg/min IV (1 to 4 mg/min).
  2. Cough 1 mg/kg IV.

C. Effect: Decreases conductance of sodium channels. Antiarrhythmic effect, sedation, neural blockade.
D. Comments
1. May cause dizziness, seizures, disorientation, heart block (with myocardial conduction defect), or hypotension.
2. Crosses the placenta.
3. Caution in patients with Wolff-Parkinson-White syndrome.

XLVI. LOW–MOLECULAR-WEIGHT HEPARIN
Please see entry for enoxaparin (Lovenox).

XLVII. MAGNESIUM SULFATE
A. Indications
1. Preeclampsia/eclampsia.
2. Hypomagnesemia.
3. Polymorphic VT (torsade de pointes).

B. Dosage
1. Obstetrics, 1 to 8 g IV, then 1 to 4 g/h.
2. Hypomagnesemia, 1 to 2 g q6–8h, prn.
3. Polymorphic VT, 1 to 2 g in 10 mL D5W over 1 to 2 minutes; 5 to 10 g may be administered for refractory arrhythmias.

C. Effect: Treatment and prevention of hypomagnesemia; prevents and treats seizures or hyperreflexia associated with preeclampsia/eclampsia.

D. Comments
1. Potentiates neuromuscular blockade.
2. Potentiates CNS effects of anesthetics, hypnotics, and opioids.
3. Toxicity occurs with serum concentration greater than or equal to 10 mEq/L.
4. May alter cardiac conduction in digitalized patients. Avoid in patients with heart block. May cause hypotension with rapid IV administration.
5. Caution in patients with renal failure.

XLVIII. MANNITOL
A. Indications
1. Increased intracranial pressure.
2. Oliguria or anuria associated with acute renal injury.

B. Dosage
1. ICP, 0.25 to 1.0 g/kg IV as 20% solution over 30 to 60 minutes (in acute situation, can give bolus of 1.25 to 25.0 g over 5 to 10 minutes).
2. Renal, 12.5 to 25 g at kidney revascularization.

C. Effect: Increases serum osmolality, which reduces cerebral edema and lowers intracranial and intraocular pressure; also causes osmotic diuresis and transient expansion of intravascular volume.

D. Comments
1. Rapid administration may cause vasodilation and hypotension.
2. May worsen or cause pulmonary edema, intracranial hemorrhage, systemic hypertension, or rebound intracranial hypertension.

XLIX. METHYLENE BLUE
A. Indications
1. Surgical marker for genitourinary surgery.
2. Methemoglobinemia.
3. Vasoplegic syndrome.

B. **Dosage**
  1. Genitourinary, 100 mg (10 mL of 1% solution) IV.
  2. Methemoglobinemia, 1 to 2 mg/kg IV of 1% solution over 10 minutes; repeat q1h prn.
  3. Vasoplegia, 2 mg/kg IV.
  C. **Effect:** Low dose promotes conversion of methemoglobin to hemoglobin. High dose promotes conversion of hemoglobin to methemoglobin.
  D. **Comments**
  1. May cause red blood cell destruction (prolonged use), hypertension, bladder irritation, nausea, diaphoresis.
  2. May inhibit nitrate-induced coronary artery relaxation.
  3. Interferes with pulse oximetry for 1 to 2 minutes.
  4. Can cause hemolysis in patients with glucose-6-phosphate dehydrogenase deficiency.

L. METHYLERGONOVINE (METHERGINE)
  A. **Indication:** Postpartum hemorrhage due to uterine atony.
  B. **Dosage**
  1. IV (*emergency only*, after delivery of placenta): 0.2 mg in 5 mL of NS over ≥1 minute.
  2. IM: 0.2 mg q2–4h, prn (<5 doses).
  C. **Effect:** Methylergonovine increases the tone, rate of, and amplitude of uterine contraction causing sustained contraction of the uterus.
  D. **Comments:** Caution in patients with hypertension.

LI. METHYLPREDNISOLONE (SOLU-MEDROL)
  A. **Indications:** See Hydrocortisone. Spinal cord injury; status asthmaticus.
  B. **Dosage**
  1. 40 to 60 mg IV q6h. Higher doses in transplant patients.
  2. Status asthmaticus, 2 mg/kg; then 0.5 to 1 mg/kg q6h.
  3. Spinal cord injury, 30 mg/kg IV over 15 minutes; after 45 minutes begin 5.4 mg/kg/h × 23 or 47 hours.
  C. **Effect:** See Hydrocortisone; has five times the glucocorticoid potency of hydrocortisone with almost no mineralocorticoid activity.
  D. **Comments**
  1. See Hydrocortisone.
  2. Evidence for benefit in acute spinal cord injury is limited.
  3. Can cause perineal pruritus after IV administration.

LII. METOCLOPRAMIDE (REGLAN)
  A. **Indications:** Gastroesophageal reflux, diabetic gastroparesis, pulmonary aspiration prophylaxis, and antiemetic.
  B. **Dosage:** 10 to 20 mg IV q6–8h.
  C. **Effect**
  1. Facilitates gastric emptying by increasing gastric motility; relaxes pyloric sphincter and increases peristalsis in the duodenum and jejunum.
  2. Increases resting tone of the lower esophageal sphincter.
  3. Weak antiemetic effects appear secondary to antagonism of central and peripheral dopamine receptors.
  4. Can cause neuroleptic malignant syndrome.
  D. **Comments**
  1. Avoid in patients with GI obstruction, pheochromocytoma, or Parkinson's disease.
  2. Extrapyramidal reactions occur in 0.2% to 1% of patients.

LIII. METOPROLOL (LOPRESSOR)
- **A. Indications:** Hypertension, angina pectoris, dysrhythmia, hypertrophic cardiomyopathy, MI, and pheochromocytoma.
- **B. Dosage:** 1 to 5 mg IV q2min, prn, up to 15 mg
- **C. Effect:** β_1-Adrenergic blockade (β_2-adrenergic antagonism at high doses).
- **D. Comments**
    1. May cause symptomatic bradycardia.
    2. Can increase the risk of heart block.

LIV. MILRINONE
- **A. Indication:** Myocardial depression requiring inotropy.
- **B. Dosage:** 50 μg/kg IV over 10 minutes, then titrate 0.375 to 0.75 μg/kg/min to effect.
- **C. Effect:** Phosphodiesterase inhibition causing positive inotropy and vasodilation.
- **D. Comments**
    1. May increase ventricular ectopy.
    2. Possible worsening of outflow tract obstruction in hypertrophic obstructive cardiomyopathy (HOCM).
    3. Hypotension is common.

LV. NALOXONE (NARCAN)
- **A. Indication:** Reversal of systemic opioid effects.
- **B. Dosage:** Adult: 0.02 to 0.4 mg doses IV, titrated q2–3min. Pediatric: 1 to 10 μg/kg IV (in increments) q2–3min (up to 0.4 mg).
- **C. Effect:** Antagonizes effects of opioids by competitive inhibition.
- **D. Comments**
    1. May cause hypertension, dysrhythmias, rare pulmonary edema, and delirium usually if given in high doses.
    2. Reversal of analgesia.
    3. Withdrawal syndrome in opioid-dependent patients.
    4. Renarcotization may occur because antagonist has shorter duration than opiates.

LVI. NICARDIPINE (CARDENE)
- **A. Indication:** Hypertension.
- **B. Dosage:** 2.5 to 5 mg/h
- **C. Effect:** IV antihypertensive calcium channel blocker.
- **D. Comments**
    1. Steady state achieved in 3 to 5 hours.
    2. Maximum dose limit: 15 mg/h.
    3. My cause hypoxemia secondary to inhibition of hypoxic pulmonary vasoconstriction (HPV).

LVII. NITROGLYCERIN
- **A. Indications**
    1. Angina, myocardial ischemia, or infarction.
    2. Hypertension.
    3. Congestive heart failure.
    4. Controlled hypotension.
    5. Esophageal spasm.
- **B. Dosage**
    1. Initial IV infusion at 50 μg/min, then titrate to effect.
    2. Sublingual (SL): 0.15 to 0.6 mg/dose.
    3. Topical: 2% ointment, 0.5 to 2.5 in q6–8h.

C. Effect
1. Produces smooth muscle relaxation by enzymatic release of NO, causing systemic, coronary, and pulmonary vasodilatation (veins more than arteries).
2. Bronchodilation, biliary, GI, and genitourinary tract relaxation.

D. Comments
1. May cause reflex tachycardia, hypotension, or headache.
2. Tolerance with chronic use may be avoided with a 10- to 12-hour nitrate-free period.
3. May be adsorbed by plastic in IV tubing.
4. My cause hypoxemia secondary to inhibition of HPV.

LVIII. NITROPRUSSIDE (NIPRIDE)
A. Indications: Hypertension, controlled hypotension, and congestive heart failure.
B. Dosage: IV infusion initially at 0.1 μg/kg/min, then titrated to patient response to a maximum 10 μg/kg/min.
C. Effect: Direct NO donor causing smooth muscle relaxation in both arterioles and veins.
D. Comments
1. May cause excessive hypotension if not titrated slowly.
2. Reflex tachycardia.
3. Accumulation of cyanide with liver dysfunction; thiocyanate with kidney dysfunction. Cyanide/thiocyanate buildup with prolonged infusion.
4. Avoid with Leber hereditary optic atrophy, hypothyroidism, or vitamin B_{12} deficiency.
5. Solution and powder are light-sensitive and must be wrapped in opaque material.
6. My cause hypoxemia secondary to inhibition of HPV.

LIX. NOREPINEPHRINE (LEVOPHED)
A. Indication: Hypotension, myocardial depression.
B. Dosage
1. 1 to 30 μg/min IV, titrated to desired effect.
2. Administered through central venous catheter.
3. Dilute (8 μg/mL) can be administered via peripheral line.

C. Effect: Both α- and β-adrenergic activity, with α-adrenergic activity predominating.
D. Comments
1. May cause tachycardia and dysrhythmias in some patients.
2. Increased uterine contractility.
3. Constricted microcirculation.

LX. OCTREOTIDE (SANDOSTATIN)
A. Indications
1. Upper GI tract bleeding and acute variceal hemorrhage.
2. Treatment of symptomatic carcinoid.

B. Dosage: 25- to 50-μg IV bolus followed by continuous IV infusion of 25 to 50 μg/h. Higher doses may be needed for carcinoid syndrome.
C. Effect: Somatostatin analogue that suppresses the release of serotonin, gastrin, vasoactive intestinal peptide, insulin, glucagon, and secretin.
D. Comments: May cause nausea, decreased GI motility, and transient hyperglycemia.

LXI. ONDANSETRON (ZOFRAN)
  A. **Indications**: Prophylaxis and treatment of perioperative nausea and vomiting.
  B. **Dosage**: Adult: 4 mg IV over greater than 30 seconds or 8 mg PO q4–8h. Pediatric: 0.05 to 0.1 mg/kg IV max 4 mg.
  C. **Effect**: Selective 5-HT_3 receptor antagonist.
  D. **Comments**: Used in much higher doses for chemotherapy-induced nausea. Mild side effects include headache and reversible transaminase elevation.

LXII. OXYTOCIN (PITOCIN)
  A. **Indications**: Postpartum hemorrhage, uterine atony, and augmentation of labor.
  B. **Dosage**
   1. Hemorrhage, 10 units IM or 10 to 40 units in 1000 mL of crystalloid-infused IV at a rate necessary to control atony (eg, 0.02 to 0.04 units/min).
   2. Labor induction: 0.0005 to 0.002 units/min, increasing until contraction pattern established or maximum dose of 20 milliunits/min reached.
  C. **Effect**: Reduces postpartum blood loss by contraction of uterine smooth muscle. Renal, coronary, and cerebral vasodilation.
  D. **Comments**
   1. May cause uterine tetany and rupture, fetal distress, or anaphylaxis.
   2. IV bolus can cause hypotension, tachycardia, and dysrhythmia.

LXIII. PHENOBARBITAL
  A. **Indication**: Seizure suppression.
  B. **Dosage**: 10 to 20 mg/kg IV, additional 5 mg/kg doses q15–30min for control of status epilepticus, then 3 to 5 mg/kg/d PO or IV in divided doses.
  C. **Comments**
   1. May cause hypotension.
   2. Multiple drug interactions through induction of hepatic enzyme systems.
   3. Therapeutic anticonvulsant concentration 15 to 40 µg/mL at trough (just before next dose).

LXIV. PHENOXYBENZAMINE
  A. **Indication**: Preoperative preparation for pheochromocytoma resection.
  B. **Dosage**: 10 to 40 mg/d PO (start at 10 mg/d and increase dosage by 10 mg/d every 4 days prn).
  C. **Effect**: Nonselective and noncompetitive α-adrenergic antagonist.
  D. **Comments**: May cause orthostatic hypotension (which may be refractory to norepinephrine) and reflex tachycardia.

LXV. PHENYLEPHRINE
  A. **Indication**: Hypotension.
  B. **Dosage**: 10 µg/min IV initially, then titrated to response; IV bolus 40 to 100 µg/dose. Customary mix: 10 to 30 mg in 250 mL of D5W or NS.
  C. **Effect**: α_1-Adrenergic agonist.
  D. **Clearance**: Hepatic metabolism; renal elimination.
  E. **Comments**: May cause hypertension, reflex bradycardia, microcirculatory constriction, uterine contraction, or uterine vasoconstriction.

LXVI. PHENYTOIN (DILANTIN)
A. **Indications**: Seizure prophylaxis, treatment of seizures.
B. **Dosage**: 10 to 15 mg/kg IV at less than 50 mg/min (up to 1000 mg cautiously, with ECG monitoring); for neurosurgical prophylaxis, then 100 to 200 mg IV q4h (at <50 mg/min).
C. **Effect**
   1. Anticonvulsant effect via membrane stabilization.
   2. Antidysrhythmic effects similar to those of quinidine or procainamide.
D. **Comments**
   1. IV bolus may cause bradycardia, hypotension, respiratory arrest, cardiac arrest, or CNS depression.
   2. Nystagmus, diplopia, ataxia, drowsiness, gingival hyperplasia, GI upset, hyperglycemia, or hepatic microsomal enzyme induction.
   3. Crosses the placenta.
   4. Significant interpatient variation in dose needed to achieve a therapeutic concentration of 7.5 to 20.0 μg/mL.
   5. Determination of unbound phenytoin levels may be helpful in patients with renal failure or hypoalbuminemia.
   6. Fosphenytoin is generally preferred over phenytoin due its improved safety and tolerability (see XXXII. Fosphenytoin).

LXVII. PHOSPHORUS (SODIUM PHOSPHATE)
A. **Indications**
   1. Treatment and prevention of hypophosphatemia.
B. **Dosage**: 0.15 to 0.25 mmol/kg IV over 6 to 12 hours.
C. **Effect**: Electrolyte replacement.
D. **Comments**
   1. Infuse doses of IV phosphate over a 4- to 6-hour period since risks of rapid IV infusion include hypocalcemia, hypotension, muscular irritability, calcium deposition, renal function deterioration, and hyperkalemia.
   2. Use with caution in patients with cardiac disease and renal insufficiency.

LXVIII. PHYSOSTIGMINE (ANTILIRIUM)
A. **Indications**: Postoperative delirium, tricyclic antidepressant overdose, and reversal of CNS effects of anticholinergic drugs.
B. **Dosage**: 0.5 to 2.0 mg IV q15min prn. May repeat q10–30min until response occurs.
C. **Effect**: Central and peripheral cholinergic effects; inhibits cholinesterase.
D. **Comments**: Rarely may cause bradycardia, tremor, convulsions, hallucinations, CNS depression, mild ganglionic blockade, or cholinergic crisis.

LXIX. POTASSIUM (KCL) (SEE APPENDIX I)

LXX. PROCHLORPERAZINE (COMPAZINE)
A. **Indications**: Nausea and vomiting.
B. **Dosage**: 5 to 10 mg IV (≤40 mg/d); 5 to 10 mg IM q2–4h prn; 25 mg PR q12h prn.
C. **Effect**: Central dopamine (D_2) antagonist with neuroleptic and antiemetic effects, with antimuscarinic and antihistaminic (H_1) actions.
D. **Comments**: May cause hypotension (especially when given IV), extrapyramidal reactions, neuroleptic malignant syndrome, leukopenia, and cholestatic jaundice.

LXXI. PROMETHAZINE (PHENERGAN)
   A. Indications: Nausea and vomiting.
   B. Dosage: Adult: 12.5 to 25 mg PO, PR q4–6h prn.
   C. Effect: Antagonist of H_1 and muscarinic receptors.
   D. Comments: May cause mild hypotension or mild anticholinergic effects.

LXXII. PROPRANOLOL (INDERAL)
   A. Indications
   1. Hypertension, atrial and ventricular dysrhythmias, myocardial ischemia, or infarction.
   2. Junctional rhythm.
   3. Hypertrophic cardiomyopathy.
   4. Thyrotoxicosis.
   5. Migraine headache.

   B. Dosage: 0.5 to 1 mg IV, then titrate to effect; 0.5 mg IV for junctional rhythm.
   C. Effect: Nonspecific β-adrenergic blockade.
   D. Comments: May cause bradycardia, AV dissociation.

LXXIII. PROSTAGLANDIN E$_1$ (ALPROSTADIL) (SEE APPENDIX I)

LXXIV. PROTAMINE
   A. Indication: Reversal of the effects of heparin.
   B. Dosage: 1 mg/100 units of heparin activity IV at less than or equal to 5 mg/min.
   C. Effect: Polybasic compound forms complex with polyacidic heparin.
   D. Comments
   1. May cause myocardial depression and peripheral vasodilation with sudden hypotension or bradycardia.
   2. May cause severe pulmonary hypertension, particularly in the setting of cardiopulmonary bypass (CPB).
   3. Concern for allergic reaction/anaphylaxis for patients taking neutral protamine Hagedorn (NPH) insulin.
   4. Transient reversal of heparin may be followed by rebound heparinization.
   5. Monitor response with a partial thromboplastin time or activated clotting time (ACT).

LXXV. RYANODEX (SEE DANTROLENE)

LXXVI. SCOPOLAMINE
   A. Indications: nausea/vomiting, motion sickness, amnesia.
   B. Dosage: 0.3 to 0.6 mg IV/IM, 1.5-mg transdermal patch.
   C. Effect: Peripheral and central cholinergic (muscarinic) antagonism.
   D. Comments
   1. Excessive CNS depression can be reversed by physostigmine.
   2. May cause excitement, delirium, transient tachycardia, hyperthermia, or urinary retention.
   3. Care when handling patch because contact with eyes may cause long-lasting mydriasis and cycloplegia.
   4. Crosses the blood–brain barrier and placenta.

LXXVII. TRANEXAMIC ACID
   A. Indications: Prevention of bleeding due to fibrinolysis.

- **B. Dosage:** Intermittent IV infusion: 1000 mg over 10 minutes not to exceed 100 mg/min. Continuous IV infusion: 1 to 16 mg/kg/h not to exceed 100 mg/min.
- **C. Effect:** Stabilizes the formed clot by inhibiting plasminogen activators and plasmin.
- **D. Comments**
  1. May cause hypotension with rapid administration.
  2. Commonly used for trauma, epistaxis, spine surgery, and joint arthroplasty.
  3. Used for management of postpartum hemorrhage.
  4. Cleared by the kidneys. Caution in patients with renal insufficiency, accumulation of drug may result in increased risk of seizure.
  5. Tranexamic acid is an antifibrinolytic and may increase risk of thromboembolic events in certain high-risk patients.

LXXVIII. VASOPRESSIN (ANTIDIURETIC HORMONE, PITRESSIN)
- **A. Indications**
  1. Diabetes insipidus (DI).
  2. Upper gastrointestinal (GI) hemorrhage.
  3. Shock refractory to fluid and vasopressor therapy.
- **B. Dosage**
  1. DI, 5 to 10 units IM/SC q8–12h.
  2. GI, 0.1 to 0.4 units/min IV infusion.
  3. Shock, 0.04 units/min IV infusion titrated as required.
- **C. Effect**
  1. Increases urine osmolality and decreases urine volume.
  2. Smooth muscle constriction; vasoconstriction of splanchnic, coronary, muscular, and cutaneous vasculature.
- **D. Comments**
  1. May cause oliguria, water intoxication, pulmonary edema; hypertension, arrhythmias, myocardial ischemia; abdominal cramps (from increased peristalsis); contraction of gallbladder, urinary bladder, or uterus; vertigo or nausea.
  2. Patients with coronary artery disease are often treated with concurrent nitroglycerin.
  3. Useful in shock states as the effect of drug is not pH-dependent.

LXXIX. VERAPAMIL
- **A. Indications:** Supraventricular tachycardia, atrial fibrillation or flutter.
- **B. Dosage:** 2.5 to 10 mg IV over ≥2 minutes, repeat once if no response in 30 minutes.
- **C. Effect:** Blocks slow calcium channels in the heart. Prolongs PR interval. Negative inotrope and chronotrope; systemic and coronary vasodilator.
- **D. Comments**
  1. May cause severe bradycardia, AV block (especially with concomitant β-adrenergic blockade), excessive hypotension, or congestive heart failure.
  2. May increase ventricular response to atrial fibrillation or flutter in patients with accessory tracts.
  3. Active metabolite has 20% of the antihypertensive effect of the parent compound.
  4. Contraindicated in Wolff-Parkinson-White Syndrome when atrial fibrillation or atrial flutter exists with preexcitation due to risk of causing malignant ventricular arrhythmias.

LXXX. VITAMIN K (PHYTONADIONE)
   A. **Indications**: Deficiency of vitamin K–dependent clotting factors, reversal of warfarin anticoagulation.
   B. **Dosage**: 2.5 to 10 mg IM/SC/PO or 1 to 10 mg IV at less than or equal to 1 mg/min (with caution). If prothrombin time is not improved 8 hours after initial dose, repeat prn.
   C. **Effect**: Increases the levels of clotting factors II, VII, IX, and X by regeneration of vitamin K–dependent epoxide reductase blocked by warfarin.
   D. **Comments**
      1. Excessive doses can make the patient refractory to further oral anticoagulation.
      2. Rapid IV bolus can cause profound hypotension, fever, diaphoresis, bronchospasm, anaphylaxis, and pain at the injection site.

LXXXI. WARFARIN (COUMADIN)
   A. **Indication**: Anticoagulation.
   B. **Dosage**: 5 mg PO × 2 to 5 days, then 2 to 10 mg PO, titrated to INR (INR should be 2 to 3, based on indication).
   C. **Effect**: Inhibits vitamin K epoxide reductase effectively lowering vitamin K levels to inhibit synthesis of factors II, VII, IX, and X and proteins C and S.
   D. **Comments**
      1. May be potentiated by ethanol, antibiotics, dextran, thyroxine, diazoxide, ethacrynic acid, glucagon, methyldopa, MAOI, phenytoin, prolonged use of narcotics, quinidine, sulfonamides, congestive heart failure, hyperthermia, liver disease, and malabsorption.
      2. May be antagonized by barbiturates, chlordiazepoxide, haloperidol, oral contraceptives, hypothyroidism, and hyperlipidemia.

Common Intravenous Antibiotics

Parita A. Chowatia

The antibiotics listed in this appendix are those usually given for surgical prophylaxis in the perioperative period. Start administration of these antibiotics within 1 hour prior to incision unless indicated in comments below.

Drug	Dose[a]	First Intraoperative Dosing Interval (hours after preoperative dose)	Subsequent Intraoperative Dosing Interval (hours after first intraoperative dose)[b,c]	Comments
Ampicillin-sulbactam (Unasyn)[d]	3 g	4 h	every 6 h	Not effective against *Pseudomonas* spp.
Aztreonam[d]	2 g	4 h	every 8 h	
Cefoxitin[d]	2 g	2 h	every 6 h	All cephalosporins require adjustment for renal function when dosed for prolonged periods to prevent seizures in high concentrations.
Cefazolin (Ancef)[d]	<60 kg = 1 g 60–120 kg = 2 g >120 kg = 3 g	4 h	every 8 h	1% of penicillin-allergic patients will cross-react to cefazolin.
Ceftazidime	2 g	4 h	every 8 h	Preferred for *Pseudomonas aeruginosa* infections and neutropenic patients with fever.
Ceftriaxone[d]	2 g	10 h	every 24 h	Preferred for empiric coverage for bacterial meningitis.
Cefuroxime[d]	1.5 g	4 h	every 8 h	Preferred for community-acquired pneumonia.

Drug	Dose[a]	First Intraoperative Dosing Interval (hours after preoperative dose)	Subsequent Intraoperative Dosing Interval (hours after first intraoperative dose)[b,c]	Comments
Ciprofloxacin[d]	400 mg	12 h	every 12 h	Start administration within 2 h prior to incision.
Clindamycin[d]	900 mg	6 h	every 6 h	Associated with *Clostridium difficile* colitis. May prolong neuromuscular blockade.
Doxycycline	200 mg	12 h	every 12 h	
Fluconazole[d]	400 mg	24 h	every 24 h	
Gentamicin[d]	5 mg/kg based on actual body weight	24 h	every 24 h	If BMI >30, use adjusted body weight, otherwise use actual body weight. Initial dose unchanged for renal failure. Renal toxicity and ototoxicity. Precipitates with heparin. May prolong neuromuscular blockade.
Imipenem-cilastatin	500 mg	2 h	every 6 h	Preferred for multiple-drug–resistant gram-negative bacterial infections. Renal adjustment to prevent seizures.
Levofloxacin[d]	750 mg	24 h	every 24 h	Start administration within 2 h prior to incision.

(*continued*)

Drug	Dose[a]	First Intraoperative Dosing Interval (hours after preoperative dose)	Subsequent Intraoperative Dosing Interval (hours after first intraoperative dose)[b,c]	Comments
Linezolid	600 mg	12 h	every 12 h	Treatment of VRE. >7–10 d of use may cause myelosuppression. **Do not give with meperidine or methylene blue. MAO inhibition may cause serotonin syndrome.**
Meropenem	0.5–1 g	2 h	every 8 h	Adjust for renal insufficiency to prevent seizures.
Metronidazole (Flagyl)[d]	500 mg	8 h	every 8 h	
Nafcillin	1–2 g	2 h	every 4–6 h	Preferred for antistaphylococcal coverage.
Penicillin G Potassium	500,000–2,000,000 Units	2 h	every 4–6 h	Hypersensitivity is common. May induce seizures at high doses and induce interstitial nephritis.
Piperacillin-tazobactam (Zosyn)[d]	3.375 g	4 h	every 6 h	Tazobactam expands the activity of piperacillin to include β-lactamase–producing strains of *Staphylococcus aureus, Haemophilus influenzae, Enterobacteriaceae, Pseudomonas, Klebsiella, Citrobacter, Serratia, Bacteroides,* and other gram-negative anaerobes.

Appendix III Common Intravenous Antibiotics

Drug	Dose[a]	First Intraoperative Dosing Interval (hours after preoperative dose)	Subsequent Intraoperative Dosing Interval (hours after first intraoperative dose)[b,c]	Comments
Vancomycin[d]	<75 kg = 1 g 75–100 kg = 1.5 g >100 kg = 2 g Give no faster than 1 g/h	12 h	every 12 h	Preferred over clindamycin for MRSA patients. Increase dose interval in renal disease. Histamine release ("Vancomycin infusion reaction") correlates with infusion rate and concentration. May precipitate with other medications. Start administration within 2 h prior to incision.

BMI, body mass index; g, gram; h, hour; IBW, ideal body weight; kg, kilogram; mg, milligram; MAO, monoamine oxidase; MRSA, methicillin-resistant *Staphylococcus aureus*; VRE, vancomycin-resistant enterococci.

[a]For adult and pediatric patients <50 kg, please refer to a pediatric weight based dosing resource.

[b]In patients with normal renal function.

[c]Consider more frequent dosing during procedures with large blood loss (>1500 mL).

[d]Drugs recommended by the Massachusetts General Hospital (MGH) Infectious Disease service for standard surgical prophylaxis.

INDEX

Note: Page numbers followed by "f" indicate figures and "t" indicate tables.

A

AAA. *See* Abdominal aortic aneurysm (AAA)
Abbott AVEIR, 64
Abciximab (Reopro), 342t, 355, 514t, 699
Abdomen
  gunshot wounds, 665
  physical examination, 8
Abdominal aortic aneurysm (AAA), 494–496, 499–500
Abdominal aortic repair
  emergency in
    hemodynamically stable patients, 499–500
    hemodynamically unstable patients, 499–500
  endovascular abdominal aortic repair (EVAR), 494–496, 497f
  open abdominal aortic surgery, 496–499
Abdominal compartment syndrome (ACS), 666
Abdominal surgery
  anesthesia management
    enhanced recovery after surgery (ERAS), 451–452
    fluid losses, 450
    fluid replacement, 449
    induction, 449
    maintenance, 449–452
    muscle relaxation, 450–451
    nasogastric (NG) tubes, 451
    nitrous oxide, use of, 451
    protocol-based strategy, 449–450
  anesthetic considerations
    after brain death, recovery of organs for transplantation, 460–462
    biliary tract procedures, 457
    esophageal surgery, 454–455
    gastric surgery, 455
    hepatic surgery, 456–457
    intestinal and peritoneal surgery, 455–456
    intraoperative radiation therapy, 458
    laparoscopic surgery, 452–454
    pancreatic surgery, 457
    robotic surgery, 454
    splenectomy, 457
    surgery for obese patient, 458–460
  anesthetic techniques
    caudal anesthesia, 448–449
    combined technique, 449
    erector spinae plane (ESP) block, 448
    general anesthesia (GA), 447
    monitored anesthesia care (MAC), 447
    rectus sheath blocks, 449
    regional anesthetic techniques, 447–448
    transversus abdominis plane (TAP) blocks, 448
  preanesthetic considerations
    emergency abdominal procedures, 447
    hypovolemia, etiology of, 446
    length of surgery, 447
    metabolic derangements, 447
    preoperative volume status, 446
ABG. *See* Arterial blood gas (ABG)
Abortion, 585
Access-related complications, 141–143
Acetaminophen, 14, 100, 106, 178, 292, 429, 452, 475, 549, 557, 607, 609, 621, 635, 693, 720, 727–728, 729t, 732, 733t
Acetazolamide, 544–545
Acetylcholine (ACh), 227, 228f

Acetylcholine receptor (AChR), 227
Acetylcholinesterase (AChE), 227, 228f
α1-Acid glycoprotein, 99
ACh. *See* Acetylcholine (Ach)
AChE. *See* Acetylcholinesterase (AChE)
Achondroplasia, 208
AChR. *See* Acetylcholine receptor (AChR)
Acid–base management, 522
ACM. *See* Alcoholic cardiomyopathy (ACM)
Acromegaly, airways, 207
ACS. *See* Acute coronary syndrome (ACS)
ACT. *See* Activated clotting time (ACT)
ACTH. *See* Adrenocorticotropic hormone (ACTH)
Activated clotting time (ACT), 519
Activated partial thromboplastin time (aPTT), 683
Acupuncture, 743
Acute coronary syndrome (ACS), 49–50
Acute kidney injury
  classification, 83, 83t–84t
  clinical features, 84
  diagnosis, 84, 84t
  epidemiology, 82
  etiology, 82
  prevention, 84
  management
    continuous renal replacement therapy (CRRT), 85
    hemodialysis, 85
    hemofiltration, 85
    medications, 84
    optimization, 84
    renal replacement therapy (RRT), 85
    ultrafiltration, 85
Acute liver failure, 109
Acute pain
  pharmacologic treatment
    acetaminophen, 728
    definitions, 725
    ketamine, 728, 731
    nonsteroidal anti-inflammatory drugs (NSAIDs), 726–728, 726t–727t
    opiates and opioids, 731–733, 733t, 735t, 737t, 740t
  treatment modalities
    acute pain management, 740–742, 741t
    continuous peripheral nerve blocks, 739–740, 740t
    neuraxial analgesia, 735–739, 737t–739t
    patient-controlled analgesia (PCA), 735, 735t
Acute respiratory distress syndrome (ARDS), 44–45, 73–75
  clinical diagnosis and severity grading criteria, 74t
  pulmonary disease, 74t
    intraoperative considerations, 75
    pneumonia, 76
    postoperative considerations, 75
    pulmonary contusion, 75–76
  risk factors, 74t
Addison disease, 128, 133–134
Adductor canal block, 377, 378f
Adenosine, 319, 627
  comments, 781
  dosage, 319, 781
  effect, 781
  hemodynamic control, perioperative, 319
  indications, 781
Adrenal cortical disease
  glucocorticoid excess
    anesthetic considerations, 127
    clinical features, 127
  physiology
    androgens, 126–127
    glucocorticoids, 126
    mineralocorticoids, 126
    primary hyperaldosteronism, 127. *See also* Conn syndrome
Adrenal cortical hypofunction
  anesthetic considerations, 128
  clinical features
    acute adrenal insufficiency, 128
    primary adrenal insufficiency, 128–129
    secondary adrenal insufficiency, 128–129
  treatment, 128
Adrenal crisis, 128
Adrenal medullary disease, 129–131
  pheochromocytoma
    clinical features, 129
    preoperative evaluation and preparation, 130
  physiology, 129
Adrenergic(s)
  agonists, 308t, 406
  α-agonists, 54, 59, 308–310, 776
  β-agonists, 310

mixed agonists, 310–312
nonadrenergic agents, 312–313
β-antagonists, 126, 294, 313–315, 314t, 572
catecholamines, 305
controlled hypotension, 320
drug dosage calculations, 320–321
receptors, perioperative hemodynamic control, 306t–307t
α1 receptors, 305
α2 receptors, 305, 308
β1 receptors, 308
β2 receptors, 308
β3 receptors, 308
dopamine receptors, 308
receptor regulation, 308
vasodilators, 315–320, 315t
Adrenergic agonists, 308–313, 308t, 406
β-Adrenergic antagonists, 572
blockers, 313
esmolol, 314t, 313, 315
labetalol, 314t, 315
metoprolol, 314t, 313
propranolol, 314t, 313
β-Adrenergic blockers, 313
α-Adrenergic receptors, 305, 308
β-Adrenergic receptors, 308
Adrenocorticotropic hormone (ACTH), 126
Adult resuscitation
advanced cardiac life support (ACLS)
advanced airway, 753
defibrillation, 753, 754f, 760f
drugs, 756
pacing, 754–755, 755f
vascular access, 755
basic life support (BLS), 749–750
airway and breathing, 751–752
circulation, 750–751
defibrillation, 752
reassessment, 752
Advanced cardiac life support (ACLS), adult resuscitation
advanced airway, 753
defibrillation
cardioversion, 754, 760f
defibrillators, 753–754
ventricular fibrillation, 754f
drugs, 756–760
adenosine, 756
β-adrenergic–blocking drugs, 757
algorithm, 755f

amiodarone, 756–757
atropine, 757
calcium, 757
calcium channel blockers, 757–758
cardiopulmonary resuscitation (CPR) termination, 761
diltiazem, 757
Do Not Resuscitate (DNR), 761
dopamine, 758
epinephrine, 758
extracorporeal membrane oxygenation (ECMO), 750–751
isoproterenol, 758
lidocaine, 758
magnesium, 759
open-chest direct cardiac compression, 760
oxygen, 759
procainamide, 759
sotalol, 759
sodium bicarbonate, 759
vasopressin, 759–760
verapamil, 757
pacing, 754–755, 755f
vascular access, 755
Advance directive, 17
Adverse anesthesia event, guidelines
anesthesiologist, 163
objectives, 163
Adverse reactions and side effects, anesthesia, 2–3
Agitation, 722
AI. *See* Aortic insufficiency (AI)
Airway(s)
anesthesia for otorhinolaryngologic procedures, 558–559
applied anatomy of, 205–207, 206f
awake intubation
complications, 225
indications, 224
techniques, 225
difficult, 221–222, 222f
emergency airway techniques
cricothyroidotomy, 223
percutaneous needle cricothyroidotomy, 223
rigid bronchoscopy, 223
tracheostomy, 223
endotracheal intubation of
alternative intubation techniques, 220–221
bronchoscopic intubation, 219–220

Airway(s) (*Continued*)
  nasotracheal, 219
  orotracheal, 215–219, 217f, 218f
  endotracheal tube (ETT) changes, 225–226
  evaluation
    achondroplasia, 208
    acromegaly, 207
    arterial blood gas tensions, 211
    arthritis, 207
    body mass index, 207
    burns/radiation/surgery, 207
    cervical disk disease, 207
    cervical spine mobility, 209
    chest/cervical imaging, 211
    congenital anomalies, 208
    head/neck, 209, 210f, 211
    history, 207–208
    infections, 207
    inhalational injury, 208
    laryngoscopy, 211
    Mallampati classification, 209, 211, 211f
    obstructive sleep apnea, 207
    osteogenesis imperfect, 208
    physical examination, 208–211, 208t, 210f–211f
    pulmonary function tests, 211
    scleroderma, 207
    snoring, 207
    tracheal tomograms, 211
    trauma, 207
    trisomy 21 patients, 208
    tumors, 207
    Wilson score, 208, 208t
  laryngeal mask airway (LMA), 213–215, 214f–215f
    adverse effects, 215
    contraindications, 213
    indications, 213
    second generation, 214–215
    use of, 213–214
  management, 3, 12, 180–181, 459
    in anterior pituitary hyperfunction, 132–133
    C-A-B sequence, 750
    in DM, 116
    endotracheal intubation, 180–181, 394
    laryngeal mask airway (LMA), 213–215
    metabolic syndrome and DM2, 116
    in obesity, 459
    in patient undergoing general anesthesia, 178
    pituitary disease, 132–133
    in radical neck dissection, 553–554
    supraglottic airways, 181
  mask
    complications, 213
    indications, 212
    techniques, 212–213
    ventilation, 213
  obesity, 116
  obstruction, 212
  patency, 212–213
  patient evaluation, 12
  protection, respiratory system, 101–102
  rapid sequence induction
    equipment/technique, 224
    indications, 224
  secretion clearance, 241
  sleep apnea, 5, 116
Airway-related complications, 143
Albumin, 99
Albuterol, 781–782
Aldosterone, 78, 126–129, 593, 672
Alfentanil, 95, 197–198, 197t
Alkalosis/acidosis, 104
Allergies
  and drug reactions, anesthesia, 2–3
  local anesthetics and, 2, 328
  medication errors, 156–157
  toxicity of, 328–330
  transfusion reactions, 692–694
  true reactions, 2
Alpha-2-adrenergic agonists, 328
Alprostadil (PGE1)
  administration guidelines, 777
  indications, 777
Alteplase (Activase)
  administration guidelines
    acute myocardial infarction, 777–778
    peripheral arterial, 778
    pulmonary embolus, 778
    venous and arterial thrombosis catheter-directed thrombolysis, 778
    venous thrombosis, 778
  indications, 777
Alveolar–interstitial syndromes, 43–45
Alveolar ventilation, in pulmonary disease, 68

American College of Cardiology and American Heart Association (ACC/AHA), 49
American Heart Association (AHA), 146, 747
  ACLS algorithm for cardiac arrest in pregnancy, 585
  guidelines for β-blockers, 313
  guidelines for CEA, 491
American Society of Anesthesiologists (ASA), 470, 632, 718
  algorithm, difficult airway, 222f
  continuous blood pressure monitoring, 427
  continuum of depth of sedation, 177
  guidelines for preoperative fasting, 14t
  physical status classification system, 13t
  standards and practice guidelines, 162
  standards for basic anesthetic monitoring, 243
  use of β-blockers, 335
Amides, 323–324, 326t
Aminocaproic acid (Amicar), 426, 443, 520, 782
Aminoglycosides, 8, 87–88, 103, 115, 148, 238, 623
Amiodarone (Cordarone), 120–122, 133, 282, 287, 330, 517, 523–524, 535, 715, 754f, 756, 758–759, 760f, 764f, 766f, 782
Amlodipine, 316
Analgesia
  labor and vaginal delivery, 574–578
  pediatric pain evaluation, 607
  postoperative, 475
Anaphylactic and anaphylactoid reactions, 301–302
Anaphylaxis, 301
Anemia, 86, 104, 296, 433, 566, 681
  sickle cell, 702
Anesthesia
  for abdominal surgery
    after brain death, recovery of organs for transplantation, 460–462
    anesthetic techniques, 447–449
    biliary tract procedures, 457
    esophageal surgery, 454–455
    gastric surgery, 455
    hepatic surgery, 456–457
    intestinal and peritoneal surgery, 455–456
    intraoperative radiation therapy, 458
    laparoscopic surgery, 452–454
    management, 449–452
    pancreatic surgery, 457
    preanesthetic considerations, 446–447
    robotic surgery, 454
    splenectomy, 457
    surgery for obese patient, 458–460
  assessment and plan, 12
  for cardiac surgery
    anesthetic management, 515–517
    cardiac tamponade, 536
    cardiac transplantation, 536–537
    cardiopulmonary bypass (CBP), 510
    constrictive pericarditis, 536
    deep hypothermic circulatory arrest (DHCA), 535–536
    extracorporeal membrane oxygenation (ECMO), 538–539
    lung transplantation, 537–538
    induction, 517–526, 520t, 523t, 525t
    off-bypass coronary artery bypass grafting (CABG), 534–535
    "off-site" cardiac procedures, 541–542
    pediatric cardiac anesthesia, 527–530, 534, 531t–533t
    percutaneous mitral valve (MV) repair, 540–541
    postoperative care, 526–527
    postoperative management, 538
    preoperative assessment, 511–515, 512t–514t
    "redo" cardiac surgery, 535
    transcatheter aortic valve replacement (TAVR), 540
    ventricular assist devices (VADs), 538–539
  for cesarean delivery, 578–579
  chest radiography before, 9
  effects on kidney, 92–93
  electrocardiogram before, 9
  ethical considerations, patient care, 17–18
  general, 265
    airway management, 180–181
    disposition, 183
    emergence, 182–183

Anesthesia (*Continued*)
   extubation, 183
   indications, 177–178
   induction of, 179–180
   intraoperative adverse effects, 183–186
   maintenance of, 181–182
   postoperative adverse effects, 185
   pre-op evaluation and planning, 178–179, 14t
   transport of, 183
  gynecologic surgery, 587
  for head and neck surgery
   ophthalmic surgery, 544–548, 546f
   otorhinolaryngologic procedures, 548–553
   procedures of neck, 553–554, 555f
  hematological studies before, 8
  history
   allergies and drug reactions, 2–3
   anesthetic records, 3
   family history, 3
   medications, 1
   presenting illness, 1
   social history and habits, 3–4
  informed consent, 14–15
  laboratory studies before, 8–9
  liver disease, 100–106
  neuraxial anesthesia, 332–333
  neurologic examination before, 8
  for neurosurgery
   electrophysiologic monitoring, 407–409
   intraoperative management, 410–413
   pharmacology, 405–407, 405t
   physiology, 402–405, 403f–404f
   preoperative considerations, 409–410
   specific neurosurgical procedures, 413–420, 413t
   spine and spinal cord, 420–421
  nil per os (NPO) status, 12
  non-operating room anesthesia (NORA)
   cardiac procedures, 651
   contrast media, 635–636
   CT-guided thermal ablations, 638–640
   diagnostic radiology, 636–638
   electroconvulsive therapy (ECT), 648–650
   ergonomics, 633
   gastrointestinal/genitourinary, 644–647
   gastrointestinal procedures, 650–651
   neurointerventions, 640–644
   patient access, 633
   proton beam radiation therapy, 647
   radiation safety, 633
   radiation therapy, 647–648
   remote locations equipment, 632–633
   safety in, 655
   techniques, 633–635
   vascular radiology procedures, 644–647
  for oocyte retrieval, 587
  non-operating room anesthesia (NORA)for computed tomography (CT), 619–620
   contrast media, 635–636
   diagnostic radiology, 636–638
   for electroconvulsive therapy (ECT), 648–650
   ergonomics, 633
   for gastrointestinal procedures, 644–647, 650–651
   genitourinary procedures, 644–647
   neurointerventions, 640–644
   for proton beam therapy and radiation therapy, 647
   radiation safety, 633
   remote locations, 632–633
   techniques, 633–635
   vascular procedures, 644–647
  orthopedic surgery
   elbow and upper arm surgery, 395–396
   foot and ankle surgery, 394–395
   forearm and hand surgery, 394–395
   orthopedic oncology, 396–397
   orthopedic trauma, 397–400, 398f, 399t
   shoulder surgery, 392–394, 393f
   spine surgery, 400
   total hip arthroplasty (THA), 390–392
   total knee arthroplasty (TKA), 390–392
  patent discussion, 12–14, 13t–14t
  physical examination for
   abdomen, 8
   back, 8

extremities, 8
head and neck, 7
height and weight measurement, 7
lungs, 7
neurologic examination, 8
precordium, 7
vital signs, 7
premedication
anticholinergics, 16
antiemetics, 16, 16t
aspiration risk-mitigating agents, 16
sedatives and analgesics, 15–16
preoperative medical optimization
anticoagulation therapy, 10
aspiration risk, 12
asthma, 11
coronary artery disease (CAD), 10
diabetes mellitus, 11
hypertension (HTN), 9
medications, 12
nonsteroidal anti-inflammatory drug (NSAID), 10
opioid tolerance, 10–11
pulmonary function tests, 9
review of systems
cardiovascular, 4–5
endocrine, 5–6
gastrointestinal, 6
hematology, 6
musculoskeletal, 6
neurological, 5
obstetric/gynecologic, 6
renal, 5
respiratory, 5
safety in, 155–163
adverse anesthesia event, guidelines, 163
cognitive errors, 157, 158t–159t, 159
communication errors, 160
crisis resource management (CRM), 160–162, 161t, 162f
documentation, 163
handoff errors, 159–160
human factors errors, 159
medication errors, 156–157
procedure errors, 157
quality assurance, 162–163
safety training, 162
standards and guidelines, 156, 162
teamwork, 160
transition errors, 159–160

segmental level/surgery and, 332, 333f, 334t
serum chemistry studies before, 8–9
for spine surgery
airway, 423–424
blood loss, 426
direct, 351–352
disposition, 428
monitoring, 425–426
postoperative pain management, 428–429
prone position, 424–425
spinal cord injury, 421, 423
spinal cord perfusion, 427–428, 428t
surgical procedures, delay, 17
for thoracic surgery
bronchopleural fistula, 483
diagnostic procedures, 470–473
esophageal surgery, 476–478
interventional pulmonary procedures, 481–482
intraoperative extracorporeal life support, 483–484
intrapulmonary hemorrhage, 482–483
laryngeal surgery, 480–481
lung isolation, 466–468
mediastinal mass resection, 475–476
one-lung ventilation, 469–470
preoperative evaluation, 465–466
preoperative preparation, 465
pulmonary resection, 473–475
tracheal injury, 483
tracheal surgery, 478–480
transplant surgery
ethical considerations, 431–432
kidney transplantation, 432–435
liver transplantation, 438–443, 442f
organ procurement, 443–445, 444t
pancreas transplantation, 435–437
for urologic surgery
cystectomy, 561–562
cystoscopy and ureteroscopy, 557
laser resection of prostate, 559–560
lithotripsy, 563
nephrectomy, 561
orchidopexy, 562
orchiectomy, 562

Anesthesia (*Continued*)
    radical retropubic prostatectomy (RRP), 560–561
    renal transplantation, 562–563
    spinal cord injury, 564
    TURBT, 557
    TURP, 557–559
    urogenital plastic surgery procedures, 562
  for vascular surgery
    abdominal aortic repair, 494–500, 497f
    amputations, 506
    carotid revascularization, 491–494
    peripheral arterial surgery, 489–491
    preoperative assessment and management, 486–489
    thoracoabdominal aortic aneurysm repair, 500–506, 501f, 505t

Anesthesia machines
  bacterial and viral contamination of, 141, 165
  breathing systems, 168–169
  circle system, 169, 170f
  checkout recommendations for, 174–175
  emergency manual ventilator, 175
  gas analysis
    infrared analysis, 174
    oxygen analyzers, 173–174
  gas delivery system, 166f
    desflurane, 168
    flow control valves and flowmeters, 167
    gas outlet, 168
    medical gas supply, 165, 167
    pressure regulators, 167
    oxygen flush valve, 168
    vaporizers, 167–168
  safety features of, 171, 173
  scavenging systems, 173
  servo-based, 171, 172f
  ventilators, 169, 171

Anesthetics
  inhalation, 200–204, 200t, 405–407, 405t
  inhalational, induction of, 180
  local anesthetics, 608–609

Anesthetists, 12
  infection control, 138
  responsibilities, 138

Angiography
  cerebral, 641–642
  spinal, 641–642
Angiotensin-converting enzyme (ACE) inhibitors, 78, 126, 312, 512–513
Angiotensin II, 78, 88, 126, 318
AngioVac device, 541
Ankle block, 380–381, 380f, 395
Antacids, 12, 447, 671
Anterior pituitary gland, 131
Anterior spinal artery syndrome, 502
Antiarrhythmics, 12, 316, 512, 524, 574, 714, 756, 758
Antibiotic resistant bacteria, 151
Antibiotics
  intravenous, 800–803
  in operating room
    aminoglycosides, 148
    clindamycin, 147
    endocarditis, 146
    fluoroquinolones, 148
    indications for, 144
    β-lactams, 147
    metronidazole, 148
    prophylaxis principles, 144–145
    Surgical Care Improvement Project (SCIP), 144–146, 145t
    surgical wound classification, 146–147
    timing and administration, 145–146
    vancomycin, 147
Anticholinergics, 16
Anticholinesterases, 61, 237–238, 240, 283, 313, 545, 710
Anticoagulation, 10, 511, 523
  neuraxial anesthesia, 353–355
Antiemetic agents, 16, 16t
Antihistamines, 643, 693, 719
Antimicrobial preservatives, 324
Antioxidants, 324, 328
Antiplatelet drugs, 341, 355, 487, 506, 513, 514t, 685, 699, 749
Antiplatelet therapy, 487, 491
Anxiolytics, 52, 102, 111, 156, 178–179, 409, 642, 743–745
Aortic cross-clamping, 283, 408, 445, 462, 487, 498
Aortic dissection, 49, 298, 498, 518, 521, 535–536, 697
Aortic insufficiency (AI), 128–129, 512, 522, 540
Aortic regurgitation, 55

Aortic stenosis (AS)
  anesthetic considerations, 55, 517
  cardiac pacing, 55
  etiology, 55
  ischemia treatment, 55
  nitrates and peripheral vasodilators, 55
  normal sinus rhythm, 55
  pathophysiology, 55
  symptoms, 54–55
Aortic unclamping, 498–499
APCs. *See* Atrial premature contractions (APCs)
Apgar scores, 766–767
  neonatal resuscitation, 761–762, 762t
Apixaban, 513, 700
Apnea, 44
Appendectomy, 455
Aprepitant, 719
aPTT. *See* Activated partial thromboplastin time (aPTT)
Aqueous vasopressin, 413
Argatroban, 342t, 489, 520t, 700
  administration guidelines, 778
  indications, 778
Arginine vasopressin (AVP), 78, 309t
  hemodynamic control, perioperative and, 312
Arndt blocker, 468
Arterial blood gas (ABG), 72, 461–462
Arterial blood pressure, cardiovascular system
  arterial cannulation, 245–247, 246f
  automated noninvasive blood pressure, 244–245
  invasive blood pressure, 245
  mean arterial pressure (MAP), 244
  systolic, 244–245
Arterial cannulation
  complications, 247
  considerations for placement, 247
  locations, 245
  procedure, 245–246, 246f
Arterial carbon dioxide tension, 469, 731
Arterial catheter, 245–247, 249, 259, 409, 439, 443, 446, 492, 504, 536, 542, 625, 655, 665, 707
Arteriovenous malformation (AVM), 415
Artery of Adamkiewicz, 502
Arthritis, airways, 207
AS. *See* Aortic stenosis (AS)

ASA. *See* American Society of Anesthesiologists (ASA)
"As low as reasonably achievable" (ALARA), 633
Ascending nociceptive (pain) pathway, 265
Ascites, 103
Aspiration, 294–295, 447, 455–456, 461
  pneumonia/pneumonitis, 143–144
  prophylaxis, 578
  risk, 12
  risk-mitigating agents, 16
  thrombectomy, 541
Aspirin, 10, 52–53, 115, 133, 292, 297, 355, 487, 513, 514t, 520, 641, 699, 715, 726t, 727, 729t
Asthma, 5, 11, 70
Atenolol, 314t, 757, 782–783
Atherosclerotic aneurysm, 500
Atracurium, 106, 229t, 230t, 234, 237
Atrial fibrillation, 285–286
Atrial flutter, 286
Atrial natriuretic peptide, 78
Atrial premature contractions (APCs), 285
Atrial-to-left-femoral-artery bypass shunt, 505t
Atropine, 60, 231, 284–285, 292, 344, 415, 421, 462, 470, 544–545, 605–606, 669, 714, 757
Audible oxygen alarm, 171
Autonomic dysreflexia, 564
AVM. *See* Arteriovenous malformation (AVM)
AVP. *See* Arginine vasopressin (AVP)
Awake craniotomy, 416–417
Axillary block, 369–370, 370f
Axillofemoral bypass grafting, 491

B

Back pain, spinal anesthesia, 341
Backup atrial pacing, 536
Baclofen, 734t
Bacteria
  antibiotic resistant, 151
  contamination of anesthesia machine, 141
  Mycobacterium tuberculosis, 151
  sepsis, 696
Balloon
  angioplasty and stenting, 52, 489
  test occlusion, 640
Balloon-occluded retrograde transvenous obliteration (BRTO), 645

Baralyme, 169, 203
Barbiturates, 68–69, 94t, 95, 100, 106, 118, 194, 280, 289, 294, 300, 406
  as inhalation anesthetic, 200–204, 200t, 201f
  as intravenous (IV) anesthetics, 406
    action mode of, 190
    adverse effects, 191
    cardiovascular system, 191
    central nervous system (CNS), 191
    dosage and administration, 190t, 191
    pharmacodynamics of, 191
    pharmacokinetics of, 190
    respiratory system, 191
Bare metal coronary stents (BMS), 52
Bariatric surgery, 452, 459, 733
Basic life support (BLS)
  adult resuscitation, 749–752
  pediatric resuscitation, 761–762
Basilic vein, 772, 773f, 775–776
Benzodiazepines, 3–4, 15–16, 69, 93–95, 94t, 101, 106, 178, 182, 186, 191, 194–196, 199, 241, 280, 289, 300–301, 330, 406, 409, 466, 499, 516, 616, 636, 649, 707, 709, 717, 720, 728, 731, 733
  as inhalation anesthetic, 200–204, 200t, 201f
  as intravenous (IV) anesthetics
    action mode of, 192
    adverse effects, 193
    cardiovascular system, 192
    central nervous system (CNS), 192
    dosage and administration, 190t, 193
    pharmacodynamics of, 192–193
    pharmacokinetics of, 192
    respiratory system, 193
Bernoulli equation, 34, 34f
Bevacizumab, 628
Bicarbonate, sodium (NaHCO$_3$), 89–90, 104, 125, 325, 328, 349, 488, 522–523, 530, 562, 579, 625, 770
  administration, 300, 759
  for aortic unclamping, 498–499
  for CIN, 635
  comments, 783
  dosage, 783
  effect, 783
  indications, 783
  for hypervolemic hypernatremia, 80
  neonatal preparation, 770
  for PALS, 759

Biliary drainage procedures, 457
Biliary injury, 109
Biliary tract procedures, abdominal surgery, 457
Bispectral index (BIS), 266
Bivalirudin (Angiomax), 489, 520, 520t, 700, 778
  administration guidelines, 778–779
  indication, 778
Bladder, spinal anesthesia, 336
Bleeding
  abdominal surgery, 446
  vascular surgery, 496
β-Blockers, 9, 52, 81, 122–123, 130–131, 282, 285–286, 296, 312–313, 318, 320, 330, 335, 348, 534
  in ACLS protocols, 757
  contraindications, 313, 316
  for fetal tachycardia, 570
  obstructive pulmonary disease, 313
  for sinus tachycardia, 313, 714
  for stable ventricular tachycardia, 715
β-Blocker therapy, 487
Blood
  component therapy, 687–689
  pressure, 244–245, 247, 305
  substitutes, 689
  typing and cross-matching, 686–687, 686t
  volumes (BVs), estimating, 683
Blood–brain barrier, 95, 409, 411–412
Blood pressure, 244–245, 247, 305
  arterial, 244–247
  arterial cannulation, 245–247, 246f
  invasive, 245
  mean arterial pressure (MAP), 244
  noninvasive, automated, 244–245
  systolic, 89, 244–245, 247, 281, 298, 445, 494, 520, 537, 643, 656
Blood transfusions
  infectious complications, 695–696
  metabolic complications, 694–695
  transfusion reactions, 692–694, 692t
  transfusion-related immunomodulation, 696–697
Bloody tap
  epidural anesthesia, 350
  spinal anesthesia, 341
Blood urea nitrogen, 87–88
BLS. *See* Basic life support (BLS)
BMI. *See* Body mass index (BMI)
BMS. *See* Bare metal coronary stents (BMS)

Body mass index (BMI), 71, 207, 329, 458, 507, 570, 683
Bone cement embolism, 427
Bosentan, 320
Bowel, manipulation, 281, 497
BPD. *See* Bronchopulmonary dysplasia (BPD)
Brachial plexus, blockade, 365
Bradycardia, 344
Brain death, 443, 444t
Brainstem–auditory evoked potentials (BAEPs), 408
Breathing systems, 168–169
 circle system, 169, 170f
Bronchopulmonary dysplasia (BPD), 619
Bronchoscopy
 aspiration, 295
 flexible, 470–471
 rigid, 471–472
Bronchospasm
 histamine-releasing drugs, 294
 reflex bronchiolar constriction, 293–294
 treatment, 294
 wheezing, 294
Brooke formula, 676
BRTO. *See* Balloon-occluded retrograde transvenous obliteration (BRTO)
Buprenorphine, 197t, 741, 741t, 742
Burn(s)
 anesthetic considerations, 677–679, 677t, 678f
 chemical burns, 672
 classification of, 673, 674f
 deep thermal injury
  acute renal failure, 672
  capillary leakage, 671–672
  cardiovascular effects, 671
  gastrointestinal function, 672
  hemoconcentration, 671
  infection, 672
  metabolic effects, 671
  thrombocytopenia, 672
 electrical burns, 672
 electrosurgical units, 303
 initial evaluation
  airway and breathing, 673–675
  cardiovascular resuscitation, 676
 injuries
  classification, 673
  clinical evaluation, 673–676
  physical implications, 670–671
  physiologic implications, 671–673
 management of, 676–677
 physical implications, 670–671
 physiologic implications, 671–673
Butorphanol, 197t, 573
Butyrophenones, 719

C

CABG. *See* Coronary artery bypass grafting (CABG)
CAD. *See* Coronary artery disease (CAD)
Calcitonin, 123–124
Calcium channel blockers, 9, 54, 56, 59, 122, 130–131, 280, 282–283, 286, 315, 330, 406, 512, 574, 580, 714–715, 757–758
Calcium chloride (calcium gluconate), 81, 125, 443, 517, 757–758, 783
Calcium metabolism and parathyroid disease
 hypercalcemia
  anesthetic considerations, 124
  bisphosphonates, 124
  calcitonin, 125
  cinacalcet, 124
  clinical features of, 124
  denosumab, 124
  etiologies of, 123–124
  glucocorticoid therapy, 124
  hydration, 124
  treatment of, 124
 hypocalcemia
  anesthetic considerations, 125–126
  clinical features of, 125
  etiologies of, 125
  treatment of, 125
 physiology, 123
 serum calcium, 123
CAM. *See* Complementary and alternative medicine (CAM)
Cangrelor, 513, 514t, 518, 699
Carbonic anhydrase inhibitors, 92t
Carbon monoxide, 675–676
Carboprost (prostaglandin F2α; Hemabate), 573, 783–784
Carcinoid
 anesthetic considerations, 135–136
 clinical features, 134
 crisis, 136
 syndrome, 134
 treatment, 135
 tumors, 134–136

Cardiac arrest, 199, 330, 748–749
    diagnosis, 748–749
    during pregnancy, 586–587
    epidemiology, 749
    etiologies, 749
    pathophysiology, 749
Cardiac catheterization, 51, 511–512, 529
Cardiac disease
    cardiac transplant
        anesthetic considerations, 61
        monitoring, 61
        physiology, 60–61
    congenital heart disease (CHD), 59–60
    congestive heart failure
        anesthetic considerations, 57–58
        etiologies, 57
        pathophysiology, 57
        ventricular assist devices (VADs), 57–58
    hypertrophic cardiomyopathy, 59
    ischemic heart disease, 53–54
    pacemakers
        cardiac implantable electronic devices (CIEDs), 61–63
        emergency external cardioversion/defibrillation, 66
        intraoperative management, 65
        leadless, 63–64
        nomenclature, 62
        postoperative management, 66
        preoperative evaluation and preparation, 64–65
        subcutaneous ICDs (S-ICDs), 64
        temporary perioperative pacing and cardioversion-defibrillation options, 65–66
    preanesthetic considerations, 52–53
    preoperative cardiovascular evaluation, noncardiac surgery
        cardiac catheterization and consultation, 51
        coronary artery bypass grafting, 52
        echocardiography, 50
        functional capacity, 50
        initial screening, 49–50
        12-lead electrocardiogram (ECG), 50
        major adverse cardiac event (MACE) risk, 50
        percutaneous coronary intervention (PCI), 52
        stress testing, 50–51
        supplemental cardiac evaluation, 50–51
    valvular heart disease
        aortic regurgitation, 55
        aortic stenosis, 54–55
        mitral regurgitation, 56
        mitral stenosis, 56
Cardiac dysrhythmias, 230–231
Cardiac evaluation, 511–512, 512t–513t
Cardiac fill status assessment, 34–38
Cardiac glycosides, 312
Cardiac implantable electronic devices (CIEDs), 61–62
Cardiac ischemia, 324
Cardiac medications, 512–515, 514t
Cardiac output, 293, 691. *See also* Central venous pressure (CVP)
    modified Fick technique, 259
    pulse contour analysis, 259
    thermodilution, 258
    thoracic bioimpedance, 259
    thoracic bioreactance, 59
Cardiac point-of-care ultrasound (POCUS), 21–26, 22f–26f
    purpose, 21
    technical aspects, 21
    views
        apical five-chamber (A5C) view, 24–25, 25f
        apical four-chamber (A4C) view, 22, 24f–25f
        parasternal long-axis (PLAX) view, 21–22, 22f
        parasternal short-axis (PSAX) view, 22, 23f–24f
        subcostal four-chamber (S4C) view, 25, 26f
        subcostal inferior vena cava (IVC) view, 26, 27f–28f
Cardiac surgery
    anesthetic management
        monitoring, 515–516
        preinduction, 516–517
    cardiac tamponade and constrictive pericarditis, 536
    cardiac transplantation, 536–537
    cardiopulmonary bypass (CBP)
        components of circuit, 510
        pathophysiology, 510
        pharmacokinetics, 510
    deep hypothermic circulatory arrest (DHCA), 535–536
    enhanced recovery after surgery (ERAS) for, 527
    extracorporeal membrane oxygenation (ECMO), 537

induction
  anesthetic management of patient, 517–518
  cardiopulmonary bypass, 521–522
  discontinuing cardiopulmonary bypass, 522–524
  post-bypass period, 525–526
  pre-bypass period, 519–521, 520t
  time of separation from CPB, 524–525
  transfer to intensive care unit, 526
lung transplantation, 537–538
mechanical circulatory support (MCS), 538–540
off-bypass coronary artery bypass grafting (CABG), 534–535
off-site cardiac procedures
  aspiration thrombectomy, 541
  cardioversion, 542
  implantable cardioverter defibrillator (ICD), 541–542
  intra-aortic balloon pump (IABP), 516
  transcatheter ablation and electrophysiology, 542
pediatric cardiac anesthesia
  anesthetic management, 529–530
  balanced shunts, 534
  cardiopulmonary bypass, 530
  congenital heart disease (CHD), 528–529
  congenital heart disease (CHD) lesions, management of, 530, 534, 531t–533t
  neonatal *vs.* adult cardiac physiology, 528
  patent ductus arteriosus (PDA) ligation, 534
  transition from fetal to adult circulation, 527–528
postoperative care
  complications, 526–527
  warming, 526
preoperative assessment
  cardiac evaluation, 511–512, 512t–513t
  cardiac medications, 512–515, 514t
  pertinent to cardiac procedure, 511
  "redo" cardiac surgery, 535
ventricular assist device (VAD), 538–539
Cardiac tamponade, 298–299, 526–527, 536
Cardiac transplantation, 536–537
Cardiopulmonary bypass (CBP)
  cardiac surgery
    components of circuit, 510
    discontinuing, 522–524
    induction, 521–522, 523t
    pathophysiology, 510
    pharmacokinetics, 510
  coagulopathy, 698
  pediatric cardiac anesthesia, 530
Cardiopulmonary resuscitation (CPR), 577, 747
  adult and pediatric, 762t, 764f
  DNR order and, 761
  termination of, 761
Cardioselective, 316
Cardiovascular instability, 415
Cardiovascular system (CVS)
  anesthesia, 4–5
  liver disease, 101
  monitoring
    arterial blood pressure, 244–247
    electrocardiogram (ECG), 243–244
    ischemia detection, 244
    mechanism of, 243–244
    rhythm detection, 244
Cardioverter-defibrillator device, 4
Carotid artery stenting (CAS), 491–492, 642
Carotid endarterectomy (CEA), 492–493
Carotid sinus, 493
CARP trial. *See* Coronary Artery Revascularization Prophylaxis (CARP) trial
Catecholamines, 95t, 126, 129–130, 134, 195, 203, 280, 286, 294, 302, 305, 308, 312, 528, 575, 581, 672, 749, 757, 770
Catheter, Foley, 666
Caudal anesthesia, 352–353, 448–449, 611–612
  anatomy, 353
  complications, 353
  physiology, 353
  technique, 353, 354f
CBF. *See* Cerebral blood flow (CBF)
CDH. *See* Congenital diaphragmatic hernia (CDH)
CEA. *See* Carotid endarterectomy (CEA)
Cefazolin, 2, 145, 147
Cefepime, 147
Cefotetan, 145t, 147
Cefoxitin, 145t, 147

Ceftazidime, 147
Ceftriaxone, 147
Celecoxib, 10, 14, 429, 452, 635, 726, 726t, 730t
Cell salvage, 691
Central line-associated blood stream infection (CLABSI), 142
Central nervous system (CNS)
 local anesthetics and, 329
 vascular surgery, preoperative assessment, 488
Central venous catheters (CVCs), 87, 141–142, 530
Central venous pressure (CVP), 402
 analysis for, 247–248
 cardiac output
  echocardiography, 259–260
  modified Fick technique, 259
  pulse contour analysis, 259
  thermodilution, 258
  thoracic bioimpedance, 259
  thoracic bioreactance, 259
 echocardiography, 259–260
 indications of, 247–248
 pathology and, 248–249
 positive-pressure ventilation, 249
 procedure
  catheter insertion, 249–253, 251f
  complications, 253–254
  femoral vein, 253
  internal jugular Seldinger technique, 251f
  landmark-based technique, 250
  locations, 249
  materials, 249
  position and preparation, 249
  SCV, 252–253
  ultrasound-guided technique, 250–252, 251f
 pulmonary artery catheter
  procedure and indications, 254
  complications, 258
  indications, 254
  materials/catheter types, 256
  mechanism, 254
  pathology, 256
  procedure, 256–258, 255f, 257f
  securing, 257
 waveform and, 248, 248f
Cephalosporin, 2, 147
Cerebral angiography, 641–642
Cerebral blood flow (CBF), 402, 403f
Cerebral hyperperfusion syndrome (CHS), 494
Cerebral metabolic rate ($CMRO_2$), 402–403
Cerebral perfusion pressure (CPP), 189, 283, 402
Cerebral protection, 406–407
Cerebral salt wasting syndrome, 413
Cerebral vasospasm, 643–644
Cerebrospinal fluid (CSF), 402
 drainage, 502
 pH, 569
 protein, 569
 rhinorrhea, 264, 661
 shunts, 419–420
 spinal anesthesia, 335
Cervical disk disease, airways, 207
Cervical plexus block (CPB)
 deep, 493
 regional anesthesia, for neck, 493, 367f
 superficial, 493
Cervical spinal cord injury, 418
Cervical spine, 209, 654, 659
Chamberlain procedure, 473
CHD. *See* Congenital heart disease (CHD)
Chest trauma, 663–664
Child-Turcotte-Pugh (CTP), 107, 107t
Chloral hydrate, 629
Cholecystectomy, 457
Cholecystojejunostomy, 457
Choledochojejunostomy, 457
Cholestasis, 100, 105
Cholinergic receptors, 227–228
Cholinesterase
 activity, reduced, 324
 atypical, 232–233, 324
Cholinesterase inhibitors, 95t, 96
Christmas disease (hemophilia B), 700
Chronic hypoxemia, respiratory system, 102
Chronic kidney disease (CKD)
 anesthetic management, 87
 clinical features, 85–86
 epidemiology, 85, 86t
 etiology, 85
 management, 86
Chronic obstructive pulmonary disease (COPD), 70–71, 133, 295, 336, 397, 481, 553, 707
CHS. *See* Cerebral hyperperfusion syndrome (CHS)
Cholinesterase inhibitors, 95t, 96
Cilostazol, 342t, 514t, 699–700
Cimetidine (Tagamet), 12

CIN. *See* Contrast-induced nephropathy (CIN)
Cinacalcet, 124
Cirrhotic cardiomyopathy, 101
Cisatracurium, 5, 95, 106, 180, 228, 229t, 229, 230t, 231, 234, 237, 240, 434, 437, 440, 517, 562, 607
CKD. *See* Chronic kidney disease (CKD)
CLABSI. *See* Central line-associated blood stream infection (CLABSI)
Cleft lip and palate (CLP) repair, 551–552
Clevidipine (Cleviprex), 131, 283, 315t, 316, 504, 784
Clindamycin, 147–148, 238, 623
Clonidine, 9, 129, 196, 280, 283, 310, 315, 328, 344, 391–392, 607, 611–612
Clopidogrel (Plavix), 342t, 355, 487, 513, 514t, 641, 699
Closed-loop communication, errors, 160
Clothesline injury, 663
Clotting factors, 99, 656, 685, 691, 697–698, 700
CMV. *See* Cytomegalovirus (CMV)
CNS. *See* Central nervous system (CNS)
Coagulopathy, 17, 104–105, 684–685
  clinical management, 657
  in liver failure, 104–105
Colectomy/hemicolectomy, 455
Colloids, 450
Colonoscopy, 651
Color Doppler, 33, 362
Combined spinal-epidural analgesia (CSE), 352, 577–578
Complementary and alternative medicine (CAM)
  categories, 743
  definitions, 742
  hypnosis, 743–744
  mindfulness meditation, 744
  music medicine and music therapy, 744–745
  perioperative acupuncture, 743
  virtual reality (VR), 745
Complete global ischemia, 406
Computed tomography (CT), 409, 439, 466, 632
Computed tomography pulmonary angiography (CTPA), 31–32
Congenital anomalies, airways, 208
Congenital diaphragmatic hernia (CDH), 589, 624–625
Congenital heart disease (CHD), 59–60, 528–529, 625

Congestive heart failure
  anesthetic considerations, 57–59
  etiologies, 57
  pathophysiology, 57
Conjugated estrogens, 91
Conn syndrome
  anesthetic considerations, 127
  clinical features, 127
  treatment, 127
Consolidated lung, 42
Constrictive pericarditis, 536
Contact precautions, 139–141
Contamination, bacteria in anesthesia machine, 141
Context-sensitive half-time (CSHT), 188, 198
Continuous positive airway pressure (CPAP), 617–618
Continuous renal replacement therapy (CRRT), 85
Contrast-induced nephropathy (CIN), 635
Controlled hypotension, 495, 691–692
COPD. *See* Chronic obstructive pulmonary disease (COPD)
Coronary anatomy, 47–49, 47f
Coronary artery bypass grafting (CABG), 52, 145t
Coronary artery disease (CAD), 4, 10, 49–53, 61, 438, 512–513, 515–518, 681, 683
Coronary Artery Revascularization Prophylaxis (CARP) trial, 487
Corticosteroids, 121, 152, 239–240, 302, 409, 419, 553, 693, 719
Coughing, 69, 545, 562
COVID-19, 141–142, 148, 723
CPAP. *See* Continuous positive airway pressure (CPAP)
CPP. *See* Cerebral perfusion pressure (CPP)
Crawford classification, thoracoabdominal aneurysms, 501, 501f
Creatinine clearance, 87, 237, 569
Creutzfeldt-Jakob disease, 151
Cricoid cartilage, of larynx, 205–206, 206f, 223–224, 365, 367, 591, 662–663
Cricothyroid membrane, of larynx, 205
Cricothyroidotomy, 223, 654, 669
Crisis resource management, 160–162, 161t

CRRT. *See* Continuous renal replacement therapy (CRRT)
Cryoprecipitate, 90, 426, 443, 643, 688, 693, 695, 697–698, 700–702
CSF. *See* Cerebrospinal fluid (CSF)
CSHT. *See* Context-sensitive half-time (CSHT)
CTP. *See* Child-Turcotte-Pugh (CTP)
Curtain sign, 43
Cushing syndrome, 127, 417
CVCs. *See* Central venous catheters (CVCs)
CVP. *See* Central venous pressure (CVP)
CVS. *See* Cardiovascular system (CVS)
Cyanide toxicity, 317
Cyclobenzaprine, 720, 733, 734t
Cyclodextrin-NMB complex, 96
Cyclopentolate, 545
Cystatin C, 87
Cystectomy, 561–562
Cystoscopy, 557
Cytokines, 89, 692
Cytomegalovirus (CMV), 100, 150, 432, 530, 688

D

Dabigatran, 700
DDD pacemaker, 62
Dalteparin (Fragmin), 342t
Damage control surgery, 657
Dantrolene, 299–300, 785
DCD. *See* Donation after cardiac death (DCD)
Deep brain stimulators, 417–418
Deep peroneal nerve, 374, 380, 380f, 395
Defibrillation, 62, 65–66, 523, 586, 752–753, 763–764
Delirium, 4, 15, 186, 277, 310, 394, 527, 604, 614, 717
Denosumab, 124
Dentistry and oral and maxillofacial surgery, 554–556
Dentition, 7
DES. *See* Drug-eluting stents (DES)
Desflurane, 69, 73, 131, 168, 182, 186, 200t, 201–203, 280, 284, 299, 405t, 426, 604, 629, 721
 effects, on brain, 272
Desmopressin, 79, 133, 413, 417, 445, 462, 690
Desmopressin acetate (DDAVP), 86, 785

Dexamethasone (Decadron), 16t, 122, 126–127, 185, 328, 410, 429, 548, 552, 617, 635–636, 711, 719, 722, 785
Dexmedetomidine, 131, 182, 190t
 hemodynamic control, perioperative and, 273–274, 274f, 310
 as inhalation anesthetic, 200–204, 200t, 201f
 as intravenous (IV) anesthetics
  action mode of, 196
  adverse effects, 197
  cardiovascular system, 196
  central nervous system (CNS), 196
  dosage and administration, 197t, 197
  endocrine system, 196
  pharmacodynamics of, 196
  pharmacokinetics of, 196
  respiratory system, 196
DI. *See* Diabetes insipidus (DI)
Diabetes insipidus (DI), 80, 133, 413, 417
Diabetes mellitus (DM), 5–6, 11, 52–53, 85–86, 91, 113
 acute complications
  diabetic ketoacidosis (DKA), 114
  hyperglycemic hyperosmolar syndrome (HHS), 114–115
 anesthetic considerations
  airway management, 116
  diabetic ketoacidosis (DKA), hyperglycemic hyperosmolar syndrome, and metabolic abnormalities, 114–115
  fixed ratio insulin combinations, 117
  neuropathy, 115–116
  oral hypoglycemic agents, 117–119
  vascular disease, 115
 diabetic autonomic neuropathy, 115
 oral hypoglycemic agents, 117–119
 peripheral neuropathy, 115
 physiology of, 113
 types of
  gestational, 113
  secondary, 113
  type 1, 113
  type 2, 113
Diabetic autonomic neuropathy, 115
Diabetic ketoacidosis (DKA), 114–115
Diaphoresis, 293
Diazepam, 12, 93, 192–193, 629, 717, 733, 734t

Diameter Index Safety System (DISS), 165
DIC. *See* Disseminated intravascular coagulation (DIC)
Diclofenac, 728, 730t
Differential blockade, nerve fibers, 323–324
Digoxin (Lanoxin), 8, 56, 95t, 96, 283, 312, 523
Dihydropyridine (DHP), 315
Diltiazem (Cardizem), 122, 286, 316, 715, 757, 785
Dimenhydrinate, 719
Dipeptidyl peptidase IV (DPP-IV) inhibitors, 118
Dipyridamole, 51, 514t, 699–700, 756
Direct factor Xa inhibitors, 700
Direct laryngoscopy, 552
Direct thrombin inhibitors (DTIs), 700
Disseminated intravascular coagulation (DIC), 105, 298, 300, 419, 559, 582, 623, 670, 672, 684
Diuretics, 8, 52, 54, 79–81, 84, 87, 91–92, 92t, 103–104, 118, 124, 290, 409, 412, 512, 544, 563, 694, 708, 716
    effect on potassium, 81
    KDIGO guidelines 2012, 91
DKA. *See* Diabetic ketoacidosis (DKA)
DM. *See* Diabetes mellitus (DM)
DNR. *See* Do Not Resuscitate (DNR)
Dobutamine, 51, 56, 282, 296, 309t, 311, 530, 584, 758, 786
    hemodynamic control, perioperative and, 311
    stress echocardiography, 439, 486, 511
DOE. *See* Dyspnea on exertion (DOE)
Donation after brain death (DBD), 443, 444t
Donation after cardiac death (DCD), 443, 461
DNR, Do Not Resuscitate, 761
Dopamine (Intropin), 12, 61, 84, 92, 129, 134, 282, 284, 296, 309t, 319, 321, 462, 504, 530, 537, 562, 758, 786
    hemodynamic control, perioperative and, 311
Dopamine receptors, 308
Dopaminergic, 305, 418, 758
Doppler ultrasound, 33, 416, 492
Doxazosin, 130, 319
Droperidol, 16t, 185, 280, 719
Drug(s) for gastric acid/volume, 12, 447, 599, 605

Drug-eluting stents (DES), 53
3D spectrogram, 270, 271f
DTIs. *See* Direct thrombin inhibitors (DTIs)
Duchene muscular dystrophy, 240–241
Dural puncture, 576
Dural puncture epidural (DPE), 578
Dysphagia/odynophagia, 6
Dyspnea, 344
Dyspnea on exertion (DOE), 4
Dysrhythmias, 462
    delaying surgical procedures, 8
    heart block, 284–285
    hemodynamic complications
        stable ventricular dysrhythmias, 715
        supraventricular dysrhythmias, 714–715
        unstable ventricular tachycardia and ventricular fibrillation, 715
    sinus bradycardia, 283–284
    sinus tachycardia, 284
    supraventricular tachycardias (SVTs), 285–287
    ventricular dysrhythmias, 287–288

E

EABL. *See* Estimated allowable blood loss (EABL)
Ear surgery, 549
Ebola, 150
Echocardiography, 51, 259–260, 511, 540
    cardiac fill status assessment, 34–38
    cardiac function assessment, 28–33, 28t, 30f
    cardiac point-of-care ultrasound (POCUS), 21–26, 22f–26f
    echocardiographic parameters, 36
    hemodynamic measurements and fluid responsiveness
        Bernoulli equation, 34, 34f
        Doppler ultrasound, 33
        flow measurements, 33
        fluid responsiveness, 35–38
        right ventricular systolic pressure (RVSP), 34
        pressure gradient assessment, 33–34
        stroke volume measurement, 33, 36
    inferior vena cava (IVC), 34–35, 35t, 36–37
    left atrial pressure (LAP) estimation, 35
    left ventricular assessment, 28–29, 30f, 28t, 37t

Echocardiography (*Continued*)
  pericardial effusion and cardiac tamponade, 32–33
  pulmonary embolism, 31–32
  rest, 50
  right ventricular assessment, 29–31
  severity, 54
  transesophageal (TEE), 26–28, 27f, 249, 252, 259–260
  transthoracic (TTE) image acquisition, 22f–25f, 49, 71, 102, 249, 252, 259–260, 282, 438, 540, 706
Eclampsia, 580
ECT. *See* Electroconvulsive therapy (ECT)
Edentulous patients, 212
EEG. *See* Electroencephalogram (EEG)
Electrical hazards, 302–303
Electroconvulsive therapy (ECT)
  anesthetic goals, 648
  anesthetic management, 649
  contraindications, 648–649
  physiologic effects of, 648
  psychiatric drug interactions during, 649–650
Electroencephalogram (EEG), 265, 647
  age-related changes, 276–277, 277f–278f
  biophysics of, 266, 266f
  bispectral index, 266
  clinical monitoring of, 278
  CNS monitoring, 492
  electrophysiologic monitoring, 407–408
  entropy, 268
  narcotrend, 267
  patient state index (PSI), 266–267
  spectral analysis of, 269–270, 269f, 271f
Electrolyte balance, 78–82, 592
Electromyography (EMG), 408–409
Embolization, 415, 453, 483
  for control of epistaxis/extracranial vascular lesions, 641
  distal, 489
  endovascular, 640–641
  for gastrointestinal bleeding and hemoptysis, 644
Emergency airway techniques
  cricothyroidotomy, 223, 661
  difficult airway
    laryngeal mask airways (LMAs), 221
    regional anesthesia, 222–223
    percutaneous needle cricothyroidotomy, 223
    rigid bronchoscopy, 223
    tracheostomy, 223
Emesis, 446
EMG. *See* Electromyography (EMG)
EMLA. *See* Eutectic mixture of local anesthetics (EMLA)
Enalaprilat, 318
  hemodynamic control, perioperative, 318
Endobronchial tubes, 473
  double-lumen, 466–468
Endobronchial ultrasound, 471
Endocarditis prophylaxis, 146
Endocrine disease
  adrenal cortical disease, 126
    glucocorticoid excess, 127
    pharmacology, 126
    physiology, 126
    primary hyperaldosteronism, 127. *See also* Conn syndrome
  adrenal cortical hypofunction, 128
  adrenal medullary disease, 129–131
  calcium metabolism and parathyroid disease, 123–126
  carcinoid, 134–136
  diabetes mellitus
    acute complications, 113–115
    anesthetic considerations, 114–119
    obsolete terminology, 113
    physiology of, 113
    therapeutics, 117–119
    types of, 113
  hypoglycemia, 114
  parathyroid disease. *See* Parathyroid disease
  pituitary disease
    anterior pituitary gland, 131–132
    posterior pituitary gland, 133–134
  thyroid disease, 120
    evaluation and laboratory studies, 120
    Graves disease, 123
    hyperthyroidism, 120–122
    hypothyroidism, 120–121
    myxedema coma, 121
    physiology, 120
    thyroid storm, 122–123
    thyroid surgery, 120, 124, 554
    thyrotoxicosis, 121–122
  vascular surgery, preoperative assessment, 488

Endoscopic procedures
  endobronchial ultrasound, 471
  flexible bronchoscopy, 470–471
  flexible esophagoscopy, 476
  laser surgery, 472
  mediastinoscopy, 472–473
  rigid bronchoscopy, 471–472
  rigid esophagoscopy, 476
Endoscopic retrograde cholangiopancreatography (ERCP), 650–651
Endoscopic sleeve gastroplasty (ESG), 651
Endoscopy, upper/lower anesthesia, 650
Endotracheal intubation, 180–181
  airway management in, 180–181
  alternative intubation techniques
    gum elastic bougie, 220–221
    laryngoscope, 220
    light wand, 221
    retrograde tracheal intubation, 221
  bronchoscopic, 219–220
  nasotracheal, 219
  orotracheal, 215–219, 217f–218f
Endotracheal tubes (ETTs), 215–221, 223–226, 471, 475–477, 479–480, 482–483, 504, 548, 551–555, 751, 753, 756, 763, 769
Energy- and biofield-based therapies, 743
End-tidal anesthetic criterion, 268–269
Enhanced recovery after surgery (ERAS) abdominal surgery, 451–452
Enoxaparin (Lovenox), 342t, 355, 699, 786
Entropy, 268
Ephedrine, 60, 131, 181, 283–285, 309t, 344, 415, 571, 575, 650, 786
  hemodynamic control, perioperative and, 312
Epidural analgesia, 110–111, 345, 349, 455, 475–477, 575–576, 710, 720, 737–738, 738t
Epidural anesthesia
  anatomy, 344–345
  anticoagulation and, 342t–343t
  for cesarean delivery, 574
  combined spinal, 352
  complications, 350–352
  confirmatory methods, 349–350
  epidural blockade
    bloody tap, 350
    catheter complications, 350–351
    direct spinal cord injury, 351–352
    dural puncture, 350
    epidural abscess, 352
    epidural hematoma, 352
    Horner syndrome, 352
    intravascular injection, 351
    levels of, 348–349
    local anesthetic overdose, 351
    onset and duration of, 349
    postdural puncture headache (PDPH), 352
    unintentional subarachnoid injection, 351
  physiology of, 345
  techniques
    catheter placement, 347–350
    epidural needles, 345
    injection of, 348
    lumbar, 346–347
    monitoring, 346
    patient position, 345
    test dose, 348
    thoracic, 347
Epidural blood patch (EBP), 343, 577
Epidural hematoma, 352
Epidural opioids, 736–737
Epiglottitis, 207
Epilepsy surgery, 418–419
Epinephrine (Adrenalin), 70, 104, 122, 203, 282–285, 294, 299, 305, 309t, 310–312, 324–325, 328, 330, 340, 344–345, 349, 351, 359, 392–393, 530, 537, 542, 545, 550, 552, 576, 579, 584, 610–613, 636, 643, 647, 711, 713, 753, 758–760, 769–770
  comments, 787
  dosage, 787
  effect, 786–787
  hemodynamic control, perioperative and, 302
  indications, 786
  local anesthetics and, 324–325, 328
Episcleral block, 547
E-point septal separation (EPSS), 29
Epoprostenol, 58, 319–320, 779
Eptifibatide (Integrilin), 342t, 355, 514t, 641, 699, 779
ERCP. *See* Endoscopic retrograde cholangiopancreatography (ERCP)
Ergonovine (Ergotrate), 573, 787. *See also* Methylergonovine (methergine)
Ergot alkaloids, 573

Errors, anesthesia safety
  cognitive, 157, 159, 158t–159t
  handoff, 159–160
  human factors in, 159
  medication. *See* Medication errors
  procedure type, 157
  teamwork and communication type, 160
Erythropoietin (EPO), 82, 90, 396, 689
Esmolol (Brevibloc), 131, 232, 283, 286, 410–411, 462, 524, 581, 649, 757, 787
  hemodynamic control, perioperative and, 313, 314t
Esophageal bougie, 455
Esophageal manometry, 262
Esophageal surgery
  anesthetic considerations for abdominal procedures, 454–455
  general considerations, 477
  operative approach and anesthesia, 477–478
Esophageal varices, 102–103
Esophagogastroduodenoscopy (EGD), 102, 476, 650
Esters, 323
Estimated allowable blood loss (EABL), 683
Ether-derived anesthetics, on brain, 272, 273f
Ethical considerations, in patient care, 17–18
Ethical issues, anesthetist, 18
Etomidate, 68, 94t, 95, 106, 127–128, 180, 188, 190, 280, 406, 410, 418, 426, 499, 517, 536, 605, 649, 665, 679
  as intravenous (IV) anesthetics
    action mode of, 193
    adverse effects, 193
    cardiovascular system, 192
    central nervous system (CNS), 192
    dosage and administration, 190t
    pharmacodynamics of, 194
    pharmacokinetics of, 193
    respiratory system, 192–193
ETTs. *See* Endotracheal tubes (ETTs)
Eutectic mixture of local anesthetics (EMLA), 325
Evoked potential monitoring
  neurosurgery, 408–409
Exercise stress testing, cardiac evaluation, 51
Exparel, 324

Extracorporeal cooling, 292
Extracorporeal membrane oxygenation (ECMO), 483–484, 518, 537–538, 584, 625, 760
Extubation, 183, 547, 549, 614, 713

F

Fascia iliaca block, 374
Fetal well-being, 585
Febrile nonhemolytic transfusion reactions (FNHTR), 693
Femoral-femoral bypass grafting, 490
Femoral herniorrhaphies, 456
Femoral nerve block, 372, 375, 376f
Femoral pseudoaneurysm, 490–491
Fenoldopam, 84, 92, 290, 315t, 318, 498, 500, 787
Fentanyl, 16, 95, 108, 180, 197, 197t, 198, 225, 283, 293, 325, 340, 349, 358, 410–411, 429, 434–435, 517, 534, 542, 545, 549, 575–579, 586, 587, 608t, 612, 614, 627, 634, 643, 646, 720, 731–732, 735t, 736–737
Ferromagnetic objects, 637
Fetal acidosis, 324
Fetal development
  body composition, 590–591
  cardiovascular development, 590
  organogenesis, 589
  respiratory development, 589
Fetal heart rate (FHR) monitoring, 570–572
FFP. *See* Fresh frozen plasma (FFP)
Fiberoptic bronchoscopy, 178, 469, 482, 708
Fibrinogen, 355, 426, 511, 581, 584, 657, 670, 684–685, 688–690, 697, 700
Fibrinolytic and thrombolytic agents, 355
Fire hazards, 302
Flail chest, 663
Flexible bronchoscopy, 470–471
Flow control valves, 167
Flowmeters, 167
Fludrocortisone, 126
Fluid challenge, 38
Fluid management, 497–498
Fluid resuscitation, 655, 671, 676, 712, 772
  in abdominal surgery, 449–450
  in HRS, 104
  in hyperkalemia, 81
  in hypovolemia, 281
  in pancreatic surgery, 457

Fluid status and responsiveness, 35
Flumazenil (Mazicon), 193, 709, 788
Fluoroquinolones, 144–145, 148
FNHTR. *See* Febrile nonhemolytic transfusion reactions (FNHTR)
Focal ischemia, 406
Foley catheter, 289–290, 300, 496, 666
Fondaparinux, 342t
Fosphenytoin, 413, 788
Fospropofol, 188
FRC. *See* Functional residual capacity (FRC)
Fractional area change (FAC), 28, 37t
Fresh frozen plasma (FFP), 105, 440, 443, 515, 614, 685
Functional residual capacity (FRC), 68
Fundoplication, 452, 454–455, 478, 611
Furosemide (Lasix), 788

G

GA. *See* General anesthesia (GA)
Gabapentin, 14, 178, 397, 429, 607, 733
Gadolinium, 635
Galvanic or fuel cell analyzers, 174
Galvanic oxygen monitors, 174
Gas analysis, 173–174
Gas delivery system, 166f
  desflurane, 168
  flow control valves and flowmeters, 167
  gas outlet, 168
  medical gas supplies, 165–167
  oxygen flush valve, 168
  pressure regulators, 167
  vaporizers, 167–168
Gas exchange, in pulmonary disease, 68–69
Gastric surgery, 455
Gastroesophageal reflux disease (GERD), 6
Gastroparesis, 116
General anesthesia (GA), 265
  abdominal surgery, 447
  airway management, 178, 180–181
  for cesarean delivery, 574
  emergence and extubation, 182–183
  head and neck surgery, 547
  indications, 177–178
  induction of
    inhalational anesthetics, 182
    intravenous (IV) medications, 179–180, 182
    patient position, 180
    preoxygenation, 179
  intraoperative adverse effects
    upper airway obstruction, 185
    cardiovascular, 184
    cognitive, 186
    hypotension, 185
    neuromuscular blockade complications, 185–186
    PONV, 185
    respiratory, 183–184
    thermoregulation, 184–185
  maintenance of, 181–182
    balanced anesthesia, 182
    total intravenous anesthesia (TIVA), 182
    volatile agents, 182
  postoperative adverse effects, 185–186
  pre-perioperative evaluation and planning
    anxiety medications, 178–179
    gastric acid and gastric volume, 178
    history and interview, 178
    intravenous (IV) access, 179
    pain management, 178–179
    physical examination, 178
    team huddle, 179
  transport and disposition, 183
GH. *See* Growth hormone (GH)
Glaucoma, 544
Glossopharyngeal nerve, 205
Glottis, 206
Glucagon, 101, 131, 646, 788
Glucagon-like–peptide 1 (GLP-1) agonists, 11, 118, 178, 434, 488
Glucocorticoids, 122, 126, 128–129, 232
Gluconeogenesis, 105
Gluteal/subgluteal approach, 378–379
Glyburide, 117
Glycopyrrolate, 16, 195, 233, 237, 288, 344, 415, 449, 466, 470, 481, 492, 529, 537, 544, 552, 555, 574, 585, 605, 607, 616, 710, 712, 714, 728, 789
Graft *versus* host disease (GVHD), 688, 694
Growth hormone (GH), 129
Gum elastic bougie, 220

H

Haloperidol (Haldol), 16t, 133, 185, 292, 548, 717, 719, 789
Halothane hepatitis, 203
Handoff checklist, 160

Handoff errors, 159
HBV. *See* Hepatitis B virus (HBV)
HCV. *See* Hepatitis C virus (HCV)
Head and neck examination, 7
Head and neck surgery
  airways, 209–211, 210f–211f
  dentistry and oral and maxillofacial surgery, 554–556
  ophthalmic surgery
    anesthetic management, 545–547, 546f
    general considerations, 544–545
    procedures, 547–548
  otorhinolaryngologic procedures
    ear surgery, 549
    general considerations, 548–549
    nasal surgery, 549–550
    upper airway surgery, 550–553
  procedures of neck
    general considerations, 553
    radical neck dissection, 553–554
    thyroid and parathyroid surgery, 554, 555f
Head trauma, 418–419
Health care proxy, 17
Heart block, 284–285
Heart transplant, 57. *See also* Cardiac disease
Height and weight measurements, 7
Heliox, 466, 711
HELLP syndrome, 580
Hematologic system, 6
  vascular surgery, preoperative assessment, 488–489
Hemicolectomy, 455
Hemodialysis, 85–87, 89, 91, 232, 400, 434, 438, 635, 646, 772
  end-stage renal disease (ESRD), 5
  intermittent, 82
Hemodilution, 643
Hemodynamic(s)
  anesthetic considerations, 452–453
  cardiac catheterization, 511–512
  complications, 713–716
  controlled hypotension, 495, 556, 691–692
  control, perioperative
    β-adrenergic antagonists, 313–315, 314t
    adrenergic receptor physiology, 305–308, 306t–307t
    autoregulation, 305
    blood pressure, 305
    drug dosage calculations, 320–321
  instability, 534–535, 712–713
  measurements
    flow measurements, 33
    pressure gradient assessment, 33–34
    using Doppler, 33
  mitral stenosis (MS), 517–518
  monitoring, 521–522
  stability, 525
  vasodilators, 315–320, 315t
Hemofiltration, 85
Hemophilia, 701
Hemorrhage, 109, 482–483, 548, 551, 581–583, 619, 628–629, 667, 670
Hemorrhoidectomy, 455
Hemostasis, 60, 525–526
Heparin, 8, 10, 81, 86, 91, 191, 256, 280, 297, 342t, 445, 461, 487, 492–493, 498, 510, 512, 515, 517, 519–520, 522–523, 525–526, 530, 534–535, 539, 640, 684–685, 691, 699
  perioperative coagulopathy, 699
Heparin-induced thrombocytopenia (HIT), 488–489, 511
  type 2, 519
Heparin–unfractionated, 355, 489, 789
Hepatic encephalopathy, 100–101
Hepatic function
  degradation
    carbohydrates, 99
    lipids, 99
    heme and bile, 99
    proteins, 99
  drug metabolism, 100
    enzyme induction/cytochrome P450, 100
Hepatic surgery, 456–457
Hepatitis, 100, 144, 696
Hepatitis B virus (HBV), 149–150, 696
Hepatitis C virus (HCV), 150, 696
Hepatopulmonary syndrome, 102, 439
Hepatorenal syndrome (HRS), 82, 103–104
Herbal medications, 355
Herpes simplex viruses (HSV) I and II, 150
HFJV. *See* High-frequency jet ventilation (HFJV)
HHS. *See* Hyperglycemic hyperosmolar syndrome (HHS)
High-frequency jet ventilation (HFJV), 483, 634
History
  allergic and drug reactions, 2–3
  anesthetic, 3
  family, 3

habits and social, 3–4
medications, 1
of presenting illness, 1
HIT. *See* Heparin-induced thrombocytopenia (HIT)
HIV. *See* Human immunodeficiency virus (HIV)
Homeostasis, disorders of
potassium, 80–82
sodium, 78–80
Hormonal therapy, 461
Horner syndrome, 352
HTN. *See* Hypertension (HTN)
Human immunodeficiency virus (HIV), 149, 696
Hydralazine, 131, 280, 283, 318, 406, 494, 580, 789
Hydrocephalus, 628
Hydrocortisone, 122, 126, 128, 302, 636, 693, 790
Hydromorphone, 197t, 735t
Hydrophilic opioids, 340, 736
Hygiene standards, operating room, 141
Hypercalcemia, 123–124, 133
Hypercarbia, 289
Hyperdynamic circulatory state, 101
Hyperglycemia, 114–115, 131, 407, 412, 419, 437, 458, 522, 573, 644
Hyperglycemic hyperosmolar syndrome (HHS), 115
Hyperkalemia, 9, 81–82, 86, 104, 128, 231, 300, 443, 523, 646, 694, 716
Hypernatremia, 79–80
Hypertension (HTN), 4, 9, 127, 462, 498
etiologies, 282–283
treatment of, 283
Hyperthermia, 292, 407, 720
Hypertrophic cardiomyopathy, 59
Hypervolemia, 85, 412, 642
Hypervolemic hypernatremia, 80
Hypervolemic hyponatremia, 79
Hypnosis
applications, 744
definition of, 743
mechanism, 744
Hypocalcemia, 86, 125–126, 694–695
Hypoglycemia, 105, 119–120, 594
Hypoglycemic agents, 117–119
Hypokalemia, 8, 80–81, 412, 716
Hypomagnesemia, 716
Hyponatremia, 9, 78–79, 86, 104, 128, 412
Hypotension, 335, 343–344, 462, 498
contractility, 280

decreased systemic vascular resistance (SVR), 280–282
dysrhythmias, 282
general anesthesia (GA), 185
hemodynamic complications
cardiac output, 714
hypovolemia, 713
impaired venous return, 713
vasodilation, 713–714
inadequate venous return, 282
myocardial ischemia, 296
treatment of, 282
Hypotensive anesthesia, 556
Hypotensive reactions, 689
Hypothermia, 184, 407, 414, 500, 503, 521, 535, 695, 713, 720
anesthetic effects, 291
heat loss, 290–291
prevention and treatment of, 291–292
severe, physiologic changes caused by, 291
Hypovolemia, 281, 446, 713
Hypervolemic hyponatremia, 79
Hypovolemic hyponatremia, 79
Hypoxemia, 73–74, 102, 296, 461–462, 469–470, 482, 538, 587, 708–709
intraoperative etiologies, 288
treatment of, 288–289
Hypoxia, delaying surgical procedures, 17

I

Ibuprofen, 133, 626, 720, 726t, 729t
ICP. *See* Intracranial pressure (ICP)
ICU. *See* Intensive care unit (ICU)
Ilioinguinal–iliohypogastric block, 372, 387, 495–496, 607
Immunomodulation, blood transfusions, 696–697
Immunosuppression, 679
Impaired hypoxic pulmonary vasoconstriction, 102
Implantable cardioverter-defibrillator (ICD), 61–64
Implantable devices, 539
Indigo carmine, 261, 283, 304, 561
Indomethacin, 573, 626
Induction, of general anesthesia (GA)
inhalational anesthetics, 182
intravenous (IV) medications, 179–180, 182
patient position, 180
preoxygenation, 179

Inhalational injury, 208–209
Infectious complications, blood transfusions, 695–696
Infectious diseases and infection control
 air exchanges, 141
 anesthetist responsibilities, 152
 antibiotics
  aminoglycosides, 148
  clindamycin, 147
  endocarditis, 146
  fluoroquinolones, 148
  indications for, 144
  β-lactams, 147
  metronidazole, 148
  prophylaxis principles, 144–146
  Surgical Care Improvement Project (SCIP), 144–145, 145t
  surgical wounds, 146–147
  vancomycin, 147
 aspiration pneumonia, 143–144
 bacteria
  antibiotic resistant bacteria, 151
  contamination of anesthesia machine, 141
  Mycobacterium tuberculosis, 151
 bactericidal cleaning agents, 141
 central venous catheter (CVC), 141–142
 clean workstation standards, 141
 exposure
  management, 152
  prevention, 151–152
 methods, infection spread, 151
 peripheral intravenous lines, 141
 prevention, infection spread, 151–152
 prion diseases, 151
 standard precautions, 139
 sterilization
  of reusable equipment, 141
  techniques of, 141
 transfusion-related infections, 144
 transmission-based precautions
  airborne precautions, 141
  contact precautions, 139–141
  droplet precautions, 141
 virus exposure
  cytomegalovirus (CMV), 150
  ebola, 150
  hepatitis B virus (HBV), 149–150
  hepatitis C virus (HCV), 150
  herpes simplex virus (HSV) I and II, 150
  human immunodeficiency virus (HIV), 149
  influenza virus, 148
  Mpox, 151
  novel coronaviruses, 148
  varicella-zoster virus (VZV), 150
Inferior laryngeal nerve, 205
Inferior vena cava (IVC) estimation, 34–35, 35t
 diameter variation, 36–37, 37t
Influenza virus, 148
Informed consent anesthesia, 14–15
Infrared analysis, 174
Inguinal herniorrhaphies, 456
Inhalational anesthetics, 182
Inhalation anesthetic(s)
 action mode of, 200, 200t
 adverse effects, 203–204
 desflurane, problems associated with, 203
 diffusion hypoxia, 203
 minimum alveolar concentration (MAC) and, 200
 nitrous oxide as
  cardiovascular system, 202
  central nervous system (CNS), 202
  respiratory system, 202
 pharmacodynamics of, 202–203
 pharmacokinetics of, 200–202, 201f
 sevoflurane, problems associated with, 203–204
 volatile anesthetics
  cardiovascular system, 202–203
  central nervous system (CNS), 202
  hepatic system, 203
  neuromuscular system, 203
  renal system, 203
  respiratory system, 203
Inhalation anesthetics, 405–406
Inotropes, 56, 59, 91, 121, 296–298, 309t, 312, 517–518, 526, 530, 534, 540–541, 577, 584, 757
INR. *See* International normalized ratio (INR)
Insulin, 11, 81, 113–119, 300, 308, 336, 435–437, 443, 458, 522–523, 525, 527, 644
 pumps, 6–7, 117
 resistance, 126–127, 695
Insulin-like growth factor binding protein 7 (IGRBP7), 96
Insulinomas, 119–120, 134
Intensive care unit (ICU), 239

International normalized ratio (INR), 105, 355, 426, 438, 584, 657, 684
Interstitial lung disease (ILD), 76
Interventricular septal morphology, 31
Intestinal and peritoneal surgery, 455–456
Intestine, spinal anesthesia, 336
Intra-anesthetic problems
 anaphylactic and anaphylactoid reactions, 301–302
 aspiration, 294–295
 bronchospasm, 293–294
 cardiac tamponade, 298–299
 diaphoresis (sweating), 293
 dysrhythmias
  heart block, 284–285
  sinus bradycardia, 283–284
  sinus tachycardia, 284
  supraventricular tachycardias (SVTs), 285–287
  ventricular dysrhythmias, 287–288
 electrical hazards in, 302–303
 equipment malfunctions, 303–304
 fire hazards in, 302
 hypercarbia, 289
 hypertension, 282–283
 hyperthermia, 290–292
 hypotension, 280–282
 hypothermia, 290–292
 hypoxemia, 288–289
 laryngospasm, 293
 malignant hyperthermia, 299–301
 myocardial ischemia, 296–297
 pneumothorax, 295–296
 pulmonary embolism (PE), 297–298
 urine output, abnormal, 289–290
Intra-arterial infusion, 643–644
Intracardiac defibrillator (ICD), 715–716
Intracranial aneurysms, 413–414, 413t
Intracranial compliance, 403, 404f, 405, 409
Intracranial hemorrhage, 628
Intracranial normotension, 643
Intracranial pressure (ICP), 231, 283, 317, 402–405, 404f
Intraocular pressure (IOP), 231, 544
Intraoperative blood transfusion, 691
Intraoperative radiation therapy, 458
Intrapulmonary hemorrhage, 482–483
Intrathecal opioids, 736
Intravenous (IV) anesthetics, 389
 Barbiturates, 95
  action mode of, 190
  adverse effects, 191
  cardiovascular system, 191
  central nervous system (CNS), 191
  dosage and administration, 190t, 191
  pharmacodynamics of, 191
  pharmacokinetics of, 190
  respiratory system, 191
 benzodiazepines, 93
  action mode of, 192
  adverse effects, 193
  cardiovascular system, 192
  central nervous system (CNS), 192
  dosage and administration, 190t, 193
  pharmacodynamics of, 192–193
  pharmacokinetics of, 192
  respiratory system, 192–193
 dexmedetomidine, 190t, 196–197
 etomidate, 190t, 193–194
 ketamine
  action mode of, 194
  adverse effects, 195–196
  cardiovascular system, 195
  central nervous system (CNS), 195
  dosage and administration, 190t, 195
  pharmacodynamics of, 195
  pharmacokinetics of, 194–195
  respiratory system, 195
 opioids, 95
  action mode of, 197
  adverse effects, 199
  cardiovascular system, 198
  central nervous system (CNS), 198
  dosage and administration, 199
  gastrointestinal system, 198–199
  pharmacodynamics of, 198–199
  pharmacokinetics of, 197–198, 197t
  respiratory system, 198
 propofol
  action mode of, 188
  adverse effects, 189–190
  cardiovascular system, 189
  central nervous system (CNS), 188–189
  dosage and administration, 189, 190t
  pharmacodynamics of, 188–189
  pharmacokinetics of, 188
  respiratory system, 189
Intravenous antibiotics, 800–803
Intravenous (IV) regional anesthesia (Bier block), 359

Intraventricular hemorrhage, 628
Intubation
  alternative
    gum elastic bougie, 220–221
    laryngoscope, 220
    light wand, 221
    retrograde tracheal intubation, 221
  bronchoscopic, 219–220
  fiberoptic, 16, 132, 178, 180, 211, 424
  nasotracheal, 219
  orotracheal, 215–219, 217f–218f
Ionized drugs, 94t, 95
Ion-trapping, 324
IOP. See Intraocular pressure (IOP)
Ipratroprium bromide, 790
Iron overload, 694
Ischemic heart disease, 53–54
Isoflurane, 69, 168, 182, 200, 200t, 201–202, 272, 275, 276f, 280, 299, 405t, 406, 426, 510, 604, 629
Isoproterenol (Isuprel), 61, 305, 309t 310, 537, 758, 790
  hemodynamic control, perioperative and, 310
Isotonic salt solution, 450
Ivor Lewis esophagectomy, 478

J

Jehovah's Witness (JW), 680–681
Joint disease, stiff, 119
Just culture, anesthesia safety, 155

K

Ketamine, 16, 68–70, 94t, 122, 131, 180, 182, 186, 190t, 224, 268, 280, 294, 391, 406, 418, 426, 429, 499, 529, 536, 544, 547, 554, 582, 604–605, 607, 629, 665, 679, 717, 722, 728, 731
  effects on brain, 274–275, 275f
  as intravenous (IV) anesthetics
    action mode of, 194
    adverse effects, 195–196
    cardiovascular system, 195
    central nervous system (CNS), 195
    dosage and administration, 190t, 195
    pharmacodynamics of, 195
    pharmacokinetics of, 194–195
    respiratory system, 195
  postoperative pain, 429
Ketorolac (Toradol), 392, 429, 607, 649, 720, 726t, 727–728, 730t, 790

Kidney disease(s)
  anesthetic management
    blood urea nitrogen, 87–88
    fluid replacement, 90
    hematologic disturbances, 90–91
    history, 87
    induction agents, 89
    intraoperative management, 89–91
    laboratory studies, 87–88
    narcotics and volatile anesthetics, 93–96, 94t–95t
    optimization, 84–85
    physical examination, 87
    positioning, 89
    postoperative management, 91
    premedication, 89
    preoperative assessment, 86–89
    renal transplantation, 91
    rhabdomyolysis, 90
    risk assessment, 88–89
    urinalysis, 88
    urine electrolytes, 88
    ventilation, 89–90
  electrolyte balance
    potassium homeostasis disorders, 80–82
    sodium homeostasis disorders, 78–80
  extrarenal regulatory and metabolic functions, 82
  fluid regulation, 78
  Kidney Disease. Improving Global Outcomes (KDIGO), 84
  pharmacology
    ionized drugs, 95, 94t–95t
    kidney, 91–93, 92t
    lipid-soluble drugs, 93, 94t
    renal failure, 93–96, 94t–95t
  physiology
    electrolyte balance, 77–79
    fluid regulation, 77
  renal failure
    acute kidney injury (AKI), 82–85
    chronic kidney disease (CKD), 85–86
Kidney failure
  acute kidney injury (AKI)
    classification system, 83, 83t
    clinical feature, 84
    criteria for, 83t
    diagnosis, 84, 84t
    epidemiology, 82
    etiology, 82

prevention, 84
treatment, 84–85
chronic kidney disease (CKD)
clinical features, 85–86
epidemiology, 85
etiology, 85
management, 86
transplantation, anesthetic management, 86
King-Denborough syndrome, 301
Kinins, 78
Kleihauer-Betke analysis, 670
Kuru disease, 151
Kyphoplasty, 642

L

Labetalol, 131, 280, 283, 649
hemodynamic control, perioperative and, 306t–307t, 314t, 315, 411, 494, 580, 649, 790–791
Labor
analgesia for, 574–578
definition, 570
intrapartum fetal evaluation, 570–572, 571f
medications, 572–574
pain, 570
placental transfer of drugs, 574
Laboratory studies
chest radiography, 9
ECG, 9
hematologic studies, 8
pulmonary function tests (PFTs), 9
serum chemistry, 8–9
β-Lactams, 147
Laparoscopic prostatectomies (LRPs), 560
Laparoscopy
anesthetic considerations, 452
anesthetic management, 452–454
operative technique, 452–453
Trendelenburg or reverse Trendelenburg positioning, 453–454
Laryngeal mask airway (LMA), 141, 178, 213
adverse effects, 215
classic, 214
contraindications, 213
flexible-reinforced, 214–215
indications, 213
intubating, 214
removal of, 214
second-generation, 214–215
use of, 213–214, 214f–215f

Laryngeal muscles, 205
Laryngoscope, 180
intubation and, 180
Laryngospasm, 212–213, 293, 614, 711
Larynx, 205, 206f
Laser resection of prostate, 559–560
LAST. *See* Local anesthetic systemic toxicity (LAST)
Leadless pacemakers, 63–64
Lefort classification, 661–662, 662f
Left atrial pressure (LAP) estimation, 35
Left ventricular (LV) assessment, 28–29, 28t
regional function, 29, 30f
Left ventricular end-diastolic area (LVEDA), 36
Left ventricular end-systolic area (LVESA), 36
Levetiracetam (Keppra), 791
Lidocaine (Xylocaine), 12, 180, 182, 189, 219, 225, 329–330, 406, 470, 517, 523, 546, 550, 576, 605, 616, 734–735, 758
comments, 791
dosage, 791
effect, 791
indications, 791
Light wand, 221
Line isolation monitors, 303
Lipid-soluble drugs, 93, 94t
Lipophilic opioids, 340
Liposomal bupivacaine, 324–325
Lithotripsy
anesthesia, 563
anesthetic options, 563
complications, 563
extracorporeal shockwave lithotripsy (ESWL), 563
percutaneous nephrolithotomy (PCNL), 563
Liver
anatomy, 98–99
blood supply, 98
structure, 98, 98f
function. *See* Hepatic function
pathology, 100
physiology, 99–100
Liver disease
anesthesia, 106–107
ascites, 103
cardiovascular system manifestations
hyperdynamic circulatory state, 101

Liver disease (*Continued*)
  central nervous system (CNS), 100–101
  cholestasis, 100
  coagulopathy, 104–105
  endocrine system manifestations, 105
  gastrointestinal system manifestations, 102–103
  glycemic control, 105
  nutritional deficiency, 103
  parenchymal
    acute hepatocellular injury, 100
    chronic parenchymal disease, 101
  postoperative liver dysfunction, 106, 110–111
  renal system manifestations
    electrolyte balance, 104
    hepatorenal syndrome, 103–104
    prerenal azotemia, 103
  respiratory system manifestations
    airway protection, 101–102
    chronic hypoxemia, 102
    hepatopulmonary syndrome, 102
    impaired hypoxic pulmonary vasoconstriction, 102
    portopulmonary hypertension, 102
  skin trauma, 106
Liver dysfunction, 511
Liver resection, 110
  enhanced recovery after surgery (ERAS) protocols for, 111
  methods to reduce blood loss, 110–111
Liver transplantation, 111, 438–443, 442f
Living will, 17
LMWH. *See* Low molecular weight heparin (LMWH)
Local anesthetics
  clinical uses of, 326t–327t
    alpha-2-adrenergic agonists, 328
    combinations of, 325
    dexamethasone, 328
    epinephrine, 325
    opioids, 325
    sodium bicarbonate, 325, 328
  commercial preparations, 324
  complications, 359
  liposomal bupivacaine, 324–325
  placental transfer, 574
  principles
    chemistry, 323
    commercial preparations of, 324
    mechanism of action, 323–324
    regional anesthesia (RA), 357–358
    sodium channel blockers, 323
  toxicity of
    allergic reactions, 328
    intravascular injection, 328
    local, 328
    local anesthetic systemic toxicity (LAST), 328–330
    methohemoglobinemia, 330
Local anesthetic systemic toxicity (LAST), 328–330
Lorazepam (Ativan), 16, 192–193, 413, 717
Lower airway, 206–207
Lower-extremity bypass grafting, 490
Lower extremity, regional anesthesia
  anatomy, 372–374, 373f
  complications, 374
  indications, 374
  techniques
    adductor canal block, 377, 378f
    ankle block, 380–381, 380f
    fascia iliaca block, 376–377, 376f–377f
    femoral nerve block, 375–376, 376f
    gluteal/subgluteal approach, 378–379
    ilioinguinal–iliohypogastric block, 372, 387
    lateral femoral cutaneous (LFC) nerve block, 375
    lumbar plexus block (psoas block), 374–375, 375f
    obturator nerve block, 378
    PENG block using UGRA, 377, 377f
    periarticular IPACK, 378
    popliteal approach using UGRA, 379–380, 379f
    saphenous nerve block, 378
    sciatic nerve (SCN) block, 378–379, 379f
Low molecular weight heparin (LMWH), 343, 766.
  See also Dalteparin (Fragmin); Enoxaparin (Lovenox)
Lumbar, epidural anesthesia and
  hanging drop technique, 347
  loss-of-resistance techniques, 346–347
Lumbar plexus, 372, 373f, 375f
Lung isolation techniques, 466–468, 473, 634

Lung protective ventilation, 655
Lung ultrasound (LUS), 38–45
　A-lines, 40–41, 41f
　B-lines, 42, 45
　examination, 38–39, 39f
　findings, 40, 40f
　limitations of, 45
　lung sliding, 41–42, 42f
Lung transplantation, 537–538
Lysine analogues, 690

M

Macintosh blade, 216
Macroshock, 302
Magnesium, 70, 123, 125, 131, 156, 182, 287, 523, 580–581, 598, 607, 716, 759
　depletion, 80
Magnesium sulfate, 125, 131, 288, 391, 574, 580, 791
Magnetic resonance imaging (MRI), 130, 303, 341, 409, 421, 439, 466, 511, 516, 607, 632, 637
Major adverse cardiac event (MACE) risk, 50, 486, 683
Malignant hyperthermia, 203, 720
　anesthesia for, 300
　clinical features, 299
　early sign of, 261
　etiology, 292, 299
　history of, 231
　neuroleptic malignant syndrome (NMS), 301
　syndromes, 301
　temperature monitoring, 263
　treatment, 292, 299–300
Mallampati classification, of airways, 7, 209, 211f, 213
Mandibular fractures, 662
Manipulative therapies, 743
Mannitol, 92t, 290, 300, 405, 410–412, 435, 462, 498, 500, 504, 522, 530, 544, 562–563, 791–792
MAOIs. *See* Monoamine oxidase inhibitors (MAOIs)
MAP. *See* Mean arterial pressure (MAP)
Mask airway
　complications, 213
　indications, 212
　techniques, 212–213
　ventilation, 213
Mass spectrometry, 173–174
Massive transfusion, 688

Mean arterial pressure (MAP), 58, 244, 305, 402, 427, 435, 656, 691
　in CPB, 521
　HRS treatment, 103–104
　hypotensive anesthesia, 556
　in spinal cord protection strategies, 503
　vasopressors and, 84, 152
Meconium aspiration syndrome, 620
Median minimal alveolar concentration (MAC) value, 268–269
Median nerve block, 371
Median sternotomy, 479
Mediastinal mass resection, 475–476
Mediastinoscopy, 472–473, 710
Medication errors, 156–157
　handoff errors, 159–160
　modification strategies, 156–157
Medications, patient evaluation, 1
Medtronic Micra leadless system, 63
MELD. *See* Model for end-stage liver disease (MELD)
Meningocele, 628
Mental status, 101, 492
Meperidine, local anesthetics, 95, 123, 197–199, 325, 344, 427, 435, 574, 86, 608t, 650, 693, 720, 735t
MEPs. *See* Motor-evoked potentials (MEPs)
Metabolic acidosis, 522
Metabolic complications, blood transfusions
　acid-base status, 695
　hyperkalemia, 694
　hypocalcemia, 694–695
　hypothermia, 695
　iron overload, 695
　stored blood, 695
Metallic implants, 637
Metformin, 117, 488
Methadone, 10, 197, 197t, 428, 608t, 709, 732–733, 741–742
Methemoglobinemia, 261, 312, 318, 326t, 330
Methohexital, 180, 190–191, 190t, 418, 649
Methylene blue, 261, 330, 561, 792
　hemodynamic control, perioperative and, 312
Methylergonovine (methergine), 573, 792
Methylparaben, 324, 328
Methylprednisolone (Solu-medrol), 126, 302, 421, 434, 437, 441, 461, 504, 636, 643, 693, 719, 792

Metoclopramide (Reglan), 12, 16t, 131, 185, 569, 578, 599, 605, 717, 793
Metoprolol (Lopressor), 283, 285–286, 296, 757, 793
  hemodynamic control, perioperative and, 313, 314t
Metronidazole, 145t, 148, 623
MG. *See* Myasthenia gravis (MG)
MH. *See* Malignant hyperthermia (MH)
MI. *See* Myocardial infarction (MI)
Microprocessor-controlled ventilators, 169
Microshock, 302–303
Midazolam, 15–16, 225, 358, 409–410, 413, 417, 529, 542, 545, 554, 579, 587, 603–605, 629, 634, 643, 646, 721
  dosage and administration, 190t
  elimination half-lives for, 192
  onset of CNS effects, 192
Middle East respiratory syndrome (MERS), 148
Midodrine, 308, 310
Miller blade, 216
Milrinone, 56, 58, 280, 282, 296, 309t, 313, 584, 793
Mind–body interventions, 743
Mindfulness meditation, 743–744
Mind–body interventions, 743
Minimum alveolar concentration (MAC), 569, 634
Miotics, 545
Mitral regurgitation (MR), 56, 518
Mitral stenosis (MS), 517–518
  anesthetic considerations, 56
  etiology, 56
  pathophysiology, 56
Mivacurium, 106, 180, 228–229, 229t–230t, 234, 280–281, 294
Model for end-stage liver disease (MELD), 107, 438
Monitored anesthesia care (MAC), 447, 634
Monitoring
  cardiovascular system
    arterial blood pressure, 245
    electrocardiogram (ECG), 243
    ischemia detection, 244
    mechanism of, 243–244
    rhythm detection, 244
  of central venous pressure (CVP)
    analysis for, 248
    cardiac output, 258–259
    complications, 253–254
    echocardiography, 259–260
    indications of, 247–248
    pathology and, 248–249
    positive-pressure ventilation, 249
    procedure, 249–252, 251f
    pulmonary artery catheter procedure and, 256–258, 257f
    waveform and, 248, 248f
  of respiratory system
    mandatory respiratory monitors, 260
    oxygenation, 260–261
    ventilation, 261–263
    standard monitoring, 243
    temperature monitoring, 263–264
Monoamine oxidase inhibitors (MAOIs), 232, 283, 292, 312, 650, 720
Morphine, 95, 131, 197, 197t, 198–199, 234, 280–281, 294, 325, 340, 411, 434–435, 437, 550, 575, 578–579, 608t, 612, 720, 733t, 734, 735t, 736–737, 743
  metabolism, 731
  side effects, 731–732
  tolerance, 732
Motion sickness, 6
Motor-evoked potentials (MEPs), 177, 182, 189, 408, 426, 503
Mouth, airways, 209
Multimodal analgesia, 742
Muscle
  laryngeal, 205
  during induction, 517, 606–607
  placental transfer, 574
  relaxants, 94t, 95, 124, 291, 301, 341, 406, 411, 455, 460, 621, 627, 679, 706–707, 714
    abdominal surgery, 450–451
    for muscle spasm, 733, 734t
Muscular dystrophies, 240–241, 301
Musculocutaneous nerve block, 395
Music medicine and music therapy, 744–745
Myalgia, 230
Myasthenia gravis (MG), 240
Mydriatics, 544–545
Myocardial dysfunction, 60
Myocardial infarction (MI), 486, 518
Myocardial ischemia, 296–297
  and infarction, 715
Myocardial protection, 521
Mycobacterium tuberculosis, 151
Myelodysplasia, 628–629
Myelomeningocele, 628

Myotonic dystrophy, 241
Myotonic syndromes, 241
Myxedema coma, 121

N

N95 respirators, 151
N-acetylcysteine (NAC), 84, 89, 488, 635
Nalbuphine, 197t, 574
Naloxone (Narcan), 199, 389, 344, 411, 709, 741, 744, 750, 750, 770, 793
Naproxen, 720, 726t, 729t
Narcotics, 71, 73, 89, 283, 293, 410–411, 477, 560, 617, 625, 627, 636, 640, 770
Narcotrend, 266–267, 269
Nasal cosmetic surgery, 550
Nasal surgery
  anesthetic technique, 549–550
  blood loss, 550
  nasal cosmetic surgery, 550
  severe epistaxis, 550
Nasotracheal intubation, 219, 661–662, 669
Natriuretic peptides, 92
Nausea and vomiting, 194, 344, 651, 718–719
Neck
  airways, 208
  cervical spine mobility and, 209
  circumference, 209
  trauma, 662–663
  thyromental distance, 209
Negative pressure pulmonary edema (NPPE), 293, 708
Neonate
  airway, 591
  analgesia, 607
  body composition, 590–591
  cardiovascular development
    anatomic, 590
    fetal circulation, 590
  cardiovascular disorders
    congenital heart disease, 625
    cyanosis, 625–626
    dysrhythmias, 627
    patent ductus arteriosus (PDA), 626–627
    persistent pulmonary hypertension of the newborn (PPHN), 627
  electrolytes, 597–598
  endotracheal intubation, 606–607
  fluids, 593, 597
    management, 613–614
  gastrointestinal disorders
    anesthetic considerations, 621–623
    duodenal atresia, 621
    gastroschisis, 621–622
    hyperbilirubinemia, 594
    necrotizing enterocolitis (NEC), 622–623
    omphalocele, 621–622
    pyloric stenosis, 621
    tracheoesophageal fistula (TEF), 589, 623–624
    volvulus, 623
  glucose, 598
  head and neck procedures, 627
  hematologic system, 594
  induction techniques, 603–605
  laboratory studies, 597
  maternal disorders, 595
  neurologic disorders
    intracranial hemorrhage, 628
    myelodysplasia, 628–629
    neurotoxicity of general anesthetics, 629–630
    retinopathy of prematurity (ROP), 629
  nutrition, 598
  organogenesis, 589
  perinatal history, 595
  pharmacotherapy, 607–613
  physical examination, 595–597
  postanesthesia care, 614–615
  preparation for surgery, 600–603
  pulmonary system, 591–593, 592t
  respiratory development
    anatomic, 589
    persistent pulmonary hypertension of the newborn (PPHN), 589
    physiologic, 589
    respiratory distress syndrome (RDS), 589
  respiratory disorders
    apnea, 592–593, 617–618
    bronchopulmonary dysplasia (BPD), 619
    differential diagnosis, 617
    meconium aspiration syndrome, 620
    pneumothorax, 619–620
    respiratory distress syndrome (RDS), 618–619
    upper respiratory infection, 620

Neonate (*Continued*)
resuscitation, 748, 791
assessment, 766–767, 767f
chest compressions, 769
drugs and fluids, 769–770
guidelines for withholding and discontinuing, 770–771
post-resuscitation care, 770
ventilation, 768–769
thermoregulation, 598–599
thoracic disorders
congenital diaphragmatic hernia (CDH), 624–625
esophageal atresia (EA) and TEF, 623–624
vital signs, 595, 593t
Neostigmine, 60, 156, 185, 232–233, 237–238, 240, 585, 607, 710, 712
Nephrectomy, 561
Nephrogenic diabetes insipidus, 290
Nephrogenic systemic fibrosis, 635
Nephropathy, 115
contrast-induced, 635
salt wasting, 79
Nerve(s)
fibers, local anesthetics and, 323–324, 324t
localization techniques, in regional anesthesia, 360–362
Neuraxial analgesia, 735–736
acute pain management
buprenorphine maintenance therapy, 741, 741t
methadone maintenance therapy, 741–742
naltrexone therapy, 742
perioperative management, 740, 741t
continuous peripheral nerve blocks, 739–740, 740t
epidural opioids, 736–737
algorithm, 737
checklist, 737, 738t
complications, 738–739
patient-controlled epidural analgesia (PCEA), 737
pharmacologic management of, 737, 737t
intrathecal opioids
hydrophilic, 736
lipophilic, 736–737
Neuraxial anesthesia, 324, 332–333, 580, 721
Neuroleptic malignant syndrome (NMS), 292
Neurologic deficits, 492, 494
Neuromuscular blockade (NMB), 5, 471, 684, 687
clinical choice of, 235t
complications, 185–186
depolarizing, 230–233, 232f
disorders, 239–241
effects of, 239
general pharmacology
cholinergic receptors, 227–228
neuromuscular-blocking drugs (NMBDs), 228, 229t, 230t
monitoring, 234
clinical assessment, 235t
double-burst stimulation, 236–237
peripheral nerve stimulators, 234–235
post-tetanic count, 236
post-tetanic single twitch, 236
single twitch, 235–236
tetanic stimulus, 236
train of four (TOF), 236
neuromuscular junction (NMJ), 227, 228f, 229t, 230t
nondepolarizing, 231, 233–234
atracurium, 229, 230t, 234
cardiovascular side effects, 230t
cisatracurium, 229, 230t, 234
clinical pharmacology, 229t, 233–234
mivacurium, 229t, 229, 230t
pancuronium, 230t
rocuronium, 230t, 234
vecuronium, 230t, 234
reversal of, 237–239
succinylcholine (SCh), 228, 229t, 230t, 230–231
upregulation and downregulation of acetylcholine receptor (AChRs), 228
Neuromuscular blocking drugs, 5, 68, 96, 106, 181, 227–229, 233–234, 236–238
Illnesses affecting response of, 239–241
Neuromuscular junction (NMJ), 227, 228f, 229t, 230t
Neuroradiologic procedures, anesthesia, 421
Neurosurgery
anesthetic considerations, 414–415
arteriovenous malformation (AVM), 415
awake craniotomy, 416–417
CSF shunts, 419–420

deep brain stimulators, 417–418
electrophysiologic monitoring
  EEG, 407–408
  evoked potential monitoring, 408–409
epilepsy surgery, 418
head trauma, 418–419
intracranial aneurysms, 413–414, 413t
intraoperative management
  emergence, 411
  immediate postoperative care, 412–413
  induction of anesthesia, 410
  maintenance, 410–411
  perioperative fluid management, 411–412
pharmacology
  cerebral protection, 406–407
  inhalation anesthetics, 405–406, 405t
  IV anesthetics, 406
  muscle relaxants, 406
  vasoactive drugs, 406
physiology
  cerebral blood flow (CBF), 402
  $CMRO_2$, 402–403
  intracranial pressure (ICP), 403–405, 404f
pituitary gland, transsphenoidal resection of, 417
posterior fossa surgery, 415–416
preoperative considerations, 409–410
of spine and spinal cord, 420–421
stereotactic surgery, 417
Neurotoxicity, 339, 629–630
Nicardipine, 69, 131, 283, 315t, 316, 406, 414, 494, 643–644, 793–794
Nifedipine, 316
Nimodipine, 316, 406, 414
Nissen fundoplication, 478, 611
Nitroglycerin, 69, 131, 280–281, 283, 292, 296, 315t, 317–318, 320, 406, 411, 494, 504, 512, 517–518, 564, 582–583, 641, 715, 794
Nitroprusside (Nipride), 69, 280, 283, 292, 315t, 316–317, 320, 462, 504, 564, 641, 794
Nitrous oxide (N_2O), 69, 157, 165, 167, 171, 173, 175, 181–183, 185, 199–203, 200t, 268, 275–276, 275f, 296, 298, 300, 302, 405–406, 416, 451, 548–549, 552, 575, 584–585, 587, 604, 621, 623, 625, 640, 664, 668, 708, 718

Nitrous oxide effects, on brain, 200, 200t, 275, 276f
NK-1 receptor antagonists, 719
NMJ. *See* Neuromuscular junction (NMJ)
NMS. *See* Neuroleptic malignant syndrome (NMS)
Nociceptive–medullary–autonomic (NMA) circuit, 265
Non–heart-beating organ donation, 461
Noninvasive positive pressure ventilation (NPPV), 78
Non-operating room anesthesia (NORA)
  anesthesia techniques, 633–635
  cardiac procedures, 651
  contrast media, 635–636
  CT-guided thermal ablations, 638–640
  diagnostic radiology, 636–638
  electroconvulsive therapy (ECT), 648–650
  enhanced recovery after procedure (ERAP), 635
  equipments in remote locations, 632–633
  ergonomics, 633
  gastrointestinal/genitourinary, 644–647
  gastrointestinal procedures, 650–651
  general anesthesia, 634
  high-frequency jet ventilation (HFJV), 634
  lung isolation techniques, 634
  MAC service, 634
  neurointerventions, 640–644
  patient access, 633
  peripheral nerve blocks (PNBs), 634
  proton beam radiation therapy, 647–648
  radiation safety, 633
  radiation therapy, 647–648
  safety in, 652
  sedation and analgesia, 633–634
  vascular radiology procedures, 644–647
Nonosmotic loop, 92t
Nonsteroidal anti-inflammatory drugs (NSAIDs), 5, 10, 81, 87–88, 103, 106, 133, 178, 341, 355, 429, 435, 475, 699, 765
  clinical uses, 728
  COX inhibition, 726t
  diclofenac, 728

Nonsteroidal anti-inflammatory drugs (NSAIDs) (*Continued*)
  formulations, 728
  GI toxicity, 727t
  ketorolac, 720, 726
  mechanism, 726
  nonopioid analgesics, 729t–730t
  renal toxicity, 727t
  toxicity, 726–728
Norepinephrine (Levophed), 61, 126, 129, 130, 152, 184, 273, 282, 285, 296, 298, 302, 308, 309t, 310–312, 319, 462, 504, 540, 572, 578, 594, 644, 649–650, 713, 742–743, 794–795
  hemodynamic control, perioperative and, 305
Normothermic regional perfusion (NRP), 432
Normovolemic hemodilution, acute, 519, 691
Normovolemic hypernatremia, 80
Normovolemic hyponatremia, 79
Nose, airways, 209
Novel coronaviruses, 148
NPPE. *See* Negative pressure pulmonary edema (NPPE)
NPPV. *See* Noninvasive positive pressure ventilation (NPPV)
NSAIDs. *See* Nonsteroidal anti-inflammatory drugs (NSAIDs)
Nutritional deficiency, 103

O
Obesity, 71–73
  diabetes mellitus, 116
  pulmonary disease, 71
    intraoperative issues, 72
    maintenance of anesthesia, 72–73
    mechanical ventilation, 73
    preoperative evaluation, 72
    respiratory pathophysiology, 71
Obstetrics and gynecology, 566–586. *See also* Labor; Pregnancy
Obstructive sleep apnea (OSA), 5, 115, 185, 207, 458, 548, 615, 707
  GLP1-RA and, 118
  in obesity, 71
Obturator nerve block, 378
Occupational TB, 151
OCR. *See* Oculocardiac reflex (OCR)
Octreotide (Sandostatin), 132, 134–135, 644, 650, 795
Ocular trauma, 662
Oculocardiac reflex (OCR), 544

Ondansetron, 16t
Odynophagia, 6
Ohm's law, 259
Oliguria, 289–290, 462, 522, 644, 716
Omalizumab, 70
Ondansetron (Zofran), 16t, 185, 344, 548, 605, 649, 719, 722, 795
One-lung ventilation, 289
  anesthetic management, 469–470
  hypoxemia management, 469–470
  oxygenation, 469
    difficulties, 469–470
  ventilation and perfusion, 469
Open-eye injury, 547–548
Operating room (OR)
  anesthetist, infection control, 138
  antibiotics
    aminoglycosides, 148
    clindamycin, 147
    endocarditis, 146
    fluoroquinolones, 148
    indications for, 144
    β-lactams, 147
    metronidazole, 148
    prophylaxis principles, 144–146
    SCIP, 144–146, 145t
    surgical wounds, 146–147
    vancomycin, 147
  infection control
    aspiration pneumonitis, 143–144
    CVC, 141–142
    hygiene standards, 141
    infection spread methods, 138
    infection spread prevention, 138
    standard precautions, 138–139
    transfusion-related infections, 144
    transmission-based precautions, 139–141, 140t
Ondansetron, 16t
Opioid(s), 16, 94t, 95, 197–198, 340, 349, 406, 410, 426, 475, 517, 574–575, 679, 707, 709, 719–720, 731–738
  α2-agonists, 733
  gabapentin, 733
  as inhalation anesthetic, 200–204, 200t
  as intravenous (IV) anesthetics, 732–733
    action mode of, 197
    adverse effects, 199
    cardiovascular system, 189
    CNS, 188–189
    dosage and administration, 199
    gastrointestinal system, 187
    pharmacodynamics of, 198–199

pharmacokinetics of, 197–198, 197t
respiratory system, 189
lidocaine, 734–735
local anesthetics and, 325
metabolism, 731
muscle relaxants, 733
neuraxial analgesia
  epidural, 736–737
  intrathecal, 736
oral, 732, 733t
in pediatric patients, 607–608, 608t, 612
physical dependence, 732
side effects, 731–732
tolerance, 10–11, 732
Opioid-induced hyperalgesia (OIH), 732
OR. *See* Operating room (OR)
Oral anticoagulants, 355
OrganOx metra device, 431
Orotracheal intubation
  complications of, 218–219
  indications, 215–216
  techniques, 216–218, 217f–218f, 219
Orthopedic disorders, 666–668
Orthopedic oncology, 396–397
Orthopedic surgery
  elbow and upper arm surgery, 395–396
  foot and ankle surgery, 394–395
  forearm and hand surgery, 395–396
  general consideration, 390
  lower extremity surgery, 394–395, 668
  orthopedic oncology, 396–397
  orthopedic trauma, 397–400, 666–668
  shoulder surgery, 392–394, 393f
  spine surgery, 423–429
  total hip arthroplasty (THA), 390–392
  total knee arthroplasty (TKA), 390–392
  upper extremity surgery, 667
Orthopedic trauma, 397–400
OSA. *See* Obstructive sleep apnea (OSA)
Osmotic diuresis, 114–115, 118
Osteogenesis imperfecta, 208
Oxygen
  analyzers, 174
  audible alarm, 171
  flush valve, 168
  ratio control, 171
  supply-demand balance, 54
Oxygenation, 260–261, 469

Oxymorphone, 197t
Oxytocin (Pitocin), 133, 572–573, 582, 584, 795

P

Pacemakers
  five-letter code, 62
  implanted cardioverter defibrillators (ICD), 62
  indications, 62
  intraoperative management, 62
  leadless, 63–64
  nomenclature, 62–63
  pacing options, perioperative, 62
  permanent, preoperative evaluation, 61
Pain
  acute. *See* Acute pain
  chronic, 725
  definitions, 725
  inflammatory, 725
  neuropathic, 725
  nociceptive, 725
  somatic, 725
  visceral, 725
PALS. *See* Pediatric advanced life support (PALS)
Pancreatic surgery, 457
Pancreaticojejunostomy, 457
Pancuronium, 131, 228, 229t, 230t, 237, 240, 284, 593, 607
Panhypopituitarism, 129
PAOP. *See* Pulmonary artery occlusion pressure (PAOP)
PAP. *See* Pulmonary artery pressure (PAP)
Papillary muscle rupture after myocardial infarction, 518
Paragangliomas, 129–131
Paramagnetic analyzers, 174
Parathyroid disease
  hypercalcemia
    acute, 125
    anesthetic considerations, 125–126
    bisphosphonates, 124
    chronic, 125
    clinical features of, 125
    denosumab, 124
    etiologies of, 125
    glucocorticoid therapy, 124
    hydration, 124
    salmon calcitonin, 124
    treatment of, 125

Parathyroid disease (*Continued*)
  hypocalcemia
    anesthetic considerations, 124
    clinical features of, 124
    etiologies of, 123–124
    treatment of, 124
  physiology, 123
  serum calcium, 123
Parathyroid hormone, 82
Paravertebral nerve block (PVB), 634
Parkinson disease, 5, 417
Parkland formula, 676
Paroxysmal supraventricular tachydysrhythmias, 715, 754
Partial hepatectomy, 456
Partial pressure of carbon dioxide ($PaCO_2$), 69, 184, 391, 402, 403f, 404
Partial pressure of oxygen (PaO_2), 74, 402
Patent ductus arteriosus (PDA), 528, 591, 626–627
Patient autonomy, 17
Patient-controlled analgesia (PCA), 735, 735t
Patient-controlled epidural analgesia (PCEA), 737
Patient state index (PSI), 266–267
PCEA. *See* Patient-controlled epidural analgesia (PCEA)
PCI. *See* Percutaneous coronary intervention (PCI)
PDA. *See* Patent ductus arteriosus (PDA)
PDPH. *See* Postdural puncture headache (PDPH)
Pediatric advanced life support (PALS), 162, 748, 763–765, 765f
Pediatric resuscitation, 761
  airway and breathing, 762
  bradycardia algorithm, 765f
  circulation, 762–765
Pediatric surgery
  analgesia, 607
  anatomy and physiology
    cardiovascular system, 593, 593t
    endocrine system, 594
    fluid and electrolyte balance, 593
    hematologic system, 594
    hepatobiliary system, 594
    pulmonary system, 591–593
    temperature regulation, 594
    upper airway, 591
  compromised airway, 615–617
  emergence and post-anesthesia care
    extubation, 614
    post-anesthesia care unit (PACU), 615
    during transport, 614
  endotracheal intubation
    laryngeal mask airway, 607
    muscle relaxants, 606–607
    nasal approach, 606
    oral approach, 606
  fluid management
    blood losses, 613–614
    estimated blood volume (EBV), 613–614
    estimated fluid deficit, 614
    maintenance fluid requirements, 613
    third-space losses, 614
  induction techniques
    full stomachs, 605
    inhalation induction, 604–605
    intramuscular induction, 605
    IV induction, 605
    sedation options, 603–604
  intra-abdominal malformations, 621
  neurotoxicity, 629–630
  operating room preparation
    airway equipment, 601–602, 601t, 602t
    anesthetic circuit, 600–601
    IV setup and supplies, 603
    monitoring, 602–603
    perioperative/procedure huddle, 600
    temperature control, 602
  periprocedural considerations and fasting guidelines
    fasting guidelines, 599, 600t
    periprocedural considerations, 599
  pharmacotherapy, 607–613
    additional regional blocks, 609
    brachial plexus block, 609
    caudal and epidural anesthesia, 611–612
    local anesthetics, pharmacology of, 608–609
    nonopioid pharmacotherapeutic agents, 607
    opioid therapy, 607–608
    regional and neuraxial anesthesia, 608
    spinal anesthesia, 609–611

preanesthetic visit, 594
 history, 595
 laboratory data, 597
 physical examination, 595–597
 upper respiratory infection, 620
PEEP. *See* Positive end-expiratory pressure (PEEP)
Pelvis trauma, 667
Penicillin, cephalosporin cross-reactivity, 147
Pentazocine, 197t
Percutaneous coronary intervention (PCI), 52–53, 784
Perfusion pressure, 305
Peribulbar block, 546–547, 546f
Pericardial tamponade, 518
Pericardiocentesis, 299, 536, 664
Perioperative cardiac assessment, 48f
 for noncardiac surgery, 49–52
 supplemental cardiac evaluation, 50–52
Perioperative coagulopathy
 cardiopulmonary bypass (CPB), 698
 chronic liver disease, 698
 disseminated intravascular coagulopathy (DIC)
  causes of, 697
  clinical features, 697
  laboratory features, 697–698
  treatment of, 698
 massive transfusion
  clotting factors, 697
  thrombocytopenia, 697
 pharmacologic intervention
  abciximab, 699
  aspirin, 699
  cangrelor, 699
  clopidogrel (Plavix), 699
  direct factor Xa inhibitors, 700
  direct thrombin inhibitors (DTIs), 700
  eptifibatide, 699
  heparin, 699
  low molecular weight heparins (LMWHs), 699
  nonsteroidal anti-inflammatory drugs (NSAIDs), 699
  platelet inhibitors, 699
  prasugrel, 699
  thrombolytic agents, 700
  ticagrelo, 699
  ticlopidine, 699
  tirofiban, 699
  warfarin (Coumadin), 699
 vitamin K deficiency, 698

Perioperative hemodynamic control
 adrenergic pharmacology
  α-agonists, 308, 310
  β-agonists, 310
  mixed agonists, 310–312
  nonadrenergic agents, 312–313
 adrenergic receptor physiology, 306t–307t
  $\alpha 1$ receptors, 305
  $\alpha 2$ receptors, 305, 308
  $\beta 1$ receptors, 308
  $\beta 2$ receptors, 308
  $\beta 3$ receptors, 308
  dopaminergic receptors, 308
  receptor regulation, 308
 autoregulation, 305
 β-adrenergic antagonists, 313, 314t, 315
 blood pressure, 305
 drug dosage calculations, 320–321
 induced hypotension, 320
 vasodilators
  adenosine, 319
  α-adrenergic antagonists, 319
  bosentan, 320
  calcium channel antagonists, 315–316
  enalaprilat, 318
  fenoldopam, 318
  hydralazine, 318
  nitric oxide, 320
  nitroglycerin, 317–318
  phentolamine, 319
  prostaglandin E_1, 319
  pulmonary, 319–320
  sildenafil, 320
  sodium nitroprusside, 316–317
Peripheral aneurysms, 491
Peripheral embolectomy, 490
Peripheral nerves, 323, 324t
 blocks, 3, 6, 143, 739
 catheters, 739
 injury, 15, 180, 427–428, 717
 neuropathic pain, 725
 stimulators, 234–235
Peripheral neurologic lesions, 717–718
Perirectal abscess, 455–456
Perirectal abscess drainage, 455–456
Permanent pacemaker (PPM), 4, 61, 516, 715–716
Perimortem cesarean delivery (PMCD), 577, 587
Perioperative acupuncture, 743
Perphenazine, 719

Persistent pulmonary hypertension of the newborn (PPHN), 589, 627
PFTs. *See* Pulmonary function tests (PFTs)
Phantom limb pain (PLP), 506
Pharmacologic stress testing, cardiac evaluation, 51
Pharynx, 205
Phenobarbital, 795
Phenothiazines, 292, 719
Phenoxybenzamine, 796
Phentolamine, 191, 280, 319, 776
Phenylephrine (Neosynephrine), 55, 58, 61, 184, 219, 282, 284, 296, 308, 309t, 319, 414, 490, 494, 504, 516, 521, 534, 544–545, 562, 572, 574, 576, 640, 644, 713, 796
Phenytoin (Dilantin), 100, 156, 411, 796
Pheochromocytomas, 129–131
Physical examination, 7–8
Phosphodiesterase III inhibitors, 313
Phosphorus (sodium phosphate), 123, 125, 672, 796
Physician orders for life-sustaining treatment (POLST), 17
Physostigmine (Antilirium), 717, 796
Pilocarpine, 545
Pilonidal cystectomy, 455
Piston ventilator, 171
Pituitary adenomas, 417
Pituitary disease
 anterior pituitary gland
  hyperfunction, 132
  hypofunction, 132–133
  physiology, 131–132
 posterior pituitary gland
  diabetes insipidus (DI), 133
  physiology, 133
  syndrome of inappropriate antidiuretic hormone secretion (SIADH), 133–134
Plasma substitutes
 albumin, 667
 hydroxyethyl starch, 667
Platelet counts, 685
Platelet function tests, 685
Pleural effusions, 32, 42–44, 44f, 102, 121, 710
PLR test, 38
PM. *See* Pringle maneuver (PM)
Pneumomediastinum, 453, 483
Pneumonia and pneumonitis, 76
Pneumopericardium, 453
Pneumoperitoneum, 69–70
Pneumothorax, 253–254, 281, 295–296, 709–711
Poikilothermia, 462
Polarographic oxygen analyzers, 174
Polycystic kidney diseases, 85
Polyuria, 413, 462, 716
PONV. *See* Postoperative nausea and vomiting (PONV)
Porphyria, 191
Portal hypertension, 102
Portal-systemic shunting, 100
Portal vein flow (PVF), 98
Portopulmonary hypertension, 102, 438
Positive end-expiratory pressure (PEEP), 169, 453, 469, 618, 655, 707
Post-anesthesia Care Unit (PACU), 183, 550
 admission, 705–706
 anesthetics, 706–707
 body temperature changes, 720
 definition, 705
 discharge criteria, 721
 fast-track recovery, 721
 enhanced recovery after surgery (ERAS), 722
 extubation guidelines, 713
 general complications, 706
 hemodynamic complications
  dysrhythmias, 714–715
  hypertension, 714
  hypotension, 713–714
  intracardiac defibrillator (ICD), 715–716
  myocardial ischemia and infarction, 715
  permanent pacemaker, 715–716
 hypoventilation
  pulmonary and respiratory muscle insufficiency, 710
  ventilatory drive, decreased, 709
 hypoxemia
  atelectasis, 708
  bronchospasm, 708
  diffusion hypoxia, 708
  hypoventilation, 708
  pneumothorax, 709
  pulmonary edema, 708–709
  pulmonary embolism, 709
  upper airway obstruction, 708
 intubated patient, 712–713
 monitoring, 706
 neurological complications
  delayed awakening, 716–717

emergence delirium, 717
intraoperative awareness and recall, 718
local anesthetic systemic toxicity (LAST), 717
neurological damage, 717
peripheral neurological lesions, 717–718
pain management principles
adjuvant analgesics, 720
continuous epidural analgesia, 720
IV patient-controlled analgesia, 720
nonsteroidal anti-inflammatory drugs (NSAIDs), 720
opioids, 719–720
regional sensory blocks, 720
pediatric recovery considerations
agitation, 722
airway obstruction, 722
postoperative nausea and vomiting (PONV), 722
post-anesthesia recovery unit, critical care, 722–723
postoperative nausea and vomiting, 718
antihistamines, 719
butyrophenones, 719
corticosteroids, 719
dexamethasone, 719
NK-1 receptor antagonists, 719
phenothiazines, 719
propofol, 719
serotonin antagonists, 719
transdermal scopolamine, 719
regional and neuraxial anesthesia, recovery from, 721
renal complications
electrolyte disturbances, 716
oliguria, 716
polyuria, 716
respiratory and airway complications, 707–713
sedatives, 706–707
upper airway obstruction, 711–712
Post-cardiopulmonary bypass (CPB) pulmonary dysfunction, 511
Postdural puncture headache (PDPH), 577
Posterior fossa tumors, 415
Posterior pituitary gland, 133
Posterior tibial nerve, 381, 408, 380f
Postexposure prophylaxis (PEP), 149

Postobstructive diuresis, 716
Postoperative analgesia, 475
Postoperative cognitive dysfunction (POCD), 186
Postoperative nausea and vomiting (PONV), 6, 547, 716, 718–719, 722
general anesthesia (GA), 182
Postoperative pulmonary complications (PPCs), 143
Postoperative respiratory failure (PRF), 53
Postoperative visual loss (POVL), 15, 427
Post spinal pain syndrome (PSPS), 328
Post-tetanic potentiation (PTP), 231–233, 236
Post-tonsillectomy hemorrhage, 551
Potassium chloride (KCl)
administration guidelines, 780
indication, 780
Potassium homeostasis disorders, 80–82
POVL. *See* Postoperative visual loss (POVL)
Power spectrum, 269, 269f
Preanesthetic considerations, abdominal surgery
full stomachs as, 447
hypovolemia, 446
length of surgery, 447
metabolic derangements, 447
preoperative volume status, 446
Preanesthetic evaluation, 52–53
Precedex effects, on brain, 273–274
Precordium, 7
Preeclampsia, 579–581
Preexcited atrial fibrillation, 288
Preexisting medical conditions, 9–12
Pregabalin, 429, 733
Pregnancy
amniotic fluid embolism (AFE), 583–584
cardiopulmonary resuscitation (CPR), 586–587
cardiovascular system, 566
cesarean section, 578–579
gastrointestinal system, 569
gynecologic surgery, 587
hematology, 566, 569
labor and delivery
analgesia for, 574–578
definition, 570
intrapartum fetal evaluation, 570–572, 571f
medications, 572–574

Pregnancy (*Continued*)
  pain, 570
  placental transfer of drugs, 574
  musculoskeletal, 569–570
  nervous system, 569
  nonobstetric surgery, 584–586, 585t
  oocyte retrieval, 587
  peripartum hemorrhage, 581–583
  physiologic changes, 566–570, 567t–568t
  preeclampsia, 579–581
  renal system, 569
  respiratory system, 566
Premedication(s), 529
  anesthesia
    antiemetic agents, 16, 16t
    glycopyrrolate, 16
    sedatives and analgesics, 15–16
  pulmonary disease, 15
  renal disease, 89
  surgery, 15–16, 16t
Prerenal azotemia, 103
Pressure alarms, 173
Pressure regulators, 167
Pringle maneuver (PM), 110–111, 456
Prion diseases, 151, 687
Processed electroencephalography, 181, 434, 440
Prochlorperazine (Compazine), 797
Promethazine (Phenergan), 16t, 185, 719, 797
Propofol, 68, 94t, 95, 190t, 421, 617
  as intravenous (IV) anesthetics
    action mode of, 188
    adverse effects, 189–190
    cardiovascular system, 189
    CNS, 188–189
    dosage and administration, 189, 190t
    pharmacodynamics of, 188–189
    pharmacokinetics of, 188
    respiratory system, 189
Propofol effects, on brain, 270–272
Propofol infusion syndrome, 190
Propranolol (Inderal), 313, 797
Prostaglandin E_1, 319, 573, 777
Prostaglandin 15-methyl $F_2\alpha$ (carboprost, Hemabate), 573
Protamine, 515, 517, 525–526, 698, 797–798
Prothrombin complex concentrate (PCCs), 105, 513, 515, 698, 701
Prothrombin time, 105, 426, 512, 581, 657, 659, 684

Proton beam radiation therapy, 647
Proton pump inhibitors, 12, 455, 672
Pseudohyponatremia, 79
Pseudocholinesterase, 99, 106, 230, 313, 323, 460
PSI. *See* Patient state index (PSI)
PSPS. *See* Post spinal pain syndrome (PSPS)
PTP. *See* Posttetanic potentiation (PTP)
Pulmonary artery catheters, 66, 90, 179, 659–660, 706
  cardiac output, 258–259
  echocardiography, 259–260
  indications, 254
  materials/catheter types, 256
  mechanism, 254
  pulmonary artery occlusion pressure (PAOP), 254–256, 255f
  pulmonary artery pressure (PAP), 254
  pathology, 256
  procedure, 256–258, 257f
  securing, 257
Pulmonary artery occlusion pressure (PAOP), 254–256, 255f
Pulmonary artery pressure (PAP), 254
Pulmonary aspiration, 102
Pulmonary contusion, 75–76
Pulmonary disease
  acute respiratory distress syndrome (ARDS), 73–74, 74t
    intraoperative considerations, 75
    perioperative considerations, 74–75
    postoperative considerations, 75
  asthma, 70
  chronic obstructive pulmonary disease (COPD), 70–71
  interstitial lung disease (ILD), 76
  obesity, 71
    extubation, 73
    intraoperative issues, 72
    maintenance of anesthesia, 72–73
    mechanical ventilation, 73
    preoperative evaluation, 72
    respiratory pathophysiology, 71
  PH, 76
  pneumonia, 76
  pulmonary contusion, 75–76
  pulmonary function
    ciliary function, 69
    coughing, 69

functional residual capacity (FRC), 68
gas exchange, 68–69
minute ventilation and alveolar ventilation, 68–69
respiratory reflexes, 69
rib fractures, 76
Pulmonary edema, 38, 44, 56, 199, 708–709
Pulmonary embolism, 256, 282, 709
air embolism, 297–298
amniotic fluid emboli, 298
fat embolism, 298
thromboemboli, 297
Pulmonary embolus, 518, 778
Pulmonary fibrosis, 44–45, 537, 710
Pulmonary function tests (PFTs), 211, 465, 512
before anesthesia, 9
Pulmonary hypertension (PH), 56, 71, 76
Pulmonary interstitial emphysema, 619
Pulmonary resection
anesthetic technique, 473–474
bronchial blockers, 468
emergence and extubation, 474–475
endobronchial tubes
choice of tube, 466–467
double-lumen tubes range, 466–468
insertion, 467
right-and left- sided double- lumen tubes, 466
lung isolation techniques, 466–468, 473
lung resections, 473
one-lung ventilation, 469–470, 473
positioning, 474
postoperative analgesia, 475
surgical techniques, 473
univent tubes, 468
Pulmonary vascular resistance (PVR), 56, 311, 439, 517, 584, 589, 624–626
Pulmonary vasodilators, 319–320
Pulse oximeters, 58, 65, 260, 304, 615, 626, 637
Pulse wave Doppler, 33, 35–36
PVF. *See* Portal vein flow (PVF)
PVR. *See* Pulmonary vascular resistance (PVR)

Q

Quincke needle, 336

R

Radical neck dissection, 553–554
Radial nerve block, 371
Radiation therapy, intraoperative, 458
Radical neck dissection, 553–554
Radical retropubic prostatectomy (RRP), 560–561
Remifentanil, 197t, 575
Ranitidine (Zantac), 12, 302, 599, 605, 693
RAP. *See* Retrograde autologous priming (RAP)
Rapid sequence induction, 6, 91, 108, 181, 231, 234, 418–419, 434, 437, 440, 447, 477–478, 547, 551, 562, 605, 617, 622–623, 654, 669
airways
equipment/technique, 224
indications, 224
Recombinant erythropoietin, 82, 90
Recombinant factor VIIa (rFVIIa), 700–701
Recovery of spontaneous circulation (ROSC), 747, 751–753, 759, 761
Rectus sheath block, abdomen, 386–687, 386f, 448
Red cell mass, 681–683
Reflex bradycardia, 284
Regional anesthesia, 13, 107, 291, 300, 332, 357–387
for abdominal surgery, 447–448
for cesarean delivery, 578–579
complications, 359
considerations, 357–358
contraindications, 358
equipments, 359–360
of lower extremity. 372–381
of neck, 362–365
nerve localization techniques, 360–362
of trunk, 381–387
of upper extremity, 365–372
Remifentanil, 95, 106, 131, 180–181, 197, 197t, 198, 224, 283, 320, 391, 409–411, 416, 421, 426, 460, 480, 545, 549, 552, 554, 562, 575, 581, 587, 608t, 617, 721
Renal blood flow, 92–93, 311
Renal insufficiency, 94t–95t, 511
Renal protection, 91–92, 504
Renal replacement therapy (RRT), 85
Renal system
diseases of. *See* Kidney disease(s)
failure. *See* Kidney failure

Renal system (*Continued*)
  liver disease manifestations
    hepatorenal syndrome (HRS), 103–104
    prerenal azotemia, 103
  transplantation, anesthetic management, 91
  vascular surgery, preoperative assessment, 487–488
Renal transplantation, 562–563
Renin-angiotensin-aldosterone system (RAAS), 78
Reperfusion, 443
Respiratory reflexes, in pulmonary disease, 69
Respiratory system
  liver disease, 101–102
  monitoring
    end-tidal carbon dioxide, 261–262
    mandatory respiratory monitors, 260
    oxygenation, 260–261
    ventilation, 261–263
  vascular surgery, preoperative assessment, 487
Response entropy (RE), 268
Rest echocardiography, 50
Restrictive pulmonary disease, 262f, 710
Resuscitation
  adult
    advanced cardiac life support (ACLS), 752–761, 754f–755f, 760f
    basic life support (BLS), 749–752
  neonatal
    assessment, 766–767
    chest compressions, 769
    drugs and fluids, 769
    guidelines for withholding and discontinuing resuscitation, 770–771
    medications and volume expansion, 769–770
    post-resuscitation care, 770
    ventilation, 768–769
  pediatric, advanced life support, 763–765
  pediatric, basic life support, 761, 762t
    airway and breathing, 762
    bradycardia algorithm, 765f
    circulation, 762–763
    PALS, 763–765
Retinopathy of prematurity (ROP), 629
Retrobulbar block, 546, 546f
Retrograde autologous priming (RAP), 520–521
Retrograde tracheal intubation, 221
Retroperitoneal (RP) approach, 496, 561
Retroperitoneal insufflation of carbon dioxide, 560
Review of systems (ROS)
  cardiovascular, 4–5
  endocrine, 5–6
  gastrointestinal, 6
  hematologic, 6
  musculoskeletal, 6
  neurological, 5
  obstetric/gynecologic, 6
  PONV, 6
  renal, 5
  respiratory, 5
Rh immune globulin, 687
Rh surface antigens, 687
Rhabdomyolysis, 90
Rib fractures, 76, 382–383, 663–664, 736
Right heart catheterization, 439
Right ventricular (RV) assessment, 29–31
  systolic function, 31
  systolic pressure (RVSP), 34, 438–439, 465–466
Rigid bronchoscopy, 223, 471–472, 479–480, 616
Rima glottidis, 206
Rivaroxaban, 513, 700
Robotic surgery, 454
Rocuronium, 95, 106, 180, 228, 229t, 230t, 231, 234, 237, 437, 441, 517, 547, 562, 593, 607, 712
Roux-en-Y gastric bypass, 459
RRP. *See* Radical retropubic prostatectomy (RRP)
Rule of nines, 673, 674f
Ryanodex. *See* Dantrolene

S

SARS-CoV-2 infection, 148
Sacral plexus, 372–374, 373f
Sacrococcygeal membrane, 344, 353
Saphenous nerve, 372
Saphenous nerve block, 374, 378, 395
SBP. *See* Systemic blood pressure (SBP)
Scavenging system, 173
SCh. *See* Succinylcholine (SCh)
SCIP. *See* Surgical Care Improvement Project (SCIP)
Scleroderma, airways, 207

Scopolamine, 499, 545, 717, 798
SCV. *See* Subclavian vein (SCV)
Second gas effect, 201
Sedation, procedural, 188, 310, 633–634
Sedatives, 15–16, 706–707
Seizures, 330, 403, 413, 419
Seldinger technique, internal jugular, 223, 246, 246f, 247
Selective internal radiation therapy (SIRT), 645
Selective serotonin reuptake inhibitors (SSRIs), 312, 650
Sellick maneuver, 224
Sensory-evoked potentials (SEPs), 408
Sepsis, 152, 281, 292, 324, 677, 696
Serotonin antagonists, 719
Serum
　creatine kinase, 301
　osmolality, 404–405
Serum creatinine (SCr), 438
　degree of muscle damage, 400
　in HRS, 103
　in liver dysfunction, 107
　in renal disease, 83–84, 87, 487–488, 569
　in rhabdomyolysis, 90
Servo-based anesthesia machines, 171
Severe acute respiratory syndrome (SARS), 148
Severe hepatic disease, 324
Sevoflurane, 73, 93, 131, 168, 182, 186, 200t, 202, 272, 273f, 275–276, 277f–278f, 280, 299, 405t, 604–605, 615–616, 629–630, 721
　effects, on brain, 203–204
Shivering, 344
Shoulder surgery, 392–394, 393f
Shunting, 288
　CNS monitoring, 492
　hypoxemia, 288
　transjugular intrahepatic portosystemic, 644–645
SIADH. *See* Syndrome of inappropriate antidiuretic hormone secretion (SIADH)
Sickle cell anemia
　anesthetic management, 702
　clinical features, 702
Sildenafil, 320, 584
Silver nitrate, 677
Silver sulfadiazine, 677
Sinus bradycardia, 283–284, 714
Sinus tachycardia, 284

Sleep apnea, obstructive, 5, 207, 458, 548
Smoking cessation, 4, 16
Sniffing position, 180, 214, 215f, 216, 606
Snoring, 207
Sodium bicarbonate (NAHCO$_3$), 80–81, 300, 325, 328
　pH adjustment of solution, 349
　vascular surgery, preoperative assessment, 488
Sodium bicarbonate infusion (SBI), 89
Sodium-glucose cotransporter 2 (SGLT2) inhibitors, 11, 118
Sodium homeostasis disorders, 78–80
Sodium nitroprusside, 95t, 316–317
Somatosensory-evoked potentials (SSEPs), 189, 408, 425, 503
Sotalol, 759
Spectral analysis, of EEG, 269–270, 269f
Spinal-epidural anesthesia, 352
Spinal anesthesia
　anatomy
　　cerebrospinal fluid (CSF), 335
　　interlaminar ligaments, 334
　　interspinous ligament, 334
　　ligamentum flavum, 335
　　meninges, 335
　　spinal canal in, 333–334, 334f
　　spinal cord, 335
　　subarachnoid space, 335
　for cesarean delivery, 577
　complications and side effects
　　cardiovascular system, 343–344
　　infections, 344
　　neurological, 340–343, 342t–343t
　　pruritis, 344
　　respiratory system, 344
　　shivering, 344
　　visceral, 344
　determinants of spinal blockade
　　cerebrospinal fluid (CSF) turbulence, 339
　　cerebrospinal fluid (CSF) volume, 340
　　drug dose, 339, 339t
　　drug volume, 339
　　hyperbaric solutions, 339, 339t
　　hypobaric solutions, 339
　　intra-abdominal pressure, 340
　　isobaric solutions, 339
　　spinal curvatures, 340, 339f
　durational determinants of spinal blockade in
　　drugs and dose, 340
　　vasoconstrictors, 340

Spinal anesthesia (*Continued*)
  physiological changes
    cardiovascular system, 335
    central nervous system effects (CNS), 336
    neural blockade, 335
    neuroendocrine, 336
    respiratory system, 336
    thermoregulation, 336
    visceral effects, 336
  preeclampsia, 580
  suggested minimum cutaneous levels, 334t
  techniques
    patient position, 337
    procedural, 337–338, 338f
    spinal needle, 336
Spinal blockade, determinants of
  cerebrospinal fluid (CSF) turbulence, 339–340
  cerebrospinal fluid (CSF) volume, 340
  drug dose, 339
  drugs and dose, 339
  drug volume, 339
  hyperbaric solutions, 339, 339t
  hypobaric solutions, 339
  intra-abdominal pressure, 340
  isobaric solutions, 339
  spinal curvatures, 340, 339f
  vasoconstrictors, 340
Spinal cord injury, 207, 351–352, 418, 421, 423, 428, 564
Spinal cord pathology, 564
Spinal cord perfusion pressure (SCPP), 420, 427, 503
Spinal curvatures, 340, 339f
Spinal hematoma, 341
Spine surgery, 384
  airway, 423–424
  blood loss, 426
  disposition, 411
  monitoring, 425–426
  postoperative pain management, 428–429
  prone position, 424–425
  spinal cord injury, 423
  spinal cord perfusion
    bone cement embolism, 427
    complications, 427–428
    peripheral nerve injury, 427–428
    postoperative visual loss (POVL), 427
    spinal cord injury, 428
    VAE, 427
    vascular injury, 428, 428t
Splenectomy, 457
Sprotte needle, 336, 352
SSRIs. *See* Selective serotonin reuptake inhibitors (SSRIs)
State entropy (SE), 268
Static echocardiograph parameters, 36
Statins, 52
Stent-related complications, 110
Stereotactic surgery, 417
Sterile water, 556
Sterilization, infectious diseases
  reusable equipment, 148
  techniques of, 143
Steroids, 302, 405, 406, 409
  stress-dose, 128, 129b
  synthetic, 126
Stomach, full abdominal surgery, 447
Strabismus repair, 548
Streptokinase, 700
Stress testing, cardiac disease, 50–51
Strokes
  hemorrhagic, 717
  ischemic, 642–643, 717
Stroke volume variation (SVV), 36
Subarachnoid injection, 351
Subarachnoid space, in spinal anesthesia, 335
Subclavian vein (SCV), 252–253, 257
Subcutaneous emphysema, 663
Subcutaneous ICDs (S-ICDs), 64
Succinylcholine (SCh), 91, 95, 185, 224, 229t, 230t, 283, 606–607
  allergy, 2
  laryngospasm, 293
  neuromuscular blockade, 230–233
Sudden cardiac arrest (SCA), 747
Sufentanil, 197t
Sugammadex, 96, 237–238, 454, 562, 585, 607, 632, 710, 712
Sulfonylureas, 117–118
Superficial neck, 7
Superficial peroneal nerve, 374, 381
Superior laryngeal nerve, 205, 206f, 225, 494
Supraglottic airways, 181
Supraventricular tachycardias (SVT)
  atrial fibrillation, 285–286
  atrial flutter, 286
  atrial premature contractions (APCs), 285
  junctional/atrioventricular (AV) nodal rhythms, 285

paroxysmal supraventricular tachycardia (SVT), 286–287
Sural nerve, 374, 381
Surgery
  biliary tract procedures, 457
  delaying surgical procedures, 17
  esophageal, 454–455
  gastric, 455
  hepatic, 456–457
  intestinal and peritoneal, 455–456
  laparoscopic, 452–454
  for obese, 458–460
    anesthetic management, 459–460
    preanesthetic considerations, 458–459
    surgical techniques, 459
  pancreatic, 457
  premedication, 15–16, 16t
  pulmonary function, 69–70
    ciliary function effect, 69
  robotic, 454
  splenectomy, 457
  transplantation
    ethical considerations, 431–432
    kidney transplantation, 432–435, 433t
    liver transplantation, 438–443, 441f
    organ procurement, 443–445, 444t
    pancreas transplantation, 435–437
Surgical Care Improvement Project (SCIP), 144–145, 145t
Surgical wound classification, 146–147
Surrogate, 17, 262
SVR. *See* Systemic vascular resistance (SVR)
SVT. *See* Supraventricular tachycardias (SVT)
Sympathetic blockade, 281
Sympathomimetics, for pulmonary disease, 292
Synaptic vesicles, 227
Synchronized cardioversion, 286, 626, 715, 753–754, 763
Syndrome of inappropriate antidiuretic hormone secretion (SIADH), 133–134, 290, 412–413
Synthetic steroids, 126
Systemic acidosis, 505
Systemic air emboli, 60
Systemic blood pressure (SBP), 305, 318, 420, 472, 516, 524, 528–529, 626, 644, 655, 706

Systemic vascular resistance (SVR), 198
  caval compression, 281
  decreased
    allergic reactions, 281
    sepsis, 281
    sympathetic blockade, 281
    vasoactive metabolites, 281
  hypovolemia, 281
  inadequate venous return, 281
  intrathoracic pressure, 281
  venous capacitance, 281

T

Tachycardias
  sinus, 284
  supraventricular
    atrial fibrillation, 285–286
    atrial flutter, 286
    atrial premature contractions (APCs), 285
    junctional/atrioventricular (AV) nodal rhythms, 285
    paroxysmal supraventricular tachycardia (SVT), 286–287
    ventricular dysrhythmias, 287–288
Tachydysrhythmias, 282, 715
Tachypnea, 231, 294, 297, 299, 596
TACO. *See* Transfusion-associated circulatory overload (TACO)
Tamponade diagnosis, 32–33
Tamsulosin, 319
TBSA. *See* Total body surface area (TBSA)
TBW. *See* Total body water (TBW)
TEG. *See* Thromboelastography (TEG)
Temperature
  body, 184–185, 263, 336
  monitoring, 263
Tension pneumocephalus, 413
Tension pneumothorax, 655
Tetanic stimulus, neuromuscular function and, 236
Tetracaine (Pontocaine), 323, 326t, 327t, 339t, 341, 605, 610
Tetralogy of Fallot, 532t, 534
Terazosin, 319
TEVAR. *See* Thoracoabdominal aortic aneurysm repair (TEVAR)
Thermal ablations, CT-guided, 638–640
Thermal injuries, 670
Thermodilution, 258
Thermoregulation, 184–185, 336
Thiazides (chlorothiazide, dyazide, and metolazone), 92t

Thiazolidinediones, 118
Thigh
  anterior, 372
  operations of, 372
Thiocyanate, 317, 675
Thoracic aortic disease, etiology of, 500
Thoracic epidural anesthesia, 347, 436–437
Thoracic paravertebral block, 382–383, 382f
Thoracic surgery
  bronchopleural fistula
    anesthetic management, 483
    general considerations, 483
  endoscopic procedures
    endobronchial ultrasound, 471
    flexible bronchoscopy, 470–471
    flexible esophagoscopy, 476
    laser surgery, 472
    mediastinoscopy, 472–473
    rigid bronchoscopy, 471–472
    rigid esophagoscopy, 476
  esophageal surgery, 476–478
    anesthesia, 477–478
    general considerations, 477
    operative approach, 477–478
  intrapulmonary hemorrhage, 482–483
  mediastinal operations
    anesthesia, 472–473
    chamberlain procedure, 473
    mediastinal surgery, 472–473
  mediastinoscopy, 472–473
  monitoring, 476
  preoperative evaluation
    arterial blood gas (ABG), 465
    cardiac screening, 465–466
    chest radiography, 466
    computed tomography (CT), 466
    magnetic resonance imaging (MRI), 466
    patients schedule, 465
    pulmonary function tests (PFT), 465
    sedation, 466
    three-dimensional reconstruction, 466
  preoperative preparation
    airway obstruction, 466
    glycopyrrolate, 466
    heavy sedation, 466
    preoperative sedation, 466
  pulmonary resection
    anesthetic technique, 473–474
    bronchial blockers, 468
    emergence and extubation, 474–475
    endobronchial tubes, 466–468
    lung isolation techniques, 466–468, 473
    one-lung ventilation, 469–470
    positioning, 474
    postoperative analgesia, 475
    surgical techniques, 473
    univent tubes, 468
  tracheal resection and reconstruction
    emergence and extubation, 480
    general considerations, 478–479
    intraoperative management, 479–480
    tracheal disruption, 471, 483
Thoracoabdominal aortic aneurysm repair (TEVAR)
  associated findings, 501
  Crawford classification, 501, 501f
  endovascular thoracic, 505–506
  open thoracic aortic aneurysm repair, 502–504, 505t
  thoracic aortic disease, etiology of, 500
Thoracotomies, 722
Thrombectomies, 647
Thrombocytopenia, 104, 672, 683–684, 697
Thromboelastography (TEG), 443, 526, 685–686, 686f
Thromboembolism, 789
  pulmonary embolism, 355
Thrombolytic agents, 355, 700
Thrombophlebitis, superficial, 193
Thymectomy, 240
Thyroid disease
  anesthesia, 5
  cartilage of larynx, 205
  evaluation and laboratory studies, 120
  hypothyroidism
    anesthetic considerations, 120–121
    clinical features, 120
    etiologies of, 120
    hypermetabolic state, 120
    myxedema coma, treatment, 121
    treatment, 121
  parathyroid surgery, 124, 554
  physiology, 120
  thyroid surgery, 554
  thyrotoxicosis (hyperthyroidism)
    anesthetic considerations, 122
    etiologies of, 121

hypermetabolic state, 121
  symptoms, 121
  thyroid storm, treatment, 122–123
  treatment, 121–122
Thyroid-stimulating hormone (TSH), 120
Thyroid storm treatment, 122–123
Thyroid surgery, 124, 554
Thyromental distance, 7, 178, 207, 209
Thyrotoxicosis
  anesthetic considerations, 122
  etiologies of, 121
  hypermetabolic state, 121
  thyroid storm, treatment, 122–123
  treatment, 121–122
Ticagrelor, 343t
Ticlopidine, 355, 514t, 698
Timolol (Blocadren), hemodynamic control, perioperative, 314t, 545
TIPS. *See* Transjugular intrahepatic portosystemic shunts (TIPS)
Tirofiban, 343t
Tissue plasminogen activator, 443, 490, 690, 700
TIVA. *See* Total intravenous anesthesia (TIVA)
Tizanidine, 734t
TNS. *See* Transient neurologic syndrome (TNS)
Tocolytics, 573–574
TOF. *See* Train-of-four (TOF)
Tonsillar or parapharyngeal abscess, 551
Tonsillar rebleeding, 551
Total body surface area (TBSA), 673
Total body water (TBW), 592
Total hepatic vascular exclusion (TVE), 110
Total hip arthroplasty (THA), 390–392
Total intravenous anesthesia (TIVA), 6, 72, 146, 181, 269, 470, 503
Total knee arthroplasty (TKA), 390–392
Tourniquet pain, 372, 391
Trachea, 206, 206f
Tracheal disruption, 471, 483
Tracheal stenosis, 465, 483, 601, 615
Tracheostomy, 209, 223, 654
  elective, 553–555
Train-of-four (TOF), 72, 183, 185, 232f–233f, 235t, 441, 710
TRALI. *See* Transfusion-related acute lung injury (TRALI)
Tranexamic acid (TXA), 391–392, 798
Transabdominal approach, 496–497, 561

Transarterial chemoembolization (TACE), 635, 645
Transcatheter aortic valve replacement (TAVR), 55, 540
Transcatheter MV replacement (TMVR) and repair (TMVRep), 540–541
Transdermal scopolamine, 719
Transduodenal sphincteroplasty, 457
Transesophageal echocardiography (TEE), 26–28, 439
Transfusion-associated circulatory overload (TACO), 694
Transfusion compatibility, 686, 686t
Transfusion reactions
  acute hemolytic transfusion reactions, 692–693, 692t
  allergic transfusion reactions, 693
  delayed hemolytic transfusion reactions, 693
  febrile nonhemolytic transfusion reactions (FNHTR), 693
  graft *versus* host disease (GVHD), 694
  infectious complications, 695–696
  metabolic complications, 694–695
  transfusion-associated circulatory overload (TACO), 694
  transfusion-related acute lung injury (TRALI), 693–694
  transfusion-related immunomodulation, 696–697
Transfusion-related acute lung injury (TRALI), 693–694
Transfusion therapy
  blood component therapy
    cryoprecipitate, 688
    fresh frozen plasma (FFP), 688
    massive transfusion, 689
    substitutes, 689
    technical considerations, 688–689
  blood typing and cross-matching
    donor blood and recipient blood, 686–687, 686t
    emergency, transfusion, 687
    recipient antibodies, 687
    Rh surface antigens, 687
  coagulation studies
    activated clotting time (ACT), 685
    activated partial thromboplastin time (aPTT), 684
    fibrinogen, 685
    international normalized ratio (INR), 685
    platelet counts, 685

Transfusion therapy (*Continued*)
    platelet function tests, 685
    prothrombin time (PT), 684
    thromboelastography (TEG), 685–686, 686f
  coagulopathy, 684
  complications, blood
    immunomodulation by, 696–697
    infectious complications, 695
    metabolic complications, 694–695
    reactions, 692–694, 692t
  conservation and salvage techniques
    acute normovolemic hemodilution (ANH), 691
    autologous donation, 691
    intraoperative autotransfusion, 691
    controlled hypotension, 691–692
  factors deciding transfusion, 681–684
  hemophilia, 701
  Jehovah's witness (JW), 702–703
  oxygen-carrying ability, 681–683
  perioperative coagulopathy
    associated with CPB, 698
    chronic liver disease, 698
    disseminated intravascular coagulopathy (DIC), 697–698
    massive transfusion, 697
    pharmacologic intervention, 699–700
    reversal of, 700–701
    vitamin K deficiency, 698
  pharmacologic therapy
    desmopressin (DDAVP), 690
    erythropoietin (EPO), 690
    lysine analogues, 690
    serpins, 690
    topical hemostatic agents, 690
  plasma substitutes
    albumin, 689
    hydroxyethyl starch, 689
  recombinant factor VIIa, 688, 700–701
  red cell mass, 681–683
  sickle cell anemia, 702
  thrombocytopenia, 683–684
  von Willebrand disease, 701–702
Transfusion-transmitted infections, 144
Transient neurologic syndrome (TNS), 341
Transient paresthesias, 340
Transjugular intrahepatic portosystemic shunts (TIPS), 107, 456–457, 644–645
TransMedics Organ Care System (OCS), 431
Transplantation
  cardiac, 536–537
  kidney, 432–435
  liver, 111, 438–443, 442f
  lung, 537–538
    anesthetic management, 537–538
    indications, 537
    surgical technique, 537
  renal, 562–563
  surgery, anesthesia for
    ethical considerations, 431–432
    kidney transplantation, 432–435, 433t
    liver transplantation, 438–443, 442f
    organ procurement, 443–445, 444t
    pancreas transplantation, 435–437
Transpulmonary thermodilution, 258
Transthoracic echocardiogram, 5, 260, 438, 540, 713
Transurethral resection of the prostate (TURP)
  anesthesia, 558
  bacteremia, 559
  bladder perforation, 559
  blood loss and coagulopathy, 559
  complications, 558–559
  cystectomy, 561
  laser resection of prostate, 559
  nephrectomy, 561–562
  orchidopexy, 562
  orchiectomy, 562
  prostatic venous sinuses, 558
  radical retropubic prostatectomy (RRP), 560–561
  renal transplantation, 562–563
  urogenital plastic surgery procedures, 562
Transversus abdominis plane (TAP), 381–382, 387, 434
Trauma
  abdominal, 665–666
  airway, 654–655
  anesthetic management, 662–665, 668
  blunt, 665–666
  breathing, 655
  cardiac and major vascular trauma, 664–665
  chest, 663–664
  circulation, 655–657
  clothesline injuries, 663

diagnostic studies, 659
disability/neurologic evaluation, 658–659
exposure, 659
facial
 anesthetic management, 662
 mandibular fractures, 662
 maxillary fractures, 661–662, 661f
 ocular, 662
genitourinary, 666
head, 418–419
intracranial and spinal cord, 421
maxillary fractures, 661–662, 661f
monitoring, 659–660
neck, 662–663, 662f
orthopedic
 extremity reimplantation, 668
 fractures/dislocations, 666–667
 lower extremity, 668
 pelvis, 667
 upper extremity, 667
in pediatrics, 668–669
peripheral vascular, 665
pregnant, 669–670
Traumatic disruption, 500
Tricuspid annular plane systolic excursion (TAPSE), 31
Tricuspid regurgitation, 258
Tricyclic antidepressants, 283, 397, 649
Trigeminal nerve, 544
Trisomy 21 patients, 208
True allergic reactions, anesthesia, 2
TSH. *See* Thyroid-stimulating hormone (TSH)
Tubulointerstitial diseases, 85
Tumors
 airway, 207, 482
 carcinoid, 134–136
Tuohy/Weiss needle, 345
TURP. *See* Transurethral resection of the prostate (TURP)
TVE. *See* Total hepatic vascular exclusion (TVE)

U

Ulnar nerve block, 371
Ulnar nerve injury, 427, 718
Ultrafiltration, 85
Ultrasound, 347
 for central venous catheter placement, 249
 guided vascular access, 772–775
 reusable ultrasound equipment, 143

Unfractionated heparin, 355
United Network for Organ Sharing (UNOS), 431, 433t
Univent tubes, 468
Upper airway obstruction, 708
Upper airway surgery
 cleft lip and palate (CLP) repair, 551–552
 direct laryngoscopy, 552
 laser, 552–553
 tonsillar or parapharyngeal abscess, 551
 tonsillar rebleeding, 551
 tonsillectomy and adenoidectomy, 550–551
Upper endoscopy, 439
Upper extremity
 regional anesthesia
  anatomy, 365–366, 364f, 365f
  complications, 367–371, 367f–370f
  indications, 366–367
  techniques, 367–371, 367f–370f.
   See also Regional anesthesia
 vascular surgery of, 491
Upper respiratory infection (URI), 5
Ureter, 557, 562
Ureteroscopy, 557
Urethra, 666
URI. *See* Upper respiratory infection (URI)
Urinalysis, 88
Urinary retention, 199, 344
Urine
 electrolytes, 88
 output
  abnormal, 289–290
  anuria, 290
  high, 290
  oliguria, 289–290
 vascular access
  depth setting, 773
  gain, 773
  imaging the bevel, 774
  linear array probe, 772–773
Urologic surgery
 cystectomy, 561–562
 cystoscopy and ureteroscopy, 557
 laser resection of prostate, 559–560
 lithotripsy, 563
 nephrectomy, 561
 orchidopexy, 562
 orchiectomy, 562
 radical retropubic prostatectomy (RRP), 560–561

Urologic surgery (*Continued*)
  renal transplantation, 562–563
  spinal cord injury, 564
  transurethral resection of the bladder tumor (TURBT), 557
  transurethral resection of the prostate (TURP), 557–559
  urogenital plastic surgery procedures, 562
Uterotonics, 572–573

V

VAD. *See* Ventricular assist device (VADs)
Vagus nerve block, 365
Vagal nerve stimulators (VNS), 418
Vagal tone, dysrhythmias and, 283–284
Valvular heart disease, 517
  aortic regurgitation, 55
  aortic stenosis
    anesthetic considerations, 55, 517
    cardiac pacing, 55
    etiology, 54
    ischemia treatment, 55
    nitrates and peripheral vasodilators, 55
    normal sinus rhythm, 55
    pathophysiology, 55
    symptoms, 54–55
    ventricle, 55
  mitral regurgitation, 56
  mitral stenosis
    anesthetic considerations, 56
    etiology, 56
    pathophysiology, 56
Valvular lesions, mixed, 518
Vancomycin, 95t, 144–147, 234, 294, 776
  resistant Enterococcus (VRE), 139
  resistant *Staphylococcus aureus* (VRSA), 139
Vaporizers, 167–168
Varicella-Zoster virus (VZV), 150
Vascular access, 755
  anatomy, 772, 773f
  devices, 773t
    IV catheter, 772
    structure, 772
  image-guided vascular access procedure, 774–775
    ultrasound, 772–774, 773f
  issues, 775–776
  troubleshooting, 775–776
Vascular cannulation, 15

Vascular diseases, diabetes mellitus (DM) and, 115
Vascular injury, 428, 428t, 662–663
Vascular occlusion catheters, 468
Vascular surgery
  abdominal aortic repair
    endovascular abdominal aortic repair (EVAR), 494–496, 497f
    open abdominal aortic surgery, 496–499
    ruptured abdominal aortic aneurysm, emergent repair of, 499–500
  amputations
    general considerations, 506
    phantom limb pain (PLP), 506
  carotid revascularization
    carotid artery stenting, 491–492
    carotid endarterectomy, 492–494
    general considerations, 491
    postoperative complications, 494
  peripheral arterial surgery
    axillofemoral bypass grafting, 491
    catheter-directed thrombolysis (CDT), 490
    femoral pseudoaneurysm, 490–491
    general considerations, 489
    lower-extremity bypass grafting, 490
    percutaneous balloon angioplasty and stenting, 489
    peripheral aneurysms, 491
    peripheral embolectomy, 490
    upper extremity, 491
  postoperative considerations, 494
  preoperative assessment and management
    cardiovascular system, 486–487
    central nervous system (CNS), 488
    endocrine system, 488
    hematologic system, 488–489
    renal system, 487–488
    respiratory system, 487
  thoracoabdominal aortic aneurysm repair (TEVAR)
    associated findings, 501
    Crawford classification, 501, 501f
    endovascular thoracic, 505–506
    open thoracic aortic aneurysm repair, 502–505, 505t
    thoracic aortic disease, etiology of, 500
Vasoactive agents, 89, 311, 402, 541

Vasoactive drugs, 406
Vasoconstrictors, 55, 101, 219, 518, 554, 668
 local anesthetic toxicity and, 351
 spinal anesthesia, 340
 systemic absorption of, 283
Vasodilation, 690–691
Vasodilators, 315, 315t
 perioperative hemodynamic control
  adenosine, 319
  α-adrenergic antagonists, 319
  amlodipine, 316
  bosentan, 320
  calcium channel antagonists, 315–316
  clevidipine, 316
  dihydropyridine (DHP), 315
  doxazosin, 320
  enalaprilat, 318
  fenoldopam, 318
  hydralazine, 318
  inhaled nitric oxide, 320
  nicardipine, 316
  nifedipine, 316
  nimodipine, 316
  nitroglycerin, 317–318
  phentolamine, 319
  prostaglandin E_1, 319
  pulmonary, 319–320
  sildenafil, 320
  sodium nitroprusside, 316–317
  tamsulosin, 319
  terazosin, 319
Vasopressin (antidiuretic hormone, Pitressin), 58, 80, 105, 131, 133–134, 136, 152, 282, 302, 413, 445, 461–462, 540, 591, 672, 690, 753, 759–760, 798–799
Vasopressors, 89, 309t, 312, 504, 572
Vecuronium, 230t, 234
Venous air embolism, 416
Venous capacitance, increased, 281
Venous gas embolism, 453
Venous return
 cannulas, 520
 inadequate, 281
Venovenous bypass (VVBP), 110–111, 440
Ventilation
 airway mask, 213
 alveolar, 68, 200
 assessment of, 37t
 controlled, 289, 469, 592
 hypercarbia, 289
 hypoventilation, 709–711
 lung protection, 75, 654
 minute, 69, 498, 566, 592, 592t
 for patients with obesity, 73
 positive-pressure, 249, 281, 295, 483, 558, 655, 713, 768–769
 renal protection, 89–90
 spontaneous/assisted, 592
Ventilators
 anesthesia machines, 165, 167, 169–171
 microprocessor-controlled, 169
Ventilator-associated events (VAEs), 143
Ventral herniorrhaphies, 456
Ventricular assist devices (VAD), 57–58, 536, 539–540
 care team, 57–58
 intraoperative challenges, 58
 parameters, 58
 pump thrombosis, 59
Ventricular dysrhythmias
 preexcited atrial fibrillation, 288
 ventricular fibrillation, 288
 ventricular premature contractions (VPCs), 287
 ventricular tachycardia, 287–288
Ventricular fibrillation (VF), 288, 715, 747, 754f
Ventricular preexcitation, ventricular dysrhythmias, 288
Ventricular septal defect (VSD), 288, 518
Ventricular tachycardia, 287–288
 pulseless, 747
 unstable, 715
Venturi masks, 173
Verapamil, 316, 799
Vertebroplasty, 427, 2
Video laryngoscopy, 220, 424, 601
Virtual reality (VR), 744–745
Viruses, infection control in OR
 cytomegalovirus (CMV), 150
 Ebola, 150
 hepatitis B virus (HBV), 149
 hepatitis C virus (HCV), 150
 herpes simplex virus (HSV) I and II, 150
 human immunodeficiency virus (HIV), 149
 influenza virus, 148
 Mpox, 151
 Varicella-zoster virus (VZV), 150
Vital signs, 7
Vitamin D, 82
Vitamin K, 698–699, 701, 799

VNS. *See* Vagal nerve stimulators (VNS)
Vocal cords
 laryngospasm, 293
 paralysis, 501, 554, 712
Volatile anesthetics, 94t, 605, 640, 707
 inhalation anesthetics and, 200
 cardiovascular system, 202–203
 CNS, 202
 hepatic system, 203
 neuromuscular system, 203
 renal system, 203
 respiratory system, 203
 narcotics and, 89
Vomiting
 aspiration, 294–295
 postoperative, 182, 547, 716, 718–719, 722
von Willebrand disease, 698
VSD. *See* Ventricular septal defect (VSD)
VVIRV pacemaker, 62
VZV. *See* Varicella-Zoster virus (VZV)

W

Wake-up test, 408, 420–421

Warfarin (Coumadin), 10, 343t, 355, 487, 489, 513, 515, 520, 685, 688, 698–701, 799
Waste gas scavenging, 173
Water, intake, daily, 80
Weiss needles, 345
West Nile virus (WNV), 696
Wheezing, 294
Whitacre needle, 336
White lung, 43
Wireless ultrasound endocardial pacing, 64
WNV. *See* West Nile virus (WNV)
Wolff–Parkinson–White syndrome, 286, 313, 756
Wound, infection control in OR, 146–147
Wrists, 366, 365f

Y

Y-piece adapter, 169
Y-shaped EZ-blocker, 468

Z

Zenker diverticulum, 477